EMERGENCY MEDICAL THERAPY

FOURTH
EDITION

TERRY J. MENGERT, M.D.

Assistant Professor of Medicine
Attending Physician
Emergency Medicine Service
University of Washington Medical Center
Seattle, Washington

MICKEY S. EISENBERG, M.D., Ph.D.

Professor of Medicine
Director, Emergency Medicine Service
University of Washington Medical Center
Seattle, Washington

MICHAEL K. COPASS, M.D.

Professor, Department of Medicine, Division of Neurology
Director, Emergency Trauma Center
Harborview Medical Center
Medical Director, Seattle Medic I Program
Seattle, Washington

W. B. SAUNDERS COI
Division of Harcourt Brace & Company
PHILADELPHIA, LONDON, TORONTO, N

D1005033

W. B. SAUNDERS COMPANY
A Division of Harcourt Brace & Company

The Curtis Center
Independence Square West
Philadelphia, Pennsylvania 19106

Library of Congress Cataloging-in-Publication Data

Emergency medical therapy/[edited by] Terry J. Mengert, Mickey S.
  Eisenberg, Michael K. Copass.—4th ed.
      p.   cm.
   Includes bibliographical references and index.
   ISBN 0-7216-5162-3
      1. Medical emergencies—Handbooks, manuals, etc.   2. Therapeutics—
Handbooks, manuals, etc.   I. Mengert, Terry J.   II. Eisenberg,
Mickey S.   III. Copass, Michael K.
   [DNLM: 1. Emergencies—handbook.   2. Therapeutics—handbook. WB
39 E527 1996]
   RC86.7.E578 1996
   616.02′5—dc20
   DNLM/DLC   94-39975

EMERGENCY MEDICAL THERAPY   ISBN   0-7216-5162-3

Printed in the United States of America.

Last digit is the print number: 9   8   7   6   5   4   3   2   1

CONTRIBUTORS

ROY COLVEN, M.D.

Department of Medicine, Duke University Medical Center, Durham, North Carolina

Cardiovascular Emergencies (Congestive Heart Failure), (Hypertensive Emergencies), (Pericarditis); Infectious Disease Emergencies (Common Hand Infections), (Pediculosis and Scabies), (Sexually Transmitted Diseases), (Tetanus Prophylaxis)

WILLIAM M. COPLIN, M.D.

Acting Instructor, Neurology/Medicine Senior Fellow, Pulmonary and Critical Care Medicine, University of Washington School of Medicine, Seattle, Washington

Toxicologic Emergencies (Management of Specific Poisonings)

D.C. DUGDALE, M.D.

Assistant Professor of Medicine, University of Washington School of Medicine, Seattle, Washington

Infectious Mononucleosis; Low Back Pain

SUSAN EGAAS, M.D.

Assistant Professor of Medicine, Department of Medicine, University of Washington School of Medicine, Seattle, Washington

Cardiovascular Emergencies (Thoracic Aortic Dissection); Infectious Disease Emergencies (Adult Epiglottitis), (Food-Borne Disease); Gynecologic Emergencies (Abnormal Vaginal Bleeding), (Ectopic Pregnancy)

MICKEY S. EISENBERG, M.D., Ph.D.

Professor of Medicine
University of Washington School of Medicine, Seattle, Washington

Cardiovascular Emergencies (Cardiac Arrest), Infectious Disease Emergencies (Botulism), (Meningitis and Encephalitis), (Otitis Media and Otitis Externa), (Pharyngitis), (Viral Hepatitis)

GREGORY C. GARDNER, M.D.

Assistant Professor of Medicine, Division of Rheumatology, Adjunct Assistant Professor of Orthopedics and Rehabilitation Medicine, University of Washington School of Medicine, Seattle, Washington

Rheumatologic Emergencies (Evaluation of the Patient with Arthritis), (Infectious Causes of Arthritis), (Crystal-Associated Arthritis), (Spondyloarthropathies, (Miscellaneous Rheumatologic Diseases)

ALISON J. GUILE, M.D.

Attending Physician, Champlain Valley Physicians Hospital, Plattsburgh, New York

Dysuria

IRL B. HIRSCH, M.D.

Associate Professor of Medicine, University of Washington School of Medicine, Seattle, Washington

Endocrine Emergencies (Hyperglycemia Without Significant Ketosis), (Diabetic Ketoacidosis), (Hyperglycemic Hyperosmolar Coma), (Hypoglycemia)

MARY T. HO, M.D., M.P.H.

Physician, Group Health Cooperative of Puget Sound, Eastside Hospital, Redmond, Washington

Chest Pain

KATHLEEN A. JOBE, M.D.

Assistant Professor of Medicine, University of Washington School of Medicine, Seattle, Washington

Airway Management; Gastrointestinal Emergencies (Appendicitis), (Gallbladder Disease), (Gastrointestinal Hemorrhage), (Hepatic Failure), (Pancreatitis)

MICHAEL B. KIMMEY, M.D.

Associate Professor of Medicine, University of Washington School of Medicine, Seattle, Washington

Abdominal Pain, Diarrhea

KEITH LEYDEN, M.D.

Physician, Emergency Medical Service, Group Health Cooperative, Seattle, Washington

Cardiovascular Emergencies (Myocardial Infarction); Infectious Disease Emergencies (Animal Bites), (Pneumonia), (Sinusitis); Gynecologic Emergencies (Pelvic Inflammatory Disease), (Vaginitis)

RUSSELL McMULLEN, M.D.

Associate Professor of Medicine, University of Washington School of Medicine, Seattle, Washington

Infectious Disease Emergencies (Viral Hepatitis)

TERRY J. MENGERT, M.D.

Assistant Professor of Medicine, University of Washington School of Medicine, Seattle, Washington

Diarrhea; Dizziness; General Care of the Emergency Department Patient; Infectious Disease Emergencies (Viral Hepatitis); Pulmonary Emergencies (Asthma), (Chronic Obstructive Pulmonary Disease), (Deep Venous Thrombosis and Pulmonary Embolism); Renal Emergencies (Electrolyte

Disorders); Shock; Syncope; Toxicologic Emergencies (Standard Therapy of the Poisoned/Overdose Patient), (Management of Specific Poisonings)

DOUGLAS S. PAAUW, M.D.

Associate Professor of Medicine, Division of General Internal Medicine, Department of Medicine, University of Washington School of Medicine, Seattle, Washington

Infectious Disease Emergencies (Acquired Immunodeficiency Syndrome), (Cellulitis), (Tuberculosis), (Urinary Tract Infections)

STEPHEN H. PETERSDORF, M.D.

Assistant Professor, Department of Medicine, University of Washington School of Medicine, Seattle, Washington

Hematologic and Oncologic Emergencies (Anemia), (Sickle Cell Disease), (Bleeding Disorders), (Blood Component Therapy), (Epidural Spinal Cord Compression), (Superior Vena Cava Syndrome)

DOMINIC F. REILLY, M.D.

Assistant Professor, Department of Medicine, University of Washington School of Medicine, Seattle, Washington

Cardiovascular Emergencies (Cardiac Arrhythmias)

TIM SCEARCE, M.D.

Attending Neurologist, Department of Neurology, Group Health Cooperative at Puget Sound, Redmond, Washington 98052

Headache; Neurologic Emergencies (Coma), (Stroke), (Seizures), (Subarachnoid Hemorrhage)

C. SCOTT SMITH, M.D.

Assistant Professor of Medicine, Adjunct Assistant Professor of Medical Education, University of Washington School of Medicine, Seattle, Washington

Infectious Disease Emergencies (Infective Endocarditis)

DAVID H. SPACH, M.D.

Assistant Professor of Medicine, Division of Infectious Diseases, Department of Medicine, University of Washington, Seattle, Washington

Infectious Disease Emergencies (Lyme Disease), (Tuberculosis)

MARGARET THORNTON, M.D.

Affiliate Faculty, University of Montana, Missoula, Montana

Renal Emergencies (Acid-Base Disorders)

EUGENE A. TROWERS, M.D., M.P.H.

Associate Professor of Medicine, Director of Endoscopy Services, Texas Tech University School of Medicine, Department of Internal Medicine, Division of Gastroenterology, Lubbock, Texas

Diarrhea

DAVID SCOTT WEIGLE, M.D.

Associate Professor of Medicine, University of Washington School of Medicine, Seattle, Washington

Endocrine Emergencies (Adrenal Crisis), (Myxedema Coma), (Thyroid Storm)

STEVEN M. WEISS, M.D.

Senior Pulmonary Fellow, University of Washington School of Medicine, Seattle, Washington

Dyspnea; Pulmonary Emergencies (Acute Respiratory Failure), (Hemoptysis), (Spontaneous Pneumothorax)

BESSIE A. YOUNG, M.D.

Acting Instructor, Division of Nephrology, University of Washington School of Medicine, Seattle, Washington

Renal Emergencies (Acute Renal Failure), (Nephrolithiasis)

PREFACE

For the physician in training, whether medical student or house officer, the rotation in the emergency department (ED) is always stressful. This stress is appropriate. It is a measure of the challenges facing the physician: multiple patients must be managed simultaneously, at least some of whom are critically ill; this patient care must be done in an expert and expeditious manner, with often little time for reflection or review; and the depth and breadth of presenting patient problems may involve every known medical specialty. This manual, like its three previous editions over the past sixteen years, has been written with these challenges in mind. It is a resource that will rapidly assist the physician confronting an adult patient with a common or life-threatening medical problem in the hectic environment of emergency medicine. It is a convenient, practical, current, and readily usable source of emergency diagnostic and therapeutic information.

This new edition has been completely revised and updated. All of the contents have been entirely rewritten and their reference lists thoroughly updated as well. The first section of the book is entirely new and presents in detail important principles in the general care of the ED patient, including use of consultants, the most recent COBRA transfer requirements, pain management, and the technique of conscious sedation. This material should help the student and houseofficer in their transition from routine outpatient and hospital ward care to the new and busy environment of the ED. Section II is also new, and it includes chapters on selected significant, common symptoms in the adult patient with an emergency medical problem (from abdominal pain to syncope). The third section of this manual presents common medical emergencies and their therapy. The format of the chapters in this section includes: Essential Facts, Clinical Evaluation, Differential Diagnosis, Therapy, Disposition, "Pearls and Pitfalls," and References. Extensive use has been made of tables to summarize information and "flow diagrams" to assist in diagnostic and therapeutic decision making.

A manual, by its very definition, is not encyclopedic. The information presented here will allow the busy student, house officer, and practitioner of emergency medicine to begin the task of expertly managing the most common adult medical problems and emergencies encountered in the ED. The focus of the manual is *adult medical emergencies.* Selected surgical conditions (e.g., appendicitis, ectopic pregnancy) are included, however, because of their significance and prevalence. We have purposely not addressed issues related to major trauma, in part because it is our desire to keep the book a manageable size, and in part because we feel the information presented in the Advanced Trauma Life Support Course and Syllabus by the American College of Surgeons can be little improved upon. This in no way reflects our lack of concern for the epidemic in trauma that has seized our nation.

It is our sincere wish that the following information will help physicians everywhere more effectively and expeditiously relieve the human suffering and prevent the untimely deaths of their patients who present with an emergency medical problem.

TERRY J. MENGERT
MICKEY S. EISENBERG
MICHAEL K. COPASS

To the emergency medicine patient;
thank you for your continuous instruction.

THE EDITORS

CONTENTS

I
INTRODUCTION

1   **General Care of the Emergency Department Patient**............1
    Terry J. Mengert

II
MEDICAL CHIEF COMPLAINTS

2   **Abdominal Pain**...**29**
    Michael B. Kimmey

3   **Low Back Pain**...**39**
    D.C. Dugdale

4   **Chest Pain**...**56**
    Mary T. Ho

5   **Diarrhea**..**73**
    Eugene A. Trowers and Michael B. Kimmey

6   **Dizziness**..**82**
    Terry J. Mengert

7   **Dyspnea**..**96**
    Steven M. Weiss

8   **Dysuria**..**104**
    Alison J. Guile

9   **Headache**..**109**
    Tim Scearce

10   **Syncope**...**128**
    Terry J. Mengert

III
MEDICAL EMERGENCIES

11 Airway Management 139
      Kathleen A. Jobe

12 Shock 167
      Terry J. Mengert

13 Cardiovascular Emergencies

      CARDIAC ARREST 194
          Mickey S. Eisenberg

      CARDIAC ARRHYTHMIAS 210
          Dominic F. Reilly

      CONGESTIVE HEART FAILURE...238
          Roy Colven

      HYPERTENSIVE EMERGENCIES 245
          Roy Colven

      MYOCARDIAL INFARCTION 252
          Keith Leyden

      PERICARDITIS 277
          Roy Colven

      THORACIC AORTIC DISSECTION 283
          Susan Egaas

14 Pulmonary Emergencies

      ACUTE RESPIRATORY FAILURE...289
          Steven M. Weiss

      ASTHMA 300
          Terry J. Mengert

      CHRONIC OBSTRUCTIVE PULMONARY DISEASE............................316
          Terry J. Mengert

      HEMOPTYSIS 329
          Steven M. Weiss

      DEEP VENOUS THROMBOSIS AND PULMONARY EMBOLISM 337
          Terry J. Mengert

Spontaneous Pneumothorax 350
    Steven M. Weiss

15 Infectious Disease Emergencies

Acquired Immunodeficiency Syndrome 359
    Douglas S. Paauw

Animal Bites 383
    Keith Leyden

Botulism 393
    Mickey S. Eisenberg

Cellulitis 396
    Douglas S. Paauw

Infective Endocarditis 402
    C. Scott Smith

Adult Epiglottitis 409
    Susan Egaas

Food-Borne Disease 415
    Susan Egaas

Common Hand Infections 423
    Roy Colven

Viral Hepatitis 429
    Russell McMullen, Terry J. Mengert, and Mickey S. Eisenberg

Lyme Disease 443
    David H. Spach

Meningitis and Encephalitis 452
    Mickey S. Eisenberg

Infectious Mononucleosis 462
    D.C. Dugdale

Otitis Media and Otitis Externa 468
    Mickey S. Eisenberg

Pediculosis and Scabies 472
    Roy Colven

Pharyngitis 477
    Mickey S. Eisenberg

PNEUMONIA...484
        Keith Leyden

SEXUALLY TRANSMITTED DISEASES.........................501
        Roy Colven

SINUSITIS 512
        Keith Leyden

TETANUS PROPHYLAXIS 520
        Roy Colven

TUBERCULOSIS..521
        David H. Spach and Douglas S. Paauw

URINARY TRACT INFECTIONS 533
        Douglas S. Paauw

16   Gastrointestinal Emergencies
        Kathleen A. Jobe

APPENDICITIS...540

GALLBLADDER DISEASE...545

GASTROINTESTINAL HEMORRHAGE.......................................553

HEPATIC FAILURE 561

PANCREATITIS 574

17   Renal Emergencies

ACID-BASE DISORDERS..581
        Margaret Thornton

ACUTE RENAL FAILURE..593
        Bessie A. Young

ELECTROLYTE DISORDERS..608
        Terry J. Mengert

NEPHROLITHIASIS 629
        Bessie A. Young

18   Gynecologic Emergencies

ABNORMAL VAGINAL BLEEDING...638
        Susan Egaas

ECTOPIC PREGNANCY.......................................651
    Susan Egaas

PELVIC INFLAMMATORY DISEASE 661
    Keith Leyden

VAGINITIS..666
    Keith Leyden

19 **Endocrine Emergencies**

ADRENAL CRISIS 673
    David Scott Weigle

HYPERGLYCEMIA WITHOUT SIGNIFICANT KETOSIS 681
    Irl B. Hirsch

DIABETIC KETOACIDOSIS....................................687
    Irl B. Hirsch

HYPERGLYCEMIC HYPEROSMOLAR COMA..................699
    Irl B. Hirsch

HYPOGLYCEMIA..707
    Irl B. Hirsch

MYXEDEMA COMA...714
    David Scott Weigle

THYROID STORM 723
    David Scott Weigle

20 **Neurologic Emergencies**
    Tim Scearce

COMA...734

STROKE...752

SEIZURES 766

SUBARACHNOID HEMORRHAGE 778

21 **Hematologic and Oncologic Emergencies**
    Stephen H. Petersdorf

ANEMIA...788

SICKLE CELL DISEASE 797

BLEEDING DISORDERS...805

BLOOD COMPONENT THERAPY...814

EPIDURAL SPINAL CORD COMPRESSION 822

SUPERIOR VENA CAVA SYNDROME..828

22 Rheumatologic Emergencies
Gregory C. Gardner

EVALUATION OF THE PATIENT WITH ARTHRITIS 833

INFECTIOUS CAUSES OF ARTHRITIS 840

CRYSTAL-ASSOCIATED ARTHRITIS 846

SPONDYLOARTHROPATHIES..848

MISCELLANEOUS RHEUMATOLOGIC DISEASES..............................852

23 Toxicologic Emergencies

STANDARD THERAPY OF THE POISONED/OVERDOSE PATIENT 860
    Terry J. Mengert

MANAGEMENT OF SPECIFIC POISONINGS
    William M. Coplin and Terry J. Mengert

ACETAMINOPHEN 885

ANTICHOLINGERGIC AGENTS 891

ANTICONVULSANTS
PHENYTOIN 894

CARBAMAZEPINE..896

VALPROIC ACID 898

ANTIPSYCHOTIC AGENTS 900

BARBITURATES 904

BENZODIAZEPINES 906

CALCIUM CHANNEL BLOCKERS 908

CARBON MONOXIDE 910

COCAINE..913

CYCLIC ANTIDEPRESSANTS 918

DIGITALIS..926

ETHANOL 929

OTHER ALCOHOLS
ETHYLENE GLYCOL 933

ISOPROPYL ALCOHOL...935

METHANOL 937

LITHIUM 940

MONOAMINE OXIDASE INHIBITORS..942

OPIOIDS..945

SALICYLATES 950

STIMULANTS 958

THEOPHYLLINE...960

INDEX..965

NOTICE

Emergency medicine is an ever-changing field. Standard safety precautions must be followed, but as new research and clinical experience broaden our knowledge, changes in treatment and drug therapy become necessary or appropriate. The editors of this work have carefully checked the generic and trade drug names and verified drug dosages to ensure that the dosage information in this work is accurate and in accord with the standards accepted at the time of publication. Readers are advised, however, to check the product information currently provided by the manufacturer of each drug to be administered to be certain that changes have not been made in the recommended dose or in the contraindications for administration. This is of particular importance in regard to new or infrequently used drugs. It is the responsibility of the treating physician, relying on experience and knowledge of the patient, to determine dosages and the best treatment for the patient. The editors cannot be responsible for misuse or misapplication of the material in this work.

THE PUBLISHER

I

INTRODUCTION

1

General Care of The Emergency Department Patient

"Returning, resuming, I thread my way through the hospitals,
The hurt and wounded I pacify with soothing hand,
I sit by the restless all the dark night, some are so young,
Some suffer so much, I recall the experience sweet and sad . . ."

WALT WHITMAN (The Wound Dresser)

I. ESSENTIAL FACTS

A. Definition

Emergency medicine is the specialty that encompasses all medical knowledge, techniques, and associated skills used in the care of patients within the emergency department (ED) and the extensions of that department. The specialty also includes the important subjects of prehospital first aid, field resuscitation and stabilization, emergency transport, environmental medicine, disaster medicine, and toxicology.

1. The emergency medicine provider cares for any and all patients who present to the ED requesting, or in need of, medical evaluation and treatment. This patient population is unrestricted, arrives unscheduled, occurs in unpredictable numbers, and may suffer from illnesses and injuries of any severity and involving any organ or body system.

2. ED patient care occurs 24 hours a day, 7 days a week, 365 days a year. It occurs in an expert and, whenever possible, expeditious manner irrespective of patient age, gender, race, faith, income, or nature of the patient's perceived illness or injury. Because it is the patient who initiates contact with the ED, *it is the patient who defines the "emergency."*

3. Every year in this country, more than 26,000 emergency physicians, in over 5600 EDs, provide health care for 90 million patient visits.

4. The ED is the primary source of medical care for the victims of violence, prehospital cardiac arrest, poisoning, and community disasters. For many Americans, the ED is their initial point of access to this nation's health care system; for many, including the uninsured, it is frequently their only available source of medical care.

5. Though emergency medicine is considered "expensive," the overall cost of ED care represents only 2% of the national health care dollar.

B. Important Definitions in Emergency Medicine

1. Prehospital Care

Prehospital care includes all medical care that takes place *prior to* the patient's ED arrival. It is an extension of the specialty of emergency medicine into the community and includes first aid, cardiopulmonary resuscitation (CPR), 911 emergency telephone number access, emergency medical services response, emergency medical technician and/or paramedic patient evaluation and treatment, safe and expedient patient transport to the ED, and disaster response.

2. Triage

Triage is the sorting and ordering of patients on the basis of their need for treatment and the resources available to provide that treatment. Under most circumstances, the ED is able to render appropriate and necessary initial care to all presenting patients; those with real or potentially life-threatening problems are treated first. In a community disaster, however, the number of patients and the severity of their presenting complaints *exceeds* the capabilities of the ED; in this situation, patients with the greatest chance of survival, who require the least expenditure of limited resources (including time, personnel, and equipment), are treated first.

3. Prioritization of Illness and/or Injury

Emergency medicine involves the simultaneous management of multiple patients with varying degrees of acuity and illness severity, and successful patient care requires prioritization of the patient's health problems beyond initial triage decisions. The ED physician must remain flexible and capable of reprioritizing treatment as time and diagnostic efforts reveal more information. The following schema is useful in ranking patient conditions:

- *Exigent,* an immediately life-threatening condition requiring *instantaneous* intervention. Examples include airway obstruction, ventricular fibrillation, pulseless ventricular tachycardia, and pulseless electrical activity.

- *Emergent,* a life-threatening condition that requires *immediate* intervention within minutes. Examples include acute myocardial infarction, an unstable patient with an arrhythmia, and tension pneumothorax.
- *Urgent,* a potentially life-threatening condition, or one otherwise associated with significant morbidity, requiring *rapid* evaluation and treatment. Examples include an acute asthma exacerbation, gastrointestinal hemorrhage, and many poisonings.
- *Nonurgent or minor,* a condition that benefits from medical care, but is not life-threatening, and in which patient morbidity is not increased by unavoidable delays in care. Examples include minor infections, minor lacerations, abrasions, simple extremity fractures, and simple sprains.

4. Primary Survey

The *primary survey* is the rapid assessment of the patient's airway, breathing, vital signs, and neurologic status. The primary survey, combined with patient resuscitation, is often referred to as the "ABCs" of emergency care:

A Airway with cervical spine stabilization

B Breathing and ventilation

C Circulation with hemorrhage control

D Disability or "deficits"—a rapid assessment of the neurologic status obtained by evaluating the patient's level of consciousness, pupillary size and reactivity, and any gross lateralized deficits

E Exposure and environmental control—the patient is undressed, further illness or injury prevented, and body temperature (e.g., hypo- or hyperthermia) assessed and managed as necessary

In practice, any life-threatening condition encountered during the primary survey is managed *immediately;* resuscitation, therefore, takes place *simultaneously* with the primary survey. All critically ill, seriously ill, or multiply injured patients are initially approached with the primary survey (*note:* the only exception to this rule is the patient with a monitored cardiac arrest secondary to either pulseless ventricular tachycardia or ventricular fibrillation. In that circumstance, immediate cardioversion/defibrillation takes priority over the primary survey).

5. Resuscitation

Resuscitation is the restoration of airway, breathing, oxygenation, ventilation, and reasonable vital signs to the critically ill patient. It takes place simultaneously with the primary survey, as described. Applying oxygen to the patient, obtaining intravenous access, and rapidly initiating necessary monitoring (including electrocardiographic and continuous pulse oximetry) are vital components of any resuscitation (*important concept:* consider *oxygen—IV—monitor* as "one word").

6. Secondary Survey

The *secondary survey* is the head-to-toe evaluation of the ED patient, including laboratory, radiographic, and/or other needed diagnostic testing. In the critically or seriously ill individual, the secondary survey takes place only *after* the primary survey has been completed, immediate and necessary resuscitation measures initiated, and airway, breathing, circulation, and vital signs reassessed.

7. Stabilization

Stabilization is the restoration of biologic homeostasis to the patient. It includes all diagnostic and therapeutic interventions necessary to ensure that deterioration of the patient's condition will not occur.

8. Definitive Care

Definitive care encompasses all aspects of medical care, including evaluation, testing, diagnosis, procedures, and treatment necessary to completely manage the patient's presenting problem(s). In many cases, the ED is capable of providing complete definitive care. In other circumstances, the ED *initiates* definitive care, but its completion will require consultation, further primary care or specialty referral, and/or hospitalization.

9. Disposition

Disposition is the patient's destination after ED evaluation and treatment. It may include discharge to home, hospitalization, or transfer to another facility more optimally equipped to provide the required level of definitive care.

C. Principles of Emergency Department Patient Care

The traditional medical approach to evaluating and caring for a patient is to take a complete history, perform a thorough physical examination, order and review appropriate laboratory work and diagnostic tests, and initiate needed therapy based upon the identified or reasonably suspected diagnoses. This approach is comprehensive and reasonable in the *stable* hospitalized patient. In the ED, however, it fails to take into account the frequent need to institute immediate therapy with limited information in an emergency; it fails to prioritize information-gathering and treatment needs; and it is not time-efficient. The following principles are useful in assisting the medical student and house officer in making the transition from hospital ward care to ED patient care:

1. The ED patient is presumed to have a life-threatening condition until proven otherwise.

2. Regardless of the patient's complaint, the ED physician must approach the patient with the following questions foremost in mind:
   - What is the *immediate* threat to life? What therapy must be instantaneously initiated to manage this life threat?
   - Is there a *potential* threat to life? What therapy and/or further evaluation is necessary to immediately manage this potential threat or reasonably exclude it as a possibility?
   - What diagnostic steps and therapy are necessary to completely evaluate, stabilize, and adequately treat the patient's condition?
   - Is there a condition that requires specialist consultation, urgent operative intervention, or hospitalization?
   - Is there a condition that requires patient transfer (after adequate evaluation and necessary stabilization) to a facility more capable of providing the optimal level of required care?

3. The threat to life is identified on the basis of the patient's
   a. Chief complaint(s).
   b. Primary survey (see I.B.4. above).
   c. Vital signs.
   d. Directed examination/diagnostic evaluation.

4. Resuscitation and other therapy needed to stabilize the patient's condition are administered simultaneously with the patient's evaluation.

5. Routine vital signs are pulse, blood pressure, respiratory rate, and temperature. Additional "vital signs" include the following:
   a. Blood glucose level in the patient with diabetes mellitus.
   b. Body weight in the pediatric patient.
   c. Cardiac rhythm and oxygen saturation in any patient with a significant cardiac or respiratory complaint.
   d. Electrocardiogram, cardiac rhythm, and SaO_2 in the critically ill patient, seriously ill patient, multiple-trauma patient, arrhythmia patient, and/or individual with chest pain suspicious of cardiac ischemia.
   e. Fetal heart tones in the pregnant patient.
   f. Mental status in all patients.
   g. Visual acuity in the patient with an eye complaint.

6. An abnormal vital sign is always cause for concern. It must be rechecked and accounted for over the course of the patient's ED evaluation and treatment.

7. The leading conditions in the differential diagnosis of the patient's presenting complaint(s) are those posing the greatest threat to life and those with significant morbidity. The evaluation of the patient must be oriented so that these conditions are reasonably excluded before the patient's final disposition is considered. *Assume the worst.*

8. Worrisome situations, or potential "red flags," include any of the following:
   a. Abnormal vital signs.
   b. Altered mentation.
   c. Age extreme (the very young or the very old).
   d. Failure to improve with reasonable treatment.
   e. Inadequate or no home situation.
   f. Multiple and significant chronic health problems.
   g. Potential or known immunocompromise (e.g., asplenic, cancer, severe diabetes mellitus, human immunodeficiency virus infection, injection drug use, and/or treatment with immunosuppressive medications).
   h. Potential or known multiple injury.
   i. Return visit to the ED.
   j. Inability to take medication by mouth.
   k. Inability to walk.

9. A diagnosis is not always possible in the ED, and the ED physician should not try to "force" a diagnosis on the patient's presenting complaint. Firm diagnoses may often take days to weeks of outpatient or inpatient evaluation. Some patients present to the ED with an illness (i.e., a perceived state of less-than-optimal health) without a specific diagnosis ever possible (i.e., no recognized disease state adequately explains or describes the patient's perceived dysfunctional health). Remember, the primary responsibility of the ED physician is to accurately identify and expertly initiate treatment for all true emergencies and to rule out conditions that are life-threatening or associated with significant morbidity. The goal of ED evaluation and treatment is *not* to arrive at a definitive diagnosis in every patient encounter.

10. The responsibility of the ED physician is first and foremost to the patient. This sometimes will necessitate uncomfortable disagreements with hospital administrators, admitting services, consultants, health care plans, and even the patient's primary care physician. All ED decisions should err on the side of the patient.

II. EMERGENCY DEPARTMENT PATIENT CARE

The following evaluation and treatment outline is based on the assumption that the patient has a real or potential life-threatening problem. In patients who are awake, alert, talking, and with normal vital signs and a nonurgent or minor presenting complaint, it is generally reasonable to proceed with a directed examination and definitive care.

A. Primary Survey and Resuscitation

1. Guard and secure the **airway** as necessary (see Chapter 11), and provide supplemental oxygen to ensure $\geq 95\%$ SaO_2. (*Caution:* in the patient with known chronic obstructive pulmonary disease who may be at risk for carbon dioxide retention with high-flow oxygen, an SaO_2 of 90% is an appropriate goal). If there is any possibility of cervical spine injury, rapidly immobilize the spine with a hard cervical collar, bolstering around the head to prevent movement, and secure the patient to a full-length backboard. Have airway suction capability at the bedside.

2. Quickly assess **breathing and ventilation.** Assist and manage as necessary depending on the specific cause of the compromise (see Chapters 13 and 14). Intubation is appropriate if *any* of the following conditions apply:
   a. The patient is unable to protect his/her airway.
   b. Spontaneous ventilations are inadequate.
   c. Oxygenation is inadequate ($< 90\%$ SaO_2 despite 100% oxygen supplementation).
   d. The patient is in profound shock.
   e. Hyperventilation (to a PCO_2 of 25–30 mmHg) is required to emergently reduce increased intracranial pressure (e.g., from a space-occupying lesion).

   Continuous *electrocardiography* and *pulse oximetry* should be routine in all critically or seriously ill individuals. An *arterial blood gas* determination may be necessary to assess PCO_2 and systemic pH, and to further assess PO_2.

3. Quickly assess **circulation and control hemorrhage.** Apply direct pressure to any external bleeding sites.
   a. Simultaneously, supporting ED staff should obtain the following:
      i. Vital signs.
      ii. Intravenous access (at least two "large-bore" lines, preferably in the upper extremities, in the setting of suspected hemorrhage or significant volume loss).
      iii. Fingerstick glucose level (if mental status is altered).
      iv. Electrocardiogram.
      v. Appropriate laboratory studies (including emergent blood typing and cross-matching in the setting of suspected significant hemorrhage or symptomatic anemia).
   b. Immediately manage any *cardiac arrhythmia* that is causing patient instability (see Chapter 13 for specific details). The *unstable* arrhythmia patient is defined by the presence of any of the following: ischemic chest pain, hypotension, altered mentation, hypoperfusion, or significant dyspnea.

c. *Hypotension* (systolic blood pressure < 90–100 mmHg) and/or *hypoperfusion* is usually secondary to a volume deficit and should generally be treated with a rapid infusion of 1–2 L normal saline or lactated Ringer's solution in the adult; monitor pulmonary status and cardiac function closely (see Chapter 12).

d. *Vasopressors* may be required if clinical evidence of pulmonary edema (cardiogenic or noncardiogenic) contraindicates crystalloid administration in the hypotensive/ hypoperfused patient. In most instances, dopamine will be the drug of choice (dose: begin with 2–5 µg/kg/min IV infusion and adjust as necessary to achieve a systolic blood pressure of approximately 95–100 mmHg). A central venous catheter and/or Swan–Ganz catheter may ultimately be necessary to optimally manage volume status in uncertain situations (see Chapter 12).

4. Look for **disability** or **deficits.** Perform a directed neurologic examination by assessing the level of consciousness, pupillary response, and any gross lateralized deficits.

a. Thiamine (100 mg IV), glucose (25–50 g D50W IV), and naloxone (≥ 0.4–2 mg IV) should be *routinely* administered to the patient with an altered level of consciousness or frank coma. If the fingerstick glucose level is ≥ 80 mg/dL, however, immediate parenteral glucose is unnecessary.

b. Administer other antidotes as required in the setting of a known toxin exposure (see Chapter 23).

c. Immediately control ongoing seizure activity (see Chapter 20).

5. **Undress the patient and obtain environmental control.** Remove the patient's clothing to allow for a complete examination, assess body temperature, initiate necessary therapy for hypo- or hyperthermia, and protect the patient from further harm.

a. In the comatose or critically ill patient place the following:

i. Foley catheter (to monitor urine output). (*Caution:* Foley catheterization is contraindicated in the trauma patient with blood at the urethral meatus, a perineal/ scrotal hematoma, and/or a high-riding prostate on rectal examination.)

ii. Nasogastric tube (to decompress the stomach). (*Caution:* a nasogastric tube should be placed orally *instead* of nasally in the patient with significant midface trauma, suspected basilar skull fracture, or known severe coagulopathy.)

b. In the comatose patient, protect the eyes from desiccation and injury (consider applying an ophthalmic lubricant [e.g., Lacrilube] and gently taping the eyelids closed).

c. Keep the guardrails up on the patient's stretcher.

d. Soft restraints should be placed to prevent patient self-harm if the patient's mental status is altered.

e. Never leave a critically ill, seriously ill, or comatose patient alone in the ED. A physician or nursing personnel should accompany the patient outside of the ED if further diagnostic studies are needed away from the department.

Note: at this point, the primary survey has been completed, and all immediate and necessary resuscitation measures have been initiated. The patient's ABCs and vital signs should now be reassessed.

B. Secondary Survey

1. Perform a comprehensive **physical examination,** including assessment of the following:
   a. Vital signs (also see comments under I.C.5, above).
   b. Skin.
   c. HEENT (Head, eyes, ears, nose, mouth, pharynx, and throat).
   d. Neck, back, and spine.
   e. Chest.
   f. Heart.
   g. Abdomen.
   h. Genitourinary tract, including
      i. Genital examination.
      ii. Pelvic examination in females.
      iii. Rectal examination.
   i. Extremities
   j. Musculoskeletal system, including
      i. Muscle bulk and tone.
      ii. Joint range of motion.
      iii. Strength assessment.
      iv. Deep tendon reflexes (DTRs).
   k. Nervous system, including
      i. Mental status.
      ii. Cranial nerves II–XII.
      iii. Sensation.
      iv. Cerebellar function.

Note: the above-outlined complete physical examination is appropriate in the ED patient who is comatose, critically ill, in shock, multiply injured, or otherwise seriously ill. In most other patients, however, the examination can be streamlined and focused on the relevant body/system areas as directed by the patient's presentation.

2. Obtain required **laboratory studies** and perform **further diagnostic testing.**
   a. The specific studies/tests necessary depend on the chief complaint and overall condition of the patient. To optimize time use, blood for laboratory evaluation should be obtained at the time of intravenous access during the primary survey.

Consider the following studies *initially* in the **critically ill patient:**

    i. Arterial blood gas values.

    ii. Blood type and crossmatch (in the patient at risk for, or known to be suffering from, significant blood loss; see Chapter 21 for further information).

    iii. Chest radiograph (portable).

    iv. Complete blood count (CBC), including platelets.

    v. Electrocardiogram.

    vi. Electrolytes, glucose, blood urea nitrogen (BUN), creatinine.

    vii. Pregnancy test (in reproductive-age females deemed at risk for pregnancy).

    viii. Prothrombin time/partial thromboplastin time (PT/PTT) (in the bleeding patient and/or those at risk for a coagulation disorder).

    ix. Urinalysis.

b. Recommendations for appropriate laboratory studies are presented in subsequent chapters on specific emergency conditions. No laboratory work or diagnostic tests may be needed in otherwise healthy patients with simple and nonurgent problems.

c. Before ordering any test, the ED physician should consider the usefulness of the test with respect to

    i. Establishing a diagnosis.

    ii. Ruling out a serious or significant condition.

    iii. Assisting in treatment.

Table 1–1 presents appropriate and inappropriate reasons for obtaining a variety of frequently ordered ED laboratory and radiographic studies.

C. Definitive Care

1. Continued Therapy

Treatment has already been initiated in the resuscitation and stabilization steps described above. *Specific therapy* of the identified disease process(es) should also be started as soon as possible. See the relevant chapters in this manual for further treatment recommendations.

2. Continued Patient Evaluation

This may include repeat examination, patient observation, additional laboratory work, and/or specific diagnostic procedures beyond those outlined in the primary and secondary surveys.

3. Specialty Consultation

a. The ED physician should use every needed and available resource to provide adequate patient care. This frequently necessitates consultation with one or more specialists. In

Table 1–1. TEST ORDERING IN THE EMERGENCY DEPARTMENT: REASONABLE AND INAPPROPRIATE USES

TEST	REASONABLE USES	INAPPROPRIATE USES
Abdominal radiographs	Evaluation of moderate or worse abdominal tenderness Radiopaque foreign-body localization (ingested or penetrating) Suspected abdominal free air Suspected bowel ischemia Suspected intestinal obstruction	Isolated gastroenteritis symptoms (nausea, vomiting, and/or diarrhea) Suspected appendicitis or biliary tract disease Routine evaluation of abdominal pain
Arterial blood gas levels (ABGs)	Asthmatic patient who is clinically developing respiratory failure or is otherwise critically ill COPD patient at risk for carbon dioxide retention Cyanosis, unexplained mental status changes, and/or coma Shock or other states of hypoperfusion Significant dyspnea and acute pulmonary disease Suspected acid–base disturbance Symptomatic smoke inhalation Unexplained anxiety, behavior changes, dyspnea, and/or restlessness	Patients with normal peripheral perfusion who have a reasonable SaO_2 by pulse oximetry and are without a suspected acid–base or ventilatory disorder Uncomplicated acute myocardial infarction or patients who are candidates for thrombolytic therapy Uncomplicated asthma (including the pediatric patient)
Blood ethanol level	Altered mental status of undetermined cause Clinically intoxicated patient in whom the blood ethanol level is useful in treatment and/or disposition Unconscious patient	Mildly intoxicated individual in whom neither treatment nor disposition is affected by the blood ethanol level
Chest radiographs	Acute MI patient or individual with symptomatic ischemic heart disease Admission radiograph in patients with any of the following: altered mental status, age > 65 yrs, cigarette use, congestive heart failure, HIV infection, history of cancer Asthma patient with any of the following (the "four Fs"): first episode of asthma, fever, focal findings on pulmonary examination, or failure to respond to reasonable ED therapy. Cough and fever in a patient > 40 yrs Febrile, neutropenic patient Evaluation of hemoptysis Pediatric ICU admission Reasonable clinical suspicion of pneumonia on the basis of symptoms and at least one vital sign abnormality Sickle cell patients with chest symptoms and/or fever Symptoms of congestive heart failure	Pediatric patient with chest pain and an unremarkable examination Routine admission radiograph in patient without chest symptoms, who does not fall into any of the high-risk groups listed at left Uncomplicated asthma exacerbation

MI, myocardial infarction; ICU, intensive care unit; hCG, human chorionic gonadotropin.
Adapted from Cantrill SV, and Karas S Jr. Cost-effective Diagnostic Testing in Emergency Medicine. Dallas: Am. Coll Emerg Phys, 1994. *Table continued on following page*

Table 1-1. TEST ORDERING IN THE EMERGENCY DEPARTMENT: REASONABLE AND INAPPROPRIATE USES *Continued*

TEST	REASONABLE USES	INAPPROPRIATE USES
Lumbar spine radiographs	**Low back pain and any of the following conditions:** Age > 50 yrs Alcohol abuse Cancer history Chronic corticosteroid use Clinically suspected ankylosing spondylitis Failure of back pain to resolve after 4 weeks of appropriate therapy Intravenous and other drug abuse Motor deficit on neurologic examination Suspected litigation Trauma history Unexplained weight loss or fever Worker's compensation	Otherwise healthy individual with back pain after lifting, bending, or other exertion
Complete blood count (CBC)	Evaluation of the patient with abdominal pain Fever of undetermined source in infants and children Other situations where the CBC is important in either diagnosis or therapy	"Routine" admission labs in the absence of specific clinical indications Uncomplicated acute gastroenteritis Uncomplicated acute upper respiratory tract infection When all that is needed is either a hemoglobin level or hematocrit
Pregnancy test (Beta-hCG)	**Reproductive age females with any of the following:** Abdominal pain (or other presentations worrisome for possible ectopic pregnancy) Abnormal vaginal bleeding Acute pelvic pain Clinical suspicion of pregnancy ED evaluation of the female sexual assault victim Patient with suspected gestational trophoblastic disease Suspected threatened or spontaneous abortion To rule out pregnancy prior to diagnostic or therapeutic interventions that are a real or potential risk to the fetus	Already documented reliable pregnancy test (note: does not include patient report of a positive home pregnancy test!) Posthysterectomy patient Postmenopausal patient Pregnancy already demonstrated clinically (e.g., positive ultrasound, fetal heart tones) When pregnancy is not an issue in either patient diagnosis or treatment
Serum electrolyte panel	Age ≥ 55 yrs Alcohol abuse Altered mental status Chronic hypertension Diabetes mellitus Diuretic use Muscle weakness New onset seizures Poor oral intake Recent electrolyte abnormality Renal disease Significant volume loss Vomiting	Healthy patients with uncomplicated gastroenteritis Routine ordering in the absence of specific clinical criteria Uncomplicated seizure in a patient with a known seizure disorder without other historical or examination findings suggesting a new electrolyte abnormality

Table 1–1. TEST ORDERING IN THE EMERGENCY DEPARTMENT:
REASONABLE AND INAPPROPRIATE USES *Continued*

TEST	REASONABLE USES	INAPPROPRIATE USES
Toxicology screens (*Caution:* remember, a negative toxicology screen does not rule out a life-threatening ingestion of a substance *NOT* detected by that screen.)	Patient has severe clinical or biochemical abnormalities possibly secondary to a drug or poison Patient has seizures, coma, or a head injury and there is suspicion of a drug ingestion To help differentiate functional psychosis from a drug effect To help differentiate hypoxic brain death from a prolonged drug effect Patient presents with a confusing clinical picture, atypical symptoms or signs, and historical clues are lacking	Diagnosis is already clear based on the history and physical examination Minimal or no symptoms and an unremarkable examination in an otherwise healthy patient When specific serum levels for the known toxin(s) are available
Urine cultures	Patients with signs and/or symptoms of a urinary tract infection; urinalysis is positive for white blood cells, leukocyte esterase, or bacteria, and one or more of the following conditions apply: Children (age ≤ 15 yrs) Diabetes mellitus Females > 50 yrs Immunocompromised (including renal dialysis patients) Males Other significant health problems Patient suspected of bacteremia, pyelonephritis, or urosepsis Pregnant Recent hospitalization or recent antibiotic course Renal disease or known urinary tract abnormalities (including indwelling catheters, neurogenic bladder, or obstructive lesions) Urinary tract symptoms for ≥ 6 days	Uncomplicated cystitis in an otherwise healthy nonpregnant female ≤ 50 yrs

MI, myocardial infarction; ICU, intensive care unit; hCG, human chorionic gonadotropin.
Adapted from Cantrill and Karas; 1994.

exigent and emergent situations, *immediate* specialist consultation may be an essential part of the patient's primary survey and resuscitation (e.g., urgent general surgery consultation in the hemodynamically unstable multiple trauma patient). *Failure to obtain necessary and appropriate specialist consultation may be considered negligent ED care!*

    b. Ideally, the consultant should respond within 30 minutes of the ED physician's call. Presentations to the consultant should be succinct! The initial one to two sentences of the presentation should
       i. Introduce the ED physician to the consultant.
      ii. Identify the patient's age and sex.
      iii. Describe the patient's condition (e.g., stable, serious, or critically ill).
      iv. Give the reason for the consultation.

After giving this preliminary information, pause to see if the consultant has any questions or if a *brief,* accurate, and to-the-point case description is wanted.

    c. Sometimes, the ED physician may not agree with the consultant's recommendations. It must be emphasized that the ED care provider is the patient's advocate, and his/her primary responsibility is always to the patient.
      i. If the difference in opinion occurs during a phone consultation, request that the consultant come to the ED to evaluate the patient directly.
      ii. If the difference in opinion occurs with a *resident* consultant, the case should be discussed with the attending specialist.
      iii. If the difference in opinion occurs with an *attending* consultant, every attempt should be made to resolve the dispute reasonably. If this is not possible, the patient should be informed of the differences in opinion and a second specialist consulted. If no second specialist is available, the director of the ED and the chief of the consulting specialty should be notified in an attempt to resolve the situation.
    d. Whenever possible, the patient's primary care physician (if there is one) should be identified and notified of the patient's ED visit and should facilitate continued care and necessary follow-up.

4. *Disposition*

Care of the ED patient continues until the diagnosis and all ED treatment is completed, all presenting complaints have been addressed, and the patient is discharged from the department. The ED physician's responsibility for the patient is not concluded until the patient safely leaves the ED. Departmental "discharge" may include any of the following:

    a. DISCHARGE TO HOME
    This disposition is reasonable when the patient's health problem does not necessitate further inpatient evaluation and/or treatment. Usual requirements for home discharge include *all* of the following:
      i. ED care is completed.

    ii. Vital signs are normal. If one or more vital signs have been persistently abnormal (e.g., mild to moderately elevated BP), the abnormal vital sign(s) should be rechecked and at the patient's "baseline" prior to discharge. In addition, the vital sign abnormality must not be serious. A plan for rechecking the abnormal vital sign(s) as an outpatient should be clearly described in the discharge instructions.

    iii. The patient is awake and alert. If the patient's mental status is chronically abnormal (e.g., from dementia), the patient must be at his/her "normal" baseline as identified by family members or caretakers.

    iv. The medical condition is satisfactory and stable.

    v. No life-threatening problem is present.

    vi. No problem necessitating hospitalization or urgent operation is present.

    vii. The patient is safely ambulatory or at "baseline" mobility.

    viii. The patient has been educated with respect to the nature of his/her illness or complaint, its evaluation and treatment in the ED, and further expected course or outcome.

    ix. The patient has received appropriate instruction (including written discharge instructions) with respect to continued required care and medication use. Discharge instructions should always include a clear statement to the patient of the absolute need for return to the ED should the patient's condition worsen or fail to improve.

    x. Outpatient follow-up (including resumption of primary care) is arranged and/or is clearly recommended in the written discharge instructions.

b. ADMISSION TO THE HOSPITAL

When one or more of the above "discharge to home" criteria cannot be met, hospitalization is appropriate. Indications for hospital admission vary with the specific condition and are covered in greater detail in subsequent chapters.

c. PATIENT TRANSFER

A patient's condition may necessitate transfer to another institution more capable of providing the required level of definitive care. Interhospital transfer is a reasonable consideration *only* when it is made in the interests of the patient and his/her health. Prior to transfer from the ED, the patient must receive (1) an adequate screening examination, and (2) adequate stabilization of the emergency medical condition to the full capabilities of the transferring institution (including diagnostic and therapeutic interventions and specialist consultation if indicated). In addition to these requirements, Consolidated Omnibus Budget

Reconciliation Act (COBRA) legislation mandates *all* of the following (and stiff penalties for violations):

   i. The medical benefits of care at the receiving facility must outweigh any increased risks associated with the transfer.

   ii. The receiving facility must be capable of providing the level of care that is necessitating the transfer (including space, personnel, and required diagnostic and treatment capabilities).

   iii. A physician at the receiving facility has been personally contacted, is informed of the patient's condition and reason(s) for the transfer, and *accepts* the patient at the receiving facility.

   iv. All relevant medical information (including the patient's history, physical examination, vital signs, laboratory and other diagnostic test results, treatment provided, responses to that treatment, consultations obtained, and condition at the time of transfer) is copied and accompanies the patient.

   v. The patient is informed of the reason(s) for the transfer and the risks and benefits of the transfer, and accepts the transfer.

   vi. A list of the risks and benefits associated with the transfer is signed by the patient and the transferring physician.

   vii. Necessary skilled personnel and equipment accompany the patient to ensure medical stability throughout the transfer.

   viii. The transferring facility has arranged an appropriate mode of transportation for the patient.

The medical record must carefully document the medical screening examination, the diagnostic and therapeutic interventions that were necessary to ensure patient stability, and the above-described transfer requirements. A competent patient may refuse the transfer, but the patient must be informed of the risks and benefits he/she is undertaking by that refusal; a written informed consent of the transfer refusal should be obtained.

III. MEDICAL RECORD DOCUMENTATION

A. General Concepts

1. The ED medical record is the written documentation of all medical information obtained and care the patient received while in the department (including prehospital field evaluation and care by paramedic and/or ambulance personnel).

2. Meticulous documentation is crucial:
   a. It conveys important information that assists all subsequent care providers in optimally treating and managing the patient's medical condition.

b. A well-documented medical record facilitates fair and appropriate ED billing and subsequent reimbursement by the patient, insurance companies, and/or governmental agencies (e.g., Medicare).

c. Careful documentation is a specific requirement of the Joint Commission for the Accreditation of Healthcare Organizations (JCAHO), the Professional Review Organization (PRO), the Health Care Financing Administration (HCFA), federal legislation (including COBRA), and many individual state statutes.

d. A well-documented medical record facilitates subsequent appropriate legal intervention and justice on behalf of patients who are victims of violence, other trauma, sexual assault, child abuse, and/or hazardous conditions.

e. It is the written proof of the expert care provided the patient by the ED physician and staff. As such, it is the first and best defense of that care in the setting of a malpractice lawsuit.

B. Specific Recommendations in Chart Documentation

1. The medical record must be legible. If the signature of the physician is not readable, his/her name should be printed legibly next to the signature.

2. The chief complaint of the patient, as documented by prehospital care providers and/or nursing staff, must also be addressed in the physician's write-up.

3. The history and physical examination should carefully address the patient's presenting complaint(s) and any potential life-threatening or serious conditions suggested by that (those) complaint(s).

4. All vital signs must be carefully recorded, and abnormal vital signs rechecked to document their return to normal over the course of the patient's ED stay. A persistently abnormal vital sign should be discussed in the write-up, and a plan for follow-up documented and included in the discharge instructions.

5. All laboratory, radiographic, and electrocardiographic results should be carefully recorded and special note made of abnormalities. Whenever possible, current abnormal findings should be compared with prior studies, and that comparison documented (e.g., "chest x-ray unchanged from prior chest radiograph 2 years previously").

6. Document the patient's ED course, including response to therapy, and the condition at the time of discharge. The patient's mode of transportation from the ED is a relevant consideration in the setting of alcohol use, other drug use, or

ED medications that may alter judgment and make driving unsafe for either the patient or society.

7. The medical record must make sense and be internally consistent. The patient's assessment (and diagnosis when a diagnosis is possible) must be logical and appropriate given the documented prehospital care, triage and nursing notes, chief complaint, history, physical examination, vital signs, and diagnostic studies.

8. The patient's disposition must be consistent with the assessment and/or diagnosis. Never discharge a patient when the diagnosis is a life-threatening, potentially life-threatening, or serious condition that mandates hospitalization.

9. The patient should be given written discharge instructions that specify needed continued care, medication use, necessary follow-up, and the need for ED return should the patient's condition worsen or fail to improve.

10. Miscellaneous recommendations:
    a. Date and time all entries.
    b. Number the pages of the write-up (e.g., "page 1 of 2," "page 2 of 2").
    c. Never use derogatory or demeaning statements.
    d. If something is written in error, draw a single line through it, and initial the correction.
    e. Document not only drug allergies, but also what that allergic reaction was (e.g., "Allergies: penicillin—rash").
    f. Document immunization status in any pediatric patient; if not current, address this issue in the patient's discharge instructions.
    g. Document tetanus immunization status, and update if indicated, in any patient with a break in his/her integument (including corneal abrasions).
    h. Consider the possibility of pregnancy in any reproductive-age female. Document last normal menstrual period, birth control method, and whether the patient believes she may be pregnant. A serum or urine pregnancy test is indicated if diagnosis or therapy are directly influenced by a positive test result.
    i. Document a careful neurovascular and functional examination in any patient with an extremity injury.
    j. Measure and record the length of lacerations or other significant skin abnormalities (e.g., abrasions, burns, hematomas).
    k. Document the dominant hand and patient occupation in any patient with an upper-extremity injury.
    l. Record the number of pills dispensed when prescribing opioids or any schedule II medications.
    m. Write a formal procedure note for any procedure performed.

n. Never alter the medical record after its completion. Additional information may be added by a dated and timed addendum.

IV. PAIN MANAGEMENT

Pain is the most common presenting symptom in emergency medicine. It may be secondary to an acute process, chronic pain of a terminal illness (most often cancer), or chronic pain not related to malignancy. The optimal management of pain depends on the accurate diagnosis and treatment of its cause, but even when this is possible, diagnosis, treatment, and response to therapy take time. The appropriate use of medications in the symptomatic treatment of pain is an essential skill of all physicians, including the ED practitioner.

A. General Concepts

1. Acute pain is *undertreated.* In the ED, patients frequently wait unnecessarily long before their acute pain and its management are addressed.

2. Opioids are *underutilized* in the management of acute pain.

3. When prompt analgesia is required to control moderate to severe acute pain, opioid analgesics are the drugs of choice, and intravenous administration is the route of choice.

4. Acetaminophen, aspirin, or other nonsteroidal anti-inflammatory drugs (NSAIDs) can be combined with opioids to achieve an additive analgesic effect.

5. Psychic dependence or addiction is extremely uncommon in patients who are appropriately given opioids for acute pain or cancer pain.

6. Opioid analgesia is *not* contraindicated in the patient with undiagnosed abdominal pain. It is reasonable to ameliorate moderate to severe pain with a carefully titrated parenteral analgesic agent while an expeditious workup proceeds. The ED physician should work with his/her surgical colleagues to develop a reasonable plan in this setting to minimize patient suffering.

7. Carefully titrated parenteral analgesia *does not* preclude an informed consent for a procedure (e.g., surgery) from an awake and competent patient.

8. Patients with a known narcotic addiction still require analgesia before any painful procedure.

9. Clinically significant physical dependence to opioids requires at least several weeks of chronic treatment with large doses of morphine-like medications.

10. Opioids are *overutilized* in the management of chronic pain not related to malignancy. They should be avoided in this setting.

B. Specific Medications

All doses are for adult patients.

1. Acetaminophen

a. **Dose.** 650 mg PO q 4–6 hr (maximum dose 1 g PO q 6 hr).
b. **Comments.** Acetaminophen has combined analgesic and antipyretic effects; antiinflammatory activity is minimal. It is especially useful in patients who are unable to take NSAIDs because of drug allergy, bleeding disorders, warfarin therapy, peptic ulcer disease, or gastrointestinal intolerance.
c. **Caution.** Some patients with active liver disease, or significant alcohol abuse and chronic hepatic injury, may develop hepatic toxicity with the 4–g/day dose.

2. Salicylates

a. **Dose.** See Table 1–2 for a list of salicylates and their dosing. Aspirin is also available in enteric-coated preparations (e.g., Ecotrin) or in combination with antacids (e.g., Ascriptin).
b. **Comments**
   i. Salicylates have analgesic, anti-inflammatory, and antipyretic effects.
   ii. Therapeutic salicylate serum levels are 10–30 mg/dL.
   iii. Adverse effects can include dose-related dizziness, hearing loss, and tinnitus; asthma exacerbation and/or anaphylaxis in asthmatics who are sensitive to salicylates or other NSAIDs; impaired platelet function and a prolonged bleeding time (most pronounced with aspirin, which irreversibly impairs platelet function for the 7-day lifetime of a platelet); Reye's syndrome in children and teenagers with influenza and varicella infections; and gastric mucosal injury (which may result in severe bleeding).
   iv. The nonacetylated aspirins (e.g., choline magnesium trisalicylate and salsalate), lack the antiplatelet effects of aspirin and are less injurious to the gastric mucosa, but have a slower onset of action.
c. **Caution.** Avoid aspirin and other salicylates in the presence of any of the following: active peptic ulcer disease, asthma and a history of aspirin or NSAID sensitivity, bleeding disorders, viral syndromes (in pediatric or young adult patients), pregnancy, renal insufficiency, or warfarin therapy.

3. Other NSAIDs

a. **Dose.** See Table 1–2 for a list of these agents and their dosing.

Table 1–2. NONSTEROIDAL ANTI-INFLAMMATORY DRUGS AND THEIR DOSING

Drug	Dose	Maximum Dose
Carboxylic Acids		
Acetylsalicylic acid (aspirin) Tablets: 325, 500 mg	325–975 mg PO q 4-6 hr	4000 mg/24 hr
Choline magnesium trisalicylate (Trilisate) Tablets: 500, 750, 1000 mg	500–1000 mg PO q 12 hr	3000 mg/24 hr
Diflunisal (Dolobid) Tablets: 250, 500 mg	1000 mg PO initially, then 500 mg PO q 8–12 hr	1500 mg/24 hr
Salsalate (Disalcid) Tablets: 500, 750 mg Capsules: 500 mg	1000 mg PO tid, or 1500 mg PO bid	3000 mg/24 hr
Acetic Acids		
Diclofenac sodium (Voltaren) Tablets: 25, 50, 75 mg	25–50 mg PO tid or qid, or 75 mg PO bid	200 mg/24 hr
Etodolac (Lodine) Capsules: 200, 300 mg	200–400 mg PO q 6–8 hr	1200 mg/24 hr in patients ≥ 60 kg
Ketorolac (Toradol) Prefilled syringes: 15 mg/mL (1 mL) or 30 mg/mL (1,2 mL) Tablets: 10 mg	30–60 mg IM initially (use lower dose for patients < 50 kg or > 65 yrs), then 30 mg IM q 6 hr or 10 mg PO q 6 hr	IM: 120 mg/24 hr, do not use daily for longer than 5 days PO: 40 mg/24 hr, for short-term use only
Indomethacin (Indocin) Capsules: 25, 50 mg SR capsules: 75 mg Suppositories: 50 mg	25–50 mg PO or PR bid–tid (start at lower dose); or slow–release (SR) capsules, 75 mg PO q day (may increase to bid if necessary)	200 mg/24 hr
Sulindac (Clinoril) Tablets: 150, 200 mg	150–200 mg PO bid	400 mg/24 hr
Tolmetin (Tolectin) Tablets: 200, 600 mg Capsules: 400 mg	400 mg PO q 8 hr	1800 mg/24 hr
Propionic and Phenylpropionic Acids		
Fenoprofen (Nalfon) Tablets: 600 mg Capsules: 200, 300 mg	200 mg PO q 4–6 hr; up to 300–600 mg PO tid or qid	1200 mg/24 hr for moderate pain; 3200 mg/24 hr for arthritis
Flurbiprofen (Ansaid) Tablets: 50, 100 mg	50–100 mg PO bid–tid	300 mg/24 hr
Ketoprofen (Orudis) Capsules: 25, 50, 75 mg	25–50 mg PO q 6–8 hr; up to 75 mg tid	300 mg/24 hr
Ibuprofen (Motrin, Rufen) Tablets: 300, 400, 600, 800 mg	300 mg PO qid; 400–600 mg PO q 6–8 hr; or maximum dose of 800 mg PO tid	2400 mg/24 hr
Naproxen (Naprosyn) Tablets: 250, 375, 500 mg	250, 375, or 500 mg PO bid	1250 mg/24 hr

Table continued on following page

Table 1–2. NONSTEROIDAL ANTI-INFLAMMATORY DRUGS AND THEIR DOSING *Continued*

DRUG	DOSE	MAXIMUM DOSE
Naproxen sodium (Anaprox) Tablets: 275, 550 mg	550 mg PO initially, then 275 mg PO q 6–8 hr; up to 550 mg PO bid	1375 mg/24 hr
Fenamic Acids		
Meclofenamate sodium (Meclomen) Capsules: 50, 100 mg	50 mg PO q 4–6 hr	400 mg/24 hr
Mefanamic acid (Ponstel) Tablets: 250, 500 mg	500 mg initially, then 250 mg PO q 6–8 hr	1250 mg/24 hr; duration of use ≤ 1 week
Enolic Acids		
Piroxicam (Feldene) Capsules: 10, 20 mg	10 mg PO bid or 20 mg PO q am	20 mg/24 hr

b. **Comments**

   i. A patient should take only a single NSAID at a time (i.e., there is no advantage to combining different agents, and toxicity is increased). Some patients may respond better to one NSAID than to another.

   ii. NSAIDs have analgesic, anti-inflammatory, and anti-pyretic effects. There is an analgesic "ceiling" with these agents: giving more than the maximum recommended dose does not improve analgesia.

   iii. Most of these medications are more potent analgesic agents than aspirin or acetaminophen; many are also more conveniently dosed.

   iv. NSAIDs should always be administered with food. Do not prescribe them to patients with active peptic ulcer disease. Avoid their use in patients with a prior history of complicated peptic ulcer disease; if this is not possible, consider simultaneous "prophylactic" anti-ulcer therapy (e.g., with ranitidine 150 mg PO bid).

   v. Lithium excretion is decreased with many of these agents.

   vi. NSAIDs can impair the antihypertensive actions of angiotensin-converting enzyme inhibitors, beta-blockers, and diuretics.

   vii. Adverse reactions are similar to those of salicylates, with the most common being gastrointestinal side effects (including significant gastrointestinal hemorrhage) and worsened renal function (including frank renal failure). Risk factors for renal injury include ascites, chronic renal insufficiency, congestive heart failure, diuretic therapy, old age, and/or volume depletion. Nephrotoxicity may be less with sulindac (Clinoril).

      viii. Miscellaneous side effects may include hepatic transaminase elevation, acute hepatitis, bone marrow toxicity, mental status changes (most frequently reported in the elderly, most significant with indomethacin), skin rashes, and/or pulmonary toxicity.

      ix. In patients using NSAIDs for extended periods, monitor renal, hepatic, and hematologic function.

  c. *Caution.* Avoid NSAIDs in the presence of any of the following: active peptic ulcer disease, asthma and a history of aspirin and/or NSAID sensitivity, bleeding disorders, lithium therapy, hepatic insufficiency, renal insufficiency (or those at significant risk for same), or warfarin therapy. They are contraindicated in patients receiving high-dose methotrexate therapy ($\geq$ 50 mg/week).

4. Opioids

  a. **Dose.** See Table 1–3 for oral agents and Table 1–4 for parenteral agents, including dosing.

  b. **Comments**

      i. *Opium* is a mixture of alkaloids extracted from the opium poppy. Both codeine and morphine are found in opium. An *opioid* is a drug with opium-like activity. The words "opioid" and "narcotic" are commonly used interchangeably, but, strictly speaking, "narcotic" is a nonspecific term referring to any drug capable of producing sleep.

      ii. Opioids are the drugs of choice for severe acute pain or chronic, malignancy-related pain. Intravenous administration is the route of choice in the ED for the patient in significant pain.

      iii. The analgesic effect of opioids may be augmented with acetaminophen, salicylates, or other NSAIDs, as described above.

      iv. The appropriate dosing of opioids varies widely between individuals. The goal of therapy is adequate analgesia without undue sedation or respiratory depression; the dosing interval should be frequent enough to prevent recurrence of moderate to severe pain.

      v. In the inpatient management of pain, repeat dosing of opioids should be on a *time* basis rather than a prn basis to minimize both pain recurrence and pain behavior. The medication can be withheld for excessive somnolence or respiratory depression.

      vi. Unfortunately, opioids are relatively ineffective in the treatment of neuropathic pain (e.g., pain secondary to amputation [phantom limb pain], cordotomy, nerve avulsion, and/or peripheral neuropathy).

      vii. Opioids should be *avoided* in patients with chronic pain unrelated to malignancy because of the real potential for addiction, conditioned pain behavior,

Table 1–3. COMMONLY USED ORAL OPIOIDS AND RECOMMENDED INITIAL DOSING

Drug	Oral Dose Equivalent to 10 MG IM Morphine	Initial Dosing	Comments
Codeine [Tylenol #3 (30 mg codeine and 300 mg acetaminophen); others]	180 mg	30–60 mg PO q 4–6 hr	Small abuse potential. Good antitussive. Prominent side effects include constipation, nausea, and sedation
Meperidine (Demerol)	160–240 mg (oral meperidine has 1/2 to 1/3 the potency of the parenteral preparation)	50–150 mg PO q 3–4 hr	Contraindicated in patients on monoamine oxidase inhibitors or in renal failure. Poor oral availability
Hydrocodone [Vicodin (5 mg hydrocodone and 500 mg acetaminophen); Vicodin ES (7.5 mg hydrocodone and 750 mg acetaminophen); others]	30 mg	5–10 mg PO q 4–6 hr	More effective than codeine with fewer side effects. Keep dose of acetaminophen component < 4 g/24 hr
Oxycodone [Percocet (5 mg oxycodone and 325 mg acetaminophen); Percodan (5 mg oxycodone and 325 mg aspirin); Tylox (5 mg oxycodone and 500 mg acetaminophen); others]	25 mg	5 mg PO q 4–6 hr	More effective than codeine with fewer side effects. Keep dose of acetaminophen component < 4 g/24 hr. Euphoria may increase abuse potential
Hydromorphone (Dilaudid)	7.5 mg (oral preparation has less bioavailability than the parenteral preparation)	2 mg PO q 4–6 hr	Potent opioid with high abuse potential and high "street value". Also available as a suppository (3 mg PR q 6–8 hr)

significant physical dependence, and overall *increased* patient suffering in this setting.

viii. Unlike NSAIDs, these agents do not have an analgesic "ceiling," although the adverse effects of respiratory depression and/or hypotension do impose a maximum safe dosage in any given patient. Tolerance develops over time.

Table 1–4. PARENTERAL OPIOIDS COMMONLY USED IN EMERGENCY MEDICINE

Drug	Parenteral Dose Equivalent to 10 mg IM Morphine	Common Dosing	Comments
Meperidine (Demerol)	80 mg	IV: 25–50 mg q 15–60 min prn IM: 50–125 mg q 3–4 hr	Contraindicated in patients on monoamine oxidase inhibitors or those in renal failure Long-acting metabolite may cause seizures; avoid multiple repeat doses
Nalbuphine (Nubain)	12 mg	IV: 10 mg in 70 kg patient; may repeat dose in 60 min IM, SC: 10 mg in 70 kg patient q 3–6 hr prn	Mixed agonist/antagonist with less risk of either abuse or respiratory depression. May cause symptoms/signs of opioid withdrawal in the opioid dependent patient
Morphine	10 mg	IV: 2–5 mg q 10 min prn IM, SC: 5–10 mg q 4 hr prn	Half-life is 2–3 hr in healthy young adults when administered IV
Butorphanol (Stadol)	1.5–2.5 mg	IV: 0.5–2 mg q 3–4 hr prn IM: 1–4 mg q 3–4 hr prn Intranasal (metered dose spray): one spray to one nostril q 3–4 hr	Mixed agonist/antagonist; may cause significant postural hypotension May cause symptoms/signs of opioid withdrawal in the opioid dependent patient
Hydromorphone (Dilaudid)	1.3 mg	IV: 1–2 mg q 4–6 hr IM, SC: 1–2 mg q 4–6 hr	Potent analgesic agent
Fentanyl (Sublimaze)	0.1 mg (100 μg)	IV: 1–2 μg/kg initially, then 1 μg/kg q 5–10 min prn IM: 100 μg q 1–2 hr	Short half-life (90 min) after IV administration makes it advantageous for analgesia during painful procedures It does not cause histamine release (unlike most other opioids)

      ix. Adverse effects include constipation, histamine release, hypotension, nausea and vomiting, sedation, other mental status changes, and respiratory depression. The latter is the most significant adverse effect.

      x. An antiemetic is frequently administered with an opioid (e.g., promethazine hydrochloride [Phenergan] 12.5–25 mg PO, PR, IM, or IV).

      xi. Opioids may be reversed with the antagonist naloxone (dose: 0.1–0.2 mg IV q 2 min as needed to reverse a *therapeutically administered* opioid, 2 mg IV as needed in the suspected opioid-poisoned patient).

  c. **Cautions**

      i. Beware of the respiratory depressant effects of opioids, especially in the elderly or patients with altered respiratory drive, asthma, chronic lung disease, hepatic insufficiency, and/or otherwise limited respiratory reserve.

      ii. The elderly patient or the individual with hepatic insufficiency should initially be given one-half the usual recommended dose of an opioid and the interval between doses should be increased by at least 50%.

      iii. The combination of opioids with alcohol, general anesthetics, phenothiazines, sedative-hypnotics, tranquilizers, and/or tricyclic antidepressants increases the risk of respiratory depression and should be avoided. Patients discharged from the ED should be cautioned to not combine a prescribed opioid with any of these medications. In addition, the patient must be cautioned against driving, operating heavy machinery, or engaging in any potentially hazardous activities while taking an opioid.

C. Conscious Sedation-Analgesia for Procedures

Emergency medicine is a procedure-oriented specialty, and adequate care of the ED patient during any procedure includes appropriate pain management. *Conscious sedation-analgesia* refers to the administration of both sedative and analgesic medications in a controlled fashion to achieve excellent pain control without compromising the patient's airway, oxygenation, or vital signs. Procedures for which conscious sedation-analgesia should be strongly considered include abscess drainage, burn care, central line insertion, chest tube insertion, dislocation or fracture reduction, and wound care.

Technique of Conscious Sedation-Analgesia*

STEP 1: PREPARATION

1. Place patient on a stretcher, administer supplemental oxygen via nasal cannula, and obtain baseline vital signs. Obtain informed

*Adapted from Yealy, Dunmire, and Paris. In Roberts JP, Hedges JR (eds): Clinical Procedures in Emergency Medicine. Philadelphia: W.B. Saunders, 1991, p. 507.

consent for both conscious sedation-analgesia and the procedure to be performed.

2. Establish intravenous access and keep the intravenous line open with a crystalloid solution.

3. Continuously monitor both cardiac rhythm and pulse oximetry. Maintain SaO_2 at $\geq 95\%$ throughout procedure.

4. Have the following immediately available at the bedside:
   - Airway suction capability.
   - Bag–valve–mask.
   - Nasopharyngeal and oropharyngeal airways.
   - Necessary equipment for intubation.
   - Cardioverter/defibrillator.
   - Resuscitation cart with all necessary drugs and equipment.
   - Benzodiazepine antagonist: flumazenil (0.1 mg/mL in 5-mL vials) Dose (if required): 0.2 mg (2 mL) IV over 15 sec. May administer subsequent doses every minute as needed to reverse excessive sedation. Maximum cumulative recommended dose in this setting is 1 mg.
   - Opioid antagonist: naloxone (0.4 mg/mL in 10-mL vials) Dose (if required): 0.1–0.2 mg IV q 2–3 min as needed to reverse respiratory depression.

5. Throughout procedure (at least every 5–10 minutes) have nursing staff check and record
   - Respiratory rate.
   - Pulse oximetry (monitor continuously, document every 5-10 minutes).
   - Pulse.
   - Blood pressure.
   - Level of consciousness.

STEP 2: ESTABLISH SEDATION

Midazolam (1 mg/mL in 2-mL vials).

1. Dosing:
   - Adult < 60 years old: 1–2.5 mg IV over 30 sec, subsequent doses of 1 mg q 3–5 min as required.
   - Adult $\geq$ 60 years old or otherwise debilitated patient: 1 mg IV over 30 sec, subsequent doses of 0.5–1.0 mg q 5 min as required.
   - Maximum recommended dose over time: $\leq$ 0.1 mg/kg.

2. Goal of sedation: a drowsy, but easily arousable patient who is able to speak with a normal or minimally altered voice.

STEP 3: ESTABLISH ANALGESIA

Fentanyl (50 µg/mL in 2-mL vials).

1. Dosing:
   - 100 µg IV over 60 sec; subsequent doses of 50–100 µg q 3–5 min. (Use one half of the above recommended dosage in patients $\geq$ 60 years old).
   - Maximum recommended dose over time: $\leq$ 5–6 µg/kg.

2. Goal of analgesia: a patient drowsy, with slightly slurred speech, and ptosis. The patient readily responds to loud verbal stimuli; respiratory rate > 10/min, $SaO_2 \geq 95\%$.

STEP 4: PROCEED WITH PROCEDURE

1. Administer local anesthesia if appropriate. Wait approximately 5 minutes after last dose of fentanyl before beginning the procedure.
2. Additional doses of fentanyl may be required depending on the patient's response.

STEP 5: POSTPROCEDURE CARE

1. Monitor the patient for at least 1 hour after the procedure is completed or until the patient is awake and can ambulate safely.
2. Caution the patient not to drive, operate heavy machinery, or engage in any hazardous activities for at least 12–24 hours after the procedure.

BIBLIOGRAPHY

American College of Surgeons Committee on Trauma: Initial assessment and management. In Advanced Trauma Life Support Student Manual. American College of Surgeons, Chicago, 1989.

Cantrill SV, Karas S Jr (eds): Cost-Effective Diagnostic Testing in Emergency Medicine. Dallas, American College of Emergency Physicians, 1994.

Dailey RH: Approach to the patient in the emergency department. In Rosen P, Barkin RM (eds): Emergency Medicine: Concepts and Clinical Practice. St. Louis, Mosby-Year Book, 1992, pp. 22–37.

Drugs for pain. Med Lett 1993; 35(887): 1–6.

Dufel SE: Lesson 25. COBRA and the Courts: Patient Transfer Legislation Update. In Critical Decisions in Emergency Medicine, vol. 8: Clinical and Management Controversies. Dallas, American College of Emergency Physicians, 1993.

Dugdale DC, Ramsey PG, EB Larson: General medical care. In Ramsy PG, Larson EB (eds): Medical Therapeutics. 2nd ed. Philadelphia, WB Saunders, 1993, pp. 2–45.

Gentile NT: Lesson 29. Consultants to the Emergency Department. In Critical Decisions in Emergency Medicine, vol 8: Clinical and Management Controversies. Dallas, American College of Emergency Physicians, 1993.

George JE: The emergency department medical record. Emerg Med Clinics North Am 1993; 11(4): 889–903.

Markovchick V: Decision making in emergency medicine. In Karkovchick VJ, Pons PT, Wolfe RE (eds): Emergency Medicine Secrets. Philadelphia, Hanley and Belfus, 1993.

Wrenn K, Slovis CM: The 'Ten Commandments' of emergency medicine (editorial). Ann Emerg Med 1991; October: 137–138.

Yealy DM, Dunmire SM, Paris PM: Pharmacologic adjuncts to painful procedures. In Roberts JR, Hedges JR (eds): Clinical Procedures in Emergency Medicine. Philadelphia, WB Saunders, 1991, pp. 504–508.

II

MEDICAL CHIEF COMPLAINTS

2

Abdominal Pain

"For philosophers, pain is a problem of metaphysics,
and exercise for stoics;
For mystics it is an ecstasy;
For the religious, a travail meekly to be borne;
For clinicians a symptom to be understood and an ill to be relieved."

CHARLES F.W. ILLINGWORTH

I. GUIDING PRINCIPLES

A. The first priority is to determine which patients need urgent surgical attention. This decision is usually made based on the physical examination of the abdomen.

B. Determine whether the patient needs further inpatient observation and evaluation. This often depends on the severity of the pain and the presence of other patient factors such as ability to follow up as an outpatient and the presence of other medical illnesses.

C. Repeated examinations of the patient over several hours in the ED can be useful for diagnosis and determining disposition.

D. Recalling the differences between general types of pain can be helpful diagnostically:

1. *Somatic* pain is well localized and caused by stimulation of pain receptors within the abdominal wall or peritoneum.

2. *Visceral* pain from abdominal organs is usually poorly localized, in the midline of the abdomen, and often associated with signs of increased autonomic activity.

3. Pain can be *referred* to a distant site mediated by nerves originating at or near the same spinal level.

E. Realize that a cause will not be found in approximately 40% of patients with abdominal pain who come to the ED.

29

II. CLINICAL EVALUATION

A. History

1. Obtain an accurate and thorough description of the pain from the patient. Answers to the following questions are helpful in formulating a differential diagnosis:
   a. Where in the abdomen is the pain concentrated? Although imperfect, this feature can suggest certain diagnoses (see Table 2–2).
   b. Does the pain move to another location from where it is concentrated? For example, right-upper-quadrant pain that radiates to the scapula suggests gallbladder pain; radiation from an upper quadrant or flank to the ipsilateral groin suggests ureteral pain.
   c. Did the pain begin suddenly, rapidly (over several minutes), or gradually (over hours)? Severe pain of sudden onset that does not diminish over time suggests an infarcted or perforated viscus, torsion, or hemorrhage.
   d. Describe the character of the pain; what does the pain feel like? Crampy pain suggests smooth muscle contraction, such as in renal colic, intestinal obstruction or hyperactivity (e.g., gastroenteritis), ectopic pregnancy, and sometimes biliary colic.
   e. How severe is the pain? The answer to this question depends on individual patient factors and past history as well as the severity of the underlying problem. Nevertheless, the most severe pain is seen with intestinal perforation or infarction, aortic dissection, and renal colic.
   f. What makes the pain worse? What makes the pain better? This may direct attention to a specific organ system (e.g., epigastric pain that is aggravated by fasting and relieved by eating suggests a duodenal ulcer).
   g. A directed review of systems can be based on the relationship of the pain to specific bodily functions: eating, defecating, urinating, sexual functioning. A menstrual history should always be obtained.
   h. What symptoms are associated with the pain? The presence of nausea, vomiting, hematemesis, diarrhea, melena or hematochezia, dysuria, or dyspareunia may narrow the differential diagnosis.
2. Obtain a general medical history.
   a. Chronic medical illness may give a clue (e.g., the presence of ischemic cardiovascular disease or chronic atrial fibrillation raises the question of ischemic bowel disease).
   b. Inquiring about current medications is another way to check for underlying illness that may be relevant to the pain.
   c. Habits also may provide diagnostic clues (e.g., chronic alcohol consumption raises the suspicion of pancreatitis or alcoholic hepatitis).
   d. Family history (e.g., sickle cell anemia, acute intermittent porphyria) may be relevant.

B. Physical Examination

1. Vital Signs

Blood pressure and pulse, including assessment of postural changes, and temperature are essential.

2. General Appearance

a. Signs of excessive autonomic activity, including diaphoresis, flushing, and dilated pupils, may contribute to the diagnosis of visceral pain.

b. Body posture can also be diagnostically helpful (e.g., patients with peritonitis often lie very still, while those with renal or intestinal colic writhe; those with pancreatitis prefer to sit up and lean forward).

3. Chest Examination

Asymmetric findings on percussion and auscultation of the lungs may be found in patients with pneumonia, some of whom occasionally present with upper-abdominal pain.

4. Abdominal Examination

a. INSPECTION

Scars from previous surgery, abdominal distension with gas or fluid, visible pulsation and peristalsis, engorged superficial veins, organomegaly, and incarcerated hernias can be detected.

b. AUSCULTATION

Murmurs from aortic or renal artery turbulence, hepatic rubs and bruits, and a gastric succussion splash can be heard; the absence of bowel sounds may be due to paralytic ileus or advanced obstruction; bowel sounds that are increased in pitch, frequency, or intensity signify increased intestinal activity from enteritis, excessive luminal blood or fluid, or early obstruction.

c. PERCUSSION

When light percussion elicits severe pain, peritonitis should be suspected and more vigorous palpation avoided. Liver and spleen size and shifting dullness in the presence of ascites can also be assessed.

d. PALPATION

Gentle palpation of the abdomen while observing the patient's face for signs of pain is more useful than forceful and deep palpation. The presence of rebound tenderness, voluntary and involuntary guarding, and the presence of abnormal structures are also assessed with palpation. Hernias in the inguinal and femoral canals, and around the umbilicus and surgical scars, should also be sought.

5. Rectal Examination

  a. The presence of tenderness on one side of the rectum, or anteriorly associated with the prostate or motion of the cervix, can be diagnostically useful.
  b. Polyps, masses, and gross or occult fecal blood can also be detected.

6. Pelvic Examination

  Lower-abdominal pain in females must be investigated by bimanual examination of the pelvis for cervical motion tenderness, ovarian cysts and masses, and tubal pregnancies.

C. Laboratory Tests and Radiography

  Laboratory tests and radiographs (Table 2–1) should be ordered based on the patient's history and physical examination. It is not necessary or advisable to order all tests for all patients.

III. DIFFERENTIAL DIAGNOSIS

The clinician should begin formulating a differential diagnosis for the patient's abdominal pain as soon as the first patient contact is made. The possible diagnoses are constantly modified as additional historical information is gathered, the physical examination performed, and laboratory and radiography data collected. The major causes of acute abdominal pain are listed in Table 2–2 according to the predominant location of the pain. The clinician should be alert for atypical presentations of these common problems and for uncommon problems that are not listed.

IV. DISPOSITION

  A. Patients with severe abdominal pain should be examined immediately upon entering the ED. If percussion and rebound tenderness are found, emergent surgical consultation is mandatory. Screening laboratory tests and chest and abdominal radiographs should be expedited and the patient given opioid analgesics while awaiting operation.

  B. Patients with moderate to severe pain whose diagnosis is in doubt after a 4–6-hour stay in the ED should be admitted for observation and further testing in most situations. Others with significant dehydration, infants, the elderly, and those with significant concomitant medical illnesses should also be considered for admission.

  C. Specific treatment and release is appropriate for most patients after a cause for the pain is elucidated. For example, infectious gastroenteritis may be treated with antidiarrheal agents and antibiotics, or peptic ulcer disease with histamine-2 receptor antagonists. The short-term use of opioid analgesics is appropriate for some causes of self-limited abdominal pain (e.g., kidney stone,

Table 2-1. LABORATORY AND RADIOLOGIC EVALUATION OF ABDOMINAL PAIN

TEST	USEFULNESS/RESULTS	PITFALLS
Hematocrit	Low with GI bleeding, ruptured aneurysm; high with dehydration	Abnormal value may be chronic
WBC	Can be elevated in infectious and inflammatory conditions	Can be normal with infection or elevated because of pain
WBC and differential	Most useful if total WBC is abnormally low or high	
Electrolytes and glucose	May be abnormal with dehydration, diarrhea, vomiting, ketoacidosis	
BUN and creatinine	Volume depletion, renal disease, upper GI bleeding	
Amylase	Useful if suspicious of acute or chronic pancreatitis; elevated amylase values should be split into pancreatic and salivary components or confirmed with an elevated lipase level	Salivary hyperamylasemia may be due to alcoholism and other causes
Bilirubin	Quantifies apparent and detects subclinical (levels between 1.5 and 4 mg/dL) jaundice. May suggest biliary cause of pain or pancreatitis	Elevated levels may be unrelated to cause of pain (e.g., Gilbert's syndrome)
Urinalysis	Hematuria with kidney stones or UTI. Pyuria wth UTI, prostatitis, inflammatory focus near ureter (e.g., Crohn's, diverticulitis); specific gravity helps with assessing state of hydration	Hematuria can be absent with kidney stones or present from menses
Pregnancy test	Ectopic pregnancy	
Abdominal radiography	Helpful if suspicious of bowel obstruction, ischemia, or perforation; kidney stone; or in patients with severe pain	Contraindicated if patient may be pregnant

WBC, white blood cell count; GI, gastrointestinal; BUN, blood urea nitrogen, UTI, urinary tract infection.

ruptured ovarian cyst). Opioids should be avoided for the treatment of acute abdominal pain of uncertain cause and of chronic abdominal pain.

D. Outpatient follow-up is recommended for most patients with abdominal pain to ascertain that the pain has resolved and to

Table 2–2. DIFFERENTIAL DIAGNOSIS OF ABDOMINAL PAIN

LOCATION AND DIAGNOSIS	CLINICAL EVALUATION AND CLUES
Entire Abdomen (Diffuse)	
Peritonitis (perforated ulcer or intestine, late course of intestinal infarction, other)	Sudden onset of severe, constant pain worsened by any movement; hypotension and tachycardia common; abdomen tender to light palpation and on rebound; leukocytosis with subdiaphragmatic air or paralytic ileus on radiograph; requires urgent surgery
Rupturing abdominal aortic aneurysm	Sudden onset of severe tearing pain in mid-abdomen and back followed by symptoms and signs of shock; requires emergent surgical management
Gastroenteritis	Diffuse abdominal or periumbilical cramping pain, often relieved by passage of diarrheal stools; physical examination and laboratory findings variable (see Chapter 5)
Diabetic ketoacidosis	Steady diffuse abdominal pain associated with hyperglycemia, acidemia, and glycosuria; pancreatic amylase may be elevated, but does not necessarily signify acute pancreatitis
Lead intoxication	Usually found in children with other findings of lead poisoning such as anemia and peripheral neuropathy
Sickle cell crisis	Abdominal pain can be steady and severe, located anywhere within the abdomen, and mimic numerous other causes of pain; personal and family history as well as examination of a peripheral blood smear for sickled cells crucial
Opioid withdrawal	Invariably accompanied by other symptoms, including sweating, nausea, diarrhea, lacrimation, rhinorrhea, and twitching muscles; elevated temperature, blood pressure, and respiratory rate frequent
Acute intermittent porphyria	Periumbilical or lower-abdominal cramping pain accompanied by signs of increased autonomic activity; autosomal dominant trait diagnosed by urinary porphyrin screen
Right Upper Quadrant	
Biliary colic	Epigastric or right-upper-quadrant pain of increasing intensity over minutes to a few hours, usually postprandial, may radiate to right scapula; most laboratory findings normal; abdominal ultrasound shows gallstones
Acute cholecystitis	Pain of biliary colic that lasts for several hours; fever, right-upper-quadrant tenderness aggravated by deep inspiration (Murphy's sign); may have elevated temperature, WBC, bilirubin, and liver enzymes
Acute cholangitis	Usually caused by common bile duct stone and accompanied by fever, jaundice, right upper quadrant tenderness, and leukocytosis; ultrasound shows gallstones and sometimes a dilated bile duct

34

Acute hepatitis	Aching pain caused by liver capsule distention is insidious in onset and usually accompanied by other obvious symptoms and signs of hepatitis
Perihepatitis (Fitz-Hugh–Curtis syndrome)	Associated with gonococcal and chlamydial PID; symptoms and signs of underlying PID and prominant right-upper-quadrant pain that is worsened by inspiration may be apparent; diagnosed by clinical syndrome and laparoscopy
Retrocecal appendicitis	See comments under Appendicitis, but pain localizes to right upper quadrant rather than right lower quadrant
Pyelonephritis	Aching pain usually more prominent in flank and accompanied by dysuria, pyuria, fever, leukocytosis
Pneumonia	Productive cough with findings in lower lung field on auscultation and chest radiography
Kidney stone	Severe cramping or steady pain, usually in flank, with radiation to groin as stone moves; hematuria not always present
Epigastric	
Pancreatitis (acute or chronic)	Severe pain coming on over hours usually associated with nausea and vomiting; alcoholism history or gallstones on ultrasound in 80%; elevated pancreatic amylase and localized ileus on radiographs; requires admission for analgesia and hydration
Duodenal ulcer	Aching or burning pain occurring 1–2 hours after eating and awakening the patient at night; relief by eating and antacids
Gastric ulcer	Similar to duodenal ulcer, but postprandial occurrence and relief by eating less constant
Nonulcer dyspepsia	Similar to duodenal and gastric ulcer pain, but ulcer not found on radiography or endoscopy; may be related to excessive acid or dysmotility
Myocardial infarction	Sudden onset of severe pain with signs of increased autonomic activity; diagnosed by high clinical suspicion and electrocardiogram
Left Upper Quadrant	
Splenic rupture	Sudden onset of left-upper-quadrant pain, usually following trauma, and may result in syncope, hypotension, and falling hematocrit; usually requires urgent surgical intervention
Splenic infarction	Sudden onset of pain without history of trauma
Pyelonephritis	See corresponding diagnosis under Right-Upper-Quadrant Pain

PID, pelvic inflammatory disease; WBC, white blood cell count.

Table continued on following page

35

Table 2–2. DIFFERENTIAL DIAGNOSIS OF ABDOMINAL PAIN *Continued*

LOCATION AND DIAGNOSIS	CLINICAL EVALUATION AND CLUES
Pneumonia	See corresponding diagnosis under Right-Upper-Quadrant Pain
Kidney stone	See corresponding diagnosis under Right-Upper-Quadrant Pain
Periumbilical	
Small-bowel obstruction	Cramping pain aggravated by eating and associated with progressive abdominal distention, nausea and vomiting; diagnosed by multiple air fluid levels on radiograph; requires hospital admission
Intestinal ischemia or infarction	Postprandial pain out of proportion to physical findings until peritonitis ensues; often seen in patients with diabetes or cardiovascular disease; laboratory findings and radiographs may be normal until infarction occurs
Early appendicitis	Moderate to severe, steady pain that precedes nausea, vomiting, and localization to right lower quadrant; see below
Right Lower Quadrant	
Evolving appendicitis	Fever, rebound pain and guarding, leukocytosis; requires surgical intervention; diagnosis by compression ultrasonography may help in ambiguous cases
Mesenteric adenitis	Similar presentation to appendicitis and often found at laparotomy: may be found in epidemics and associated with *Yersinia* infection
Regional enteritis	Usually presents with diarrhea and symptoms of partial intestinal obstruction; avoid surgery unless there are signs of intestinal perforation
Cecal or Meckel's diverticulitis	See comments regarding Diverticulitis, below
Left Lower Quadrant	
Diverticulitis	Steady or cramping pain of moderate severity associated with local tenderness; radiographs nonspecific
Irritable bowel syndrome	A common cause of chronic recurrent lower abdominal pain, usually relieved by bowel movements, that rarely awakens patient at night; common history of diarrhea and constipation, flatulence, and mucus in stools; radiographic and laboratory findings normal

Right or Left Lower Quadrant (Depends on Side Involved)

Pelvic inflammatory disease — Lower midline, bilateral, or unilateral pain associated with vaginal discharge; fever, cervical motion tenderness, leukocytosis, and leukocytes on Gram stain of cervical mucus

Ruptured ovarian cyst — Sudden onset of acute, severe pain during mid to late menstrual cycle or early pregnancy; may have local peritoneal signs on examination; spontaneous resolution over 6–24 hours

Ovarian torsion — Similar to ruptured cyst, but pain does not diminish, and may be associated with palpable adnexal mass; early diagnostic laparoscopy indicated

Ruptured ectopic pregnancy — Mild cramping pain that can generalize and radiate to shoulder following rupture; may have history of PID and recently missed or irregular menstrual period; positive serum pregnancy test in over 95%; compression ultrasonography and culdocentesis helpful

Ureteral stone — Radiation of pain to anterior groin associated with previous flank pain and hematuria; pain can be severe

Incarcerated inguinal hernia — Symptoms of intestinal obstruction accompanied by presence of tender mass in region of hernia; requires early surgery to avoid infarction

Lower Midline

Irritable bowel syndrome — See comments above

arrange further evaluation if a diagnosis has not been made and the pain continues. In some cases, the ED physician can establish follow-up contact by telephone or in person. In other situations, it is more appropriate to refer the patient to an internist, surgeon, or gynecologist, depending on the best assessment of the cause of the pain.

V. PEARLS AND PITFALLS

A. The highest *diagnostic* priorities are to

1. Identify a life-threatening process (e.g., acute myocardial infarction, aneurysm dissection).

2. Identify a surgical abdomen.

B. A thorough history and physical examination, augmented by appropriate laboratory evaluation, are key in making a diagnosis.

C. Repeat abdominal examinations over time are crucial in uncertain cases.

D. Beware of the very young patient, the elderly patient, and the pregnant patient, in whom a surgical abdomen or abdominal catastrophe may present very atypically.

E. The female patient of reproductive age (approximately 12–45 years old) is considered pregnant until proven otherwise.

F. Obtain an electrocardiogram on the patient with abdominal pain who is ≥ 40 years old or who has other coronary artery disease risk factors.

G. A thorough genitourinary (including pelvic examination in females) and rectal examination is a mandatory component of the physical examination in the adult patient with abdominal pain.

H. In up to 40% of patients with abdominal pain in the ED, no clear cause will be identified. If the patient is discharged, the discharge diagnosis should be "abdominal pain—cause unclear." Do not give an inaccurate diagnostic label (e.g., "peptic ulcer disease"). Follow-up evaluation by a physician in 24–48 hours is appropriate.

I. Patients should not be diagnosed as having gastroenteritis unless both vomiting and diarrhea are prominent symptoms, and a surgical abdomen has been clearly excluded. Infectious enteritis may occur with diarrhea but no vomiting.

BIBLIOGRAPHY

Halsey J, Kimmey M: Abdominal pain. In Dugdale DC, Eisenberg MS (eds): Medical Diagnostics. Philadelphia, WB Saunders, 1992, p. 279.
Silen W: Cope's Early Diagnosis of the Acute Abdomen, 18th ed. New York, Oxford University Press, 1991.

3

Low Back Pain

*"As to pain, I am almost ready to say
that the physician who has not felt it
is imperfectly educated."*

S. WEIR MITCHELL

I. ESSENTIAL FACTS

A. Definition

Low back pain is discomfort that occurs in the lumbar region of the spine or paraspinous structures. It may be accompanied by pain elsewhere, such as the chest, abdomen, or extremities. Soft tissues irritated by inflammation or trauma may *refer* pain to the low back, even in the absence of spinal pathology. When pain follows the course of a spinal nerve root, it is often due to nerve root irritation or inflammation and is called *radicular* pain.

1. The ED physician must rapidly and accurately diagnose and treat the serious or life-threatening conditions that cause *referred* low back pain; he/she must also identify and initiate appropriate consultation/treatment for the back-pain patient with a neurosurgical emergency (e.g., cauda equina syndrome, spinal cord compression).

2. Fortunately, most low back pain is mechanical in nature, and in 90% of patients the symptoms are self-limited and resolve within 1 month.

B. Serious or Life-Threatening Conditions That Can Refer Pain to the Back

1. Abdominal aortic aneurysm
2. Bowel obstruction
3. Pancreatic disease (inflammation or neoplasm)
4. Pelvic disease (infection, ectopic pregnancy)
5. Pleural effusion
6. Prostatitis
7. Retrocecal appendicitis
8. Retroperitoneal pathology (hemorrhage, neoplasm)
9. Perforated viscus
10. Urinary tract infection

11. Thoracic aortic dissection

12. Urolithiasis

C. Importance

1. Low back pain is the fourth most common adult ambulatory complaint in this country, and it affects 80% of persons at some point in their lives. The peak incidence of acute low back pain occurs in patients 30 to 50 years of age.

2. Low back pain is the leading cause of activity restriction in persons < 45 years old; it is the third leading cause of restricted activity, after heart disease and arthritis, in patients > 45 years old.

3. Approximately 25 billion dollars are spent annually on low back pain in the United States.

II. CLINICAL EVALUATION

A directed history and physical examination will allow the physician to determine whether emergent evaluation and simultaneous therapy for a catastrophic illness are necessary. Low back pain that is associated with hemodynamic instability, paralysis, or bowel/bladder dysfunction requires expedited management as part of the initial clinical evaluation.

A. History

1. General

Obtain information with respect to the following:
a. Patient's age.
b. Known current health problems.
c. Occupation.
d. Prior episodes of back pain and their treatment.
e. Prior medical and surgical history.
f. Current medications.
g. Habits (including history of drug and alcohol abuse).
h. Allergies.

2. Current Back Pain History

In addition to determining the exact circumstances pertaining to the onset of pain, ask about the following:
a. *Location of pain.* Diffuse back pain is usually muscular in origin. Sacroiliac pain may be produced by soft tissue or sacroiliac joint pathology (e.g., patients with lumbar strain or a seronegative spondyloarthropathy [these latter include ankylosing spondylitis, Reiter's syndrome, psoriatic arthritis, and the arthropathy associated with inflammatory bowel disease]).
b. *Radiation.* Pain due to nerve root compression is often unilateral and radiates over the peripheral distribution of the

involved nerve root into the leg and foot ("sciatica"). The most commonly involved nerve roots are L5 (from L4–5 disc herniation) and S1 (from L5–S1 disc herniation).

  c. *Onset.* Acute pain after minor injury or physical activity suggests a primary musculoskeletal condition that is likely to be benign. Infectious and inflammatory conditions usually have a more insidious onset.

  d. *Aggravating and ameliorating factors.* Activity may improve pain due to inflammatory diseases but worsen that due to degenerative disease or muscle strain. Forward bending, coughing, and sneezing all increase the pain of a herniated disc. Slight forward bending may improve the pain of spinal stenosis, which may be aggravated by standing or walking.

  e. *Neurologic symptoms.* Pain due to nerve root irritation is classically associated with paresthesia or hypesthesia. More significant lesions may be associated with weakness or bladder, bowel, or sexual dysfunction. *Caution:* the new onset of bladder, anal sphincter, or sexual dysfunction associated with back pain indicates a neurosurgical emergency.

  f. *Other symptoms.* Chest, abdominal, flank, costovertebral angle, or pelvic pain increases the chance that the low back pain is referred pain. Many infectious or inflammatory conditions that affect the lower back have associated symptoms such as fever, rash, or arthritis of the peripheral joints.

B. Physical Examination

In order to conduct a proper examination for back pain, the patient must be undressed.

1. General Examination

Complete vital signs are mandatory. A screening examination of the lungs, heart, abdomen, and peripheral pulses should be done, and may indicate life-threatening pathology.

2. Back Examination

  a. VISUAL INSPECTION

Inspection of the back (including cervical and thoracic spine) may reveal evidence of trauma or deformities. An exaggerated lumbar lordosis occurs in pregnancy and obesity; a diminished lordosis occurs in ankylosing spondylitis and muscle spasm. With flexion of the spine, the lumbar lordosis should disappear; failure to do so indicates decreased spinal motion. The normal range of motion of the lumbar spine is 90 degrees of flexion, 15 degrees of extension, and 45 degrees of lateral bending.

  b. PALPATION

Palpation of the spine and paraspinous tissues may elicit bony tenderness or evidence of muscle spasm.

c. SPECIFIC TESTS
   i. Straight-Leg-Raising (SLR) Test. With the patient supine, the straight leg on the involved side (i.e., the side with radicular symptoms) should be raised slowly. Nerve root tension begins to occur at 30 degrees of elevation. A positive test must reproduce the patient's radicular symptoms into the leg or foot (exacerbation of back pain, without radicular symptoms, is not a positive SLR test). This test is used to detect irritation of the L5–S1 nerve roots, usually from a herniated disc.
   ii. Crossed SLR Test. The examiner elevates the straight leg of the supine patient on the uninvolved side. A positive test results in radicular symptoms on the involved side. This test is less sensitive but more specific for disc herniation than is the SLR test.
   iii. Sitting Root Test. The patient sits upright with the knees bent and the lower legs hanging over the edge of the bed. The examiner slowly straightens the leg on the involved side to determine exacerbation of radicular symptoms. This test is physiologically equivalent to the SLR test.
   iv. Femoral Stretch Test. The examiner passively extends the hip joint on the involved side in the prone patient. Anterior thigh pain indicates L3 nerve root irritation; medial thigh pain suggests L4 nerve root irritation.
   v. Bilateral SLR Test. The examiner raises both straight legs in the supine patient. This places strain on the sacroiliac joints prior to the lumbar nerve roots because of pelvic tilt.
   vi. Faber (Patrick) Test. With the patient supine, the foot of the uninvolved side is placed over the opposite knee and the flexed knee of the uninvolved side is then abducted. Pain in the inguinal area on the abducted side suggests hip joint involvement; pain in the sacroiliac joint on the other side indicates disease in that joint.

d. NEUROLOGIC EXAMINATION (TABLE 3–1)

   A screening examination for strength and reflex abnormalities is sufficient in patients with no complaints of radiating pain or neurologic dysfunction. For patients with leg pain or neurologic complaints, a more detailed examination is mandatory:
   i. Sensation. Evaluation of sharp–dull discrimination and light touch should be done, especially in the foot and lower leg. Corresponding dermatomes in the two legs should be compared.
   ii. Motor. Weakness and fatigability (inability to hold strength > 5 seconds) should be assessed. Test strength with intervening joints in a neutral position and do both sides simultaneously if possible. Longstanding weakness is associated with muscle atrophy.

Table 3–1. NEUROLOGIC EXAMINATION OF PERSONS WITH LUMBAR PAIN

NERVE ROOT	SENSORY CHANGE	MOTOR CHANGE	REFLEX CHANGE
L3	Upper buttock to anterior thigh	Iliopsoas; quadriceps	Patellar
L4	Medial foot; medial calf	Tibialis anterior; quadriceps	Patellar
L5	Dorsum of foot; lateral calf	Extensor hallucis	Superficial gluteal
S1	Sole; lateral foot	Gastrocnemius	Achilles
S2	Posteromedial upper leg	Flexor hallucis longus	—
S3	Medial buttocks	—	—
S4	Perianal	—	—

iii. Reflexes. Patient relaxation is important for checking deep tendon reflexes. The superficial gluteal reflex (contraction with stroking of the skin over the buttock) is used to assess the L5 dermatome. The plantar (Babinski) reflex assesses for nerve lesions above the cauda equina.

e. GENITOURINARY EXAMINATION

The examiner should assess both perianal sensation and rectal tone. The medial buttocks and perianal region are innervated by S3–5 roots. Urinary retention has a 90% sensitivity for the cauda equina syndrome and anal sphincter tone is decreased in 60–80% of cauda equina syndrome cases.

f. SIGNS SUGGESTING PSYCHOLOGICAL FACTORS (WADDELL'S SIGNS)

The presence of three or more of the following signs suggests a psychological overlay to the patient's complaints:
   i. Overreaction during the examination, including disproportionate verbalization, bizarre expressions, exaggerated muscle tremor, or tension.
   ii. Superficial, nonanatomic, and/or variable tenderness.
   iii. Simulation testing that indicates inorganic disease: axial loading (pushing on skull of standing patient) and simulated rotation (passive rotation of shoulder and pelvis simultaneously) should not cause low back pain.
   iv. Distraction testing that indicates inconsistencies in the patient's responses.
   v. Nonanatomic motor and/or sensory disturbances.

C. Laboratory Evaluation

1. For otherwise healthy patients with acute musculoskeletal back pain, a laboratory evaluation is usually unnecessary. Patients with a suspected medical or surgical condition and referred

back pain, however, will require selected tests, depending on the working diagnosis.

2. Laboratory tests sometimes of use include the following:
   a. Hematocrit. Malignancy may be associated with anemia.
   b. White blood cell count. Leukocytosis may be seen in the setting of osteomyelitis or discitis.
   c. Erythrocyte sedimentation rate (ESR). An ESR > 20 mm/hr correlates with the presence of malignancy as a cause of back pain. Patients with a seronegative spondyloarthropathy (e.g., ankylosing spondylitis) generally have an elevated ESR.
   d. Serum pregnancy test. Ectopic pregnancy may be a cause of referred back pain in the female patient of reproductive age.
   e. Urinalysis. Low back pain that is referred pain from the genitourinary tract (infection and/or obstruction) is usually associated with an abnormal urinalysis.

3. *Note:* the patient >50 years old with nonacute or recurrent low back pain should *minimally* have the following laboratory tests performed:
   a. Complete blood count (CBC)
   b. ESR
   c. Urinalysis
   d. Lumbosacral spinal films (see below)

4. Imaging studies include the following:
   a. Lumbosacral (LS) Radiography. LS spine films should *not* be routinely ordered on most back pain patients. They are reasonable, however, if any of the conditions listed in Table 3–2 are present. The standard views include an anteroposterior and lateral film. Additional views may be necessary depending on initial findings.
   b. Radionuclide Imaging. Bone scans are very sensitive in the detection of both malignant disease and infectious lesions. A radionuclide bone scan, after plain films, is appropriate in

Table 3–2. CLINICAL INDICATIONS FOR LUMBOSACRAL SPINAL RADIOGRAPHY IN PATIENTS WITH LOW BACK PAIN

New-onset low back pain in a patient age <15 years or >50 years
Alcohol or drug abuse
Altered mental status
Corticosteroid use
Elevated ESR
Fever, weight loss, adenopathy, or other systemic signs of infection or malignancy
Findings suggestive of ankylosing spondylitis
History of malignancy
History of significant trauma
Motor neurologic deficit
Patient actively seeking compensation
Previous vertebral fracture or back surgery
Progressive symptoms or those not relieved by appropriate conservative therapy
Spinal deformity

the patient with back pain and fever, unexplained weight loss, an elevated ESR, or other signs that indicate cancer or occult infection; or in the patient > age 50 whose back pain is unresponsive to 4 weeks of conservative therapy.

  c. Advanced Body Imaging Procedures. These should be reserved for patients who are likely to require surgical intervention (e.g., patients with lower-extremity weakness, bowel/bladder dysfunction, suspected spinal epidural metastasis, or an epidural abscess).

    i. Computed Tomography (CT). CT scanning of the lumbar spine has an 80–95% sensitivity and an 68–88% specificity for herniated discs. It is superior to myelography for the diagnosis of lateral disc herniations, paraspinous abnormalities, and subtle bony abnormalities. Approximately 20% of patients without back pain will have disc herniations diagnosed by CT scanning.

    ii. Myelography. This is the time-honored technique for diagnosing disc herniation. It has an advantage over CT scanning in that it can detect intradural abnormalities of the spinal cord and cauda equina. As with CT scanning, approximately 20% of patients without back pain will have disc herniations diagnosed by myelography. Headaches, nausea, vomiting, and seizures are occasional side effects.

    iii. Magnetic Resonance Imaging (MRI). MRI is the procedure of choice for imaging the lumbar spine when a need for emergent surgical intervention is suspected. Its advantages include its ability to accurately detect tumors of the spinal cord and cauda equina and involvement of the vertebral marrow space by infection or tumor. Its disadvantages are increased scanning times, high cost, and limited availability. Ten percent of asymptomatic young women have disc herniation diagnosed by MRI and 45% have bulging discs.

III. DIFFERENTIAL DIAGNOSIS

The many causes of low back pain are presented in Table 3-3.

A. Major Musculoskeletal Causes

1. Lumbar Strain

This is usually a diagnosis of exclusion.

  a. HISTORY

Most patients can identify an activity or event that precipitated their symptoms; current symptoms are often a recurrence of previous ones. Pain is usually lumbar in location and of maximum intensity in the paraspinous muscles, and it does not radiate below the mid-buttock. There are no neurologic symptoms.

Table 3–3. CAUSES OF LOW BACK PAIN

Nonmusculoskeletal Disease

Gastrointestinal
  Cholecystitis
  Pancreatitis
  Perforated ulcer (posterior)
Vascular
  Aortic aneurysm
  Aortic dissection
Urinary
  Pyelonephritis
  Nephrolithiasis
  Perinephric abscess
  Prostatitis
Gynecologic
  Ovarian cyst
  Endometriosis
  Pregnancy (intrauterine or ectopic)

Primary Musculoskeletal Disease

Noninflammatory
  Lumbar strain
  Vertebral fracture
  Disc herniation
  Osteoarthritis
  Spinal stenosis
  Spondylosis
  Facet syndrome
  Paget's disease
  Spondylolisthesis
  Kyphosis
  Scoliosis
Inflammatory
  Seronegative spondyloarthropathies
    Ankylosing spondylitis
    Psoriatic arthritis
    Arthropathy associated with chronic inflammatory bowel disease
    Reiter's syndrome
  Rheumatoid arthritis
Infectious
  Osteomyelitis
  Discitis
  Epidural abscess
  Paraspinous abscess
Neoplastic
  Metastatic cancer (breast, lung, prostate, renal cell)
  Multiple myeloma
  Leukemia
  Lymphoma
  Sarcoma
  Spinal cord tumor

b. PHYSICAL EXAMINATION

Often shows paraspinal muscle spasm, limited lumbar range of motion secondary to pain, and an inability to reverse the lumbar lordosis. There is no spinous process tenderness, and the neurologic examination is normal.

c. Management

If spinal films are obtained, they are commonly normal or may demonstrate nonspecific findings of degenerative disc disease or degenerative disease of the posterior facet joints. Treatment should be symptomatic with analgesics with or without muscle relaxants. Limited bedrest may hasten pain resolution.

2. Disc Herniation

a. History

This condition is often heralded by a "popping" sound with a mechanically stressful activity. The typical pain complaint is lumbar pain radiating to the leg, ankle, foot, or toes. There may be paresthesias and muscle weakness in a radiculopathic distribution. The pain is usually worse with flexion of the lumbar spine, coughing, sneezing, or other activities that raise intra-abdominal pressure.

b. Physical Examination

Evidence of nerve root impingement is frequently found (see Table 3–1). Most disc herniations are lateral, in the L4–5 interspace (L5 nerve root) or L5–S1 interspace (S1 nerve root). A central disc herniation may affect multiple roots in the cauda equina and is associated with "saddle" paresthesia, bilateral leg weakness, and bowel or bladder dysfunction (cauda equina syndrome).

c. Management

Rapidly evaluate for a potential surgical emergency (e.g., the cauda equina syndrome). More typical disc herniations affecting a single nerve root may initially be managed by bedrest, analgesics, muscle relaxants, and referral for follow-up within 3 days. Patients should eat standing (to avoid sitting), and get up to walk for 20 minutes for every 3 hours of bedrest to minimize deconditioning.

3. Spinal Stenosis

The underlying anatomic abnormality is usually multilevel disc degeneration, facet joint osteoarthritis with hypertrophic spurs, or spondylolisthesis (see number 4, below). Occasionally, a congenitally narrowed spinal canal or tumor is found.

a. History

Symptoms include pseudoclaudication (pain worse with standing, walking, or extension of the back) and bilateral lower extremity numbness and/or pain. The pain is usually not radicular in nature.

b. Physical Examination

Pain is relieved with flexion and exacerbated by hyperextension. Lower extremity numbness and weakness may occur only with walking. Objective weakness is found in only one third of patients.

c. Management

Most patients with spinal stenosis can be treated without surgery (anti-inflammatory drugs, activity modification). Referral is appropriate. Patients who are incapacitated with spinal stenosis should be considered for operative therapy.

4. Spondylolisthesis

Slippage of one vertebra on another; usually it is L5 that displaces anteriorly with respect to S1. *Spondylolysis* is the defect in the pars interarticularis (the section of the posterior arch between the inferior and superior articular processes) that allows for this slippage.

a. History

Spondylolisthesis may be noted on lumber radiographs and is usually asymptomatic. It is graded according to the slippage of the superior vertebral body with respect to the inferior vertebral body: grade I (up to 25% displacement), grade II (25–50% slippage), grade III (50–75% slippage), and grade 4 (75–100% slippage). When symptoms occur, they may include low back pain, fatigue, and/or pain referred to the sacroiliac joints, hips, thighs, and lower legs. Nerve root irritation is uncommon.

b. Physical Examination

Clinical characteristics of one or more of the above described conditions may be present.

c. Management

Usually consists of analgesics, activity modification, and referral for follow-up. Surgical fixation should be considered if nerve dysfunction is present or if slippage exceeds 50% (grade III or IV spondylolisthesis). Cauda equina syndrome associated with spondylolisthesis is a neurosurgical emergency but is fortunately very rare.

B. Spinal Cord Compression

1. Causes

a. Most Common
   i. Tumor, usually secondary to metastatic disease to the vertebral column with secondary epidural compression.
   ii. Infection, usually an epidural abscess.

b. OTHER

Mechanical compression by disc herniation or vertebral fracture; but disc herniation at such a high level (L2 or above) is rare, and vertebral fracture usually requires significant trauma (except in the setting of osteoporosis or metastatic tumor).

2. Clinical Presentation

a. The initial symptom is usually pain (axial, radicular, or referred in a pattern that may not clearly suggest the spine as the source of symptoms). The pain may be aggravated by Valsalva and SLR maneuvers; the pain is often made worse by lying down (in distinction to the pain of disc disease).
b. Weakness, sensory loss, and sphincter disturbances occur after pain. Once a neurologic deficit has developed, paraplegia may occur in hours to days.

3. Diagnosis

Rapid diagnostic work-up is mandatory! In patients known to have cancer and radicular symptoms, metastatic epidural compression is present in 25% of those with normal radiographs. MRI or myelography is the diagnostic procedure of choice and early specialist consultation is appropriate.

4. Therapy

Therapy consists of surgery in the setting of infection (i.e., epidural abscess), and high-dose corticosteroids and emergency radiotherapy for malignancy. Also, see Chapter 21.

IV. THERAPY OF LOW BACK PAIN (GENERAL PRINCIPLES; FIGURE 3-1)

A. Step 1: Secure and Support Airway, Breathing, and Circulation

Patients with pain referred to the low back from another anatomic site may be suffering from a life-threatening cause (e.g., abdominal aortic aneurysm or[31] ectopic pregnancy; see section I. B). Management should be directed at supporting vital signs (i.e., oxygen supplementation, cardiac monitoring, intravenous crystalloid infusion, type and crossmatch blood), rapid diagnostic evaluation, emergency consultation, and expedited appropriate definitive care.

B. Step 2: Diagnose and Initiate Treatment of Neurologic Emergencies

Patients who have a primary musculoskeletal disease with evidence of infection or neurologic compromise (spinal cord compression or cauda equina syndrome) need a rapid clinical examination, appropriate laboratory evaluation [e.g., CBC, elec-

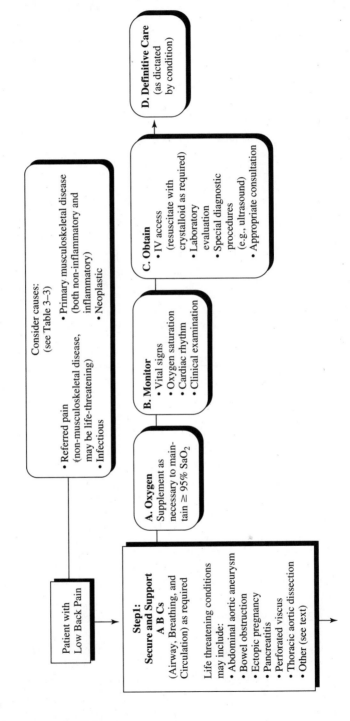

Patient with Low Back Pain

Step1:
Secure and Support
A B Cs
(Airway, Breathing, and Circulation) as required

Life threatening conditions may include:
• Abdominal aortic aneurysm
• Bowel obstruction
• Ectopic pregnancy
• Pancreatitis
• Perforated viscus
• Thoracic aortic dissection
• Other (see text)

A. Oxygen
Supplement as necessary to maintain ≥ 95% SaO$_2$

B. Monitor
• Vital signs
• Oxygen saturation
• Cardiac rhythm
• Clinical examination

C. Obtain
• IV access (resuscitate with crystalloid as required)
• Laboratory evaluation
• Special diagnostic procedures (e.g., ultrasound)
• Appropriate consultation

D. Definitive Care
(as dictated by condition)

Consider causes:
(see Table 3–3)
• Referred pain (non-musculoskeletal disease, may be life-threatening)
• Infectious
• Primary musculoskeletal disease (both non-inflammatory and inflammatory)
• Neoplastic

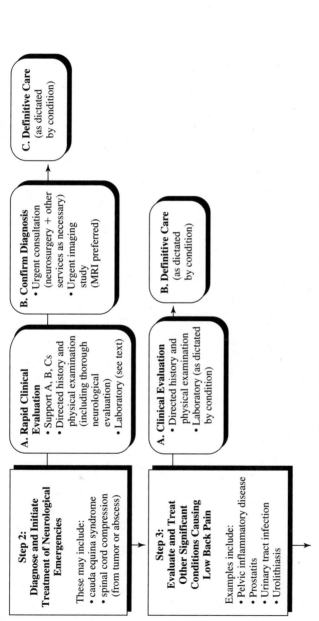

Figure 3–1. Emergency evaluation of the patient with low back pain

Illustration continued on following page.

Step 2:
Diagnose and Initiate Treatment of Neurological Emergencies

These may include:
• cauda equina syndrome
• spinal cord compression (from tumor or abscess)

A. Rapid Clinical Evaluation
• Support A, B, Cs
• Directed history and physical examination (including thorough neurological evaluation)
• Laboratory (see text)

B. Confirm Diagnosis
• Urgent consultation (neurosurgery + other services as necessary)
• Urgent imaging study (MRI preferred)

C. Definitive Care (as dictated by condition)

Step 3:
Evaluate and Treat Other Significant Conditions Causing Low Back Pain

Examples include:
• Pelvic inflammatory disease
• Prostatits
• Urinary tract infection
• Urolithiasis

A. Clinical Evaluation
• Directed history and physical examination
• Laboratory (as dictated by condition)

B. Definitive Care (as dictated by condition)

Step 4:
Diagnose and Treat
Mechanical Low Back Pain

(Most acute back pain will be in this category)

Causes include:
• Lumbar strain
• Disc herniation
• Spinal stenosis
• Spondylolisthesis
• Osteoarthritis
• Inflammatory spondyloarthopathies
• Other (see text)

A. Clinical Evaluation
• Directed history and physical examination
• Laboratory as required by condition (most acute mechanical low back pain in the otherwise healthy adult will not require radiographs or other tests)

B. Definitive Care
• Rest, followed by rehabilitation
• Analgesia
• ± Referral and follow-up as dictated by condition

Figure 3–1. *Continued*

trolyte panel, glucose, blood urea nitrogen (BUN), creatinine, urinalysis, ESR, prothrombin time/partial thromboplastin time (PT/PTT)], and urgent imaging (MRI). Emergent consultation (e.g., neurosurgery and radiation oncology in the setting of cord compression by a tumor) is mandatory.

C. Step 3: Evaluate and Treat Other Conditions Causing Referred Pain

Therapy will be dependent on the condition responsible for the referred pain (e.g., for pyelonephritis, administer antibiotics).

D. Step 4: Treat Mechanical Back Pain

The great majority of patients seen in the ED with low back pain have a primary musculoskeletal disease with either no neurologic findings or findings that do not warrant urgent surgical evaluation or hospital admission. The most likely diagnoses are lumbar strain, disc herniation, degenerative joint disease of the spinal joints, or inflammatory spondyloarthropathy (see also III, above). There are three categories of therapeutic intervention for this very large group of patients:

1. Rest, Followed by Rehabilitation

a. The duration of rest should be relatively short (2 days for most patients). The patient should attempt to walk for 20-minute periods for every 3 hours spent in bed to minimize deconditioning.
b. Initially, the sitting position should be avoided (this is especially important in the patient with a suspected disc herniation).
c. After a 2-day period of bedrest, reconditioning should begin even though most patients will not yet be pain free. Walking is a good initial aerobic exercise. Patients with spinal stenosis and pseudoclaudication may need an alternate form of aerobic exercise.
d. As pain becomes less severe, patients should begin flexibility exercises (aimed especially at the hamstrings) and isometric exercises to strengthen the abdominal and paraspinous musculature. Referral to a qualified physical therapist will facilitate recovery.

2. Analgesics

See Chapter 1 (section IV) for a discussion of pain medication use in the ED.
a. Most patients will benefit from an anti-inflammatory agent, but limit the quantity supplied to $\leq$ 2 weeks. Table 1–2 presents nonsteroidal anti-inflammatory drugs and their dosing.
b. Acetaminophen (650 mg PO q 4 hr) is a useful medication when an anti-inflammatory agent is contraindicated.

c. Narcotics (opioids) should be avoided in the treatment of back pain if possible. If severe pain necessitates their use, prescribe only a 3-day supply. Table 1–3 presents commonly used oral opioids and their dosing.

3. Muscle Relaxation

In some patients, paraspinous muscle spasm is a major cause of pain.

a. Acutely, ice packs to the painful area can be used intermittently for the first 48 hours. After 48 hours, moist heat should be used.

b. Muscle relaxants and their dosages are presented in Table 3–4. Faster symptomatic relief occurs when these agents are combined with analgesics. Use of muscle relaxants should be for a specific period of time rather than based on symptoms. All of these medications are sedating.

V. DISPOSITION

A. Discharge

The great majority of patients who present with mechanical low back pain may be safely discharged to home. For patients with pain confined to the back, management by the ED physician is often definitive, but follow-up should be recommended if there is not significant improvement in 1 week and near resolution of symptoms in 1 month. Follow-up care should be arranged in approximately 3 days for the patient with symptoms or signs of nerve root irritation from a suspected disc herniation (though 80% of these patients will respond eventually to conservative therapy).

B. Admit

Patients with low back pain and *any* of the following clinical features should be admitted to the hospital for completion of diagnosis and/or definitive care:

1. Hemodynamic instability.

2. Fever not explained by an identified focus.

3. Single-level radiculopathy in a patient with cancer.

4. Multilevel radiculopathy of new onset.

Table 3–4. MUSCLE RELAXANTS

NAME	USUAL DOSE	TYPICAL ADVERSE EFFECTS
Carisoprodol (Soma, Rela)	350 mg qid	Sedation
Cyclobenzaprine (Flexeril)	10 mg tid	Sedation, dry mouth
Methocarbamol (Robaxin)	1500 mg qid	Sedation, dizziness
Orphenadrine (Norflex)	100 mg bid	Anticholinergic effects

5. Progressive neurologic symptoms.

6. Bowel or bladder dysfunction.

7. Severe pain or a living situation that precludes outpatient therapy.

VI. PEARLS AND PITFALLS

A. The highest diagnostic priority in the patient with low back pain is to rule out a life-threatening condition that is referring pain to the back. The next highest diagnostic priority is to rule out a neurosurgical emergency.

B. The clinical evaluation of the patient (history, physical examination, and limited laboratory testing) should allow for an accurate assessment of the risk that the back pain is referred, or secondary to an infection or neoplastic process.

C. Women of child-bearing age are considered pregnant until proven otherwise; a pregnancy test is appropriate.

D. A screening neurologic examination should be performed in all patients with back pain.

E. Perianal sensation and rectal sphincter function should be checked in patients with neurologic complaints or persistent/recurrent symptoms.

F. Low back pain patients should have appropriate and timely follow-up arranged.

G. Do *not* do any of the following:

1. Obtain lumbosacral radiographs on all patients.

2. Prescribe medications for > 2 weeks.

3. Routinely prescribe opioids.

BIBLIOGRAPHY

Deyo RA, Loeser JD, Bigos SJ: Herniated lumbar intervertebral disc. Ann Intern Med 1990;112:598-603.
Hamilton GC, Trott AT, Sanders AB, Strange GR (eds): Emergency Medicine: An Approach to Clinical Problem-Solving. Philadelphia, WB Saunders, 1991.
Rosen P, Baker FJ, Barkin RM, Braen CR, Dailey RH, Levy RC (eds): Emergency Medicine: Concepts and Clinical Practice, 2nd ed. St. Louis, CV Mosby, 1988.
Vukmir RB: Low back pain: Review of diagnosis and therapy. Am J Emerg Med 1991;9:328-335.

4

Chest Pain

*"Pain, messenger of harm
Nature's poignant alarm
Often man's wily friend
To signal means to mend."*

DAVID SEEGAL

I. ESSENTIAL FACTS

A. Definition

Chest pain is a discomfort or abnormal sensation in the thorax. It accounts for 5–7% of patient visits to the ED. Chest pain is of crucial importance to both the patient and the ED physician because its cause may be life-threatening. *It should be assumed to have a serious cause until proven otherwise.*

B. Etiology

The many possible etiologies of chest pain are presented in Table 4–1.
1. The significant life-threatening causes of acute chest pain include:
   a. Acute myocardial infarction (MI).
   b. Unstable angina (defined as angina of new onset, angina at rest or with minimal activity, or angina of increasing severity/duration/frequency).
   c. Aortic dissection.
   d. Pulmonary embolism.
   e. Pneumothorax.
   f. Esophageal rupture.
Of the above, acute MI and unstable angina are the most common. Over 1.5 million patients with *suspected* acute MI are admitted to hospitals annually in the United States (30% of these patients subsequently have confirmation of infarction).
2. The most common causes of chest pain in the ED include:
   a. Coronary artery disease (including acute MI, unstable angina, and stable angina).
   b. Gastrointestinal disorders.
   c. Musculoskeletal disorders.
   d. Psychogenic disorders.

II. CLINICAL EVALUATION

A. Diagnostic Considerations

Table 4–2 presents diagnostic clues to the many potential causes of chest pain.

Table 4–1. CAUSES OF CHEST PAIN

Cardiovascular Disorders

Angina pectoris
Myocardial infarction
Tachyarrhythmia
Bradyarrhythmia
Aortic stenosis and insufficiency
Mitral valve prolapse
Mitral stenosis
Hypertrophic cardiomyopathy (idiopathic hypertrophic subaortic stenosis)
Pericarditis
Postmyocardial infarction syndrome
Aortic dissection
Aortic aneurysm, leaking
Superficial thrombophlebitis (Mondor's syndrome)

Pulmonary Disorders

Pneumothorax
Pneumomediastinum
Pleurisy and pleurodynia
Pulmonary embolus or infarction
Pulmonary hypertension
Pneumonia

Gastrointestinal Disorders

Esophageal disorders (esophageal spasm, esophagitis, hiatal hernia)
Perforated esophagus, stomach, or duodenum
Peptic ulcer disease
Pancreatitis
Cholecystitis
Splenic flexure syndrome

Musculoskeletal Disorders

Costochondrodynia
Cervical and thoracic disc or joint disease
Tietze's syndrome
Thoracic outlet syndrome
Muscle spasm and fibrositis
Chest wall tenderness (nonspecific)

Miscellaneous Disorders

Anxiety states (hyperventilation syndrome)
Herpes zoster
Intrathoracic neoplasm

Data from Ho MT: Chest pain and angina. In Dugdale DC, Eisenberg MS (eds): Medical Diagnostics. Philadelphia, WB Saunders, 1992, p. 60.

B. History

A carefully elicited, thorough history is the most useful step in diagnosing the cause of chest pain. Physical examination and routine laboratory tests are often nonspecific or useful mainly to confirm the diagnosis already suspected from the history.

1. Quality of Pain

a. The typical pain of ischemic heart disease is described as squeezing, strangling, crushing, a tightness, pressure,

Table 4-2. DIAGNOSTIC CLUES TO CAUSES OF CHEST PAIN

Cause	Previous Attacks of Similar Pain	HISTORY			Common Associated Findings	Signs	Other Abnormalities	Other Comments
		Pain						
		Location	Character	Onset	Duration				
Angina	Usually	Retrosternal, radiating to left arm	Squeezing, oppressive	With stress or exercise	2–10 min up to 20–30 min	Occasionally dyspnea; dizziness and syncope rare	Often none; S_4 occasionally	ECG often normal between attacks.	Relieved by nitroglycerin.
Acute myocardial infarction	In some cases	Retrosternal, radiating to left arm, neck; rarely in back	Squeezing, oppressive, increases with time	No precipitating factor necessary	> 20 min	Nausea and vomiting, diaphoresis, dyspnea	Heart failure, restlessness, shock; cardiac examination often normal	ECG may be diagnostic or normal.	Elevated CK, LDH, or CK MB isoenzymes. Normal isoenzyme levels on one determination do not exclude diagnosis.

Mitral valve prolapse	Usually	Variable	Variable	Variable	Variable; usually hours	Dyspnea, dizziness common; syncope in some	Midsystolic click or murmur in most cases	ECG may show inverted T waves on leads II, III, and aVF. Echocardiogram is diagnostic	Usually seen in young women. High-arched palate or chest or spine deformities may be present.
Aortic stenosis	May have occurred	Like angina	Like angina	Like angina	Like angina	Syncope, dyspnea	Systolic ejection murmur transmitted to carotid arteries; delayed carotid pulse	ECG usually shows left ventricular hypertrophy. Echocardiography and angiocardiography are diagnostic	More common in older men.

From Mills J, Ho MT, Saunders CE (eds): Current Emergency Diagnosis and Treatment 4th ed. Norwalk, CT: Appleton & Lange, 1990, pp 100–101.
Table continued on following page

Table 4–2. DIAGNOSTIC CLUES TO CAUSES OF CHEST PAIN *Continued*

		HISTORY						
	Previous Attacks of	*Pain*				*Common Associated*		*Other Abnor-*	*Other*
Cause	*Similar Pain*	*Location*	*Character*	*Onset*	*Duration*	*Findings*	*Signs*	*malities*	*Comments*
Aortic insufficiency	In some cases	Like angina	Like angina	Like angina	May be prolonged	Dyspnea	Diastolic murmur transmitted to carotid arteries; water-hammer and Quincke's pulse; wide arterial pulse pressure	ECG may be normal or may show left ventricular hypertrophy. Echocardiography and angiocardiography are diagnostic.	History of rheumatic heart disease, connective tissue disease, or syphilis
Pericarditis	In some cases	Retrosternal	Variable; often pleuritic and relieved by sitting	Variable	Hours to days	Variable	Pericardial friction rub in many	ECG may be diagnostic, nonspecific, or normal	Relieved by sitting. Perform echocardiography to detect fluid.
Aortic dissection	No	Retrosternal and back	Tearing, maximal at onset	Sudden	Variable	Myocardial infarction, stroke, limb ischemia, syncope	Stroke, absent pulses, hematuria, shock	Chest x-ray shows widened mediastinum. ECG may show acute myocardial infarction.	Angiography or CT scan is definitive. Hypertension or connective tissue disease may be present.

Pleurisy	No	Variable, usually lateral thorax	Pleuritic	Usually sudden	Variable	Subjective dyspnea	Often none; occasionally friction rub, low-grade fever	Occasionally pleural effusion.	Negative lung scan or pulmonary angiogram
Pneumothorax	In some cases	Variable	Variable; often pleuritic	Usually sudden	Variable	Dyspnea and cough; shock if tension pneumothorax is present	Tachycardia, lung collapse with or without mediastinal shift	Chest x-ray is diagnostic but needs careful examination.	
Pneumomediastinum	No	Retrosternal	Variable; often pleuritic	Usually sudden	Variable	Dyspnea	Medastinal crunch	Chest x-ray is diagnostic.	Frequently associated with pneumothorax.
Pulmonary hypertension	Usually	Retrosternal	Like angina	Like angina	Variable	Dyspnea, fatigue, exercise syncope	Loud P_2, right ventricular lift	ECG shows right heart strain. Chest x-ray shows signs of pulmonary hypertension.	

Table continued on following page

61

Table 4–2. DIAGNOSTIC CLUES TO CAUSES OF CHEST PAIN *Continued*

			HISTORY					
	Previous Attacks of Similar Pain		*Pain*			*Common Associated Findings*	*Signs*	*Other Abnormalities*	*Other Comments*
Cause		*Location*	*Character*	*Onset*	*Duration*				
Pulmonary embolism	In some cases	Variable, usually lateral thorax	Usually strong pleuritic component	Usually sudden	Minutes to hours	Dyspnea, cough, and tachypnea; hemoptysis sometimes	Friction rub or splinting in some	Hypoxia and hypocapnia. Chest x-ray usually abnormal, but findings are not specific.	Abnormal lung scan or pulmonary angiogram.
Pneumonia	Rare	Over affected lobe	Pleuritic	Variable	Variable	Fever and chills, cough, dyspnea, sputum production	Fever, rales with or without consolidation, friction rub	Infiltrates on chest x-ray; purulent sputum.	
Esophagitis, esophageal spasm, hiatal hernia	Usually	Retrosternal or epigastrium	Changes with eating	Usually gradual	Variable	Gastrointestinal symptoms; flushing, sweating	None	Positive barium swallow and Bernstein (acid perfusion) test.	Relieved by antacids or topical anesthesia.

Perforated duodenal ulcer	No, or milder pain of ulcer	Retrosternal to epigastrium	Severe	Variable	Variable	Variable	Epigastric pain	Free air in peritoneum; elevated amylase.	Rare as cause of chest pain.
Pancreatitis	In some cases	Retrosternal to epigastrium	Variable	Variable	Hours to days	Vomiting, anorexia	Epigastric or upper quadrant tenderness	Markedly elevated urine or serum amylase.	Rare as cause of chest pain.
Cholecystitis	Usually	Right upper quadrant; occasionally epigastrium or retrosternal	Variable	Usually sudden	Hours to days	Vomiting, anorexia	Epigastric or right upper quadrant tenderness	Abnormal liver function tests. Sonography is diagnostic.	Rare as cause of chest pain.
Musculoskeletal disorder (Tietze's syndrome, stitch, etc.), rib fracture	Variable	Costochondral junctions; retrosternal and lateral	Pleuritic ache, "sticking" sensation	Gradual to sudden	Variable; fleeting for stitch	Splinting	Tender costosternal junctions, especially first and second ribs, or over affected ribs; rarey swelling over joints	None.	Relieved by anti-inflammatory medications.

heaviness, or more vaguely as a "funny feeling." The discomfort of angina or MI may not be perceived as pain by many patients.

b. A sharp, knifelike pain is not typical of myocardial ischemia but must be interpreted with caution, since patients may be referring to severity rather than the quality of pain.

2. Location of Pain

a. Discomfort related to myocardial ischemia is most commonly centered in the retrosternal region. The pain may radiate to the axilla, down the arms (more often the left), to the jaw, or to the back. Less commonly the pain may be confined to one of the areas in the usual path of radiation.

b. Pain of MI is often retrosternal, although up to 35% of patients may have pain located elsewhere, especially in the epigastric region. In patients with MI who have a history of angina, 94% experience the myocardial pain in the same location as the angina pain, even if the site of angina pain is atypical.

c. Esophageal dysfunction is the most common cause of central chest pain that is confused with myocardial ischemia. Fifty percent of patients with esophageal dysfunction have central chest pain, and one-third have "angina-like" chest pain.

3. Duration of Pain

Pain caused by angina usually lasts 2 to 10 minutes but can last up to 20 to 30 minutes especially when it is precipitated by emotional stress. Pain lasting a few seconds or less is not caused by myocardial ischemia.

4. Provocation of Pain

a. Angina is often precipitated by exertion, emotional stress, cold weather, food, or drink. Pain begins during the stress as opposed to after the event. Prinzmetal's or variant angina is caused by coronary artery spasm and usually occurs at rest, often at the same time each day.

b. Pain of MI often occurs without any identifiable precipitating event and begins during rest or sleep in 20–40% of patients.

c. Pain on swallowing, eating, or lying down is more frequently caused by esophageal dysfunction but may also occur with pericarditis or, less commonly, with angina.

d. Pleuritic pain or pain with movement usually suggests pulmonary, musculoskeletal, or mediastinal involvement. Pain of pericarditis may be pleuritic.

5. Relief of Pain

a. Pain caused by angina usually subsides within 1 to 15 minutes of the patient's cessation of the activity provoking the pain. Esophageal spasm, however, can be similarly relieved.

b. Patients with pericarditis or esophageal dysfunction usually report improvement or relief of symptoms upon assuming the sitting position. Patients with dyspnea related to myocardial ischemia or pulmonary disease also feel better in a more upright position.

c. Nitroglycerin usually relieves chest pain caused by angina within 5 to 10 minutes. Unfortunately, nitroglycerin is also very effective in relieving pain related to esophageal spasm within the same time period. Moreover, almost a fifth of patients with myocardial infarction also experience pain relief.

d. Rapid relief with antacids is reported by only a quarter of patients with reflux esophagitis. Conversely, up to 4% of patients with myocardial ischemia may experience relief.

6. Associated Symptoms

a. Complaints of nausea, vomiting, diaphoresis, or dyspnea are commonly associated with chest pain caused by myocardial ischemia but are nonspecific and occur frequently in patients with other conditions.

b. Absence of associated symptoms does not exclude ischemic heart disease.

7. Risk Factors for Ischemic Heart Disease (IHD)

a. Age > 30 years old
b. Male sex
c. Cigarette smoking
d. Hypertension
e. Diabetes mellitus
f. Positive family history for IHD
g. Hypercholesterolemia

The presence of risk factors for IHD is of concern in the patient presenting with chest pain, but their absence does not exclude the possibility of chest pain of myocardial origin.

C. Physical Examination

Special attention should be paid to features of the physical examination that can rule in or exclude certain diagnoses. Occasionally, more than one disease process may be present. For example, the stress of pneumonia may precipitate angina in a patient with aortic stenosis.

1. Patients with angina, unstable angina, uncomplicated acute MI, esophageal disorders, pulmonary embolus, or psychogenic chest pain usually have no diagnostic abnormalities detectable by physical examination.

2. Examine the fundus for diabetic or hypertensive changes and the pharynx for the high-arched palate often seen in patients

with Marfan's syndrome and occasionally in mitral valve prolapse.

3. Examine the chest wall carefully by inspection and palpation.
    a. The rash of herpes zoster (cluster of vesicles in a dermatome distribution) or Tietze's syndrome (erythematous nodules over the costochondral junction) are diagnostic.
    b. Pain on palpation of the chest wall may indicate musculoskeletal disorders such as costochondritis, rib fracture or contusion, thoracic outlet syndrome, or cervical or thoracic radicular syndrome. *Caution:* care must be taken to ascertain that the pain elicited by palpation of the chest wall is identical to that of the patient's chief complaint.

4. Percuss and auscultate over both the anterior and posterior lung fields and mediastinum, while listening for any abnormal sounds.

5. Cardiovascular system evaluation should include the following steps:
    a. Assess central venous pressure with the patient's upper body elevated 30°.
    b. Inspect and palpate for heaves, lifts, or thrills.
    c. Auscultate for any abnormality in S_1 or S_2 and for any abnormal sounds such as S_3, S_4, click, murmur, or rub.
    d. Determine the intensity and amplitude of carotid, femoral, and other peripheral pulses.

6. Examine the abdomen carefully, looking especially for bruits, abnormal aortic pulse, or any evidence of intraabdominal disease.

7. Examine the patient's legs for evidence of thrombophlebitis such as swelling, redness, tenderness, increased warmth, and the presence of cords.

D. Diagnostic Studies

Diagnostic tests should be tailored to the individual situation; the limitations in the interpretation of test results must be recognized. In general, a positive test result is useful in a population with a high prevalence of disease; a negative test result is useful in a population with a low prevalence of disease. In the converse situations, some tests may actually contribute to the uncertainty of a diagnosis.

1. Electrocardiography

The electrocardiogram (ECG) is the single most important study to obtain in the chest pain patient. Depending on the disease process, findings may include the following:
    a. **Angina.** During a symptomatic episode of angina characteristic ECG changes include transient ST-segment depres-

Sections II. A–C modified from Ho MT: Chest pain and angina. In Dugdale DC, Eisenberg MS (eds): Medical Diagnostics. Philadelphia, WB Saunders, 1992, pp. 59–61, 70–72.

sions or T-wave inversions. A normal ECG, nonspecific changes, or transient bundle-branch blocks may also occur.

b. **Prinzmetal's angina.** Coronary artery vasospasm causes transient ST-segment elevation.

c. **Acute MI.** Classic ECG changes include new Q waves in leads I, AVL, or in two or more diaphragmatic or precordial leads, $\geq$ 1-mm ST-segment elevation or depression in the same lead combinations, and/or T-wave abnormalities (peaked upright or symmetrically inverted). A new, complete left bundle-branch block (LBBB) may sometimes occur.

d. **Pericarditis.** Many leads will show ST-segment elevation with an upward concavity; T waves are initially upright but will invert with time.

e. **Pulmonary Embolism.** Sinus tachycardia is the most common ECG finding. Less frequent, but more specific, changes include new-onset right bundle-branch block (RBBB), intraventricular conduction defects (of a RBBB pattern), or an S1-Q3-T3 pattern (S wave in lead I, Q wave and inverted T wave in lead III).

f. **Aortic Dissection.** The ECG may be normal, or may show sinus tachycardia, ischemia, or various infarct patterns (depending on the coronary artery(s) occluded by the torn intimal flap).

Cautions: comparison with previous ECGs is essential (if available) to determine the presence and extent of changes; absence of characteristic changes does *not* exclude acute ischemia in patients presenting with a consistent history (6–21% of admission ECGs are normal in patients suffering from an acute MI).

2. Chest Radiography

Radiography of the chest is commonly ordered and is occasionally helpful. Findings may include the following:

a. **Ischemic Heart Disease.** Radiographs may be normal or show evidence of cardiac decompensation and congestive heart failure.

b. **Pulmonary Embolism.** Radiographic findings are nonspecific and insensitive, but may include focal infiltrates, pleural effusions, elevated hemidiaphragm, atelectasis, Hampton's hump (a pleural-based triangular infiltrate whose apex points toward the hilum), or Westermark's sign (proximally dilated pulmonary vessels with collapse or sharp cutoff of those same vessels distally).

c. **Aortic Dissection.** Chest radiographs are abnormal in 80–90% of cases. The most common abnormality is a widened mediastinum; other findings may include obliteration of the aortic knob, a localized bulge in an otherwise smooth aortic contour, "calcium sign" (displacement of intimal calcification from the outer border of the aorta by > 5 mm), double-density appearance of the aorta, displacement of the trachea or nasogastric tube to the right, pleural effusions, and/or an apical cap.

d. **Pneumothorax.** Diagnosed definitively by the chest radiograph. The well-demarcated lung edge is noted approximately parallel to the chest wall, separated from the chest wall by a radiolucent band without pulmonary markings. Findings may be more apparent on an expiratory film.

3. Echocardiography

Echocardiography readily detects regional wall motion abnormalities, measures global systolic function of the left and right ventricles, and is useful in the evaluation of cardiac valve dysfunction. Sensitivity is 70–95% and specificity is 85–100% in the early diagnosis of acute MI. Its positive predictive value for detecting acute MI in the ED setting, however, is only 50% given the low prevalence of acute MI in patients presenting with chest pain. In the emergency medicine setting, echocardiography is most useful in detecting conditions that mimic MI (e.g., pericarditis, aortic dissection) or in diagnosing the complications of MI (e.g., right ventricular infarction, papillary muscle rupture, ventricular septal rupture, left ventricular aneurysm, and/or mural thrombus).

4. Cardiac Enzyme Analysis (Creatine Phosphokinase [CPK] ± Lactate Dehydrogenase [LDH] with Isoenzymes)

Elevation of serum levels of cardiac enzymes over time in hospitalized patients is the most specific test available for the detection of an acute MI. Despite this, initial enzyme determinations are only 40–50% sensitive and are *not* useful in excluding ischemic heart disease in the ED. In addition, myocardial ischemia in the absence of infarction (e.g., unstable angina) is not associated with cardiac enzyme elevations, yet is a true emergency mandating hospitalization.

5. Miscellaneous Studies

a. **Ventilation–Perfusion (V/Q) Scan.** The initial diagnostic procedure of choice in the patient suspected to have a pulmonary embolism. A perfusion scan alone is highly sensitive for detecting pulmonary embolism. A normal V/Q scan reliably excludes this disease. Specificity of V/Q scanning is low and pulmonary angiography may be required for definitive assessment.

b. **Gastrointestinal Studies.** Multiple studies are available to further evaluate the patient with a suspected gastrointestinal cause of chest pain, including barium swallow, upper gastrointestinal series, upper tract endoscopy, esophageal manometry, and/or Bernstein's test (esophageal acid perfusion test). These studies are almost never performed in the ED but may be ordered by a consultant or referral specialist *after* the possibility of cardiac disease as a cause of chest pain has thoroughly been considered and ruled out. An esophageal disorder is the most common cause of chest pain in such patients.

   c. **Transesophageal Echocardiography (TEE), Chest Computed Tomography (CT) Scanning, or Aortography.** May be obtained to evaluate the emergency patient with chest pain suspected secondary to thoracic aortic dissection. The study ordered depends on the capabilities of the institution and the preferences of the cardiothoracic surgery consultant. At many major medical centers, TEE is the initial diagnostic procedure of choice in this setting.

   d. **Specialist Studies (Cardiology).** Additional tests that may be ordered by the internal medicine or cardiology consultant *after* hospitalization for chest pain of presumed cardiac origin include exercise electrocardiography ("stress" testing), radionuclide imaging, and/or coronary artery catheterization.

III. DIAGNOSTIC/TREATMENT APPROACH

Caution: assume the chest pain patient is suffering from a life-threatening disorder until proven otherwise.

A. Initial Assessment

Secure and support airway, breathing, and circulation as necessary.

1. Place the patient on oxygen (2–5 L/min via nasal cannula) and continuously monitor the cardiac rhythm and oxygen saturation. In the setting of pulmonary edema or cardiogenic shock, supplement oxygen with a 100% non-rebreather mask if necessary to ensure $\geq 95\%$ SaO_2.

2. Rapidly obtain vital signs (including blood pressure in both arms), ECG, intravenous access, and chest roentgenography.

3. Simultaneously with the above, obtain a relevant history (with special emphasis on risk factors for IHD and the location, duration, and quality of the chest pain) and perform a directed physical examination.

B. Treatment and Further Diagnostic Testing (As Appropriate)

On the basis of the above, the physician often has a probable or definite diagnostic opinion as to the cause of the patient's chest complaints. If a life-threatening process is present, further ED management should include immediate and appropriate therapy, necessary consultation, and admission to the ICU.

1. Acute MI

a. Treatment may include the following:
   i. Nitroglycerin.
   ii. Morphine sulfate.
   iii. Aspirin.
   iv. Thrombolytic therapy (e.g., tissue plasminogen activator, streptokinase, or anistreplase) or mechanical reperfusion (e.g., coronary angiography with percutaneous coronary angioplasty or emergent coronary artery bypass grafting).
   v. Heparin.
   vi. Beta-blockers (e.g., metoprolol, propranolol, or atenolol).
   vii. Magnesium sulfate (in the patient with hypomagnesemia).
   viii. Antiarrhythmic therapy (e.g., lidocaine) as indicated.
b. Diagnostic confirmation of acute MI will occur in the ICU with serial ECG and cardiac enzyme analysis. Other studies that may be obtained include echocardiography, radionuclide scans, and/or coronary angiography.

2. Unstable Angina

a. Treatment may include the following:
   i. Nitroglycerin.
   ii. Morphine sulfate.
   iii. Aspirin.
   iv. Heparin.
   v. Beta-blockers (e.g., metoprolol, propranolol, or atenolol).
   vi. Antiarrhythmic therapy (e.g., lidocaine) as indicated.
b. The patient with unstable angina must be admitted to a monitored bed for serial ECG and cardiac enzyme analysis.

3. Aortic Dissection

Type A dissections involve the ascending aorta, type B dissections do not.
a. Treatment may include the following:
   i. If patient is hypotensive: resuscitate with intravenous fluids and blood.
   ii. If patient is hypertensive: control blood pressure and shear forces with intravenous sodium nitroprusside and beta-blocker therapy (e.g., esmolol).
   iii. Morphine sulfate (for pain relief).
b. Confirmation of suspected acute aortic dissection will require TEE, emergent chest CT, and/or aortography. A cardiothoracic surgeon should be consulted on an urgent basis. The patient should be admitted to an ICU bed. Type A dissections require surgical treatment.

4. Pulmonary Embolism

a. Treatment may include:
   i. Anticoagulation: heparin (followed by warfarin as an inpatient).
   ii. Thrombolytic therapy (in the setting of a massive pulmonary embolus with hemodynamic compromise).
   iii. Surgical interventions (e.g., vena cava filter placement in the patient with contraindications to anticoagulation).
b. Diagnostic confirmation of pulmonary embolism will require V/Q lung scanning, documentation of an extremity deep venous thrombosis (e.g., with duplex ultrasound or impedance plethysmography), and/or pulmonary angiography. Admission is mandatory.

5. Pneumothorax

Treatment may include the following:
   i. Tension pneumothorax: immediate decompression is mandated with needle thoracostomy (second intercostal space mid-clavicular line), followed by chest tube thoracostomy.
   ii. Simple pneumothorax: treatment will vary with the size of the pneumothorax and the patient's characteristics. Therapeutic options include observation (*caution:* observation should be considered only if the patient is healthy, reliable, has no underlying lung disease, and the simple nontraumatic pneumothorax is < 10% size), catheter aspiration, or tube thoracostomy.

6. Esophageal Rupture

a. Treatment includes the following:
   i. Intravenous crystalloid resuscitation as necessary.
   ii. Morphine sulfate (for pain).
   iii. Broadspectrum intravenous antibiotics (e.g., ticarcillin/clavulanate).
   iv. NPO patient status and nasogastric suction.
   v. Urgent surgical consultation.
b. The classic chest radiographic findings of esophageal perforation include mediastinal air (with or without subcutaneous emphysema), left-sided pleural effusion, pneumothorax, and/or widened mediastinum. Confirmation of the esophageal tear can be made with water-soluble contrast (Gastrograffin) esophagram and/or endoscopy. Urgent surgical repair of the perforation is mandatory.

7. Miscellaneous Disorders

a. Musculoskeletal Disorders. Treat with nonsteroidal anti-inflammatory medications (e.g., ibuprofen, naproxen).
b. Nonsurgical Gastrointestinal Disorders. Antacids and/or histamine-2 blockers (e.g., ranitidine or cimetidine).

IV. DISPOSITION

A. Discharge

Patients whose chest pain is clearly secondary to a benign condition (e.g., musculoskeletal strain) may be discharged to home with appropriate follow-up.

B. Admit

All patients with a potentially life-threatening cause of chest pain must be admitted to the hospital. Patients suffering from on-going myocardial ischemia must be admitted to the ICU. If myocardial ischemia cannot be ruled out in the ED, and the cause of chest pain remains uncertain, it is wisest to admit the patient to a monitored bed for observation until a more definitive diagnosis can be made.

V. PEARLS AND PITFALLS

A. Assume chest pain is caused by a potentially life-threatening disorder until proven otherwise.

B. The most important tool in evaluating the patient with chest pain is the history. The ECG may provide useful adjunctive information.

C. A normal ECG, absence of risk factors for ischemic heart disease, or relief of chest pain with a "GI cocktail" (e.g., antacid ± viscous lidocaine) do not rule out myocardial ischemia when the history is suggestive of same.

D. The elderly patient and the diabetic patient may present with on-going myocardial ischemia and very atypical symptoms (e.g., nausea and vomiting only, profound fatigue, abdominal complaints, dyspnea, confusion).

E. Consider the possibility of myocardial ischemia and obtain an ECG in the adult patient with upper-abdominal complaints.

F. When in doubt as to the cause of chest pain, admit for cardiac monitoring and further evaluation.

G. Patients who clearly have chest pain of a benign cause may be discharged, but document the chart carefully, and provide for appropriate follow-up.

H. Never work in a vacuum. Compare current ECG with prior ECGs in the patient's medical record. Obtain consultation whenever necessary.

BIBLIOGRAPHY

Brooks TA: Chest pain. In Hamilton GC (ed): Presenting Signs and Symptoms in the Emergency Department. Evaluation and Treatment. Baltimore, Williams & Wilkins, 1993, pp. 106–114.

Craddock LD: The physical examination in acute cardiac ischemic syndromes. J Emerg Med 1991;9:55-60.

Howell JM, Hedges JR: Differential diagnosis of chest discomfort and general approach to myocardial ischemia decision making. Am J Emerg Med 1991;9:579.

McLaughlin T, GC Hamilton. Chest pain. In Markovchick VJ, Pons PT, Wolfe RE (eds): Emergency Medicine Secrets. Philadelphia, Hanley and Belfus, 1993.

Mills J, Ho MT: Chest pain. In Mills J, Ho MT, Trunkey DD (eds): Current Emergency Diagnosis and Treatment. Los Altos, CA, Lange Medical Publishing, 1983, pp 55-72.

5

Diarrhea

"I am poured out like water, and all my bones are out of joint: my heart is like wax; it is melted in the midst of my bowels."

PSALMS 22:14

I. GUIDING PRINCIPLES

A. Most acute diarrhea is self-limited.

B. The very young and very old are at risk for dehydration and may require hospital admission.

C. The evaluation of chronic diarrhea is usually done on an outpatient basis.

II. CLINICAL EVALUATION

A. History

1. How long has the diarrhea been present? Diarrhea lasting < 3 weeks is arbitrarily defined as acute diarrhea.

2. How much stool is passed in a 24-hour period? An estimate of stool number and volume is helpful, although a 24-hour stool collection weighing more than 200 g provides a more precise definition of diarrhea.

3. Is there any blood in the stool? The presence of grossly visible blood suggests an invasive pathogen, inflammation, colitis, or a mucosal lesion. Stool cultures should be obtained, and if negative, a follow-up sigmoidoscopy performed.

4. Does the diarrhea awaken the patient from sleep? Functional bowel disturbances usually do not awaken patients from sleep.

5. Is there anything that brings on the diarrhea or helps to relieve it? Questions pertaining to dietary, sexual, or toxin exposure are relevant.

6. How is the diarrhea affected by fasting? Endogenous secretory diarrhea due to a tumor (e.g., VIPoma) will not abate with fasting, while osmotic diarrhea due to laxatives and dietary causes will cease with fasting.

7. Does the patient relate the onset of diarrhea to travel or ingesting a particular foodstuff or potentially contaminated water? Giardiasis, amebiasis, and other causes of traveler's diarrhea such as enterotoxigenic *Escherichia coli* and *Vibrio parahaemolyticus* should be sought, especially if others with similar exposure are also ill.

8. Are there associated symptoms suggesting a systemic viral syndrome (e.g., myalgias, arthralgias, cough, and other upper-respiratory symptoms)?

9. Has there been any fever or shaking chills? Invasive bacterial pathogens are more likely to cause fever.

10. Is there any associated nausea or vomiting? These symptoms are more common with viral gastroenteritis and staphylococcal food poisoning.

11. Is there associated abdominal pain or urgency to defecate? Cramping abdominal pain relieved by diarrhea is common with all causes of diarrhea. A sense of urgency without significant amounts of associated diarrhea (tenesmus) suggests rectal inflammation.

12. Has there been any change of diet? Ask about diet foods containing sorbitol, caffeine, and dairy products.

13. Has there been any recent weight loss? Significant weight loss suggests either a severe acute process or a chronic debilitating illness.

14. Are there symptoms of hyperthyroidism such as heat intolerance, palpitations, or excessive sweating?

15. Are there any new medications? Ask specifically about antibiotics, laxatives, diuretics, quinidine, beta-blockers, and theophylline (Table 5–1).

16. Has there been any recent or previous surgery? Bowel or gastric resection, vagotomy, and cholecystectomy alone or in combination may cause diarrhea.

17. Are there any chronic bowel problems in other family members? Inflammatory bowel disease is more frequent in patients with a family history of Crohn's disease or ulcerative colitis.

B. Physical Examination

Obtain vital signs and examine skin, HEENT and neck, chest, heart, abdomen (including rectal examination and stool heme test), and neurologic status.

Table 5–1. MEDICATIONS ASSOCIATED WITH DIARRHEA

MEDICATION	PATHOPHYSIOLOGY OF DIARRHEA
Antacids (containing magnesium)	Osmotic diarrhea
Laxatives (milk of magnesia, Epsom salts, neutral phosphate)	Osmotic diarrhea
Artificial sweeteners (mannitol, xylitol, sorbitol)	Osmotic diarrhea
Diuretics (ethacrynic acid, furosemide)	Secretory diarrhea
Asthma medication (theophylline)	Secretory diarrhea
Antiarrhythmic drugs (digitalis, quinidine)	Secretory diarrhea
Antibiotics	*Clostridium difficile* toxin or altered gut flora

C. Laboratory and Radiographic Evaluation

1. These tests are not indicated in all cases and should be ordered based on the patient's history and physical examination. For example, patients with acute viral gastroenteritis have a self-limited illness and usually require no laboratory tests.

2. A complete blood count (CBC) may be useful in patients with fever and other signs of systemic inflammation, abdominal pain, or significant rectal bleeding.

3. Electrolyte values should be obtained to assess severity and guide rehydration in patients with dehydration.

4. Fecal leukocyte levels should be obtained in all patients with significant diarrhea.

5. Stool cultures should be obtained if fecal leukocytes are present or if the patient has fever, bloody stools, dehydration, and/or diarrhea that has persisted for longer than 48–72 hours.

6. Stool should be obtained to test for ova and parasites when diarrhea has been present for more than 1 week or when a particular parasite (e.g., *Entamoeba histolytica* or *Giardia*) is suspected because of a travel or exposure history.

7. Sigmoidoscopy is indicated in patients with persistent rectal bleeding and those with bloody diarrhea and negative stool cultures. Mucosal neoplasms and inflammatory bowel disease may be detected.

8. Twenty-four-hour stool collection for weight and fat content is useful in the evaluation of patients with chronic diarrhea to measure stool volume and detect steatorrhea.

III. DIFFERENTIAL DIAGNOSIS

Table 5–2 lists the major causes of diarrhea according to duration and categories, in addition to useful diagnostic clues.

Table 5-2. DIFFERENTIAL DIAGNOSIS OF DIARRHEA

DURATION	CATEGORY	SPECIFIC CAUSE	DIAGNOSTIC STUDIES	DIAGNOSTIC CLUES
Acute (< 3 weeks)	Infectious	*Salmonella, Campylobacter, Shigella*	Fecal leukocyte count; stool culture	Watery or bloody diarrhea; may have history of recent travel or exposure to others with diarrhea
		Yersinia enterocolitica	Culture on selective media	Right lower quadrant pain may be prominent
		Vibrio	Stool culture	Recent exposure to seafood, especially oysters
		Clostridium difficile	Stool culture and toxin	Recent antibiotic therapy
		Entamoeba histolytica	Stool ova and parasites; serology	Recent travel to underdeveloped countries
		Giardia lamblia	Stool ova and parasites	Water ingestion from mountain stream or lake; travel; daycare center exposure
		Rotavirus	Stool assay	Wintertime epidemics, especially in children
	Osmotic	Medications (see Table 5–1)	Stool magnesium	History of specific drug exposure
		Lactose	Stool, electrolytes, and osmoles	Dietary history
	Secretory	Medications (see Table 5–1)	None, except KOH test for phenolphthalein laxatives	History of specific drug exposure

Duration	Category	Specific Cause	Diagnostic Studies	Diagnostic Clues
Chronic (> 3 weeks)	Infectious	*Giardia*, amoeba	See above	See above
	Drug-induced	See above	See above	Pertinent drug exposure; surreptitious chronic laxative abuse
	Systemic illness	Diabetes, hyperthyroidism, scleroderma, carcinoid	Serum glucose, thyroid screen, urinary 5-HIAA	Other symptoms and signs of specific disease
	Neoplasm	Colon cancer or polyps	(+) Fecal occult blood test	Bloody diarrhea, weight loss
Chronic (> 3 weeks)	Inflammatory bowel disease	Crohn's disease	Sigmoidoscopy with biopsy; small-bowel radiographs	Watery, bloody, or fatty diarrhea; intermittent small-bowel obstruction; arthritis; perianal diseases
		Ulcerative colitis	Sigmoidoscopy with biopsy	Bloody diarrhea
	Malabsorption	Small-bowel disease	Fecal fat stain	Large volume nonbloody diarrhea; surgical history
		Pancreatic disease	Fecal fat stain	History of chronic alcohol abuse; recurrent pancreatitis; or surgical removal of a portion of the pancreas

Table 5-3. SPECIFIC ORAL ANTIMICROBIAL THERAPY FOR COMMON ENTERIC PATHOGENS

PATHOGEN	DRUG	ADULT DOSAGE
Campylobacter jejuni	Ciprofloxacin, or	500 mg PO bid × 3 days
	ofloxacin, or	300 mg PO bid × 3 days
	erythromycin	500 mg PO qid × 5 days
Salmonella sp.	1. Treatment not recommended for uncomplicated acute gastroenteritis in nonimmunosuppressed patients without bacteremia unless a typhoid strain is present.	
Enteric (typhoid) fever is usually caused by *S. typhi* or *S. paratyphi.* Symptoms include fever, anorexia, headache, malaise, relative bradycardia, and diarrhea or obstipation.	2. If the patient is systemically ill, hospitalize for initial intravenous antibiotic administration. Antibiotic choices for typhoid fever include the following:	
	Ciprofloxacin, or	400 mg IV q 12 hr
	Chloramphenicol, or	50–100 mg/kg/day IV in divided doses q 6 hr (4 g/day maximum)
	Ceftriaxone, or	3–4 g/day IV in 2 divided doses
	Trimethoprim-sulfamethoxazole, or	320 mg/1600 mg IV q 12 hr
	Ampicillin	1–2 g IV q 6 hr
	3. Uncomplicated septicemia should be treated for at least 2 weeks (changing from IV to PO therapy as clinical condition allows).	
	4. Patients with suspected typhoid fever and shock or mental status changes should also be treated with corticosteroids (dexamethasone: 3 mg/kg initially, followed by 1 mg/kg q 6 hr × 8 doses).	
	5. Chronic carriers (excretion of *Salmonella* in the stool for > 3 months after recovery) generally require:	
	Ampicillin and probenicid	1–1.5 g and 500 mg (respectively) PO qid × 4–6 weeks
	or	
	Ciprofloxacin	750 mg PO bid × 3 weeks
	Cholecystectomy may be required to eradicate the carrier state.	

Shigella sp.	Ciprofloxacin, or	500 mg PO bid × 3 days
or	Ofloxacin, or	300 mg PO bid × 3 days
Enterotoxigenic *Escherichia coli*	Trimethoprim-sulfamethoxazole	160 mg–800 mg (respectively) bid × 5 days
Clostridium difficile	Metronidazole, or	250 mg PO tid × 7–10 days
	Vancomycin	125 mg PO qid × 7–10 days
Giardia lamblia	Quinacrine, or	100 mg PO tid × 5–7 days
	Metronidazole	250 mg–500 mg PO tid × 5–7 days
Entamoeba histolytica	Metronidazole and	750 mg PO tid × 10 days
	Iodoquinol	650 mg PO tid × 20 days

IV. THERAPY

A. Carefully evaluate the patient for moderate or worse volume depletion and replace deficits as indicated with intravenous crystalloid solutions (normal saline or lactated Ringer's solution). Simultaneously, consider and correct any detected electrolyte deficiencies (including potassium and magnesium).

B. Oral rehydration solutions are also appropriate and may be continued after ED discharge. Solutions that contain glucose and electrolytes promote fluid absorption and are preferred over simple juices or water. Commercial preparations are available (e.g., Pedialyte). A practical "home-made" electrolyte solution is as follows: 4 tablespoons sugar + ¾ teaspoons salt + 1 teaspoon sodium bicarbonate (baking soda) + 1 cup orange juice + 1 quart water. Patients must be instructed to measure these ingredients carefully (e.g., not to confuse measurement of salt for sugar).

C. Empiric antidiarrhea therapy in the adult may also include the following:

1. *PeptoBismol:* 2 tablespoons PO q 30 min until diarrhea stops, up to 8 doses in a 24-hour period. This agent is effective for most episodes of acute infectious diarrhea.

2. *Diphenoxylate-atropine* (Lomotil) or *loperamide* (Imodium), up to 8 tablets daily, are alternatives, but they should not be used in the patient with abdominal pain, fever, or bloody diarrhea.

D. Antibiotic therapy should generally be guided by stool culture results (Table 5–3). Empiric antibiotics (e.g., ciprofloxacin 500 mg PO bid for 3–5 days) are somewhat controversial, but many consider them reasonable in the setting of bloody diarrhea, fecal leukocytes, or diarrhea with a fever. Disadvantages to empiric antibiotics may include promotion of bacterial resistance and the risk of prolonging asymptomatic carriage of *Salmonella.*

E. Severely ill patients, especially at the extremes of age, should generally be admitted to the hospital for intravenous hydration and observation along with empiric antibiotic coverage.

V. DISPOSITION

A. Patients with significant dehydration who are unable to maintain hydration orally because of vomiting, other medical problems, or social problems should be admitted. Infants and the elderly require special consideration for admission.

B. Fit patients with acute diarrhea of unknown cause should be contacted in several days to see if the diarrhea has resolved; if it has not, follow-up evaluation should be recommended.

C. Referral for sigmoidoscopy or specialty consultation is indicated if diarrhea has been present for more than 2 weeks, if the patient has bloody diarrhea with negative stool cultures, or if the diagnosis is unclear and the patient is not responding to current therapy.

VI. PEARLS AND PITFALLS

A. The patient with diarrhea may be seriously volume depleted and may have significant electrolyte abnormalities (including hypomagnesemia). Assessing volume status and instituting aggressive intravenous crystalloid replacement is a top priority.

B. The key to diagnosis is a careful history (including description of stools, medication use, travel history, and sexual habits), a directed physical examination, and a selective laboratory evaluation.

C. Stool should be examined for fecal leukocytes and sent for enteric pathogen culture in all patients with diarrhea for ≥ 48–72 hours or diarrhea accompanied by fever, abdominal pain, or blood in stool. Send stool for ova and parasite examination (multiple specimens may be required) when diarrhea has been present for ≥ 1 week or when parasites are otherwise expected because of travel or exposure history.

D. Patients with diarrhea who have been taking antibiotics at any time during the previous 6 weeks should also have their stool evaluated for *Clostridium difficile* toxin.

E. Whether to empirically treat presumed bacterial enteritis or wait for definitive culture results remains controversial. If empiric antibiotic therapy is prescribed, ciprofloxacin is a good initial choice. Remember, however, that the quinolones (ciprofloxacin, norfloxacin, ofloxacin) should not be used in patients < 18 years old or in pregnant patients.

F. Referral for sigmoidoscopy is appropriate in patients with persistent rectal bleeding or bloody diarrhea and negative stool cultures.

G. Do not prescribe antimotility agents (diphenoxylate-atropine or loperamide) to patients with inflammatory diarrhea (e.g., fever, abdominal pain, or bloody diarrhea).

BIBLIOGRAPHY

Bell BP, Goldoft M, Griffin PM, Davis MA, et al: A multistate outbreak of *Escherichia coli* 0157:H7—associated bloody diarrhea and hemolytic uremic syndrome from hamburgers. JAMA 1994;272:1349–1353.
Bruckstein AH: Diagnosis and therapy of acute and chronic diarrhea. Postgrad Med 1989;86:151.
DuPont HL, Edelman R, Kimmey MB: Infectious diarrhea: from *E. coli* to *Vibrio*. Patient Care 1991;25:18.
Fry RD: Infectious enteritis: a collective review. Dis Colon Rectum 1990;33:520-527.
Pickering LK: Therapy for acute infectious diarrhea in children. J Pediatr 1991;118:S118.
Powell DW: Approach to the patient with diarrhea. In Kelly WN (ed): Textbook of Internal Medicine. Philadelphia, JB Lippincott, 1991.

6

Dizziness

"Prithee do not turn me about. My stomach is not constant."

WILLIAM SHAKESPEARE

I. ESSENTIAL FACTS

A. Definition

Dizziness is defined as a disturbed state of spatial awareness. From the patient's perspective, it is an uncomfortable sensation of motion, unsteadiness, giddiness, or lightheadedness. Normal balance requires the appropriate input and integration of the vestibular, visual, and proprioceptive systems; dizziness may result from dysfunction in one or more of these systems or their central integration, impaired cerebral blood flow, altered brain metabolism, or a psychogenic disorder.

B. Causes

A patient whose chief complaint is "dizziness" should have that complaint more specifically categorized as *presyncope, vertigo, dysequilibrium,* or *unclassified dizziness.*

1. Presyncope

a. DEFINITION

Presyncope is the sensation of an imminent faint *without* actual loss of consciousness; it occurs secondary to inadequate cerebral blood flow. The patient may report lightheadedness, visual blurring or darkening, and the need to sit or lie down to improve symptoms and avoid loss of consciousness.

b. CAUSES

Anemia, autonomic insufficiency, cardiovascular disease (e.g., aortic stenosis, cardiomyopathy, carotid sinus hypersensitivity, arrhythmias, or otherwise impaired cardiac output), hypovolemia, drugs, and vasovagal responses. Presyncope is not caused by cerebrovascular disease.

2. Vertigo

a. DEFINITION

Vertigo is the sensation of *abnormal motion* of the body or its environment; the patient may complain of a spinning or turning sensation, or that the "room is moving." Vertigo may occur secondary to central, peripheral, or systemic disorders.

b. CENTRAL CAUSES

In these disorders, vertigo occurs secondary to dysfunction of the brainstem, cerebellum, or cerebral cortex, and the patient's neurologic examination is usually abnormal. Brainstem symptoms and signs include compromised cranial nerve function (e.g., diplopia, dysarthria, dysphagia, impaired corneal reflex, and/or facial weakness), motor weakness or paralysis, and/or sensory abnormalities. Cerebellar signs include gait ataxia, finger-to-nose ataxia, and/or difficulty with rapid alternating movements.

    i. **Acoustic Neuroma.** This tumor begins as a peripheral lesion in the sheath cells of the vestibular portion of cranial nerve VIII, and early symptoms include tinnitus, altered hearing, and dizziness. The acoustic neuroma subsequently grows into the cerebellopontine angle, resulting in an impaired corneal reflex, facial weakness, and cerebellar signs.

    ii. **Brainstem Hemorrhage or Infarction.** The patient presents with the sudden onset of brainstem symptoms and signs.

    iii. **Cerebellar Hemorrhage or Infarction.** The patient presents with the sudden onset of dizziness, headache, vomiting, and ataxia. Pupils are usually of normal size and reactivity, but the patient may be *unable* to look to the side of the lesion. *Caution:* a computed tomography (CT) scan may miss cerebellar lesions, necessitating more sensitive magnetic resonance imaging (MRI). Emergent neurosurgical consultation is indicated; without rapid intervention, death may occur secondary to brainstem compression.

    iv. **Geniculate Ganglionitis.** Presents with ear pain, vertigo, and facial paralysis. The Ramsay Hunt syndrome is geniculate ganglionitis secondary to herpes zoster (in which case herpetic lesions are seen in the external auditory canal).

    v. **Head Trauma.** Headache, dizziness, and vertigo are common complaints after head trauma (including the postconcussion syndrome).

    vi. **Infections.** Vertigo may be a prominent complaint in the patient with a serious central nervous system (CNS) infection (e.g., brain abscess, encephalitis, or meningitis).

    vii. **Lateral Medullary Syndrome** (Wallenberg's syndrome). Patients present with vertigo, ataxia (patient falls toward the lesion), diplopia, dysphagia, hoarseness (from vocal cord paralysis), and nausea. In addition, ipsilateral to the lesion there is facial numbness, Horner's syndrome (anhidrosis, miosis, and ptosis), and limb ataxia; contralateral to the lesion the patient has decreased or absent extremity pinprick and temperature sensation. The lateral medullary syndrome occurs secondary to occlusion of the vertebral or posterior inferior cerebellar artery.

viii. **Posterior Fossa Tumors.** These present with symptoms and signs of brainstem and/or cerebellar dysfunction, including vertigo. Fundoscopic examination may reveal evidence (e.g., absence of venous pulsations, papilledema) of increased intracranial pressure.

ix. **Subclavian Steal Syndrome.** May occur when the subclavian artery has a narrowing proximal to the origin of the vertebral artery. Exercise of the upper extremity "steals" blood from the vertebral artery, resulting in symptoms and signs of vertebrobasilar insufficiency (see below). On examination, upper-extremity blood pressures may be asymmetrical and a subclavian bruit sometimes is auscultated.

x. **Vertebrobasilar Insufficiency.** Symptoms may include vertigo, diplopia, dysphagia, numbness, and slurred speech, accompanied by brainstem and cerebellar signs. Certain head positions may mechanically worsen vascular compromise and intensify symptoms. Drop attacks (sudden loss of motor tone resulting in a fall, but not associated with altered consciousness) may also rarely occur. Most patients are elderly, and the vascular insufficiency is secondary to arteriosclerosis, cervical arthritis, or vascular malformations.

xi. **Other Causes.** Basilar artery migraine, drugs, multiple sclerosis, temporal lobe epilepsy, and toxins may cause vertigo.

c. PERIPHERAL CAUSES

In these disorders, vertigo occurs secondary to dysfunction of the external auditory canal, middle ear, inner ear, or cranial nerve VIII. Most vertigo (> 80% of cases) is of peripheral origin.

i. **Acute Labyrinthitis.** Symptoms include one or more days of intense vertigo, generally accompanied by hearing loss. Limited caloric testing is usually normal. Acute labyrinthitis occurs in the setting of a middle/inner ear infection, mastoiditis, or a systemic viral infection (e.g., influenza, measles, or mumps).

ii. **Acute Vestibular Neuronitis.** This self-limited disorder results in sudden and severe vertigo of one or more days duration. Tinnitus may occur, but, unlike acute labyrinthitis described above, hearing loss does not. Symptoms are aggravated by certain head or eye movements. Limited caloric testing reveals hypofunction on the involved side. In the ED, acute vestibular neuronitis is frequently mislabeled as acute labyrinthitis.

iii. **Benign Positional Vertigo.** In this condition, changing head position (e.g., when turning over in bed) results in sudden but self-limited vertigo. Hearing is not affected, and calorics are normal. Most cases are idiopathic, but some may occur after infection or trauma. Benign positional vertigo is the most common cause of vertigo, and it typically occurs in middle-aged or elderly patients.

iv. **Drugs.** The following agents may affect inner ear function and result in peripheral vertigo: alcohol, aminoglycosides, aspirin, caffeine, cisplatin, loop diuretics, and phenytoin.

v. **External Auditory Canal Abnormalities.** Vertigo may result from excess or impacted cerumen and foreign bodies.

vi. **Middle-Ear Abnormalities.** May cause vertigo, including cholesteatoma (a cystlike mass filled with desquamating cholesterol-laden debris), impaired eustachian tube function; serous, suppurative, or chronic otitis media; otosclerosis (where deposition of spongy bone immobilizes the stapes and results in conductive hearing loss); and trauma.

vii. **Meniere's Disease.** Classic paroxysmal symptoms include vertigo, tinnitus, and hearing loss. The attacks of vertigo are sudden, severe, accompanied by nausea and vomiting, and last 1–2 hours. Multiple episodes may result in permanent hearing loss. Meniere's disease is uncommon and usually occurs in individuals aged 30–60 years.

viii. **Motion Sickness.** Patients with intense vestibular stimuli, or contrary visual and vestibular inputs, may suffer symptoms of dizziness, diaphoresis, and vomiting.

ix. **Trauma.** Any of the following may result in vertigo: ruptured tympanic membrane, dislocated ossicles, labyrinthine concussion, middle-ear fractures (which may be accompanied by a cerebrospinal fluid leak), and perilymphatic fistula.

d. SYSTEMIC DISORDERS

Occasionally, vertigo occurs secondary to systemic disease, including hypoglycemia (e.g., as a complication of the treatment of diabetes mellitus), hypothyroidism, and syphilis.

3. *Disequilibrium*

a. DEFINITION

Disequilibrium is a sense of imbalance or unsteadiness, generally accompanied by ataxia or an abnormal gait. Disequilibrium is usually only noticed by the patient when walking. It may be described as "dizziness in the legs and feet" rather than "dizziness in the head."

b. CAUSES

Disequilibrium occurs secondary to multiple sensory deficits (e.g., auditory, proprioceptive, vestibular, and visual), CNS disease (e.g., cerebellar disease, frontal-lobe apraxia, parkinsonism), drugs, muscle disorders, osteoarthritis, and/or spinal disease.

4. *Unclassified Dizziness*

a. DEFINITION

Dizziness that is not adequately classified into one of the above specific categories should be considered "unclassified."

b. CAUSES

May include anxiety disorder, depression, hyperventilation, and panic attacks.

C. Important Principles

1. Dizziness may be the manifestation of a *life-threatening* disorder, including one or more of the following:
   a. Anemia.
   b. Aortic stenosis.
   c. Brainstem hemorrhage or ischemia (including vertebrobasilar insufficiency).
   d. Cardiomyopathy.
   e. Cerebellar hemorrhage or ischemia.
   f. Arrhythmia.
   g. Heat illness.
   h. Hypertension.
   i. Hypoglycemia.
   j. Hypoxia.
   k. Hypovolemia.
   l. Infection (including brain abscess, encephalitis, and meningitis).
   m. Poisoning.
   n. Posterior fossa tumor.
   o. Trauma.
2. The ED physician must carefully evaluate the dizzy patient for any life-threatening or serious disease, initiate appropriate

Table 6–1. CHARACTERISTICS OF CENTRAL AND PERIPHERAL VERTIGO

CHARACTERISTIC	CENTRAL VERTIGO	PERIPHERAL VERTIGO
Caloric testing	Symmetrical, but not necessarily normal response	Reproduces patient's "dizziness" and/or decreased response in the affected ear
Changes with head position	Vertigo not positional	Vertigo positional and/or worsened by head movement
Direction patient falls	Falls to the side of the central lesion and *toward* the fast component of nystagmus	Falls to the side of the peripheral lesion and *away* from the fast component of nystagmus
Duration	Long (>10 sec) and not fatiguable	Brief (usually ≤ 10 sec) and fatiguable
Hearing loss	Unusual	Possible hearing loss and/or tinnitus
Intensity of vertigo and associated symptoms	Less intense Mild or no associated symptoms	Very intense motion sensation; nausea, vomiting, and diaphoresis common, and may be incapacitating
Latency	None	3–10 sec
Neurologic symptoms and signs	Brainstem and/or cerebellar symptoms/signs common, including one or more of the following: ataxia, cranial nerve abnormalities, diplopia, dysarthria, dysphagia, hemiparesis, or papilledema	None (except for cranial nerve VIII abnormalities)
Nystagmus	May be present without vertigo May be of any direction, including vertical Not inhibited by ocular fixation	Always accompanied by vertigo Frequently rotatory, may be horizontal; never vertical (unless secondary to a drug effect) Inhibited by ocular fixation
Onset	Usually insidious (sudden onset, however, if secondary to an acute vascular event)	Begins suddenly

treatment for these conditions, and arrange for any indicated consultation and/or hospitalization. It is not necessary or possible to diagnose the cause of dizziness in every patient (case series have reported no diagnosis in 10-37% of ED patients with the chief complaint of dizziness).

3. If the patient is suffering from vertigo, it is essential to determine whether the vertigo is central or peripheral (Table 6–1):
   a. Central vertigo may be insidious in onset (it is of sudden onset in the setting of an acute vascular event), usually produces less dramatic motion-related symptoms, is uncommon (15% of cases), and often has a serious cause

that mandates neuroimaging, consultation, and hospitalization.

b. Peripheral vertigo is usually of sudden and dramatic onset, is symptomatically more intense than central vertigo, is more common (85% of cases), and generally has a benign cause.

4. Patients with vertigo usually manifest *nystagmus,* which is a rhythmic, to-and-fro, involuntary movement of the eyes. The characteristics of nystagmus provide important information as to the cause of vertigo. Nystagmus has a slow component (directed away from an excited semicircular canal) and a fast component. This latter is a "corrective" movement occurring secondary to input from the cerebral cortex; the "direction" of nystagmus is named for the fast component. Nystagmus may be horizontal, vertical, rotatory, or a mixture of these.

a. When a central lesion causes central vertigo
   i. Nystagmus is most prominent when looking *toward* the lesion.
   ii. Nystagmus may be in any direction. Vertical nystagmus is a sign of brainstem disease, except in the setting of a drug effect (including barbiturates, phencyclidine, and phenytoin toxicity).
   iii. The direction of the slow and fast components *varies* with the direction of gaze.
   iv. The patient may have nystagmus without experiencing vertigo.

b. When a peripheral lesion causes peripheral vertigo
   i. Nystagmus is most prominent when the patient looks *away from* the lesion (i.e., looks away from the affected ear).
   ii. Nystagmus is rotatory or horizontal (never vertical).
   iii. The slow component of nystagmus is toward the affected ear and the fast component away from it.
   iv. The patient experiences vertigo when nystagmus is present.

5. Beware of the dizzy, elderly patient! Dizziness, regardless of its cause, represents a significant danger because of the risks associated with falling and concomitant injury. Injuries secondary to falls cause two-thirds of all accidental deaths in the elderly, and 50% of elderly patients who require hospitalization after a fall die within 1 year.

D. Epidemiology

1. In primary care practice, dizziness is the chief complaint for 1% of patients > 25 years old; its frequency increases to 3.7% of all chief complaints for patients > 85 years old.
2. One-third of all people by age 65 have experienced at least one episode of dizziness.
3. In the ED, the most common causes of dizziness are peripheral vestibular disorders and cardiovascular diseases.

II. CLINICAL EVALUATION

A. History

1. Have the patient carefully describe symptoms without using the word "dizzy," and attempt to better categorize the complaint as presyncope, vertigo, disequilibrium, or unclassified (see I.B, above).

2. Ask the following questions:
   a. Are symptoms of sudden or gradual onset? Is the dizziness complaint new for the patient or a recurrent problem?
   b. Are symptoms made worse with certain head positions, body positions, or body movements?
   c. Are there other symptoms associated with the dizziness, such as headache, fever, chills, nausea, vomiting, and/or diaphoresis?
   d. Are there complaints associated with central disease, such as ataxia, diplopia, dysarthria, dysphagia, facial numbness, headache, limb weakness, sensory abnormalities, or bilateral visual blurring?
   e. Are there ear complaints suggesting peripheral disease, such as ear pain, fullness, tinnitus, and/or altered or decreased hearing?

3. Determine if the patient has
   a. Cardiovascular symptoms (such as chest pain, palpitations, and dyspnea) and/or a prior history of cardiac disease.
   b. A history of bleeding (such as hematemesis, hematochezia, or melena) or anemia.
   c. Volume loss (poor oral intake, vomiting, diarrhea).
   d. A history of cerebrovascular disease.
   e. Gait problems and prior history of falls. Are there complaints of chronic visual loss, auditory dysfunction, or known sensory deficits that contribute to disequilibrium?

4. Obtain a careful medication history, including any recent changes in drug dosing.
   a. Drugs that may cause *orthostatic hypotension* include antidepressants, antihypertensives, nitrates, phenothiazines, and tranquilizers.
   b. Drugs or toxins known to *affect the inner ear* include alcohol, antibiotics (aminoglycosides, chloramphenicol, erythromycin, minocycline, and vancomycin), anticonvulsants (barbiturates, carbamazepine, ethosuximide, and phenytoin), aspirin and other nonsteroidal antiinflammatory drugs, chemotherapeutic agents (cisplatin and vinblastine), diuretics (bumetanide, ethacrynic acid, and furosemide), and miscellaneous agents (including chloroquine, methanol, mercury, phencyclidine, phenothiazines, propylene glycol, quinidine, and quinine).
   c. Drugs that may cause *disequilibrium* include anticonvulsants, benzodiazepines, haloperidol, lithium, and other psychotropic medications.

5. Accurately identify any pre-existing significant medical problems (e.g., alcoholism, cancer, congestive heart failure,
diabetes mellitus, pulmonary disease, renal insufficiency,
thyroid dysfunction, valvular heart disease, spinal disease).

B. Physical Examination

Carefully evaluate the following: vital signs, HEENT examination, neck, chest, heart, abdomen (including rectal examination
and stool hemoccult test), and neurologic examination.

C. Provocative Testing

One or more of the following maneuvers may assist the ED
physician in determining the cause of the patient's dizziness
complaint.

1. **Postural Vital Signs.** These should regularly be obtained when
   presyncope is clinically suspected.

2. **Carotid Sinus Massage.** This test is reasonable when carotid
   sinus hypersensitivity is the suspected cause of presyncope. A
   positive test reproduces the patient's symptoms and is
   associated with either 3 sec of asystole on the rhythm monitor
   or a drop in systolic blood pressure $\geq$ 50 mmHg.
   Caution: monitor cardiac rhythm throughout carotid sinus massage. An intravenous line should be in place and atropine immediately available if prolonged sinus arrest or hypotension occurs
   with massage. Do not perform this test if the patient has carotid
   bruits, a history of cerebrovascular disease, or is $\geq$ 65 years old.

3. **Valsalva Maneuver.** This maneuver is performed to further
   evaluate a cardiac murmur suggestive of a valve abnormality
   (e.g., aortic stenosis, hypertrophic cardiomyopathy) responsible for presyncope. Performing a valsalva maneuver for
   approximately 15 sec results in decreased return to the right
   heart followed by decreased left ventricular volume and blood
   pressure. The murmur of aortic stenosis decreases and that of
   hypertrophic cardiomyopathy increases with valsalva.

4. **Nylen–Barany (Dix–Hallpike) Maneuver.** This test is useful
   in eliciting nystagmus in the patient with vertigo. The
   characteristics of nystagmus frequently assist in differentiating
   vertigo of central origin from that of peripheral origin (see
   Table 6–1).
   Technique (Figure 6–1). The patient is rapidly taken from a
   sitting to supine position, with the head 30° below the examining
   table and rotated 30–45° to one side. Observe the eyes carefully
   for nystagmus for at least 15 sec; the maneuver should then be
   repeated with the head turned in the opposite direction.

5. **"Limited" Caloric Testing.** Consider limited caloric testing
   when it otherwise cannot be determined whether vertigo is of
   central or peripheral origin (also see Table 6–1). The stimulated

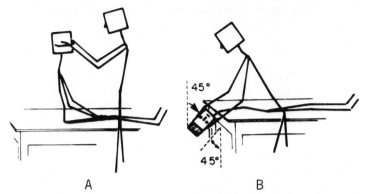

Figure 6–1. The Nylen-Bárány maneuver for positional vertigo and nystagmus. The patient is moved abruptly from a seated (A) to a supine (B) position, with his head hanging 30° below the horizontal and rotated 30–45° to one side. He is observed for the development of nystagmus and vertigo. (From Drachman DA, Hart CW: An approach to the dizzy patient. Neurology 1972;22:323.)

nystagmus and vertigo may be intense and uncomfortable for the patient. Limited caloric testing is contraindicated in the setting of a ruptured tympanic membrane.

Technique. The patient is placed supine with head elevated to 30°. Gently irrigate one ear at a time with 0.2 mL of ice water using a tuberculin syringe and observe nystagmus. Normally, the fast component of nystagmus is away from the irrigated ear, lasting approximately 1 min, and the caloric response is symmetrical.

6. **The "Fistula" Test.** This test is appropriate when either a cholesteatoma or perilymphatic fistula is the suspected cause of vertigo.

Technique. Gently and passively extend the supine patient's head to 60° below horizontal and use a pneumatic otoscope with an appropriately snug fit. Vertigo and nystagmus with insufflation constitutes a positive test. When a labyrinthine fistula is present, the patient's eyes deviate to one side and then the other with positive and negative insufflation pressures, respectively.

7. **Hyperventilation.** Dizziness or lightheadedness may occur secondary to hyperventilation. This can be tested by noting if symptoms are reproduced by having the seated patient hyperventilate for 3 min.

D. Laboratory and Other Diagnostic Evaluations

Further diagnostic testing of the dizzy patient must be individualized to the category of dizziness and the diagnostic possibilities suggested by the above history and physical examination findings.

1. If patient has presyncope:
   a. Monitor cardiac rhythm.

     b. Obtain an electrocardiogram if any of the following apply:
       i. Cardiac rhythm is abnormal.
       ii. Age ≥ 40 years.
       iii. The patient is at risk for ischemic heart disease.
       iv. Cardiac symptoms are present.
       v. The patient is known to have ischemic heart disease.
     c. Check SaO_2 and continuously monitor if abnormal.
     d. Minimal laboratory evaluation should include hematocrit.
     e. Consider one or more of the following, depending on the clinical situation:
       i. Serum electrolytes, glucose, blood urea nitrogen, creatinine.
       ii. Inpatient cardiac monitoring (for patients at high risk for a arrhythmia; see Chapter 10).
       iii. Outpatient cardiac (Holter) monitoring (for stable patients deemed appropriate for outpatient arrhythmia evaluation).
       iv. Echocardiography (if aortic stenosis or hypertrophic cardiomyopathy are clinically suspected).
       v. Other studies if indicated (e.g., arterial blood gas values, blood type and crossmatch, chest radiograph, ethanol level, serum pregnancy test).

2. If patient has central vertigo:
     a. Neuroimaging is indicated! CT is usually performed because of its availability, but MRI is more sensitive in the diagnosis of posterior fossa and brainstem lesions.
     b. Other studies may include one or more of the following as indicated: further blood work (e.g., serum glucose, thyroid function tests, serum VDRL test), angiography (vertebrobasilar insufficiency), lumbar puncture (suspected meningitis), electroencephalography (suspected temporal lobe epilepsy), Doppler studies with or without angiography (subclavian steal syndrome), or referral for electronystagmography.

3. If patient has vertigo of uncertain cause, consider neurology and/or otolaryngology consultation. Useful outpatient studies may include complete audiometric evaluation, brainstem auditory evoked responses, or electronystagmography.

4. In patients with disequilibrium:
     a. Neuroimaging (CT or MRI) is indicated if the neurologic examination reveals focal findings.
     b. Further testing may include one or more of the following: formal visual field and acuity testing, audiography, serum B_{12} level, glucose, serum VDRL test, and heavy-metal and/or toxicologic screening.

III. DIAGNOSTIC AND THERAPEUTIC APPROACHES

A. Assess, secure, and support airway, breathing, and circulation as indicated (see Chapter 1. II).

1. Administer supplemental oxygen, establish intravenous access, and monitor both cardiac rhythm and SaO_2. Continuous electrocardiographic monitoring is reasonable until a presyncopal or otherwise potentially serious disorder has been excluded.
2. Manage any symptomatic cardiac arrhythmia.
3. Control any identified source of hemorrhage or volume loss. Replace identified volume deficits with intravenous crystalloid.

B. Perform a directed history and physical examination. Attempt to establish not only the general cause of the patient's dizziness (e.g., presyncope, vertigo, disequilibrium, or unclassified) but also its specific cause whenever possible (see section II, above).

C. Provide specific therapy for the identified cause(s) of dizziness.

1. Optimal treatment of the dizzy patient depends on the cause of this chief complaint (see the relevant chapter(s) in this manual addressing therapy of the specific identified condition(s)).
2. Obtain specialty consultation when indicated:
   a. Otolaryngology (e.g., patients with cholesteatoma, dislocated ossicles, mastoiditis, middle- or inner-ear trauma, a perilymphatic fistula, or purulent labyrinthitis).
   b. Neurosurgery (e.g., patients with acoustic neuroma, cerebellar or brainstem hemorrhage, or suspected brain tumors).
   c. Neurology (e.g., patients with other central causes of vertigo, including CNS infection and vertebrobasilar insufficiency).
3. Provide symptomatic relief to the patient with *peripheral vertigo:*
   a. Useful drugs include the following:
      i. **First-Line Agent**
         • **Diazepam** (Valium)
            Dose: IV: begin with 2–10 mg, no faster than 2 mg/min; followed by 2–10 mg q 6–8 hr as necessary.
            PO: 2–10 mg q 8–12 hr.
      ii. **Second-Line Agents**
         • **Prochlorperazine** (Compazine)
            Dose: IV: 2.5–10 mg by slow injection or infusion (no faster than 5 mg/min). May repeat q 3–4 hr as needed.
            IM: 5–10 mg q 3–4 hr as needed
            PO: 5–10 mg q 6–8 hr as needed
            PR: 25 mg q 12 hr as needed
         or
         • **Promethazine** (Phenergan)
            Dose: IV or IM (deeply): 12.5–25 mg q 4 hr
            PO or PR: 25 mg to start, followed by 12.5–25 mg q 4–6 hr
         or

- **Meclizine** (Antivert)
    - *Dose:* 25–50 mg PO to start, followed by 25 mg q 6–8 hr

    or

- **Scopolamine** (Transderm Scop). This is an effective agent for motion sickness.
    - *Dose:* 0.5-mg patch applied to postauricular skin q 3 days

    or

- **Dimenhydrinate** (Dramamine)
    - *Dose:* PO: 50–100 mg q 6 hr

  b. Patients with *acute vestibular neuronitis* (see section I. B. 2. c, above) may benefit from corticosteroids (125 mg **methylprednisolone** IV initially; followed by 30 mg **prednisone** bid for 4 days; then taper off prednisone over the subsequent 4 days).

  c. Patients with *Meniere's disease* (see section I. B. 2. c, above) may benefit from salt restriction and diuretic therapy.

  d. Nonpharmacologic adjuncts to improve symptoms of peripheral vertigo include patient reassurance, rest, visual fixation to inhibit nystagmus, and instruction to make all movements in a slow and deliberate fashion.

IV. DISPOSITION

A. Discharge

Patients with the chief complaint of dizziness who meet *all* of the following criteria may be considered for ED discharge:

1. Vital signs are normal.

2. ED evaluation has been completed, and dizziness symptoms are now minor or completely gone.

3. No serious cause for dizziness mandating hospitalization is present (see below).

4. If the patient is suffering from vertigo, it is of peripheral origin and has been well controlled in the ED with symptomatic treatment.

5. The patient is safely ambulatory.

6. The patient has been carefully informed of the risks associated with dizziness while driving, ambulating, operating hazardous equipment, and engaging in otherwise hazardous activities.

7. Appropriate follow-up has been arranged. This is especially important for patients with hearing loss, undiagnosed vertigo, or disequilibrium.

B. Admit

Patients who do not meet all of the above discharge criteria, or individuals with *any* of the following, should be hospitalized for further diagnosis and treatment:

1. Central vertigo (especially CNS ischemia, infection, hemorrhage, trauma, or tumor).
2. Inability to safely ambulate.
3. Vertigo with persistent vomiting despite appropriate symptomatic therapy.
4. Presyncope of serious cause (especially severe anemia, significant autonomic or cardiac dysfunction, arrhythmia, or hemorrhage).
5. Other potentially serious disorder requiring hospitalization or surgery.

V. PEARLS AND PITFALLS

A. Blood loss, arrhythmias, hypoxia, poisoning, life-threatening CNS disorders, serious infections, significant cardiovascular disease, trauma, or volume depletion may all present as dizziness.

B. Drugs may be causing or exacerbating the patient's symptoms. Review all medications carefully; also inquire about over-the-counter preparations.

C. Central causes of vertigo require neuroimaging, consultation (neurology or neurosurgery), and hospitalization.

D. Vertical nystagmus is a sign of brainstem disease (except in the setting of drug toxicity with barbiturates, phencyclidine, or phenytoin).

E. A normal CT scan does not rule out serious brainstem or posterior fossa disease.

F. Cerebellar hemorrhage presents as headache, vomiting, and ataxia. Consult neurosurgery immediately!

G. Elderly patients with recent onset of vertigo of undetermined cause should be suspected of suffering from vertebrobasilar insufficiency until proven otherwise. Consult neurology.

H. A fall in any patient, especially the elderly individual, may be associated with significant morbidity and mortality. Do not discharge the dizzy patient who is unable to safely ambulate.

BIBLIOGRAPHY

Ariyasu L, Byl FM, Sprague MS, Adour KK: The beneficial effect of methylprednisolone in acute vestibular vertigo. Arch Otolaryngol Head Neck Surg 1990;116:700–703.

Garrison TE, Frey JK. Vertigo and dizziness. In Hamilton GC (senior ed): Presenting Signs and Symptoms in the Emergency Department. Baltimore, Williams & Wilkins, 1993, pp. 537–547.

Herr RD, Zun L, Mathews JJ: A directed approach to the dizzy patient. Ann Emerg Med 1989;18(6):664–672.

Warner EA, Wallach PM, Adelman HM, Sahlin-Hughs K: Dizziness in primary care patients. J Gen Int Medicine 1992;7:454–463.

7

Dyspnea

"Some folk seem glad even to draw their breath."

WILLIAM MORRIS

I. ESSENTIAL FACTS

A. Definition

The term *dyspnea* refers to the subjective, abnormal, and uncomfortable sensation of breathlessness. Dyspnea is difficult to quantify and patients may use different terms to describe the sensation. For example, some patients may describe dyspnea as a feeling of "chest tightness," or a "choking" or "suffocating" sensation. Other patients may complain that they are "winded," "out of breath," "not getting enough air," or "unable to take a deep breath." Patterns of dyspnea include the following:

1. **Orthopnea.** The development of dyspnea or worsening of dyspnea in the supine position.

2. **Platypnea.** The development of dyspnea or worsening of dyspnea in the upright position.

3. **Trepopnea.** The development of dyspnea or worsening of dyspnea in the right or left lateral decubitus position.

4. **Paroxysmal Nocturnal Dyspnea** (PND). The sudden occurrence of breathlessness that wakes a patient from sleep.

B. Epidemiology

Precise data on the epidemiology of dyspnea are difficult to obtain because dyspnea is a subjective experience and difficult to define quantitatively. Nevertheless, it is estimated that 5–10% of patients seen in the ED complain of dyspnea as either their primary symptom or a part of their overall symptom complex.

C. Causes

Dyspnea may be caused by a wide variety of conditions. In previously healthy patients, dyspnea may be the result of an acute event such as a pneumothorax or pulmonary embolism; in other patients dyspnea may result from an exacerbation of underlying cardiac or pulmonary disease. A careful history and physical examination, followed by appropriate laboratory evaluation, should allow the clinician to narrow the differential diagnosis in individual cases. A differential diagnosis for dyspnea is given in Table 7–1.

II. CLINICAL EVALUATION

A. History

The patient's history is a key element in defining the cause of dyspnea.

1. Particular attention should be paid to the *onset, severity,* and *pattern* of symptoms.
   a. *Acute* onset of dyspnea suggests pulmonary embolism, pneumothorax, myocardial infarction, or arrhythmia.
   b. Dyspnea that develops *over several hours* is common with asthma, pneumonia, or congestive heart failure (CHF).
   c. *Chronic dyspnea* is more likely to be related to underlying pulmonary or neuromuscular disease.

2. The patient's *past medical history, exposure history,* and *medications* should also be evaluated.

3. *Concomitant* symptoms or *character of dyspnea* may suggest an underlying cause of the patient's symptoms:
   a. *Orthopnea* and *PND* suggest left ventricular dysfunction, but may also accompany chronic obstructive pulmonary disease (COPD).
   b. *Exertional dyspnea* may be secondary to cardiac disease or underlying pulmonary interstitial disease.
   c. *Platypnea* may be associated with neuromuscular disease (e.g., quadriplegia) and abdominal muscle weakness.
   d. *Wheezing* suggests asthma, COPD, or localized airway obstruction.
   e. *Cough* may accompany pneumonia, bronchitis, asthma, or heart failure.
   f. *Fever* and *purulent sputum* suggest pneumonia.
   g. *Hemoptysis* may be a sign of respiratory tract infection, pulmonary embolism, heart failure, mitral valve disease, pulmonary vasculitis, or an endobronchial tumor.
   h. Burning or *crushing chest pain* accompanying dyspnea suggests myocardial ischemia or myocardial infarction.
   i. *Pleuritic chest pain* is more commonly associated with pneumonia, pulmonary embolism, or pneumothorax.

B. Physical Examination

Physical examination findings in dyspneic patients may vary depending on the underlying cause of the patient's dyspnea. Signs associated with dyspnea may include the following:

1. **Vital Signs.** *Tachycardia, tachypnea, hypertension.*

2. **Skin.** *Diaphoresis* usually indicates the patient is in moderate to severe distress. *Cyanosis* is an important, although late, sign of tissue hypoxia.

3. **HEENT.** *Nasal flaring, dry mucous membranes.*

Table 7–1. DIFFERENTIAL DIAGNOSIS OF DYSPNEA

I. *Respiratory Disease*

1. Exacerbation of COPD
   a. Emphysema
   b. Chronic bronchitis
2. Asthma
3. Pleural disease
   a. Pleural effusion
   b. Pneumothorax/hemothorax
   c. Pleurisy
4. Pulmonary embolism
   a. Pulmonary thromboembolism
   b. Amniotic fluid embolism
   c. Fat embolism
   d. Septic embolism (e.g., infective right-sided endocarditis)
5. Pulmonary infarction (e.g., sickle cell crisis)
6. Pneumonia
7. Interstitial lung disease
   a. Pulmonary fibrosis
   b. Pulmonary vasculitis
   c. Sarcoidosis
   d. Hypersensitivity pneumonitis
8. Non-cardiogenic pulmonary edema (e.g., adult respiratory disease syndrome)
9. Acute inhalation injury
   a. Aspiration
   b. Toxic gas inhalation
10. Alveolar hemorrhage syndromes
    a. Goodpasture's syndrome
    b. Wegener's granulomatosis
    c. Idiopathic pulmonary hemosiderosis
11. Airway obstruction
    a. Endobronchial tumor
    b. Laryngospasm
    c. Epiglottitis
    d. Foreign-body aspiration

II. *Cardiac Disease*

1. Left ventricular failure
2. Valvular heart disease
   a. Mitral stenosis or regurgitation
   b. Aortic stenosis or regurgitation
3. Pericardial disease
   a. Pericardial effusion or tamponade
   b. Pericarditis
4. Sustained arrhythmia
5. Pulmonary hypertension and cor pulmonale

III. *Chest Wall or Neuromuscular Disease*

1. Primary myopathies (e.g., polymyositis)
2. Primary neuropathies (e.g., Guillain-Barré syndrome)
3. Phrenic nerve injury and diaphragmatic paralysis
4. Severe electrolyte disturbance (e.g., hypokalemia)
5. Central nervous system respiratory center dysfunction
6. Obesity

IV. *Miscellaneous Conditions*

1. Shock
2. Severe anemia
3. Metabolic acidosis
4. Hyperthyroidism
5. Psychogenic dyspnea
6. Medications (e.g., beta-blockers in patient with asthma)

4. **Neck.** *Accessory muscle use* during respiration generally indicates excessive work of breathing. *Jugular venous distention* may be present in cases of right heart failure.

5. **Lungs.** Patients with COPD may have evidence of *hyperinflation* with *hyperresonant tones* noted on chest percussion. *Wheezing* is a sign of airflow obstruction, whereas *rales* may be present in patients with congestive heart failure, pneumonia, or interstitial lung disease. A *pleural rub* may be detected in patients with pleurisy, pulmonary infarction, or pneumonia. *Bronchial breath sounds* can often be heard overlying an area of consolidated lung in cases of pneumonia. *Diminished breath sounds* and *dullness to percussion* are often noted overlying a pleural effusion. *Diminished or absent breath* accompanied by *hyperresonance to percussion* suggests a pneumothorax. *Egophony* ("ee" to "ay") may be appreciated by auscultating near the top of a pleural effusion. *Stridor* may be present with epiglottitis, and *localized wheezing* may indicate focal endobronchial obstruction.

6. **Heart.** In addition to rales, patients with dyspnea secondary to left ventricular dysfunction may have an S_3 *gallop*. A *cardiac murmur* may give important clues to the cause of a patient's dyspnea. A systolic murmur suggests aortic stenosis, mitral regurgitation, ventricular septal defect, or idiopathic hypertrophic subaortic stenosis, whereas a diastolic murmur suggests aortic regurgitation or mitral stenosis. *Muffled heart tones* or a *pericardial friction rub* may be present in patients with dyspnea from pericardial disease.

7. **Abdomen.** *Ascites,* either secondary to liver disease or CHF, may cause severe dyspnea. *Hepatomegaly* accompanied by a *hepatojugular reflex* suggests the presence of congestive heart failure. *Paradoxical movement of the diaphragm or abdominal muscles* during respiration may indicate spinal cord injury or phrenic nerve damage.

8. **Extremities.** *Peripheral edema* may be a sign of cor pulmonale. *Clubbing* suggests chronic disease such as bronchiectasis, pulmonary fibrosis, or cancer. *Swelling, warmth, erythema,* or *tenderness* of a lower extremity may accompany a deep venous thrombosis, however, these findings are neither sensitive nor specific.

9. **Neurologic Signs.** A neuromuscular or humoral cause of dyspnea is suggested by signs of *muscle weakness.* A careful assessment of the dyspneic patient's *mental status* is important, since agitation may be a sign of hypoxia and lethargy may accompany hypercarbia and indicate respiratory failure.

C. Laboratory Data

1. *Routine laboratory tests* in the dyspneic patient should include
   a. *Complete blood count (CBC).*

   b. *Electrolytes, blood urea nitrogen (BUN), creatinine, and glucose.*
   c. Arterial blood gas levels (ABG).
   d. Chest roentgenogram.
   e. Electrocardiogram (ECG).

2. *Further evaluation* should be directed according to individual clinical circumstances. For example:
   a. *Spirometry* may indicate airflow obstruction (decreased FEV_1, FVC, and FEV_1/FVC ratio) or suggest restrictive lung disease (decreased FEV_1, and FVC with normal or high FEV_1/FVC ratio).

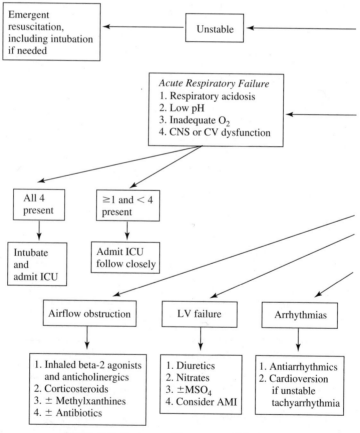

Figure 7–1. Emergency Management of Dyspnea

b. *Flow-volume loops* may differentiate between obstructive and restrictive disease as well as diagnose upper airway obstruction (e.g., tracheal stenosis).

c. A *ventilation/perfusion (V/Q) nuclear scan,* lower extremity *duplex examination,* or *pulmonary angiogram* should be considered in cases of suspected pulmonary embolism.

d. *Sputum Gram stain* may be helpful in diagnosing bacterial pneumonia.

III. TREATMENT

Emergency management of dyspnea is outlined in Figure 7–1.

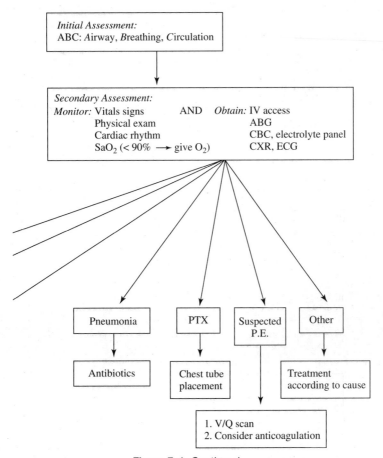

Figure 7–1. *Continued*

A. General Measures

1. *Vital signs*

2. *Cardiac monitoring*

3. *Intravenous access*

4. *SaO_2 monitoring*

5. *Supplemental oxygen* as needed to maintain SaO_2 above 90%.

6. Endotracheal intubation and mechanical ventilation are indicated in patients with severe hypoxemia despite high concentrations of supplemental oxygen, ventilatory failure (pH < 7.25–7.32), or inability to adequately protect their airway (see Chapter 11).

B. Therapy Directed at Specific Causes of Dyspnea

1. **Airflow Obstruction.** Inhaled beta-2 agonists and anticholinergic agents, corticosteroids, ± methylxanthines.

2. **Left Ventricular Failure.** Diuretics, nitrates, ± morphine sulfate. Consider and specifically treat acute myocardial infection (AMI).

3. **Pneumonia.** Antibiotics.

4. **Pulmonary Embolism.** Anticoagulants.

5. **Pneumothorax.** Thoracostomy tube placement.

6. **Large Pleural Effusion.** Consider thoracentesis.

7. **Acute Toxic Inhalation Injury.** Consider specific antidotes in certain circumstances (e.g., high-flow oxygen ± hyperbaric oxygen for carbon monoxide inhalation).

8. **Arrhythmias.** Treatment should be quickly initiated with appropriate antiarrhythmics or cardioversion in hemodynamically unstable patients with tachyarrhythmias (see Chapter 13).

IV. DISPOSITION

A. Discharge

Discharge from the ED should be considered under the following circumstances:

1. The cause of dyspnea is identified and symptoms rapidly improve with therapy in the ED (e.g., a patient with known asthma that improves to baseline with treatment in ED).

2. The vital signs, ABGs, chest roentgenogram, and ECG are normal or at patient's baseline, appropriate medical follow-up is arranged, and the patient is prescribed appropriate medication depending on the cause of the dyspnea.

3. The work-up in the ED is negative for any worrisome cause of dyspnea (i.e., *no* evidence for pneumonia, pneumothorax, CHF, myocardial infarction, or pulmonary embolism).

B. Admit

1. The clinically unstable patient or individual with a substantial change in their baseline level of dyspnea.

2. The patient exhibiting evidence of acute respiratory failure (represents a change in patient's baseline condition):
   a. $PaO_2 < 60$ mmHg while breathing room air.
   b. $PaCO_2 > 50$ mmHg.
   c. pH < 7.32.

3. The patient exhibiting evidence of significant respiratory distress or potential for significant respiratory compromise:
   a. Respiratory alkalosis, $PaCO_2 < 30$ mm/Hg, and/or (A–a) oxygen gradient > 30 mm/Hg.
   b. Inability to protect airway.

4. The patient suspected of having a myocardial infarction, pulmonary embolism, or arrhythmia.

5. The patient with pneumonia, CHF, COPD, or asthma exacerbation that cannot be adequately treated in the ED and would benefit from inpatient management.

6. Select patients following inhalation of certain toxic chemicals for observation for possible delayed reactions.

   Note: most patients presenting to the ED with dyspnea require hospitalization. Whether the patient should be admitted to the ICU, telemetry unit, or general medicine ward depends on the cause of the patient's dyspnea, the severity of symptoms, and the response to therapy in the ED.

V. PEARLS AND PITFALLS

A. Ensure adequate airway, oxygenation, ventilation, and hemodynamic stability for all patients presenting with dyspnea.

B. Remember the extensive differential diagnosis of dyspnea, and thoroughly investigate all possible causes of the patient's complaint.

C. Try to quantify degree of respiratory failure with ABG measurements, spirometry, or other objective parameters instead of relying solely on the patient's subjective descriptions.

D. Aggressively use inhaled beta-adrenergic agonists and anticholinergics in the ED in patients with dyspnea from COPD or asthma exacerbations.

E. Quickly identify patients with dyspnea due to left ventricular dysfunction and treat with supplemental oxygen, nitrates, and morphine sulfate. Patients with suspected myocardial infarction should be quickly evaluated for appropriateness of thrombolytic therapy.

Do not do any of the following:

A. Fail to obtain an ABG to determine a dyspneic patient's pH and pCO_2, even if the hemoglobin saturation is normal.

B. Withhold supplemental oxygen in a hypoxemic patient with respiratory distress, even if the patient has a respiratory acidosis. However, be prepared to treat ventilatory failure if it occurs.

C. Administer sedation to a severely dyspneic patient or a patient with respiratory acidosis.

D. Fail to recognize that a rising PCO_2 in a dyspneic patient who had been hyperventilating may signify fatigue and impending respiratory failure.

E. Discharge a patient from the ED unless the cause of the dyspnea is known, improvement to the baseline level of functioning has occurred, and adequate medical follow-up has been arranged.

BIBLIOGRAPHY

Mahler DA: Dyspnea: diagnosis and management. Clin Chest Med 1987;8(2):215-230.
Nisell O: Causes and mechanisms of breathlessness. Clin Physiol 1992;12(1):1-17.
Sweer L, Zwillich CW: Dyspnea in the patient with chronic obstructive pulmonary disease. Etiology and management. Clin Chest Med 1990;11(3):417-445.
Tobin MJ: Dyspnea. Pathophysiologic basis, clinical presentation, and management. Arch Intern Med 1990;150(8):1604-1613.

8

Dysuria

"Not again."
ANONYMOUS

I. ESSENTIAL FACTS

A. Definition

Painful urination, or *dysuria,* is sometimes characterized as internal (pain experienced at the urethral meatus) or external (pain experienced external to the urethral meatus). External dysuria is often the result of urine irritating inflamed skin, such as occurs with vaginitis.

B. Etiology

Painful urination results from disorders that cause inflammation or irritation in the urogenital tract. The differential diagnosis depends on the sex and age of the patient.

C. Differential Diagnosis

1. Women who present to the ED with the isolated complaint of dysuria will have a urinary tract infection (UTI), urethral syndrome (dysuria and frequency without evident pathology), or vaginitis. Vulvar trauma, atrophy, or infections can also cause dysuria when urine flows over the labia.

2. Men with dysuria will likely have urethritis, a UTI, or irritative symptoms from prostatic hypertrophy. Patients with prostatitis, epididymitis, orchitis, and early pyelonephritis may have prominent dysuria as well as regional symptoms.

3. In either sex, bladder diverticuli and interstitial cystitis are occasional causes of dysuria. Sterile urine containing irritative substances (excessive calcium or crystals) can sometimes cause painful urination. Foreign bodies, whether iatrogenic (catheters, cystoscopes), or patient placed, can cause dysuria with or without accompanying infection. At times dysuria from foreign bodies may not present until weeks to months after placement. Very rarely, bowel disorders, including appendicitis, diverticulitis, and Crohn's disease, may present as dysuria with bacteriuria.

D. Workup

The workup for dysuria should define whether the patient has uncomplicated cystitis, urethritis, or vaginitis, or a more complicated disorder. Upper UTI in men mandates a workup for structural abnormalities. Women who present for emergency care of vaginitis should generally be screened for a sexually transmitted disease.

II. CLINICAL EVALUATION

A. History

Details to elicit include the following:

1. Duration of symptoms. Frequent recurrence of symptoms suggests that the patient is being reinfected, usually by an untreated sexual partner. Otherwise, recurrence despite adequate treatment raises the likelihood that the patient has one of the more esoteric underlying causes of dysuria.

2. Accompanying *local* symptoms. Frequent voiding of small volumes of urine and hesitancy in starting the stream of urine are classic symptoms of cystitis and the urethral syndrome (the distinction is made by culture of the urine). Vaginal discharge may signify vaginitis. Penile discharge is diagnostic of

urethritis, but is not present in all patients. Hematuria can be seen in simple UTIs, but should also prompt consideration of nephrolithiasis and urinary tract tumors, especially in older patients. *Pneumaturia,* passage of air or gas with urination, is indicative of an enterovesical fistula (e.g., as a complication of Crohn's disease or diverticulitis).

3. Accompanying *regional* symptoms. Pain in the back, flank, or scrotum may reflect extention of disease into the kidneys, pelvis, prostate, or testes.

4. Accompanying *systemic* symptoms. Fever, chills, or severe malaise implies more extensive genitourinary tract disease or the presence of another disease process.

5. Sexual activity. Most men who are evaluated for dysuria in the ED will have a sexually transmitted disease (STD). Having multiple partners or contact with prostitutes increases the likelihood of STDs and should also prompt counseling and evaluation regarding human immunodeficiency virus exposure. Patients who are diagnosed with a STD should be advised to have their partners examined as well. Sexual abuse may explain otherwise confusing episodes of cystitis or vaginitis in young girls.

6. Accompanying medical conditions. Ask about:
   a. Pregnancy. It will affect choice of drugs used in treatment as well as threshold for treatment of bacteriuria.
   b. Intrinsic renal disease, especially if actual urinary obstruction is suspected, because obstruction may more quickly compromise damaged kidneys.
   c. Conditions in which immune function is compromised, including diabetes, acquired immunodeficiency syndrome, and chronic steroid use.
   d. Conditions in which there is a high likelihood of recurrent or chronic symptoms (e.g., neurogenic bladder with an indwelling Foley catheter).

B. Physical Examination

1. Fever, tachycardia, and hypotension should be noted, because any of these may reflect systemic or severe regional disease.

2. Costovertebral tenderness, if elicited with gentle pressure, likely represents pyelonephritis. This sign is often overinterpreted by inexperienced examiners because patients with minor musculoskeletal complaints will report bilateral discomfort.

3. In women, a pelvic examination should be performed unless a reliable patient gives a history unequivocal for an uncomplicated UTI.
   a. Look for vulvar erythema, and, in postmenopausal women, atrophic changes (shiny, pale mucosa with loss of rugae).
   b. Bartholin's gland abscesses present as painful swellings along the posterolateral aspect of the vaginal opening.

    c. On speculum examination, look for abnormal vaginal discharge and put samples of it on slides for wet preparation and KOH evaluation. Remember that the speculum examination in a patient with vaginitis may be quite painful.

    d. Simple cervicitis should not produce dysuria (consider taking endocervical samples for Gram stain and cultures for gonococci and chlamydiae). Cervical motion tenderness is a nonspecific indicator of pelvic peritoneal irritation; by itself it is not diagnostic of PID.

    e. Adnexal masses or tenderness should prompt pregnancy testing to assess the possibility of ectopic pregnancy.

4. In men, squeeze the urethral opening to look for discharge. If none is evident, milk the urethra by drawing your gloved hand along the shaft of the penis, exerting firm traction from the root to the glans. Any expressed exudate should be examined on Gram stain.

    a. Cultures for gonococci and chlamydiae are obtained using swabs made specifically for the male urethra. Because chlamydiae are intracellular organisms, cultures can only be positive if the urethra is scraped firmly enough to obtain cells lining the urethra. Warn the patient in advance that this will be mildly painful: Hold the penis in an erect position and insert a swab 2–3 cm into the urethra. Do this once for the gonococci culture and again for the Gram stain and chlamydiae culture. Obtain these specimens before the urine specimen.

    b. Examine the scrotal contents. Dysuria is almost never the sole or major complaint in patients who have epididymitis or orchitis, but untreated urethritis can result in either condition. Epididymitis causes tenderness and induration of the epididymis, the spaghetti-like tube that lies at the superior pole of the testicle. Orchitis causes exquisite tenderness of the testes, with or without associated edema. Note any testicular masses.

    c. Examine the prostate. A boggy or abnormally tender gland suggests prostatitis. In older men, prostatic hypertrophy may or may not be evident on examination, because the periurethral tissue that is most prone to enlargement is not directly palpable. In acute prostatitis the gland will be extremely tender and should not be firmly palpated, as vigorous palpation may cause bacteremia.

C. Urine Examination

1. Examination of the urine is necessary in the evaluation of dysuria. The patient should clean the genital area with antiseptic, and void the initial urine into the toilet. Midstream urine is then collected. The presence of squamous cells defines contamination and the presence of bacteria in a contaminated sample is not meaningful. A patient who is not able to collect the specimen appropriately should be in-and-out catheterized.

2. In men, it may be useful to collect the urine in three fractions (the "three-glass test"). The first 10 mL voided is from the urethra; the subsequent urine is from the bladder. The last few milliliters of urine excreted before the bladder is completely empty contain relatively high concentrations of prostatic fluid, which can be increased by prostatic massage after the second fraction is urinated.

3. Unspun urine is analyzed by dipstick. Urine should be examined promptly, because bacteria will multiply, the pH will rise, and cellular detail will be lost as the urine sits.
   a. Note the pH (very alkaline urine in the 8–9 range suggests infection with urea-splitting organisms such as *Proteus*). Occasionally, the presence of leukocyte esterase on dipstick evaluation may be the only evidence for pyuria, because leukocytes left to sit in hypotonic urine may lyse within an hour. If the urine is heme positive, examine microscopically for erythrocytes: heme-positive urine without erythrocytes on microscopic examination suggests myoglobinuria. Nitrite positivity correlates with the presence of bacteriuria. The combined presence of leukocyte esterase and nitrite positivity is > 90% sensitive and specific for UTI. Microscopic urinalysis will increase the yield of nonbacterial causes of dysuria.

4. Examine the urine microscopically.
   a. The presence of leukocytes suggests infection. A quick way to determine this is to examine *unspun* urine in a hemocytometer chamber. The presence of > 8 leukocytes/mm in women is empiric evidence for inflammation (and thus infection). Greater than 2 leukocytes/high-power field on a regular glass slide is also empiric evidence for infection. In clinical situations of uncomplicated UTI no further laboratory tests are indicated.
   b. If a fractionated specimen is collected from a male patient, pyuria in the first fraction only is diagnostic of urethritis; increased pyuria in the third fraction only supports prostatitis. In UTI or pyelonephritis, pyuria is seen in all three fractions. In practice there may be significant overlap in leukocyte content among the three specimens.
   c. The presence of bacteria is less important because a urine specimen may grow out abundant bacteria even if the Gram stain is negative. However, pyuria in the absence of bacteriuria (including a negative nitrite test by dipstick) should raise the index of suspicion for chlamydiae, viral causes, and acid-fast bacilla. Leukocyte casts are suggestive of pyelonephritis.
   d. Crystals precipitate when the urine is supersaturated with any of several substances, most commonly calcium, oxalate, struvite, and uric acid. The presence of occasional crystals on urinalysis is not abnormal. Do not confuse true urinary crystals with contaminating talc from latex gloves.

e. Parasites, usually trichomonads, are common. Young children may have *Enterobius* in their urine; schistosomes will sometimes cause dysuria in patients who have lived or traveled in the Middle East.

5. The decision to culture the urine is a clinical one. Most otherwise healthy women with only local symptoms can be treated empirically with good results. In patients with significant regional symptoms, or complicated UTI (see Chapter 15), who will need a longer course of therapy, a culture should generally be performed. Quantitative culture of the different fractions of urine obtained in the three-glass test can help diagnose male patients in borderline cases.

BIBLIOGRAPHY

Brumfitt, Hamilton-Miller: Urinary infection in the 1990's. Infection 1990;18 Suppl 2:S34-39.
Richardson DA: Dysuria and urinary tract infections. Obstet Gynecol Clin N Am 1990;17(4):881-888.
Sapira JD: The Art and Science of Bedside Diagnosis. Baltimore: Urban & Schwarzenberg, 1990.

9

Headache

"Lord, how my head aches! What a head have I!
It beats as it would fall into twenty pieces."

WILLIAM SHAKESPEARE

(Romeo and Juliet, II, v, 49)

I. ESSENTIAL FACTS

A. Epidemiology

1. Up to 10% of the general population seeks medical care annually for headache.

2. Approximately 1–2% of patients presenting to the ED indicate headache as their chief complaint.

3. The incidence of headache is inversely proportional to age.

B. Pathophysiology

1. Traditional teaching has held that migraine headaches result from dilation of intracranial vessels, and tension headaches are due to sustained contraction of the skeletal muscles of the head and neck.

2. Recent studies cast doubts on these theories and suggest a continuum between migraine and muscle tension. The common pathophysiologic mechanism involves a disturbance in serotonin-mediated central pain pathways.

3. While migraine and tension headaches may share similar diagnostic and therapeutic features, cluster headaches appear to have unique clinical features that warrant different evaluation and treatment.

II. CLINICAL EVALUATION (TABLES 9–1 AND 9–2)

A. *Certain clinical presentations suggest secondary headaches and should prompt further aggressive diagnostic investigation:*

1. Any headache occurring suddenly or for the first time in a patient over age 50.

2. A change in the character of a chronic or recurrent headache syndrome.

3. Any headache described by the patient as "the worst of my life," especially if associated with a stiff neck and/or focal neurologic signs.

4. Headaches associated with a change in personality.

5. Headaches associated with hypertension.

6. Headaches associated with fever, photophobia, and/or neck stiffness.

7. Any headache of increasing severity over days to weeks.

B. History

1. A careful history helps establish a therapeutic rapport and serves as the single most useful tool for arriving at a correct diagnosis. Inquire with respect to:
   a. Acuity of onset.
   b. Pain: location, character, severity, and duration.
   c. Prodromal symptoms: waving or jagged lines, flashing lights, autonomic symptoms, yawning, irritability, or depression.
   d. Associated symptoms: nausea, vomiting, rhinorrhea, tearing, photophobia, neck stiffness, fever, aphasia, or any focal neurologic deficit.
   e. Prior history of headache, including family history (although the absence of a family history does not exclude the diagnosis of migraine).
   f. Prior evaluation, including diagnostic studies and medication trials. Carefully note the maximal dose and duration of any medication previously tried.

2. The time course may be of value in distinguishing between various headache types (Fig. 9–1).

Table 9-1. EPIDEMIOLOGY AND PROFILE OF PRIMARY HEADACHES

	MIGRAINE WITHOUT AURA	MIGRAINE WITH AURA	CLUSTER HEADACHE (HORTON'S HISTAMINE CEPHALALGIA, MIGRAINOUS CRANIAL NEURALGIA)	TENSION HEADACHE (MUSCLE CONTRACTION HEADACHE, PSYCHOGENIC HEADACHE)
Epidemiology				
Male:female ratio	1:3	1:3	9:1	1:3
Onset	25% in childhood	25% in childhood	Onset in adult life (peak prevalence in 4th–6th decades)	
Familial associations				
Incidence	Strong	Strong	None	Weak
	Common	Less common than common migraine 1:7	Relatively unusual	Very common
Attack profile prodrome	Vague prodrome; may have autonomic symptoms, depression, irritability, yawning	Scotoma; semianesthesia, aphasia, or other neurologic symptoms	None	None
Duration	Builds over several hours; lasts hours to days	One hour to reach peak; lasts hours to days	Groups of attacks over days, weeks, or months; attacks last 30–90 min	Variable
Type of pain	Severe; may be confined to one side	Severe, often throbbing; may be confined to one side	Excruciating, sudden onset; steady or throbbing usually unilateral	Moderate, bilateral band of constriction or tightness, often occipital
Associated symptoms	Nausea, vomiting, chills, polyuria, nasal congestion, tearing	Nausea, vomiting, photophobia	Autonomic symptoms; bizarre behavior (perhaps due to excruciating pain)	Contraction of neck and scalp muscles sometimes present
Precipitants	Life stress (headache tends to occur at the ending of a stressful time); certain foods, drugs, menses; decreases during pregnancy	Life stress, pregnancy, certain foods, drugs, menses	During cluster attacks, may be precipitated by alcohol, nitroglycerine	Stress, fixed positions (such as typing)
Other	Tends to disappear or decrease in frequency in middle age	Tends to disappear or decrease in frequency in middle age	Leonine facies, cutaneous telangiectases common	

From Eisenberg and Capass: "Epidemiology and Profile of Primary Headaches," in Emergency Medical Therapy, 3rd ed. Philadelphia: W. B. Saunders, Table 10-5, p. 294.

111

Table 9–2. CLINICAL CHARACTERISTICS OF SECONDARY HEADACHES

	SUBARACHNOID HEMORRHAGE	MENINGITIS	TEMPORAL ARTERITIS	HYPERTENSIVE	TRIGEMINAL NEURALGIA
Onset	Acute	Acute or chronic	Acute or chronic	Acute or chronic	Acute and recurrent
Location	Global	Global	Localized	Occipital and/or frontal	Hemifacial
Associated symptoms	Nausea Vomiting Meningismus Focal neurologic deficit	Fever Nausea Vomiting Photophobia Meningismus Seizures	Temporal tenderness Jaw claudication Ipsilateral monocular visual loss Fever Myalgias Weight loss	Nausea Vomiting Focal neurologic deficits	Trigger points (e.g., while shaving, chewing, or brushing teeth)
Pain character	Usually (but not always) severe "Worst headache of my life"	Severe throbbing	Moderate or worse headache	Throbbing	Sharp, lancing
Duration	Brief	Usually brief	Prolonged	Brief	Recurring bursts and clusters
Prior history	(−)	(−)	(−)	(+)	(+)
Physical examination	Focal signs Decreased level of consciousness Meningismus Fundoscopic exam may be abnormal	Meningismus Decreased level of consciousness Fever Rash	Tender temporal, other cranial, or cervical arteries Fever Myalgias	Elevated blood pressure Abnormal fundi (e.g., papilledema) Decreased level of consciousness	Usually normal
Diagnosis	Lumbar puncture most sensitive diagnostic procedure; CT is 85–95% sensitive	Lumbar puncture	ESR usually ≥ 50 mm/hr in relevent clinical setting	Clinical picture; consider head CT to evaluate for other possibilities (e.g., intracranial hemorrhage)	Clinical picture; suspect multiple sclerosis if patient young (consider MRI in that setting)

3. Direct inquiries about anxiety or depression may reveal a primary psychiatric or psychosocial cause for the headaches. Some patients may be unable or unwilling to provide this information spontaneously.

C. Physical Examination

1. Perform a directed examination with specific attention to the head, neck, and throat.

2. A careful and complete neurologic examination is essential. Carefully evaluate the fundi.

3. Assess for signs of meningeal irritation.

D. Laboratory Studies

1. Routine studies will not usually establish the diagnosis in the majority of headache patients. Specific tests should be ordered as dictated by the clinical situation:
   a. A complete blood count (CBC) if infection or severe anemia is suspected.
   b. An erythrocyte sedimentation rate (ESR) should be considered in the evaluation of most patients older than age 50 with a new-onset headache. Initiation of steroid therapy for temporal arteritis should be considered if the ESR is $\geq$ 50 mm/hr. Temporal artery biopsy should be scheduled as soon as possible but should not delay treatment.

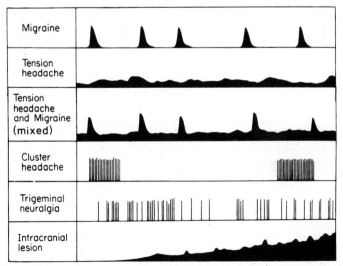

Figure 9–1. Temporal patterns of headache. (From Lance JW: Mechanism and Management of Headache, 4th ed. London, Butterworths, 1982.)

     c. Electrolytes, glucose, blood urea nitrogen (BUN), and creatinine levels should be obtained if an abnormality is suspected (e.g., secondary to vomiting).

     d. Pregnancy testing prior to administering ergotamine therapy should be considered in all women of reproductive age.

2. Lumbar puncture (LP) should be performed in any patient in whom meningitis or subarachnoid hemorrhage is suspected (even if an initial head computed tomography (CT) scan for the latter is negative). Head CT scanning should be done prior to the LP in any patient with focal neurologic deficits, with signs of elevated intracranial pressure, or known to be human immunodeficiency virus (HIV) positive.

3. CT should be considered emergently in any of the following clinical situations:

     a. Headache of abrupt onset described as the worst headache of the patient's life, or associated with depressed sensorium or focal neurologic deficits.

     b. Headache associated with fever, nuchal rigidity, and/or photophobia.

     c. Clinical suspicion of cerebellar hemorrhage or infarct (nausea, vomiting, ataxia).

     d. A significant change in the character of headaches in a patient with a chronic headache disorder.

     e. Headache in association with signs of increased intracranial pressure (papilledema, somnolence, vomiting).

     f. Head injury with an open or depressed skull fracture, a history of loss of consciousness, amnesia for event, and/or an abnormal Glasgow Coma Score.

     g. Headache associated with focal neurologic deficits (unless part of a stable complicated migraine syndrome) or recent personality change.

     h. Steadily progressing headache, especially if associated with headaches awakening the patient in the early morning.

III. HEADACHE CLASSIFICATION

A. Primary Headache Syndromes

1. "Migraine" Headache

     a. Migraine with aura
     b. Migraine without aura
     c. Atypical migraine
     d. Perimenstrual headache

2. "Tension or Muscle Contraction" Headache

     a. Tension, stress, or depression related
     b. Mixed tension and migraine

    c. Eyestrain
    d. Post-traumatic
    e. Cervical spine disease

3. Cluster Headache

B. Secondary Headaches

1. Underlying Vascular Disease

    a. Hypertension
    b. Ischemic stroke (especially embolic)
    c. Vascular dissection

2. Inflammation or Meningeal Irritation

    a. Secondary to sinus, ocular, or ear disease
    b. Intraparenchymal hemorrhage
    c. Subarachnoid hemorrhage
    d. Subdural or epidural hematoma
    e. Meningitis or encephalitis
    f. Mass lesion (tumor/abscess)
    g. Vasculitis (especially temporal arteritis)
    h. Pseudotumor cerebri
    i. Post–lumbar–puncture headache

3. Underlying Metabolic Causes

    a. Opioid and/or analgesic drug withdrawal
    b. Fever
    c. Hypoxia
    d. Hypoglycemia
    e. Drugs (including alcohol, nitrates, nitrites, hydralazine)
    f. Poisoning (including arsenic, benzene, carbon monoxide, carbon tetrachloride, carbon disulfide, and lead)
    g. Pheochromocytoma

4. Miscellaneous

    a. Glaucoma
    b. Temporomandibular joint disease
    c. Dental disease
    d. Exercise induced
    e. Coital

IV. THERAPY

A. General Measures

1. Be empathetic: the majority of patients with headaches are not seeking opioids. Often, reassurance that there is nothing wrong inside the patient's head will go a long way in relieving unspoken anxieties.

2. Provide a quiet, dimly lit environment with as little distraction as possible.

3. Education with respect to inciting factors (e.g., stress, lack of sleep, alcohol use, tyramine-containing food consumption) should be offered. A handout containing a list of foods associated with migraine and a referral number for tension/stress management training should be made available to every patient.

B. Migraine and Tension Headaches

1. Abortive Drug Therapy (Fig. 9–2; Tables 9–3 and 9–4)

a. *Standard analgesics* (e.g., *aspirin* or *acetaminophen*) are often effective for mild to moderate headaches, but usually have already been tried by the patient prior to ED arrival.

b. *Nonsteroidal anti-inflammatory drugs* (NSAIDs) are useful for both abortive and prophylactic therapy, but response may be idiosyncratic. If one medication is ineffective, a different class of NSAID should be tried.

   i. *Naproxen* and *naproxen sodium* have been extensively evaluated and are appropriate first choices.

   ii. *Indomethacin* appears uniquely effective for treatment of episodic and chronic paroxysmal hemicrania, ice-pick headaches, and benign orgasmic, exertional, or cough headaches.

   iii. *Ketorolac* is a parenteral NSAID that is generally as effective as morphine and meperidine in moderate to severe postoperative pain without the respiratory suppression and habituating problems of the opioids.

c. *Combination drugs* such as *Midrin* (acetaminophen, isometheptene [a mild vasoconstrictor], and dichloralphenazone [a mild sedative]) can be effective in patients with mild to moderate headache in whom ergotamines and NSAIDs are not tolerated.

d. *Ergot alkaloids* are extremely effective in the management of severe headache pain. When given within 1–2 hours of headache onset, effectiveness rates of 90% (intravenously), 80% (intramuscularly), and 50% (orally) have been achieved. Their use must be monitored, as dependency and rebound headache are not uncommon.

   i. Contraindications to the use of these agents include hypertension; peripheral vascular disease; ischemic heart disease; collagen vascular, renal, or hepatic disease; thrombophlebitis; pregnancy; or age > 60.

   ii. *Intravenous dihydroergotamine* (DHE) has become a standard therapy for treatment of severe or intractable primary headaches. Success rates of 70–90% have been achieved in several studies. Premedication with an antiemetic (e.g., prochlorperazine) is appropriate before administering intravenous DHE.

e. *Phenothiazines* are effective as primary therapy in treating both nausea and pain and as a premedication for ergotamine therapy. The hypotensive effect of these medications usually necessitates intravenous hydration, especially in individuals dehydrated because of vomiting.

f. *Sumatriptan succinate* is a selective agonist of the 5HT-1D receptor and acts by modulating serotonin-mediated central pain pathways.

   i. In several double-blinded trials, a single 6-mg subcutaneous dose has been shown to significantly reduce or eliminate headache in up to 90% of patients. Repeat doses were not effective in nonresponders.

   ii. Contraindications to sumatriptan include ischemic heart disease, Prinzmetal's angina, uncontrolled hypertension, known sumatriptan hypersensitivity, complicated migraines (i.e., hemiplegic or basilar artery migraines), pregnancy, and concurrent ergotamine derivative therapy.

   iii. There have been reports of myocardial infarction and severe arrhythmias in otherwise healthy patients, using sumatriptan.

g. *Corticosteroids* have been recommended for severe or refractory migraine. Most protocols recommend high-dose therapy followed by a rapid taper.

h. *Opioids* should be used only as a last resort. Many patients with severe daily "migraine" are actually experiencing analgesic and/or opioid-withdrawal headache. Consider using a long-acting preparation such as *methadone* (10 mg) or *butorphanol* (2 mg) so that the drug does not wear off before the headache ends. Meperidine is an appropriate choice for pregnant women with migraine.

i. *Calcium channel antagonists:* in patients with complicated migraine (in whom ergotamines are contraindicated), *nifedipine* (10 mg bite and swallow) may help abort the hemiparesis. Long-term therapy with *verapamil* may be helpful as a prophylactic treatment.

2. Preventive Therapy (Table 9–5)

Note: in most circumstances, preventive therapy should be prescribed by the referral physician.

a. Indications for daily prophylactic therapy include 3 or more days of disabling headaches per month, frequent headaches that cause excessive use of abortive medications, a suboptimal response to abortive medications, complicated migraines or migraines with prolonged auras, and concomitant medical conditions that preclude the use of abortive medications.

b. Each medication should be started at a low dose and gradually increased until a favorable response is achieved or side effects develop. Each medication should be given an adequate trial (1–2 months). Successful therapies should be tapered slowly after 3–6 months.

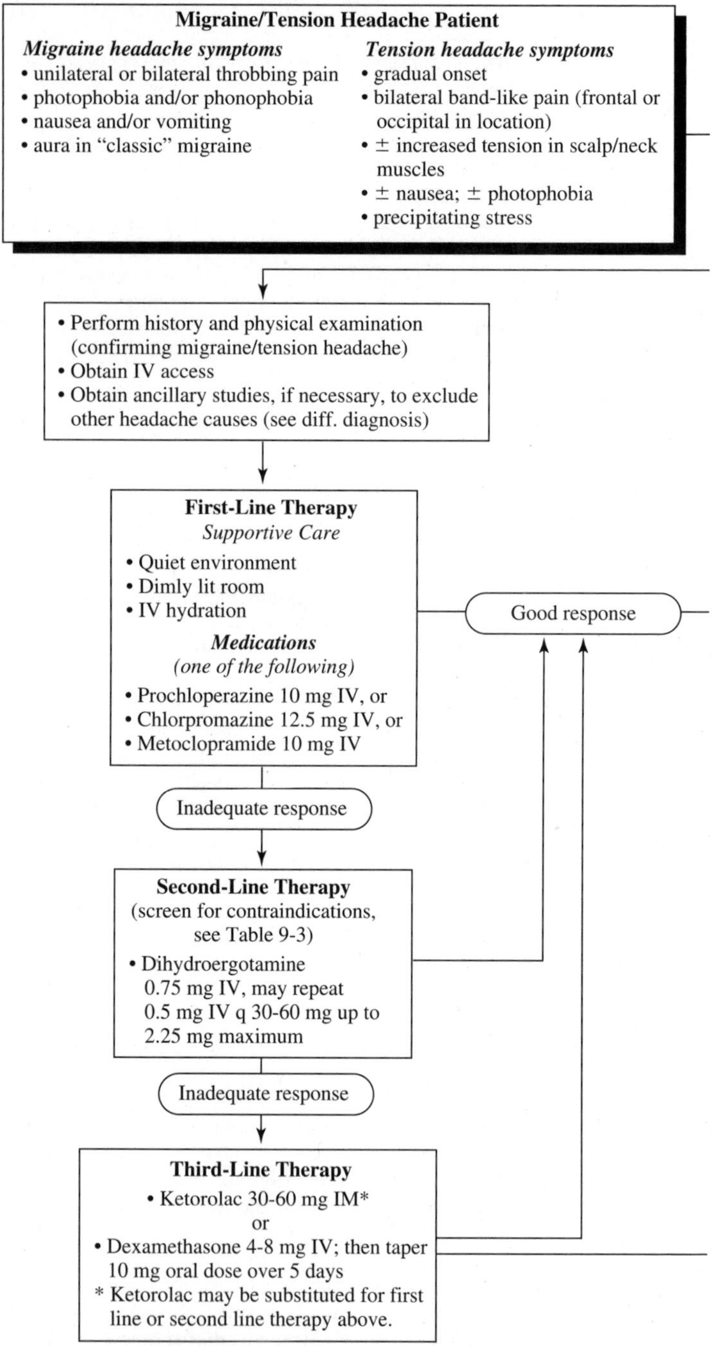

Figure 9–2. Emergency medical therapy of the moderate to severe migraine/ tension headache.

Consider Differential Diagnosis, including:

- Carbon monoxide or other toxin
- Cerebrovascular accident
- Dental, ear, eye, or sinus infection
- Epidural/subdural hematoma
- Encephalitis/meningitis
- Exercise-induced or coital headache
- Glaucoma
- Intracranial mass lesion
- Hypertension
- Hypoglycemia
- Hypoxia
- Subarachnoid hemorrhage
- Temporal arteritis (age ≥ 50 years)
- Temporal mandibular joint disease
- Vasculitis

Discharge patient from ED

- Patient should not drive themselves home.
- Arrange for followup with primary care physician.
- Consider naproxen (500 mg PO q 12 hr for 3-5 days) to prevent headache recurrence.
- Discuss diet/lifestyle adjustments to reduce headache triggers.

If patient still with poor response:

- Reconsider diagnosis
- Consider neurology consultation
- Admission appropriate for persistent severe pain, moderate to severe dehydration, severe nausea/vomiting, and/or needed drug detoxification

Figure 9–2. *Continued*

Table 9-3. PARENTERAL ABORTIVE THERAPY FOR MIGRAINE AND TENSION HEADACHES

Drug	Trade Name	Dose	Side Effects	Comments
Chlorpromazine	Thorazine	12.5 mg IV or 25 mg IM	Sedation, hypotension, extrapyramidal reactions	Do not give to the hypotensive patient
Dexamethasone	Decadron	4-8 mg IV	Dyspepsia, hyperglycemia; mental status changes in some elderly patients	Useful in severe refractory migraine
Dihydroergotamine	DHE	1 mg IV or IM; repeat every 60 min up to 3 mg IM or 2 mg IV; do not exceed 6 mg/week	Nausea and vomiting	Drug of choice for severe migraine; premedicate with an antiemetic 10 min before administration; contraindicated if coronary artery disease, peripheral vascular disease, hypertension, pregnancy, hepatic or renal failure
Ketorolac	Toradol	30-60 mg IM; subsequent doses of 15-30 mg IM q 6 hrs.	Dyspepsia, nausea, sweating, drowsiness	Use smaller doses in the elderly; useful drug to assist with pain in narcotic withdrawal
Metoclopramide	Reglan	10 mg IV	Extrapyramidal reactions; worsened Parkinson's disease	
Prochlorperazine	Compazine	5-10 mg IV	See chlorpromazine above	See chlorpromazine above
Sumatriptan	Imitrex	6 mg SQ once only	Angina, dizziness, nausea, vomiting	Expensive; repeat doses not helpful; contraindicated in patient with coronary artery disease, Prinzmetal's angina, hypertension, or while receiving concurrent ergotamine derivatives

Table 9–4. ORAL ABORTIVE THERAPY FOR MIGRAINE AND TENSION HEADACHES

Drug	Trade Name	Dose	Side Effects	Comments
Ergotamine (1 mg)/caffeine (100 mg)	Cafergot (oral)	1–2 capsules immediately, repeat q 30 min; max. dose 5/day or 10/week	Nausea, vomiting, angina, cramps, numbness	Contraindications include coronary artery disease, peripheral vascular disease, hypertension, pregnancy, hepatic or renal failure
Ergotamine (2 mg)/Caffeine (100 mg)	Cafergot (rectal)	1 suppository PR immediately; may repeat in 60 min if necessary; do not exceed 2 suppositories per attack or 5/week	See above	See above; PR route is useful if vomiting is prominent
Ergotamine (2 mg) for SL administration	Ergostat	1 tablet sublingual (SL) immediately; may repeat q 30 min if necessary; do not exceed 3/day or 5/week.	See above	See contraindications above
Isometheptene (65 mg) Dichloralphenazone (100 mg)/ Acetaminophen (325 mg)/	Midrin	2 capsules immediately; may repeat in 1 hr; do not exceed 5/day or 10/week	Dizziness	Contraindicated in patients with severe cardiac/hepatic/renal disease or glaucoma; useful drug, however, in patients intolerant of ergotamines
Naproxen or naproxen sodium	Naprosyn, Anaprox	500 mg PO q 8–12 hr; do not exceed 1500 mg/day	Constipation, heart burn, abdominal pain, dyspepsia	Useful drug in migraine headache prophylaxis as well

121

Table 9–5. PROPHYLACTIC HEADACHE THERAPIES

MIGRAINE AND/OR TENSION HEADACHES	DOSE (RANGE)	SIDE EFFECTS	CONTRAINDICATIONS	COMMENTS
Nonsteroidal Antiinflammatory Drugs				
Diflunisal	500 mg bid	Nausea	Active ulcer disease	Response may be idiosyncratic; excellent for menstrual migraines
Ibuprofen	400–2400 mg/day (in 3–4 divided doses)	Dyspepsia Constipation Dizziness Somnolence Tinnitus	Renal insufficiency	
Naproxen	500 mg bid–tid	Hepatotoxicity		Indomethacin is the drug of choice for chronic paroxysmal hemicrania, cough headache, orgasmic headache, and "ice-pick" headache
Indomethacin	25–200 mg/day (in 2–3 divided doses)	Nephrotoxicity		
Sulindac	150–200 mg bid			
Meclofenamate	100–400 mg/day (in 3–4 divided doses)			
Beta-Blockers				
Propranolol	40–320 mg/day	Drowsiness	Diabetes mellitus	Dose must be gradually increased to maximum recommended or tolerated dose before changing to an alternative medication
Nadolol	40–240 mg/day	Depression Memory disturbance Insomnia	Asthma COPD Congestive heart failure	

Drug	Dose	Side effects	Contraindications	Comments
Calcium Channel Blockers				
Verapamil	240–720 mg/day	Hypotension Atrial-ventricular block CHF Nausea	CHF Heartblock Sick sinus syndrome Hypotension	Beneficial effect may take 3–4 weeks to appear
Nifedipine	30–180 mg/day		Hypotension	
Tricyclic Antidepressants				
Amitriptyline	10–300 mg/day	Drowsiness Urinary retention Constipation Mania	Glaucoma Urinary retention	Headache relief is independent of antidepressant effect. Excellent first choice, start with low dose.
Nortriptyline	20–150 mg/day			
Fluoxetine	20–80 mg/day	Nausea Jitteriness	Concurrent use of MAO inhibitors	Fewer anticholinergic effects than the tricyclic agents above
Cyproheptadine	2–4 mg qid	Drowsiness Weight gain	Narrow-angle glaucoma Prostatic hypertrophy Advanced age	Antiserotoninergic; may be more efficacious in children and young adults
Methysergide	2–4 mg bid–tid (allow for a 4-week drug-free period at least every 6 months to minimize risks of fibrosis)	Nausea Cramps Weight gain	Pregnancy Peripheral vascular disease Cardiac valvular disease Coronary artery disease	Highly effective and serotoninergic; risk of retroperitoneal, endocardial, or pulmonary fibrosis (1/5000)

Table continued on following page

CHF, congestive heart failure; COPD, chronic obstructive pulmonary disease; MAO, monoamine oxidase

Table 9-5. PROPHYLACTIC HEADACHE THERAPIES *Continued*

Cluster Headaches	Dose (Range)	Side Effects	Contraindications	Comments
Cluster Headaches				
Verapamil	240–720 mg/day	As above	As above	Effect may take 1–5 weeks to appear
Lithium	300 mg bid–tid	Tremor Goiter Nausea Weight gain		Maintain level 0.6–1.2 mEq/mL; effect seen within 1–2 weeks
Ergotomine	1–2 mg daily (do NOT exceed 6 mg/24 hr or 10 mg/week)	See Table 9-4	See Table 9-4	Use qhs for nocturnal attacks

C. Cluster Headaches: Abortive Therapy
(Table 9–6)

1. *Oxygen* 6–8 L/min by simple face mask for 10–20 minutes is effective in aborting cluster headaches in approximately 70% of adults. The patient should sit with the head bent forward.

2. *Ergotamines* are second only to oxygen in efficacy for treatment of cluster headache. Unfortunately, subcutaneous absorption is erratic and suppositories are inconvenient.

3. *Dihydroergotamine* (DHE) is effective in most patients in ≤ 30 minutes. Relief is achieved faster with intravenous as opposed to intramuscular administration. Premedication with an anti-emetic is appropriate. Intranasal DHE may become available in the near future.

4. *Sumatriptan* has recently been shown to be effective and well-tolerated in a multicenter trial.

5. *Intranasal lidocaine* (1 mL of a 4% solution ipsilateral to the side of the pain) is effective in some patients. Premedication with *phenylephrine* 0.5% is helpful if nasal congestion is present.

6. All patients with cluster headaches should be strongly urged to quit smoking.

D. Status Migrainosis

1. This is defined as a severe persistent primary headache refractory to standard therapies for at least 48 hours.

2. Treatment usually requires hospitalization for rehydration and detoxification from opioids, ergotamine preparations, and/or analgesics.

3. Therapy should be administered in a controlled and consistent manner so as to allow adequate assessment of the response to individual interventions.
   a. *Intravenous DHE* is the initial drug of choice. Administer 1 mg IV q 8 hours for 72 hours. Premedication with prochlorperazine (10 mg IV) or metoclopramide (10 mg IV) 10–30 minutes prior to DHE may help reduce nausea.
   b. *Ketorolac* 60 mg IM followed by 30 mg IM q 8 hours is an appropriate second-line therapy.
   c. *Neuroleptics* (e.g., haloperidol, thiothixine, chlorpromazine, or prochlorperazine) should be considered. Care must be taken to avoid hypotension and extrapyramidal reactions.
   d. Corticosteroids are often useful when other therapies have failed. One protocol calls for *hydrocortisone* 100 mg IV q 6 hours for 24 hours, then q 8 hours for 24 hours, then q 12 hours for 24 hours. *Prednisone* (80 mg) or *dexamethasone* (10 mg) with a rapid taper over 3–5 days has also been recommended.

Table 9-6. ABORTIVE THERAPY FOR CLUSTER HEADACHES

THERAPY	TRADE NAME	DOSE	SIDE EFFECTS	COMMENTS
Oxygen		Close-fitting oxygen mask 8 L/min for 15–20 min; have patient bend head forward	Avoid high-flow oxygen in the COPD patient with CO_2 retention	Rebound headache may occur when oxygen is discontinued
Dexamethasone	Decadron	4–8 mg IV, IM, or PO	Dyspepsia, hyperglycemia; possible steroid-induced mental status changes in the elderly	Single dose may provide necessary relief for days
Dihydroergotamine	DHE	1 mg IM or IV; may repeat q 60 min; do not exceed 3 doses/day	Nausea, vomiting, angina, cramps, numbness	Contraindicated in patient with coronary artery disease, moderate or worse hypertension, peripheral vascular disease, pregnancy, hepatic or renal failure
Lidocaine (4% solution)		1 mL sprayed into nostril ipsilateral to pain	Minimal when dosed appropriately unless patient hypersensitive to drug	
Sumatriptan	Imitrex	6 mg SQ once only	Angina exacerbation, dizziness, nausea, vomiting, tingling	Repeat doses not effective; contraindicated in patients with known coronary artery disease or Prinzmetal's angina

COPD, chronic obstructive pulmonary disease.

V. DISPOSITION

A. Discharge

1. Patients with a benign headache that has responded to ED therapy may be considered for discharge. Their vital signs should be normal, they should be able to take liquids orally, and they should have a safe means of transportation from the ED if any sedating medications were administered.
2. Discharge instructions should include the following:
   a. Counseling and literature on awareness of lifestyle and dietary factors influencing headache occurrence.
   b. Arrangement for follow-up with a primary care provider.
   c. Encouragement of the use of a headache calendar to document headache occurrence, inciting factors, duration, and response to therapy.
   d. Information about support groups. A helpful resource for the headache patient is the National Headache Foundation. There is a small membership fee:

   National Headache Foundation
   5252 N. Western Avenue
   Chicago, IL 60625

B. Admission

Consider admission for further workup and/or therapy, the headache patient with any of the following:

1. A history or physical examination suggestive of a rapidly progressive symptomatic headache in whom a definitive diagnosis cannot be readily established.
2. Status migrainosis.
3. Evidence of habituation to opioids, ergotamines, or analgesics, in whom inpatient detoxification is required to prevent daily severe rebound headaches.
   a. Education, support, and long-term follow-up should be made available to these patients to prevent recurrence.
   b. Suggested therapies include IV hydration, DHE, phenothiazines, neuroleptics, clonidine (0.1 mg bid), or ketorolac (30 mg IM q 8 hours).

BIBLIOGRAPHY

Baumel B, Eisner LS: Diagnosis and treatment of headache in the elderly. Med Clin N Am 1991; 75: 661-675.

Diamond ML: Emergency department treatment of the headache patient. Headache Quart 1992; 3 (Suppl. 1): 28-33.

Headache Classification Committee of the International Headache Society: Classification and diagnostic criteria for headache disorders, cranial neuralgia and facial pain. Cephalgia 1988; 8 (Suppl.): 1–96.

Mathew NT: Cluster headache. Neurology 1992;42 (Suppl. 2): 22-31.

Silberstein SD (ed): Intractable headache: inpatient and outpatient treatment strategies. Neurology 1992;42 (Suppl. 2): 1-51.

The Subcutaneous Sumatriptan International Study Group: Treatment of migraine attacks with sumatriptan. N Engl J Med 1991; 325: 316-321.

10

Syncope

"Persons who have had frequent and severe attacks of swooning, without any manifest cause, die suddenly."

HIPPOCRATES

I. ESSENTIAL FACTS

A. Definition

Syncope is a sudden and temporary loss of consciousness. Inherent elements of the definition are (1) the patient is unable to maintain postural tone during the episode, (2) the patient regains consciousness spontaneously, and (3) the loss of consciousness was not due to either head trauma or a seizure. Syncope is a symptom whose proximate cause is usually cerebral hypoperfusion. This hypoperfusion may be secondary to a vast number of disorders (Table 10–1), some of which are potentially life-threatening.

B. Epidemiology

Syncope accounts for 3% of ED visits and 1% of hospital admissions. One-third of people will complain of at least one episode of syncope in their lifetime, and the prevalence of syncope increases with age.

C. Prognosis

The prognosis depends on the cause. When the cause is benign, the patient's mortality is the same as that of the general population. If syncope results from underlying cardiovascular disease (cardiac syncope), annual mortality is as high as 33%, with a 24% annual incidence of sudden death.

D. Difficulties in the Diagnosis of Syncope

1. It is a common complaint.
2. It may be caused by many different disorders.
3. A large array of expensive diagnostic tests may be used in an attempt at diagnosis.
4. Even with an aggressive and expensive workup, the etiology may still *not* be apparent in up to 50% of patients.

E. Goal of the ED Physician

The goal of the ED physician in the evaluation of the syncopal patient is to correctly identify and aggressively evaluate and admit

Table 10–1. CAUSES OF SYNCOPE

Vagal Causes

"Simple faint"
Carotid sinus hypersensitivity
Glossopharyngeal syncope
Micturition syncope
Swallow syncope
Postpain (trigeminal neuralgia) syncope

Cardiovascular Causes

Arrhythmias
  Sick-sinus syndrome
  Bradycardia
  Atrioventricular block (Mobitz type II or complete heart block)
  Pacemaker malfunction
  Supraventricular tachycardia
  Ventricular tachycardia
  Drug-induced arrhythmias
  Congenital prolonged QT-interval
Valvular heart disease
  Aortic stenosis
  Mitral stenosis
  Pulmonic stenosis
  Tricuspid stenosis
  Mitral valve prolapse
  Prosthetic valve thrombosis or malfunction
Cardiomyopathy
  Obstructive cardiomyopathy
  Restrictive cardiomyopathy
Ischemic heart disease
  Angina pectoris
  Myocardial infarction
Nonvalvular obstructive disease
  Atrial myxoma
  Pulmonary hypertension
  Pulmonary embolus
Other cardiovascular causes
  Aortic artery dissection
  Pericardial disease
  Anemia

Continued

those patients with a cardiovascular or other life-threatening cause of the patient's symptoms. The goal is not to correctly diagnose the cause of syncope in every patient.

II. CLINICAL EVALUATION

The most important component of the clinical evaluation is the history and physical examination; in cases in which a diagnosis of syncope is possible, a thorough history and physical examination usually provide the key to that diagnosis.

A. History

1. Inquire about the patient's activities minutes to hours prior to the episode, including general state of health, amount

Table 10–1. CAUSES OF SYNCOPE *Continued*

Orthostatic Hypotension

Drug-induced
Hypovolemia (including hemorrhage [e.g., gastrointestinal bleed, ectopic pregnancy])
Autonomic insufficiency
Adrenal insufficiency
Idiopathic

Metabolic Causes

Hypoxemia
Hypocapnia
Poisoning (e.g., carbon monoxide)
Other drug toxicity

Neurologic Causes

Posterior circulation transient ischemic attack
Migraine
Imminent stroke
Subclavian steal syndrome
Neurocirculatory asthenia
Multiple sclerosis
Hypertensive encephalopathy
Subarachnoid hemorrhage

Miscellaneous Causes

Hyperventilation
Hysteria
Allergic reaction

Unknown Cause

of sleep, last meal, alcohol or other drug use, and medication use.

2. Obtain a thorough description of the episode from the patient, family, and witnesses (if possible). Important aspects include
   a. Immediate preceding events (e.g., change in body position, fearful or painful stimuli, hyperventilation, coughing, micturition, swallowing, use of medication, exertion).
   b. Body habitus and movements during the unconscious episode. Was the patient upright or supine when syncope occurred? Were there any unusual or abnormal muscular movements? What was the patient's facial color? What was the breathing like? Did the patient strike any objects in the fall, bite the tongue, or lose bowel or bladder continence?
   c. Duration of unconsciousness.
   d. Return to consciousness (immediate or prolonged). True syncope is associated with a rapid and spontaneous return to baseline mental status in the supine patient.

3. Have similar episodes occurred before, and under what circumstances?

4. What other symptoms accompanied the loss of consciousness (e.g., facial pain, throat pain, chest pain, palpitations, headache, visual changes, nausea, dizziness, dyspnea, weakness, and/or paralysis)?

5. What other health problems does the patient have (e.g., coronary artery disease, valvular heart disease, cerebrovascular disease, known risk factors for pulmonary embolism, diabetes mellitus)?

6. Was the patient injured during the episode?

7. Obtain a thorough medication history, including over-the-counter medications. Antihypertensive medications, nitrates, and other drugs known to cause orthostatic hypotension are potential causes of syncope. Be especially alert to any recently started drugs or medications whose dosage has just been changed.

B. Physical Examination

1. **General.** Observe the patient closely. Is he/she awake, oriented, and acting appropriately? Postictal?

2. **Vital Signs.** Note tachycardia, tachypnea, blood pressure instability, and hypothermia or fever. Obtain postural vital signs if the patient's condition allows. Up to 30% of elderly patients, however, have postural vital sign changes "normally."

3. **Skin.** Note diaphoresis, cyanosis, and/or clamminess.

4. **HEENT.** Assess for trauma, including oral mucosa and tongue lacerations (e.g., sustained during seizure activity).

5. **Neck.** Assess jugular venous distention and carotid artery pulses, and auscultate for carotid bruits.

6. **Chest.** Listen for overall air movement, wheezes, rales, and/or rhonchi.

7. **Heart.** Note whether the patient is bradycardic or tachycardic. Palpate the precordium and then listen carefully to the heart sounds, searching for murmurs, rubs, and/or gallops.

8. **Pulses.** Palpate radial, femoral, dorsalis pedis, and posterior tibial pulses.

9. **Abdomen.** Look for distention, bowel sounds, masses, palpable aortic abnormalities, or findings of localized peritoneal irritation that suggest intra-abdominal pathology. Include a rectal examination and stool heme test if occult gastrointestinal bleeding is suspected.

10. **Extremities.** Assess peripheral edema and extremity perfusion.

11. **Neurologic Examination.** Carefully evaluate the patient's mental status, cranial nerve function (including a fundoscopic

evaluation), musculoskeletal system (range of motion, muscle bulk and tone, strength, and deep tendon reflexes), cerebellar function, and sensation.

C. Laboratory Studies

1. Routinely perform the following:
   a. Electrocardiography (ECG). (An electrocardiogram is mandatory in the syncopal patient ≥ 40 years old or the patient with *any* risk factors for cardiac disease.)
   b. Continuous cardiac rhythm monitoring while the patient is in the ED.

2. Additional studies are not routinely necessary. Specific tests should be ordered only as indicated by suggestive findings in the history and physical examination:
   a. Complete blood count: consider in the postural patient, patient with history of blood or volume loss, or patient clinically suspected of being anemic.
   b. Glucose level: mandatory in the diabetic or the alcoholic patient.
   c. Electrolyte levels: mandatory in the patient who is postural, has a history of volume loss, or who takes a diuretic. Electrolyte levels are also reasonable in the elderly patient or when alcohol or other drug abuse is suspected.
   d. Calcium, magnesium, phosphorus levels: should not be routinely ordered unless the history and physical examination reveal a concomitant medical condition likely to result in an abnormality in one of these (e.g., starvation, alcoholism, parenteral nutrition); or if, after a thorough history and physical examination, a seizure disorder is a likely possibility.
   e. Chest roentgenography: unlikely to be helpful unless the history and physical examination suggest a cardiopulmonary abnormality (e.g., pulmonary hypertension).
   f. Arterial blood gas (ABG) levels: unlikely to be helpful unless the history and physical examination suggest a cardiopulmonary abnormality (e.g., pulmonary embolus).
   g. Continuous (ambulatory) ECG is appropriate in the patient with syncope and known or suspected cardiac disease. It may be ordered by either the ED physician or the internal medicine or cardiology consultant. In many cases, the patient should initially be monitored in the hospital (see section IV, below). Outpatient (Holter) monitoring should then be done for 48–72 hours. Special devices are available for more prolonged monitoring.
   h. Echocardiography is usually ordered to further evaluate a cardiac abnormality suspected on the basis of history (e.g., exertional or postexertional syncope) or identified on physical examination (e.g., aortic stenosis). Other cardiac causes of syncope that may be silent on examination, but present on echocardiography, include asymmetric septal

hypertrophy, pericardial effusions, and atrial myxomas or thrombi.

i. Ventilation/perfusion lung scanning is appropriate when pulmonary embolism is a suspected cause of syncope on the basis of history, physical examination, and suggestive ABG levels.

j. Carotid sinus massage can be performed at the bedside in patients in whom carotid sinus hypersensitivity is suspected (e.g., syncope that occurs, usually in the older individual, with neck hyperextension or head turning). The patient must have both blood pressure and pulse continuously monitored, intravenous access established, atropine at the bedside, and *no* carotid bruits or history of cerebrovascular disease. There are two types of carotid hypersensitivity: (1) cardioinhibitory (ventricular asystole > 3 seconds with carotid massage), and (2) vasodepressor (≥ 50-mmHg drop in systolic blood pressure with carotid massage). Documenting carotid sinus hypersensitivity does not necessarily prove it is the cause of syncope. Important questions include the following: Did it reproduce the patient's symptoms? Was the clinical setting in which the syncope occurred compatible with a carotid sinus hypersensitivity mechanism?

3. None of the many and often expensive specialist studies, below, are routine or mandatory in the majority of patients presenting with syncope; one or more may be ordered by the referral or consultant physician, however, as clinical circumstances dictate.

a. Signal-averaged ECG is used to detect patient susceptibility to malignant ventricular arrhythmias. It evaluates the surface ECG for high-frequency, low-amplitude signals in the terminal portion of the QRS complex. These signals correlate with an increased risk of sustained ventricular arrhythmias.

b. Stress testing can provide evidence of stress induced heart block or other arrhythmias. It may also be useful in the occasional patient with syncope induced by severe ischemic heart disease.

c. Head-up tilt table testing has proven useful in demonstrating a vasovagal cause of syncope in patients who have eluded diagnosis. A special motorized tilt table with a footplate support is used to travel from 0° (supine) to 60° (reverse Trendelenburg) in 15 seconds. Electrocardiographic monitoring is performed continuously; blood pressure is measured every 5 minutes with an automatic sphygmomanometer. This head-up tilt is maintained for a maximum time of 45 minutes (or until syncope and bradycardia are reproduced in a shorter time period).

d. Electrophysiologic (EPS) testing is expensive and invasive. Its use is recommended in the patient with recurrent syncope, a negative noninvasive workup, and a suspected cardiac arrhythmia. It is uncertain, however, whether medical management of arrhythmias identified by EPS testing reduces subsequent mortality in syncopal patients.

  e. Cardiac catheterization may be pursued in the setting of a highly abnormal stress test or when echocardiography reveals significant aortic stenosis.

  f. Electroencephalography is reasonable when a seizure disorder is suspected as the cause of transient loss of consciousness.

  g. Computed tomography is a very low-yield procedure in the workup of syncope. It is reasonable in the patient who describes focal neurologic symptoms in association with syncope, or when the neurologic examination reveals focal abnormalities.

  h. Skull films and/or lumbar puncture are generally unhelpful in the workup of the syncope patient.

II. DIFFERENTIAL DIAGNOSIS

A. Syncope

1. Syncope is the most common cause of transient loss of consciousness (LOC).
2. Vasovagal mechanisms are the most common identified cause.
3. Syncope of cardiovascular origin has a significant mortality.

B. Other Causes of Temporary LOC

The patient who presents to the ED with a transient LOC may or may not have syncope. The many causes of temporary LOC are presented in Table 10–2.

1. Differentiating a Seizure from Syncope

  a. With both seizures and syncope, the patient may lose bladder control and may have myoclonic jerking. Convulsive movements in the setting of cerebral hypoperfusion (in the absence of an underlying seizure disorder) have been well described. Unusual muscular movements during the episode of unconsciousness do *not* necessarily mean the patient has suffered a seizure.

  b. The most reliable indication that a patient has had a true seizure rather than a syncopal episode is a delayed return of an alert mental status (i.e., a postictal state) or the occurrence of a Todd's paralysis. The syncopal patient may not feel well or normal immediately after the event, but should be alert with clear mentation.

  c. Additional indications that a seizure has occurred include brief aura (déjà vu, olfactory, gustatory, or visual) just prior to the event; preceding stimulus of monotonous music or blinking lights; occurrence of the event during sleep; cyanosis or stertorous breathing during the episode; and/or tongue-biting.

Table 10–2. CAUSES OF TRANSIENT LOSS OF CONSCIOUSNESS

Syncope (the most common category of transient loss of consciousness)

Seizures

  Generalized seizures
   Absence
   Myoclonic
   Clonic, tonic, and tonic–clonic
   Atonic
  Partial complex seizures
  Status epilepticus

Drug-Induced

  Alcoholic blackouts
  Sedatives
  Other

Metabolic–Hypoglycemia

Head Trauma

Other Central Nervous System

  Cerebral vascular insufficiency
  Subarachnoid hemorrhage
  Narcolepsy and other sleep disorders
  Brain tumors/metastasis

Hysterical–Psychogenic

---

d. Partial seizures, absence seizures, and atonic or akinetic seizures occur with little or no motor activity. Therefore, the absence of convulsive movements with the loss of consciousness does *not* exclude a seizure disorder.

2. Syncope versus Other Causes of LOC (Besides Seizures)

To assist in differentiating syncope from the other items listed in Table 10–2, the clinician must rely on historical information, a high index of suspicion, and the physical examination. Frequently it becomes crucial to obtain further data from family, friends, witnesses, and/or ambulance personnel. Always attempt to obtain information from witnesses or relatives before ordering diagnostic tests when evaluating a patient with transient LOC.

III. DIAGNOSTIC AND THERAPEUTIC APPROACH

A. Step 1: Assess, Secure, and Support the Airway, Breathing, and Circulation as Indicated (See Chapter 1.II)

Syncope may be the presenting symptom of a life-threatening disorder (e.g., cardiac arrhythmia, myocardial infarction, pulmonary embolus, aortic dissection, acute hemorrhage). The first step in patient management should be a primary survey and simultaneous resuscitation as required.

1. If there is any possibility of cervical spine injury, appropriately immobilize the patient. Administer supplemental oxygen, establish intravenous access, and monitor both cardiac rhythm and SaO_2.

2. Manage any symptomatic cardiac arrhythmia.

3. Control any identified source of hemorrhage or volume loss. Replace identified volume deficits with intravenous crystalloid.

4. Evaluate and treat any trauma sustained during the syncopal event.

B. Step 2: Complete a Careful History, Physical Examination, and Directed Laboratory Evaluation (Secondary Survey)

After immediate threats to life have been identified and their treatment initiated, the ED physician should undertake a thorough history and physical examination as outlined under section II, above.

1. Be precise: make certain at the outset that the patient had syncope. Was there actual loss of consciousness, postural tone, and spontaneous recovery of consciousness?

2. Keep the differential diagnosis of both transient loss of consciousness and syncope in mind while proceeding with the history and physical examination. Special emphasis should be placed on the cardiopulmonary and neurologic systems. Obtain postural vital signs in the stable patient.

3. Perform ECG and rhythm monitoring: this is the only routine diagnostic test.

C. Step 3: Treat Specific Identified Cause of Syncope

When a diagnosis of syncope is possible, the information obtained with the above simple steps will provide that diagnosis in the majority of patients. Definitive therapy of the patient depends on the identified cause of the symptom (see Table 10–1). Unfortunately, in as many as 50% of patients no cause will be identified.

D. Step 4: Make an Appropriate Disposition

See Disposition, below.

IV. DISPOSITION

Whether to discharge or admit the ED patient with syncope depends on the clinically suspected or identified cause of the symptom. If the cause of syncope remains unknown despite a meticulous history and physical examination, the patient should be risk stratified as outlined below:

A. Low-Risk Patients

Patients with *either* of the following characteristics may be discharged to home; appropriate follow-up is *recommended.*

1. Patients ≤ 30 years of age with no past history of syncope and no evidence of cardiac syncope.

2. Patients ≤ 70 years of age with vasovagal syncope.

B. Intermediate-Risk Patients

Patients with the following characteristics may also be discharged to home, but follow-up is *mandatory.* Further diagnostic testing should be individualized, but 48 hours of continuous ambulatory ECG monitoring is reasonable.

1. Patients with a prior history of cardiac disease but no current evidence of cardiac syncope.

2. Patients aged 30–70 years with no findings suggestive of cardiac syncope, but whose cause of syncope is otherwise undetermined.

3. Patients > 70 years old with clearly noncardiac syncope.

C. High-Risk Patients

Patients with syncope from a cardiac cause have an annual mortality as high as 33%. *Any* of the following characteristics is suspicious for cardiac syncope and *mandates hospital admission* to a monitored bed. Cardiology consultation is also appropriate.

1. Frequent episodes of syncope that occur with little or no warning.

2. Syncope that occurred while the patient was recumbent.

3. Syncope with concomitant cardiac symptoms (e.g., palpitations, chest pain, dyspnea).

4. Abnormal electrocardiogram.

5. Elderly patients whose syncope cannot be explained as clearly noncardiac.

V. "PEARLS AND PITFALLS"

A. Syncope is a symptom, not a disease. It has many potential causes, some of which are life-threatening.

B. The cause of syncope can not be determined in up to 50% of patients. When a cause is identified, however, a meticulously obtained history and physical examination are usually the key to the diagnosis. Further diagnostic testing, when necessary, should be guided by the history and physical examination.

C. Routinely obtain postural vital signs and perform ECG and rhythm monitoring on the syncopal patient.

D. Patients with suspected cardiac syncope should be admitted to a monitored bed.

E. Patients with noncardiac syncope who are discharged from the ED should have follow-up arranged.

BIBLIOGRAPHY

Branch WT Jr: Approach to syncope. J Gen Intern Med 1986; 1: 49–58.

Fitzpatrick A, Sutton R: Tilting towards a diagnosis in recurrent unexplained syncope. Lancet 1989; March 25: 658–660.

Kapoor WN: Evaluation and outcome of patients with syncope. Medicine 1990; May/June 69: 160–175.

Kapoor WN: Evaluation and management of the patient with syncope. JAMA 1992; 268(18): 2553–2560.

Manolis AS, Linzer M, Salem D, Estes NAM III. Syncope: Current diagnostic evaluation and management. Ann Intern Med 1990; 112: 850–863.

III

MEDICAL EMERGENCIES

11

Airway Management

*"Treatment is to be always directed
to the part which is mostly in trouble."*

CELSUS

I. GENERAL CONCEPTS

Airway management is of paramount importance in emergency medicine: it is the *A* of the *ABC*s of emergency patient care. Complete airway obstruction results in cardiac arrest in as little as 4 minutes, and profound hypoxia results in irreversible brain injury in only 3–5 minutes. Meticulous airway management is often the key to improving patient outcome. Conversely, inattention to the basics of airway management can have disastrous consequences.

A. Components of the Upper Airway

1. The *nose* and *mouth*.

2. The *pharynx* is the musculomembranous passage between the mouth and posterior nares and the larynx and esophagus. The pharynx is subdivided into the nasopharynx (the part of the pharynx above the soft palate), the oropharynx (the area between the soft palate and the larynx), and the hypopharynx (the area posterior to the larynx and superior to the beginning of the esophagus).

3. The *larynx* is the musculocartilaginous structure between the pharynx and the trachea. It guards the entrance to the trachea, and it is the organ of voice generation. The glottis is the vocal apparatus of the larynx. The narrowest portion of the adult airway is the glottic opening (at the level of the true vocal cords).

4. The *trachea* is the cartilaginous and membranous tube that descends inferiorly from the larynx and divides at the carina

into the right and left main bronchi. The narrowest portion of the pediatric airway is in the proximal trachea at the level of the cricoid ring. The adult trachea is 9–16 mm in diameter, and its length is 10–15 cm from the inferior aspect of the cricoid cartilage to the carina.

B. Symptoms and Signs of an Inadequate Airway

1. An *abnormal mental status* may be a consequence of hypoxia, carbon dioxide retention, or both. Conversely, altered mentation of any cause may result in the patient's inability to maintain or protect his/her own airway. The patient with altered mentation has a compromised airway until proven otherwise.

2. *Aphonia* is the loss of voice. It may occur because of inadequate airflow, severe vocal cord dysfunction, or complete airway obstruction.

3. *Apnea* is the cessation of breathing. It mandates immediate assisted ventilation on the patient's behalf.

4. A *cough* may be voluntary or reflexive secondary to stimulation of airway cough receptors. A barking cough suggests subglottic abnormalities; a harsh, brassy, or productive cough suggests tracheobronchial disease.

5. *Cyanosis* is a bluish discoloration of the skin and mucous membranes. Cyanosis is a late finding indicative of severe hypoxia. It requires at least 5 g/100 mL of desaturated hemoglobin. In the setting of poisoning, cyanosis occurs with 0.5 g/100 mL of sulfhemoglobin or 1.5 g/100 mL of methemoglobin. Aggressive and appropriate airway intervention and assisted ventilation should occur *before* the patient becomes cyanotic.

6. *Diaphoresis,* or abnormal sweating, may occur secondary to any stressful state, including hypoxia, hypercapnea, and/or respiratory acidosis. Beware of the diaphoretic ED patient!

7. The *inability to handle oral secretions (drooling)* in the setting of respiratory distress suggests impending upper-airway compromise.

8. A *gurgling* sound indicates foreign material or significant secretions in the upper airway.

9. *Hoarseness* indicates an abnormality of the larynx (e.g., from edema or unilateral vocal cord dysfunction).

10. The conscious patient in *respiratory distress* is anxious, agitated, dyspneic, frequently diaphoretic and tachycardic, and demonstrates increased respiratory efforts.

11. *Stridor* is a high-pitched, harsh respiratory sound usually occurring during inspiration. It is louder in the neck than over

the chest wall, and it indicates partial airway obstruction at the level of the larynx or trachea. Expiratory wheezing suggests obstruction at the level of the bronchi and smaller airways.

C. Causes of Upper-Airway Compromise

1. *Declining consciousness* of any cause will eventually compromise oropharyngeal muscle tone and allow the tongue to fall posteriorly, resulting in an impaired airway. The tongue is the leading cause of upper-airway obstruction in both the trauma and the nontrauma patient. In addition, the patient with altered mentation may lose normal airway protective mechanisms, predisposing to aspiration.

2. *Aspirated foreign bodies* can cause mechanical obstruction. Aspirated materials may also damage airway structures, with resulting laryngospasm or inflammation.

3. *Congenital abnormalities.*

4. *Soft-tissue swelling* of airway-related structures may result from an anaphylactic or anaphylactoid response, infection, inhalational injury, or trauma.

5. *Infectious causes* of upper-airway compromise include epiglottitis, laryngotracheobronchitis (croup), Ludwig's angina (a diffuse, purulent infection of the floor of the mouth), retropharyngeal abscess, and peritonsillar abscess.

6. *Neoplasms.*

7. *Trauma* may result in direct injury to the structures of the upper airway or secondarily cause airway compromise as a consequence of altered mentation, aspiration, hematoma formation, hemorrhage, foreign bodies (e.g., teeth), soft-tissue edema, or neurovascular injury.

8. *Vocal cord dysfunction.* Abnormalities that can result in airway compromise include laryngospasm (spasmodic closure of the larynx), neoplasms, and recurrent laryngeal nerve injury.

II. BASIC AIRWAY MANAGEMENT

A. Foreign-Body Airway Obstruction

1. The sudden onset of acute respiratory distress, especially while or immediately after eating, suggests foreign-body airway obstruction.

2. It is managed in the following manner:
   a. If the patient can cough and is able to maintain adequate air exchange, then only partial obstruction is present. Proceed as follows:
      i. Do not actively intervene in the patient's own efforts to dislodge the foreign body with forceful coughing.

    ii. Stay with the patient at all times!

    iii. Supply supplemental oxygen and provide reassurance and encouragement.

    iv. Be prepared for any clinical deterioration and have the following immediately available at the bedside: suction, necessary equipment for intubation and emergency cricothyrotomy, required monitoring devices, and cardiac arrest medications.

b. Further patient deterioration, as evidenced by declining air exchange, inability to cough, or complete absence of airflow, mandates urgent intervention. Proceed as follows:

    i. Provide sequential subdiaphragmatic abdominal thrusts (the Heimlich maneuver) in patients >1 year of age until successful or the patient loses consciousness:

- *In the standing patient:* stand behind the patient and wrap your arms around the patient's waist. Make a fist, thumb side toward the patient, half-way between the patient's navel and xiphoid process. Grasp your fist with the other hand and quickly and forcefully thrust inward and upward against the patient's abdomen.

- *In the supine patient:* kneel astride the patient, and place the heel of your hand halfway between the patient's navel and xiphoid process. Place your other hand on top of the first and make a forceful thrust inward and cephalad against the patient's abdomen.

- *In patients with advanced pregnancy or significant obesity:* perform chest thrusts instead of abdominal thrusts.

    ii. If the patient loses consciousness:

- Optimally position the patient's airway and attempt to ventilate (see below). If unable to ventilate, reposition the patient's airway and try again.

- If still unable to ventilate, repeat a series of abdominal thrusts.

- Attempt to visualize the foreign body in the open mouth. Perform a blind finger sweep (wrap your finger with gauze to prevent salivary slippage) in an attempt to dislodge any foreign body. *Caution:* do not perform blind finger sweeps in children or in a conscious patient.

- Attempt to ventilate again.

- If still unable to ventilate, perform direct laryngoscopy and use either suction or Magill forceps to remove the foreign body under direct visualization (many experienced emergency medicine providers prefer proceeding immediately to this step after abdominal thrusts and attempted and unsuccessful ventilation in the unconscious patient with foreign-body obstruction).

B. Airway Control: Proper Positioning

Regardless of the cause of airway compromise, proper opening of the airway is the crucial initial management step. Remember, the most common cause of airway obstruction in the unconscious patient is the tongue and/or epiglottis.

1. **Head Tilt-Chin Lift**

    a. This maneuver is recommended in the *nontrauma* patient.
    b. *Technique.* Place one hand on the supine patient's forehead and tilt the head backward sufficiently to open the airway. Simultaneously, place the fingers of your other hand under the patient's mandible and displace the chin forward. The jaw thrust (see II. B. 2, below) may also be added if the head tilt-chin lift is unsuccessful.

       Cautions: avoid excessive neck hyperextension or pressure with your fingers on the patient's soft tissues beneath the chin, as either may actually worsen airway obstruction. The head tilt maneuver should be avoided in the trauma patient with a suspected cervical spine injury. Patients with advanced rheumatoid arthritis, psoriatic arthritis, Reiter's syndrome, or ankylosing spondylitis may suffer from atlantoaxial subluxation and potential spinal cord injury with cervical hyperextension.

2. **Jaw Thrust**

    a. The head tilt component of the head tilt-chin lift should not be performed in patients with a suspected cervical spine injury. Under these circumstances, appropriately immobilize the spine. The airway should be opened with the chin lift alone (as described above) or the jaw thrust.
    b. *Technique.* Grasp the rami of the patient's mandible and lift the jaw anteriorly to open the airway. If the patient cannot be ventilated with an appropriately applied chin lift-jaw thrust, consider *cautiously* applying the minimal amount of head tilt necessary to open the airway and allow for ventilation.

C. Basic Airway Adjuncts

1. **Nasopharyngeal Airway.**

    This is an uncuffed tube made of soft rubber or plastic (Fig. 11–1). It provides a passage from the external naris to the oropharynx and helps prevent the tongue from occluding the airway. The nasopharyngeal airway is better tolerated than an oropharyngeal airway in the semiconscious patient, and it can be placed when insertion of the latter is difficult or impossible (e.g., actively seizing patient, trismus, mandibular trauma). The nasopharyngeal airway may also be used to facilitate placement of a nasogastric tube.

Oropharyngeal airway

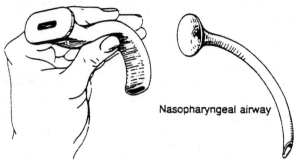

Nasopharyngeal airway

Figure 11–1. Nasopharyngeal and oropharyngeal airways. (From Clinton JE, Ruiz E: Emergency airway management procedures. Chapter 1. In Roberts JR, Hedges JR (eds): Clinical Procedures in Emergency Medicine. 2nd Ed. Philadelphia, WB Saunders, 1991, p. 5. [Courtesy of "From Clinton JE, Ruiz E: Trauma Life Support Manual, 1982."])

    a. **Airway Sizing.** Hold the tube by the side of the patient's face; the flange should be at the external naris and the tip at the tragus of the patient's ear.

    b. **Insertion Technique.** Lubricate the proper-sized airway with 2% lidocaine jelly. Preapplication of a topical vasoconstrictor (e.g., two or three sprays of 0.05% oxymetazoline [Afrin]) may shrink the nasal mucosal and decrease the risk of epistaxis. Gently insert the airway along the floor of the naris toward the nasopharynx until the external flange of the airway is at the nasal orifice. If resistance is encountered, slight rotation of the tube will assist insertion. Do not force the airway.

    Cautions: proper airway positioning (e.g., head tilt-chin lift in the nontrauma patient) must be maintained. A nasopharyngeal airway that is too long may precipitate vomiting and/or laryngospasm. An airway that is too short is ineffective. Nasal mucosal injury from forceful or careless airway insertion may result in significant hemorrhage. Nasopharyngeal airways should not be used in patients with mid-facial fractures (LeFort II or III) or suspected basilar skull fractures.

  2. **Oropharyngeal Airway.**

    This stiff, curved device holds the tongue away from the posterior pharyngeal wall (Fig. 11–1). Several types are available: the Guedel is tubular and the Berman is channeled along its sides. The oropharyngeal airway is appropriate only in unconscious patients.

    a. **Airway Sizing.** Hold the airway by the side of the patient's face; the flange should be at the central incisors and the tip at the angle of the jaw.

b. **Insertion Technique.** Suction the mouth and pharynx as necessary. Insert the airway upside-down (curved tip pointing cephalad) and rotate the device 180° during insertion until it is properly placed and the flange is just distal to the central incisors. Alternatively, this airway may be placed under direct visualization using a tongue depressor to hold the tongue to the floor of the mouth during insertion. If the patient resists airway insertion, the oropharyngeal airway is neither necessary nor appropriate.

Cautions: proper airway positioning (e.g., head tilt-chin lift in the nontrauma patient) must be maintained. If the oropharyngeal airway is too long it may depress the epiglottis and completely occlude the airway. An airway that is too short is ineffective. The oropharyngeal airway should only be used in unconscious patients or vomiting and/or laryngospasm may result. Improper placement may posteriorly displace the tongue and actually worsen airway obstruction.

c. An oropharyngeal airway that is well tolerated by the unconscious patient indicates complete absence of airway protective reflexes and the need for subsequent endotracheal intubation.

D. Rescue Breathing

1. After opening the airway, carefully assess the patient's breathing by *looking* for chest wall expansion with respiration, *listening* for air movement, and *feeling* for the patient's exhaled breath against the examiner's cheek.

2. If the patient is breathing *adequately:*
   a. Supply supplemental oxygen.
   b. Continue to protect the airway.
   c. Proceed with the primary survey (see Chapter 1. II).

3. If the patient's respiratory efforts are *inadequate,* or *if frank apnea is present:*
   a. Provide assisted positive-pressure ventilation.
      i. The technique used depends on the situation, but may include mouth-to-mouth (with barrier protection), mouth-to-mask, or the bag-valve-mask device (which includes a self-inflating bag, a nonrebreathing valve, an oxygen reservoir, and a face mask). In the ED, the bag-valve-mask unit attached to high-flow oxygen (≥ 15 L/min) is used most commonly. Optimal use of the bag-valve-mask device requires two individuals: one to squeeze the bag to provide adequate tidal volumes and the other to manage the airway and hold the mask to the patient's face.
      ii. If the patient wears dentures and they are loose, remove them. If the dentures are snug, leave them in place to help support the mouth, which makes it easier to obtain a good orofacial seal while ventilating the patient.

      iii. Ventilate the adult at a respiratory rate of 12–20 breaths/min and a tidal volume of 10–15 mL/kg; allow for complete exhalation between delivered breaths. During ventilation, the patient's chest should rise and fall and adequate bilateral breath sounds should be auscultated.

  b. Have suction at the bedside and prepare all necessary equipment for more definitive airway management with intubation. Consider the Trendelenburg position to minimize the risks of aspiration.

  c. In the setting of a cardiorespiratory arrest:

      i. Confirm patient unresponsiveness.

      ii. Immediately activate a "code" response, including a call for a cardioverter-defibrillator and additional bedside help.

      iii. Establish an airway (e.g., with the head tilt-chin lift maneuver in the nontrauma patient).

      iv. Assess breathing (remember: look, listen, and feel, as outlined under II. D. 1, above). If the patient is apneic, deliver two slow full breaths (e.g., with a bag-valve-mask device attached to high-flow oxygen). Allow for adequate exhalation between breaths.

      v. Assess circulation by palpating for a carotid pulse. If the patient is pulseless, initiate cardiopulmonary resuscitation (CPR). In the adult, the chest compression rate should be 80–100/minute, and the sternum should be compressed by 1.5–2 inches with each compression. After every five chest compressions, pause for 1–1.5 seconds to allow a second rescuer to deliver a ventilatory breath.

      vi. Upon arrival of the cardioverter-defibrillator at the patient's bedside, *immediately* determine the patient's cardiac rhythm and manage as indicated (see Chapter 13, part 1).

      vii. Orotracheal intubation is appropriate in the cardiac-arrest patient, unless immediate return of a perfusing rhythm and consciousness occurs with initial arrhythmia management.

E. Oxygen Administration

1. All seriously ill or multiply injured patients should receive supplemental oxygen.

2. The types of oxygen delivery systems, along with their advantages and disadvantages, are presented in Table 11–1.

3. Maximal oxygen may be administered with any of the following:

  a. *Nonrebreather reservoir mask* (oxygen flow rate > 12 L/min) in the spontaneously breathing patient.

Table 11–1. OXYGEN DELIVERY SYSTEMS[a]

SYSTEM	ADVANTAGES	DISADVANTAGES	COMMENTS
Nasal cannula (prongs)	Simple; fairly comfortable; can be used during airway care, eating, and drinking	Limited Fio_2 capability; exact Fio_2 quite variable (dependent on inspiratory flow rate and minute ventilation); may dry or irritate mucous membranes	Each liter/minute raises Fio_2 about 3%; humidify if flow rate > 4 L/min (for two prongs), a water-soluble lubricant may help avoid mucous membrane irritation
Simple oxygen mask	Provides higher Fio_2 than nasal cannula	Uncomfortable and must be removed when eating, drinking, and expectorating; Fio_2 is variable, dependent on inspiratory flow and minute ventilation	Fio_2 of about 35% at 6 L/min flow; Fio_2 about 55% at 10 L/min flow; because of CO_2 entrapment, dead space may be increased (with increased work of breathing)
Nonrebreather reservoir mask (the reservoir is attached to the base of the mask, but a one-way valve prevents rebreathing of expired gas)	Provides highest Fio_2 short of intubation (approximately 90–95%)	See "Simple oxygen mask," above	The reservoir *must* remain filled; because of high Fio_2, absorption atelectasis and oxygen toxicity may occur; if reservoir bag collapse occurs, oxygen delivery will be insufficient to maintain adequate ventilation
Continuous positive airway pressure (CPAP) mask	Increases pulmonary volume, opens previously closed alveoli (reducing shunt); may improve V/Q mismatch	Uncomfortable; risk of aspiration if patient vomits	May improve PaO_2 in intrapulmonary arterialvenous shunt for given Fio_2
Jet-mixing "Venturi" mask	Provides more exact Fio_2 than other methods described above	Uncomfortable; must be removed when eating, drinking, and so forth	Most accurate Fio_2 at 24% (flow of 4 L/min) and 28% (flow of 6 L/min); other Fio_2's available (31%, 35%, 40%, and 50%) are less accurate
Open face tent	May be better tolerated in some patients than nasal cannula or face masks; communication and expectoration not impeded	Fio_2 varies with flow rate and minute ventilation; eating impaired	May be able to provide Fio_2 as high as 70%

Table continued on following page

Table 11–1. OXYGEN DELIVERY SYSTEMS[a] *Continued*

SYSTEM	ADVANTAGES	DISADVANTAGES	COMMENTS
T tube	Exact Fio$_2$ possible up to 100%; humidification excellent	Requires endotracheal tube or tracheostomy	Maintain flow rate at least two times minute ventilation; humidification is mandatory because upper airway has been bypassed

[a]Medical gases do not contain water vapor. Humidification is appropriate at flow rates greater than 4 L/min. Humidification options include pass-over type, bubble, jet, and heated units. The last-named is the most efficient.

From Mengert T, Albert R: In Ramsey P, Larson E (eds): Medical Therapeutics. 2nd Ed. Philadelphia, WB Saunders, 1993, pp. 246–247.

    b. *Bag-valve-mask device* (oxygen flow rate ≥ 15 L/min) in the patient requiring assisted ventilation.

    c. *Patient intubation and ventilation* via a bag-valve device (oxygen flow rate ≥ 15 L/min) or ventilation via a mechanical ventilator with an FiO$_2$ of 100%.

F. Patient Monitoring

1. Continuous *electrocardiographic* and *pulse oximetry monitoring* should be routine in all seriously or critically ill individuals (remember the concept: oxygen–IV–monitor is "one word").

    a. Optimal airway management with oxygen supplementation should maintain the patient's SaO$_2$ at ≥ 95% (*Caution:* in the patient with known chronic obstructive pulmonary disease (COPD) who may be at risk for carbon dioxide retention with high-flow oxygen, an hemoglobin saturation (SaO$_2$) of 90% is appropriate).

    b. The pulse oximeter determines the concentration of oxyhemoglobin in the blood by means of a spectrophotometer that measures the absorbance of light due to oxyhemoglobin. Oximetry may provide inaccurate readings in the setting of poor tissue perfusion, other skin or blood pigments (e.g., jaundice), carboxyhemoglobin > 3%, or an abnormal hemoglobin level.

2. An *arterial blood gas level* is appropriate in all seriously ill patients and in those individuals suspected of having a significant carbon dioxide, pH, and/or oxygen abnormality.

III. PREHOSPITAL AIRWAY DEVICES

The ED physician may encounter a patient whose airway has been managed in the field using other devices in communities where prehospital personnel are not allowed to perform endotracheal intubation.

A. Esophageal Airways

1. The esophageal obturator airway (EOA) is a large-bore tube connected to a clear plastic oronasal mask proximally; the tube ends in a closed rounded tip with an inflatable cuff (Fig. 11–2). Multiple fenestrations along the sides of the tube allow for ventilation of the hypopharynx and unoccluded trachea when the cuffed end of the EOA occludes the esophagus (below the level of the carina). The theoretical advantage of the EOA is that placement does not require laryngeal visualization by prehospital personnel. The EOA should be used only as a *temporary* device in unconscious, apneic patients who are > 16 years old. The EOA should not be used in patients with known esophageal disease or after caustic ingestions. Inadvertent placement of the blind cuff in the trachea is fatal unless recognized immediately.

2. Other esophageal airway devices include the esophageal gastric tube airway (EGTA), the tracheoesophageal airway, the pharyngotracheal lumen airway (PTL), and the esophageal tracheal combitube (ETC).

B. Additional Comments

1. Use of the devices above in the prehospital setting remains controversial.

2. Regardless of the particular device, it is critical to rapidly assess the patient for correct placement and adequate ventilation. The patient's chest should rise and fall and good breath sounds should be auscultated bilaterally with assisted ventilation.

3. Prior to removing one of these devices in the ED, it is absolutely essential to protect the patient's airway against an aspiration event. Endotracheal intubation and gastric decompression should take place prior to airway removal whenever possible:
    a. In the unconscious patient with an EOA in place, intubate the trachea with a cuffed endotracheal tube prior to removing the EOA.
    b. In the patient who has regained consciousness and adequate spontaneous ventilations en route to the hospital, evaluate the airway protective reflexes. If these are absent, proceed with rapid-sequence intubation before removing the EOA. If airway reflexes are present, place the patient in the Trendelenburg position, turn him/her onto the left side, have suction on and at the bedside, deflate the EOA cuff, and quickly remove the tube.

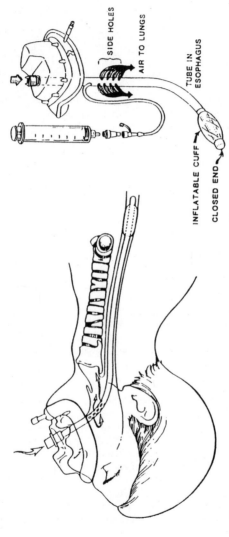

Figure 11–2. The esophageal obturator airway and its correct placement in the patient. (From Clinton JE, Ruiz E: Emergency airway management procedures. Chapter 1. In Roberts JR, Hedges JR (eds): Clinical Procedures in Emergency Medicine. 2nd Ed. Philadelphia, WB Saunders, 1991, p. 7. [Courtesy of "From Clinton JE, Ruiz E: Trauma Life Support Manual. 1982" and "From Jacobs LM: The importance of airway management in trauma. J Natl Med Assoc 80:873, 1988."])

IV. ADVANCED AIRWAY MANAGEMENT

A. Endotracheal Intubation: General Concepts

Endotracheal intubation is the placement of a tube, via the nose or the mouth, into the trachea. Endotracheal intubation isolates the airway, keeps it patent, and allows for the optimal delivery of a selected tidal volume (10–15 mL/kg) to the patient. Its many advantages include airway protection with decreased risk of aspiration, facilitated tracheal suctioning, and optimal delivery of high oxygen concentrations to the lungs. The endotracheal route may also be used to administer the following drugs when intravenous access is unavailable: *n*aloxone, *a*tropine, *v*alium, *e*pinephrine, and *l*idocaine (note the mneumonic "navel").

1. **Indications for Intubation**

    a. Apnea.
    b. Inability to clear significant pulmonary secretions.
    c. Inability to maintain $PaO_2 \geq 55$ mmHg despite an $FiO_2 > 0.5$–0.6.
    d. Loss of airway protective mechanisms or an inadequate upper airway.
    e. Major chest-wall trauma.
    f. Profound shock.
    g. Progressive hypoventilation and worsening respiratory acidosis despite aggressive medical management ($PaCO_2 > 50$ mmHg with arterial pH < 7.3).
    h. When controlled hyperventilation is required (e.g., in the setting of increased intracranial pressure).
    i. When heavy sedation or paralysis of the patient is necessary for diagnosis or treatment.
    j. When respiratory failure is imminent (e.g., respiratory muscle fatigue or exhaustion, respiratory rate < 10 or > 30–40/min in the adult, or inspiratory pressure < 25 cmH$_2$O).

2. **Intubation Route**

    a. **Orotracheal Intubation.** This is the most common, technically easier, and generally preferred intubation route for the emergency patient. It also allows for placement of a larger-diameter tube than with nasotracheal intubation. Relative contraindications include epiglottitis, suspected atlantoaxial instability (e.g., in the setting of advanced rheumatoid arthritis or ankylosing spondylitis), major maxillofacial trauma, significant supraglottic bleeding, and potential cervical spine injury.
    b. **Nasotracheal Intubation.** This is technically more difficult than orotracheal intubation, generally necessitates a smaller-diameter endotracheal tube, and should not be used in the apneic patient (except when intubation is fiberoptically guided). Its advantages include the following: the tube

is more easily stabilized and cared for, and is better tolerated by the awake patient; intubation is possible in the sitting patient; it can be performed when access to the oral cavity is not possible (e.g., because of trismus or distorted anatomy), and intubation may be accomplished using only local anesthetic agents, obviating the need for excessive sedation and paralysis in the patient with marked respiratory distress. Nasotracheal intubation has been traditionally considered the intubation route of choice in the nonapneic trauma patient with a suspected cervical spine injury. It is contraindicated in patients with apnea, coagulopathies, severe nasal or midface trauma (including LeForte II or III fractures), nasal or nasopharyngeal obstruction, foreign-body airway obstruction, suspected basilar skull fractures, or closed head injury with suspected or potential increased intracranial pressure. Whether these are absolute or relative contraindications depends on the specific clinical situation and the skills of the intubator.

c. **The Trauma Patient: Nasal versus Oral Intubation.** This area is controversial. As mentioned above, nasotracheal intubation has traditionally been recommended in the nonapneic trauma patient with suspected cervical spine injury, but much recent literature has questioned this recommendation. Oral intubation is possible in the trauma patient *without* cervical spine compromise provided *all* of the following precautions are carefully adhered to:

   i. Intubation under direct laryngoscopy is performed in a careful, controlled, and atraumatic manner.

   ii. The cervical spine is meticulously immobilized manually by an assistant throughout the procedure.

   iii. Rapid-sequence intubation techniques are used, including appropriate neuromuscular blockade (see IV. B, below, and Table 11–2).

   iv. If the attempt at orotracheal intubation is unsuccessful, a surgical airway (e.g., cricothyrotomy) should be rapidly obtained.

3. **Intubation Equipment.** The following equipment should be immediately available for emergent intubations:

   a. Bag-valve-mask device attached to supplemental oxygen (≥ 15 L/min).

   b. Colorimetric end-tidal carbon dioxide detector. This device changes color on exposure to exhaled carbon dioxide, and it is useful in the assessment of endotracheal tube placement. Lack of color change with ventilation immediately after intubation generally indicates esophageal intubation. Under some circumstances (e.g., cardiac arrest with poor pulmonary blood flow or massive pulmonary embolus) color change may not occur even with correct placement of the endotracheal tube.

Table 11–2. RAPID-SEQUENCE INTUBATION

Step 1: Preoxygenate the patient with 100% oxygen. ⎤
Step 2: Prepare equipment.   ⎦ Perform simultaneously

Step 3: Administer adjunctive medications as indicated.
For example:
- Defasciculation with minidose **succinylcholine, vecuronium,** or **pancuronium** (defasciculation is necessary only if succinylcholine will be used for neuromuscular blockade in Step 5, below).
- Vagolysis with **atropine**
- Blunt the intracranial hypertensive response with **lidocaine.**
See text for indications and dosing. These medications should be given approximately *3 minutes* prior to neuromuscular blockade.

Step 4: Establish anesthesia.
Administer one of the following:
- Thiopental
- Methohexital
- Minidose thiopental
- Fentanyl with midazolam
- Ketamine with midazolam
See text for indications and Table 11–3 for dosing. Cricoid pressure should be applied simultaneously with administration of the above.

Step 5: Establish neuromuscular blockade.
Administer one of the following:
- Succinylcholine
- Vecuronium
- Pancuronium
See Table 11–4 for dosing.

Step 6: Intubate the patient.

Step 7: Immediately confirm correct tube placement.
Cricoid pressure should not be discontinued until the endotracheal tube is properly placed and the cuff on the tube inflated.

---

   c. Endotracheal tubes in the appropriate sizes. Usual sizes for women age 7.0–8.0 mm internal diameter, and usual sizes for men are 7.5–8.5 mm internal diameter. A 7.5-mm tube is reasonable in either sex in an emergency. A water-soluble lubricant should be used to lubricate the distal portion of the tube prior to intubation. A 10-mL syringe should be available to inflate the cuff on the endotracheal tube immediately after successful intubation (uncuffed tubes are used in children < 6 years old).

   d. Flexible stylet. The stylet is used to shape the endotracheal tube as desired to assist with its insertion. Lubrication of the stylet with a water-soluble lubricant aids in stylet removal after intubation. *Caution:* the end of the stylet must be recessed at least ½ inch from the distal end of the endotracheal tube.

   e. Intubation drugs in syringes (see IV. B, below, and Tables 11–3 and 11–4).

   f. Laryngoscope with several blades. Blades come in different sizes and are of two common types: curved blade (MacIntosh) and straight blade (Miller). When a curved blade is

Table 11–3. ANESTHETIC MEDICATIONS USED IN RAPID-SEQUENCE INTUBATION

Drug	Dose	Onset & Duration	Comments
Thiopental (short-acting barbiturate)	3–5 mg/kg IV, no faster than 2 mg/kg/min (use 0.5–1 mg/kg IV if patient hypotensive)	*Onset:* within 1 min *Duration:* 5–10 min	*Advantages:* rapid onset, short duration of action, high potency; decreases intracranial pressure. *Disadvantages:* vasomotor and myocardial depression may result in significant hypotension, especially in the hypovolemic patient. May exacerbate bronchospasm.
Methohexital (short-acting barbiturate)	1–2 mg/kg IV over 30–60 sec	*Onset:* within 1 min *Duration:* 4–6 min	See thiopental, above.
Fentanyl (short-acting, potent, synthetic opioid)	3–5 µg/kg IV, at a rate of 1–2 µg/kg/min	*Onset:* within 2 min *Duration:* 30–40 min	*Advantages:* reversible and unlikely to cause hypotension. Does not cause histamine release. May be used to establish effective analgesia in awake patients. *Disadvantages:* may cause respiratory depression. Dosage must be titrated. May require concomitant administration of midazolam to achieve adequate relaxation for intubation purposes. Muscular rigidity may occur with rapid infusion of large doses.
Midazolam (short-acting benzodiazepine)	0.02–0.04 mg/kg IV in 1 mg boluses, no faster than 2.5 mg every 2 min	*Onset:* 1–2 min *Duration:* emergence within 15–20 min	*Advantages:* relatively rapid onset, short duration, and reversible. Good muscle relaxation and event amnesia. *Disadvantages:* dosage must be titrated. Mild hypotension may occur, especially in hypovolemic patients. Optimal use frequently necessitates concomitant **fentanyl** administration.
Ketamine (dissociative anesthetic)	1–2 mg/kg IV over 1 min	*Onset:* anesthesia within 1 min *Duration:* approximately 15 min	*Advantages:* produces good analgesia with increased cardiac output, blood pressure, and bronchodilation. Does not produce respiratory depression. *Disadvantages:* postanesthesia emergence reactions may be problematic in adults and necessitate concomitant benzodiazepine administration. Increases intragastric, intraocular, and intracranial pressures. Increases myocardial oxygen consumption. Does not relax skeletal muscles.

Table 11–4. NEUROMUSCULAR BLOCKING AGENTS USED IN RAPID-SEQUENCE INTUBATION

DRUG	DOSE	ONSET & DURATION	COMMENTS
Succinylcholine	1.5 mg/kg IV	*Onset:* within 1 min *Duration:* 3–5 min	*Advantages:* rapid onset and short duration of action. *Disadvantages:* increased intragastric, intraocular, and intracranial pressure. Fasciculations require premedication in patients >5 years old (see text). Bradyarrhythmias may also occur. Increased potassium levels (by 0.5 mEq/L) occur with routine administration. Histamine release occurs. Uncommon complications may include malignant hyperthermia, masseter muscle spasm, and prolonged apnea in patients with cholinesterase deficiency. *See text for other warnings and contraindications.*
Vecuronium	Low dose: 0.1 mg/kg IV	*Onset:* 2.5–3 min *Duration:* 30–35 min	*Advantages:* lacks the many disadvantages of succinylcholine, above. No cardiovascular side effects or histamine release.
	High dose: 0.25 mg/kg IV	*Onset:* 1–1.5 min *Duration:* 60–120 min	*Disadvantages:* low dose has a longer onset than succinylcholine. Duration of action is prolonged (especially with high-dose).
Pancuronium	0.1 mg/kg IV	*Onset:* 2–5 min *Duration:* 40–60 min	*Advantages:* lacks many of the disadvantages of succinylcholine, above. *Disadvantages:* slower onset and prolonged duration of action as compared to succinylcholine. Unlike vecuronium, above, vagolytic effect may increase heart rate, blood pressure, and cardiac output; tachycardias are a potential complication. Also unlike vecuronium, histamine release may occur.

used, the tip of the blade is inserted in the vallecula, and upward traction is used to lift the epiglottis anteriorly. When a straight blade is used, the blade is actually placed over the epiglottis, and the epiglottis is then lifted anteriorly (Fig. 11–3).

g. Magill forceps. These may be used to remove foreign debris as well as to help direct the tip of the endotracheal tube into the larynx if necessary.

h. Monitoring equipment. Both cardiac rhythm and SaO_2 should be monitored.

i. Oral and nasopharyngeal airways. One of these can be used to help maintain the airway while preoxygenating the patient prior to intubation.

j. Suction. Accompanying equipment should include a rigid pharyngeal suction-tip (Yankauer) and tracheal suction catheters.

B. Orotracheal Intubation

The ED patient requiring endotracheal intubation must be assumed to have a full stomach and to be at risk for aspiration. The following steps outline an approach to rapid-sequence intubation and are summarized in Table 11–2. These steps should be conducted in a controlled, efficient, and expeditious manner. It is also appropriate to adapt the steps as indicated to the clinical situation. For example, in a cardiac-arrest patient in need of endotracheal intubation, an assistant should preoxygenate the patient while the intubator rapidly prepares equipment, proceeds with endotracheal intubation, and immediately confirms tube placement. In this case, the administration of sedating drugs or a neuromuscular blocking agent is unnecessary.

Caution: prior to administering any sedative and/or paralytic drugs to a patient, quickly evaluate the patient's anatomy to anticipate intubation difficulties. Patients with a short, muscular

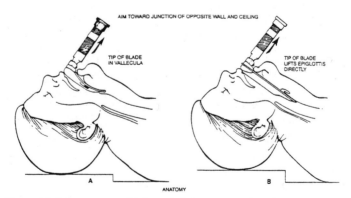

Figure 11–3. Laryngoscope blades and their correct use in the patient. *A.* Use of the curved laryngoscope blade. *B.* Use of the straight laryngoscope blade. (From Clinton JE, Ruiz E: Emergency airway management procedures. Chapter 1. In Roberts JR, Hedges JR (eds): Clinical Procedures in Emergency Medicine. 2nd Ed. Philadelphia, WB Saunders, 1991, p. 12. [Courtesy of "From Clinton JE, Ruiz E: Trauma Life Support Manual, 1982."])

neck, receding chin, abnormal or poorly mobile mandible or neck, or who, for whatever reason, have a distorted airway may pose significant challenges to intubation. Neuromuscular blocking agents should *never* be administered unless the physician is absolutely sure the patient can be intubated. Neuromuscular paralysis should also be avoided in patients who cannot be preoxygenated (e.g., severe asthma or COPD exacerbation).

1. **Step 1: Preoxygenate the Patient.** Administer 100% oxygen to the patient via either a nonrebreather mask or a bag-valve-mask device for at least *several minutes* while preparing the necessary equipment (Step 2, below). Avoid positive-pressure ventilation in the breathing patient because of the associated risks of gastric distention, emesis, and aspiration. If positive-pressure ventilation is necessary because of hypoventilation or apnea, apply manual cricoid pressure at this time, and avoid excessive airway pressures with ventilation.

2. **Step 2: Prepare Equipment.** Rapidly prepare all necessary equipment (see IV. A. 3, above) simultaneously with preoxygenation.
   a. Establish adequate intravenous (IV) access, and monitor both the cardiac rhythm and SaO_2.
   b. Have suction on and at the bedside.
   c. Check the laryngoscope light and have extra laryngoscope blades immediately available.
   d. Check the endotracheal tube and its cuff and lubricate the tube.
   e. If a stylet is used, lubricate it, insert it in the endotracheal tube, make sure the tip of the stylet is recessed at least ½ inch from the cuffed end of the tube, and shape it as desired.
   f. All needed drugs should be predrawn and instantly available.

3. **Step 3: Administer Adjunctive Medications as Indicated**
   a. **Defasciculation.** If the depolarizing neuromuscular blocker succinylcholine (Anectine) is to be used for neuromuscular blockade (Step 5, below), its administration may be accompanied by elevated intracranial, intraocular, and intragastric pressure, muscle fasciculations, and emesis (with the associated increased risk of aspiration). Fasciculations may be prevented by administering minidose succinylcholine (0.1 mg/kg IV) at this time *or* by administering a defasciculating dose of one of the nondepolarizing neuromuscular blocking agents:
      • Vecuronium (Norcuron): 0.01 mg/kg IV, or
      • Pancuronium (Pavulon): 0.01 mg/kg IV.
      The defasciculating drug should be given 3 minutes prior to the paralytic dose of succinylcholine. Defasciculation is not necessary in children < 5 years old.
   b. **Vagolysis.** Vagolysis is not routinely necessary in the adult patient, but atropine is a mandatory premedication in infants

≤ 1 year old, and it should be considered in children ≤ age 5 to help prevent bradycardia associated with muscle paralysis and intubation. Consult a pediatric manual for appropriate dosing in the pediatric patient. Some vagotonic adults may also benefit from premedication with atropine (minimal adult dose: 0.5 mg IV given 2–3 minutes prior to paralysis and intubation).

   c. **Blunt Increased Intracranial Pressure.** Premedication with lidocaine (1.5–2.0 mg/kg IV) 2–3 minutes before intubation attenuates the associated rise in intracranial pressure that occurs with intubation. Administration of lidocaine should be routine in the adult patient at risk for elevated intracranial pressure (e.g., suspected intracerebral lesion, hemorrhage, or head injury).

4. **Step 4: Establish Anesthesia.** Administration of one of the medications listed in Table 11–3 allows for a comfortable and well-tolerated intubation. Simultaneously with sedation/analgesia, apply firm posterior pressure over the cricoid cartilage (the Sellick maneuver) to occlude the esophagus until intubation is completed and the endotracheal tube cuff is inflated. The specific agent(s) chosen depend on the clinical setting:

   a. If the patient is hemodynamically stable without reactive airway disease: use thiopental or methohexital.

   b. If the patient has suspected increased intracranial pressure: use thiopental or methohexital.

   c. If the patient has both elevated intracranial pressure and hypotension: consider low-dose thiopental (0.5–1 mg/kg IV).

   d. If the patient is hemodynamically unstable: use fentanyl or ketamine supplemented with midazolam.

   e. If the patient has severe reactive airway disease: use ketamine or fentanyl supplemented with midazolam.

5. **Step 5: Establish Neuromuscular Blockade.** Immediately after performing Step 4, administer one of the neuromuscular blockers outlined in Table 11–4. Under most circumstances, succinylcholine is the drug of choice because of its rapid onset and short duration of action.

   Caution: succinylcholine should not be used in patients with angle-closure glaucoma or penetrating eye injuries, central nervous system diseases/injuries associated with extensive skeletal muscle denervation, degenerative or dystrophic neuromuscular diseases, disorders of plasma pseudocholinesterase, known hypersensitivity to the drug, malignant hyperthermia, myopathies associated with elevated serum creatinine, paraplegia, pre-existent hyperkalemia, or in patients several days to weeks after severe burns or major skeletal muscle injury.

6. **Step 6: Intubate the Patient (Fig. 11–4).** Proceed with intubation when muscle relaxation is maximal.

a. In the nontrauma patient, the head should be extended and the neck slightly flexed (consider placing a folded towel under the patient's occiput to help with neck flexion). In the trauma patient, do not allow motion of the cervical spine (an assistant must manually maintain the cervical spine in alignment and prevent any flexion or extension of the spine throughout the procedure).

b. Suction the mouth and pharynx as necessary. Remove any dentures if they were not removed earlier.

c. Use the fingers of the right hand to open the patient's mouth; the lighted laryngoscope is held in the left hand.

d. Insert the laryngoscope blade in the right side of the patient's mouth, moving the blade to the midline as it is advanced, which will displace the tongue to the left. A curved blade should be advanced into the vallecula; a straight blade is placed posterior to the epiglottis. Upward traction on the laryngoscope handle is then used to visualize the vocal cords. The intubator's left arm and back should be kept straight as the laryngoscope is used to "lift" the epiglottis anteriorly to bring the vocal cords into view. *Caution:* do not use the laryngoscope as a prying instrument, and never use the teeth as a fulcrum!

e. With your right hand, now advance the endotracheal tube along the right side of the mouth and observe its tip pass through the vocal cords. Advance the tube further until the proximal end of the deflated cuff is approximately 1–2.5 cm past the vocal cords. Remove the stylet, and inflate the endotracheal cuff with 10 mL of air.

Caution: an intubation attempt should ideally be ≤ 15 seconds in duration, and it should *never* exceed 30 seconds. The intubator should hold his/her breath throughout the intubation attempt; if tube placement is not accomplished by the time the intubator needs to take a breath, abort the attempt, and reventilate and oxygenate the patient for 15–30 seconds while preparing for the next attempt.

7. **Step 7: Immediately Confirm Correct Tube Placement**
   a. Immediately attach an end-tidal carbon dioxide detector to the proximal end of the endotracheal tube along with a bag-valve device connected to a high-flow oxygen source (> 15 L/min).
   b. Begin ventilating the patient. Observe the appropriate color change in the end-tidal carbon dioxide detector confirming tracheal placement, listen carefully over the lateral chest bilaterally for equal breath sounds, watch the chest rise and fall with ventilation, and listen over the epigastrium to ensure the absence of gastric bubbling.
   c. Cricoid pressure may be released now that correct tube placement is confirmed.
   d. Adjust the volume of air in the endotracheal tube cuff to just eliminate any air leak around the cuff with ventilation. Note

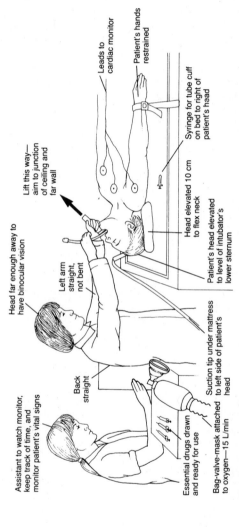

Figure 11-4. Orotracheal intubation of the adult patient. (From Clinton JE, Ruiz E: Emergency airway management procedures. Chapter 1. In Roberts JR, Hedges JR (eds): Clinical Procedures in Emergency Medicine. 2nd Ed. Philadelphia, WB Saunders, 1991, p. 10.)

Assistant to watch monitor, keep track of time, and monitor patient's vital signs

Head far enough away to have binocular vision

Left arm straight, not bent

Lift this way—aim to junction of ceiling and far wall

Leads to cardiac monitor

Patient's hands restrained

Syringe for tube cuff on bed to right of patient's head

Head elevated 10 cm to flex neck

Patient's head elevated to level of intubator's lower sternum

Back straight

Suction tip under mattress to left side of patient's head

Essential drugs drawn and ready for use

Bag-valve-mask attached to oxygen—15 L/min

the centimeter markings on the side of the endotracheal tube. These depth markings should be between 19 and 23 cm at the central incisors for an orally intubated adult patient, with the depth of the tube in males greater than that in females.

  e. Appropriately secure the tube in place.
  f. Order a stat portable chest radiograph to further confirm correct tube position. The tip of the endotracheal tube should be halfway between the vocal cords and the carina.

  Caution: incorrect placement of the endotracheal tube in the esophagus may not be immediately apparent. Breath sounds can be falsely interpreted as "normal" with a misplaced tube, especially when auscultation is incorrectly performed over the anterior chest instead of laterally. The "gold standard" for reliable intratracheal tube placement is direct observation of the tube passing through the vocal cords at the time of laryngoscopy; end-tidal carbon dioxide detectors provide further confirmation. Careful, meticulous assessment and reassessment of tube position and patient oxygenation and ventilation will help prevent the catastrophic and fatal complication of unrecognized esophageal intubation.

C. Nasotracheal Intubation

Nasotracheal intubation is less commonly performed in the ED than orotracheal intubation. Its advantages and contraindications have already been described (see IV. A. 2. b, above). As time allows, the physician should evaluate the nose, nasal passages, oral cavity, and neck prior to proceeding with the steps outlined below. The procedure should also be carefully explained to the awake patient before proceeding.

1. **Step 1: Preoxygenate the Patient.** See comments under IV. B. 1, above.

2. **Step 2: Prepare Equipment**

   See comments under IV. B. 2, above. The endotracheal tube should be 0.5–1.0 mm smaller in internal diameter than the size of the optimal tube for oral intubation. Lubricate the tube with 2% **lidocaine** anesthetic jelly. A stylet is not used.

3. **Step 3: Establish Topical Anesthesia and Vasoconstriction**
   a. Topical anesthesia and vasoconstriction should be applied to both nasal passages. Medication choices include
     • 10% lidocaine spray and 0.05% oxymetazoline nasal spray. With this regimen, topical anesthesia occurs after 1 minute.
     • 4% cocaine solution (may be sprayed in the nares or applied to the nasal mucosa with saturated cotton pledgets; do not exceed 1 mg/kg total dose). Topical

anesthesia and vasoconstriction requires approximately 5 minutes. *Caution:* avoid cocaine in patients with hypertension, active cardiovascular disease, or severely traumatized nasal mucosa.

- Benzocaine, butyl aminobenzoate, tetracaine, and benzalkonium chloride (Cetacaine) spray and 0.05% oxymetazoline nasal spray. Topical anesthesia occurs after 1 minute.

b. In addition to the above, some physicians recommend "priming" the nasopharynx by temporarily inserting an appropriately sized nasopharyngeal airway lubricated with 2% lidocaine jelly and leaving this airway in the nostril for 4–5 minutes.

c. In patients with intact airway protective reflexes, consider translaryngeal anesthesia. *Technique:* in a sterile fashion and with local anesthesia, puncture the inferior border of the cricothyroid membrane with a 25-gauge needle attached to a 5-mL syringe containing 2 mL of sterile 4% lidocaine solution. Aspirate air to confirm intratracheal penetration and then rapidly inject the anesthetic solution into the trachea. Withdraw the needle and apply firm pressure for at least one minute.

d. Depending on clinical circumstances, topical anesthesia as outlined above may be supplemented with parenteral analgesia/sedation (e.g., fentanyl with or without midazolam; see Table 11–3 for dosing).

4. **Step 4: Intubate the Patient Nasotracheally.** The technique of blind nasotracheal intubation is described here.

a. The endotracheal tube should be placed in the naris with the tube's bevel toward the nasal septum. At this time, the curvature of the tube is directed superiorly.

b. Advance the tube along the floor of the nasal cavity by applying steady forward pressure and gently rotating the tube as necessary. Do not force the tube!

c. When the tip of the tube enters the pharynx, rotate it 180° so that the tube's curvature is now directed inferiorly. The endotracheal tube will begin to function as a nasopharyngeal airway when its tip is in the posterior pharynx.

d. Continue to advance the endotracheal tube, gently rotating it as necessary, while listening for maximal airflow through the tube. Use the breath sounds heard through the tube as a guide to the appropriate direction of tube advance.

e. When airflow through the tube is maximal, have an assistant apply cricoid pressure, and quickly pass the tube into the trachea during the patient's inspiration.

f. Inflate the cuff of the endotracheal tube with 5–10 mL of air and release cricoid pressure.

5. **Step 5: Immediately Confirm Correct Tube Placement.** See comments under IV. B. 7, above.

D. Other Intubation Techniques

Other intubation techniques include nasotracheal intubation under direct vision, digital intubation, lighted stylet intubation, bronchoscopically guided intubation, and retrograde orotracheal intubation. Descriptions of these techniques are beyond the scope of this manual. The reader is encouraged to consult one or more of the reference works in the bibliography.

V. SURGICAL AIRWAYS

When a definitive airway cannot be established by any other means, a surgical airway is indicated. There are two ED possibilities: percutaneous translaryngeal ventilation and cricothyrotomy.

A. Percutaneous Translaryngeal Ventilation (Needle Cricothyrotomy)

This procedure is only a temporary alternative to more definitive airway control (e.g., cricothyrotomy or tracheostomy) when endotracheal intubation is either unsuccessful or contraindicated.

1. **Advantages**
   a. It is a simple and rapid procedure.
   b. It is easier to perform and the risk of bleeding is less than with cricothyrotomy.
   c. It does not require surgical skills to perform.
   d. There is less risk of scar formation or subglottic or glottic stenosis post procedure.
   e. It may be used to bypass a more proximal partial tracheal obstruction.

2. **Contraindications**
   a. Tracheal transection with retraction of the distal trachea into the mediastinum.
   b. Significant cricoid cartilage injury.
   c. Complete tracheal obstruction.
   d. When endotracheal intubation is otherwise possible and easily performed.

3. **Equipment**
   a. Betadine swabs, 1–2% lidocaine with epinephrine (1:200,000), #11 scalpel blade, syringes, and 2–4% lidocaine.
   b. High-pressure oxygen source capable of providing 50 psi (this may include the wall oxygen outlet in the ED or a standard oxygen cylinder). If an oxygen wall source is used, open the flow meter completely (i.e., set it on "flush"); if an oxygen cylinder is used, do not use a regulator valve (demand valve devices do not provide sufficient flow for patient ventilation using this technique).
   c. High-pressure tubing to connect the oxygen source with the

catheter used for ventilation. There must be a method to intermittently interrupt oxygen flow to the patient to allow for exhalation. This interruption may include a Y-connector on the high-pressure line, a trigger-type interrupter, or even a small hole cut in the side of the oxygen tubing.

d. Large-bore (14-gauge or larger) 1.25-inch needle with intravenous (IV) cannula. Avoid longer cannulas because of their increased tendency to kink.

e. Commercial kits are available that have the above necessary equipment prepackaged. It is appropriate to stock these kits on the "crash cart" or in the "difficult intubation tray" within the ED.

4. **Technique**

a. Place 2 mL of 2–4% lidocaine in a 10-mL syringe and attach this to the large-bore IV needle with cannula.

b. Locate the cricothyroid membrane between the cricoid cartilage (inferiorly) and the prominent thyroid cartilage superiorly.

c. Prepare the skin with povidone-iodine, and in a sterile fashion anesthetize the skin over the puncture site with a small amount of lidocaine with epinephrine. Use a #11 scalpel blade to make a small puncture in the skin in the midline over the inferior aspect of the cricothyroid membrane (just superior to the cricoid cartilage).

d. Use your nondominant hand to steady the cricoid cartilage and overlying skin.

e. In your dominant hand hold the 10-mL syringe attached to the large-bore needle with cannula. Insert the needle through the skin puncture and the cricothyroid membrane at a 45° angle, the tip of the needle and its cannula directed inferiorly. Continually aspirate on the syringe while advancing the needle with cannula.

f. Aspiration of air indicates the tip is now in the trachea. Forcefully inject the 2 mL of lidocaine in the syringe to topically anesthetize the trachea and then advance the cannula over and off the inner needle till the hub of the cannula lies against the skin. The needle is now completely removed, and the 10-mL syringe reattached to the cannula hub. Reaspirate to confirm the cannula tip is still in the trachea.

g. Attach the high-pressure oxygen tubing to the hub of the cannula and begin oxygenating and ventilating the patient. The appropriate rate is 12–20 ventilations/minute: allow oxygen inflow to the patient for 1 second, then interrupt the inflow for 2 seconds to allow for exhalation (some authors recommend oxygen inflow for 2 seconds and watching for chest expansion, then allowing 4–5 seconds for exhalation). Hold the hub of the cannula in place until it is adequately secured.

h. Suture the cannula hub in place while continuing patient ventilation.

Cautions: definitive airway control must be secured as soon as possible to prevent hypercarbia, which may develop in as little as 30 minutes using percutaneous translaryngeal ventilation. Ventilating the patient with this technique will cause upper-airway secretions to blow out of the nose and mouth; ED staff should be warned to stand clear. Place the patient in the Trendelenburg position to minimize aspiration. Do not use this technique in the setting of complete airway obstruction because significant barotrauma (including fatal air embolism) may result. (In a desperate situation, when complete airway obstruction is proximal to the cricothyroid membrane, a second large-bore cannula may be placed through the cricothyroid membrane to allow for exhalation between oxygen insufflations).

B. Cricothyrotomy

Cricothyrotomy is the establishment of an airway via an incision through the cricothyroid membrane. It is the surgical airway of choice when a definitive airway is required in the adult patient and endotracheal intubation is otherwise not possible.

1. **Absolute Contraindications**
   a. Tracheal transection with retraction of the distal trachea into the mediastinum.
   b. Fractured larynx.
   c. Significant other laryngeal or cricoid injury.
   d. When endotracheal intubation is otherwise possible and easily performed.

2. **Relative Contraindications**
   a. Bleeding diathesis.
   b. Massive neck edema.
   c. Acute laryngeal disease.
   d. Pediatric patients < age 10–12 years old. (Remember, the cricoid cartilage is the narrowest portion of the pediatric airway; postcricothyrotomy scarring and granuloma formation may result in the devastating complication of tracheal stenosis in the child. When a surgical airway is required in the pediatric patient [age < 10–12 years], percutaneous translaryngeal ventilation is the initial procedure of choice, followed by tracheostomy performed in the operating suite.)

3. **Equipment**
   a. Betadine swabs, small syringe with a 25-gauge needle, 2% lidocaine with epinephrine (for local anesthesia), a #11 and #15 scalpel blade, extra syringes, and gauze pads.
   b. Curved hemostats (two), curved Mayo scissors, tracheal dilator (Trousseau) or spreader, and tracheal hook.

c. Suction apparatus and tubing (including tracheal suction catheter).
d. Cuffed tracheostomy tube (usually a No. 4 Shiley in adults; inner diameter 5 mm and outer diameter 8.5 mm).
e. Tape, suture, and needle holder for securing the tube in place after the procedure.

4. **Technique**
a. Locate the cricothyroid membrane between the cricoid cartilage (inferiorly) and the prominent thyroid cartilage (superiorly). In the nontrauma patient without cervical spinal injury, slight hyperextension of the head assists in exposing landmarks.
b. As time allows, prepare the skin with betadine. In the conscious patient, establish local anesthesia in the midline with lidocaine with epinephrine.
c. Stabilize the larynx with the nondominant hand. With the dominant hand, use the #15 scalpel blade and make a *vertical* midline incision (3–4 cm long) in the skin overlying the cricothyroid membrane to expose the membrane.
d. Continue to stabilize the larynx with the nondominant hand or a tracheal hook. Now make a 1-cm *horizontal* stabbing incision through the anterior-inferior portion of the exposed cricothyroid membrane with the #11 scalpel blade. Insert curved Mayo scissors alongside the scalpel and spread the scissors to widen the space. Remove the scalpel.
e. Insert either a tracheal dilator or curved hemostat into the opening and remove the scissors.
f. Insert the tracheostomy tube into the opening so the cuffed portion is completely within the trachea. Use the tracheal hook as necessary to keep the larynx from moving posteriorly during tube insertion.
g. Inflate the cuff on the tube, initiate and confirm ventilation, and secure the airway in place.

BIBLIOGRAPHY

Clinton JE, Ruiz E: Emergency airway management procedures. Chapter 1. In Roberts JR, JR Hedges (eds): Clinical Procedures in Emergency Medicine, 2nd Ed. Philadelphia, WB Saunders, 1991, pp. 1-29.
Dailey RH, Simon B, Young GP, Stewart RD: The Airway: Emergency Management. St. Louis, Mosby-Year Book, 1992.
Dronen SC. Pharmacologic adjuncts to intubation. Chapter 2. In Roberts JR, Hedges JR (eds): Clinical Procedures in Emergency Medicine. 2nd Ed. Philadelphia, WB Saunders, 1991, pp. 29-40.
Grande CM, Stene JK, Bernhard WN: Airway management: considerations in trauma patients. Crit Care Clin 1990;6(1):37–59.
Mace SE: Cricothyrotomy. Chapter 3. In Roberts JR, Hedges JR (eds): Clinical Procedures in Emergency Medicine. 2nd ed. Philadelphia, WB Saunders, 1991, pp. 40-59.
Morris IR: Pharmacological aids to intubation and the rapid sequence induction. Emerg Med Clin N Am 1988;6(4):753-768.
Walls RM: Rapid-sequence intubation in head trauma. Ann Emerg Med 1993;22(6):1008–1013.
Walls RM: Airway management. Emerg Med Clin N Am 1993;11(1):53–60.

12

Shock

"All the deeper problems of physiology turn on the mutual action of the tissues and the blood, as the stream of the latter sweeps among the elements of the former."

SIR MICHAEL FOSTER

GENERAL CONCEPTS

I. DEFINITION

Shock is a condition of inadequate tissue perfusion with resultant insufficient oxygen and metabolic substrate delivery. Its consequences include impaired energy production and utilization, altered cellular metabolism, acidosis, cellular injury and loss of cellular integrity, tissue and organ dysfunction, and, ultimately, death unless early and aggressive treatment is initiated. Shock is the final common pathway by which many disease processes result in death.

II. BEDSIDE CLINICAL FINDINGS INDICATIVE OF SHOCK

A. **Vital Signs.** Pulse, blood pressure (BP), respiratory rate, and temperature.

1. Tachycardia is the most sensitive vital sign abnormality indicative of volume depletion.

2. As the clinical condition worsens, hypotension (systolic BP < 90 mmHg) eventually occurs. (*Caution:* in the setting of hemorrhagic shock, the otherwise healthy supine adult patient does not become hypotensive until as much as 30% of the blood volume is lost; impending shock should be treated *before* the patient becomes hypotensive!).

3. Both pulse and BP can be incorporated into a recently described ratio, the *shock index* (SI = heart rate/systolic BP). The SI may prove to be a useful marker of acute critical illness. Normally, the SI is 0.5–0.7. Values > 0.9 have been associated with illnesses requiring immediate treatment, hospitalization, and intensive therapy.

4. If supine vital signs are normal and the presenting condition allows (e.g., mental status is normal; no spinal or pelvic trauma), evaluate for orthostatic changes.
   Technique. Obtain pulse and BP after the patient has been supine for 2–3 minutes; have the patient then assume an upright

posture and note symptoms, pulse, and BP after 1 minute. Symptoms of hypovolemia (e.g., dizziness or near-syncope) are abnormal, constitute a positive test, and should terminate the test. Other positive test findings in adults include a pulse change of 30 beats/min (some consider a 20-beats/min change significant), a drop in systolic BP of ≥ 25 mmHg, or a drop in diastolic BP of ≥ 10 mmHg.

5. Additional "vital signs" should include oxygen saturation (SaO_2) (via pulse oximetry) and cardiac rhythm.

B. **Skin.** In the normothermic patient with shock, capillary refill is usually prolonged (> 2 seconds); patients are also frequently cool, clammy, and/or diaphoretic (patients in early septic shock or with neurogenic shock, however, are usually warm and dry).

C. **Urine Output.** In early compensated shock, urine is concentrated and urine output is decreased. As the condition progresses, significant oliguria (≤ 0.5 mL/kg/hr) will eventually be followed by anuria.

D. **Mental Status.** This may initially be normal. As the clinical condition deteriorates, the patient may become confused, agitated, restless, and, eventually, lethargic and/or comatose.

III. THE CARDIOVASCULAR TRIAD

The *cardiovascular triad* is a valuable tool in initially evaluating and treating the patient in impending or actual shock. All forms of shock ultimately result from one or more of the following three basic mechanisms:

A. **Rate/Rhythm Problem.** A cardiac arrhythmia, or an inappropriate heart rate given the clinical situation, may result in hemodynamic compromise and shock. The rate/rhythm can be quickly assessed from the cardiac monitor and the electrocardiogram (ECG).

Examples:

1. Rhythm too slow: sinus bradycardia, slow junctional rhythm, slow idioventricular rhythm, second- or third-degree heart block, and pacemaker failure.

2. Rhythm too fast: inappropriately rapid sinus tachycardia, atrial flutter, atrial fibrillation, multifocal atrial tachycardia, paroxysmal supraventricular tachycardia (PSVT), other atrial tachycardia, and ventricular tachycardia.

B. **Pump Problem.** Myocardial dysfunction from any cause may result in hemodynamic compromise.

Examples

1. Primary causes of cardiac dysfunction: acute myocardial infarction (MI), cardiac contusion, cardiomyopathy, conges-

tive heart failure (CHF) of any cause, myocarditis, ruptured intraventricular septum, and valvular dysfunction (e.g., acute aortic insufficiency, chordae tendineae rupture, papillary muscle dysfunction, prosthetic valve thrombus or other prosthetic valve dysfunction, and severe aortic stenosis).

2. Secondary causes of cardiac dysfunction: atrial myxoma, cardiac tamponade, medications, pulmonary embolism, severe hypertension, systemic toxins or myocardial depressant factors, tension pneumothorax, and vena cava obstruction.

C. **Volume or Vascular Resistance Problems ("Tank" Problems).** Intravascular volume depletion (i.e., an "empty tank") or inappropriate vascular tone given the clinical situation (i.e., an inappropriately "sized tank") may cause shock.

Examples

1. Volume loss: acute hemorrhage, adrenal insufficiency (aldosterone deficiency), altered capillary permeability (e.g., anaphylaxis, prolonged hypoxia/ischemia of any cause, tissue injury, sepsis), insensible losses (e.g., diaphoresis, significant skin disease, burns), gastrointestinal losses (e.g., vomiting or diarrhea), inadequate oral intake, third spacing (e.g., ascites, intestinal obstruction, pancreatitis, peritonitis, splanchnic ischemia), and urinary losses (e.g., diabetes insipidus, diabetes mellitus, diuretic use, renal disease).

2. Altered vascular resistance: adrenal insufficiency (cortisol deficiency), anaphylaxis, central nervous system (CNS) injury, drugs or toxins, sepsis, prolonged shock of any cause, and spinal cord injury.

IV. PATIENT MONITORING

A. Closely monitor the following in all hemodynamically unstable patients:

1. Vital signs.

2. Cardiac rhythm.

3. SaO_2 (via continuous pulse oximetry).

4. Repeated physical examination (i.e., continual patient reassessment).

5. Urine output (via bladder catheterization).

B. Invasive monitoring is frequently of assistance and may include one or more of the following (*note:* depending on ED capabilities, invasive monitoring may be started in the ED or after the patient's admission to the ICU):

1. Systemic artery catheterization for intra-arterial BP monitoring.

2. Central vein catheterization (i.e., superior vena cava catheterization via the antecubital, internal jugular, or subclavian veins) for central venous pressure (CVP) monitoring. The CVP is determined by blood volume, intrathoracic pressure, right-ventricular (RV) function, and venomotor tone. Normal values are 6–12 cmH_2O. A low CVP (< 6 cmH_2O) generally indicates hypovolemia. An elevated CVP, however, does *not* rule out a volume deficit. For example, patients with RV infarction or pulmonary embolism may have a high CVP despite low left-ventricular (LV) filling pressures and needed volume infusion. Trends in CVP measurement with volume challenge are more helpful than absolute numbers. For example, if the CVP is low and volume challenge results in a minimal change in the CVP, then the patient is significantly hypovolemic and further aggressive crystalloid infusion is indicated. If the CVP is normal, however, and volume challenge results in a rapid increase in the CVP with no improvement or a deterioration in hemodynamic status, then the cause of the shock state is pump dysfunction and further volume infusion is not indicated.

3. Pulmonary artery catheterization with a balloon-flotation catheter (Swan-Ganz catheter). This allows for measurement of the following:
   a. Central venous pressure.
   b. Mean pulmonary artery pressure (PAP; normal 9–19 mmHg).
   c. Pulmonary artery end-diastolic pressure (PAEDP; normal = 4–13 mmHg). This measurement will closely approximate PAOP (see below) unless the patient is tachycardic or has pulmonary hypertension.
   d. Pulmonary artery occlusive pressure (PAOP; normal = 4.5–13 mmHg). PAOP (also called pulmonary capillary wedge pressure) is used as an indirect measurement of LV filling pressure. Measurements should be made at end exhalation. In patients with normal cardiac function, the PAOP should generally be maintained in the upper range of normal. In patients with cardiac dysfunction, however, volume status should be adjusted to maintain the PAOP in the 18–20 mmHg range to optimize cardiac performance. A PAOP > 20–25 mmHg generally indicates volume overload and the need for diuresis (if the patient is hypotensive, vasoactive agents will be required in this setting for BP support).
   e. Thermodilution cardiac output (CO; normal adult = 4–8 L/min). The cardiac index (CI) is the CO divided by the patient's body surface area (normal CI = 2.8–4.2 L/min/m^2).
   f. Mixed venous oxygen tension (should be maintained > 35 mmHg) and mixed venous oxygen saturation (should be maintained > 65%).

V. INITIAL CARE OF THE PATIENT IN SHOCK

Regardless of the specific cause(s) of the impending or actual shock state, initially proceed as follows:

A. Assess, secure, and support the *airway, breathing,* and *circulation* as indicated. (See Chapter 1. II.)

B. Simultaneously, administer supplemental oxygen, establish intravenous (IV) access, and continuously monitor both cardiac rhythm and SaO_2.

C. Rapidly obtain vital signs, an ECG, arterial blood gas (ABG) levels, and a directed history, and perform an appropriate physical examination. Recheck vital signs frequently.

D. Obtain a portable chest roentgenogram and relevant laboratory values.

ANAPHYLACTIC SHOCK

I. ESSENTIAL FACTS

A. Definition

Anaphylactic shock is an acute shock state caused by an allergic reaction. It usually occurs within 60 minutes of antigen exposure; circulatory and/or respiratory failure and death may result.

1. *Anaphylaxis* is a type I immune response (hypersensitivity reaction) involving three components: an allergen or antigen, IgE antibodies to the antigen, and mediator synthesis and release from effector cells (mast cells and basophils).

2. An *anaphylactoid* reaction presents similarly to anaphylaxis, but an IgE-mediated mechanism is not involved. Examples include radiocontrast media and aspirin or nonsteroidal anti-inflammatory drug (NSAID)-induced reactions.

B. Mediators of Anaphylaxis

The primary chemical mediators from mast cells are stored in granules or may be newly synthesized on antigen exposure. Known mediators include histamine, prostaglandin D2, leukotrienes (including C4, D4, and E4), platelet-activating factor, tryptase, chymase, heparin, vasodilatory cytokines, tumor necrosis factor, and chondroitin sulfate. Physiologically, mediators cause increased vascular permeability, systemic vasodilation, pulmonary vasoconstriction, bronchoconstriction, arrhythmias, and a negative inotropic effect.

C. Incidence

In the United States, anaphylaxis occurs at rates at high as 1 in every 3000 inpatients, and it may be responsible for as many as 500 deaths per year. Antibiotics are the most common cause of anaphylaxis, and penicillin is responsible for as many as 75% of anaphylactic deaths. Sixty percent of deaths occur within 60 minutes of antigen exposure.

D. Etiologic Agents

Etiologic agents are given in Table 12–1.

II. CLINICAL PRESENTATION

A. Signs and Symptoms

Clinical features can occur independently or concomitantly in each involved organ system (Table 12–2).

1. The most common clinical manifestations are cutaneous and include erythema, flushing, pruritis, urticaria, and, in severe cases, angioedema.

2. The potentially life-threatening manifestations are upper-airway compromise secondary to soft-tissue edema (early symptoms may include hoarseness, dysphagia, or a "lump" in

Table 12–1. INITIATORS OF ANAPHYLAXIS

IgE-Mediated

Proteins
    Foods (nuts, fish, shellfish, eggs)
    Antiserum (tetanus and diphtheria antitoxins)
    Hormones, enzymes (insulin, ACTH, TSH)
    Venom (*Hymenoptera* sting [bee, wasp, hornet, or bite of fire ant])
    Allergen extract (ragweed, Bermuda grass, buckwheat, egg white, cottonseed)
    Vaccines (tetanus toxoid, influenza, measles and other egg-containing vaccines)
Polysaccharides
    Dextran
    Iron dextran
Haptens
    Antibiotics (penicillin, tetracycline, nitrofurantoin, streptomycin)
    Vitamins (thiamine, folic acid)

Complement-Mediated

Transfusion reaction with IgA deficiency; methotrexate

Arachidonate-Mediated

Aspirin and other nonsteroidal anti-inflammatory agents

Direct Mast Cell–Releasing Agent

Exercise, opiates, tubocurarine, radiocontrast media, hydralazine

Idiopathic

Melphalan, procarbazine, chlorambucil, hydroxyurea, 5-fluorouracil, busulfan, mitomycin

ACTH, adrenocorticotropic hormone; TSH, thyroid-stimulating hormone.

Table 12–2. SIGNS AND SYMPTOMS OF ANAPHYLAXIS[a]

EARLY SYMPTOMS	CUTANEOUS	RESPIRATORY	CARDIO-VASCULAR	GASTRO-INTESTINAL
Headache of sudden onset Itching palms and soles Apprehension Sensation of warmth	Pruritus Urticaria (hives) Angioedema Flushing (vasodilation) Dermatographism Cyanosis (hypoxia)	Shortness of breath Upper-airway obstruction: "lump in throat" (angioedema of epiglottis) stridor choking } laryngeal edema hoarseness and loss of voice } laryngospasm Lower airway obstruction: wheezing "chest" tightness } bronchospasm Complete airway obstruction	Hypotension Diaphoresis Lightheadedness Syncope Cardiac arrhythmias (hypoxia, hypotension)	Nausea Vomiting Abdominal cramps Diarrhea (may be bloody) Dysphagia (food antigen)

[a]From Bonnin M: In Eisenberg MS (ed): Critical Emergencies. Philadelphia, Hanley & Belfus, 1986, p. 16.

the throat), dyspnea and wheezing secondary to bronchoconstriction, vascular collapse secondary to vasodilation and increased vascular permeability, and/or cardiac arrhythmias secondary to hypoxia, acidosis, or myocardial hypoperfusion.

3. *Caution:* patients taking beta-adrenergic-blocking drugs or those with asthma may suffer worsened airway responses to anaphylaxis and may be more difficult to treat.

B. Laboratory Studies

1. Routine tests are generally not diagnostic. An elevated serum histamine level may be useful in confirming the clinical diagnosis. A prolonged coagulation time and reduction in complement may be found in special cases.

2. Electrocardiographic changes may include T-wave inversion or flattening, bundle-branch blocks, supraventricular tachycardia (SVT) or other arrhythmias, and intraventricular conduction delays.

III. DIAGNOSIS

The diagnosis of anaphylaxis is based on the acute onset of typical symptoms and signs after exposure to an initiating substance. The *differential diagnosis* includes asthma, carcinoid syndrome, hereditary angioedema (C1 esterase inhibitor deficiency), monosodium glutamate reaction, scombroid fish poisoning, systemic mastocytosis, vasovagal reactions, and viral or bacterial infections of the upper airway.

IV. THERAPY

A. *Provide initial care of the patient in impending or actual shock* (see General Concepts, earlier in this chapter). Administer supplemental oxygen and meticulously maintain an adequate upper airway. Angioedema of the lips, tongue, uvula, or soft palate is a concerning finding indicative of potential airway compromise.

1. Posterior pharyngeal and early laryngeal angioedema may be treated with inhaled racemic epinephrine 2.25% (*dose:* 0.5 mL in 2 mL normal saline [NS] nebulized; do not exceed three treatments in 60 minutes).

2. Be prepared for immediate endotracheal intubation in the setting of impending upper-airway compromise, inadequate oxygenation, or profound shock.

3. Cricothyrotomy may be necessary if severe angioedema precludes intubation via the oral route.

B. *Stop further antigen exposure.*

1. If the antigenic stimulus is located in an extremity (e.g., *Hymenoptera* sting, subcutaneously (SQ) or intramuscularly (IM) administered medication, chemical exposure), proceed as follows:
   a. Apply a relatively loose tourniquet on the extremity proximal to the antigen site to impede lymphatic and venous flow. Remove the tourniquet periodically (e.g., 1 minute every 10 minutes). Keep the extremity in a dependent position.
   b. Carefully flick off a retained *Hymenoptera* stinger without squeezing the stinger to avoid further venom release.
   c. Cleanse the skin of any chemical with water and a mild soap.
   d. Apply ice locally to the site for 15 minutes every 30 minutes.

2. If the reaction occurs secondary to an IV medication, immediately stop the drug infusion, and completely replace all IV tubing.

C. *Administer epinephrine* (accomplish simultaneously with the above). Epinephrine is the drug of choice in the treatment of anaphylactic reactions. Its potent alpha- and beta-adrenergic actions counteract the angioedema, bronchoconstriction, vasodilation, and other mediator effects. Epinephrine also inhibits further mediator release from mast cells and basophils. It may be given SQ, IM, IV, or endotracheally (ET). The route of administration depends on the severity of the patient's anaphylactic response:

1. SQ or IM administration: this is the appropriate route in the setting of early and minimal airway edema, mild bronchospasm, or isolated cutaneous anaphylactic responses. Administer 0.3–0.5 mg of 1:1000 dilution (0.3–0.5 mL) SQ or IM every 10–20 minutes as indicated. If the site of antigen exposure can be isolated (e.g., insect sting or allergen injection site), a portion of the administered epinephrine dose (0.1–0.2 mg) can be injected SQ directly into that site.

2. IV administration: this is the appropriate route in the setting of laryngeal edema, severe bronchospasm, or vasodilatory anaphylactic responses with hypotension. Place 0.1 mg (1 mL of 1:10,000 solution) in 10 mL NS and give as a slow IV push over 5 minutes. This dose may be repeated once or twice every 10 minutes as required. Alternatively, a continuous epinephrine IV infusion may be started (dose: 0.5–10 µg/min).

3. Use epinephrine cautiously in elderly patients, or in individuals with diabetes mellitus, cardiovascular disease, thyroid disease, cerebral arteriosclerosis, or Parkinson's disease (consider using one-half the above recommended doses initially in these patients). Patients taking beta-adrenergic-blocking agents may suffer unopposed alpha-adrenergic stimulation and marked hypertension with epinephrine administration.

D. *Administer antihistamines.* Antihistamines should be given to help combat the effects of mediator release; they are second-line drugs after epinephrine. Many deleterious effects in the setting of anaphylaxis are mediated through the H1 receptor. Combined therapy with H1 and H2 antagonists, however, is more effective than either one alone in preventing hypotension.

1. H1-blocking antihistamines:
   a. Diphenhydramine (Benadryl) 50 mg IV or IM every 6–8 hours as needed (in severe anaphylaxis, administer 100 mg IV initially); *or*
   b. Hydroxyzine (Vistaril) 25–50 mg IM every 6–8 hours as needed.

2. H2-blocking antihistamines:
   a. Cimetidine 300 mg IV every 6 hours; *or*
   b. Ranitidine 50 mg IV every 6–8 hours.

E. *Treat bronchospasm as necessary* (accomplish simultaneously with the above-outlined therapy).

1. Albuterol (2.5 mg in 3 mL saline) 2.5–5 mg nebulized every 20 minutes as necessary.

2. Aminophylline 6 mg/kg IV loading dose (if patient is not currently taking aminophylline or theophylline) over 20–30 minutes followed by a continuous IV infusion (0.7 mg/kg/hr in otherwise healthy nonsmoking adults).

F. *Provide circulatory support as necessary* (accomplish simultaneously with the above-outlined therapy).

1. Place the hypotensive patient in the Trendelenburg position if airway and respiratory status allow.

2. Rapidly adminster crystalloid volume infusion (1 L every 20–30 minutes as needed) with NS or lactated Ringer's solution (LR).

3. Carefully monitor cardiac rhythm, volume status, and urine output.

4. Hypotension refractory to the above therapy (including epinephrine administration) may require treatment with one of the following agents (the pneumatic antishock garment [PASG] may also be considered in the absence of pulmonary edema):

    a. Norepinephrine (Levophed 1 mg/mL in 4 mL ampules) 2–12 µg/min IV infusion; or

    b. Phenylephrine (Neosynephrine 10 mg/mL in 1 mL ampules) 0.1–0.5 mg IV bolus every 10–15 minutes as necessary or 100–180 µg/min continuous IV infusion; decrease infusion to 40–60 µg/min after BP has stabilized; or

    c. Glucagon: place 1 mg in 1 L 5% dextrose in water (D5W) and administer IV at the rate of 5–15 µg/min (i.e., 5–15 mL/min). A prominent side effect of glucagon therapy is nausea, and much higher doses than the above may sometimes be necessary (e.g., 1–2 mg IV over 5 minutes). Glugacon may be especially useful in patients who are taking beta-adrenergic-blocking agents because it can stimulate both cardiac inotropic and chronotropic function independent of beta blockade. Patients taking beta blockers may also benefit from terbutaline (0.25 mg SQ, not to exceed 0.5 mg SQ every 4 hours).

G. *Administer corticosteroids.* These agents are appropriate in any potential or actual life-threatening anaphylactic reaction involving airway edema, bronchospasm, or hypotension. They are useful in shortening or reducing prolonged reactions, and they may help prevent a recurrence.

1. Methylprednisolone (Solu-Medrol) 125 mg IV; may repeat dose every 6–8 hours as necessary; or

2. Hydrocortisone 250 mg IV; may repeat dose every 6–8 hours as necessary.

V. DISPOSITION

A. Discharge

Patients who present with a mild anaphylactic response, and who have had complete resolution of their symptoms in the ED with appropriate management, may be discharged to home after a prolonged period of observation (recommended observation times vary from 3 to 8 hours depending on the circumstances).

1. At the time of ED discharge, prudent discharge medications should include an antihistamine (e.g., diphenhydramine 25–50 mg PO every 6–8 hours as needed) ± several days of a corticosteroid (e.g., prednisone 60 mg PO daily).

2. Patients must be carefully instructed on the sedating nature of antihistamines, to avoid exposure to the initiating antigen in the future, and to follow up with a primary care physician.

3. Patients with a serious anaphylactic reaction should be

prescribed a kit for the self-administration of epinephrine (e.g., Epi-Pen or Ana-Kit) and instructed in its use.

4. Those patients with a generalized or other potentially serious reaction to an antigen for which immunotherapy is available (e.g., *Hymenoptera* venom) should be referred to an allergist.

B. Admit

Patients with a potentially life-threatening anaphylactic reaction on ED presentation (e.g., severe bronchospasm, upper airway obstruction, or shock), or those who do not adequately improve with ED therapy, should be hospitalized in an ICU. Hospitalization should also be strongly considered in the elderly, those who live alone, those who do not have ready access to medical care after ED discharge, or individuals with other significant comorbid conditions (e.g., pulmonary disease, cardiac disease).

CARDIOGENIC SHOCK

I. ESSENTIAL FACTS

A. Definition

Cardiogenic shock is inadequate tissue perfusion and oxygenation secondary to cardiac pathology. Mortality is as high as 70–90% unless aggressive and highly technical care is rapidly utilized in managing the patient.

B. Etiology

See General Concepts, earlier in this chapter. Loss of ≥ 40% of the LV myocardium in the setting of ischemic heart disease is associated with cardiogenic shock.

C. Incidence

Six to twenty percent of acute MI patients who survive to hospital admission will suffer cardiogenic shock. Cardiogenic shock patients tend to be older than acute MI patients without shock, more frequently suffer anterior MIs and/or have had a prior MI, and more commonly have a history of either CHF or angina.

II. CLINICAL PRESENTATION

A. Signs and Symptoms

1. Symptoms will vary with the cause of cardiac pathology. Nonspecific clinical findings include cool and clammy skin, decreased pulse pressure with weak peripheral pulses, diaphoresis, fatigue, hypotension, and weakness. In severe cases, mental status may be altered.

2. Pulmonary vascular congestion is frequently present and may manifest as dyspnea, labored respirations, rales, and tachypnea. In severe cases, frothy sputum or cyanosis may occur (*note:* the patient with RV infarction may present in cardiogenic shock with clear lung fields).

3. Cardiac auscultation often reveals significant abormalities. A prominent S4 indicates decreased ventricular compliance and suggests myocardial ischemia in the setting of on-going chest pain. An S3 indicates increased ventricular diastolic pressure and CHF. Hemodynamically significant mitral regurgitation (from papillary muscle dysfunction or rupture) usually causes a prominent and typical holosystolic murmur. Ventricular septal rupture is associated with a systolic thrill and a holosystolic murmur heard best at the lower left sternal border.

4. Elevated venous pressure is frequently present. Its differential diagnosis includes constrictive pericarditis, pericardial tamponade, pulmonary hypertension, RV infarction, superior vena cava obstruction, tension pneumothorax, and tricuspid valve disease (either insufficiency or stenosis).

B. Findings With Invasive Monitoring

1. Hypotension (systolic BP < 90 mmHg or ≥ 30 mmHg below normal baseline BP for ≥ 30 minutes).

2. Elevated PAOP (> 15 mmHg).

3. Decreased CI (< 2.2 $L/min/m^2$ body surface area).

4. Elevated arteriovenous oxygen difference (> 5.5 mL O_2 /dL).

C. Laboratory Studies

Immediately obtain an ECG, portable chest roentgenogram, arterial blood gas values (ABG), complete blood count (CBC), and blood urea nitrogen (BUN), creatinine, glucose, calcium, magnesium, phosphorus, and serum electrolyte levels. Additional studies obtained (e.g., prothrombin time, partial thromboplastin time, creatinine phosphokinase, lactate dehydrogenase) depend on the clinical situation. The ECG usually reveals significant abnormalities. The chest roentgenogram frequently shows pulmonary vascular congestion or frank pulmonary edema. Echocardiography may be extremely valuable (e.g., by visualizing valve dysfunction, global systolic function, wall-motion abnormalities, or pericardial effusions) if the cause of cardiogenic shock is otherwise not clinically apparent.

III. DIAGNOSIS

The diagnosis of cardiogenic shock is based on the clinical syndrome of tissue hypoperfusion (inadequate peripheral perfusion, hypotension, oliguria, and, possibly, mental status changes) in the setting of *adequate* intravascular volume and a primary or secondary cause of cardiac dysfunction.

IV. THERAPY

A. *Provide initial care of the patient in impending or actual shock* (see General Concepts, earlier in this chapter).

    1. Allow the awake patient in acute pulmonary edema to assume an upright posture unless hypotension is severe.

    2. Endotracheal intubation is sometimes necessary (e.g., in the setting of airway compromise, inadequate oxygenation or ventilation, severe pulmonary edema, or profound shock [see Chapter 11]).

    3. Tension pneumothorax (as a secondary cause of cardiac dysfunction) should be identified immediately at the time of the primary survey and treated with needle decompression followed by chest tube thoracostomy.

B. *Immediately treat cardiac arrhythmias responsible for, or contributing to, the impending or actual shock state.* Assess the patient's cardiac rhythm from the cardiac monitor and the ECG. Immediately manage any arrhythmias per Advanced Cardiac Life Support (ACLS) guidelines (see arrhythmia management in Chapter 13).

C. *Identify any volume deficit that may be contributing to the shock state and treat as appropriate.*

    1. The patient with acute or chronic cardiac disease may simultaneously be suffering from a volume deficit. This may be suspected on the basis of the history (e.g., poor oral intake, nausea/vomiting/or diarrhea, profuse diaphoresis, acute hemorrhage), physical examination (e.g., poor peripheral perfusion despite clear lung fields and normal heart sounds), and laboratory studies (e.g., clear chest roentgenogram).

    2. In the absence of acute pulmonary edema, administer a fluid bolus of NS (250–500 mL) and note the patient's response. Repeat boluses are indicated if the patient clinically improves and lung fields remain clear. If invasive central monitoring has been accomplished, a PAOP of 18-20 mmHg in most situations indicates an appropriate intravascular volume (i.e., a "full tank").

    3. Nearly one-half of all acute *inferior MIs* result in RV infarction. Obtain a reverse ECG; look carefully at the right precordial lead *V4R* for ST-segment elevation, which is 70% sensitive and 100% specific for RV infarction. Cardiogenic shock in these patients is frequently responsive to volume loading with normal saline and dobutamine therapy (see IV. D, below).

    4. *Caution:* in the setting of acute pulmonary edema, do *not* administer further volume to the patient. Proceed directly to

vasopressors as outlined below. Vasopressor therapy is also appropriate if the patient with clear lung fields and hypotension fails to respond, or deteriorates, with volume challenge in the setting of known cardiac decompensation.

D. *Administer vasopressors if volume infusion* (see IV. C, above) is either contraindicated or ineffectual. The systolic BP should generally be maintained at 100 mmHg with vasopressor therapy if myocardial ischemia is suspected. Medication choices include the following:

1. Dopamine
   a. The effects of dopamine depend on its dosing. At low doses (1–2 μg/kg/min IV) dopamine dilates renal and mesenteric blood vessels. At intermediate doses (2–10 μg/kg/min IV) it maintains its splanchnic effects but has significant beta-adrenergic receptor (inotropic) effects, which result in increased cardiac output. At high doses (> 10 μg/kg/min IV) increasing alpha-adrenergic receptor effects and peripheral vasoconstriction occur.
   b. Dopamine is usually the vasopressor of choice in the patient with signs and symptoms of cardiogenic shock when the systolic BP is < 90–100 mmHg. A reasonable starting dose is 5 μg/kg/min IV, with subsequent dose titration as necessary to maintain adequate perfusion pressure.
   c. *Caution:* heart rate and PAOP usually increase with use. Dopamine may also precipitate arrhythmias, and extravasation can cause tissue necrosis. It is contraindicated in patients with pheochromocytoma or a hypersensitivity to sulfites.
2. Norepinephrine
   a. Norepinephrine has largely alpha-adrenergic receptor (vasoconstricting) properties with some minimal beta-adrenergic receptor effects as well. The starting dose is 0.5–1.0 μg/min IV, with subsequent titration to the desired effect (doses as high as 30 μg/min may be necessary).
   b. Norepinephrine should be considered in the profoundly hypotensive patient (systolic BP < 70 mmHg) in cardiogenic shock. When the patient's blood pressure improves to > 70 mmHg, dopamine should be added and the norepinephrine gradually decreased and discontinued if possible.
   c. Norepinephrine is also indicated if the cardiogenic shock patient initially started on dopamine (as described under IV. D. 1, above) fails to show an appropriate clinical and BP response.
   d. *Cautions:* peripheral or mesenteric vascular ischemia may occur with use. Increase in afterload may cause deterioration in cardiac function. Extravasation can cause severe tissue necrosis. Norepinephrine is contraindicated in patients with a hypersensitivity to sulfites.

3. Dobutamine
   a. This beta-1 adrenergic agonist (inotrope) is used in the treatment of significant CHF. The usual starting dose is 2–5 μg/kg/min IV, with titration upward (to 20 μg/kg/min) if necessary.
   b. Dobutamine is an appropriate initial agent in the *nonhypotensive* patient (systolic BP ≥ 90–100 mmHg) with significant cardiac failure. If the patient is also hypotensive, first support the BP with dopamine (see IV. D. 1, above) *before* beginning dobutamine.
   c. Dobutamine is preferred over dopamine as a vasopressor in the setting of RV infarction.
   d. Invasive hemodynamic monitoring, with measurement of CO, PAOP, and systemic vascular resistance (SVR), assists with the appropriate management and titration of dobutamine.
   e. *Cautions:* heart rate usually increases with dobutamine use, and it may precipitate arrhythmias. It is contraindicated in patients with idiopathic hypertrophic subaortic stenosis or in individuals with a hypersensitivity to sulfites.

4. Phosphodiesterase Inhibitors (Amrinone or Milrinone)
   a. These agents result in increased cardiac contractility without adrenergic stimulation. They should be considered in patients who have failed to improve with catecholamine therapy as outlined above or when arrhythmias or worsened ischemia limit effective catecholamine use. Unfortunately, long-term studies show *increased* mortality in heart failure patients treated with phosphodiesterase inhibitors.
   b. Amrinone dosing: 0.75 mg/kg IV over 2–3 min followed by a maintenance infusion of 5–10 μg/kg/min (not to exceed a total dose of 10 mg/kg/day). The initial bolus may need to be repeated in 30 minutes. Reduce dose by 50–75% in patients with renal failure and a creatinine clearance of < 10 mL/min.
   c. Milrinone dosing: 50 μg/kg IV loading dose over 10 minutes followed by 0.375–0.75 μg/kg/min continuous infusion (total daily dose is between 0.59–1.13 mg/kg).

E. *Consider vasodilator therapy (with nitroglycerin or sodium nitroprusside)* **after** *the patient's BP has been stabilized (systolic BP 100 mmHg) with the above steps.*

1. Vasodilators reduce afterload and can improve pump function. They are especially useful when:
   a. The cause of the pump problem is severe hypertension;
   b. The patient is in significant pulmonary edema; or
   c. Valvular decompensation (e.g., severe acute mitral regurgitation) is present. Ideally, invasive hemodynamic monitoring should be initiated *before* beginning vasodilator therapy in the setting of cardiogenic shock.

2. Nitroglycerin
   a. Nitroglycerin is a smooth muscle relaxant; it dilates both veins and arteries (more prominent venodilation at lower doses). In the setting of myocardial ischemia, it is the preferred vasodilator.
   b. *Dose:* begin at 10 μg/min IV and increase by 5–10 μg/min every 5–10 minutes as BP allows, to a maximum dose of 200 μg/min.
   c. *Cautions:* nitroglycerin may result in systemic hypotension (systolic BP < 100 mmHg), especially in patients with volume depletion (e.g., profuse diaphoresis, vomiting) or those with RV infarction. Under no circumstances should the systolic BP fall below 100 mmHg in the setting of ongoing myocardial ischemia. Other potential complications of nitroglycerin therapy include headache, tachycardia, paradoxical bradycardia, pulmonary ventilation-perfusion mismatch, and methemoglobinemia.

3. Sodium nitroprusside
   a. Sodium nitroprusside is a potent peripheral vasodilator affecting both arteries and veins.
   b. *Dose:* begin IV infusion at 0.5–2.0 μg/kg/min and titrate as necessary (maximum dose 10 μg/kg/min).
   c. *Cautions:* complications of therapy include coronary "steal" (preferential blood flow to nonischemic coronary vascular beds), hypotension, headaches, abdominal cramping, nausea/vomiting, worsened pulmonary ventilation-perfusion mismatch, and eventual accumulation of cyanide and thiocyanate (byproducts of sodium nitroprusside metabolism). Invasive central monitoring will assist with the appropriate titration of this medication in the patient with cardiac dysfunction.

F. *Provide definitive therapy for the cause of cardiac dysfunction.* This should take place simultaneously with the above-outlined therapy.

1. **Acute Myocardial Infarction.** See "Myocardial Infarction" in Chapter 13. Treatment generally includes oxygen, aspirin, and reperfusion therapy with or without heparin. Morphine and nitroglycerin may also be administered once the patient's BP has been stabilized as outlined in IV. C and IV. D above. Indications for an intra-aortic balloon pump in this setting (as a "bridge" to reperfusion therapy) include cardiogenic shock or severe CHF unresponsive to maximal medical therapy or persistent ischemic pain despite maximal medical intervention.
   a. In the setting of cardiogenic shock, emergent coronary angiography and angioplasty are preferred over peripherally administered thrombolytic therapy. If this level of cardiac care is not available at the given institution, thrombolytic therapy should be administered to appropriate candidates and the patient transferred to a center capable of coronary

artery angiography and mechanical reperfusion (angioplasty or bypass surgery).

b. Patients suffering a right ventricular infarction should be treated with oxygen, aspirin, volume loading (see IV. C, above), dobutamine (see IV. D. 3, above), and reperfusion therapy. Nitrates and diuretics should be avoided because of the risks of significantly worsening hypotension.

2. **Acute Pulmonary Edema.** See "Congestive Heart Failure" in Chapter 13.

   a. Initial therapy generally includes upright posture (unless the patient is significantly hypotensive), oxygen, morphine, furosemide, and nitroglycerin. The hypotensive patient should not be given morphine, furosemide, or nitroglycerin until the BP has been stabilized with a vasopressor (dopamine with or without dobutamine) as outlined in IV. D, above. Ongoing myocardial ischemia should be treated simultaneously.

   b. Additional therapy for acute pulmonary edema may include dobutamine (if not started earlier), dopamine (if not started earlier), sodium nitroprusside, continuous positive airway pressure (CPAP), or positive end-expiratory pressure (PEEP) if the patient has been intubated.

   c. Third-line actions may include amrinone, aminophylline (if the patient is wheezing), and/or an intra-aortic balloon pump (as a "bridge" to definitive care of the underlying cardiac condition responsible for CHF).

3. **Acute Valvular Decompensation.** Patients with acute severe mitral regurgitation or ventricular septal rupture require immediate treatment with oxygen, invasive monitoring, precise volume management (to a PAOP of 18 mmHg), vasopressor therapy (see IV. D, above), afterload reduction (see IV. E, above), and an intra-aortic balloon pump (as a "bridge" to definitive surgery). Emergently consult a cardiothoracic surgeon.

4. **Cardiac Tamponade**

   a. Clinical findings may include tachycardia, normal or decreased BP, elevated jugular venous pressure, pulsus paradoxus, and distant heart sounds. Kussmaul's sign is an increase in jugular venous pressure during inspiration. Central venous pressure is elevated (unless a concomitant volume deficit is present). Echocardiography will confirm the diagnosis and should be obtained emergently.

   b. Treatment includes oxygen, aggressive saline administration augmented with dopamine for BP support, and pericardiocentesis or surgical pericardiotomy. If the clinical situation allows, pericardiocentesis should be performed with echocardiographic guidance.

   c. *Caution:* nitrates, diuretics, or other agents that may reduce preload are absolutely contraindicated in this setting.

V. DISPOSITION

Patients in cardiogenic shock must be admitted to the ICU. The admitting facility must be capable of providing the level of cardiac care the patient requires or an appropriate transfer, after necessary stabilization and consultation, should be arranged.

HYPOVOLEMIC SHOCK

I. ESSENTIAL FACTS

A. Definition

Hypovolemic shock is inadequate tissue perfusion and oxygenation secondary to volume depletion.

B. Etiology

See General Concepts, earlier in this chapter.

C. Classification of Acute Hemorrhagic Shock

Hypovolemic shock is frequently a consequence of acute blood loss. The normal circulating blood volume of a healthy adult is 7% of the ideal body weight. With acute and on-going hemorrhage, a graded physiologic response occurs as outlined in Table 12–3. The classification presented in Table 12–3, however, is a guideline

Table 12–3. CLINICAL RESPONSES TO ACUTE HEMORRHAGE

BLOOD VOLUME LOSS	MILD (< 20%)	MODERATE (20-40%)	SEVERE (> 40%)
Vital Signs	Variable tachycardia; orthostatic vital sign changes	Tachycardia; supine hypotension; tachypnea	Marked tachycardia; supine hypotension; rapid and deep respirations
Skin	Normal to cool and moist	Clammy, diaphoretic, delayed capillary refill	Pale, mouled, peripheral cyanosis, markedly delayed capillary refill
Urine Output	Normal to concentrated	Oliguria	Anuria
Mental Status	Normal to anxious	Restless, anxious to confused	Confused to obtunded

Adapted from Trunkey DD, Salber PR, Mills J. Chapter 3: Shock, Table 3-2, p. 52. *In* Saunders CE and MT Ho (eds): Current Emergency Diagnosis and Treatment, 1992, Appleton and Lange.

only; individual patient characteristics may result in variations from the expected responses. For example, the athlete, elderly individuals, or those taking beta-adrenergic blocking drugs may not mount the expected level of tachycardia for any given volume of blood loss.

II. CLINICAL PRESENTATION

A. Signs and Symptoms

1. Nonspecific clinical findings are as outlined in General Concepts, earlier in this chapter. The patient's neck veins are flat and CVP is low (unless a primary or secondary disorder of pump function is also present).

2. Other symptoms and signs depend on the specific cause of volume loss. After the initial primary survey and resuscitation, a complete head-to-toe physical examination is appropriate in all seriously or critically ill patients.

B. Laboratory Studies

1. Immediately obtain a spun hematocrit, CBC (including platelets), ABG, BUN, creatinine, glucose, serum electrolyte values, ECG, portable chest roentgenogram, prothrombin time (PT), partial thromboplastin time (PTT), and pregnancy test (in females of reproductive age).

2. Remember, the patient's initial hematocrit is *unreliable* for estimating acute blood loss or in diagnosing shock. Serial hematocrits are helpful, however, in following the patient's response to resuscitation.

3. Send a blood sample for type and crossmatch purposes in the setting of suspected hemorrhage (see blood component therapy in Chapter 21).

4. Additional studies obtained (e.g., amylase, bilirubin, abdominal computed tomography (CT) scan, diagnostic peritoneal lavage) depend on the clinical situation.

5. Arterial or central venous lactate levels may be measured and followed serially as one guide to adequate therapy. Normal lactate values are 0.3–1.3 mmol/L. In critically ill patients, blood lactate levels > 4 mmol/L, or raised levels that fail to progressively clear with appropriate therapy, are concerning and associated with a worse prognosis.

III. DIAGNOSIS

The diagnosis of hypovolemic shock is based on the clinical syndrome of tissue hypoperfusion (inadequate peripheral perfusion, tachycardia, with or without hypotension, oliguria, with or without mental status changes) in the setting of known or suspected volume loss (including hemorrhage). *The tachycardic and/or hypotensive trauma patient is bleeding and in hypovolemic shock until proven otherwise.* Patients with *undiagnosed* shock should also be assumed to be hypovolemic until proven otherwise.

IV. THERAPY

The treatment goals of the ED physician are to ensure an adequate airway, oxygenation, and ventilation, stabilize hemodynamic parameters as necessary with volume replacement (including blood products if clinically indicated), identify and treat the cause of volume loss, and arrange for definitive care.

A. *Provide initial care of the patient in impending or actual shock* (see General Concepts, earlier in this chapter).

1. Administer supplemental oxygen, and immobilize the cervical spine if clinically indicated. Endotracheal intubation is sometimes necessary (e.g., in the setting of upper-airway compromise, inadequate oxygenation or ventilation, or profound shock [see Chapter 11]).

2. Rapidly obtain vital signs, establish large bore intravenous access (at least two 14–16-gauge upper-extremity IV lines are recommended), obtain blood samples for indicated laboratory studies (see II. B, above), and continuously monitor both cardiac rhythm and SaO_2. If acute hemorrhage is a possibility, emergently order blood type and crossmatch and obtain serial hematocrits.

3. Control any obvious external hemorrhage with direct pressure.

4. Obtain an ECG and portable chest roentgenogram. In the patient suffering from multiple trauma, also obtain a bedside cervical spine series (anterior-posterior [AP], lateral, and odontoid views) and an AP pelvis film.

B. *Stabilize hemodynamic parameters by initiating volume replacement with crystalloid: either warmed NS or LR.*

1. If hemorrhage is not the cause of hypovolemia, replace volume deficits as necessary with IV crystalloid.

2. If acute hemorrhage is a possible or known cause of hypovolemia:
   a. Rapidly administer up to 2 L warmed crystalloid (*note:* in the individual in extremis secondary to acute hemorrhage, low-titer O-negative whole blood should be started emergently at the outset of the resuscitation; see Chapter 21).
   b. If the adult patient with an acute hemorrhage has not rapidly stabilized with up to 2 L crystalloid infusion, begin type-specific blood transfusion as well. Emergent operative intervention for internal (e.g., intrathoracic, intraperitoneal) hemorrhage control may be necessary depending on the

clinical circumstances; obtain an emergent surgical consultation as indicated.

   c. Maintain the patient's platelet count > 50,000/μL by transfusing platelets if necessary. If coagulation studies (i.e., PT/PTT) are abnormal, correct pre-existing coagulopathy with fresh-frozen plasma.

3. Monitor cardiopulmonary systems carefully, and avoid inducing CHF or pulmonary edema. A central venous catheter and CVP monitoring may assist in managing fluid resuscitation; consider a Swan-Ganz catheter in the patient with significant cardiopulmonary disease or renal insufficiency (see General Concepts, earlier in this chapter).

4. Consider additional interventions as indicated (e.g., nasogastric tube, Foley catheter, appropriate splinting of injured extremities; treatment of acid–base or electrolyte disorders). Remember the cardiovascular triad (see General Concepts, earlier in this chapter) and accurately identify and treat concomitant arrhythmias (see Chapter 13) and/or myocardial dysfunction. In the trauma patient, tension pneumothorax and cardiac tamponade (both "secondary" causes of pump dysfunction) should be identified and immediately treated at the time of the primary survey.

5. Continually reassess the patient's hemodynamic status throughout the ED stay.

C. *Identify and treat the cause of hypovolemia.* This should be accomplished simultaneously with the above-outlined therapy.

1. Consider the many potential causes of volume loss (see General Concepts, earlier in this chapter). Obtain a history and perform a complete physical examination with these possibilities in mind, and urgently order any additional necessary diagnostic studies.

2. Obtain appropriate consultation as clinically indicated. In the serious or critically ill patient, emergent consultant involvement should be a component of the patient's initial shock care (e.g., an obstetrician in the unstable female patient with suspected ectopic pregnancy, a general surgeon in the hemodynamically unstable trauma patient).

D. *Arrange for definitive care and hospitalization* (see V, below).

E. *Additional issues:*

1. **Hypertonic Saline.** Small-volume hypertonic saline solutions (e.g., 250 mL of 7.5% NaCl in 6% dextran 70) are under investigation as initial resuscitation fluids in the adult patient with significant hypovolemia (e.g., from thermal injury or acute trauma-related hemorrhage). These solutions result in an osmotic fluid shift from the interstitial and intracellular spaces to the intravascular compartment, improve cardiac efficiency,

and decrease SVR. Their use at this time, however, should be restricted to well-designed clinical trials.

2. **Pneumatic Anti-Shock Garment** (PASG). Application of the PASG increases peripheral vascular resistance, "auto-transfuses" blood from the lower body regions compressed by the garment to the upper body, and theoretically helps control hemorrhage in those body areas directly compressed by the garment. Its use is controversial and should generally only be considered in the patient with severe pelvic fractures and potential retroperitoneal hemorrhage while awaiting definitive care. Unfortunately, efficacy of the PASG in ultimately improving patient outcome has not been demonstrated, and many studies show an increased mortality with its prehospital use. Contraindications to the PASG include pulmonary edema, bleeding from sites outside the body regions compressed by the garment (e.g., intrathoracic hemorrhage), and diaphragmatic rupture.

3. **"Restricted" Crystalloid Resuscitation.** Actual *restriction* of crystalloid fluids may be appropriate in the hypotensive trauma patient with penetrating torso injuries until expeditious and emergent operative control of internal hemorrhage is achieved. This concept challenges the traditional recommendation for aggressive crystalloid volume resuscitation in this setting. In a recent prospective trial of 598 hypotensive adults with penetrating torso injuries, the rate of survival was 70% in the delayed fluid resuscitation group as compared to 62% in the immediate fluid resuscitation group ($P = 0.04$). Further studies are needed, however, before this practice is adopted as the standard of care in the victim of penetrating trauma.

4. **Emergency Thoracotomy and Direct ("Open") Cardiac Massage.** The patient with profound hypovolemia may suffer a cardiac arrest. Emergency thoracotomy and direct cardiac massage is indicated when the victim of penetrating chest trauma arrests in the ED. If the patient arrests at the scene or enroute to the hospital, survival is not improved with emergency thoracotomy if prolonged cardiopulmonary resuscitation (CPR) was required prior to the procedure (in one series, there were no survivors if CPR was performed for > 9.4 minutes prior to emergency thoracotomy). Emergency thoracotomy should also be considered when cardiac arrest occurs secondary to hypothermia, pulmonary embolism, or acute intraabdominal hemorrhage (e.g., secondary to penetrating abdominal trauma or other acute vascular catastrophe).

V. DISPOSITION

Patients seen in the ED with hypovolemic shock should be admitted to the hospital for definitive and intensive care.

SEPTIC SHOCK

I. GENERAL CONCEPTS

A. Definitions

The American College of Chest Physicians–Society of Critical Care Medicine Consensus Conference (1992) has defined the following terms:

1. *Bacteremia:* the presence of viable bacteria in the blood (usually confirmed by positive blood cultures).

2. *Sepsis:* clinical evidence of infection (e.g., viral, bacterial, or fungal) accompanied by a systemic response, including two or more of the following:
   a. Tachypnea (respiratory rate > 20 breaths/min or PCO_2 < 32 mmHg; if the patient is mechanically ventilated, minute ventilation is > 10 L/min);
   b. Tachycardia (heart rate > 90 beats/min);
   c. Hyperthermia or hypothermia (core or rectal body temperature > 38°C or < 36°C); and/or
   d. Elevation or reduction in the leukocyte count (> 12,000 cells/μL, or < 4,000 cells/μL, or ≥ 10% bands).

3. *Systemic inflammatory response syndrome* (SIRS): the presence of a severe clinical insult (e.g., burns, hypoxia, ischemia, pancreatitis, significant trauma) accompanied by two or more of the same systemic responses as outlined under sepsis, above.

4. *Severe sepsis:* hypoperfusion (e.g., altered mentation, lactic acidosis, and/or oliguria), hypotension, or organ dysfunction associated with sepsis.

5. *Septic shock:* sepsis accompanied by hypotension (systolic BP < 90 mmHg or ≥ 40 mmHg below normal baseline) and perfusion abnormalities despite adequate fluid resuscitation. *Refractory septic shock* is present when hypotension lasts > 1 hour despite appropriate volume replacement and high-dose vasopressor use.

6. *Multiple organ dysfunction syndrome* (MODS): syndrome of altered organ function in an acutely ill patient requiring intervention to maintain homeostasis.

B. Etiology

Septic shock begins with an infection (e.g., abscess, cellulitis, pneumonia, pyelonephritis, peritonitis) caused by gram-positive or gram-negative bacteria, or, infrequently, viruses, or fungi. Microorganism proliferation results in direct blood stream invasion and/or release of locally produced substances into the blood (e.g., exotoxins, teichoic acid antigen). This is followed by the release from plasma precursors, monocytes or macrophages, endothelial cells, and/or neutrophils of endogenous inflammatory mediators. These latter include arachidonic acid metabolites, complement C5a, coagulation factors, cytokines, endorphins, endothelium-derived relaxing factor, kinin, myocardial depressant substances, and platelet-activating factor. These mediators result in significant physiologic effects that may include direct organ injury (e.g., acute renal failure, adult respiratory distress syndrome [ARDS], hepatic failure, disseminated intravascular coagulation [DIC]), vasodilation, endothelial-cell dysfunction and altered capillary permeability, leukocyte aggregation, and myocardial depression. If aggressive therapy does not reverse the process, death ultimately results from refractory hypotension or multiple organ failure.

C. Incidence

It is estimated that 400,000 cases of sepsis and 200,000 episodes of septic shock occur annually in the United States. Septic shock is the leading cause of death in the ICU, and it is the 13th most common cause of death in this nation.

D. Mortality

Varies between 20 and 80% depending on the study and the definition of septic shock used. Roughly 50% of patients hypotensive secondary to sepsis who are admitted to the ICU ultimately die.

E. Risk Factors for Sepsis

Risk factors include age (the very young or the elderly), burn injury, chronic alcohol abuse, chronic renal failure, diabetes mellitus, endothelial disruption, hypoxia, hypotension or hypoperfusion of any cause, immunosuppression (e.g., autoimmune diseases, cancer and/or cancer chemotherapy, congenital immunodeficiency states, corticosteroid use, human immunodeficiency virus infection, immunosuppressive medication after organ transplantation, neutropenia), infection (gram-positive or gram-negative bacteria, fungi, viruses), malnutrition, and multisystem trauma.

II. CLINICAL PRESENTATION

A. Signs and Symptoms

1. Early signs of sepsis include temperature instability (hyperthermia most commonly, but hypothermia may occur, especially in the elderly or otherwise debilitated patient), tachypnea, tachycardia, oliguria, and possibly mental status changes. The skin is initially warm and flushed secondary to decreased vascular resistance.

2. Later manifestations are those of inadequate organ perfusion, including impaired capillary refill, hypotension, worsened

mental status, further decline in urine output, impaired myocardial function, and lactic acidosis.

3. Additional findings depend on the site of infection. Most commonly this is the genitourinary tract, followed by the respiratory and gastrointestinal tracts. Other sites include the skin, wounds, and indwelling catheters. After the initial primary survey and resuscitation, a complete head-to-toe physical examination is mandatory in search of the site(s) of infection or other pertinent abnormalities.

B. Laboratory Studies

1. Obtain a complete blood count (leukocytosis and/or bandemia are common; but a normal leukocyte count or leukopenia may occur), ABG, arterial lactate, BUN, creatinine, glucose, serum electrolytes, ECG, chest roentgenogram, PT, PTT, pregnancy test (in females of reproductive age), blood cultures (at least two), urinalysis, and urine culture.

2. Additional laboratory studies may also be appropriate depending on the clinical circumstances (e.g., amylase, bilirubin, liver function tests, fibrinogen level, fibrinogen degradation products).

3. Other overt foci of infection should be cultured as clinically indicated (e.g., abscesses, cerebrospinal fluid, cervix, infected or inflamed joints, skin, pharynx, rectum, stool, sputum, and/or wounds).

III. DIAGNOSIS

The diagnosis of septic shock is based on the clinical syndrome of sepsis accompanied by hypotension and other perfusion abnormalities. The differential diagnosis includes other causes of shock (including anaphylaxis, cardiogenic shock, and hypovolemic shock).

IV. THERAPY

The treatment goals of the ED physician are to insure an adequate airway, oxygenation, and ventilation; restore intravascular volume; stabilize hemodynamic parameters with vasopressor support; obtain appropriate cultures and urgently administer antibiotic therapy; and arrange for definitive care for the underlying cause of the infection (e.g., drainage of abscesses; relief of visceral obstruction).

A. *Provide initial care of the patient in impending or actual shock* (see General Concepts, earlier in this chapter). Endotracheal intubation may be necessary (e.g., in the setting of airway compromise, inadequate oxygenation or ventilation, or profound shock [see Chapter 11]).

B. *Initiate crystalloid volume replacement: either NS or LR.*

1. Begin crystalloid replacement at the rate of 250 mL IV every 15 minutes, and adjust rate as dictated by vital signs, tissue perfusion, cardiopulmonary status, and urine output. Volume deficits may be in excess of 4–6 L secondary to capillary leak phenomenon.

2. If invasive central monitoring has been accomplished, do not exceed a PAOP of approximately 15 mmHg.

3. *Caution:* monitor cardiopulmonary status closely and do not volume overload the patient. Pulmonary edema, cerebral edema, and ARDS are significant potential complications.

C. *Administer vasopressors for further hemodynamic support.* Vasopressors are appropriate in the patient with persistent hypotension and/or inadequate peripheral perfusion despite intravascular volume replacement.

1. Dopamine is the initial agent of choice under most circumstances. Begin the infusion at 5 µg/kg/min and titrate as necessary (also see Cardiogenic Shock, earlier in this chapter).

2. Norepinephrine should be considered if hypotension is profound (systolic BP < 70 mmHg) or is unresponsive to dopamine. Begin the infusion at 0.5 µg/min and titrate as necessary (also see Cardiogenic Shock, earlier in this chapter).

D. *Simultaneously with the above, obtain appropriate cultures and administer empiric antibiotic therapy.*

1. Obtain two or more blood cultures, and other cultures as indicated (e.g., sputum and urine), and promptly administer antibiotic therapy appropriate for the patient's clinical characteristics (e.g., immunocompetent or immunosuppressed) and suspected source of infection (see Chapter 15).

2. If the source of infection is unknown, but the patient is immunocompetent, consider one of the following antibiotic regimens:
   a. Imipenem 500 mg IV every 6 hours, *or*
   b. Third-generation cephalosporin (e.g., ceftazidime 2 g IV every 8 hours or ceftriaxone 2 g IV every 12 hours or cefotaxime 2 g IV every 4 hours) and an antipseudomonal aminoglycoside (e.g., gentamicin or tobramycin 2 mg/kg IV load followed by 1.5 mg/kg IV every 8-12 hours; remember potential for nephrotoxicity and ototoxicity; dose carefully and follow serum levels), *or*
   c. Antipseudomonal penicillin (e.g., mezlocillin 225–300 mg/kg/day IV in four to six divided doses, usually 4 g IV every 6 hours or 3 g IV every 4 hours; or ticarcillin 200–300 mg/kg/day IV in divided doses every 4–6 hours, usually 4

g IV every 6 hours or 3 g IV every 4 hours; or piperacillin 3–4 g IV every 4–6 hours, maximum dose 24 g/day; or ticarcillin-clavulanate 3.1 g IV every 4–6 hours) and an antipseudomonal aminoglycoside, *or*

d. Cefoxitin 2 g IV every 4 hours or 3 g IV every 6 hours or cefotetan 2 g IV every 12 hours and an antipseudomonal aminoglycoside, *or*

e. Ampicillin 2 g IV every 6 hours or ampicillin-sulbactam (Unasyn) 3 g IV every 6 hours and clindamycin 600 mg IV every 6–8 hours or 900 mg IV every 8 hours and an antipseudomonal aminoglycoside.

3. If the patient is neutropenic or otherwise immunocompromised, either of the following regimens is appropriate.

a. Imipenem, *or*

b. An antipseudomonal penicillin (e.g., mezlocillin or ticarcillin or piperacillin) or an antipseudomonal cephalosporin (e.g., ceftazidime or cefoperazone 2 g IV every 12 hours) and an antipseudomonal aminoglycoside ± vancomycin 500 mg IV every 6 hours.

4. *Caution:* do not delay antibiotic therapy if acquisition of additional cultures, other than blood, will be delayed (e.g., patient with possible meningitis who requires a head CT prior to a lumbar puncture). Under these circumstances, proceed with antibiotic therapy immediately after the blood cultures are obtained!

E. *Obtain specialist consultation (e.g., internal medicine, general surgery, infectious disease) and arrange for definitive care (including indicated drainage and/or debridement procedures).*

F. *Additional issues:*

1. **Corticosteroids.** These are unhelpful in the management of human septic shock. Their administration is necessary, however, in the patient with clinically suspected adrenal insufficiency (see Chapter 19).

2. **Monoclonal Antiendotoxin Antibody Preparations.** These have yet to be proven clearly beneficial to patients; further clinical evaluation is necessary.

3. **Naloxone.** This opioid antagonist may be helpful in reversing endotoxin-mediated hypotension. It is not FDA approved for this use, however, and further clinical evaluation is necessary. Recommended dose: 0.8 mg IV, with dose doubled and repeated every few minutes as necessary to a maximum of 4 mg total over time).

4. **Other Sepsis Mediator Inhibitors.** Examples include monoclonal antibodies to tumor necrosis factor and interleukin-1 receptor antagonists. These are currently experimental only. Recommendations on use must await the results of clinical trials now being conducted.

V. DISPOSITION

The patient in septic shock must be admitted to the ICU.

BIBLIOGRAPHY

Bickell WH, Wall MJ Jr, Pepe PE, et al: Immediate versus delayed fluid resuscitation for hypotensive patients with penetrating torso injuries. N Engl J Med 1994;331:1105–1109.
Bochner BS, Lichtenstein LM: Anaphylaxis. N Engl J Med 1991;324:1785–1790.
Bone RC: The pathogenesis of sepsis. Ann Intern Med 1991;115:457–469.
Califf RM, Benstson JR: Cardiogenic shock. N Engl J Med 1994;1724–1730.
Committee on Emergency Cardiac Care, 1991–1994: Hypotension/shock/acute pulmonary edema. Chapter 1: Essentials of ACLS. In Cummins RO (ed): Textbook of Advanced Cardiac Life Support. American Heart Association, 1994, pp. 1-40–1-47.
Jorden RC: Penetrating chest trauma. Emerg Med Clin N Am 1993;11:97–106.
Kinch JW, Ryan TJ: Right ventricular infarction. N Engl J Med 1994;330:1211–1217.
Members of the ACCP–SCCM Consensus Conference Committee: American College of Chest Physicians–Society of Critical Care Medicine Consensus Conference: Definitions for sepsis and organ failure and guidelines for the use of innovative therapies in sepsis. Crit Care Med 1992;20:864.
NIH Conference: Selected treatment strategies for septic shock based on proposed mechanisms of pathogenesis. Ann Intern Med 1994;120:771–783.
Parrillo JE: Pathogenetic mechanisms of septic shock. N Engl J Med 1993;328:1471–1477.
Rackow EC, Astiz ME: Pathophysiology and treatment of septic shock. JAMA 1991;266:548–554.
Rady MY, Smithline HA, Blake H, Nowak R: A comparison of the shock index and conventional vital signs to identify acute, critical illness in the emergency department. Ann Emerg Med 1994;24:685–690.
Reisman RE: Insect stings. N Engl J Med 1994;331:523–527.

13

Cardiovascular Emergencies

CARDIAC ARREST

"At a cardiac arrest, the first procedure is to take your own pulse."

SAMUEL SHEM

I. ESSENTIAL FACTS

A. Definition

Cardiac arrest is the absence of cardiac output with resulting loss of pulse and blood pressure (BP). *Sudden cardiac arrest* (or *sudden cardiac death)* refers to unexpected or sudden death caused by underlying heart disease occurring without symptoms or with symptoms of less than an hour's duration. Sudden cardiac arrest is the leading cause of death among adults and accounts for 400,000 deaths per year in the United States.

B. Etiology

1. Heart Disease.

Most cases of sudden cardiac arrest are associated with underlying ischemic heart disease. The actual event triggering sudden death is only partially understood, and several syndromes may be responsible. In many instances, myocardial infarction (MI) or ischemia leads to the terminal event, but in other instances a primary disturbance of the conduction system leads to ventricular fibrillation (VF) (Table 13–1).

2. Other Causes.

Causes of cardiac arrest other than ischemic heart disease are numerous. A partial list includes pulmonary embolism, prolonged QT syndrome, sepsis, hypoxia, stroke, renal failure, liver failure, electrolyte disorders, and massive blood loss.

II. THERAPY

A. Management

A discussion of the management of specific arrhythmias associated with cardiac arrest follows this section. The manage-

Table 13–1. SYNDROMES OF SUDDEN CARDIAC DEATH

	MYOCARDIAL INFARCTION	MYOCARDIAL ISCHEMIA	ELECTRICAL DISORDER
Cause of death	Infarcted area causes pump failure or may lead to rhythm disturbance	Ischemic area may trigger rhythm disturbance	Rhythm disturbance triggered by poorly understood mechanisms
Percentage of sudden cardiac death	20–30%	Unknown	Unknown
Autopsy	Coronary artery occlusion with resultant myocardial infarction	Evidence of ischemia	"Normal" heart in a small percentage of cases; usually evidence of underlying coronary artery disease
Most common rhythm	Ventricular fibrillation; other arrhythmias	Ventricular fibrillation	Ventricular fibrillation
Warning symptom prior to collapse	Minutes to hours	Minutes	None or seconds
Long-term prognosis after successful resuscitation	Good	Good	Poor

From Emergency Medical Therapy, 3rd ed, Eisenberg & Capass, eds. Table 1-17 p. 2.

ment of cardiac arrest necessitates that much be done rapidly and simultaneously. One person should assign tasks and direct therapy. Control rather than chaos can occur only if a standard approach is used. The following approach and protocols are based on the American Heart Association's 1992 Standards and Guidelines for Emergency Cardiac Care. These guidelines should not preclude flexibility in the management of cardiac arrhythmias.

1. Confirm cardiac arrest
   a. Establish unresponsiveness.
   b. Call for help or call a "code" response.
   c. Assess respirations (agonal respirations may be present for several minutes following cardiac arrest) and lack of pulse.

2. Determine cardiac rhythm with quick-look paddles or cardiac electrodes if a defibrillatory monitor is present.

3. Defibrillatory shocks, if pulseless ventricular tachycardia (VT) or VF is present, are the most important aspects of therapy. Provide these as soon as possible.

4. Initiate cardiopulmonary resuscitation (CPR) if initial shocks are unsuccessful or until a defibrillator becomes available. Establish an open airway, and ventilate with mouth-to-mouth resuscitation, a pocket mask, or a bag-valve-mask device. Supplement with 100% oxygen if possible. Verify effective ventilation by observing chest-wall motion. Give two slow breaths initially followed by 10–12 breaths/min. Start closed-chest compression with the patient on a firm surface. Place the heel of the hand over the lower half of the sternum in the midline and the heel of the other hand on top of the back of the first hand. Extend the elbows so that the arms are straight and perpendicular to the patient's sternum. Firmly depress the sternum 1½–2 inches, with compression 50% of the compression–release cycle, at a rate of 80–100/min. Verify the effectiveness of cardiac compression by palpating the femoral or carotid pulse. For two-person CPR, give one ventilation over 1 to 2 seconds after every five compressions.

5. Intubate with an endotracheal tube and check for bilateral and equal breath sounds. Each intubation attempt should take no more than 20 seconds.

6. Establish an intravenous (IV) line. Use 5% dextrose in water (D5W) unless hypovolemia as the cause of arrest is suspected. If at all possible, do not interrupt CPR.

7. Give medications and/or additional defibrillatory shocks as defined in the following sections.

8. Epinephrine, lidocaine, and atropine can be administered endotracheally when IV access cannot be obtained. The dose

should be 2–2.5 times the IV dose in a 10-mL volume for endotracheally administered drugs.

9. After each IV dose of medication, give 25 ml of D5W to flush the medication, and elevate the extremity if possible.

10. Management of the airway, adequate oxygenation, chest compression, and defibrillation take precedent over IV access and medications.

B. Additional Comments

Tachyarrhythmias, bradyarrhythmias, atrioventricular (AV) block, and hypotension (discussed in following sections) should be treated vigorously during resuscitation and during the immediate postresuscitation period.

C. Complications

Numerous complications can result from CPR. These should be anticipated, especially if CPR is prolonged or if CPR is initiated by an untrained bystander. Complications include

1. Pneumothorax or hemothorax of the lung resulting from a fractured rib puncturing the lung or a vessel.

2. Aspiration of stomach contents.

3. Laceration of the liver or spleen, with internal bleeding.

4. Contusion of the heart.

5. Puncture of the coronary artery or pneumothorax secondary to laceration of the lung, either of which may occur from intracardiac injection.

III. VENTRICULAR FIBRILLATION AND PULSELESS VENTRICULAR TACHYCARDIA

Ventricular fibrillation is the most frequently encountered rhythm in sudden cardiac death in adults, seen in approximately 60% of all cases. It may also result from hypoxia, electrolyte disorders, acidosis, drug overdose, and hypothermia. Ventricular fibrillation rarely, if ever, spontaneously changes to an organized rhythm.

Defibrillatory shocks are required to stop (defibrillate) VF. They constitute the most important aspect of therapy for VF, and the sooner the shocks are given, the more likely they are to be successful.

A. Identification

Rhythm is chaotic in appearance. There are no organized complexes. Rate is indeterminate, but frequency of fibrillation on the electrocardiogram (ECG) is fast (>300/min). Ventricular fibrillation may be coarse, regular, or fine. This distinction is arbitrary, as VF does not consist of multiple rhythms; rather, the appearance of VF depends on its duration (and probably the underlying condition of the heart). Initially, VF is coarse in appearance; as it continues, the amplitude of deflection decreases such that within several minutes VF is "regular" in appearance. As VF continues still longer, the amplitude becomes less and less. After 10–15 minutes, VF appears fine; beyond 15–20 minutes, it becomes asystole. The distinction between fine VF and asystole is difficult to determine precisely. Prognostically, the coarser the VF, the more easily defibrillation can be accomplished.

The following criteria distinguish fine, medium, and coarse VF. These are arbitrary criteria.

1. *Coarse VF.* Average amplitude >7 mm.

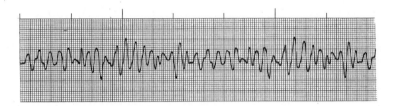

2. *Medium VF.* Average amplitude 3–≤7 mm.

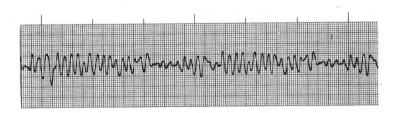

3. *Fine VF.* Average amplitude 1–<3 mm.

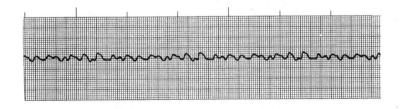

B. Clinical Evaluation

1. **History.** Frequently, collapse occurs suddenly without warning symptoms. In other cases, there may be symptoms suggestive of MI or ischemia preceding the collapse.

2. **Signs and Symptoms.** Consciousness is lost within seconds. There is no pulse or BP. Agonal respirations may be present for up to several minutes.

C. Diagnosis

See Section III. A, Identification. Ventricular fibrillation can be confused with artifact, especially if quick-look paddles are used or if leads are not fully attached.

D. Therapy

1. **General Measures.** The management of VF and pulseless VT is outlined in Figure 13–1. Drug dosages are summarized in Table 13–2.
    a. Confirm cardiac arrest by noting an unresponsive, unconscious, pulseless patient; initiate a "code" response.
    b. For witnessed cardiac arrest, give a precordial thump.
    c. Rapid defibrillation is the most important aspect of therapy and should precede CPR, establishment of an IV line, and intubation. If a defibrillator is not immediately available, perform CPR until one is. The initial three defibrillatory shocks (200 J, 300 J, and 360 J—assuming VF persists) should be given one after the other without pausing for CPR.
    d. Check the pulse and rhythm after each shock. Give the initial three shocks as rapidly as possible, assuming that VF persists.
    e. Continue CPR, intubate, and establish IV access.
    f. Give epinephrine 1 : 10,000, 1.0 mg IV, every 3–5 minutes for persistent VF. Higher subsequent doses may be considered if the initial dose of 1.0 mg is unsuccessful (Fig. 13–1).
    g. The administration of bicarbonate, 1 mEq/kg IV push, should be given if the patient has known hyperkalemia. It may possibly be helpful in other circumstances (see Fig. 13–1), but should not be given routinely. Bicarbonate, if used, may be repeated every 10 minutes (0.5 mEq/kg IV push).
    h. When defibrillation is successful a lidocaine infusion should be started at 1–4 mg/min IV. If the patient did not receive a bolus of lidocaine during the resuscitation, a 1 mg/kg bolus should be given before the infusion (and 0.5 mg/kg rebolused in 5 minutes).

2. **Refractory Ventricular Fibrillation.** Unfortunately, a significant number of people in VF, treated as outlined, either may remain in VF or may develop recurrent VF. In recurrent VF, the countershocks successfully defibrillate the myocardium but the heart soon refibrillates. The two interventions most beneficial in this situation are endotracheal intubation with administration of 100% oxygen and IV administration

200 / CARDIOVASCULAR EMERGENCIES

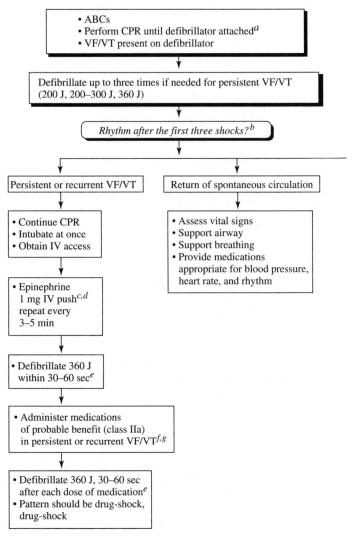

Figure 13–1. Ventricular fibrillation/pulseless ventricular tachycardia (VF/VT) treatment algorithm. PEA, pulseless electrical activity. (From Emergency Cardiac Care Committee and Subcommittees, American Heart Association: Guidelines for cardiopulmonary resuscitation and emergency cardiac care. JAMA 1992; 268:2199–2241.)

of antifibrillatory medications (see discussion of VT in the Cardiac Arrhythmias section). When refibrillation occurs, one must consider what the rhythm was during the brief period of non-VT rhythms. The therapeutic approaches may be different.

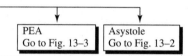

PEA Go to Fig. 13–3	Asystole Go to Fig. 13–2

Class I: definitely helpful
Class IIa: acceptable, probably helpful
Class IIb: acceptable, possibly helpful
Class III: not indicated, may be harmful

a Precordial thump is a Class IIb action in witnessed arrest, no pulse, and no defibrillator immediately available.

b Hypothermic cardiac arrest is treated differently after this point (active internal rewarming to raise core body temperature to $\geq 30°C$ before further defibrillation attempts).

c The recommended dose of epinephrine is 1 mg IV push every 3–5 min. If this approach fails, several class IIb dosing regimens can be considered:
- *Intermediate:* epinephrine 2–5 mg IV push, every 3–5 min
- *Escalating:* epinephrine 1 mg–3 mg–5 mg IV push, 3 min apart
- *High:* epinephrine 0.1 mg/kg IV push, every 3-5 min

d Sodium bicarbonate (1 mEq/kg) is class I if patient has known preexisting hyperkalemia.

e Multiple sequenced shocks (200, 200–300 J, 360 J) are acceptable here (class I), especially when medications are delayed.

f Medications:
- Lidocaine 1.5 mg/kg IV push. Repeat in 3–5 min to total loading dose of 3 mg/kg; then use
- Bretylium 5 mg/kg IV push. Repeat in 5 min at 10 mg/kg
- Magnesium sulfate 1–2 g IV in torsades de pointes or suspected hypomagnesemic state or severe refractory VF
- Procainamide 30 mg/min in refractory VF (maximum total 17 mg/kg)

g Sodium bicarbonate (1 mEq/kg IV):
Class IIa
- if known preexisting bicarbonate-responsive acidosis
- if overdose with tricyclic antidepressants
- to alkalinize the urine in certain drug overdoses
Class IIb
- if intubated and continued long arrest interval
- upon return of spontaneous circulation after long arrest interval
Class III
- hypoxic lactic acidosis

Table 13–2. MEDICATIONS USED IN CARDIAC ARREST

DRUG	INDICATION	DOSE	COMMENTS
Epinephrine	VF, PEA, asystole pulseless VT	1 mg IV push every 3–5 min	If 1-mg dose fails, consider the following regimens: *Intermediate:* 2–5 mg IV every 3–5 min *Escalating:* 1mg–3mg–5mg IV, 3 min apart *High:* 0.1 mg/kg IV every 3–5 min
Lidocaine	VF, VT	1.5 mg/kg IV push. Repeat in 3–5 min to total of 3 mg/kg	Follow success with 2–4 mg/min IV infusion.
Bretylium	VF	5 mg/kg IV push; repeat in 5 min at 10 mg/kg	Maximum dose is 30–35 mg/kg. Follow success with a 1–2-mg/min infusion.
Magnesium	Refractory VF, Torsades de pointes	1–2 g IV	
Procainamide	Refractory VF	30 mg/min IV to max of 17 mg/kg	Follow success with 1–4-mg/min infusion.
Sodium bicarbonate	Known hyperkalemia; Known pre-existing bicarbonate-responsive acidosis	1 mEq/kg IV; if necessary. Subsequent doses are 0.5 mEq/kg IV q 10 min	Should not be used routinely
Atropine	Asystole	1 mg IV; may repeat every 3–5 min to total of 0.04 mg/kg	

PEA, pulseless electrical activity.

When there is refractory or recurrent VF and defibrillation, the patient is intubated, and IV antifibrillatory agents are unsuccessful, the following conditions (listed in order of recommended consideration) should be considered as possible causes.

a. **Acidosis.** Consider improper placement of the endotracheal tube, pneumothorax, pericardial tamponade, and the need for sodium bicarbonate therapy.

b. **Alkalosis.** Alkalosis can cause or perpetuate ventricular arrhythmias. It shifts the oxyhemoglobin dissociation curve to the left, which prevents adequate delivery of oxygen to the tissues. Alkalosis can be caused by hyperventilation. If the arterial blood gas (ABG) levels demonstrate alkalosis, do *not* administer sodium bicarbonate and consider an appropriate adjustment in the rate of ventilation.

c. **Excessive Parasympathetic Stimulation.** There are occasionally patients in whom the sequence is (1) VF; (2) defibrillation to a transiently normal sinus rhythm, bradycardia, or asystole; and (3) refibrillation to VF. In this situation, excessive parasympathetic stimulation may be present. Intravenous atropine (1.0 mg) may speed up any underlying supraventricular rhythm and prevent recurrence of VF. Overdrive pacing with one of the newly available transcutaneous pacemakers may stabilize the rhythm and prevent return of VF.

d. **Excessive Catecholamine Stimulation.** If VF is defibrillated to a rapid sinus tachycardia, yet that rhythm becomes unstable and refibrillation occurs, the problem may be an excess of catecholamines. Withhold additional epinephrine, and consider IV propranolol (1.0 mg every minute up to 5 mg, if necessary). The patient with recurrent VF may then respond to repeat defibrillatory shocks when loaded with propranolol during a resuscitation attempt.

e. **Hypokalemia**. There is clinical evidence that sudden death and lethal arrhythmias in otherwise normal hypertensive patients may be triggered by diuretic-induced hypokalemia. Potassium depletion enhances automaticity, alters myocardial conduction velocity, and can cause a wide spectrum of atrial and ventricular arrhythmias. In a confirmed hypokalemic patient who is suffering recurrent VF, with only brief periods of a stable rhythm between defibrillations, consider aggressive potassium replacement: 10 mEq of potassium chloride diluted in 50 mL of D5W given over 30 minutes; repeat every 30 minutes until serum potassium measures 4.0 mEq/L.

f. **Hypomagnesemia.** Often combined with hypokalemia, hypomagnesemia is frequently observed in malnourished patients, in alcoholics, and in patients taking diuretics. Malignant rhythm disturbances, including VF, can occur with low serum magnesium levels, particularly if hypokalemia is simultaneously present. Hypomagnesemia can be corrected relatively rapidly: 1–2 g of magnesium sulfate (2–4 mL of a 50% solution) diluted in 50 ml of D5W and given IV over 1–2 minutes. Once this condition and other electrolyte abnormalities have been corrected, recurrent acute episodes of VF may disappear or additional attempts at defibrillation may be successful.

IV. VENTRICULAR FLUTTER

Ventricular flutter is a transitional rhythm between VT and VF and is usually present for a very brief time. The management is the same as that of VF.

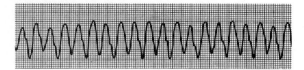

V. ASYSTOLE

A. Definition

Asystole is the end result of VF or other rhythms. On rare occasions, asystole may be the result of increased parasympathetic tone.

B. Identification

Electrical activity is absent, or the amplitude of the ECG signal is <1 mm, sometimes with occasional agonal contractions. The prognosis of successful resuscitation is extremely poor.

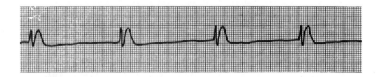

C. Clinical Evaluation

1. **History.** Usually, a history of underlying disease is obtained.
2. **Signs and symptoms.** Vital signs are absent.

D. Diagnosis

Rarely, VF may masquerade as asystole (if the VF vector is isoelectric in the particular monitoring lead). Therefore, when asystole is encountered, verify its existence with another ECG lead or by repositioning of the electrode. Always check the calibration, cables, electrodes, and cable-paddle switch, and use a low-battery indicator to confirm that asystole is not artifactual.

E. Therapy

The management of asystole is shown in Figure 13–2.

1. Confirm asystole in two leads or with repositioning of chest electrodes; maximize the "gain" dial on the monitor.
2. If it is unclear whether fine VF or asystole is present, provide a defibrillatory shock; if this is unsuccessful, proceed as indicated in Figure 13–2.
3. Repeat epinephrine and atropine every 3–5 minutes. Higher

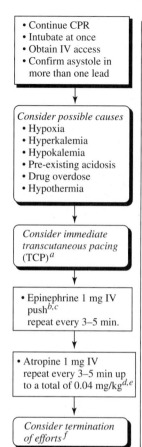

Class I: definitely helpful
Class IIa: acceptable, probably helpful
Class IIb: acceptable, possibly helpful
Class III: not indicated, may be hamful

a TCP is a Class IIb intervention. Lack of
   success may be due to delays in pacing. To
   be effective TCP must be performed early,
   simultaneously with drugs. Evidence does
   not support routine use of TCP for asystole.
b The recommended dose of epinephrine is
   1 mg IV push every 3–5 min. If this approach
   fails, several class IIb dosing regimens can
   be considered:
   • *Intermediate:* epinephrine 2–5 mg IV push,
     every 3–5 min
   • *Escalating:* epinephrine 1 mg–3 mg–5 mg IV
     push, 3 min apart
   • *High:* epinephrine 0.1 mg/kg IV push every
     3–5 min
c Sodium bicarbonate 1 mEq/kg is class I if
   patient has known preexisting hyperkalemia.
d Shorter atropine dosing intervals are class
   IIb in asystolic arrest.
e Sodium bicarbonate 1 mEq/kg:
   Class IIa
   • if known pre-existing bicarbonate-responsive
     acidosis
   • if overdose with tricyclic antidepressants
   • to alkalinize the urine in drug overdoses
   Class IIb
   • if intubated and continued long arrest
     interval
   • upon return of spontaneous circulation after
     long arrest interval
   Class III
   • hypoxic lactic acidosis
f If patient remains in asystole or other
   agonal rhythms after successful intubation
   and initial medications and no reversible
   causes are identified, consider termination of
   resuscitative efforts by a physician. Consider
   interval since arrest.

Figure 13–2. Asystole treatment algorithm. (From Emergency Cardiac Care Committee and Subcommittees, American Heart Association: Guidelines for cardiopulmonary resuscitation and emergency cardiac care. JAMA 1992; 268:2199–2241.)

doses of epinephrine can be considered (see Fig. 13–2) if there is no response to doses of 1.0 mg every 3–5 minutes.

4. Consider and treat the possible causes of asystole: hypoxia, hyperkalemia, hypokalemia, acidosis, drug overdose, or hypothermia. Bicarbonate may be useful for hyperkalemia or

acidosis. Dose: 1 mEq/kg IV push followed by 0.5 mEq/kg IV every 10 minutes as indicated.

VI. PULSELESS ELECTRICAL ACTIVITY

Pulseless electrical activity (PEA), formerly called electromechanical dissociation, is usually associated with severe myocardial damage and carries a grave prognosis.

A. Definition

Pulseless electrical activity refers to organized electrical activity (may be sinus, ventricular, or nodal) without effective cardiac contraction. In other words, an organized complex is seen on the monitor, but there is no pulse or BP.

B. Etiology

Usually, PEA is associated with underlying heart disease and frequently occurs in the setting of massive MI. It may also be the result of hypoxemia, hypovolemia, severe acidosis, pericardial tamponade, tension pneumothorax, pulmonary embolism, drug overdose, hyperkalemia and/or hypothermia.

C. Clinical Evaluation

1. **History.** Usually, a history of heart disease is obtained, but other causes (listed earlier) may be present.

2. **Signs and Symptoms.** Pulse and BP are absent.

D. Diagnosis

Pulseless electrical activity is diagnosed by the presence of organized electrical activity on the cardiac monitor with a lack of pulse and BP.

E. Therapy

1. The management of PEA is shown in Figure 13–3.
2. Administer a minimum of epinephrine 1 mg IV every 3–5 minutes.
3. If the rhythm is slow, consider atropine (1 mg IV every 3–5 minutes to a total dose of 0.04 mg/kg).
4. Consider correctable causes of PEA: hypoxemia, hypovolemia, cardiac tamponade, severe acidosis, tension pneumothorax, hyperkalemia, hypothermia, pulmonary embolism, or drug overdose.

VII. POSTRESUSCITATION CARE

The requirements of the resuscitated patient will vary from monitoring with supplemental oxygen to extensive multisystem interventions. All patients successfully resuscitated should be

Includes: • Electromechanical dissociation (EMD)
           • Pseudo-EMD
           • Idioventricular rhythms
           • Ventricular escape rhythms
           • Bradyasystolic rhythms
           • Postdefibrillation idioventricular rhythms

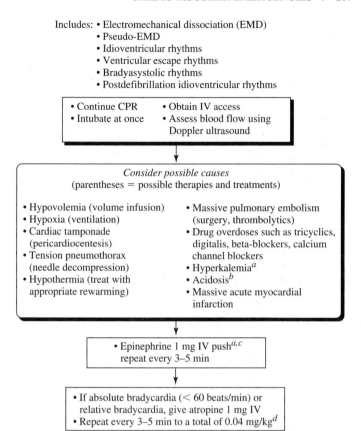

Figure 13–3. Pulseless electrical activity (electromechanical dissociation) treatment algorithm. (From Emergency Cardiac Care Committee and Subcommittees, American Heart Association: Guidelines for cardiopulmonary resuscitation and emergency cardiac care. JAMA 1992;268:2199–2241.)

Illustration continued on following page

evaluated with a 12-lead ECG and portable chest roentgenography. ABG determination, a complete blood count (CBC), electrolyte levels, magnesium, blood urea nitrogen (BUN), glucose, and cardiac enzyme levels should also be obtained (Table 13–3).

Special attention should be paid to the following:

A. Cardiovascular System

1. Patients who are hypotensive following resuscitation should receive hemodynamic monitoring to guide therapy. If hemodynamic monitoring is not possible or delayed, empiric therapy with a vasopressor may be indicated. Vasopressors are not effective if hypovolemia is present; in the absence of pulmonary edema, a fluid challenge with 250–500

Class I: definitely helpful
Class IIa: acceptable, probably helpful
Class IIb: acceptable, possibly helpful
Class III: not indicated, may be harmful

---

[a] Sodium bicarbonate 1 mEq/kg is class I if patient has known preexisting hyperkalemia
[b] Sodium bicarbonate (1 mEq/kg):
Class IIa
• if known pre-existing bicarbonate-responsive acidosis
• if overdose with tricyclic antidepressants
• to alkalinize the urine in drug overdoses
Class IIb
• if intubated and long arrest interval
• upon return of spontaneous circulation after long arrest interval
Class III
• hypoxic lactic acidosis
[c] The recommended dose of epinephrine is 1 mg IV push every 3–5 min. If this approach fails, several class IIb dosing regimens can be considered:
• Intermediate: epinephrine 2–5 mg IV push, every 3–5 min
• Escalating: epinephrine 1 mg–3 mg–5 mg IV push, 3 min apart
• High: epinephrine 0.1 mg/kg IV push, every 3–5 min
[d] Shorter atropine dosing intervals are possibly helpful in cardiac arrest (class IIb).

Figure 13–3. *Continued*

mL normal saline (NS) should be considered, and repeated as clinically indicated, before a vasopressor is given (see Chapter 12).

2. Norepinephrine bitartrate (Levophed) 4–8 mg in 500 mL D5W IV (8–16 μg/mL) may be infused (begin with 0.5–1.0 μg/min IV and titrate as necessary) to increase BP in the profoundly hypotensive patient (i.e., systolic BP < 70 mm Hg).

3. An alternative to norepinephrine is dopamine. Start dopamine 200 mg in 250 mL D5W (800 μg/mL) at 2 to 5 μg/kg/min and increase until the desired effect is achieved. Peripheral vasoconstriction generally occurs at a dosage > 10 μg/kg/min.

4. Dobutamine therapy (usual dosage 2.5–10 μg/kg/min IV) causes less systemic vasoconstriction and tachycardia and should be considered in the *nonhypotensive* patient in congestive heart failure.

B. Respiratory System

The chest roentgenogram will define the location of the tip of the endotracheal tube as well as determine pneumothorax, pulmonary edema, and fractured ribs. Patients not breathing spontaneously will require mechanical ventilation.

C. Renal System

Monitor urinary output. Bladder catheterization is appropriate.

D. Central Nervous System

Elevate the patient's head 30° to increase venous drainage. Optimal cerebral perfusion pressure is obtained by maintaining a normal or slightly elevated mean arterial pressure and a normal intracranial pressure.

E. Gastrointestinal System

Insert a nasogastric tube for patients with absent bowel sounds. Give prophylactic antacids hourly and/or antiulcer medication to prevent stress ulceration.

VIII. PEARLS AND PITFALLS

A. Continually recheck breath sounds throughout the resuscitation.

B. Appoint someone to keep the patient's family and friends informed throughout the resuscitation.

Table 13–3. POSTRESUSCITATION CARE SUMMARY

General

100% inspired oxygen
Assess electrolytes, BUN, glucose, calcium, magnesium, cardiac enzymes

Cardiovascular System

12-lead ECG
Correct hypotension:
    Fluid challenge with 250–500 mL NS, repeat if indicated
    Consider dopamine, norepinephrine (Levophed)
    Pulmonary artery flow-directed catheter for hemodynamically unstable patients
    Consider dobutamine for significant cardiac failure

Respiratory System

Mechanical ventilation, if needed
Pulse oximetry
Chest roentgenogram to confirm position of endotracheal tube and examine for
    pneumothorax
Frequent ABGs initially (intra-arterial catheter should be considered)
Carefully perform endotracheal suctioning to avoid increases in intracranial pressure;
    preoxygenate

Renal System

Catheterize bladder and monitor urine output

Central Nervous System

Elevate head of bed 30% (if BP allows)
Maintain a normal or slightly elevated mean arterial pressure
Aggressively treat seizure activity with diazepam, phenobarbital, and/or phenytoin

Gastrointestinal System

Nasogastric tube
Provide prophylactic antacids or antiulcer medications

C. A postresuscitation debriefing and review is educationally and psychologically worthwhile.

BIBLIOGRAPHY

Brooks R, McGovern BA, Garan H, et al: Current treatment of patients surviving out-of-hospital cardiac arrest. JAMA. 1991;265:762-768.

Cummins RD (ed): Textbook of Advanced Cardiac Life Support. Dallas, American Heart Association, 1994.

Emergency Cardiac Care Committee and Subcommittees, American Heart Association. Guidelines for cardiopulmonary resuscitation and emergency cardiac care. JAMA. 1992;268:2172-2302.

CARDIAC ARRHYTHMIAS

> *"My heart,*
> *Where either I must live or bear no life,*
> *The fountain from the which my current runs*
> *Or else dries up."*
>
> WILLIAM SHAKESPEARE

I. GENERAL APPROACH TO THE PATIENT

Patients presenting with new arrhythmias are frequently critically ill. Their evaluation and treatment require a calm and systematic approach with simultaneous evaluation and therapy. Successful management requires an understanding of basic life support, common arrhythmias, and their therapy. It also entails identifying and treating the precipitating cause.

Always treat primarily the patient and not the monitor. Upon initial assessment determine if the patient is *stable* or *unstable*. The following features identify the *unstable* patient:

A. Unresponsive.

B. Pulseless.

C. Anginal chest pain.

D. Hypotensive (systolic blood pressure [BP] <90 mm Hg).

E. Pulmonary edema.

F. Respiratory distress.

G. Altered mentation.

II. EVALUATION OF THE PATIENT WITH AN ARRHYTHMIA

A. Initial Management

Assess, Secure, and Support Airway, Breathing, and Circulation as indicated.

See Chapter 1. II.

1. The first step in patient management should be a primary survey and simultaneous resuscitation as required. If there is any possibility of cervical spine injury, appropriately immobilize the patient. The initial directed physical examination should include the airway, breathing (including a pulmonary examination), and circulation (including vital signs and cardiac auscultation) (the "ABCs").

2. Simultaneously with the above, administer supplemental oxygen, establish intravenous access, and monitor both cardiac rhythm and oxygen saturation (SaO_2).

3. Assess cardiac rhythm from the rhythm monitor and, in a non–cardiac-arrest situation, a 12-lead electrocardiogram (ECG).

B. History

1. Essential information to obtain includes the following:
   a. Medical illnesses, all medications, and allergies.
   b. Previous cardiac or thoracic surgery.
   c. Drug and alcohol use.

2. Identify risk factors for coronary artery disease:
   a. Smoking.
   b. Diabetes mellitus.
   c. Hypertension.
   d. Hyperlipidemia.
   e. Family history.
   f. Peripheral vascular disease.
   g. Male gender.
   h. Age.
   i. Obesity.

C. Laboratory Studies

1. Obtain routine laboratory values:
   a. Complete blood count.
   b. Electrolyte levels.
   c. Blood urea nitrogen.
   d. Creatinine.
   e. Magnesium.
   f. Therapeutic drug levels.
   g. Glucose.

2. Consider additional studies as indicated:
   a. Arterial blood gas values.
   b. Chest roentgenogram.
   c. Thyroid function.
   d. Toxicology screen.
   e. Creatinine phosphokinase with isoenzymes.
   f. Lactate dehydrogenase with isoenzymes.
   g. Calcium.

III. THERAPY

(Accomplish simultaneously with the above.)

A. Act to correct hypoxemia, hypoventilation, and electrolyte abnormalities.

B. Identify the abnormal rhythm and institute therapy.

C. Determine the underlying cause of the abnormal rhythm and initiate treatment.

IV. DISPOSITION

Many arrhythmias arise in conjunction with acute medical problems, such as pneumonia, pulmonary embolism, or myocardial infarction (MI). As a result, many patients seen in the ED with a new symptomatic arrhythmia will require admission. Hospitalization may be indicated for the management of the arrhythmia, investigation of the underlying cause, or treatment of other medical problems.

A. Admit

1. Unstable patients.

2. Those requiring electrical cardioversion or cardiopulmonary resuscitation (CPR).

3. Those begun on quinidine or procainamide.

4. Those with suspected drug toxicity.

5. Those with medical illnesses requiring inpatient therapy.

6. Patients who are unlikely to keep follow-up appointments.

B. Discharge

1. Those with a recurrence of a known paroxysmal atrial arrhythmia.

2. Those with asymptomatic sinus bradycardia.

3. Those with sinus tachycardia, when correctable.

4. Those with first-degree atrioventricular (AV) block, when otherwise asymptomatic.

V. PEARLS AND PITFALLS

A. Maintain control of the airway/oxygenation.

B. Use a cardiac monitor and pulse oximeter, and ensure that someone is watching them.

C. Search for the underlying cause of the arrhythmia.

D. Check for, and correct, electrolyte abnormalities.

E. Check all therapeutic drug levels.

F. Check the apical pulse when evaluating a patient with a slow radial pulse.

G. Inquire about eye drops containing beta adrenergic blocking drugs ("beta blockers"), as they are a frequently overlooked cause of bradycardia.

H. Monitor potassium levels when using digoxin.

Do not do any of the following:

A. Delay cardioversion in an unstable patient.

B. Use beta blockers or calcium channel blockers in hypotensive patients.

C. Obtain cardiac isoenzymes in the ED unless you plan to admit the patient.

D. Start quinidine or procainamide in outpatients.

E. Disable monitor alarms.

F. Give excessive atropine, especially with acute MI.

G. Perform carotid sinus massage in elderly patients or those with cerebrovascular disease.

Sinus Bradycardia

I. ESSENTIAL FACTS

A. Definition

Sinus bradycardia refers to a sinus rhythm with a rate < 60 beats/min. A normal P wave should precede each QRS complex.

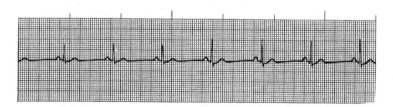

B. Etiology

1. May be normal in otherwise healthy, well-conditioned adults.

2. Drugs: beta-blockers, calcium channel blockers, lithium, clonidine, digoxin, amiodarone, beta-blocking eye drops.

3. Myocardial infarction, especially inferior MI.

4. Hypothermia.

5. Hypothyroidism.

6. Increased vagal tone (vomiting, faints).

7. Increased intracranial/intraocular pressure.

8. Electrolyte abnormalities.

9. Sick-sinus syndrome.

II. DIFFERENTIAL DIAGNOSIS

Atrioventricular block: examine the PR– interval to assess for variation in the relationship between the P wave and the QRS complex.

III. THERAPY (FIG. 13–4)

A. In the asymptomatic patient with no evidence of compromise, observation is sufficient. Consider medication changes and arrange appropriate follow-up.

B. In the symptomatic patient, raise the pulse to relieve symptoms and to keep the systolic BP > 90 mmHg.
   For specific doses and drug information, see Table 13–4.

1. Atropine 0.5–1.0 mg IV push; repeat as needed every 3–5 minutes, to a maximum of 0.04 mg/kg.

2. Transcutaneous (external) pacemaker.

3. Dopamine 5–20 µg/kg/min IV, titrated to heart rate and BP.

4. Epinephrine 2–10 µg/min IV, titrated to heart rate and BP.

5. Transvenous pacemaker.

Caution: pharmacologic agents used to increase the heart rate may increase myocardial oxygen demand (worsening ischemia), and precipitate tachyarrhythmias. They should only be used until a transvenous pacemaker can be placed.

Sinus Tachycardia

I. ESSENTIAL FACTS

A. Definition

Sinus tachycardia refers to a sinus rhythm with a rate >100 beats/min. A normal P wave precedes each QRS complex.

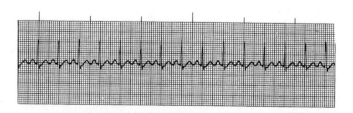

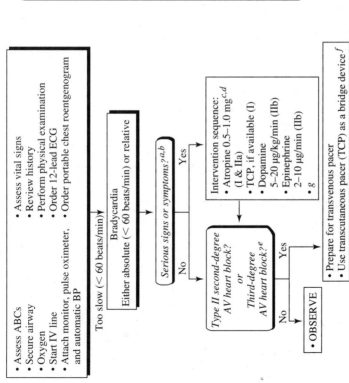

Figure 13–4. Bradycardia treatment algorithm (patient is not in cardiac arrest). (From Emergency Cardiac Care Committee and Subcommittees, American Heart Association, JAMA 1992. 268:2177–2183)

- Assess ABCs
- Secure airway
- Oxygen
- Start IV line
- Attach monitor, pulse oximeter, and automatic BP
- Assess vital signs
- Review history
- Perform physical examination
- Order 12-lead ECG
- Order portable chest roentgenogram

↓

Too slow (< 60 beats/min)

Bradycardia
Either absolute (< 60 beats/min) or relative

Serious signs or symptoms?[a,b]

No → Yes

Yes → Intervention sequence:
- Atropine 0.5–1.0 mg[c,d] (I & IIa)
- TCP, if available (I)
- Dopamine 5–20 μg/kg/min (IIb)
- Epinephrine 2–10 μg/min (IIb)
- [g]

No → *Type II second-degree AV heart block?* or *Third-degree AV heart block?*[e]

No → • OBSERVE

Yes → • Prepare for transvenous pacer
• Use transcutaneous pacer (TCP) as a bridge device[f]

---

a Serious signs or symptoms must be related to the slow rate.
   Clinical manifestations include:
   - *symptoms* (chest pain, shortness of breath, decreased level of consciousness) and/or
   - *signs* (low BP, shock, pulmonary congestion, congestive heart failure, acute MI, extremes of heart rate).
b Do not delay TCP while awaiting IV access or for atropine to take effect if patient is symptomatic.
c Denervated transplanted hearts will not respond to atropine. Go at once to pacing, cactecholamine infusion, or both.
d Atropine should be given in repeat doses in 3–5 min up to total of 0.04 mg/kg. Consider shorter dosing intervals in severe clinical conditions. It has been suggested that atropine should be used with caution in AV block at the His-Purkinje level (type II AV block and new third-degree block with wide QRS complexes) (class IIb).
e Never treat third-degree heart block plus ventricular escape beats with lidocaine.
f Verify patient tolerance and mechanical capture. Use analgesia and sedation as needed.
g Isoproterenol should be used, if at all, with extreme caution. At low doses it is class IIb (possibly helpful); at higher doses it is class III (harmful).

Table 13–4. AGENTS THAT INCREASE THE VENTRICULAR RATE

NAME	ADULT DOSAGE	INDICATIONS	CONTRAINDICATIONS AND WARNINGS
Atropine	0.5–1.0 mg IV push, repeated as needed every 3–5 minutes, titrated to heart rate. Maximum of 0.04 mg/kg	1. Symptomatic sinus bradycardia. 2. Second-degree, type I (Wenckebach) AV block.	*Warnings* 1. Excessive doses may significantly increase heart rate and myocardial oxygen consumption (worsening ischemia) and precipitate tachyarrhythmias. 2. Doses < 0.5 mg may cause paradoxical bradycardia.
Dopamine	5–20 μg/kg/min infusion, titrated to heart rate and blood pressure	1. Symptomatic bradycardia or AV block, which is unresponsive to atropine and transcutaneous (external) pacing	*Warnings* 1. Excessive doses may significantly increase heart rate and myocardial oxygen consumption (worsening ischemia) and precipitate tachyarrhythmias. 2. Avoid using, or reduce the dose to one tenth usual, in patients taking monoamine oxidase inhibitors.
Epinephrine	2–10 μg/min IV infusion, titrated to heart rate and BP		
Isoproterenol	2–10 μg/min IV infusion, titrated to rhythm response	1. Torsades de pointes, which is refractory to magnesium and overdrive pacing	*Warning* May increase myocardial oxygen consumption, worsen ischemia, and precipitate tachyarrhythmias.

B. Etiology

1. Physiologic: fear, pain, anxiety, and fever.

2. Hypovolemia: dehydration, hemorrhage, and anemia.

3. Congestive heart failure, cardiac tamponade, and cardiomyopathy.

4. Pulmonary embolism.

5. Drugs: nifedipine, vasodilators, caffeine, theophylline, anticholinergics, amphetamines, and cocaine.

6. Hyperthyroidism.

7. Myocardial infarction.

II. DIFFERENTIAL DIAGNOSIS

A. Paroxysmal supraventricular tachycardia, especially with a rate >150 beats/min.

B. Atrial flutter, particularly when the rate is 150 beats/min.

C. Atrial fibrillation: when rapid, may appear fairly regular.

D. Multifocal atrial tachycardia: look for variation in the appearance of the P waves.

III. THERAPY

A. Investigate and treat the underlying disorder:

1. Correct hypovolemia/anemia.

2. Stop offending drugs/medications.

3. Treat fever with antipyretics.

4. Treat pain and anxiety.

5. Treat congestive failure with diuretics and inotropes.

B. If the tachycardia is due to acute MI, provide intravenous (IV) beta blockers (unless contraindicated): metoprolol 5 mg IV every 2–5 minutes, to a total dose of 15 mg. An oral regimen (50 mg PO every 6 hours) is then instituted 15 minutes after the last IV dose. Other beta blockers that can be administered intravenously include propranolol, atenolol, and esmolol.

Atrial Fibrillation

I. ESSENTIAL FACTS

A. Definition

Atrial fibrillation is an irregulary irregular supraventricular rhythm without recognizable P waves. The ventricular rate is controlled by AV nodal conduction and is usually 110–150 beats/min, but may be as high as 200 beats/min.

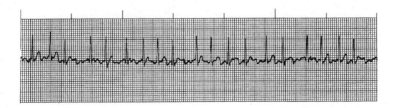

B. Etiology

1. Pulmonary disease: chronic obstructive pulmonary disease (COPD), asthma, and mechanical ventilation.

2. Hyperthyroidism.

3. Pulmonary embolism.

4. Electrolyte abnormalities.

5. Cardiac disease: coronary artery disease, congestive heart failure (CHF), and valvular (especially mitral) heart disease.

6. Alcohol abuse.

7. Accessory conduction pathway (e.g., Wolff–Parkinson–White syndrome).

II. DIFFERENTIAL DIAGNOSIS

A. Atrioventricular block: examine the P–R interval to assess variation in the relationship between the P wave and the QRS complex.

B. Atrial flutter with variable block: look for flutter waves.

C. Multifocal atrial tachycardia: look for P waves of varying morphology.

III. THERAPY

A. The duration of atrial fibrillation to some extent determines the therapeutic strategy. For patients who have been fibrillating for more than 2 days, cardioversion should be avoided (unless absolutely necessary) owing to the risk of embolism. Patients in this category should be heparanized and kept anticoagulated for 3 weeks prior to (and at least 1 week after) cardioversion.

B. In the unstable patient, perform *synchronized* cardioversion with 100 J; repeat as needed with 200 J, 300 J, and 360 J (Table 13–5).

C. In the stable patient with a narrow QRS complex (Fig. 13–5):

1. Improve oxygenation.

2. Correct electrolyte abnormalities.

3. Treat the underlying disorder.

4. Control the ventricular rate by slowing AV nodal conduction with one of the following (Table 13–6).
   a. Calcium Channel Blockers
      i. Diltiazem 0.25 mg/kg IV infusion over 2 minutes. If no response after 15 minutes, repeat at 0.35 mg/kg IV infusion over 2 minutes; and/or begin a drip at 5 to 15 mg/hr. Titrate dose to heart rate.
      ii. Verapamil 2.5–5.0 mg IV over 2–3 minutes. Repeat at

Table 13–5. SYNCHRONIZED CARDIOVERSION

Urgent cardioversion is indicated in the treatment of *unstable* patients with the following rhythms (initial energy level):
- Atrial flutter (50 J)
- Paroxysmal supraventricular tachycardia (50 J)
- Atrial fibrillation (100 J)
- Ventricular tachycardia, with a pulse (100 J)
- Ventricular tachycardia, pulseless (200 J)

Procedure

1. Obtain control of airway, administer oxygen, and attach the pulse oximeter (call an anesthesiologist, if available).
2. Obtain intravenous access.
3. Attach cardiac monitor/defibrillator.
4. Obtain suction device and intubation equipment.
5. Sedate whenever possible (adult dosages):
   a. Midazolam 1–2 mg slow IV push; repeat as needed, every 2 minutes, to a maximum of 3.5–5.0 mg

   or

   b. Diazepam 2.5–5 mg IV slow push; repeat as needed, every 2–5 minutes, to a maximum of 10–15 mg

   or

   c. Methohexital sodium 500 mg mixed in 250 mL of D5W and infused with a micro-drip IV system; the patient should become drowsy after infusion of approximately 25 mL; usual dose is 1–2 mg/kg

   Warning: These agents may cause respiratory depression and hypotension. Lower doses should be used in elderly patients. Be prepared to treat complications. Some patients may require higher doses.
6. Perform synchronized cardioversion
   a. Select the correct power and shock; repeat as needed with 100 J, 200 J, 300 J, and 360 J.
   b. Be prepared to treat asystole/ventricular fibrillation.
7. Monitor the patient closely after the procedure for potential complications (i.e., aspiration, respiratory depression, hypotension).

              15-minute intervals as needed to control rate to a maximum of 10–20 mg.

    b. Beta Blockers

        i. Propranolol 1.0–3.0 mg IV over 3–4 minutes; repeat in 5–10 minutes as needed to control rate to a maximum of 0.1 mg/kg.

        ii. Esmolol 500 µg/kg for 1 minute as a bolus, followed by a 50-µg/kg/min infusion. Repeat the bolus and increase the infusion rate by 50 µg/kg/min every 5 minutes as needed to control rate. Maximum infusion rate is 200 µg/kg/min.

    c. Digoxin 0.25–0.50 mg IV over 5 minutes, followed by additional doses of 0.25 mg every 4 hours, to a maximum of 15 µg/kg in a 24-hour period.

  D. In the stable patient with a wide QRS complex, if atrial fibrillation occurs with an underlying conduction abnormality (e.g., bundle branch block), it may be both wide and irregular. When patients with an accessory conduction pathway (e.g., Wolff-Parkinson-White syndrome) develop atrial fibrillation, the electrical impulses

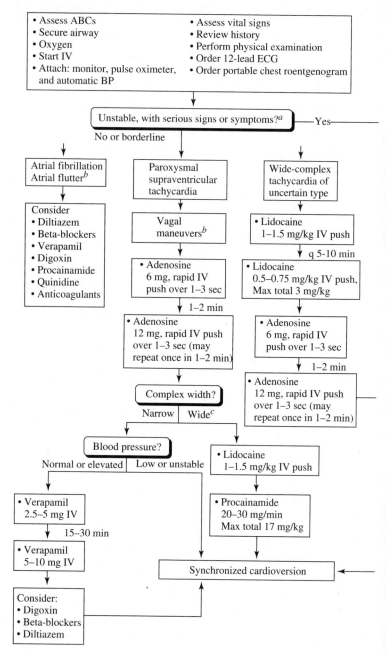

Figure 13–5. Tachycardia treatment algorithm. (From Emergency Cardiac Care Committee and Subcommittees, American Heart Association, JAMA 1992. 268:2172–2183)

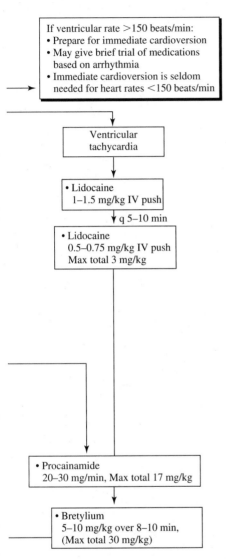

If ventricular rate >150 beats/min:
• Prepare for immediate cardioversion
• May give brief trial of medications
  based on arrhythmia
• Immediate cardioversion is seldom
  needed for heart rates <150 beats/min

Ventricular
tachycardia

• Lidocaine
  1–1.5 mg/kg IV push

q 5–10 min

• Lidocaine
  0.5–0.75 mg/kg IV push
  Max total 3 mg/kg

• Procainamide
  20–30 mg/min, Max total 17 mg/kg

• Bretylium
  5–10 mg/kg over 8–10 min,
  (Max total 30 mg/kg)

[a] Unstable condition must be related to the tachycardia. Signs and
symptoms may include chest pain, shortness of breath, decreased level
of consciousness, hypotension, shock, pulmonary congestion, CHF,
acute MI.
[b] Carotid sinus massage is contraindicated in patients with carotid bruits;
avoid ice-water immersion in patients with ischemic heart disease.
[c] If the wide-complex tachycardia is known with certainty to be
paroxysmal supraventricular tachycardia and BP is normal/elevated,
sequence can include verapamil.

Table 13–6. AGENTS THAT SLOW AV NODAL CONDUCTION

NAME	ADULT DOSAGE	INDICATIONS	CONTRAINDICATIONS AND WARNINGS
Adenosine	6 mg IV rapid push, followed by a 20-mL saline flush; repeat with 12 mg if no response (1 vial = 6 mg)	1. Paroxysmal supraventricular tachycardia. 2. Diagnosis of atrial flutter. 3. Wide-complex tachycardia of uncertain type, unresponsive to lidocaine.	*Contraindications* 1. Sick-sinus syndrome. 2. Second- or third-degree heart block, except with a functioning artificial pacemaker. *Warning* 1. May cause transient chest pain, flushing, and dyspnea.
Digoxin	0.25–0.50 mg IV over 5 min, or PO, followed by additional doses of 0.25 every 4 hr, to a maximum of 15 µg/kg (1.05 mg for a 70-kg patient) Maintenance therapy, 0.125–0.25 mg PO gD	Rate control in atrial fibrillation or flutter.	*Contraindications* 1. Hypokalemia. 2. Atrial fibrillation or flutter or wide complex tachycardia with a suspected accessory conduction pathway (i.e., Wolff-Parkinson-White syndrome). *Warnings* 1. Do not use if anticipating cardioversion. 2. Reduce dose in elderly patients or with renal insufficiency.

Calcium Channel Blockers

NAME	ADULT DOSAGE	INDICATIONS	CONTRAINDICATIONS AND WARNINGS
Verapamil	2.5–5 mg IV over 2–3 min; repeat at 15-min intervals as needed to control rate, to a maximum of 10–20 mg 40 to 80 mg PO every 6–8 hours	1. Rate control with paroxysmal atrial tachycardia, atrial fibrillation or flutter. 2. Paroxysmal supraventricular tachycardia.	*Contraindications* 1. Congestive heart failure. 2. Hypotension. 3. Atrial fibrillation or flutter or wide complex tachycardia with a suspected accessory conduction pathway (i.e., Wolff-Parkinson-White syndrome). 4. Ventricular tachycardia. 5. Sick-sinus syndrome or high-degree AV nodal block.
Diltizem	0.25 mg/kg IV over 2 min; repeat with 0.35 mg/kg if needed in 15 min to control rate, and/or begin a continuous infusion at 5–15 mg/hr 30–60 mg PO every 8 hr		*Warnings* 1. Can cause hypotension, which may respond to fluid, Trendelenburg positioning, or calcium infusion. 2. Combined use of these agents with a beta blocker may result in bradycardia or hypotension.

Beta Blockers

NAME	ADULT DOSAGE	INDICATIONS	CONTRAINDICATIONS AND WARNINGS
Propranolol	1.0–3.0 mg IV over 3–4 min, repeat in 5–10 minutes as needed to control rate, to a maximum of 0.1 mg/kg 10 to 30 mg PO every 6–8 hr	1. Rate control with paroxysmal atrial tachycardia, atrial fibrillation or flutter, and multifocal atrial tachycardia 2. Paroxysmal supraventricular tachycardia.	*Contraindications and Warnings apply to all beta blockers* *Contraindications* 1. Congestive heart failure. 2. Hypotension.

Table 13–6. AGENTS THAT SLOW AV NODAL
CONDUCTION *Continued*

NAME	ADULT DOSAGE	INDICATIONS	CONTRAINDICATIONS AND WARNINGS
Beta Blockers–cont'd			*Contraindications–cont'd*
Esmolol	500 µg/kg IV bolus over 1 minute, followed by a 50-µg/kg/min infusion. Repeat the bolus and increase the infusion by 50 µg/kg/min every 5 minutes as needed to control rate, to a maximum of 200 µg/kg/min		3. Bronchospasm. 4. Bradycardia. 5. Atrial fibrillation or flutter or wide complex tachycardia with a suspected accessory conduction pathway (i.e., Wolff-Parkinson-White syndrome).
Metoprolol	5-mg IV slow push at 2–5-min intervals to a total of 15 mg, followed by a PO dose of 50 mg every 6 hr for at least 1 day. It may then be increased to 100 mg bid PO.	MI patients	*Warnings* 1. May cause hypotension and bradycardia. 2. Combined use of these agents with verapamil or diltiazem may result in bradycardia or hypotension.

from the atria may proceed down the accessory pathway (antidromic) yielding a wide complex rhythm. Accessory pathways do not generally respond to agents that *slow* AV nodal conduction. As such, digoxin, beta blockers, and the calcium channel blockers should be *avoided* in these patients as they may paradoxically increase the ventricular rate or cause hypotension. If in doubt about the cause of a wide-complex tachycardia, treat it as ventricular tachycardia:

1. Improve oxygenation.

2. Correct electrolyte abnormalities.

3. Treat the underlying disorder.

4. Procainamide 20 mg/min IV infusion, to a maximum of 17 mg/kg (1.2 g for a 70-kg patient), followed by a continuous infusion of 1–4 mg/min (see Table 13–8).

5. Patients who do not respond to procainamide may respond to disopyramide, propafenone, flecainide, or electrical cardioversion. Cardiology consultation is indicated.

Atrial Flutter

I. ESSENTIAL FACTS

A. Definition

Atrial Flutter refers to a supraventricular rhythm with atrial flutter waves (usually at a rate of 300 beats/min). The ventricular rate is limited by AV nodal conduction, typically with a 2:1 or 4:1 block.

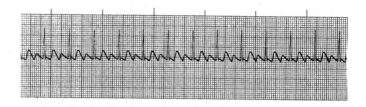

B. Etiology

1. Pulmonary disease: COPD/asthma, and mechanical ventilation.

2. Medical illness: pneumonia and sepsis.

3. Pulmonary embolism.

4. Electrolyte imbalance.

5. Cardiac disease: coronary artery disease, congestive heart failure (CHF), valvular heart disease (especially mitral), and myocarditis.

6. Drugs: quinidine, procainamide, theophylline, caffeine, and alcohol.

7. Hyperthyroidism.

II. DIFFERENTIAL DIAGNOSIS

A. Sinus tachycardia, particularly if the rate is < 140 beats/min.

B. Paroxysmal atrial tachycardia: frequently associated with digoxin therapy.

C. Paroxysmal supraventricular tachycardia: no flutter waves.

D. Atrial fibrillation: look for irregularity in the R–R interval.

III. DIAGNOSTIC MANEUVERS TO DEMONSTRATE FLUTTER

The diagnosis of atrial flutter depends on the demonstration of the flutter waves. Flutter waves are often seen in leads II, III, and AVF of the 12-lead ECG. With an atrial rate of 300 beats/min and 2:1 ventricular conduction, half of the flutter waves may fall directly within the QRS complex, making them very difficult to see. As such, atrial flutter may closely resemble sinus tachycardia or paroxysmal supraventricular tachycardia. Look for irregularities in the QRS-T complex halfway between atrial beats.

When the flutter waves cannot be clearly seen, diagnostic maneuvers may be used to better demonstrate their presence. The most common method is to slow the ventricular rate in order to better observe the atrial activity. Alternatively, an electrode may be placed in the esophagus to examine the atrial activity.

A. Physiologic Maneuvers

Increased vagal tone can cause a transient AV nodal block. This allows flutter waves that would normally be hidden by the QRS complex to be more easily seen (Table 13–7). *Caution:* some vagal maneuvers, such as carotid sinus massage, may be dangerous. Consider using adenosine.

B. Pharmacologic Maneuvers

Adenosine is an endogenous purine nucleotide that can block AV nodal conduction for 10–15 seconds, allowing the background flutter waves to be more clearly seen. Observe and record the ECG during the infusion (Table 13–6).

1. Adenosine 6 mg (1 ampule) IV rapid push (over 1–3 seconds) followed by a 20-mL saline flush. If no response, repeat with a 12-mg IV rapid push. Patients on theophylline are less sensitive to adenosine and may require larger doses. Lower doses should be used for patients on dipyridamole or carbamazepine. *Caution:* patients should be in the Trendelenburg position when adenosine is given.

Table 13–7. MANEUVERS TO INCREASE VAGAL TONE

Observe and record the ECG during:
1. Valsalva's maneuver (in which the patient exhales against a closed glottis).
2. Carotid sinus massage (*Caution:* Patient should be in Trendelenburg position. Do not perform on the patient with a history of a prior cerebrovascular accident. Use cautiously, if at all, in elderly patients)
   a. Auscultate the carotid arteries for bruits (if present, the procedure is *contraindicated*).
   b. Turn the head to the left and palpate the right carotid artery at the bifurcation, just below the angle of the jaw.
   c. Massage firmly (but do not occlude the carotid pulse) for up to 5–10 seconds while observing the ECG.
3. Trendelenburg positioning: Raise the foot of the bed while lowering the head.
4. Facial immersion: Have the patient place his/her face in a basin filled with cold water while holding breath (should only be contemplated in cooperative patients).

Indications
   a. Treatment of paroxysmal supraventricular tachycardia.
   b. In the diagnosis of atrial flutter.

Warnings
   a. Vagal maneuvers, particularly carotid sinus massage, may result in life-threatening complications (high-degree AV nodal block, stroke).
   b. They should *not* be attempted by inexperienced individuals, or with elderly patients.
   c. Pharmacologic therapy should be considered as an alternative.

C. Lewis Leads

Observe lead I while moving the left and right arm leads over the precordium, looking for clear evidence of flutter waves.

D. Esophageal Electrode

A small electrode is placed in the esophagus via a capsule or a nasogastric tube. The wires are attached to the right and left arm leads. Flutter waves are most apparent with the electrode in proximity to the atria. Placement of the electrode may evoke a vagal response, thus demonstrating flutter waves, so monitor the rhythm during placement.

IV. THERAPY

A. In the unstable patient, perform *synchronized* cardioversion with 50 J; repeat as needed with 100 J, 200 J, 300 J, and 360 J with one of the following (Table 13–5).

B. In the stable patient, follow the algorithm in Figure 13–5. Atrial flutter is frequently resistant to pharmacologic therapy. Electrical cardioversion is probably the therapy of choice for all patients. However, pharmacologic therapy may be used to slow the ventricular rate, and may convert the patient to sinus rhythm or atrial fibrillation.

1. Improve oxygenation.

2. Correct electrolyte abnormalities.

3. Treat the underlying disorder.

4. Control the ventricular rate by slowing AV nodal conduction with one of the following (Table 13–6).
   a. Calcium Channel Blockers
      i. Verapamil 2.5–5.0 mg IV over 2–3 minutes; repeat at 15-minute intervals as needed to control rate, to a maximum of 10–20 mg.
      ii. Diltiazem 0.25 mg/kg IV infusion over 2 minutes. If no response after 15 minutes, repeat increasing the IV infusion to 0.35 mg/kg over 2 minutes; or begin a drip at 5 to 15 mg/hr, titrated to heart rate.
   b. Beta Blockers
      i. Propranolol 1.0–3.0 mg IV over 3–4 minutes; repeat in 5–10 minutes as needed to control rate, to a maximum of 0.1 mg/kg.
      ii. Esmolol 500 μg/kg for 1 minute as a bolus, followed by a 50-μg/kg/min infusion. Repeat the bolus and increase the infusion rate by 50 μg/kg/min every 5 minutes as needed to control rate, to a maximum of 200 μg/kg/min.
   c. Digoxin 0.25–0.50 mg IV over 5 minutes, followed by additional doses of 0.25 mg every 4 hours, to a maximum of 15 μg/kg.

Table 13–8. ANTIARRHYTHMIC AGENTS

Name (Class)	Adult Dosage	Indications	Contraindications and Warnings
Lidocaine (IB)	1.0–1.5 mg/kg IV bolus, followed by additional doses of 0.5–0.75 mg/kg every 5–10 min, to a maximum of 3 mg/kg; once stable begin a continuous infusion at 1–4 mg/min	Life-threatening ventricular arrhythmias	*Contraindication* High-degree AV nodal block. *Warnings* 1. Lidocaine may cause altered mental status, slurred speech, muscle twitching, and seizures. 2. Use lower doses in elderly patients, or those with hepatic dysfunction. 3. Follow therapeutic levels.
Procaina-mide (IA)	20 mg/min IV to a maximum of 17 mg/kg (1.2 g for a 70-kg patient), followed by a continuous infusion of 1–4 mg/min Discontinue if 1. Hypotension develops or 2. The QRS widens by > 50%	1. Atrial fibrillation or flutter, once rate controlled 2. Ventricular arrhythmias unresponsive to lidocaine 3. Atrial fibrillation with suspected accessory pathway (i.e., Wolff-Parkinson-White syndrome)	*Contraindications* 1. Hypotension. 2. Prolonged QT interval or torsades de pointes. 3. High-degree AV nodal block. *Warnings* 1. May cause significant hypotension with rapid infusion. 2. Reduce the dose with renal insufficiency. 3. Follow therapeutic levels of procainamide and *N*-acetylprocainamide (NAPA).
Bretylium (III)	5–10 mg/kg IV over 8–10 min, repeat as needed, to a maximum of 30 mg/kg; if successful, begin a continuous infusion at 1–2 mg/min	1. Ventricular arrhythmias unresponsive to lidocaine	*Warnings* 1. May cause hypotension. 2. Use cautiously in patients with renal insufficiency. 3. May worsen digitalis-induced arrhythmias.
Phenytoin (IB)	100 mg IV every 5 min, until arrhythmia abolished or to a total of 12 mg/kg (840 mg for a 70 kg patient); maintenance therapy is 100 mg IV tid	1. Life-threatening, digitalis associated, ventricular arrhythmias unresponsive to lidocaine. Consider the use of digoxin immune Fab (see Table 13–9). 2. Torsades de pointes, which is refractory to magnesium and overdrive pacing.	*Contraindications* Sinus bradycardia, second- or third-degree AV block. *Warnings* 1. Rapid infusion may cause hypotension; monitor the patient closely. 2. Follow therapeutic levels.

5. Consider the use of a type IA antiarrhythmic once the rate is controlled (Table 13–8): procainamide 20 mg/min IV infusion, to a maximum of 17 mg/kg (1.2 g for a 70-kg patient), followed by a continuous infusion of 1–4 mg/min.

Paroxysmal Supraventricular Tachycardia

I. ESSENTIAL FACTS

A. Definition

Paroxysmal supraventricular tachycardia is a rapid supraventricular arrhythmia frequently resulting from re-entrant conduction within the AV node. The ventricular rate is generally 150–250 beats/min.

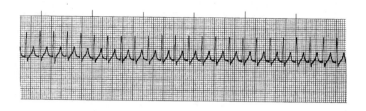

B. Etiology

1. May occur in otherwise healthy persons.

2. May occur in the presence of an accessory conduction pathway (e.g., Wolff-Parkinson-White syndrome).

3. Drugs: caffeine, alcohol, cocaine, and amphetamines.

4. Atrial septal defect.

5. Myocardial ischemia.

II. DIFFERENTIAL DIAGNOSIS

A. Sinus tachycardia, particularly if the rate is < 140 beats/min.

B. Atrial flutter, especially with a rate of 150 beats/min; look for flutter waves buried in the QRS complex (leads II, III, and AVF).

C. Paroxysmal atrial tachycardia: consider in the presence of digoxin therapy.

III. THERAPY

Paroxysmal supraventricular tachycardia frequently occurs in otherwise healthy individuals. As such, it is usually well tolerated. If the rate is particularly rapid (e.g., >180 beats/min), or the arrhythmia is sustained, congestive heart failure may occur.

A. In the unstable patient, perform *synchronized* cardioversion with 50 J; repeat as needed with 100 J, 200 J, 300 J, and 360 J (Table 13–5).

B. In the stable patient, follow the algorithm in Figure 13–5. Re-entrant arrhythmias may be abolished by slowing (or briefly abolishing) AV nodal conduction. This may be accomplished by physiologic or pharmacologic measures.

1. Improve oxygenation.
2. Correct electrolyte abnormalities.
3. Consider vagal maneuvers (Table 13–7). *Caution:* some vagal maneuvers, such as carotid sinus massage, may be dangerous. Consider using pharmacologic therapy instead.
4. Administer pharmacologic therapy (Table 13–6).
    a. Adenosine 6 mg (1 ampule) IV rapid push (over 1–3 seconds) followed by a 20-mL saline flush. If no response, repeat with a 12-mg IV rapid push. Or
    b. Verapamil 2.5–5.0 mg IV over 2–3 minutes; repeat at 15-minute intervals as needed to control rate, to a maximum of 10–20 mg. Or
    c. Diltiazem 0.25 mg/kg IV infusion over 2 minutes. If no response after 15 minutes, repeat a 0.35-mg/kg IV infusion over 2 minutes. Or
    d. Propranolol 1.0–3.0 mg IV over 3–4 minutes; repeat in 5–10 minutes as needed to control rate, to a maximum of 0.1 mg/kg. Or
    e. Esmolol 500 µg/kg for 1 minute as a bolus, followed by a 50-µg/kg/min infusion. Repeat the bolus and increase the infusion rate by 50 µg/kg/min every 5 minutes as needed, to a maximum of 200 µg/kg/min.

C. Outpatients with frequent attacks may be maintained on chronic suppressive therapy. Those with infrequent episodes can be taught to employ vagal measures (*not* carotid sinus massage) or to keep a supply of medications at home for use during epsiodes. Always observe the patient in the ED after giving the first dose of suppressive therapy (Table 13–6).

1. Verapamil 40–80 mg PO every 8 hours.
2. Propranolol 10–30 mg PO every 6–8 hours.

Caution: do not administer verapamil or propranolol as outpatient suppressive therapy to patients with the Wolff-Parkinson-White syndrome.

Paroxysmal (Automatic) Atrial Tachycardia

I. ESSENTIAL FACTS

A. Definition

Paroxysmal (automatic) atrial tachycardia refers to an atrial rate of 160–240 beats/min resulting from increased atrial automaticity. The ventricular rate is limited by AV nodal conduction. This rhythm may appear like sinus tachycardia with an altered P-wave axis. When rapid (rate >160 beats/min) it may appear indistinguishable from atrial flutter or paroxysmal supraventricular tachycardia.

B. Etiology

1. Digitalis toxicity, especially atrial tachycardia with block.
2. Acute MI.
3. Pulmonary disease/hypoxia
4. Drugs: quinidine, alcohol, cocaine, and amphetamines.
5. Electrolyte abnormalities.

II. DIFFERENTIAL DIAGNOSIS

A. Paroxysmal supraventricular tachycardia.

B. Sinus tachycardia: rate is generally < 140 beats/min.

C. Atrial flutter: look for flutter waves in leads II, III, and AVF.

III. THERAPY

A. If associated with digitalis therapy

1. Discontinue digitalis and check the serum level.
2. Correct hypoxemia/hypoventilation.
3. Check the potassium level and keep it in the normal range.
4. Consider digitalis antibodies, particularly if there are associated ventricular arrhythmias or the patient appears unstable (Table 13-9; also see Chapter 23).
5. If there is frequent ventricular ectopy, consider phenytoin 100 mg IV every 5 minutes, to a maximum of 12 mg/kg (840 mg for a 70-kg patient) (Table 13–8).
6. If there is a rapid ventricular response, consider beta blockers (Table 13–6).
   i. Propranolol 1.0–3.0 mg IV over 3–4 minutes; repeat in 5–10 minutes as needed to control rate, to a maximum of 0.1 mg/kg.
   ii. Esmolol 500 µg/kg for 1 minute as a bolus, followed by a 50-µg/kg/min infusion. Repeat the bolus and increase the infusion rate by 50 µg/kg/min every 5 minutes as needed to control rate, to a maximum of 200 µg/kg/min.

B. If the condition is not digitalis associated, treat as atrial flutter.

Multifocal Atrial Tachycardia

I. ESSENTIAL FACTS

A. Definition

Multifocal atrial tachycardia involves an atrial rate > 100 beats/min with P waves of at least three distinct morphologies, a varying P–R interval, and an isoelectric baseline.

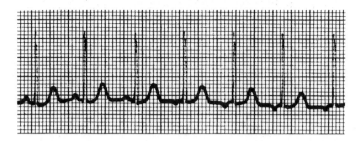

B. Etiology

1. Pulmonary disease: COPD, acute pulmonary infection, and hypoxia.
2. Cardiac disease: hypertension, coronary artery disease, and CHF.
3. Electrolyte disturbances.
4. Severe illness: sepsis, postoperative, and acidosis.
5. Drugs: bronchodilators, sympathetic amines, and alcohol.

II. DIFFERENTIAL DIAGNOSIS

A. Sinus tachycardia: less likely with rate > 140 beats/min.

B. Paroxysmal supraventricular tachycardia: generally very regular.

C. Atrial fibrillation: there should be no P waves.

D. Atrial flutter: look for flutter waves in leads II, III, and AVF.

E. Paroxysmal atrial tachycardia, especially with digoxin therapy.

III. THERAPY

Multifocal atrial tachycardia does not generally respond to pharmacologic intervention.

A. Treat the underlying disorder, i.e., COPD, pneumonia, and CHF.

B. Correct hypoxemia and electrolyte abnormalities (especially potassium and magnesium abnormalities).

C. Control the ventricular rate as needed: consider diltiazem or verapamil (Table 13–6).

Atrioventricular Block

I. ESSENTIAL FACTS

A. Definition

Atrioventricular block refers to impaired AV conduction of varying degree.

1. First-Degree AV Block
   a. PR– interval > 0.20 seconds.
   b. Usually asymptomatic.

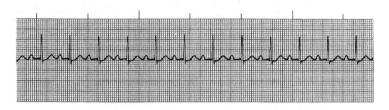

2. Second-Degree AV Block
   a. Type I (Wenckebach): progressive increases in the P–R interval of successive beats leading to a blocked atrial beat.

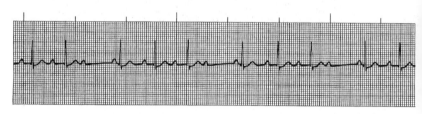

   b. Type II (Mobitz type II): Unconducted atrial beats often occurring in a fixed interval (e.g., 2:1 AV conduction).

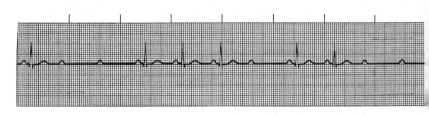

3. Third-Degree AV Block. A complete block of atrial impulses to the ventricles with disassociation of the P wave and QRS complex. There is frequently a ventricular escape rhythm at 40–60 beats/min.

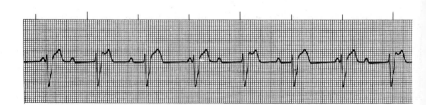

B. Etiology

1. Drugs: beta blockers, calcium channel blockers, digoxin, procainamide, and quinidine.
2. Myocardial ischemia or infarction.
3. Trauma: myocardial contusion.
4. Degenerative changes in the conduction system.
5. Cardiomyopathy, especially infiltrative diseases, sarcoidosis, hemochromatosis, and amyloidosis.
6. Infections: endocarditis, myocarditis, Lyme disease, and Chagas' disease.
7. Electrolyte abnormalities: hyperkalemia.
8. Hypoxemia.

II. DIFFERENTIAL DIAGNOSIS

Sinus bradycardia: examine the relationship between the P waves and the QRS complex. There should be no variation in the P–R interval in sinus bradycardia.

III. THERAPY (FIG. 13–4)

A. In unstable patients with second-degree, type II or third-degree AV block:

1. Transcutaneous (external) pacemaker, until
2. Transvenous (temporary) pacemaker placement.

B. In stable patients:

1. If asymptomatic (first-degree or second-degree, type I), observe if there is no evidence of compromise.
2. If symptomatic, treat as symptomatic bradycardia (Fig. 13–4).

Premature Ventricular Contractions

I. ESSENTIAL FACTS

A. Definition

Premature ventricular contractions are premature beats of ventricular origin, with a QRS complex generally longer than 0.12 seconds, without a preceding premature P wave.

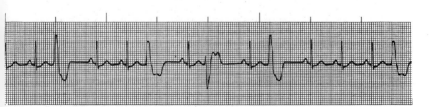

B. Etiology

1. May be normal in otherwise healthy individuals.

2. Ischemic heart disease.

3. Hypertensive heart disease.

4. Cardiomyopathy.

5. Electrolyte abnormalities.

6. Pulmonary disease, acute and chronic.

7. Drugs: procainamide, quinidine, digoxin, alcohol, cocaine, amphetamines, epinephrine, and dopamine.

II. DIFFERENTIAL DIAGNOSIS

Aberrantly conducted premature atrial contractions.

III. THERAPY

A. Correct hypoxemia and electrolyte abnormalities (especially potassium and magnesium).

B. Treat pain and anxiety.

C. Check therapeutic drug levels, and discontinue offending drugs.

D. In general, pharmacologic treatment of asymptomatic premature ventricular contractions is not indicated, unless there is evidence of ongoing myocardial ischemia.

E. For patients with suspected myocardial ischemia administer either of the following:

1. Lidocaine 1 mg/kg IV load, followed by a 1–4 mg/min IV infusion. Should be considered in patients with frequent ventricular contractions (> 6/min), R on T phenomena, or multifocal couplets (Table 13–8).

2. Magnesium sulfate 1–2 g (8–16 mEq) mixed in 50–100 mL of dextrose in water (D5W) and infused intravenously over 5–60 minutes, followed by a continuous infusion of 0.5–1.0 g/hr (Table 13–9).

Ventricular Tachycardia

I. ESSENTIAL FACTS

A. Definition

Ventricular tachycardia refers to three or more successive beats of ventricular origin with a rate > 100 beats/min. The QRS complex is usually wide, and P waves are usually not apparent.

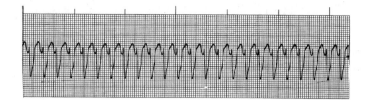

B. Etiology

1. Myocardial ischemia.

2. Cardiomyopathy.

3. Drugs: procainamide, quinidine, digoxin, alcohol, cocaine, amphetamines, epinephrine, dopamine, tricyclic antidepressants, and phenothiazines.

4. Electrolyte abnormalities.

II. DIFFERENTIAL DIAGNOSIS

When confronted with the patient with a wide-complex tachycardia (rate > 150 beats/min), particularly if unstable, treat as ventricular tachycardia.

A. Any aberrantly conducted supraventricular arrhythmia may simulate ventricular tachycardia, particularly if the patient has a pre-existing conduction abnormality (i.e., bundle branch block).

B. Atrial fibrillation with an accessory conduction pathway (e.g., Wolff-Parkinson-White syndrome).

C. Artifact.

III. THERAPY

A. In the unstable patient perform *synchronized* cardioversion with 100 J; repeat as needed with 200 J, 300 J, 360 J (Table 13–5).

B. In the stable patient (Fig. 13–5)

1. Obtain control of airway.

2. Administer oxygen

3. Obtain IV access.

4. Administer lidocaine 1–1.5 mg/kg IV bolus, followed by additional boluses of 0.5–0.75 mg/kg IV every 5–10 minutes, to a maximum of 3 mg/kg. If successful, begin a continuous IV infusion at 1–4 mg/min (Table 13–8).

5. If there is no response to lidocaine, administer procainamide 20

mg/min IV infusion, to a maximum of 17 mg/kg (1.2 g for a 70-kg patient), followed by a continuous infusion of 1–4 mg/min (Table 13–8).

6. If there is no response to procainamide, administer bretylium 5–10 mg/kg IV over 8–10 minutes; repeat if needed, to a maximum of 30 mg/kg). If successful, begin a continuous infusion at 1–2 mg/min (Table 13–8).

7. If the patient remains in a wide complex tachycardia, consider the use of adenosine to treat potential aberrantly conducted supraventricular arrhythmias (Fig. 13–5): 6 mg (1 ampule) IV rapid push (over 1–3 seconds) followed by a 20-mL saline flush. If no response, repeat with a 12-mg rapid push (Table 13–6).

8. If the patient has not responded to pharmacologic therapy, or is unstable at any point, provide synchronized cardioversion beginning at 100 J (Table 13–5).

Torsades de Pointes

I. ESSENTIAL FACTS

A. Definition

Torsades de pointes is a form of polymorphic ventricular tachycardia in which the QRS complex appears to twist about the isoelectric baseline.

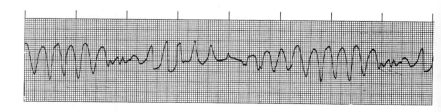

B. Etiology

1. Prolonged Q–T interval.

2. Drugs: procainamide, quinidine, disopyramide, amiodarone, phenothiazines, tricyclic antidepressants, erythromycin, trimethoprim-sulfamethoxazole, terfenadine, astemizole, and pentamidine.

3. Electrolyte abnormalities: hypokalemia and hypomagnesemia.

4. Cardiac disease: myocarditis, ischemia, and bradycardia.

5. Intracranial process: subarachnoid hemorrhage, stroke, and tumors.

II. DIFFERENTIAL DIAGNOSIS

See Ventricular Tachycardia, above.

III. THERAPY

A. In the unstable patient, perform *synchronized* cardioversion with 200 J; repeat as needed with 300 J and 360 J (Table 13–5).

B. In the stable patient

1. Obtain control of airway.

2. Administer oxygen.

3. Obtain IV access.

4. The drug of choice is magnesium sulfate 1–2 g (8–16 mEq) mixed in 50–100 mL of D5W and infused IV 1–2 minutes, followed by a continuous infusion of 0.5–1 g/hr (Table 13–9).

5. Use a transcutaneous (external) pacemaker until a transvenous pacemaker can be installed for overdrive pacing.

Table 13–9. MISCELLANEOUS AGENTS

NAME	ADULT DOSAGE	INDICATIONS	CONTRAINDICATIONS AND WARNINGS
Potassium Chloride	10 mEq IV infused over 1 hr through a peripheral IV line will usually raise the serum level by 0.1 mEq/L; repeat as needed 20–40 mEq PO; repeat every 6–8 hr	Hypokalemia	*Contraindications* 1. Hyperkalemia. 2. Use cautiously, if at all, in patients with renal insufficiency. *Warnings* 1. Infusion rates of more than 15 mEq/hr may precipitate ventricular arrhythmias. 2. Follow serum levels closely during acute therapy.
Magnesium Sulfate	1–2 g (8–16 mEq) mixed in 50–100 mL of D5W and infused IV over 5–60 minutes (may be infused over 1–2 minutes in urgent situations); follow with a continuous infusion of 0.5–1 g/hr	1. Hypomagnesemia 2. Treatment of torsades de pointes 3. Postinfarction arrhythmias	*Warnings* 1. Rapid infusion may cause hypotension and asystole. 2. Use with caution in patients with renal insufficiency. 3. Follow both potassium and magnesium levels closely.
Digoxin Immune Fab	Each 40-mg vial IV will bind approximately 0.6 mg of digoxin. (See Chapter 23 for dosing formulas.)	Serious digoxin overdose	*Contraindications* History of allergic reaction to the product or to sheep proteins. *Warnings* 1. Treatment may result in hypokalemia; monitor potassium levels closely. 2. Be prepared to treat hypersensitivity reactions.

6. Isoproterenol may be tried if magnesium and overdrive pacing are unsuccessful. Infuse at 2–10 µg/min IV, titrated to rhythm response (Table 13–4).

7. For refractory arrhythmias, administer phenytoin 100 mg IV every 5 minutes, to a maximum of 12 mg/kg (840 mg for a 70-kg patient) (Table 13–8).

8. Synchronized cardioversion, beginning at 200 J, may be tried if the above measures are unsuccessful (Table 13–5).

BIBLIOGRAPHY

Boahene K, Klein G, Yee R, et al: Atrial fibrillation in the Wolff-Parkinson-White Syndrome. In Horowitz LN (eds): Current Management of Arrhythmias. Philadelphia, BC Decker, 1991, pp. 123-129.

Canessa R, Lema G, Urzua J, et al: Anesthesia for elective cardioversion: A comparison of four anesthetic agents. J Cardiothorac Vasc Anesth 1991;5(6):556–568.

Cummins RD (ed): Textbook of Advanced Cardiac Life Support. Dallas, American Heart Association, 1994.

Drugs for cardiac arrhythmias. Med Lett 1991;33(846):55–60.

Emergency Cardiac Care Committee and Subcommittees, American Heart Association. Guidelines for cardiopulmonary resuscitation and emergency cardiac care. III: Adult advanced cardiac life support. JAMA 1992;268:2172–2183.

CONGESTIVE HEART FAILURE

"It would be difficult to overrate the value, as guides to practice, of the signs which declare themselves through the medium of the lungs in every case of unsound heart."

PETER MERE LATHAM

I. ESSENTIAL FACTS

A. Definition

Congestive heart failure (CHF) is a syndrome of inadequate forward cardiac output despite normal or supranormal circulating blood volume. This generally implies impaired systolic pump function, though states of diastolic ventricular dysfunction (e.g., hypertrophic or restrictive cardiomyopathies) and of supranormal cardiac output (e.g., anemia, thyrotoxicosis, atrioventricular [AV] shunts) can manifest with symptoms of CHF.

B. Etiology

The most common causes of CHF in the United States are hypertension and coronary artery disease. In the ED, the identification and treatment of the precipitant of heart failure in a patient with previously compensated pump function is crucial. Common precipitants include the following:

1. Myocardial infarction (MI).

2. Accelerated hypertension.

3. Arrhythmias.

4. Acute valvular dysfunction.

5. Ventricular septal rupture.

6. Infection and fever, with or without sepsis.

7. Pulmonary embolism.

8. Anemia.

9. Thyrotoxicosis.

10. Infective endocarditis.

11. Dietary indiscretion.

12. Medical noncompliance.

II. CLINICAL PRESENTATION

A. Symptoms

Symptoms and signs of CHF depend on whether right, left, or both ventricles are involved, and the acuity of pump failure.

1. Left-ventricular (LV) failure. Dyspnea is the chief symptom of LV failure. This may include
   a. Dyspnea on exertion.
   b. Orthopnea.
   c. Paroxysmal nocturnal dyspnea.
   d. Wheezing related to cardiac asthma.
   e. Frank respiratory distress.
   Other manifestations include Cheyne-Stokes breathing, chronic nonproductive cough, weakness, and fatigue.

2. Right-ventricular (RV) failure. Symptoms may include
   a. Dependent edema.
   b. Right-upper-quadrant pain and, later, jaundice due to congestive hepatomegaly.
   Symptoms of LV failure may lessen with the onset of RV failure.
   The time course and severity of the above symptoms will vary depending on the precipitating cause and acuity of disease onset.

B. Signs

1. Vital sign alterations:
   a. Tachypnea.
   b. Tachycardia.
   c. Hypo- or hypertension.

2. Left-ventricular failure:
   a. Pulmonary rales.
   b. Pleural effusion.
   c. Third and fourth heart sounds.

3. Right-ventricular failure:
   a. Jugular venous distention.
   b. Right-ventricular heave.
   c. Peripheral edema.
   d. Tender, enlarged, and pulsatile liver.

C. Laboratory and Other Studies

1. Routine studies include a complete blood count, electrolyte levels, glucose, blood urea nitrogen, creatinine, electrocardiogram, and chest roentgenogram.

2. Consider, depending on clinical circumstances, arterial blood gas (ABG), creatinine phosphokinase/lactate dehydrogenase with isoenzymes, magnesium, calcium, thryoid function tests, echocardiography, and urinalysis.

III. DIFFERENTIAL DIAGNOSIS

A. Left-ventricular failure: Consider other conditions that cause dyspnea as the primary symptom:

1. Primary pulmonary disease: chronic obstructive pulmonary disease (COPD), asthma, pneumonia, pulmonary embolism, pneumothorax, and malignancy.

2. Extrapulmonary conditions: pericardial tamponade, primary hyperventilation (central nervous system pathology or anxiety), sepsis, and metabolic acidosis.

B. Right-ventricular failure: pericardial tamponade, primary pulmonary hypertension, pulmonary embolism, nephrotic syndrome, cirrhosis, and idiopathic edema.

IV. THERAPY

As in any acute cardiopulmonary syndrome, the first step in the management of CHF is to ensure the stability of the airway, breathing, and circulation (ABCs). Not uncommonly, CHF precipitated by acute MI or pulmonary embolism may present as respiratory failure and cardiogenic shock. Therapy in these situations must be aimed at securing the ABCs and treating the precipitating cause.

A. General Measures

1. Physical rest.

2. Oxygen by nasal cannula (3–5 L/min) and assessment of adequate oxygen delivery (by pulse oximetry or ABG assessment).

3. Gain IV access.

4. Cardiac monitoring.

5. Repeated measurement of blood pressure (BP).

Treatment of specific arrhythmias is discussed in the previous section.

B. Specific Measures

Specific measures can be categorized according to their effect on preload, pump, or afterload: decreasing end-diastolic ventricular volume or pressure (preload), enhancing myocardial inotropy (pump), and decreasing systemic vascular resistance and thus systolic work (afterload). These measures will differ according to the acuity of onset of heart failure (Table 13–10).

C. Therapy of Acute Pulmonary Edema (Fig. 13–6)

1. Assess the need for endotracheal intubation and/or circulatory support.

2. Administer supplemental oxygen, establish intravenous access, and monitor both cardiac rhythm and oxygen saturation (SaO_2). Obtain an emergent ECG and portable chest roentgenogram.

3. Specific drug therapy:

   Note: if the patient is hypotensive (systolic BP < 100 mmHg), first support blood pressure with dopamine (2.5–20 µg/kg/min IV) before proceeding with the therapy outlined below. Adverse effects with dopamine include tachycardia, ventricular irritability, and increased systemic vascular resistance. If hypotension is severe (systolic BP < 70 mmHg) or refractory to dopamine, consider norepinephrine (0.5–30 µg/min IV) with

Table 13–10. SPECIFIC MEASURES USED IN THE TREATMENT OF CONGESTIVE HEART FAILURE

DECREASE PRELOAD	ENHANCE PUMP	DECREASE AFTERLOAD
Acute-Onset CHF		
Furosemide (IV)	Sympathomimetics: dopamine, dobutamine	Nitroprusside
Morphine sulfate (IV)		IV nitroglycerin
Nitroglycerin (paste, SL, IV)	Digitalis glycosides	Intra-aortic balloon pump
Intra-aortic balloon pump	Amrinone	
Dialysis	Emergent heart surgery: coronary artery bypass grafting, valve replacement	
Rotating tourniquets		
Phlebotomy	Coronary angioplasty	
Gradual-Onset and Chronic CHF		
Sodium and fluid restriction	Digitalis glycosides	Angiotensin converting enzyme inhibitors
Diuretics: furosemide, thiazides, potassium-sparing diuretics	Milrinone	Nitrates
Nitrates	Cardiac transplant	Hydralazine
Dialysis		Other peripheral vasodilators: nifedipine, prazosin, minoxidil

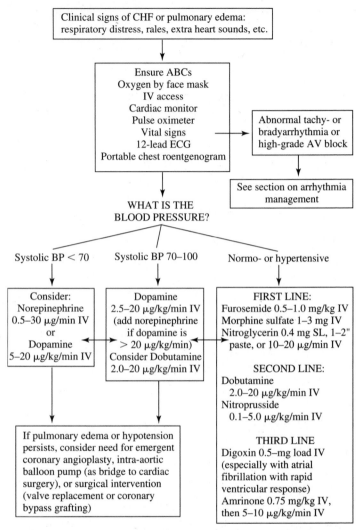

Figure 13–6. Acute pulmonary edema treatment algorithm. (Adapted from Emergency Cardiac Care Committee and Subcommittees, American Heart Association, 1992.)

or without dopamine, and emergently arrange for an intra-aortic balloon pump as a "bridge" to definitive cardiac therapy.

  a. First-Line Therapy

    i. Morphine sulfate (1–3 mg IV, repeated every 5–10 minutes as indicated): venodilator, anxiolytic, and analgesic agent.

    ii. Furosemide (0.5–1 mg/kg IV): venodilator and diuretic agent. If diuresis is not initiated in 30 minutes, consider administering twice the initial dose. Hypokalemia, hypomagnesemia, and ototoxicity are potential adverse effects. Doses of 200 mg or more IV rarely augment the response and are associated with increased ototoxicity. The addition of metolazone (5–10 mg PO) may enhance the diuretic effect of furosemide. Again, monitor potassium and magnesium levels closely.

    iii. Nitroglycerin (0.4 mg SL, 1–2 inches transdermal paste, or initially 10–20 µg/min IV infusion): vasodilation decreases both preload and afterload. Hypotension is a potential side effect.

  b. SECOND-LINE THERAPY

    i. Dobutamine (2–20 µg/kg/min IV infusion): inotropic agent and reflex vasodilator. Ventricular irritability is an adverse effect.

    ii. Nitroprusside (0.1–5 µg/kg/min IV infusion): potent vasodilator. Dosage must be carefully adjusted to avoid hypotension; invasive hemodynamic monitoring is recommended. In the setting of ongoing myocardial ischemia, coronary "steal" and decreased coronary perfusion pressures are worrisome complications. Thiocyanate toxicity may occur within 72 hours of therapy in patients with normal renal function; risks are increased in patients with renal insufficiency and this drug should be avoided in that setting.

  c. THIRD-LINE THERAPY

    i. Digoxin (0.5 mg slowly IV): useful in patients with rapid atrial fibrillation or supraventricular tachycardias complicating CHF.

    ii. Amrinone (0.75 mg/kg IV load followed by 5–10 µg/kg/min IV): this phosphodiesterase inhibitor has both inotropic and diuretic effects. Hypotension is a potential adverse effect. Dosage should be reduced in patients with a creatinine clearance < 10 mL/min.

    iii. Aminophylline (loading dose: 5 mg/kg IV over 20–30 minutes): appropriate in the patient clinically wheezing. Dose carefully and follow blood levels to avoid toxicity.

    iv. Additional interventions, depending on clinical circumstances, may include an intra-aortic balloon pump, emergent coronary artery angioplasty, or surgical intervention (e.g., valve replacement, coronary artery bypass grafting, or cardiac transplant).

4. A Foley catheter is appropriate to closely monitor urine output. Invasive hemodynamic monitoring (including an arterial line and Swan-Ganz catheter) is frequently useful in optmizing

therapy, especially when parenteral afterload reduction is needed.

5. Admit the patient to the hospital (See Disposition, below).

D. Therapy of Gradual-Onset Congestive Heart Failure

1. Gradual decompensation of chronic CHF, or progression of symptoms in a patient not previously diagnosed, usually presents with milder symptoms and shifts the emphasis of the ED physician from emergent therapeutic measures to an aggressive search for the precipitating cause (see list, above).

2. In the patient with chronic CHF and no clear new precipitant, often an additional dose of a loop diuretic either PO or IV will be all that is required to alleviate congestion. Initiation of new medications is best done after discussion of the situation with the patient's personal physician. Close follow-up for improvement of symptoms and verification of electrolyte balance is required.

3. In the patient with gradual, but new onset of CHF, hospital admission is generally warranted to search for the underlying and precipitating cause, or at least to rule out cardiac ischemia. Therapy should be directed at hypoxemia, specific arrhythmias, and electrolyte disturbances. Specific therapy with diuretics (e.g., furosemide 20 mg IV) and/or angiotensin converting enzyme (ACE) inhibitors (e.g., captopril 12.5 mg PO) may be initiated in the ED in advance of admission.

E. Therapy of Congestive Heart Failure Without Pulmonary Congestion

Acute onset of peripheral edema without pulmonary edema indicates RV decompensation. Right-ventricular infarction, pulmonary embolism, and decompensation of chronic cor pulmonale are important precipitants. A right-sided ECG will help identify RV infarction. One must maintain a high index of suspicion for pulmonary embolism in anyone with chronic peripheral edema. If the patient is hypotensive, an isotonic IV fluid challenge is appropriate. If the patient is normotensive, therapy is aimed at relieving hypoxemia, correcting electrolyte disturbances, and treating specific arrhythmias. Patients with new-onset right-sided heart failure generally warrant admission to the hospital to rule out infarction or pulmonary embolism.

V. DISPOSITION

A. Candidates for admission include

1. All patients presenting with respiratory distress in acute pulmonary edema; ICU/CCU monitoring is warranted.

2. Patients with a new arrhythmia as either a precipitant or effect

of CHF; telemetry or ICU/CCU monitoring should be dictated by the clinical situation.

3. Patients with newly diagnosed CHF with no clear underlying cause.

4. Patients with chronic CHF with moderate to severe decompensation (or mild decompensation with evidence of ischemia).

B. Candidates for discharge include patients with chronic CHF with mild decompensation without evidence of ischemia. Appropriate follow-up is mandatory.

VI. PEARLS AND PITFALLS

A. Remember, like diabetic ketoacidosis, CHF is a syndrome that is generally easily diagnosed. An aggressive search for the precipitating cause(s) should be carried out once the patient is stabilized.

B. Diffuse pneumonia in a patient with chronic CHF or COPD is at times difficult to distinguish from acute CHF. A Swan-Ganz catheter may be necessary to make the distinction.

C. If follow-up with an outpatient physician cannot be arranged, see the patient back in the ED within 24–48 hours to verify improvement and tolerance of any new medications.

BIBLIOGRAPHY

Dei Cas L, Leier CV: Initial management of acute congestive heart failure. J Crit Illness 1992;7:1612.

Emergency Cardiac Care Committee and Subcommittees, American Heart Association: Guidelines for cardiopulmonary resuscitation and emergency cardiac care: II. Adult advanced cardiac life support. JAMA 1992;268:2199.

Marantz PR, Kaplan MC, Alderman MH: Clinical diagnosis of congestive heart failure in patients with acute dyspnea. Chest 1990;97:776.

Perret C: Acute heart failure in myocardial infarction: principles of treatment. Crit Care Med 1990;18:S26.

Wuerz RC, Meador SA: Effects of prehospital medications on mortality and length of stay in congestive heart failure. Ann Emerg Med 1992;21:669.

HYPERTENSIVE EMERGENCIES

> *My fate cries out,*
> *And makes each petty artery in this body*
> *As hardy as the Newean Rion's nerve.*
>
> WILLIAM SHAKESPEARE

I. ESSENTIAL FACTS

A. Definitions

1. *Hypertensive emergency* describes a severe elevation of blood pressure (BP) in association with acute end-organ damage

requiring immediate therapy to prevent further morbidity. Organ system compromise or syndromes coming under this term are listed below; in some of these, increased BP is the result, rather than the cause, of the organ system pathology.

a. **Central Nervous System (CNS).** Intracranial hemorrhage, thrombotic stroke, subarachnoid hemorrhage, hypertensive encephalopathy (headache, irritability, alterations of consciousness, or other symptoms and signs of CNS disturbance in association with a rapid rise in BP), severe retinopathy (exudates and hemorrhages with or without papilledema), and head trauma.

b. **Cardiovascular.** Acute left-ventricular failure, unstable angina or acute myocardial infarction, and aortic dissection.

c. **Renal.** Acute renal insufficiency.

d. **Eclampsia.** Hypertension in pregnancy with edema and proteinuria, associated with convulsions, coma, and often, renal failure. Because many pre-eclamptic women are previously normotensive, eclamptic manifestations may occur at BPs as low as 150/100 mmHg.

e. **Catecholamine Crisis:** Extreme elevation in BP associated with catecholamine release, including recreational drug use (e.g., cocaine and amphetamines), pheochromocytoma, ingestion of tyramine-containing foods in conjunction with use of monoamine oxidase inhibitors (MAOI), or clonidine withdrawal. This may or may not have associated acute end-organ damage as an immediate consequence, but most authors agree emergent therapy is indicated.

2. *Hypertensive urgency* is used to describe severe elevation in diastolic BP ($\geq$ 115 mmHg), but without immediate end-organ compromise. This situation requires more gradual lowering of BP over the next 24–48 hours. Generally, treatment is initiated in the ED and continued on an outpatient basis.

II. CLINICAL PRESENTATION

A. History

The history should focus on the following:

1. Precipitating factors (e.g., acute CNS event; antihypertensive medication cessation; recreational drug, decongestant, or diet pill use; MAOI therapy and ingestion of tyramine).

2. Symptoms indicating end-organ damage, especially nervous system (e.g., headache, visual disturbance, nausea/vomiting, seizures), and cardiovascular system (e.g., chest pain, dyspnea with exertion).

3. Prior history of hypertension and its severity, duration, and control.

4. Significant past medical history.

B. Physical Examination

The physical examination should include the following:

1. Repeated BP measurements with an appropriate-sized cuff, initially taken in both arms.

2. Directed examination focusing on detection of retinopathy (papilledema, exudates, hemorrhages), congestive heart failure (CHF), aortic dissection, neurologic deficits, and mental status changes.

C. Other Studies

Other studies should generally include the following:

1. Electrocardiography (ECG) (ischemia or injury).

2. Chest roentgenography (cardiomegaly with or without CHF, widened mediastinum with aortic dissection).

3. Oximetry (consider arterial blood gas determinations).

4. Urinalysis (red-cell casts).

5. Blood urea nitrogen (BUN)/creatinine.

6. Electrolyte values (hypokalemia).

7. Glucose.

8. Complete blood count (CBC) with smear evaluation (intravascular hemolysis).

III. THERAPY FOR HYPERTENSIVE EMERGENCIES (FIG. 13–7)

A. Hypertensive emergencies should be treated with parenteral agents, as the goal of therapy is prompt and controlled lowering of BP. The choice of drug is largely dictated by the clinical situation. Table 13–11 outlines common IV medications, their mechanism of action, onset, duration of action, dosage, and adverse side effects.

B. The goal of therapy is to lower mean arterial BP (MAP) by approximately 25% or to gradually reduce diastolic BP to 100–110 mmHg. (Remember MAP is estimated by adding one-third the pulse pressure to the diastolic BP). Precipitous decrease or reduction to normotensive levels should be avoided.

C. Intravenous infusion is preferred over bolus therapy for better minute-to-minute control, but intensive BP monitoring is required. For this reason, sodium nitroprusside is the drug of choice in most situations.

D. Treatment recommendations according to type of hypertensive emergency are shown in Table 13–12.

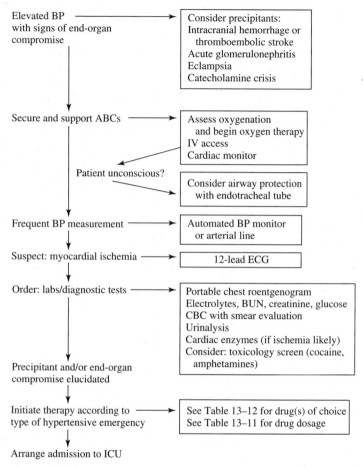

Figure 13–7. Therapy for hypertensive emergency. ABCs, airway, breathing, circulation.

IV. THERAPY FOR HYPERTENSIVE URGENCY

A. Hypertensive urgency can usually be treated with oral medications, with eventual patient discharge from the ED. Follow-up should be arranged within the next 24 hours, either back in the ED, to an appropriate clinic, or with the patient's primary care provider (Table 13–13).

B. The goal of therapy again is gradual reduction of MAP by 20%, or a diastolic BP of 100–110 mmHg. Additionally, tolerance of the medication must be observed to ensure success of therapy. Observation in the ED is necessary to ensure the reduction in BP and the medication are well tolerated.

C. The most common agents used for hypertensive urgencies are oral, buccal, or sublingual nifedipine and oral clonidine. Other agents have also been used successfully and include captopril, propranolol, or metoprolol; furosemide; and prazosin. Case reports of clinically significant myocardial ischemic events have been documented during sublingual nifedipine therapy for acute BP

Table 13–11. DRUGS USED IN THE TREATMENT OF HYPERTENSIVE EMERGENCIES

DRUG (AND MECHANISM)	DOSE	ONSET/ DURATION	ADVERSE EFFECTS/ COMMENTS
Nitroprusside (vaso-dilator)	0.25–8 µg/kg/min IV	< 1 min/ 2–3 min	Start at low dose and titrate for effect. *Adverse effects:* Excess hypotension, thiocyanate toxicity; avoid in renal failure.
Nitroglycerin (vaso- and venodilator)	5–200 µg/min IV	1 min/ 3–5 min	Start at low dose and titrate upward in 10-µg/min increments. Maintains coronary perfusion pressure.
Labetalol (alpha- and beta blocker)	20–80 mg IV bolus every 5–10 min, max 300 mg, *or* 10–30 mg/min continuous infusion IV	1–5 min/ 3–6 hr	Excess hypotension, heart block, heart failure. Avoid in asthmatics.
Esmolol (beta blocker)	500 µg/kg IV load over 1 min, then 50–200 µg/kg/min	1–2 min/ 10–30 min	As with labetalol.
Trimethaphan (ganglionic blocker)	0.5–5 mg/min IV	1–5 min/ 10 min	Excess hypotension, urinary retention.
Diazoxide (vasodilator)	50–100 mg IV every 5–10 min, up to 600 mg, *or* 10–30 mg/min IV	1–5 min/ 6–12 hr	Excess hypotension, reflex tachycardia.
Hydralazine (vasodilator)	5–10 mg IV every 20 min, up to 20 mg	10–20 min/ 3–6 hr	Excess hypotension, reflex tachycardia, local phlebitis.
Phentolamine (alpha blocker)	5–10 mg IV every 5–15 min	1–2 min/ 3–10 min	Excess hypotension, reflex tachycardia, paradoxical pressor effect.
Furosemide (loop diuretic)	10–80 mg IV	15 min/ 4 hr	Hypokalemia, hypovolemia. Adjunct to vasodilator.
Magnesium sulfate	4–6 g IV over 6–10 min, followed by an infusion of 1–2 g/hr	—	Combined with hydralazine, this is the drug of choice for pre-eclampsia and eclampsia. Monitor deep tendon reflexes; discontinue IV infusion if they disappear.

Table 13–12. TYPES OF HYPERTENSIVE EMERGENCY AND TREATMENT RECOMMENDATIONS

Type of Hypertensive Emergency	Drug(s) to Use	Drugs to Avoid
Hypertensive encephalopathy	Nitroprusside, *or* labetalol, *or* diazoxide	Beta blockers, methyldopa, clonidine
CNS event (infarction, intracerebral hemorrhage)	No treatment (*or* nitroprusside if diastolic BP > 130 mmHg)	Beta blockers, methyldopa, clonidine
Myocardial ischemia/infarction	Nitroglycerin, beta blocker	Nitroprusside, hydralazine, diazoxide
Cardiogenic pulmonary edema	Nitroglycerin, *or* nitroprusside with furosemide	Beta blockers, labetalol, hydralazine, diazoxide
Aortic dissection	Nitroprusside with beta blocker, or labetalol	Hydralazine, diazoxide
Renal failure	Loop diuretic and/or calcium channel blocker, hydralazine	Beta blockers, trimethaphan
Eclampsia/pre-eclampsia	Hydralazine and magnesium sulfate	Trimethaphan, beta blockers, diuretics
Pheochromocytoma	Phentolamine, *or* labetalol, *or* nitroprusside	Beta blockers
Other catecholamine crisis: cocaine or amphetamine-related, MAOI-related, antihypertensive withdrawal	Labetalol, *or* phentolamine, *or* nitroprusside	Beta blockers

Adapted from Calhoun DA, Oparil S: Current concepts—treatment of hypertensive crisis. N Engl J Med 1990;323(17):1177–1183.

reduction, so caution should be used in those with known coronary artery disease, or ECG evidence of ischemia or left-ventricular hypertrophy.

D. Patients requiring therapy for hypertensive urgency optimally should be continued on the same drug initiated in the ED. Both clonidine and long-acting calcium channel antagonists may be used as the primary antihypertensive or added to the patient's present regimen.

E. Depending on the severity of BP elevation, many patients with elevated BP need to be treated in the ED. In patients with a known history of hypertension, restarting previously effective drugs may be all that is required. All hypertensive patients should have a plan for follow-up and be instructed on symptoms of end-organ compromise, low-salt diet, and weight reduction.

V. DISPOSITION

A. All patients with a hypertensive emergency should be admitted to the ICU.

B. Most patients with urgent hypertension can be discharged from the ED. Exceptions to this are

1. If BP does not respond to ED therapy.

2. If appropriate follow-up cannot be ensured.

C. Hypertension in the pregnant patient warrants at least phone contact with the patient's obstetrician. Pre-eclamptic patients will need admission for maternal and fetal monitoring during antihypertensive therapy.

VI. PEARLS AND PITFALLS

A. Attempt to tailor emergent antihypertensive therapy to the organ system most prominently involved. For example, hypertension with symptoms of angina and ECG changes consistent with myocardial ischemia is best treated with nitroglycerin, morphine, and a beta blocker. Pulmonary edema in the setting of a hypertensive emergency might be best treated with a combination of a loop diuretic (e.g., furosemide 20–40 mg IV), morphine, and a nitroglycerin or nitroprusside IV infusion.

B. Meticulous BP monitoring is essential. Many authors advocate the use of an intra-arterial catheter, especially with nitroprusside therapy.

C. Blood pressure reduction in acute thromboembolic stroke is generally not recommended. A reduced systemic BP could lead to decreased cerebral blood flow. If therapy is required because of severe hypertension (i.e., diastolic BP > 120 mmHg), the BP should be gradually reduced over 24 hours (and decreasing the diastolic BP to < 105 mmHg avoided).

Table 13–13. ORAL ANTIHYPERTENSIVES USED TO TREAT HYPERTENSIVE URGENCY

Agent	Dose and Route	Onset/Duration	Adverse Effects
Nifedipine	10–20 mg bite and swallow q 15–30 min or PO q 30–60 min	5–10 min/3–6 hr 15–30 min/3–6 hr	Tachycardia, excessive hypotension, headache
Clonidine	0.2 mg PO load, then 0.1 mg PO q 1 hr up to 0.7 mg over time	30–60 min/8–12 hr	Sedation, rebound drug withdrawal
Captopril[a]	12.5–25 mg PO single dose	15–30 min/4–6 hr	Excessive hypotension
Labetalol[a]	100–300 mg PO	30–60 min/4–8 hr	Excessive hypotension, bradycardia; do not use in patients with asthma, h/o CHF, or AV block

[a]Limited experience.

BIBLIOGRAPHY

Calhoun DA, Oparil S: Current concepts—treatment of hypertensive crisis. New Engl J Med 1990;323:1177.

Gonzalez ER, et al: Dose-response evaluation of oral labetalol in patients presenting to the emergency department with accelerated hypertension. Ann Emerg Med 1991; 20:333.

Just VL, et al: Evaluation of drug therapy for treatment of hypertensive urgencies in the emergency department. Am J Emerg Med 1991;9:107.

Sand IC, Brody SL, et al: Experience with esmolol for the treatment of cocaine-associated cardiovascular complications. Am J Emerg Med 1991;9:161.

Sanders AB: Hypertensive emergencies. Am Fam Phys 1991;44:1767.

MYOCARDIAL INFARCTION

> *"Of all the ailments which may blow out life's little candle, heart disease is the chief."*
>
> WILLIAM BOYD

I. ESSENTIAL FACTS

A. Definition

1. *Myocardial infarction* (MI) is the irreversible cellular injury and necrosis of cardiac muscle caused by prolonged ischemia.

2. It results from a marked reduction or absence of blood flow through one or more coronary arteries. In the vast majority of cases, there is rupture of an atherosclerotic plaque with secondary thrombosis and coronary artery spasm. Other less common mechanisms include coronary artery dissection, embolism, vasculitis, and cocaine-induced coronary artery spasm.

B. Epidemiology

1. Heart disease (predominantly MI) was responsible for 36% of all deaths in the United States in 1986.

2. Approximately 1.25 million patients suffered an acute MI in this country in 1993, resulting in nearly 500,000 deaths. Over one-half of these deaths occurred suddenly, within 1 hour of symptom onset, and prior to the patient's hospital arrival.

3. The mortality from acute MI can be significantly reduced if the patient seeks prompt medical attention at the onset of symptoms, and if thrombolytic therapy is urgently administered to appropriate candidates upon ED arrival. Other therapeutic modalities that favorably effect both morbidity and mortality in the setting of acute MI include oxygen, intravenous (IV) nitroglycerin, aspirin, beta blockers, heparin, and angiotensin converting enzyme (ACE) inhibitors.

4. Risk factors for coronary artery disease include
   a. Male sex.
   b. Hypertension.
   c. Hyperlipidemia.
   d. Diabetes mellitus.
   e. Age > 30 years.
   f. Smoking.
   g. Family history.
   h. Obesity.
   i. Sedentary life style.

   In a patient with chest pain, however, the absence of risk factors does not exclude ischemic heart disease.

II. CLINICAL EVALUATION

A. General

1. The patient's history and electrocardiogram (ECG) are the most useful ED tools in the diagnosis of cardiac ischemia and acute MI.

2. The index of suspicion for myocardial ischemia must remain high despite vague or atypical chest and/or upper-abdominal symptoms.

B. Symptoms

1. Chest pain is the hallmark of acute ischemia, and occurs in approximately 90% of patients with an acute MI. Classically the pain is described as a pressure, heavy, cramping, burning, and/or aching sensation not affected by respiration or movement. Sharp, stabbing, positional pain, or pain reproducible by palpation, is less likely to represent acute ischemia, but the use of these descriptors does *not* exclude ischemia.
   a. **Location.** Pain is generally substernal, but may be epigastric (35% of patients). Pain is less frequently isolated in the shoulder, back, jaw, or arm.
   b. **Radiation.** Substernal or precordial chest pain may radiate to the arms, neck, or jaw.
   c. **Duration.** The pain generally persists for > 30 minutes.
   d. **Relief.** Response of pain to nitroglycerin does *not* prove myocardial ischemia (e.g., esophageal spasm also responds to nitrates). Likewise, relief of pain with oral antacids mixed with viscous lidocaine does *not* rule out myocardial ischemia (i.e., this is not a valid diagnostic test).

2. Dyspnea is the most important non–chest-pain symptom. It is present in about 33% of patients with acute infarction. In some MI patients, sudden dyspnea may be the chief presenting complaint.

3. Diaphoresis occurs in 20–50% of acute MI patients; when

associated with chest pain, it increases the likelihood of acute infarction.

4. Nausea and vomiting are a frequent symptom complex in patients with MI (especially in the setting of inferior myocardial ischemia).

5. Silent MI: as many as 25% of nonfatal MIs are unrecognized by the patient; of these, one-half are truly silent. Silent MI occurs more frequently in the elderly, patients with diabetes, hypertension, and those without antecedent angina.

C. Physical Examination

Note: the patient should be on supplemental oxygen and the cardiac rhythm continuously monitored before proceeding with the physical examination!

1. General
Note the patient's anxiety and degree of pain, color, and any respiratory difficulty.

2. Vital Signs
Quickly assess pulse and blood pressure (BP), respiratory rate, and temperature. Blood pressure should be checked and documented in *both* upper extremities. Continuous monitoring of the patient's cardiac rhythm and oxygen saturation (SaO_2), and a nursing staff-initiated ECG, should be considered additional "vital signs" in any patient suspected of ongoing myocardial ischemia.

3. Skin
Note diaphoresis, cyanosis, clamminess, and any evidence of a potential lipid disorder (e.g., *xanthomas:* local cutaneous lipid infiltrates).

4. Neck
Assess jugular venous distention and carotid pulses, and auscultate for bruits.

5. Chest
Palpate the chest for any chest-wall tenderness; listen for overall air movement, wheezes, and rales.

6. Heart
Note whether the patient is bradycardic or tachycardic. Palpate the precordium and listen carefully to the heart sounds. A prominent S4 indicates decreased ventricular compliance and is suggestive of myocardial ischemia in the setting of on-going chest pain. An S3 indicates increased ventricular diastolic pressure and congestive heart failure (CHF). A prominent and new systolic murmur may suggest acute mitral regurgitation from papillary muscle dysfunction or rupture, or ventricular septal rupture.

7. Pulses
   Palpate radial, femoral, dorsalis pedis, and posterior tibial pulses.

8. Abdomen
   Evaluate for distention, bowel sounds, masses, palpable aortic abnormalities, and/or findings of localized peritoneal irritation that suggest intra-abdominal pathology.

9. Extremities
   Assess peripheral edema and extremity perfusion.

10. Neurologic Examination
    Note the patient's mental status.

Note: the physical examination in the patient with an acute MI may be completely normal. Occasionally, the physical examination may suggest a nonischemic cause of the patient's complaints.

D. Laboratory and Diagnostic Studies

1. Routine Studies
   a. ECG (initiate concomitantly with the patient's vital signs)
   b. Chest roentgenogram (portable)
   c. Electrolyte levels
   d. Blood urea nitrogen/creatinine
   e. Complete blood count
   f. Calcium, magnesium
   g. Creatinine kinase (CK with isoenzymes)
   h. Glucose
   i. Prothrombin time/partial thromboplastin time (PT/PTT)
   j. Urinalysis

2. Additional Studies
   The following *may be required* depending on clinical circumstances:
   a. Lactate dehydrogenase (LDH with isoenzymes).
   b. Echocardiography.
   c. Emergent coronary artery angiography.

3. Laboratory and Diagnostic Test Considerations
   a. **Electrocardiogram (Table 13–14)**
      i. *The ECG is the first and most useful test to perform in patients suspected of having ischemic chest pain.* The inital ECG, however, is consistent with ischemia/infarction in only 64% of patients with acute MI; and in 6% of acute MI patients the initial ECG is normal.
      ii. Careful ECG analysis requires assessment of the following:
         • Rate.
         • Rhythm.

Table 13–14. ECG MARKERS FOR THE LOCATION OF ACUTE MI

MI LOCATION	LEADS	POSSIBLE ECG CHANGES	POTENTIAL CORONARY ARTERY INVOLVEMENT	RECIPROCAL LEADS	POSSIBLE RECIPROCAL ECG CHANGES
Inferior	II,III,AVF	Q-wave, ST↑	RCA	I,AVL,V$_{1-3}$	ST↓
Anterior	V1–4,AVL	Q-wave, ST↑ R-wave[a]	LCA	II,III,AVF	ST↓
Lateral	I,AVL	Q-wave, ST↑	LCx	V1, V3	ST↓
Posterior	V1–2	R[b]> S, ST↑	RCx	II,III,AVF	—
Apical	V3–6	Q-wave, ST↑ R wave[a]	LAD, RCA	—	—
Anterolateral	I,AVL,V5,V6	Q-wave, ST↑ R wave[a]	LAD, LCx	II,III,AVF	ST↓
Anteroseptal	V1–4	Q-wave, ST↑ R-wave[a]	LAD	—	— .

[a]Loss of R-wave progression.
[b]Followed in time by abnormally tall R waves.
LCA, left coronary artery; LCx, left circumflex; RCx, right circumflex; LAD, left anterior descending; RCA, right coronary artery.

- PR/QRS/ and QT intervals.
- R-wave axis.
- ST-segment abnormalities (ST-segment elevation ≥ 0.1 mV [1 mm] in two or more contiguous limb leads, or ≥ 0.2 mV [2 mm] in two or more precordial leads, suggests transmural myocardial ischemia/infarction; ST-segment depression may indicate subendocardial ischemia).
- T-wave abnormalities (hyperacute T-waves may be the earliest ECG finding of acute ischemia; tall peaked T-waves are also seen in hyperkalemia; T-wave inversion suggests acute ischemia).
- Q waves (may indicate prior myocardial infarction; abnormal Q waves are 0.04 seconds in duration, greater than 25% of the R-wave amplitude, and are present in more than one lead).
- Conduction disturbances (e.g., right-bundle-branch block [RBBB], left-bundle-branch block [LBBB], and/or left-anterior or posterior hemiblock).
- Evidence of right- (RV) or left-ventricular (LV) hypertrophy.
- Evidence of right or left atrial abnormality.

iii. The ECG is a static representation of a dynamic process. *Serial ECGs and ECGs with changes in the patient's pain complaints are helpful in diagnosis and assessing therapeutic effectiveness.*

b. **Cardiac Enzymes.** Elevations in the serum level of cardiac enzymes with time are the most specific tests available in the detection or exclusion of MI. Initial enzyme determinations are only 40–50% sensitive, however, so an initial normal test does *not* exclude myocardial ischemia in the ED. CK (with isoenzymes) should be routinely ordered on all MI patients in the ED, with the levels rechecked at 12 and 24 hours postpresentation while the patient is in the ICU. For MI patients presenting 24 or more hours after the onset of their symptoms, LDH with isoenzymes should *also* be obtained.

c. **Echocardiography.** May be used to detect regional wall-motion abnormalities, valvular dysfunction, pericardial effusions, and global ventricular systolic function. In the ED, echocardiography is helpful in confirming the diagnosis of RV infarction, papillary muscle rupture, ventricular septal rupture, pericardial effusion, LV aneurysm, aortic stenosis, and/or LV mural thrombus. An emergent echocardiogram may also be used to confirm a regional wall-motion abnormality suggesting transmural ischemia in a patient with atypical chest pain and a nondiagnostic ECG (echocardiography has a sensitivity of 70–95% and a specificity of 85–100% in the early diagnosis of acute MI).

d. **Cardiac Catheterization and Coronary Artery Angiography (with possible angioplasty).** Indicated emergently in the acute MI patient with cardiogenic shock, the patient who presents within 12 hours of symptom onset but who has a contraindication to thrombolytic therapy, and/or the patient with recurrent postischemia or postinfarction chest pain. See the discussion of thrombolytic therapy versus angioplasty in IV. C. 5., below.

III. DIFFERENTIAL DIAGNOSIS

The differential diagnosis of chest pain includes

A. Myocardial infarction.

B. Unstable angina.

C. Pericarditis and myocarditis.

D. Mitral valve prolapse.

E. Pulmonary hypertension.

F. Pneumothorax.

G. Esophageal spasm.

H. Esophageal rupture.

I. Peptic ulcer disease.

J. Acute cerebrovascular disease.

    K. Spinal and chest-wall diseases.

    L. Angina.

    M. Aortic stenosis.

    N. Aortic dissection.

    O. Pulmonary embolism.

    P. Pneumonia.

    Q. Pleurisy.

    R. Esophageal reflux.

    S. Gallbladder disease.

    T. Pancreatitis.

    U. Acute anxiety states.

IV. THERAPY (TABLE 13–15 AND FIG. 13–8)

A. Initial Assessment

1. Place the patient on oxygen (2–5 L/min via nasal cannula) and continuously monitor the cardiac rhythm and SaO_2. In the setting of pulmonary edema or cardiogenic shock, supplement oxygen with a 100% non-rebreather mask if necessary to ensure $\geq$ 95% hemoglobin saturation.

2. Rapidly obtain vital signs, ECG, IV access (at least two IV lines are recommended), and a directed physical examination. The ECG should be repeated every 30–60 minutes throughout the patient's ED stay or with changes in chest pain complaints/ clinical status as indicated.

3. Obtain a portable chest roentgenogram and order relevant laboratory studies (see II. D, above).

B. First-Line Therapy

Note: thrombolytic therapy (see IV. C, below) should be started as rapidly as possible in the appropriate candidate in conjunction with the medications described in this section. In the patient with unstable vital signs, hemodynamic support (rhythm management, volume management, and/or pressor use: see IV. E) should be started immediately as indicated.

1. **Nitroglycerin.** Available as sublingual tablets or spray, percutaneous paste, or IV continuous infusion.
   - a. Relieves pain by dilating epicardial arteries, increasing collateral flow to ischemic myocardium, and decreasing ventricular preload.
   - b. IV nitroglycerin may reduce infarct size, prevent ventricular aneurysm formation, decrease susceptibility to ventricular fibrillation during acute MI, and, in some studies, reduce mortality.

Text continues on page 266

Table 13–15. EMERGENCY MEDICAL THERAPY FOR THE PATIENT WITH AN ACUTE MI

DRUG	DOSE	COMMENTS
Oxygen	Begin wtih 2–5 L/min via nasal cannula	Adjust as necessary to maintain hemoglobin saturation $\geq$ 95%. Beware of patients with COPD and CO_2 retention whose respiratory drive may be diminished by high oxygen flow rates.
Nitroglycerin		
Sublingual tablets or spray	1 tablet or spray SL q 3–5 min to a total of three doses	Use SL as initial treatment until IV access is established.
Paste	½ to 2 inches to the skin q 6 hr	Titrate to pain; maintain systolic BP $\geq$ 100 mmHg.
Intravenous	Begin at 10–20 µg/min IV. Infusion may be increased by 5–10 µg/min q 5–10 min as necessary.	IV nitroglycerin is the preferred method of administration in the acute MI patient. Monitor pain and hemodynamic response. Maximum dosage is 200 µg/min.
Morphine Sulfate	2–4 mg IV q 5 min, titrated to pain and anxiety	Use small incremental doses at frequent intervals to avoid respiratory depression.
Aspirin	160–325 mg PO (chewed and swallowed)	Should be given as soon as myocardial ischemia is suspected.
Thrombolytic Agents (one of the following)		Thrombolytic therapy needs to be started in the appropriate candidate *as rapidly as possible* after ED arrival. See Table 13–16 for contraindications.
Streptokinase (SK)	1.5 million units IV over 1 hr	
Anistreplase (APSAC)	30 units IV over 2–5 min	
t-PA (alteplase)	"Front-loaded" t-PA: 15 mg IV bolus over 2 min, followed by 0.75 mg/kg (50 mg maximum dose) IV over 30 min, followed by 0.5 mg/kg (35 mg maximum dose) IV over 60 min (see text for other possible t-PA dosing regimens)	Cost of medications vary significantly: streptokinase ($300 per dose), anistreplase ($1725 per dose), t-PA ($2200 per dose).
Heparin Intravenous	80 units/kg IV bolus (rounded to the nearest 50 units) followed by a continuous infusion of 15–18 units/kg/hr IV	In the setting of thrombolytic therapy: initiate bolus and infusion simultaneously with t-PA. The use of heparin is controversial with SK (see text).

Table continued on following page

Drug	Dose	Comments
		Do *not* use heparin after anistreplase: bleeding is increased. Heparin is useful for the patient with unstable angina, anterior MIs, non-Q-wave MIs, and after angioplasty. Goal is a PTT of 60–100 sec (two times control).
Subcutaneous	5000 units SQ q 8–12 hr	Subcutaneous heparin is used for DVT prophylaxis of the patient not on IV heparin after CCU admission.
Beta blockers (one of the following)		
Metoprolol	5 mg slow IV push q 2 min as tolerated, to a total IV load of 15 mg	Contraindications to beta blockade include heart rate < 60 beats/min, systolic BP < 100 mmHg, moderate to severe LV failure, significant AV conduction abnormalities (including PR– interval > 0.24 sec, second- or third-degree heart block), or reactive airway disease.
Propranolol	0.1 mg/kg divided into three equal doses q 3–5 min	
Atenolol	5–10 mg given slowly IV over at least 5 min.	
Esmolol	250–500 µg/kg IV load over 1 min, followed by a continuous infusion of 50 µg/kg/min IV. The dose is subsequently titrated q 4 min by repeating the bolus and increasing the infusion in 50-µg/kg/min increments.	
ACE Inhibitors (one of the following)		ACE inhibitor therapy may be started in hemodynamically stable patients *as early as 3 days after admission.* Their use reduces mortality, overt heart failure, and subsequent hospitalization for CHF after MI.
Lisinopril	Begin with 5 mg PO once daily.	
Captopril	6.25 mg PO once, followed by 12.5 mg PO tid and increased to 25 mg PO tid in several days.	
Magnesium Sulfate	16 mEq (2 ampules) in 50 mL D5W IV over 15 min followed by a continuous infusion of 5.4 mEq/hr for 24 hr.	Recent data (ISIS–4) found magnesium sulfate unhelpful in reducing mortality in the acute MI patient. *Its routine use is no longer recommended.* Replacement therapy is appropriate, however, if the patient is hypomagnesemic. Do not give magnesium to the anuric patient or the patient with renal insufficiency.
Furosemide	0.5–1.0 mg/kg IV, given slowly	Use for the treatment of acute pulmonary edema. May cause hypokalemia and hypotension

Table 13–15. EMERGENCY MEDICAL THERAPY
FOR THE PATIENT WITH AN ACUTE MI *Continued*

DRUG	DOSE	COMMENTS
Lidocaine	Initial bolus of 1–1.5 mg/kg followed by a continuous infusion of 2 mg/min. Additional boluses of 0.5–1.5 mg/kg can be given q 5–10 min as needed, to a total bolus over time of 3 mg/kg. If necessary, the rate of the infusion can be increased to a maximum of 4 mg/min.	Lidocaine should be used only if necessary for the management of ventricular ectopy, ventricular tachycardia, or ventricular fibrillation. The dose of the continuous infusion should be started at 1 mg/min in patients with liver disease, age > 70, significant CHF, and shock. Therapeutic level is 1.5–5 μg/mL.
Atropine	0.5–1.0 mg IV q 3–5 min as necessary to a total dose of 0.04 mg/kg	Use only if necessary for the management of symptomatic bradycardia or bradycardia with increased ventricular ectopy.
Vasopressor Agents		A pressor agent should be used for BP support only if IV crystalloid is unsuccessful or contraindicated (see text). Dopamine is the initial pressor agent of choice.
Dopamine	Begin IV infusion at 2–5 μg/kg/min. Titrate upward as necessary to maintain systolic BP ≥ 95 mmHg. Usual dose range is 2–20 μg/kg/min.	
Norepinephrine	Begin IV infusion at 0.5–1.0 μg/min and titrate as necessary (doses as high as 30 μg/min IV are sometimes necessary).	Norepinephrine should only be used if hypotension is severe (systolic BP < 70 mmHg) or if the patient is unresponsive to dopamine. The patient should be tapered off norepinephrine as quickly as possible once the clinical situation allows.
Dobutamine	Begin IV infusion at 2–5 μg/kg/min IV and titrate as necessary. Usual dose range is 2–20 μg/kg/min.	Should be used for the treatment of significant CHF when the patient's blood pressure is ≥ 95–100 mmHg. The hypotensive patient with CHF should first have the BP stabilized with dopamine before dobutamine is started.
Vasodilating Agents		These agents are useful for the treatment of significant CHF (afterload reduction). The hypotensive patient must first have the BP stabilized with dopamine.
Nitroglycerin	(See earlier discussion in table.)	
Sodium Nitroprusside	Initial infusion rate of 0.5 μg/kg/min IV. Usual dose range is 0.5–10.0 μg/kg/min.	Thiocyanate intoxication due to nitroprusside is possible but uncommon unless large doses are infused more than 2–3 days or if patient has renal failure.

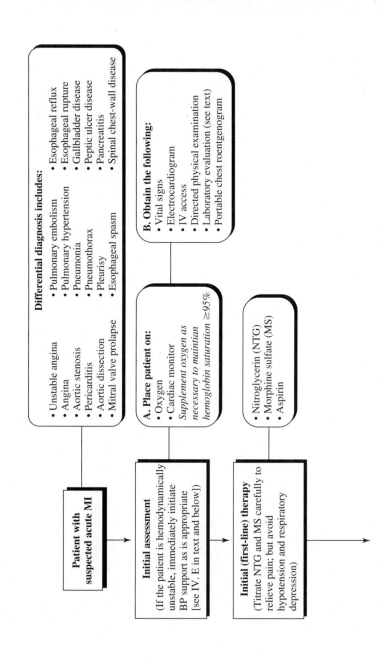

Differential diagnosis includes:

- Unstable angina
- Angina
- Aortic stenosis
- Pericarditis
- Aortic dissection
- Mitral valve prolapse

- Pulmonary embolism
- Pulmonary hypertension
- Pneumonia
- Pneumothorax
- Pleurisy
- Esophageal spasm

- Esophageal reflux
- Esophageal rupture
- Gallbladder disease
- Peptic ulcer disease
- Pancreatitis
- Spinal chest-wall disease

Patient with suspected acute MI

Initial assessment

(If the patient is hemodynamically unstable, immediately initiate BP support as is appropriate [see IV. E in text and below])

A. Place patient on:

- Oxygen
- Cardiac monitor

Supplement oxygen as necessary to maintain hemoglobin saturation ≥95%

B. Obtain the following:

- Vital signs
- Electrocardiogram
- IV access
- Directed physical examination
- Laboratory evaluation (see text)
- Portable chest roentgenogram

Initial (first-line) therapy

(Titrate NTG and MS carefully to relieve pain; but avoid hypotension and respiratory depression)

- Nitroglycerin (NTG)
- Morphine sulfate (MS)
- Aspirin

Thrombolytic Therapy
• **Streptokinase (SK)** or
• **Anistreplase** or
• **t-PA**

i. *Goal:* administer thrombolytic therapy within 30 min of ED arrival to the appropriate candidate.

ii. Do *not* administer thrombolytic therapy to the patient in cardiogenic shock: consult cardiology emergently for coronary artery angiography and mechanical reperfusion.

iii. At major centers where emergent cardiac cath + angioplasty is always available, the role of primary angioplasty vs peripheral thrombolysis for the acute MI patient is currently uncertain. Emergent cardiology consultation is appropriate at these centers prior to initiating thrombolysis, especially in the hemodynamically unstable patient.

A. Indications:
• Symptoms consistent with acute MI,
• Duration of symptoms ≤ 12 hrs,
• ST-segment elevation of ≥ 0.1 mV in two or more contiguous limb leads, or ≥ 0.2 mV in two or more contiguous precordial leads, or new LBBB, AND
• No contraindications to therapy (see Table 13–16)

In the patient with a relative contraindication to thrombolysis, or with persistent pain and ECG changes > 12 hr after symptom onset, consult cardiologist emergently.

B. Heparin:
• Initiate bolus + continuous infusion at the same time as t-PA.
• Because the use of heparin with SK is currently controversial, heparin does not need to be started in the ED in patients receiving SK unless indicated for other reasons.
• Heparin's use with antistreplase significantly increases bleeding complications, and is *not* currently recommended.

Figure 13–8. Emergency therapy of the acute MI patient (see Table 13–15 for medication dosages).

Illustration continued on following page

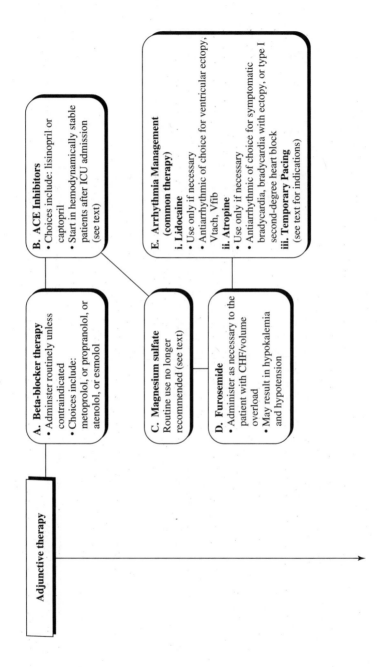

Adjunctive therapy

A. Beta-blocker therapy
- Administer routinely unless contraindicated
- Choices include: metoprolol, or propranolol, or atenolol, or esmolol

B. ACE Inhibitors
- Choices include: lisinopril or captopril
- Start in hemodynamically stable patients after ICU admission (see text)

C. Magnesium sulfate
Routine use no longer recommended (see text)

D. Furosemide
- Administer as necessary to the patient with CHF/volume overload
- May result in hypokalemia and hypotension

E. Arrhythmia Management (common therapy)
i. Lidocaine
- Use only if necessary
- Antiarrhythmic of choice for ventricular ectopy, Vtach, Vfib
ii. Atropine
- Use only if necessary
- Antiarrhythmic of choice for symptomatic bradycardia, bradycardia with ectopy, or type I second-degree heart block
iii. Temporary Pacing
(see text for indications)

Therapy of hemodynamic instability

i. The hemodynamically unstable MI patient is defined by the following:
- poor peripheral perfusion
- anuria or oliguria
- hypotension (systolic BP < 100 mm Hg)
- heart rate > 100 or < 60 beats/min

ii. Therapy of the hemodynamically unstable patient should be initiated simultaneously with earlier steps!

A. Rate/rhythm therapy
- see lidocaine/atropine/pacing, above
- manage arrhythmia as indicated per ACLS guidelines (see arrhythmia chapter)

B. Volume ("Tank") Therapy
- if no clinical evidence for CHF, consider a volume challenge (e.g., 250–500 mL IV normal saline bolus, repeated as necessary)
- titrate volume carefully to vital signs, urine output, and cardiopulmonary status

C. "Pump" Therapy

i. Identify cause of myocardial dysfunction: massive MI, acute mitral regurgitation, ventricular septal rupture, severe hypertension, LV aneurysm, cardiac tamponade

ii. If volume infusion is contraindicated or ineffective, use pressor for BP support:
- Dopamine: pressor of choice; titrate as necessary
- Norepinephrine: consider if systolic BP < 70 mm Hg or if patient's BP is unresponsive to dopamine

iii. Intra-aortic balloon pump: use if necessary to temporize till definitive care (e.g., surgery) for the patient in cardiogenic shock/CHF/persistent ischemic pain/ or acute valvular decompensation unresponsive to maximal medical therapy

iv. Moderate to severe CHF therapy:
- Dobutamine: positive inotrope. If the patient is hypotensive, first support the BP (systolic BP ≥ 95mm Hg) with dopamine and then add dobutamine.
- Furosemide: diuretic and venodilator (see "Adjunctive Therapy" above)
- Nitroglycerin: reduces preload and to a lesser extent afterload. Cannot be given to the hypotensive patient until the BP has been first appropriately supported and stabilized.
- Sodium nitroprusside: reduces afterload and improves cardiac output. In the hypotensive patient use only after the patient's BP has been appropriately supported and stabilized.

Figure 13–8. *Continued*

265

   c. Dose:
       i. Sublingual tablets or spray: 0.4 mg SL every 3–5 minutes, up to three total doses for pain relief (useful for myocardial ischemia as IV access is being established).
      ii. Paste: 0.5–2 inches to the skin every 6 hours.
     iii. IV (this is the preferred route of administration for the acute MI patient once an IV line has been established): begin at 10–20 µg/min IV and increase by 5–10 µg/min every 5–10 minutes as the patient's pain complaints dictate and BP allows.
   d. *Cautions:*
       i. May result in systemic hypotension (systolic BP ≤ 100 mmHg), especially in patients with volume depletion (e.g., profuse diaphoresis, vomiting) or those with right-ventricular infarction. In normotensive patients, nitroglycerin will result in a decline in BP. The systolic BP should *not* be allowed to decrease by > 10% in normotensive patients or > 30% in initially hypertensive patients; and under no circumstances should the systolic blood pressure fall below 100 mmHg. Do *not* start nitroglycerin in the hemodynamically unstable patient until the blood pressure has been appropriately supported with IV fluid and/or pressor therapy (see IV. E, below).
      ii. Other potential complications of nitroglycerin therapy include headache, tachycardia, paradoxical bradycardia, pulmonary ventilation–perfusion mismatch, and methemoglobinemia.

2. **Morphine Sulfate**
   a. The analgesic and anxiolytic agent of choice for the relief of ischemic cardiac pain.
   b. Blocks sympathetic efferent discharge at the central nervous system (CNS) level, resulting in peripheral venous and arterial dilation, a decrease in myocardial oxygen demand, and a decrease in pulmonary vascular congestion.
   c. Dose: 2–4 mg IV every 5 minutes, titrated till the desired effect is achieved.
   d. *Cautions:*
       i. Hypotension and bradycardia can occur as a result of vagal actions, vascular dilation, and histamine release. Do not begin morphine sulfate in the hypotensive patient until the BP has been appropriately supported with IV fluid and/or pressor therapy (see IV. E, below).
      ii. Respiratory depression is a rare side effect.

3. **Aspirin (Acetylsalicylic Acid)**
   a. Inhibits cyclooxygenase-dependent platelet aggregation.
   b. Its use in acute MI reduces mortality by 21%, and reduces mortality by 39% when used in combination with a thrombolytic agent.
   c. Dose: 160–325 mg PO (bite and swallow).

C. Thrombolytic Therapy

Note: time is muscle, and thrombolytic therapy must be initiated to appropriate candidates as rapidly as possible (ideally within 30 minutes of the patient's ED arrival).

1. **General Considerations**
   a. Thrombotic coronary occlusion causes over 85% of acute MIs.
   b. Thrombolytic therapy restores patency, salvages ischemic myocardium, improves myocardial function, and decreases mortality.
   c. Complete myocardial necrosis occurs betwen 20 minutes and 6 hours after coronary artery occlusion; the longer the occlusion, the greater the myocardial muscle damage.
   d. Mortality is reduced when thrombolytic therapy is administered within 12 hours of symptom onset, but benefits are most dramatic when thrombolysis is initiated within 2 hours of symptom onset.

2. **Indications for Thrombolytic Therapy**
   a. Symptoms consistent with an acute MI,
   b. Duration of symptoms $\leq$ 12 hours (*note:* older "duration of symptom" guidelines were $\leq$ 6 hours, but data from GISSI, ISIS-2, and ISSIS-3 suggest mortality reduction when thrombolytic therapy is used within *12 hours* of symptom onset),
   c. ST-segment elevation $\geq$ 0.1 mV (1 mm elevation with standard ECG calibration) in two or more contiguous limb leads, or $\geq$ 0.2 mV (2 mm) in two or more contiguous precordial leads, or new-onset LBBB, *and*
   d. No contraindications to thrombolytic therapy (Table 13–16).

3. **Specific Agents**
   a. **Streptokinase**
      i. Dose: 1.5 million units IV over 1 hour.
      ii. *Note:* streptokinase may not be effective if used 5 days to 12 months after the previous use of either streptokinase or anistreplase therapy or a known streptococcal infection.

      or
   b. **Anistreplase** (APSAC or Eminase)
      i. Dose: 30 units IV over 2–5 minutes.
      ii. *Note:* anistreplase may not be effective if used 5 days to 12 months after prior streptokinase or anistreplase therapy or a known streptococcal infection.

      or
   c. **Tissue Plasminogen Activator** (t-PA, Alteplase)
      i. Dose (*Note:* optimal dosing of t-PA is evolving. The manner of administration may vary from that indicated below, depending on the institution):
         • *"Front-loaded" t-PA administration:* 15 mg IV bolus over 2 minutes, followed by 0.75 mg/kg IV over 30

Table 13–16. CONTRAINDICATIONS TO THROMBOLYTIC THERAPY

Absolute Contraindications

Active internal bleeding

Altered consciousness

Cerebrovascular accident (CVA) in the past 6 months or *any* history of hemorrhagic CVA

Intracranial or intraspinal surgery within the previous 2 months

Known bleeding disorder

Known intracranial or intraspinal neoplasm, aneurysm, or AV malformation

Persistent, severe hypertension (systolic BP > 200 mmHg and/or diastolic BP > 120 mmHg)

Pregnancy

Previous allergy to a streptokinase product (does not contraindicate t-PA)

Recent (within 1 month) head trauma

Suspected aortic dissection

Suspected pericarditis

Trauma or surgery within 2 weeks, which could result in bleeding into a closed space

Relative Contraindications

Active peptic ulcer disease

Cardiopulmonary resuscitation for > 10 min

Current use of oral anticoagulants

History of chronic, uncontrolled hypertension (diastolic BP > 100 mmHg), treated or untreated

History of ischemic or embolic CVA

Significant trauma or major surgery > 2 weeks ago but < 2 months ago

Subclavian or internal jugular venous cannulation

Adapted from National Heart Attack Alert Program Coordinating Committee 60 Minutes to Treatment Working Group, 1993.

minutes (maximum dose of 50 mg), followed by 0.50 mg/kg (maximum dose of 35 mg) over the subsequent 1 hour.

or

- *"Traditional" t-PA administration:*

    —*Adult patient* < 65 kg: total dose 1.25 mg/kg to be given IV over 3 hours as follows: 60% in the first hour (6–10% as an IV bolus over the first 1–2 minutes of therapy, with the other 50–54% given IV over the first hour) followed by the remaining 40% given IV over the next 2 hours of therapy.

    —*Adult patient* ≥ 65 kg: 60 mg IV over the first hour as follows: 6–10 mg as an IV bolus over the first 1–2 minutes of therapy, with the remaining 50–54 mg given over the rest of the first hour; the subsequent 40 mg is given IV over the next 2 hours of therapy.

ii. *Note:* t-PA is the most expensive of the thrombolytic agents ($2200 per 100 mg).

iii. The GUSTO investigators (a study of 41,021 patients from 1081 centers in 15 countries) found that front-loaded t-PA with intravenous heparin resulted in a significantly reduced mortality at 30 days post-treatment (6.3% mortality) as compared to streptokinase (7.3% mortality). The benefit of t-PA over streptokinase was smaller or nonexistent, however, for the following patient subgroups: age > 75 years, inferior MIs, or patients presenting > 4 hours after symptom onset.

4. **Complications of Thrombolytic Therapy**
   a. The most significant complictions are related to hemorrhage, with the most catastrophic event being intracranial hemorrhage (0.5–1% risk in most studies).
   b. To minimize hemorrhagic complications: do *not* administer thrombolytic therapy to any patient with an absolute contraindication to its use; in patients with relative contraindications to thrombolytic therapy, carefully weigh potential benefits versus risks in consultation with cardiology; limit venous access to easily compressible sites (avoid central lines); avoid nasogastric tubes and nasotracheal intubation; and avoid all unnecessary needle sticks.
   c. Hypotension and allergic reactions may occur after either streptokinase or anistreplase administration. t-PA is not antigenic: urticaria may occur, but serious allergic reactions do not.

5. **Peripheral Thrombolysis versus Primary Angioplasty**
   a. Patients with cardiogenic shock (hypotension and poor peripheral perfusion despite adequate intravascular volume) treated medically have a 70–90% mortality. Peripherally administered thrombolytic therapy is minimally effective in these patients. Cardiogenic shock is an indication for emergent coronary artery angiography and mechanical reperfusion (e.g., angioplasty) if available. Emergent cardiology consultation is appropriate in these patients.
   b. At medical centers where *emergent* cardiac catheterization, percutaneous transluminal coronary angioplasty (PTCA), and coronary artery bypass grafting are continuously available, recent data have added controversy to the optimal therapy of the acute MI patient. Immediate angioplasty has the following advantages over peripherally administered thrombolytic therapy in the acute MI patient: higher patency of the infarct-related vessel, reduced high-grade stenosis after therapy, shorter patient hospital stays, lower follow-up costs, and fewer subsequent patient readmissions. The optimal acute MI management strategy (with respect to the ideal method of reperfusion) for

centers where cardiac catheterization is always emergently available is currently uncertain. At most hospitals, however, peripherally administered thrombolytics continue to be the treatment of choice in the suitable candidate with an acute MI.

6. **Additional Considerations.** Patients with an acute transmural MI with on-going chest pain who present 12–24 hours after symptom onset, or patients with only relative contraindications to thrombolysis, may still benefit from thrombolytic therapy. Emergently consult a cardiologist in these settings to decide on the optimal therapeutic approach.

7. **Heparin** (SQ or IV)
   a. Indications for IV heparin in the setting of acute myocardial ischemia include patients with unstable angina, patients post–t-PA therapy or angioplasty, patients with non–Q-wave MIs, and patients with large anterior MIs (ejection fraction < 30%) at risk for LV thrombus formation. *Dose:* 80 units/kg IV bolus (rounded to the nearest 50 units) followed by a continuous IV infusion of 15–18 units/kg/hr. The PTT is then checked 6 hours after initiating therapy and the heparin dose adjusted to maintain the PTT in the range of 60–100 seconds (two times control). In the setting of thrombolytic therapy, the heparin bolus and continuous infusion should be started *at the same time* that t-PA infusion is started. The use of heparin with streptokinase is currently controversial; heparin does not need to be started emergently in the ED when streptokinase is used. The use of heparin after anistreplase is of uncertain benefit and appears to increase bleeding complications: it is not recommended at this time.
   b. The patient admitted to the ICU who is not on IV heparin should be placed on SQ heparin while at bedrest to prevent the development of deep-venous thrombosis. *Dose:* 5000 units SQ every 8–12 hours.
   c. Contraindications to heparin include uncontrollable active bleeding or severe thrombocytopenia.

D. Adjunctive Therapy

1. **Beta Blockers**
   a. These agents reduce myocardial oxygen demand by decreasing heart rate and arterial pressure. Ideal candidates for beta-blocker therapy are patients with reflex tachycardia or systolic hypertension *without* signs of CHF.
   b. Long-term use in ischemic heart disease decreases mortality by 20%, reinfarction by 25% post-MI, and sudden death by 30%.
   c. In the setting of acute MI, beta-blocker therapy may reduce infarct size and the incidence of myocardial rupture when given during the first few hours of infarction.

d. Dose:
   i. Metoprolol: 5 mg slow IV push every 2 minutes as tolerated to a total IV load of 15 mg over time. A PO regimen should then be started at 50 mg PO every 6 hours when the patient is admitted to the ICU;

   or

   ii. Propranolol: 0.1 mg/kg divided into three equal doses, each dose given slowly IV every 3–5 minutes. A regimen of 20–40 mg PO every 6–8 hours may then be started in the ICU;

   or

   iii. Atenolol: 5-10 mg given slowly IV over at least 5 min. A regimen of 50–100 mg PO every day may then be started in the ICU;

   or

   iv. Esmolol: 250–500 µg/kg IV bolus over 1 minute, followed by a continuous IV infusion starting at 50 µg/kg/min. The dose is titrated, as necessary, every 4 minutes by repeating the bolus and increasing the continuous infusion in 50-µg/kg/min increments. Esmolol's short half-life (10 minutes) makes it advantageous if beta blockade is not well tolerated by the patient.

e. Contraindications include heart rate < 60 beats/min, systolic BP < 100 mmHg, moderate to severe LV failure, significant atrioventricular (AV) conduction abnormalities (PR– interval > 0.24 sec, second- or third-degree heart block), reactive airway disease, and severe chronic obstructive pulmonary disease (COPD).

2. **Angiotensin Converting Enzyme (ACE) Inhibitors**
   a. Both GISSI-3 (19,000 acute MI patients) and ISIS-4 (58,000 acute MI patients) investigators found that initiation of ACE inhibitor therapy as early as 3 days after acute MI resulted in a significant mortality reduction. The absolute benefits of ACE inhibitor therapy were greatest for high-risk patients (i.e., those with a prior MI, ejection fraction ≤ 40%, heart failure, and/or anterior MI).
   b. Specific agents (*note:* these medications should generally *not* be started in the ED, but may be initiated in 72 hours in the ICU in hemodynamically stable patients).
      i. Lisinopril: begin with 5 mg PO once daily,

      or

      ii. Captopril: 6.25 mg PO as a single dose, followed by 12.5 mg PO tid, increased over the next several days to 25 mg PO tid.

3. **Magnesium Sulfate**
   a. In the meta-analysis of many small studies and one medium-sized prospective trial (LIMIT-2), magnesium administration was associated with a 24% reduction in mortality at 28 days. In the largest study done to date

(ISIS-4, involving 58,000 acute MI patients), however, magnesium administration was associated with a 4 per 1000 patient mortality *excess* at 35 days. The routine administration of magnesium sulfate to the acute MI patient can *not* be recommended at this time, although magnesium replacement is appropriate in the hypomagnesemic patient.

b. Dose: 16 mEq (2 g) in 50 mL D5W IV over 15 minutes, followed by 5.4 mEq/hr continuous IV infusion for 24 hours. (*Note:* different institutions may use a different dosing regimen.)

c. *Cautions:* IV magnesium may cause bradycardia and hypotension. Neuromuscular blockade may rarely occur if the dose is large enough to raise serum concentration to 4–5 mmol/L. IV magnesium should not be given to the anuric patient or the patient with renal insufficiency.

4. **Furosemide**

a. This is a potent diuretic and direct venodilator when given IV.

b. It is indicated in the management of acute pulmonary edema and the treatment of cerebral edema post-cardiac arrest.

c. Dose: 0.5–1.0 mg/kg given slowly IV.

d. *Cautions:* furosemide will decrease serum potassium and may result in hypotension. Do not give furosemide to the hypotensive patient (systolic BP < 100 mmHg) in acute pulmonary edema until BP is first supported with vasopressor therapy.

5. **Lidocaine**

a. In acute MI, lidocaine is recommended in the following situations: frequent (> 6/min) premature ventricular contractions (PVCs), multiform PVCs, PVCs occurring in short bursts of three or more in succession, ventricular tachycardia, and ventricular fibrillation.

b. Routine prophylactic use of lidocaine in the absence of significant ventricular ectopy can *not* be recommended at this time. While primary ventricular fibrillation is reduced by 33%, there is no decrease in mortality. Central nervous system toxicity is a significant potential side effect.

c. Dose: initial bolus of 1.0–1.5 mg/kg IV followed by an infusion of 2 mg/min. Additional boluses of 0.5–1.5 mg/kg can be given every 5–10 minutes as needed, to a total bolus dose over time of 3 mg/kg. If necessary, the continuous infusion can be increased to a maximum of 4 mg/min.

d. *Cautions:* lidocaine is hepatically metabolized. The initial infusion should be started at 1 mg/min in the following situations: age > 70, shock, known liver disease, or significant CHF. Toxic effects may include muscle twitching, slurred speech, altered mentation, and seizures.

6. **Atropine**
   a. This agent reduces vagal tone, enhances the rate of discharge of the sinus node, and facilitates AV conduction.
   b. Atropine is recommended for sinus bradycardia with evidence of low cardiac output, bradycardia with significant ventricular ectopy, acute inferior infarction with symptomatic type I second-degree AV block, and/or when bradycardia/hypotension complicate nitroglycerin or morphine administration.
   c. Dose: 0.5–1.0 mg IV every 3–5 minutes as necessary, to a total dose over time of 0.04 mg/kg.
   d. *Cautions:* doses < 0.5 mg should not be given to adults (paradoxical worsening of bradycardia may result). Atropine will increase myocardial oxygen demand and may precipitate tachyarrhythmias. Use it cautiously in the setting of acute MI and only if absolutely necessary. Atropine may also paradoxically decrease the ventricular response in the setting of type II second-degree heart block and third-degree block with wide QRS complexes.

7. **Temporary Cardiac Pacing**
   a. In the setting of acute MI, transcutaneous pacing followed by transvenous pacing may be life-saving in the appropriate patient. Cardiology should be consulted urgently in all cases where transvenous pacing is deemed necessary.
   b. Prophylactic pacing for acute MI is indicated for symptomatic bradycardia not responsive to atropine, *anterior MI* with type II second-degree heart block or third-degree heart block, *anterior MI* with new RBBB, RBBB with left-anterior fascicular block (LAFB) or left-posterior fascicular block (LPFB), or new LBBB with first-degree AV block. The need for prophylactic pacing is controversial for isolated new LBBB or inferior MI with new RBBB.

E. Therapy of Hemodynamic Instability

1. **General Considerations**
   a. In the acute MI patient, poor tissue perfusion (e.g., cool, clammy extremities; oliguria) and/or hypotension (systolic BP < 100 mmHg) may be caused by one or more of the following three mechanisms:
      i. A rate/rhythm problem.
      ii. A volume problem.
      iii. A pump (myocardial) problem.
   b. In the ED, rapid clinical assessment of the patient must be undertaken with this "cardiovascular triad" in mind to identify the cause(s) of the patient's hemodynamic compromise and the appropriate course of therapy.
      i. The rate/rhythm must be quickly assessed from the

  ECG and cardiac monitor (is the rate inappropriately slow or fast?).

 ii. A volume problem can be identified from the history (e.g., poor PO intake; nausea, vomiting, or diarrhea; profuse diaphoresis; acute hemorrhage), physical examination (e.g., vital signs, poor peripheral perfusion, oliguria, clear lung fields, normal heart sounds), and laboratory values (e.g., clear chest roentgenogram, concentrated urine, azotemia, acute anemia).

 iii. A pump problem may also be initially identified on the basis of history (e.g., dyspnea, orthopnea, prior heart failure history), initial examination (e.g., vital signs, jugular venous distention, pulmonary rales, S3 gallop, acute mitral regurgitation) and laboratory values (e.g., cardiomegaly and/or pulmonary edema on chest roentgenogram).

 c. The following should be *routinely* monitored in the ED in all hemodynamically unstable acute MI patients:

  i. Cardiac rhythm.

  ii. SaO_2.

  iii. Vital signs.

  iv. Physical examination.

  v. Urine output via bladder catheterization.

 d. Invasive monitoring is frequently of assistance and includes intra-arterial BP monitoring and pulmonary artery catheterization for purposes of assessing central venous pressure (CVP), pulmonary artery occlusive pressure (PAOP), systemic vascular resistance (SVR), and cardiac output (CO). Indications for invasive monitoring include cardiogenic shock, severe or progressive congestive heart failure, or persistent hypotension unresponsive to appropriate initial therapy. Depending on ED capabilities, invasive monitoring may be started in the ED or after the patient's transfer to the ICU.

2. **Specific Therapy**

 a. **Rate/Rhythm Problems.** The use of lidocaine, atropine, and cardiac pacing has been discussed in IV. D, above (see also Cardiac Arrhythmias, earlier in this chapter).

 b. **Volume Problems.** These may be the consequence of either insufficient fluid ("empty tank") or inadequate vascular tone ("enlarged tank"). The highest priority in either case is to initiate crystalloid replacement (normal saline or lactated Ringer's solution). Fluid may be given in 250–500-mL IV boluses as the patient's status (especially cardiopulmonary system) is closely followed. If invasive central monitoring has been accomplished, a PAOP of 18–20 mmHg in most situations indicates an appropriate intravascular volume (a "full tank"). Patients with RV infarction and hypotension are especially responsive to volume resuscitation. *Caution:* overly aggressive fluid administration in the setting of cardiac decompensation may result in pulmonary edema, compromised pump function, and worsening oxygenation.

c. **Pump (Myocardial) Problems.** In the setting of an acute MI, pump problems occur secondary to significant myocardial injury, severe hypertension (increased afterload), ventricular septal rupture, acute mitral regurgitation, LV aneurysm formation, and/or cardiac rupture with tamponade. Often the patient's evaluation will reveal marked cardiac decompensation and acute pulmonary edema. In the setting of pulmonary edema, further fluid administration for BP support is generally contraindicated.

   i. Vasopressors: should be used in the hypotensive acute MI patient when initial volume resuscitation is ineffective or contraindicated. Drug choices include dopamine, norepinephrine, and/or dobutamine (see Table 13–15 and Chapter 12).

   ii. Vasodilators: may be used to reduce afterload and thereby improve pump function. They are especially useful when the cause of the pump problem is severe hypertension, when the patient is in significant pulmonary edema, or to temporize acute valvular decompensation (e.g, severe acute mitral regurgitation) until surgical repair can be accomplished. Drug choices include nitroglycerin and/or sodium nitroprusside (see Chapter 12 and Congestive Heart Failure, earlier in this chapter). *Caution:* these medications can not be given to the hypotensive MI patient until the blood pressure is first supported with fluids (if appropriate) and/or the pressor agents described above.

   iii. Intra-aortic balloon pump: may be used as a "bridge" to surgery or definitive care in the patient with an acute MI and significant pump dysfunction. It should be emergently considered in the patient with cardiogenic shock unresponsive to maximal pharmacologic therapy; in patients with acute ventricular septal rupture, acute mitral regurgitation, severe CHF unresponsive to maximal medical therapy; and in patients with persistent ischemic pain despite maximal medical interventions.

V. DISPOSITION

A. The patient with an acute MI must be admitted to an ICU/CCU.

B. The patient with unstable angina (defined as new-onset angina, angina at rest or with minimal activity, or angina of increasing severity, frequency, or duration) should be admitted to a monitored bed for observation, stabilization, rule out myocardial infarction (R/O MI) protocol, and further testing as deemed appropriate by either the internal medicine or cardiology consultant.

C. The patient with long-standing stable angina or atypical chest pain clearly believed *not* to be of cardiac origin may be discharged to home with mandatory follow-up by the patient's own physician within several days.

VI. PEARLS AND PITFALLS

A. Err on the side of caution when ascribing a "noncardiac" diagnosis to a patient with chest pain. (The ED physician cannot afford to "miss" even one acute MI.)

B. A patient with a good history for acute myocardial ischemia suggestive of unstable angina or an acute MI should be admitted to a monitored bed, even if the ECG is normal.

C. Candidates for thrombolytic therapy should have that therapy started as rapidly as possible after ED arrival (the goal is to start thrombolysis < 30 minutes after patient presentation). Clear-cut candidates do not need cardiology consultation or approval prior to beginning thrombolytic therapy (except at institutions where emergent cardiac catheterization and PTCA is available 24 hr/day and the role of thrombolysis versus primary PTCA is in transition).

D. Patients who have relative contraindications to thrombolytic therapy, or who would otherwise be candidates for thrombolysis but are presenting > 12 hours after symptom onset, should have an urgent cardiology consultation.

E. Patients who are presenting with an acute transmural MI but have absolute contraindications to thrombolytic therapy also mandate an emergent cardiology consultation for consideration of coronary artery angiography and mechanical reperfusion.

F. Patients presenting in cardiogenic shock should not be given peripherally administered thrombolytic therapy if cardiac catheterization is available within 60 minutes. An emergent cardiology consultation is mandatory for emergent coronary artery catheterization and mechanical reperfusion.

G. Calcium channel antagonists (e.g., verapamil, diltiazem, and nifedipine) have no role in the ED management of acute MI.

H. Anticipate and be prepared for the hemodynamic and arrhythmic complications of MI.

BIBLIOGRAPHY

Anderson HV, Willerson JT: Thrombolysis in acute myocardial infarction. N Engl J Med 1993;329(10):703–709.

Emergency Cardiac Care Committee and Subcommittee, American Heart Association: Part III: Adult Advanced Cardiac Life Support. JAMA 1992;268(16):2184–2241.

Fuster V: Coronary thrombolysis—a perspective for the practicing physician (editorial). N Engl J Med 1993;329(10):723–725.

Lange RA, Hillis LD: Immediate angioplasty for acute myocardial infarction (editorial). N Engl J Med 1993;328(10):726–728.

National Heart Attack Alert Program Coordinating Committee 60 Minutes to Treatment Working Group: Emergency department: Rapid identification and treatment of patients with acute myocardial infarction. U.S. Department of Health and Human Services; Public Health Service; National Institutes of Health; National Heart, Lung, and Blood Institute. NIH Publication No. 93-3278, September, 1993.

Scott JL, Pigman EC, Gordon GG, Silverstein S. Ischemic heart disease. In Rosen, Barkin (eds): Emergency Medicine: Concepts and Clinical Practice, 3rd ed. St.Louis, CV Mosby, 1992, pp. 1312–1372.

Woods KL, Fletcher S, Roffe C, Haider Y: Intravenous magnesium sulfate in suspected acute myocardial infarction: results of the second Leicester Intravenous Magnesium Intervention Trial (LIMIT-2). Lancet 1992;339:1553–1558.

PERICARDITIS

> *"Not only degrees of pain, but its existence, in any degree, must be taken upon the testimony of the patient."*
>
> PETER MERE LATHAM

I. ESSENTIAL FACTS

A. Definition

Pericarditis is an inflammatory process involving the parietal and visceral pericardium, usually with involvement of the epicardium and outer myocardium. The myocardial involvement causes the electrocardiographic (ECG) injury currents and arrhythmias associated with pericarditis.

B. Etiology

There are several causes of acute pericarditis (Table 13–17).

1. **Idiopathic/Viral.** This is the most common type of pericarditis in an ambulatory setting and is thought to be due to a viral infection. A viral cause, however, is identified in only 15–20% of cases. It most often occurs in young adults. Symptoms resolve in 3–6 weeks, although it will recur in 25% of cases. Complications, the most common of which is cardiac tamponade, are rare in viral pericarditis and the prognosis is good.

2. **Uremic.** Pericarditis occurs in up to one-third of patients with chronic uremia. A friction rub is common, but pain is usually absent. Large hemorrhagic pericardial effusions may occur, probably because of uremic platelet dysfunction; cardiac tamponade occurs occasionally.

3. **Myocardial Infarction-Associated Pericarditis.** In 20% of cases, acute myocardial infarction (MI) is complicated by pericarditis within the first 10 days, which is thought to be due to inflammation caused by underlying myocardial necrosis.

Table 13–17. ETIOLOGY OF PERICARDITIS

Idiopathic (no specfic cause detected or clinical condition associated)

Infectious

Viral (coxsackie virus, echovirus, mumps, varicella, adenovirus, herpes simplex, influenza, cytomegalovirus)
Pyogenic (staphylococcus, streptococcus, pneumococcus)
Mycobacterial *(M. tuberculosis, M. avium-intracellulare)*
Fungal *(Histoplasma capsulatum, Cryptococcus neoformans)*
Parasitic (toxoplasmosis)
Syphilitic

Noninfectious

Uremia
Myxedema
Neoplasm (leukemia, lymphoma, metastases from breast or lung, or melanoma, Kaposi's sarcoma, primary myocardial or percicardial tumor)
Acute MI
Trauma
Dissecting aortic aneurysm
Postradiation
Sarcoid

Autoimmune Hypersensitivity

Rheumatic fever
Collagen vascular disease (rheumatoid arthritis, systemic lupus erythematosus, scleroderma)
Drug-induced (procainamide, hydralazine, minoxidil, cromolyn, isoniazid)
Postcardiac injury (Dressler's syndrome [post-MI], postpericardiotomy, trauma)

Large effusions are rare. In general, this form of pericarditis is painless and is detected by a friction rub or an effusion seen on echocardiography. If pain occurs, the distinction between this and recurrent or persistent ischemia may be difficult.

4. **Post–cardiac-Injury Syndrome.** This syndrome may be seen after MI (Dressler's syndrome), after pericardiotomy, or after both penetrating and nonpenetrating trauma. It presents 1–4 weeks after pericardial injury and is due to an immunologic hypersensitivity reaction to myocardial antigens.

5. **Neoplastic.** Pericarditis may result from primary or, more commonly, metastatic tumors, especially lung and breast tumors, lymphoma, leukemia, and melanoma. Mediastinal radiation therapy can also cause pericarditis.

6. **Bacterial (Pyogenic or Purulent Pericarditis).** Pericardial infection usually results from extension of pulmonary or mediastinal infection through surgical or traumatic penetration. A large cardiac silhouette is seen on the chest roentgenograph, but there are often no ECG changes or friction rub.

7. **Tuberculous.** Tuberculous pericarditis is of gradual onset, characterized by weight loss and low-grade fever. It may present as cardiac tamponade or constrictive pericarditis.

II. CLINICAL PRESENTATION

A. Signs and Symptoms

1. The main features of pericarditis are chest pain, fever, and a characteristic friction rub. Patients with acute pericarditis will complain of sharp pleuritic precordial or substernal chest pain aggravated by inspiration, coughing, swallowing, twisting the trunk, and reclining. The pain is usually relieved by sitting up and leaning forward, and it may be referred to the back, the trapezius ridge, the neck, and the jaw.

2. Nonspecific findings include malaise, fever, arthralgias, dyspnea, and dysphagia.

3. Patients with chronic forms of pericarditis, such as uremic, tuberculous, or neoplastic, may have no chest pain and may present with cardiac tamponade or constrictive pericarditis (see VII, below).

B. Physical Examination

1. The pericardial friction rub associated with pericarditis is a superficial, scratchy, grating sound heard best with the diaphragm of the stethoscope at the left midsternal edge with the patient sitting up and leaning forward in held expiration. The rub has three components that are attributed to pericardial/epicardial/pleural contact during the various phases of the cardiac cycle. The presystolic component is associated with atrial systole, the systolic phase with ventricular systole, and the early diastolic phase with early ventricular filling. Because the rub is only detectable intermittently, its absence does not exclude pericarditis.

2. A pericardial effusion is almost always present; its size and hemodynamic importance, however, vary with how quickly it accumulates rather than its volume. Pulsus paradoxus should be sought if pericardial effusion is suspected.

C. Laboratory Findings

1. Complete blood count with differential: granulocytosis is usually followed by lymphocytosis.

2. Erythrocyte sedimentation rate: often elevated.

3. Creatine kinase: may be elevated, but myocardial band isozymes will not generally demonstrate myocardial damage.

4. Other laboratory studies to consider ordering:
   a. Blood urea nitrogen/creatinine: to rule out uremia.
   b. Blood cultures.
   c. Antistreptococcal serology: to rule out poststreptococcal rheumatic heart disease.

5. The chest roentgenogram is usually normal; but it may show left pleural effusion or large pericardial effusion.

6. The ECG typically goes through a four-stage evolution. All stages may not be seen, depending on the time of the patient's presentation and the frequency of serial ECGs.

   a. **Stage 1.** Acute diffuse ST-segment elevation in the precordial leads, especially V5–6, due to subepicardial inflammation. There is ST depression in AVR and V1, and P–R segment depression in II, AVF, and V4–6.

   b. **Stage 2.** After several days, the ST segments return to isoelectric (normal ECG).

   c. **Stage 3.** Isoelectric ST segment with T-wave inversion.

   d. **Stage 4.** Resolution of T waves to normal. T-wave inversion can persist for months to years.

   Atrial arrhythmias (e.g., flutter and fibrillation) may occur with acute pericarditis but are uncommon.

   With pericardial effusion, various degrees of diminished QRS voltage occur. With large effusions, electrical alternans can occur.

D. Adjuvant Studies and Procedures

1. **Echocardiography.** This is the procedure of choice for detecting pericardial effusion, although failure to detect an effusion by echocardiography does not exclude acute pericarditis.

2. **Pericardiocentesis.** An emergent life-saving procedure in cardiac tamponade, pericardiocentesis also can be an elective diagnostic procedure to culture a bacterial effusion or detect a malignant one.

3. **Surgical Biopsy of the Pericardium.** May be required to diagnose more obscure causes of pericarditis.

III. DIAGNOSIS

In hospital, the diagnosis of pericarditis is based on typical sequential ECG changes and echocardiographic evidence of pericardial effusion. In the ED setting, diagnosis must be based on a suggestive history of chest pain, the possible finding of a friction rub, and diffuse ST-segment elevation on the ECG.

IV. DIFFERENTIAL DIAGNOSIS

A. Diseases likely to present similarly to pericarditis are listed in Table 13–18.

B. Both early repolarization and acute MI may mimic acute pericarditis on the ECG. Distinctions include the following:

1. **Pericarditis Versus Early Repolarization.** Early repolarization on the ECG is a normal variant, particularly in young adult males. Tall T-wave and diffuse ST-segment elevations are typical. An ST-segment/T-wave ratio greater than 0.25 in V5 or

Table 13–18. DIFFERENTIAL DIAGNOSIS FOR PERICARDITIS

Acute MI
Angina pectoris
Dissecting aortic aneurysm
Intercostal neuralgia
Mediastinal emphysema
Pleuritic/pleurisy
Pneumonia
Prinzmetal's angina
Pulmonary embolus
Pulmonary infarction
Spontaneous pneumothorax

V6 is suggestive of acute pericarditis. Serial changes do not occur in early repolarization.

2. **Pericarditis Versus Acute Myocardial Infarction.** In pericarditis, ST-segment elevation is more diffuse, with an upward concavity, and is rarely more than 5 mm high. In pericarditis, Q waves do not evolve and T-wave inversion occurs after normalizaton of the ST segment.

V. THERAPY

A. Medical therapy for acute idiopathic or viral pericarditis consists of anti-inflammatory therapy. Indomethacin (25–75 mg PO tid) or aspirin ($\leq$ 900 mg PO qid) have been the traditional mainstays, though newer agents are also effective. Steroids can be used (prednisone 20–80 mg PO qd) for refractory cases, but only when bacterial or tuberculous causes are ruled out. Either therapy should be tapered slowly once the patient has been asymptomatic and afebrile for approximately 1 week. Relapses after withdrawal of steroid therapy are common.

B. Surgical intervention may be necessary in some cases, such as pericardiocentesis for tamponade, or pericardiectomy for bacterial or constrictive pericarditis, or for recurrent tamponade.

VI. DISPOSITION

Hospitalization for patients with pericarditis depends on the clinical situation. For example, suspected idiopathic or viral pericarditis without arrhythmic or hemodynamic complications may be managed on an outpatient basis with appropriate follow-up arranged. Uremic pericarditis in a patient on chronic dialysis generally requires intensification of dialysis, best arranged with the patient's nephrologist. When the cause is in doubt, or if life-threatening conditions such as myocardial ischemia cannot be excluded, hospitalization is indicated. Complications of pericarditis, outlined below, mandate ICU admission.

VII. COMPLICATIONS

Acute complications of pericarditis may occur and should be anticipated.

A. Myocarditis

Findings include conduction disturbances, transient Q waves, and myocardial enzyme elevation. Patients exhibiting signs of myocarditis should be monitored in an ICU.

B. Cardiac Tamponade

Signs and symptoms are due to decreased cardiac output and circulatory failure from the impaired diastolic filling caused by the increasing intrapericardial pressure of the accumulating pericardial effusion.

1. **Symptoms.** Dyspnea, orthopnea, lightheadedness, and syncope.

2. **Signs.** Pale or cyanotic skin, upright posture, extreme anxiety, hypotension with narrow pulse pressure, hepatomegaly, jugular venous distention (JVD) with clear lung fields, falling arterial pressure with rising venous pressure, distant heart sounds, Kussmaul's sign (inspiratory neck vein distention), pulses paradoxus (systolic blood pressure drop of >10 mmHg on inspiration).

3. **Electrocardiogram.** May show low QRS voltage and/or electrical alternans.

4. **Chest Roentgenogram.** May show cardiomegaly with obscured cardiophrenic angles.

5. **Echocardiogram.** Suspected tamponade is an indication for emergent echocardiography.

6. **Treatment.** Consists of early percutaneous pericardiocentesis. Definitive treatment is surgical (pericardiectomy or pericardial window placement).

C. Constrictive Pericarditis

Constrictive pericarditis can be a long-term sequela of acute pericarditis.

BIBLIOGRAPHY

Fowler NO: Pericardial disease. Heart Dis Stroke 1992;March/April:85.
Shabeti R: Acute pericarditis. Cardiol Clin 1990;8:639.
Spodick DH: Pericarditis in systemic diseases. Cardiol Clin 1990;8:709.
Spodick DH: Pericarditis, pericardial effusion, cardiac tamponade, and constriction. Crit Care Clin 1989;5:455.

THORACIC AORTIC DISSECTION

*"The physics of a man's circulation are the physics of the
waterworks of the town in which he lives, but once out of gear,
you cannot apply the same rules for the repair of the one as of the other."*

SIR WILLIAM OSLER

I. ESSENTIAL FACTS

A. Definition

Thoracic aortic dissection occurs when an intimal tear allows
arterial blood to dissect into the aortic media, resulting in a
separation of the intima from the adventitia and the creation of a
double-lumen vessel.

1. It is a life-threatening emergency: if untreated, the mortality, as
   reported in one series, is 33% within 48 hours, 75% at 2 weeks,
   and 90% at 1 year.

2. Significant complications of aortic dissection may include

   a. Occlusion of major branch vessels of the aorta (causing
      ischemia distal to the occlusion, including cerebrovascular
      accident [CVA], acute myocardial infarction [MI], and renal
      vascular compromise);

   b. Rupture into a body space (e.g., hemothorax with resultant
      hemorrhagic shock);

   c. Retrograde extension into the aortic valve (with acute aortic
      insufficiency, fulminant congestive heart failure, and/or
      cardiac tamponade); and/or

   d. Compression of adjacent structures (e.g., superior cervical
      ganglia [causing Horner's syndrome], recurrent laryngeal
      nerve [causing hoarseness], superior vena cava [causing
      superior vena cava syndrome], and/or esophagus [causing
      dysphagia]).

3. Aortic dissection has been classified according to two systems
   (Fig. 13–9):

   a. **DeBakey system**
      i. Type I (60–70% of cases): the intimal tear originates in
         the ascending aorta and the dissection extends into the
         descending aorta.
      ii. Type II (10% of cases): the dissection is confined to the
          ascending aorta.
      iii. Type III (20-30% of cases): the intimal tear originates
           distal to the left subclavian artery and the dissection
           extends caudally.

   b. **Stanford system**
      i. Type A: the dissection involves the ascending aorta.
      ii. Type B: the dissection is limited to the descending aorta.

TYPE I TYPE II TYPE III

DeBakey System:

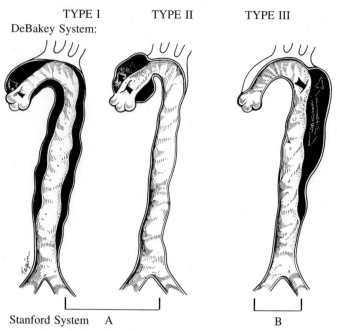

Stanford System   A   B

Figure 13–9. Classification of thoracic aortic dissections.

B. Epidemiology

1. Approximately 2000 new cases of thoracic aortic dissection are diagnosed yearly in the United States.

2. Most cases occur in patients between the ages of 40 and 70 years; the male-to-female ratio is 3:1.

3. Risk factors include hypertension (85–90% of patients), atherosclerosis, coarctation of the aorta, cystic medial necrosis, Marfan's syndrome, third trimester of pregnancy, post-cardiothoracic surgery involving pump bypass, and trauma.

II. CLINICAL EVALUATION

A. History

Acute dissection is associated with chest pain in > 95% of patients. This discomfort is frequently described as a sudden, severe, tearing or ripping sensation. Diaphoresis is common. The pain may move (e.g., from the chest to the back or into the abdomen) as the dissection extends.

1. In proximal dissection, the pain is often located in the anterior chest and may migrate to the upper back or radiate to the jaw or neck.

2. Dissection of the descending aorta may cause intrascapular pain that spreads to the abdomen or lower back.

3. Some patients may be unable to report the pain because of syncope or a CVA caused by the dissection.

B. Physical Examination

1. Carefully assess vital signs, peripheral pulses, neck veins, chest, abdomen, and perform careful cardiac and neurologic examinations.

2. Most patients are hypertensive on presentation; note any difference in the systolic blood pressures measured in the upper extremities. In the hemodynamically unstable patient, check for pulsus paradoxus (possible cardiac tamponade).

3. A proximal dissection may dilate the aortic root, causing acute aortic insufficiency.

4. Compression of the superior cervical ganglia may cause Horner's syndrome (ptosis, miosis, and anhydrosis on the involved side). Involvement of aortic arch branches may result in altered mental status (including coma) and/or a focal neurologic deficit.

C. Laboratory Studies

Minimally obtain the following:

1. Complete blood count with platelet count. Serial hematocrits are appropriate.

2. Electrolyte panel, blood urea nitrogen, creatinine, glucose levels. Prothrombin time/partial thromboplastin time.

3. Arterial blood gas levels.

4. Electrocardiogram (ECG). Evaluate carefully for arrhythmia, ischemia, infarction, or abnormally low voltage (consistent with cardiac tamponade).

5. Pregnancy test. Mandatory in reproductive-age females.

6. Emergent type and crossmatch. Order 6–8 units minimum; whole blood preferred.

7. Chest roentgenogram. Most patients (80–90%) will have an abnormal chest roentgenogram. Findings may include one or more of the following: widened mediastinum (75% of abnormal films), obliteration of the aortic knob, apical pleural capping, left-sided pleural effusion, "calcium sign" (separation of aortic intimal calcification from the outermost part of the aorta by > 5 mm), deviation of the trachea to the right, and/or deviation of the nasogastric tube to the right.

8. Urinalysis.

D. Diagnostic Imaging

Imaging is necessary to confirm dissection and define its origin and extent. A cardiothoracic surgeon should be consulted *prior to* definitive diagnostic imaging. The exact procedure chosen will vary with the experience and capabilities of the institution and the preferences of the consulting surgeon.

1. *Transesophageal echocardiography* is the diagnostic procedure of choice if available. It is sensitive, can be done at the bedside, takes < 20 minutes to perform, and does not require contrast agents or radiation exposure.

2. *Aortography* has traditionally been the diagnostic "gold standard" for aortic dissection. It is highly sensitive, very accurate in determining the origin of the intimal tear and extent of dissection, and useful in assessing branch vessel compromise secondary to the tear (all of which is important information to the thoracic surgeon). Disadvantages include the invasive nature of the procedure, high cost, radiation exposure, and the associated risks of radiographic contrast agents (including renal failure and contrast reactions).

3. *Computed tomography with contrast* is available at most institutions. The false-negative rate for thoracic aortic dissection is ≤ 5%. It is the imaging modality of choice in the stable patient with suspected thoracic aortic dissection if transesophageal echocardiography is not available.

4. *Magnetic resonance imaging* has excellent sensitivity and specificity in the setting of suspected dissection. Unfortunately, it is expensive, unavailable at many institutions, and difficult to obtain in patients who require sophisticated life-support equipment.

III. DIFFERENTIAL DIAGNOSIS

The differential diagnosis includes the following:

A. Acute MI. This is the most important alternative diagnosis to consider and exclude. Remember: thrombolytic therapy is the standard of care in the acute MI patient who is a candidate for same; but thrombolytic therapy would have disastrous consequences if given to a patient with an acute thoracic aortic dissection.

B. Pericarditis.

C. Pneumonia.

D. Pneumothorax.

E. Pulmonary embolism.

F. Cholecystitis.

G. Pancreatitis.

H. Cerebrovascular accident.

IV. THERAPY

A. Initial Assessment

Assess, secure, and support airway, breathing, and circulation as indicated (see Chapter 1. II).

1. Administer supplemental oxygen, establish IV access (at least two large-bore IV lines recommended), and continuously monitor both cardiac rhythm and oxygen saturation (SaO_2).

2. Rapidly obtain vital signs, an ECG, and a portable chest roentgenogram, and perform a directed physical examination and relevent laboratory studies (see II. C, above).

3. If the patient is hypotensive (systolic blood pressure [BP] < 90 mmHg), resuscitate with volume with or without blood products as clinically indicated and urgently consult a cardiothoracic surgeon.

B. Cardiothoracic Surgery Consultation and Hypertension Control

1. Consult a cardiothoracic surgeon emergently when thoracic aortic dissection is suspected on the basis of the initial evaluation outlined in IV. A, above.

2. Re-evaluate oxygenation, cardiac rhythm, and vital signs.

3. Control pain and anxiety with opiates (e.g., morphine sulfate 1–3 mg IV every 5 minutes, titrated as necessary).

4. Control hypertension and tachycardia: most patients are hypertensive on presentation. Treat immediately to control shear stress and prevent extension of the dissection. Maintain systolic BP between 100 and 120 mmHg (or the lowest BP possible that still provides adequate organ perfusion [e.g., clear mentation, warm perfused extremities, reasonable urine output]); maintain heart rate between 60 and 75 beats/min.

   a. **Beta-Blocker Therapy.** These should be initiated prior to or simultaneously with vasodilators as outlined below. Drug choices include:

      i. Esmolol: the short half-life of this agent is an advantage if beta-blocker therapy is not well tolerated.

      Dose: initial bolus 500 µg/kg IV over 1 minute, followed by a continuous IV infusion of 50 µg/kg/min. Titrate as necessary every 4 minutes by repeating the bolus and increasing the infusion in increments of 50 µg/kg/min. The maximum continuous infusion rate is 200 µg/kg/min IV;

or

    ii. Metoprolol: 5 mg slow IV push every 2–5 minutes as tolerated, to a total IV load of 15 mg; subsequent doses of 5–15 mg may be given IV every 4–6 hours as necessary;

or

    iii. Propranolol: 0.5–1.0 mg IV, followed by 1 mg IV every 5 minutes as required (to maximum total dose of 0.1–0.15 mg/kg). Maintenance dose may be repeated as necessary every 4–6 hours.

        Caution: beta blockers are contraindicated in the hypotensive patient or the patient in significant heart failure; they may exacerbate asthma and/or chronic obstructive pulmonary disease as well. If beta-blocker therapy is contraindicated or poorly tolerated (e.g., exacerbation of bronchospastic disease) consider heart-rate control with a calcium channel blocker (e.g., diltiazem: 0.25 mg/kg IV load, followed by continuous IV infusion of 5–15 mg/hr).

  b. **Vasodilator Therapy.** Sodium nitroprusside is the drug of choice. *Dose:* begin with 0.5 µg/kg/min IV and titrate as necessary. The maximum dose is 10 µg/kg/min. Early placement of an arterial catheter for continuous monitoring of BP is appropriate. *Caution:* in the pregnant patient, avoid sodium nitroprusside if at all possible; consult an obstetrician emergently and consider hypertension and heart rate control with labetalol (initiate at 2 mg/min IV; usual dose range is 0.5–4 mg/min IV).

C. Confirmation of diagnosis and arrangement for definitive care

Once the patient is hemodynamically stabilized, a definitive anatomic diagnosis must be made via imaging studies (see II. D, above). ICU admission is required.

V. DISPOSITION

Any patient with suspected or confirmed thoracic aortic dissection requires ICU admission. Acute proximal dissections (type A in the Stanford classification system) require operative repair, descending aortic dissections (type B in the Stanford classification system) are generally treated with medical therapy unless the patient has secondary vascular complications. If definitive surgical or medical care is not available at the given institution, the patient should be stabilized and transferred to an appropriate tertiary care facility.

VI. PEARLS AND PITFALLS

A. Suspect thoracic aortic dissection in any patient with chest pain of a tearing or ripping quality; chest pain that radiates into the back or abdomen; and/or chest pain accompanied by neurologic abnormalities, BP differences in the upper extremities, or syncope.

B. Always check and document BP in both upper extremities and carefully evaluate by palpation the following arterial pulses: carotid, radial, femoral, dorsalis pedis, and posterior tibial.

C. Evaluate neck veins and auscultate the heart carefully: consider the possibility of cardiac tamponade and/or acute aortic insufficiency.

D. Evaluate the ECG carefully for arrhythmia, acute ischemia/infarction, and/or low voltages suggestive of cardiac tamponade.

E. A normal chest roentgenogram does *not* rule out acute thoracic aortic dissection in the patient with a consistent presentation for same.

F. Consult a cardiothoracic surgeon early.

G. Aggressively manage hypertension and tachycardia immediately, even before the diagnosis is confirmed with definitive imaging. Beta-blocker therapy should be started prior to initiating vasodilator therapy.

H. *Do not* administer thrombolytic therapy for MI if thoracic aortic dissection is suggested by the history, physical examination, and/or chest roentgenogram.

BIBLIOGRAPHY

Asfoura JY, Vidt DG: Acute aortic dissection. Chest 1991;99:724–729.
Cigarroa JE, Isselbacher EM, De Sanctis RW, Eagle KA: Diagnostic imaging in the evaluation of suspected aortic dissection. N Engl J Med 1993;328(1):35–43.
Crawford S: The diagnosis and management of aortic dissection. JAMA 1990;264(19):2537–2541.

14

Pulmonary Emergencies

ACUTE RESPIRATORY FAILURE

> *"From troublous sights and sounds set free;*
> *In such a twilight hour of breath,*
> *Shall one retrace his life, or see,*
> *Through shadows, the true face of death?"*
>
> ERNEST DOWSON

I. ESSENTIAL FACTS

A. Definition

Acute respiratory failure (ARF) is defined as an impairment in gas exchange to a level that causes a significant potential for morbidity or mortality. The levels of arterial oxygen tension (PaO_2) and carbon dioxide tension ($PaCO_2$) that define ARF are arbitrary, since normal values for an individual patient vary, and are influenced by barometric pressure as well as the patient's age, underlying cardiopulmonary status, and metabolic condition. In a previously normal individual, a $PaO_2 < 60$ mmHg while breathing room air, with or without a $PaCO_2 > 50$ mmHg, is generally considered to be consistent with the diagnosis of ARF. In patients with chronic respiratory acidosis, ARF is suggested by a significant fall in the baseline PaO_2, or a rise in the baseline $PaCO_2$ accompanied by a fall in the arterial serum pH to < 7.35. By definition, ARF represents a *change* in the patient's usual or baseline condition.

B. Classification

Acute respiratory failure is usually manifested in one of two clinical presentations:

1. **Hypoxic/Hypocapnic or Normocapnic Respiratory Failure.** ($PaO_2 < 55$–60 mmHg, with a normal or low $PaCO_2$). This type of respiratory failure is often caused by acute lung injury (e.g., the adult respiratory distress syndrome [ARDS] or acute *Pneumocystis carinii* pneumonia), and generally occurs in patients without prior underlying lung disease. Both ventilation–perfusion (V/Q) mismatch and physiologic right-to-left shunt contribute to hypoxia in these cases.

2. **Hypoxic/Hypercapnic Respiratory Failure.** ($PaO_2 < 55$–60 mmHg, $PaCO_2 > 50$ mmHg). This type of respiratory failure is more common in patients with chronic underlying lung disease (e.g., chronic obstructive pulmonary disease [COPD] or interstitial lung disease) or in patients with neuromuscular disease or drug overdose. Hypercapnic respiratory failure is typically caused by alveolar hypoventilation, which is frequently superimposed on areas of V/Q mismatch.

C. Epidemiology

The precise incidence of ARF is difficult to establish, since definitions of the syndrome vary. Cases of ARF are common in the ED and are a frequent cause of admission to the ICU.

1. The 30-day mortality rate for patients with COPD presenting to the ED in ARF approaches 10%. The long-term prognosis for patients with underlying lung disease presenting with an episode of ARF is quite poor.

2. Patients without underlying lung disease have a relatively good

long-term prognosis if they survive the acute episode of ARF and the related illness.

3. The incidence of ARDS, which is an important cause of hypoxic/hypocapnic respiratory failure, is estimated at 150,000 cases per year in the United States. Despite the availability of sophisticated monitoring systems and supportive therapy, mortality for patients with ARDS remains approximately 50%.

D. Etiology

Numerous causes of ARF have been described, and a partial list of these causes is presented in Table 14–1. The four basic pathophysiologic mechanisms responsible for the clinical syndrome of ARF are described below:

1. **Alveolar Hypoventilation.** This is reflected by the presence of hypercapnia and respiratory acidosis. Hypoxia in these cases is secondary to inadequate alveolar ventilation.

    a. *Arterial hypoxemia* resulting from alveolar hypoventilation is not typically associated with an increase in the alveolar–arterial oxygen gradient $\{P(A-a)O_2\}$. The $P(A-a)O_2$ gradient is calculated by subtracting the measured arterial PO_2 from the calculated alveolar PO_2. The alveolar PO_2 can be derived from a simplified version of the alveolar–gas equation:

    $$PAO_2 = FiO_2(P_B - 47) - \frac{PaCO_2}{R}$$

    where FiO_2 = fraction of inspired oxygen, P_B = atmospheric pressure, $PaCO_2$ = pressure of carbon dioxide in mmHg from the arterial blood gas, and R = respiratory quotient (assumed to be 0.8).

    The normal $P(A-a)O_2$ gradient in a young person without underlying lung disease is 5–10 mmHg. A $P(A-a)O_2$ difference > 20 mm Hg is generally considered abnormal at any age.

    b. *Examples* of clinical conditions that may cause ARF via hypoventilation include narcotic overdoses, neuromuscular diseases (e.g., Guillain-Barré syndrome, amyotrophic lateral sclerosis), and episodes of acute airway obstruction (e.g., epiglottitis).

2. **Ventilation–Perfusion (V/Q) Mismatch.** V/Q mismatch is the most common cause of arterial hypoxemia, and occurs in areas of the lung in which there is inhomogeneity in the distribution of ventilation and perfusion.

    a. *Hypoxia* in these cases results from areas of the lung that are underventilated with respect to their blood flow. Blood traversing underventilated alveoli will reflect the low alveolar PO_2 and the high PCO_2 of these regions.

Table 14-1. COMMON CAUSES OF ACUTE RESPIRATORY FAILURE

Airflow Obstruction

Status asthmaticus
Chronic obstructive pulmonary disease in exacerbation
Foreign-body aspiration
Upper-airway obstruction
  Acute epiglottitis
  Laryngeal edema

Alveolar-Filling Processes

Pneumonia
Pulmonary edema
  Cardiogenic (e.g., left-ventricular failure, mitral valve disease, cardiac tamponade)
  Noncardiogenic (ARDS)
Intra-alveolar hemorrhage
Aspiration

Interstitial Lung Diseases

Pulmonary fibrosis
Sarcoidosis
Collagen–vascular-associated lung diseases
Hypersensitivity pneumonitis

Pulmonary Vascular Disease

Pulmonary thromboembolism
Fat embolism
Amniotic fluid embolism
Pulmonary vasculitis

Neuromuscular Disease

Narcotic/sedative drug overdose
Guillain-Barré syndrome
Amyotrophic lateral sclerosis
Phrenic nerve injury
Spinal cord injury
Stroke
Obesity/hypoventilation syndrome

Chest Wall/Pleural Disease

Pneumothorax
Hemothorax
Large pleural effusion
Flail chest

Miscellaneous

Toxic inhalation injury
  Smoke inhalation
  Carbon monoxide poisoning
Metabolic derangements
  Hypophosphatemia
  Severe hypothyroidism
Right-to-left shunts
  Pulmonary arteriovenous malformations
  Ventricular or atrial septal defects

  b. *Examples* of conditions that may cause ARF via V/Q mismatch include severe pneumonia and air-flow obstruction (e.g., status asthmaticus).

3. **Shunt.** The term *shunt* describes the passage of blood from the venous to the arterial system without traveling through any ventilated region of lung.
  a. Areas of *intrapulmonary shunt* reflect an extreme instance of V/Q mismatch in which part of the lung receives *no* ventilation, but continues to receive blood flow.
  b. *Intrapulmonary shunts* may result from anatomic abnormalities such as pulmonary arteriovenous fistulas. More commonly, shunts result from perfusion of areas of nonventilated lung tissue. Disruption of alveolar ventilation may occur when the alveoli are collapsed (e.g., atelectasis) or filled with fluid (e.g., pulmonary edema or intra-alveolar hemorrhage).
  c. In addition to intrapulmonary shunts, right to left *intracardiac shunts* can cause severe hypoxemia.
  d. In contrast to hypoxemia caused by V/Q mismatch, hypoxemia due to shunting does *not* improve with the administration of supplemental oxygen.

4. **Diffusion limitation** occurs when the PO_2 in pulmonary capillary blood fails to reach equilibrium with the alveolar gas.
  a. Diffusion limitation is an uncommon cause of clinically significant hypoxemia.
  b. Diffusion limitation occurs primarily in patients with a thickened pulmonary capillary membrane (e.g., interstitial lung disease) and/or a shortened transit time for erythrocytes to come into contact with the alveolar–capillary membrane (e.g., tachycardia).

II. CLINICAL EVALUATION

A. History

Pertinent historical information in patients presenting with ARF should include

1. Assessment of the rapidity of *symptom onset.*

2. Assessment of the presence of *underlying* pulmonary, cardiovascular, or neuromuscular disorders.

3. Information about *past episodes* of respiratory failure.

4. *Current medications.*

5. Potential *toxic exposures* (inhalation or ingestion).

6. *Recent illnesses.*

7. *Recent trauma.*

B. Symptoms

1. The most common symptom associated with ARF is *dyspnea.* Dyspnea is more common in patients with hypoxic/hypocapnic respiratory failure.

2. In contrast, patients with hypoxic/hypercapnic respiratory failure may present with *somnolence* and *lethargy* in the absence of dyspnea.

3. *Confusion* and *disorientation* may be present, especially in severely hypoxic patients.

4. Patients with severe hypercapnia may complain of a *headache,* which is probably a result of dilatation of cerebral blood vessels secondary to the increased $PaCO_2$.

5. Patients with ARF secondary to acute left-ventricular dysfunction may complain of *chest pain, nausea,* or *diaphoresis.*

6. *Pleuritic chest pain* may accompany a pneumothorax or pulmonary embolism.

7. Patients with an exacerbation of underlying COPD experiencing ARF may complain of *fever, malaise,* and *purulent sputum* production.

C. Signs

Physical examination of patients with ARF may vary depending on the severity and underlying cause of their respiratory failure. Patients in the ED with ARF should be re-examined frequently to assess any changes in their condition.

1. **Vital Signs.** In the early phase of ARF, patients are often *restless* and may demonstrate *tachypnea, tachycardia,* and *mild hypertension.* Unlike patients with hypoxic/hypocapnic respiratory failure, patients with hypercapnic respiratory failure may have very *slow respiratory rates. Fever* may be present in patients with ARF secondary to pneumonia or pulmonary embolism. *Hypotension* may accompany ARF associated with sepsis, or may indicate tension pneumothorax, cardiogenic shock, or cardiac tamponade.

2. **Skin.** *Cyanosis* may be present in patients with severe hypoxia. *Diaphoresis* is common in patients with pneumonia, myocardial infarction, or an excessive work of breathing associated with ARF.

3. **HEENT.** *Nasal flaring* is common during inspiration in patients with ARF, and mucous membranes are often dry.

4. **Neck.** Patients with ARF often demonstrate *use of accessory muscles* for respiration. *Jugular venous distention* may be present in patients with congestive heart failure, cardiac tamponade, or tension pneumothorax.

5. **Lungs.** Pulmonary examination findings in patients with ARF typically reflect the underlying cause of their acute illness. For example, patients with ARF secondary to airflow obstruction often demonstrate *wheezing* or *diminished breath sounds,* whereas patients with pneumonia may have evidence of pulmonary consolidation or *bronchial breath sounds.* Patients with a pneumothorax typically have *decreased or absent breath sounds* on auscultation of the affected side as well as *hyperresonant tones* with percussion. The presence of *crackles* or *rales* usually indicates fluid in the small airways and alveolar spaces, although similar sounds may be present in patients with pulmonary fibrosis.

6. **Heart.** An S_3 *gallop* may be present in patients with left-ventricular failure. Cardiac *murmurs* are often audible in patients with pulmonary edema secondary to valvular heart disease, whereas *muffled heart tones* or a *pericardial rub* may indicate pericardial disease.

7. **Abdomen.** *Hepatomegaly, ascites,* and/or the presence of the *hepatojugular reflex* indicates right-sided heart failure. *Paradoxical movement of the abdominal muscles* during respiration can often be observed in patients with spinal cord damage or phrenic nerve injury.

8. **Extremities.** *Clubbing* is a nonspecific finding, but may indicate chronic respiratory disease such as bronchiectasis or pulmonary fibrosis. Peripheral *edema* is a common sign of right-sided heart failure, and may indicate the presence of cor pulmonale in some patients.

9. **Mental Status.** Patients in the early stage of ARF or patients with hypoxic/hypocapnic or normocapnic respiratory failure are typically *agitated* or *restless,* whereas patients with ARF secondary to hypoventilation often develop progressive *somnolence* as hypercapnia worsens. Severely hypoxic patients may be *disoriented* as well.

D. Laboratory Studies

1. *Arterial blood gas analysis* (ABG) in patients with ARF typically demonstrates hypoxemia with or without hypercapnia. ARF can occur with a low, normal, or high arterial $PaCO_2$ level. Respiratory failure is present when the PaO_2 is < 60 mmHg, or when there is an acute rise in the $PaCO_2$ > 50 mmHg with a concomitant fall in the serum arterial pH to < 7.35. Arterial blood gas analysis should be obtained in *all* patients with suspected ARF, since the history and physical examination are very insensitive measurements of the extent of respiratory failure.

2. The *chest roentgenogram* in a patient with ARF may be helpful in establishing the cause of the respiratory compromise. A focal infiltrate suggests pneumonia, whereas a diffuse infiltrate is

more commonly associated with pulmonary edema or interstitial lung disease.

3. *Other laboratory tests* should include an *electrocardiogram* to rule out left ventricular dysfunction or arrhythmia, *complete blood count* (CBC) and *electrolyte panel. Sputum Gram stain* should be obtained in cases of suspected pneumonia. A *V/Q scan* is an appropriate diagnostic test in patients with a suspected pulmonary thromboembolism. A *carboxyhemoglobin level* should be obtained in cases of suspected carbon monoxide poisoning, since the PaO_2 is unaffected by the carbon monoxide level.

III. TREATMENT

A. Initial Priorities

1. **Airway.** First priority must be given to ensure an adequate airway for the patient in respiratory failure. Endotracheal intubation should be considered in patients with a diminished or absent gag reflex who are unable to adequately protect the airway (see Chapter 11).

2. **Ventilation.** After the patient's airway is adequately secured, priority must be given to ensuring adequate ventilation and oxygenation. Endotracheal intubation should be considered in patients with hypoventilation and acute respiratory acidosis. Additional criteria for endotracheal intubation and mechanical ventilation are presented in Chapter 11 (IV. A. 1.). Emergent intubation may be avoided in alert patients with respiratory failure secondary to COPD exacerbations who improve with low-flow supplemental oxygen and aggressive bronchodilator therapy.

3. **Oxygenation.** Patients with ARF and severe hypoxemia despite high concentrations of supplemental oxygen should be treated with endotracheal intubation and mechanical ventilation. Common mechanical ventilator settings are presented in Table 14–2. Patients with less severe oxygenation failure should receive supplemental oxygen through one of a variety of different delivery systems (e.g., nasal cannulae, Venturi masks, oxygen reservoir masks, continuous positive airway pressure [CPAP]; see Table 11–1). In general, the amount of supplemental oxygen delivered should be adjusted to achieve an oxygen hemoglobin saturation level (SaO_2) > 90%. The amount of supplemental oxygen delivered by these methods varies depending on the flow rates employed and the amount of room air entrained around the device. Tight-fitting masks should be avoided in obtunded patients because of the high risk for aspiration if they vomit while wearing the mask.

4. **Circulation.** Patients with ARF may have hemodynamic instability as either a cause or effect of their respiratory

Table 14–2. RECOMMENDED INITIAL
MECHANICAL VENTILATOR SETTINGS

PARAMETER	COMMENTS
Ventilator mode	*Assist-Control* most commonly (the ventilator senses a patient's efforts to breathe and delivers a fixed tidal volume with each effort, in addition to providing a predetermined "back-up" rate if the patient's inspiratory efforts are infrequent). Other modes may include *Intermittent Mandatory Ventilation* (IMV) and *Pressure Support.*
Tidal volume	10–15 mL/kg. In the patient with COPD, 10 mL/kg is preferred to avoid hyperinflation and the risks of barotrauma.
Respiratory rate	12–16 breaths/min. Changes in the respiratory rate may be guided by the following equation: New respiratory rate = old rate $\times$ (old $PaCO_2$/desired $PaCO_2$)
Oxygen concentration	Begin with 100% oxygen. Subsequent adjustments should be guided by ABG analysis.
Flow rates	Usually begin with 50 L/min. In general, flow rates should be set so that expiratory time exceeds inspiratory time (usually allowing twice as much time for exhalation as for inhalation). In the setting of marked air-flow obstruction, exhalation time should be increased even more.
Sensitivity	Initially 2–3 cmH_2O *Sensitivity* is the amount of negative pressure the patient must generate before the ventilator will deliver an assisted breath in the *Assist-Control* mode.
Humidifiers	100% humidifed and generally warmed to a temperature of 35° C.
Monitors and alarms	Two of the most important alarms include a pressure limit (usually $\leq$ 50 cmH_2O or set about 5–10 cmH_2O above the pressure necessary to deliver the desired tidal volume) and exhaled tidal volume monitor (to detect decreased tidal volumes delivered to the patient because of ventilator malfunction or leaks in the circuit). Additional alarms include those that sound with electrical failure or because of inadequate oxygen line pressure.
Sighs	Usually unnecessary because of the large tidal volumes that are now typically used. If, for whatever reason, the ventilator is set with a small tidal volume (< 8 mL/kg), then a sigh should be set at 1.5–2.0 times the tidal volume every 5–10 min to prevent atelectasis.
Positive end-expiratory pressure (PEEP)	Initially 0. PEEP may be useful in the patient with a diffuse pulmonary process and refractory hypoxemia despite oxygen supplementation. It increases end-expiratory and mean pressure across the walls of airways and alveoli, re-expanding collapsed alveoli and allowing them to participate in gas exchange. If PEEP is deemed appropriate and necessary, begin with 5 cmH_2O and make increments thereafter of 2.5–5.0 cmH_2O at a time. PEEP levels > 10 cmH_2O generally require the patient to have a Swan-Ganz catheter for invasive hemodynamic monitoring purposes.

298 / PULMONARY EMERGENCIES

insufficiency. After securing a patient's airway, ventilation, and oxygenation, immediate attention must be paid toward achieving hemodynamic stability. In the ED, assessment and treatment of hemodynamic problems often occurs simultaneously with treatment of respiratory failure (see Chapter 12).

B. General Measures

1. *Vital signs.*

2. *Continuous SaO$_2$.*

3. *Cardiac monitor.*

4. Intravenous access.

5. Chest roentgenogram.

6. Electrocardiogram.

7. Laboratory analysis.

    a. Arterial blood gas (ABG).
    b. Complete blood count (CBC).
    c. Electrolyte panel, renal function, glucose level.

C. Therapy Directed at Specific Causes of ARF

1. **Airflow Obstruction.** Inhaled beta-2 agonists and anticholinergic agents, corticosteroids, ± methylxanthines, ± antibiotics.

2. **Left-Ventricular Failure.** Diuretics, nitrates; morphine sulfate if indicated.

3. **Pneumonia.** Antibiotics.

4. **Pulmonary Embolism.** Anticoagulants.

5. **Pneumothorax.** Thoracostomy tube placement.

6. **Large Pleural Effusion.** Consider thoracentesis.

7. **Acute Toxic Inhalation Injury.** Consider specific antidotes in certain circumstances (e.g., high-flow oxygen; hyperbaric oxygen for carbon monoxide inhalation if indicated).

IV. DISPOSITION

Nearly all patients with evidence of ARF by ABGs in the ED should be admitted to the hospital for further evaluation and treatment. Patients with ARF should be admitted to the ICU when they meet any of the following criteria:

A. Intubated.

B. Clinically unstable requiring close nursing supervision or continuous SaO$_2$ or ECG monitoring.

C. High FiO_2 requirements in the ED (e.g., requiring an $FiO_2 > 0.50$ to maintain SaO_2 above 90%).

D. Persistent respiratory acidosis (e.g., pH < 7.30 to 7.35, and $PaCO_2$ >50 mmHg) despite treatment in the ED.

V. PEARLS AND PITFALLS

A. Ensure adequate airway, oxygenation, ventilation, and hemodynamic stability for all patients presenting with ARF.

B. Thoroughly investigate all possible causes of the patient's ARF.

C. Concentrate on treatment of the underlying cause of the patient's respiratory failure after emergent therapy has been rendered.

D. Quickly obtain an ABG in all patients suspected of having ARF instead of relying solely on the patient's history and other less objective parameters.

E. Consider early endotracheal intubation for unstable patients (see Chapter 11).

F. Admit unstable patients or those requiring close observation to the ICU.

Do not do any of the following:

A. Fail to obtain an ABG to determine the pH and $PaCO_2$ in a patient with suspected ARF, even if the SaO_2 is normal.

B. Withhold supplemental oxygen in a hypoxemic patient with respiratory distress, even if the patient has a respiratory acidosis. However, be prepared to treat ventilatory failure if it occurs.

C. Overlook the extensive list of potential causes of ARF.

D. Administer sedation to a patient with a respiratory acidosis, unless the patient is intubated and receiving mechanical ventilation.

E. Fail to recognize that a rising $PaCO_2$ in a patient that had been hyperventilating may signify fatigue and impending respiratory arrest.

F. Overventilate a patient with a chronic respiratory acidosis after the patient has been intubated for ARF, since rapid correction of the $PaCO_2$ can lead to a severe uncompensated metabolic alkalosis.

G. Use a tight-fitting oxygen mask or continuous positive airway pressure mask in an obtunded patient.

BIBLIOGRAPHY

Derenne JP, Fleury B, Pariente R: Acute respiratory failure of chronic obstructive pulmonary disease. Am Rev Respir Dis 1988;138(4):1006–1033.

Hudson LD: Chapter 140, Acute respiratory failure: overview. In Fishman AP (ed): Pulmonary Diseases and Disorders, 2nd Ed, New York, McGraw-Hill, 1988, pp. 2189–2198.

Ingbar DH, White DA: Acute respiratory failure. Crit Care Clin 1988;4(1):11–40.

Johanson WG, Peters JI: Respiratory failure: general principles and initial approach. Chapter 94. In Murray JF, Nadel JA (eds): Textbook of Respiratory Medicine. Philadelphia, WB Saunders, 1988, pp. 1973–1975.

Pingleton SK: Complications of acute respiratory failure. Am Rev Respir Dis 1988; 137(6):1463–1493.

Tobin MJ: Mechanical ventilation. N Engl J Med 1994;330(15):1056–1060.

ASTHMA

> *"All that wheezes is not asthma."*
>
> CHEVALIER JACKSON

I. ESSENTIAL FACTS

A. Definition

Asthma is an obstructive pulmonary disease in which airway inflammation and hyperresponsiveness result in episodic patient symptoms of dyspnea, wheezing, and/or cough. Pulmonary function testing during symptoms will demonstrate obstructive changes (reduced FEV_1 [forced expiration volume in 1 second] and decreased FEV_1/FVC [forced vital capacity]). Unlike chronic obstructive pulmonary disease (COPD), the obstructive changes on pulmonary function tests generally normalize with therapy or between symptomatic episodes. Status asthmaticus is a severe exacerbation of asthma unresponsive to usual outpatient treatment methods.

B. Epidemiology

1. Ten million individuals in the United States suffer with asthma.

2. Asthma is the most common chronic disease of childhood.

3. One-third of asthmatics are *not* diagnosed until after the age of 30, and those patients with the onset of their disease in adulthood may be plagued by severe and recurrent symptoms.

4. Asthma is a potentially life-threatening disease that kills over 4000 Americans annually. Unfortunately, the mortality from asthma is increasing (the death rate from 1980 to 1987 increased by 31%). Theoretically, every death from asthma is preventable.

C. Causes of Exacerbations

1. Viral or bacterial respiratory tract infections (including pneumonia and sinusitis).

2. Medication noncompliance.

3. Environmental factors: cigarette smoke, pollution, cold air, occupational exposures, and strong odors.

4. Immunologic reactions to animal dander, pollen, dust mites, molds, and food additives (e.g., sulfites).

5. Medications: beta blockers, salicylates, and other nonsteroidal anti-inflammatory drugs (NSAIDs).

6. Miscellaneous causes: gastroesophageal reflux, exercise, and emotional factors (e.g., fear, anger, anxiety).

II. CLINICAL EVALUATION

A. History

Patients frequently present to the ED with a prior diagnosis of asthma. Determine the following: duration of the patient's current symptomatic episode and "home" treatment before ED presentation; prior history of exacerbations and severity (e.g., need for oral corticosteroids, hospitalization and intubation record); use of and compliance with medications; allergic history; likely cause of current attack; and home/social situation. The patient may be so dyspneic at the time of presentation that a history will not be possible until emergent therapy for the acute attack has been started.

B. Symptoms

Asthma is a possible diagnosis in any patient who suffers from episodic cough, wheezing, chest tightness, and/or dyspnea. Nocturnal symptoms are common. Some patients will present with cough only.

C. Signs

1. *Common* signs include tachypnea, tachycardia, diaphoresis, coughing, wheezing, and a prolonged expiratory phase of respiration.

2. *Severe asthma,* with marked airway obstruction, is suggested by accessory muscle use, pulsus paradoxus, decreasing breath sounds, poor air flow, and/or a "quiet" chest. (*Reminder:* severe asthma may also be present in the absence of these signs.)

3. *Imminent respiratory arrest* is suggested by altered mental status, appearance of extreme fatigue or exhaustion, respiratory alternans (alternating rib cage and abdominal breathing), abdominal paradox (inward abdominal motion during respiration), or cyanosis.

D. Physical Examination

1. **Vital Signs.** Note degree of tachycardia, tachypnea, and fever.

2. **Skin.** Diaphoresis indicates a patient in moderate to severe distress.

3. **HEENT.** Note TMs, sinus tenderness, nasal discharge, or pharyngeal inflammation suggestive of infection.

4. **Neck.** Accessory muscle use indicates a severe attack. Check for enlarged lymph nodes.

5. **Chest.** Note air flow, wheezing, symmetry of breath sounds, duration of expiratory phase, and any localized findings suggestive of pneumonia.

6. **Heart.** Listen for murmurs, rubs, and/or gallops.

7. **Abdomen.** Look for abdominal movements with respiration that might suggest either respiratory alternans or abdominal paradox (see C. 3, above).

8. **Extremities.** Check for clubbing, cyanosis, and/or edema.

9. **Mental Status.** Note mental status changes suggestive of drug ingestion or impending respiratory failure.

The asthma patient requires continual reassessment over time as therapy proceeds.

E. Monitoring

1. **Pulmonary Function Tests**

   a. These are of utmost importance in determining the severity of the asthma attack, the patient's response to treatment, and the need for hospitalization.

   b. Bedside spirometry with either FEV_1 or PEFR (peaked expiratory flow rate) should be obtained as the patient's condition allows (patients with severe asthma may be so dyspneic on presentation that bedside spirometry will not be immediately possible).

   c. Severe airway obstruction is characterized by an $FEV_1 <$ 0.8–1.0 L ($< 25\%$ predicted) or a PEFR < 100 L/min ($< 20\%$ predicted).

2. **Routine monitoring**
   a. Vital signs.
   b. Bedside spirometry.
   c. Oxygen saturation (SaO_2): maintain $\geq 95\%$.

3. In the moderate to severe attack, also continuously monitor the cardiac rhythm.

F. Laboratory Studies

1. Obtain a *theophylline* level (for patients taking theophylline as an outpatient).

2. Additional laboratory work may occasionally be necessary depending on the clinical circumstances. Consider the following if appropriate:

   a. **Arterial Blood Gas (ABG).** This test is *not* necessary in every asthma patient. Consider it, however, in the life-threatening attack not immediately responsive to aggressive therapy. Hypoxemia is common. A normal or rising PCO_2 indicates a severe attack and potential ventilatory failure.

b. **Chest Roentgenography.** Appropriate if the patient is presenting with their *first* episode of asthma, in the *febrile* asthmatic patient, if the pulmonary examination suggests pneumonia or pneumothorax (*focal* findings), or if the patient is *failing* ED therapy (the "Four Fs").

c. **Sputum for Gram Stain and Culture.** In the asthma patient with pneumonia.

d. **Miscellaneous.** Additional studies may be necessary depending on clinical circumstances (e.g., complete blood count, sinus computed tomography, serum pregnancy test).

III. DIFFERENTIAL DIAGNOSIS

The differential diagnosis includes pulmonary edema ("cardiac asthma"), pulmonary embolism, anaphylaxis, pneumonia, aspiration, epiglottitis, pneumothorax, exacerbation of chronic bronchitis/emphysema, chest-wall injury, carcinoid tumors, eosinophilic pneumonia, drug exposure/overdose; and airway injury, foreign body, or neoplasm.

IV. THERAPY

Note: dosages given are for the adult patient (Fig. 14–1 and Table 14–3).

A. First-Line Therapy

As therapy is being initiated a history, a directed physical examination, and bedside spirometry can be performed. The patient should be monitored with a pulse oximeter. If the attack is moderate to severe, also obtain intravenous (IV) access and monitor cardiac rhythm continuously.

1. **Oxygen.** Should always be administered to the patient. Maintain $SaO_2 \geq 95\%$.

   Dose. Begin with 2–3 L/min via nasal cannula and adjust as necessary to maintain an appropriate SaO_2.

2. **Inhaled Beta Agonists.** These agents produce direct bronchodilation and are mast-cell stabilizers. Their routine use is mandatory in the ED treatment of asthma. Administer one of the following agents aggressively over the first hour of the patient's ED stay (one treatment every 20 minutes, or even near-continuous nebulization in the severe attack). As the patient responds to bronchodilation, the frequency of beta-agonist administration may be decreased. *Medication choices include* the following.

   a. Albuterol (nebulized, 0.83 mg/mL; 3 mL ampules): deliver

Table 14–3. EMERGENCY MEDICAL THERAPY OF THE PATIENT WITH AN ASTHMA EXACERBATION

Drug	Dose	Comments
First-Line Therapy		
Oxygen	Begin wtih 3–5 L/min via nasal cannula	Maintain SaO$_2$ ≥ 95% as determined with monitor.
Nebulized Beta Agonists		
Albuterol	0.83 mg/mL; 3 mL nebulized q 20 min for 3 to 6 doses	Administer all of these agents aggressively (3 treatments within the first 60 min of ED visit). Then decrease frequency of administration as patient's condition allows to one nebulized treatment q 1–6 hr. In the elderly patient, or the patient with active cardiac disease, more cautious use (decreased dosage and/or frequency) may be necessary.
or		
Terbutaline	1-mg/mL vial; put 0.5 mL in 2.5 mL NS nebulized q 20 min for 3 doses	
or		
Metaproterenol	0.4% solution; 2.5 mL nebulized q 15–20 min for 3 to 4 doses	
Corticosteroids		
Methylprednisolone	2 mg/kg IV infusion. May repeat q 6 hr	The ideal dose of corticosteroids is undetermined. Inhaled corticosteroids have no role in the ED management of the acute asthma attack (inhaled steroids may worsen the exacerbation by acting as an airway irritant). If the patient responds to therapy and is discharged home, a 7–14-day tapering dose of prednisone should be prescribed.
or		
Hydrocortisone sodium succinate	5–7 mg/kg IV infusion. May repeat q 4–6 hr	
or		
Dexamethasone	0.25 mg/kg IV infusion. May repeat q 8–12 hr	
Second-Line Therapy		
Subcutaneous Beta Agonists		
Epinephrine	0.3 mg SQ q 20 min for 3 doses	The use of beta agonists parenterally will increase unwanted side effects. *Do not* use in the cardiac patient. Avoid epinephrine in the pregnant patient.
or		
Terbutaline	0.25 mg SQ, *not* to exceed 0.5 mg SQ q 4 hr	
Third-Line Therapy		
Methylxanthines		
Aminophyline (IV therapy)	If patient is not on medications, IV load is 5–6 mg/kg over 20 min (1 mg/kg IV will raise blood level by 2 µg/mL). Follow load by IV infusion: Adult smoker 0.9 mg/kg/hr; Adult nonsmoker 0.5–0.7 mg/kg/hr; Adult > 50 yr 0.4 mg/kg/hr; Elderly/CHF/ *or* liver disease 0.2–0.3 mg/kg/hr	*Do not* administer to a patient already on these medications without first checking a blood level. Therapeutic level is between 10 and 18 µg/mL.
or		

Table 14–3. EMERGENCY MEDICAL THERAPY OF THE PATIENT WITH AN ASTHMA EXACERBATION *Continued*

DRUG	DOSE	COMMENTS
Theophylline (PO therapy)	Reasonable average oral doses (in a 70 kg patient): Nonsmoker — 900 mg/day Smoker — 1100 mg/day Cimetidine use — 500 mg/day Cor pulmonale — 400 mg/day Liver disease — 350 mg/day	Ideally, use a long-acting oral preparation that can be given PO bid. *Remember:* multiple medications will interact with methylxanthine metabolism.

Adjunctive Therapy

Anticholinergic Agents		
Ipratropium bromide	2–3 puffs via MDI. Repeat q 1–2 hr for 2 doses, then taper to 2 puffs q 6 hr as clinical condition allows	This agent has a slower onset of action and is less potent than the beta agonists.
Antibiotics		
Amoxicillin *or*	250–500 mg PO q 6 hr	Use antibiotics as necessary to treat purulent bronchitis, pneumonia, and/or sinusitis. Exact agent chosen will depend on patient's clinical setting, suspected organism, and drug allergy history. If the patient is on theophylline, keep drug interactions in mind: erythromycin and quinolone antibiotics will raise serum theophylline levels.
Trimethoprim/sulfamethoxazole *or*	1 double strength tablet (160 mg trimethoprim/800 mg sulfamethoxazole) q 12 hr	
Amoxicillin and clavulanate (Augmentin) *or*	250–500 mg PO q 6 hr	
Erythromycin *or*	250–500 mg PO q 6 hr	
Tetracycline *or*	250–500 mg PO q 6 hr	
Cefuroxime (Ceftin)	250 mg PO q 12 hr	
Magnesium Sulfate	1.2–2.0 g IV over 20 min	*Consider* in the life-threatening asthma attack unresponsive to earlier therapy. *Do not* administer to the patient with renal dysfunction.

Postintubation/Mechanical Ventilation Therapy

Sedation (Benzodiazepines)		Use as necessary to maintain patient's comfort. *Avoid* opioids, as these can result in histamine release (fentanyl does not cause histamine release).
Midazolam (Versed) *or*	1–2.5 mg IV, subsequent doses 0.5–1.0 mg IV q 2–4 min as patient's condition dictates	
Diazepam (Valium) *or*	2–5 mg IV, repeat q 10–20 min as condition dictates	
Lorazepam (Ativan)	1–2 mg IV, repeat q 10–20 min as condition dictates	

Table continued on following page

305

Table 14–3. EMERGENCY MEDICAL THERAPY OF THE PATIENT WITH AN ASTHMA EXACERBATION *Continued*

DRUG	DOSE	COMMENTS
Muscle Paralysis Pancuronium (Pavulon)	0.1 mg/kg IV load; subsequent doses of 0.025 mg/kg as needed to maintain paralysis	Muscle paralysis will minimize patient's carbon dioxide production and will eliminate the patient's tendency to "fight" the ventilator. Sedate the patient *first* with benzodiazepines. *Avoid* succinylcholine and tubocurarine because they may result in histamine release.
Ketamine	2–4.5 mg/kg IV given at the rate of 0.5 mg/kg/min. If necessary a continuous infusion can then be given at the rate of 1 mg/kg/hr.	Produces a "dissociative" state in the patient, and is a powerful bronchodilator. Use in combination with benzodiazepines to minimize emergence reactions.
General Inhalational Anesthesia	Dose and administration to be determined by the anesthesia consultant.	All inhalational anesthetic agents are potent bronchodilators. Avoid halothane because of its cardiac effects.

3 mL via aerosol every 20 minutes for three to six doses, then decrease frequency of administration to every 4–6 hours as patient's condition allows; *or*

b. Terbutaline (nebulized, 1-mg/mL solution): deliver 0.5 mL in 2.5 mL normal saline (NS) aerosol every 20 minutes for three doses, then decrease frequency as condition allows to every 4–6 hours; *or*

c. Metaproterenol (nebulized, 0.4% solution): deliver 2.5 mL aerosol every 15–20 minutes for three doses, then decrease frequency as condition allows to every 4 hours.

3. **Corticosteroids.** These agents decrease airway inflammation. Parenteral corticosteroids are the anti-inflammatory medications of choice in the ED management of the asthma exacerbation.

   a. *Parenteral corticosteroids should be started immediately* in the following circumstances: the moderate to severe attack not rapidly responsive to beta-agonist therapy; the asthmatic patient who is a revisit to the ED within 7 days of a prior attack; the patient who is currently on corticosteroids (either oral [PO] or inhaled); or the patient who was recently tapered off corticosteroids.

   b. *Medication choices include*

      i. Methylprednisolone (Solu-medrol) 2mg/kg (about 125 mg for the average patient) IV rapid infusion. May repeat every 6 hours. *Or*

      ii. Hydrocortisone sodium succinate 5–7 mg/kg IV infusion. May repeat every 4–6 hours. *Or*

      iii. Dexamethasone 0.25 mg/kg IV infusion. May repeat every 8–12 hours.

  c. The patient who will be discharged home after responding to beta agonists and parenteral corticosteroids should be prescribed a 1–2-week tapering regimen of PO prednisone (beginning with 40–60 mg PO q AM). The patient should not resume use of inhaled corticosteroids until the PO prednisone dose is reduced to approximately 20 mg/day.

  d. Patients who respond quickly to nebulized beta agonists may not require corticosteroids.

B. Second-Line Therapy: Subcutaneous Beta Agonists

1. Subcutaneous (SQ) administration of beta agonists may benefit a subset of patients who are not getting immediate benefit from the inhaled medication because of significant airway obstruction, mucus plugging, and/or inflammation.

2. *Consider* subcutaneous beta-agonist therapy in the patient with a life-threatening exacerbation or the patient not responding to first-line-therapy above.

3. *Medication choices include*
  a. Epinephrine 0.3–0.5 mg (1:1000 aqueous solution) SQ every 20 minutes up to three doses; *or*
  b. Terbutaline 0.25 mg SQ, not to exceed 0.5 mg SQ every 4 hours.

4. *Cautions:* subcutaneous use will increase systemic side effects (e.g., tremor, tachycardia) and should not be used in the pregnant patient or the patient with active cardiac disease.

C. Third-Line Therapy: Methylxanthines

1. Methylxanthines have a real role in the *chronic* management of the asthma patient. Their role in the management of the *acute* asthma exacerbation, however, remains uncertain. Many ED based studies have failed to demonstrate significant benefit from their use and have shown a definite increase in side effects.

2. *Consider* using methyxanthines in the following circumstances:
  a. Patient is already taking a methylxanthine at time of presentation to the ED.
  b. Patient is suffering from a life-threatening asthma exacerbation not responsive to the first- and second-line therapies outlined above.

3. *Medication choices include*
  a. Aminophylline (for parenteral administration): loading dose: 5–6 mg/kg IV (1 mg/kg will raise blood level by 2 µg/mL). Infuse IV load over 20 minutes. Blood level should subsequently be checked 1–2 hours after beginning maintenance infusion:

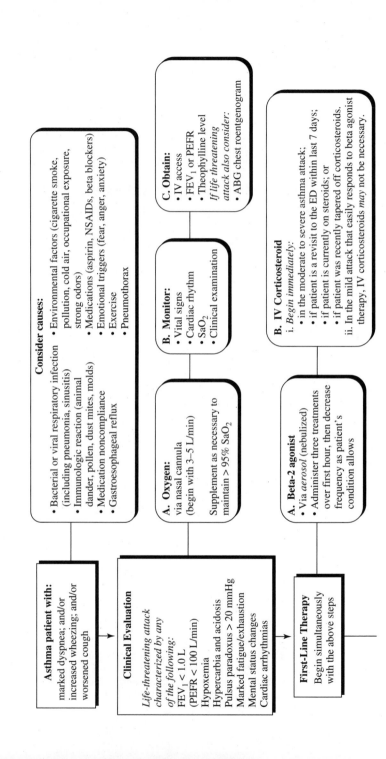

Asthma patient with: marked dyspnea; and/or increased wheezing; and/or worsened cough

Clinical Evaluation

Life-threatening attack characterized by any of the following:
FEV_1 < 1.0 L
(PEFR < 100 L/min)
Hypoxemia
Hypercarbia and acidosis
Pulsus paradoxus > 20 mmHg
Marked fatigue/exhaustion
Mental status changes
Cardiac arrhythmias

First-Line Therapy
Begin simultaneously with the above steps

Consider causes:
- Bacterial or viral respiratory infection (including pneumonia, sinusitis)
- Immunologic reaction (animal dander, pollen, dust mites, molds)
- Medication noncompliance
- Gastroesophageal reflux
- Environmental factors (cigarette smoke, pollution, cold air, occupational exposure, strong odors)
- Medications (aspirin, NSAIDs, beta blockers)
- Emotional triggers (fear, anger, anxiety)
- Exercise
- Pneumothorax

A. Oxygen:
via nasal cannula (begin with 3–5 L/min)

Supplement as necessary to maintain > 95% SaO_2

B. Monitor:
- Vital signs
- Cardiac rhythm
- SaO_2
- Clinical examination

C. Obtain:
- IV access
- FEV_1 or PEFR
- Theophylline level

If life threatening attack also consider:
- ABG chest roentgenogram

A. Beta-2 agonist
- Via *aerosol* (nebulized)
- Administer three treatments over first hour, then decrease frequency as patient's condition allows

B. IV Corticosteroid
i. *Begin immediately:*
- in the moderate to severe asthma attack;
- if patient is a revisit to the ED within last 7 days;
- if patient is currently on steroids; or
- if patient was recently tapered off corticosteroids.

ii. In the mild attack that easily responds to beta agonist therapy, IV corticosteroids *may* not be necessary.

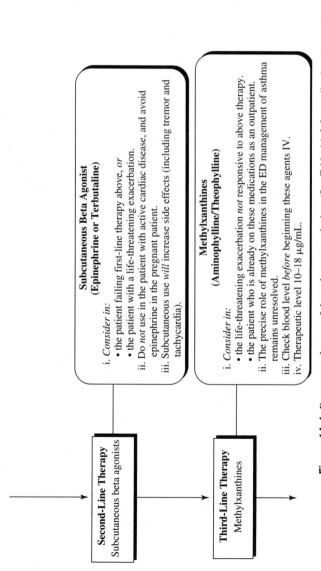

Second-Line Therapy
Subcutaneous beta agonists

Subcutaneous Beta Agonist
(Epinephrine or Terbutaline)

i. *Consider in:*
  • the patient failing first-line therapy above, *or*
  • the patient with a life-threatening exacerbation.
ii. Do *not* use in the patient with active cardiac disease, and avoid epinephrine in the pregnant patient.
iii. Subcutaneous use *will* increase side effects (including tremor and tachycardia).

Third-Line Therapy
Methylxanthines

Methylxanthines
(Aminophylline/Theophylline)

i. *Consider in:*
  • the life-threatening exacerbation *not* responsive to above therapy.
  • the patient who is already on these medications as an outpatient.
ii. The precise role of methylxanthines in the ED management of asthma remains unresolved.
iii. Check blood level *before* beginning these agents IV.
iv. Therapeutic level 10–18 μg/mL.

Figure 14–1. Emergency therapy of the asthma exacerbation. (See Table 14–3 for medication dosages.)

Illustration continued on following page

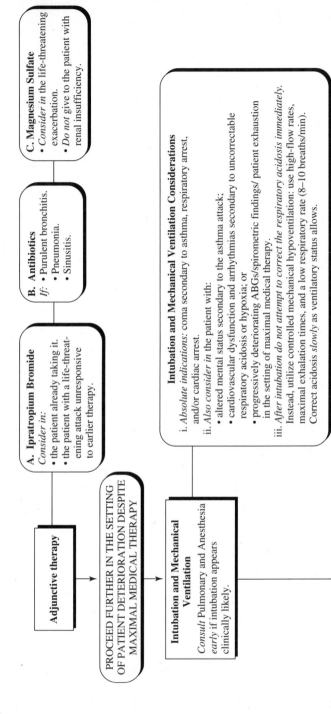

C. Magnesium Sulfate
- *Consider* in the life-threatening exacerbation.
- *Do not* give to the patient with renal insufficiency.

B. Antibiotics
If:
- Purulent bronchitis.
- Pneumonia.
- Sinusitis.

A. Ipratropium Bromide
Consider in:
- the patient already taking it.
- the patient with a life-threatening attack unresponsive to earlier therapy.

Adjunctive therapy

PROCEED FURTHER IN THE SETTING OF PATIENT DETERIORATION DESPITE MAXIMAL MEDICAL THERAPY

Intubation and Mechanical Ventilation
Consult Pulmonary and Anesthesia *early* if intubation appears clinically likely.

Intubation and Mechanical Ventilation Considerations
i. *Absolute indications*: coma secondary to asthma, respiratory arrest, and/or cardiac arrest.
ii. *Also consider* in the patient with:
   - altered mental status secondary to the asthma attack;
   - cardiovascular dysfunction and arrhythmias secondary to uncorrectable respiratory acidosis or hypoxia; or
   - progressively deteriorating ABGs/spirometric findings/ patient exhaustion in the setting of maximal medical therapy.
iii. *After intubation do not attempt to correct the respiratory acidosis immediately.* Instead, utilize controlled mechanical hypoventilation: use high-flow rates, maximal exhalation times, and a low respiratory rate (8–10 breaths/min). Correct acidosis *slowly* as ventilatory status allows.

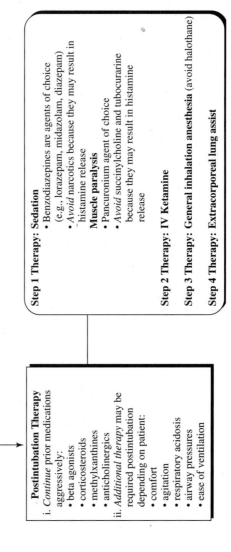

Postintubation Therapy

i. *Continue* prior medications aggressively:
- beta agonists
- corticosteroids
- methylxanthines
- anticholinergics

ii. *Additional therapy* may be required postintubation depending on patient:
- comfort
- agitation
- respiratory acidosis
- airway pressures
- ease of ventilation

Step 1 Therapy: Sedation
- Benzodiazepines are agents of choice (e.g., lorazepam, midazolam, diazepam)
- *Avoid* narcotics because they may result in histamine release

Muscle paralysis
- Pancuronium agent of choice
- *Avoid* succinylcholine and tubocurarine because they may result in histamine release

Step 2 Therapy: IV Ketamine

Step 3 Therapy: General inhalation anesthesia (avoid halothane)

Step 4 Therapy: Extracorporeal lung assist

Figure 14–1. *Continued*

311

MAINTENANCE INFUSION	(mg/kg/hr)
Nonsmokers	0.5–0.7
Smokers	0.9
Cimetidine use	0.3–0.4
Cor pulmonale	0.25–0.30
Hepatic insufficiency	0.20–0.25

(Above dosing regimen adapted from Mengert T, Albert RK, Pulmonary Conditions, Chap. 7. In Ramsey PG, Larsen EB (eds). Medical Therapeutics, Philadelphia: WB Saunders, 1993.)

b. Theophylline (for PO administration): if presenting with a therapeutic theophylline level, the patient may be maintained on his/her usual oral dose if PO intake is possible.

Dose: Average daily oral doses for theophylline in a 70-kg patient are outlined below. Generally a sustained-release preparation is used twice daily.

EVENTUAL PO DOSE	(70-kg patient, mg/day)
Nonsmokers	800 mg/day
Smokers	1100 mg/day
Cimetidine use	500 mg/day
Cor pulmonale	400 mg/day
Hepatic insufficiency	350 mg/day

(Above dosing regimen adapted from Mengert T, Albert RK, Pulmonary Conditions, Chap. 7. In Ramsey PG, Larsen EB (eds). Medical Therapeutics, Philadelphia: WB Saunders, 1993.)

4. *Cautions:*
   a. Therapeutic theophylline serum level is 10–18 µg/mL. Use these medications carefully to avoid potent toxicity.
   b. Do not give aminophylline/theophylline to a patient already on these medications without first checking the serum level.
   c. Multiple drugs may interfere with the metabolism of methylxanthines and dangerously change drug levels. Some agents known to raise levels and increase the risk of toxicity include cimetidine, oral contraceptives, erythromycin, norfloxacin, ciprofloxacin, and allopurinol.

D. Adjunctive Therapy

1. **Ipratropium Bromide.** This anticholinergic bronchodilating medication is neither as potent nor as rapid acting as the beta agonists. Still, some patients will benefit from its use. Consider using it in the patient already taking ipratropium bromide as an outpatient, and in the treatment of the life-threatening exacerbation not responsive to earlier therapy. The best route

currently for its administration in the ED is via a metered dose inhaler (MDI) with a spacer.

Dose. Three puffs delivered *after* a nebulized beta agonist. Repeat every hour twice, then taper off to two puffs every 4–6 hours.

2. **Antibiotics.** These are appropriate if the diagnosis of a bacterial infection (e.g., sinusitis, purulent bronchitis, or pneumonia) is made during the patient's ED evaluation.

3. **Magnesium Sulfate.** Parenteral magnesium sulfate inhibits smooth-muscle contraction and assists bronchodilation in asthma. Its duration of action is short, however, and its optimal use and dosing are not yet clear. Consider using it in the life-threatening exacerbation not responsive to earlier therapy.

Dose. 2.0 g IV over 20 minutes.

Cautions: do not administer magnesium to the patient with renal insufficiency.

E. Intubation and Mechanical Ventilation

In a *minority* of patients who present to the ED with a severe asthma exacerbation, impending respiratory failure will necessitate intubation and mechanical ventilation despite the appropriate use of maximal medical therapy.

1. *Absolute indications* include coma secondary to asthma, respiratory arrest, or cardiac arrest.
2. Intubation/mechanical ventilation should also be *considered* in the patient with
   a. Altered mental status secondary to severe asthma,
   b. Cardiovascular dysfunction/arrhythmias secondary to uncorrectable hypoxia/acidosis,
   c. Progressively deteriorating ABGs, spirometry, or clinical examination despite maximal medical therapy,
   d. Profound patient fatigue/exhaustion.
3. *Cautions:*
   a. After intubation immediately confirm proper endotracheal tube placement by listening to breath sounds in both axillae. Also listen over the epigastrium for sounds that suggest inappropriate esophageal placement.
   b. Intubation may result in laryngospasm, apnea, worsened bronchospasm, and cardiac arrhythmias.
   c. Obtain a postintubation chest roentgenogram to further confirm proper endotracheal tube positioning.
   d. Respiratory acidosis in the mechanically ventilated asthma patient should be corrected gradually. Begin with high flow rates, maximal exhalation times, and low respiratory rates (8–10 breaths/min); make further ventilator adjustments as the patient's condition allows. Maintain peak airway pressure $\leq$ 50 cm H_2O (this may require small tidal volumes initially).

4. *Postintubation therapy:*
   a. Continue prior medications aggressively: beta agonists, corticosteroids, methylxanthines, and anticholinergics.
   b. Additional therapy that may be of benefit in the intubated asthmatic patient to assist with patient comfort, agitation, respiratory acidosis, airway pressures, and ease of ventilation include (see Table 14–3 for dosing of these agents):
      i. *Sedation:* Benzodiazepines are the agents of choice for this purpose (e.g., lorazepam, diazepam, or midazolam). Fentanyl is a potent, short-acting opioid that does not cause histamine release; it may also be of benefit in this setting.
      ii. *Muscle paralysis:* pancuronium is the agent of choice.
      iii. *Intravenous ketamine:* a dissociative agent that is also a powerful bronchodilator.
      iv. *General Inhalational Anesthesia:* Most inhalational anesthetics are potent bronchodilators. Avoid halothane, however, because of its cardiac effects.
      v. *Extracorporeal lung assist* may ultimately be necessary when all of the above fail.

V. DISPOSITION

A. Discharge

1. Consider discharging an asthmatic patient home if *all* of the following three conditions apply:
   a. The asthma attack has responded to ED therapy within 4 hours of ED arrival as evidenced by a markedly improved clinical examination *and* an FEV_1 (or PEFR) > 60% predicted;
   b. Patient has *no* worrisome condition(s) responsible for the exacerbation; and
   c. Vital signs are normal.
2. If discharged, the patient should have the following medications prescribed (depending on exact clinical circumstance and response to ED therapy):
   a. Beta-agonist MDI (including instructions on its use; strongly consider sending the patient home with a spacer to assist in the MDI's use).
   b. Consider prednisone.
   c. Consider theophylline.
   d. Consider an ipratropium bromide MDI.
   e. Consider antibiotics.
3. Ensure follow-up in several days with the patient's private physician. The patient with moderate to severe asthma who cannot be seen by the private physician in several days should return to the ED for a follow-up clinical examination and bedside spirometry. If prednisone was

prescribed, avoid tapering it until the follow-up visit documents excellent control of the patient's asthma.

4. In asthma cases hovering between discharge and admission it is better to err on the side of admission. Poor social situation and patient reliability are relevant considerations.

B. Admit

1. Asthma patients who do not respond to ED therapy within 4 hours of presentation, as outlined above, should be hospitalized.

2. Whether to admit the patient to the general medicine ward, telemetry, or the ICU is an individual decision dependent on patient's clinical status, spirometry, ABGs (if obtained), precipitating illness, and comorbid conditions.

VI. PEARLS AND PITFALLS

A. Administer oxygen as necessary to maintain SaO_2 at 95%.

B. Aggressively use nebulized beta agonists over the first hour of the ED stay, then decrease frequency of administration as patient's condition allows.

C. Administer parenteral corticosteroids immediately in the setting of a life-threatening exacerbation.

D. Use bedside spirometry to assess the patient's condition and response to therapy.

E. Search for precipitants of the asthma attack and include their treatment in the patient's management.

F. Provide early follow-up for patients discharged.

G. Obtain early consultation in the asthma patient who is not responding to aggressive and appropriate ED treatment.

H. Review with the patient the correct use of an MDI. Use a spacer regularly.

Do not do any of the following:

A. Administer aminophylline/theophylline to the patient taking these medications without first obtaining a blood level.

B. Administer cromolyn or inhaled corticosteroids to the acute asthmatic in the ED.

C. Fail to take social situation or patient reliability into account when making discharge plans.

D. Obtain ABG in every asthma patient.

E. Obtain a chest roentgenogram on every asthma patient.

BIBLIOGRAPHY

Expert Panel on the Management of Asthma. Executive Summary: Guidelines for the Diagnosis and Management of Asthma. U.S. Department of Health and Human Services. Publication No. 91-3042A, 1991.

Green SM, Rothrock SG: Intravenous magnesium for acute asthma: Failure to decrease emergency treatment duration or need for hospitalization. Ann Emerg Med 1992; 21:260–265.

McFadden, ER Jr., Gilbert IA: Asthma. N Engl J Med 1992; 327:1928-1937.

Mengert T, Albert RK: Pulmonary Conditions. Chapter 7. In Ramsey PG, Larsen EB (eds): Medical Therapeutics. 2nd Ed. Philadelphia, WB Saunders, 1993, pp. 238–293.

Wiener C: Ventilatory management of respiratory failure in asthma. JAMA 1993; 269(16):2128–2131.

CHRONIC OBSTRUCTIVE PULMONARY DISEASE

"Each person is born to one possession which outvalues all his others—his last breath."

MARK TWAIN

I. ESSENTIAL FACTS

A. Definition

Chronic obstructive pulmonary disease (COPD) is a nonspecific term that refers to patients with chronic cough, expectoration, variable degrees of exertional dyspnea, and obstructive changes on pulmonary function testing (e.g., reduced FEV_1 [forced expiratory volume in 1 second] and decreased FEV_1/FVC [forced vital capacity] ratio). Unlike asthma, the obstructive changes on pulmonary function testing do *not* normalize with bronchodilator therapy.

The two more specific disorders *chronic bronchitis* and *emphysema* are included under the label COPD.

1. *Chronic bronchitis* is defined clinically; it is present when a patient has a chronic or recurrent productive cough on most days for at least 3 months per year for at least 2 successive years.

2. *Emphysema* is defined pathologically; it is a condition in which there are destructive changes in the alveolar walls, with air space enlargement distal to the nonrespiratory bronchioles.

Both disorders are usually present in the same patient to various degrees and both result in air-flow obstruction, exertional dyspnea, and bronchospasm.

B. Epidemiology

1. Chronic obstructive pulmonary disease is the fifth leading cause of death in the United States (in 1981, 60,000 persons

died from COPD), and over the last 20 years the death rate has increased by 22%. It affects at least 32 million Americans.

2. *Risk factors* include
   a. Cigarette smoking.
   b. Family history.
   c. Recurrent pulmonary infections.
   d. Environmental pollution.
   e. Industrial or occupational exposures.
   f. Alpha-1 antitrypsin deficiency.
   g. Cystic fibrosis.

C. Causes of Exacerbations

1. *Common causes* include upper-respiratory tract infections, noncompliance with medications, underuse of medications, drug exposure (e.g., beta blockers), environmental exposure (e.g., smoke, dust, fumes, pollen, animal danders), and weather changes.

2. *Always be alert for* other causes of acute decompensation: acute congestive heart failure (CHF), pneumonia, spontaneous pneumothorax, pulmonary embolism, metabolic acidosis, anemia, renal dysfunction.

3. *Additional causes* include aspiration, cardiac arrhythmia, electrolyte disturbances (e.g., hypophosphatemia), pleural effusion, chest-wall injury, sedation, surgery, and other systemic illness.

II. CLINICAL EVALUATION

A. History

Patients frequently present to the ED with a "known" diagnosis of COPD because it is a *chronic* disease. Determine the following: patient's prior severity of exacerbations (e.g., need for intubation), compliance with medications, exposure to inhaled irritants or noxious agents (including cigarette smoke and occupational exposures), likely cause of current exacerbation, and home/social situation.

B. Symptoms

Common symptoms include increased wheezing, worsened dyspnea (both with exertion and at rest), increased cough, changed sputum production (increased amount, changed color, changed consistency), worsened chest tightness, and/or new or increased right-sided heart failure (edema, right-upper-quadrant tenderness).

C. Signs

Common signs include tachypnea, tachycardia, accessory muscle use, wheezing, rhonchi, distant breath sounds, poor air flow, rales, jugular venous distention, edema, right-sided gallop, and sometimes cyanosis.

D. "Classic" Entities

1. **"Pink Puffers."** Patients with predominantly emphysema. These patients work hard to maintain oxygenation; are dyspneic, tachycardic, and barrel-chested; use pursed-lip breathing; have a prolonged expiratory phase; and have distant breath sounds.

2. **"Blue Bloaters."** Patients with predominantly chronic bronchitis. These patients tolerate a reduced oxygen level, retain carbon dioxide, and usually do not hyperventilate; are overweight and cyanotic; are in right-sided heart failure; and are found to have a variable assortment of rales, rhonchi, and wheezes upon lung examination.

E. Physical Examination

The directed physical examination should include the following:

1. **Skin.** Diaphoresis indicates a patient in moderate to severe distress.

2. **Accessory Muscle Use.** Also present in a patient in moderate to severe respiratory distress.

3. **Jugular Venous Distention (JVD).** Present in the setting of right-sided CHF or generalized fluid overload.

4. **Chest.** Look for stridor, wheezes, rales, rhonchi, and overall air movement. A severe exacerbation may be accompanied by a very quiet chest with few wheezes because of severe air-flow limitation.

5. **Heart.** Note bradycardia, tachycardia, murmurs, rubs, and/or gallops.

6. **Abdomen.** The presence of ascites, hepatomegaly, and/or the hepatojugular reflex indicates fluid overload or right-sided CHF.

7. **Extremities.** Note clubbing, cyanosis, and/or edema.

8. **Mental Status.** Lethargy may indicate either severe hypoxia or worsening CO_2 retention.

The COPD patient requires continual reassessment over time.

F. Monitoring

Routinely monitor the following in the patient with a COPD exacerbation:

1. Vital signs.
2. Cardiac rhythm.

3. Oxygen saturation: maintain a hemoglobin saturation (SaO_2) of 90%.

4. Arterial blood gas levels (ABGs): though not routine in the asthmatic patient, an ABG is important in the COPD patient to assess degree of respiratory failure (by evaluating PO_2, PCO_2, and pH). Comparing the current ABG with prior results in the patient's chart is very helpful.

5. Bedside spirometry: FEV_1 (forced expiratory volume in 1 second) or PEFR (peaked expiratory flow rate) from bedside spirometry may be difficult to interpret and by definition will *not* normalize in the COPD patient. Compare bedside spirometry with the patient's baseline spirometry if available in the patient's chart.

G. Laboratory Studies

1. *Routinely* obtain the following:
   a. Complete blood count (CBC).
   b. Electrolyte panel.
   c. Glucose level.
   d. Electrocardiogram.
   e. Chest roentgenogram.
   f. Arterial blood gas levels.
   g. Blood urea nitrogen, creatinine levels.
   h. Theophylline level (if patient is on same).

2. *Additional studies* may be necessary, depending on clinical circumstances (e.g., sputum Gram stain and culture in the setting of pneumonia).

III. DIFFERENTIAL DIAGNOSIS

The differential diagnosis includes asthma, pulmonary edema, pulmonary embolism, anaphylaxis, pneumonia, airway injury, aspiration, epiglottitis, pneumothorax, anemia, electrolyte disturbance, chest-wall injury, and drug exposure/overdose.

IV. THERAPY

See Figure 14–2 and Table 14–4.

A. First-Line Therapy

1. **Oxygen.** Oxygen should be administered to the patient with a COPD exacerbation. The goal is to maintain an SaO_2 of 90%. The administration of *excessive oxygen* may result in worsened carbon dioxide retention in some COPD patients, but this risk has been overstated in the past. Use oxygen carefully to maintain the appropriate SaO_2. In the tachypneic, cyanotic patient in acute respiratory failure aggressive oxygen use is appropriate.

Dose. Generally begin with oxygen 1–1.5 L/min via nasal cannula and adjust as necessary to maintain 90% SaO_2.

2. **Beta Agonists.** Their routine use is mandatory. Administer one of the following agents aggressively over the first 1 hour of the patient's ED stay, then gradually decrease the frequency of administration as the patient's clinical condition allows.
   a. Albuterol (nebulized, 0.83 mg/mL; 3-mL ampule): deliver 3 mL via aerosol every 20 minutes for three to six doses, then decrease frequency of administration to every 4–6 hours as patient's condition allows; *or*
   b. Terbutaline (nebulized, 1 mg/mL solution): deliver 0.5 mL in 2.5 mL normal saline (NS) aerosol every 20 minutes for three doses, then decrease frequency to every 4–6 hours as condition allows; *or*
   c. Metaproterenol (nebulized, 0.4% solution): deliver 2.5 mL aerosol every 15–20 minutes for three doses, then decrease frequency to every 4 hours as condition allows.

3. **Subcutaneous (SQ) Terbutaline.** Should be considered in the life-threatening situation, in addition to one of the nebulized treatments above, if the patient does *not* have active cardiac disease *and* if the patient is not responding rapidly enough to aerosol therapy.

   Dose. 0.25 mg SQ, not to exceed 0.5 mg SQ every 4 hours.

4. **Anticholinergic Agents.** There is growing evidence that, in the ED treatment of a COPD exacerbation, these agents supplement the effects of the beta agonists above. Ipratropium bromide is the preferred drug because of its lack of significant side effects. The best route currently for its administration in the ED is via a metered-dose inhaler (MDI) with a spacer.
   a. Ipratropium bromide (MDI): deliver three puffs immediately after first treatment with a nebulized beta agonist. Repeat every hour twice, then taper off to every 6 hours; *or*
   b. Atropine (nebulized): deliver 0.025 mg/kg nebulized solution every 6 hours (side effects with atropine *may be significant* and include drying of secretions, urinary retention, and mental status changes).

B. Second-Line Therapy: Corticosteroids

1. Corticosteroids are *not* as effective in COPD as they are in asthma. They should be used, however, in the following circumstances:
   a. The patient not immediately responsive to the first-line agents described above.
   b. The patient who is currently on corticosteroids, and now presents with an acute exacerbation.
   c. The patient who has just recently been tapered off corticosteroids.
   d. The patient in a life-threatening COPD exacerbation.

2. **Methylprednisolone.** The drug of choice
   Dose. The best dose to use is unclear, but a reasonable approach is to give a 1–2 mg/kg (125 mg for the average patient) intravenous (IV) bolus followed by 0.5 mg/kg IV every 6 hours.
3. The patient who will be discharged home after responding to the above therapy in the ED should be prescribed a 1–2-week (or slower) tapering regimen of oral prednisone (beginning with 60 mg PO every morning).

C. Third-Line Therapy: Methylxanthines

1. Methylxanthines have a real role in the *chronic* management of the COPD patient. Their use in the ED, however, managing the *acute* COPD exacerbation is uncertain at best. Many ED-based studies have failed to demonstrate significant benefit from their use, and a definite increase in side effects.

2. *Consider* them in the following circumstances:
   a. A patient who arrives already on a methylxanthine should be maintained on same. Use blood levels to guide dosing and administration.
   b. Consider beginning methylxanthines in the life-threatening COPD exacerbation unresponsive to maximal use of first- and second-line therapy described above.

3. *Medication choices include:*

   a. **Aminophylline** (for parenteral administration)
      Dose. Loading dose: 5–6 mg/kg IV (1 mg/kg will raise blood level by 2 µg/mL). Infuse IV load over 20 minutes. The blood level should subsequently be checked 1–2 hours after beginning maintenance infusion:

Maintenance Infusion	(mg/kg/hr)
Nonsmokers	0.5–0.7
Smokers	0.9
Cimetidine use	0.3–0.4
Cor pulmonale	0.25–0.30
Hepatic insufficiency	0.20–0.25

   (Above dosing regimen adapted from Mengert T, Albert RK, Pulmonary Conditions, Chap. 7. In Ramsey PG, Larsen EB (eds). Medical Therapeutics, Philadelphia: WB Saunders, 1993.)

   b. **Theophylline** (for PO administration). If the patient presents with a therapeutic theophylline level, he/she may be maintained on his/her usual oral dose if PO intake is possible.
      Dose. Average daily oral doses for theophylline in a 70-kg patient are outlined below. Generally a sustained-release preparation is used bid.

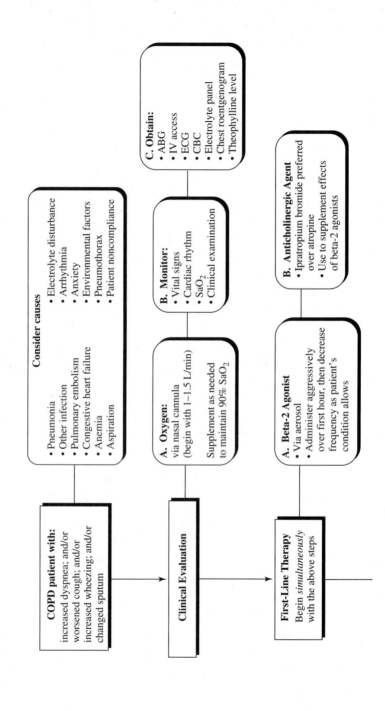

Consider causes

- Pneumonia
- Other infection
- Pulmonary embolism
- Congestive heart failure
- Anemia
- Aspiration
- Electrolyte disturbance
- Arrhythmia
- Anxiety
- Environmental factors
- Pneumothorax
- Patient noncompliance

COPD patient with:
increased dyspnea; and/or worsened cough; and/or increased wheezing; and/or changed sputum

Clinical Evaluation

First-Line Therapy
Begin *simultaneously* with the above steps

C. Obtain:
- ABG
- IV access
- ECG
- CBC
- Electrolyte panel
- Chest roentgenogram
- Theophylline level

B. Monitor:
- Vital signs
- Cardiac rhythm
- SaO_2
- Clinical examination

A. Oxygen:
via nasal cannula
(begin with 1–1.5 L/min)

Supplement as needed to maintain 90% SaO_2

B. Anticholinergic Agent
- Ipratropium bromide preferred over atropine
- Use to supplement effects of beta-2 agonists

A. Beta-2 Agonist
- Via aerosol
- Administer aggressively over first hour, then decrease frequency as patient's condition allows

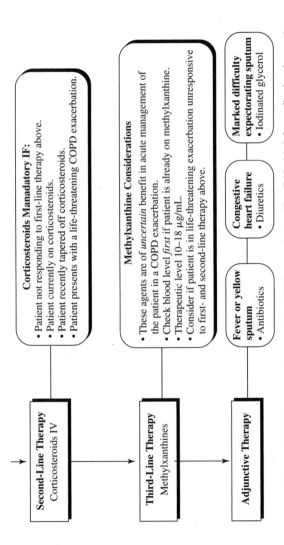

Second-Line Therapy
Corticosteroids IV

Corticosteroids Manadatory IF:
- Patient not responding to first-line therapy above.
- Patient currently on corticosteroids.
- Patient recently tapered off corticosteroids.
- Patient presents with a life-threatening COPD exacerbation.

Third-Line Therapy
Methylxanthines

Methylxanthine Considerations
- These agents are of *uncertain* benefit in acute management of the patient in a COPD exacerbation.
- Check blood level *first* if patient is already on methylxanthine.
- Therapeutic level 10–18 µg/mL.
- Consider if patient is in life-threatening exacerbation unresponsive to first- and second-line therapy above.

Adjunctive Therapy

Fever or yellow sputum
- Antibiotics

Congestive heart failure
- Diuretics

Marked difficulty expectorating sputum
- Iodinated glycerol

Figure 14–2. Emergency therapy of the COPD exacerbation. (See Table 14-4 for medication dosages.)

Table 14–4. EMERGENCY MEDICAL THERAPY OF THE PATIENT WITH A COPD EXACERBATION

DRUG	DOSE	COMMENTS
First-Line Therapy		
Oxygen	Begin with 1–1.5 L/min via nasal cannula	Administer sufficient oxygen to maintain 90% SaO$_2$.
Nebulized Beta Agonists		
Albuterol	0.83 mg/mL; 3 mL nebulized q 20 min for 3 to 6 doses	Administer all of these agents aggressively over the first 60–90 min, then decrease frequency to one nebulized treatment every 2–6 hr. In the elderly patient or the patient with active heart disease more cautious use (decreased dosage and/or frequency) may be necessary.
or		
Terbutaline	1 mg/mL; 0.5 mL in 2.5 mL NS nebulized q 20 min for 3 doses	
or		
Metaproterenol	0.4% solution; 2.5 mL nebulized q 15–20 min for 3 doses	
Anticholinergic Agents		
Ipratropium bromide	3 puffs via metered dose inhaler. Repeat every hour for 2 doses, then taper to 2–3 puffs q 6 hr	Use in combination with the inhaled beta agonists above. Ipratropium bromide is preferred because of its excellent side effect profile. The use of atropine may be accompanied by multiple and significant side effects.
or		
Atropine	0.025 mg/kg in 3 mL NS via nebulized solution every 2 hours for 2 doses, then taper to a treatment q 6 hr	
Parenteral Sympathomimetics		
Terbutaline subcutaneously	0.25 mg SQ, not to exceed 0.5 mg SQ q 4 hr	Consider in addition to the nebulized treatments above if the patient is *not* improving. *Do not* use in the setting of active cardiac disease.
Second-Line Therapy		
Corticosteroids		
Methylprednisolone	125 mg IV infusion	Subsequent doses should be 0.5 mg/kg q 6 hr IV
Third-Line Therapy		
Methylxanthines		
Aminophylline (IV therapy)	IV load is 5–6 mg/kg over 20 min. Follow load by IV infusion: *Adult smoker* 0.9 mg/kg/hr *Adult nonsmoker* 0.7 mg/kg/hr *Severe COPD/ elderly/CHF/or liver disease* 0.2–0.3 mg/kg/hr	The role of methylxanthines in the management of the COPD exacerbation is controversial. *Do not* administer to a patient already on these medications without first checking a blood level. Therapeutic level is between 10 and 18 µg/mL. Ideally, use a long acting oral preparation that can be given PO bid. Remember that multiple medications will interact with the metabolism of methylxanthines.
or		
Theophylline (PO therapy)	Reasonable average PO doses (in a 70 kg patient) *Nonsmoker* 900 mg/day *Smoker* 1100 mg/day *Cimetidine use* 500 mg/day *Cor pulmonale* 400 mg/day *Liver disease* 350 mg/day	

Table 14–4. EMERGENCY MEDICAL THERAPY OF THE PATIENT WITH A COPD EXACERBATION *Continued*

DRUG	DOSE	COMMENTS
Adjunctive Therapy		
Antibiotics		
Amoxicillin *or*	250–500 mg PO q 8 hr	Helpful even in the absence of pneumonia if: patient has increased cough with yellow sputum and worsened dyspnea.
Trimethoprim/sulfamethoxazole (Septra DS) *or*	1 PO q 12 hr	
Doxycycline *or*	200 mg PO × 1, then 100 mg PO q 12 hr	
Amoxicillin and clavulanate (Augmentin) *or*	250–500 mg PO q 6 hr	
Cefuroxime (Ceftin) *or*	250 mg PO q 12 hr	
Azithromycin	500 mg PO on day 1, then 250 mg PO on days 2–5	
Diuretics		
Furosemide	Begin with 0.5–1 mg/kg IV (or patient's usual PO dose IV)	Use as necessary to treat fluid overload/CHF.
Mucolytic Expectorants		
Iodinated glycerol	2 tablets 4×/day, *or* Elixir 1 tsp 4×/day, *or* Solution 20 drops 4×/d	Consider in the outpatient management of the patient with chronic bronchitic symptoms.

EVENTUAL PO DOSE	(70-KG PATIENT)
Nonsmokers	800 mg/day
Smokers	1100 mg/day
Cimetidine use	500 mg/day
Cor pulmonale	400 mg/day
Hepatic insufficiency	350 mg/day

(Above dosing regimen adapted from Mengert T, Albert RK, Pulmonary Conditions, Chap. 7. In Ramsey PG, Larsen EB (eds). Medical Therapeutics, Philadelphia: WB Saunders, 1993.)

4. *Cautions:*
   a. Therapeutic theophylline serum level is 10–18 µg/mL. Use these medications carefully to avoid potent toxicity.
   b. Do not give aminophylline/theophylline to a patient already on these medications without first checking the serum level.
   c. Multiple drugs may interfere with the metabolism of methylxanthines and dangerously change drug levels. Some

326 / PULMONARY EMERGENCIES

agents known to raise levels and increase the risk of toxicity include cimetidine, oral contraceptives, erythromycin, norfloxacin, ciprofloxacin, and allopurinol.

D. Adjunctive Therapy

The following agents should be considered along with the first-, second-, or third-line agents above, depending on clinical circumstances.

1. **Antibiotics.** Though literature studies are conflicting, in the setting of a COPD exacerbation accompanied by increased cough, increased volume of sputum, changed viscosity of sputum, or yellow color of sputum, antibiotics will probably help resolve symptoms even in the absence of an infiltrate on the chest roentgenogram. Any of the following are appropriate for 7–10 days (except for azithromycin, which is given for only 5 days):

   a. Amoxicillin 250–500 mg PO every 8 hours; *or*
   b. Trimethoprim/sulfamethoxazole (Septra DS), 1 PO every 12 hours; *or*
   c. Doxycycline 200 mg PO once, then 100 mg PO every 12 hours; *or*
   d. Amoxicillin/clavulanate (Augmentin) 250–500 mg PO every 8 hours; *or*
   e. Cefuroxime (Ceftin) 250 mg PO every 12 hours; *or*
   f. Azithromycin 500 mg PO once on day 1, then 250 mg once daily on days 2–5 for a total dose of 1.5 g.

2. **Diuretics.** Many patients with COPD have a component of CHF (either left or right sided) complicating their clinical presentation. Consider IV furosemide (begin with the patient's usual PO dose IV or start with 0.5–1 mg/kg IV). If there is no initiation of diuresis within 30 minutes of administration, double the dose and again administer it IV. Watch for potassium depletion.

3. **Mucolytic-Expectorants.** Cough severity, frequency, ease of expectoration, and other common subjective complaints may be improved in the COPD patient over time with iodinated glycerol (Organidin). This medication should be considered in a select group of patients who will be sent home from the ED plagued with chronic bronchitic symptoms.

   Dose: • *Tablets:* 2 tablets four times a day; *or*
   • *Elixir:* 1 tsp four times a day; *or*
   • *Solution:* 20 drops four times a day.
   (An 8-week trial may be necessary for full benefit.)

E. Intubation and Mechanical Ventilation

1. In most circumstances the decision to intubate the COPD patient will be made on the basis of close observation and

continual reassessment over time. Irwin (1991) recommends considering the following six points:

a. Is there worsening carbon dioxide retention in the setting of aggressive therapy?

b. Is the pH becoming acidotic despite aggressive therapy?

c. Can an acceptable PaO_2 (i.e., ≥ 55 mmHg with 90% SaO_2) be maintained with low-flow oxygen?

d. How is the patient's overall clinical status changing with maximal medical therapy?

e. Is the patient exhausted?

f. Is there evidence of significant central nervous system (CNS) and/or cardiovascular dysfunction?

2. According to Irwin, a COPD patient *with all four* of the following is a candidate for intubation and mechanical ventilation:

a. Acute respiratory acidosis.

b. Low arterial pH.

c. Inadequate PO_2, *and*

d. CNS and cardiovascular dysfunction.

3. In intermediate situations (with less than all four of the above present), ensure maximization of the outlined medical therapy above and *consult a pulmonary specialist* for further assistance.

V. DISPOSITION

A. Discharge

1. Consider discharging a patient home if all *five* of the following circumstances are present:

a. Exacerbation has rapidly responded to therapy in the ED;

b. Patient has *no* worrisome conditions responsible for the exacerbation (e.g., *no* pneumonia, *no* CHF, *no* pneumothorax, *no* pulmonary embolism);

c. Vital signs and respiratory status are at patient's baseline;

d. The patient has an adequate home situation; *and*

e. The patient is reliable.

2. If discharged, the patient should have the following medications prescribed (depending on exact clinical circumstance and response over the course of his/her ED stay):

a. Albuterol MDI *and* ipratropium bromide MDI (including instructions on how to use the MDI; strongly consider sending the patient home with a spacer to assist in the MDI's use).

b. Consider prednisone.

c. Consider theophylline.

d. Consider antibiotics.

e. Consider a diuretic.

f. Consider iodinated glycerol.

3. Ensure follow-up in several days with the patient's primary care physician, urgent care clinic, or return to the ED. We do not recommend tapering the prednisone (if the patient is discharged on same) until the time of the follow-up visit.

B. Admit

Most patients with an acute COPD exacerbation will require hospitalization. Whether to admit the patient to the general medicine ward, telemetry, or the ICU will depend on the patient's clinical status and response to therapy in the ED. The patient with a pH $\leq$ 7.3, altered mental status, significant cardiovascular dysfunction, clinical exhaustion, other significant comorbid conditions, *or* inadequate oxygenation despite appropriate supplementation should be monitored in an ICU setting.

VI. PEARLS AND PITFALLS

A. Administer oxygen as necessary to maintain 90% SaO_2.

B. Aggressively use beta agonists and anticholinergics over the first 1 hour of the ED stay.

C. Provide early follow-up for patients deemed fit enough to be discharged.

D. Obtain early consultation in the COPD patient who is not responding to aggressive and appropriate ED treatment.

E. Consider and diagnose the cause(s) of the exacerbation.

Do not do any of the following:

A. Administer too much oxygen when SaO_2 via pulse oximetry (or ABGs) demonstrates such administration is unnecessary. (Remember: your goal is an SaO_2 of 90%.)

B. Withhold oxygen in the patient in obvious and severe respiratory distress.

C. Withhold steroids in the patient who does not immediately improve with aggressive beta-agonist and anticholinergic therapy.

D. Administer aminophylline/theophylline to the patient on same without first obtaining a blood level.

BIBLIOGRAPHY

Hudson LD, Monti CM: Rationale and use of corticosteroids in chronic obstructive pulmonary disease. Med Clin North Am 1990; 74:661–690.

Irwin RS: Chronic obstructive pulmonary disease. Chapter 44. In Rippe JM, Irwin RS, Alpert JS, Fink MP (eds): Intensive Care Medicine. 2nd Ed. Boston,ed. Little, Brown, 1991. pp. 468-476.

Mengert T, Albert R: Pulmonary conditions. Chapter 7. In Ramsey PG, Larsen EB (eds): Medical Therapeutics. 2nd Ed. Philadelphia, WB Saunders, 1993, pp. 238-293.

Shrestha M, O'Brien T, Haddox R, et al: Decreased duration of emergency department treatment of chronic obstructive pulmonary disease exacerbations with the addition of ipratropium bromide to B-agonist therapy. Ann Emerg Med 1991; Nov.:62–65.

HEMOPTYSIS

> *"This is a mighty wonder: in the discharge from the lungs alone,*
> *which is particularly dangerous, the patients do not despair*
> *of themselves,*
> *even although near the last."*
>
> ARETAEUS OF CAPPADOCIA

I. ESSENTIAL FACTS

A. Definition

Hemoptysis is the expectoration of blood from the respiratory tract *below* the level of the larynx.

1. Hemoptysis may be mild with minimal blood-streaked sputum, or massive and life-threatening. Massive hemoptysis is defined as expectoration of ≥ 100 mL/hr of blood acutely, or ≥ 300–500 mL of blood in a 24-hour period. Lesser amounts of bleeding may also be life-threatening in patients with underlying lung disease and suboptimal physiologic reserve, or in those with an impaired ability to clear their airway.

2. The cause of death in massive hemoptysis is asphyxiation, not exsanguination.

3. True hemoptysis must be distinguished from nasopharyngeal hemorrhage and from hematemesis (vomiting of blood).

B. Etiology

Bronchitis, bronchiectasis, lung carcinoma, and tuberculosis are the most common causes of hemoptysis, accounting for > 65% of cases.

II. CLINICAL EVALUATION

A. History

1. Determine the frequency, duration, and extent of bleeding.

2. Current symptoms may suggest an underlying cause of the patient's hemoptysis:

    a. Upper respiratory tract infection symptoms (e.g., fever, cough, purulent sputum) suggest bronchitis or pneumonia.

    b. Chronic cough, weight loss, and night sweats suggest tuberculosis.

    c. Aspiration with chronic fatigue, fever, malaise, and foul sputum may be present in patients with hemoptysis from a lung abscess.

d. Dyspnea, orthopnea, and paroxysmal nocturnal dyspnea indicate congestive heart failure (CHF). A concomitant valve problem (e.g., mitral stenosis) may be present.

e. Pleuritic chest pain and dyspnea may be associated with pneumonia or pulmonary embolism.

3. Hemoptysis must be distinguished from hematemesis and nasopharyngeal bleeding.

a. Patients with hemoptysis usually give a history of coughing. Expectorated blood is frothy and bright red, and has an alkaline pH.

b. Patients with hematemesis typically complain of concomitant nausea. Vomited blood is often mixed with gastric contents, is dark red or brown, and has an acid pH.

4. Evaluate pertinent current and past medical problems, including prior episodes of hemoptysis, smoking habits, occupational exposures (e.g., asbestos), recent chest trauma; history of bronchiectasis and/or chronic bronchitis; presence of known cardiopulmonary, collagen-vascular, or other diseases; history of cancer; history of prior tuberculosis; and risk factors for deep venous thrombosis and pulmonary thromboembolism (e.g., prior thromboembolic episode, lower-extremity trauma, immobility).

5. Review all medications (e.g., anticoagulants).

B. Physical Examination

Caution: massive hemoptysis is a true medical/surgical emergency. A detailed physical examination should only take place after first securing and supporting the patient's airway, breathing, and circulation (see Chapter 1). Physical signs may then give a clue to the underlying cause.

1. **Vital Signs.** Note tachycardia, tachypnea or hypopnea, and fever.

2. **Skin.** Diaphoresis indicates a patient in moderate to severe distress. Search for telangiectasias (may be seen in Osler-Weber-Rendu syndrome or progressive systemic sclerosis) and ecchymoses or petechiae (suggesting thrombocytopenia or coagulopathy). Cyanosis is a late and ominous sign of severe tissue hypoxia.

3. **HEENT.** The nasal pharynx and oral cavity should be closely examined to exclude an upper-airway source of bleeding. Rule out foreign bodies, laryngeal masses, and mucosal telangiectasia. Sinus disease or perforation of the nasal septum may be present in patients with Wegener's granulomatosis.

4. **Neck.** Accessory muscle use during respiration indicates excessive work of breathing. Jugular venous distention may be

present in patients with mitral valve disease and/or CHF. Bronchogenic or laryngeal cancer may cause prominent adenopathy.

5. **Lungs**

   a. Patients with chronic obstructive pulmonary disease (COPD) and chronic bronchitis usually have wheezing, rhonchi, and evidence of hyperinflation.

   b. Localized wheezing suggests an endobronchial lesion or foreign body that is partially obstructing an airway.

   c. Rales may be detected in patients with mitral stenosis, CHF, or pneumonia. Fine, dry rales or crackles are typically heard in patients with interstitial lung disease; moist, coarse rales are more common overlying an area of bronchiectasis.

   d. Consolidation (e.g., pneumonia, atelectasis) is suggested by dullness to percussion and bronchial breath sounds.

   e. A pleural rub may be present in patients with pulmonary infarction or pneumonia.

6. **Heart.** An S_3 gallop indicates left-ventricular dysfunction. The classical cardiac examination findings in mitral stenosis include an accentuated S_1 at the apex, an opening snap, and a diastolic rumble.

7. **Abdomen.** Evaluate for tenderness, masses, and hepatosplenomegaly. An enlarged liver may be seen in biventricular CHF or metastatic cancer. Splenomegaly suggests an underlying malignancy, significant hepatic dysfunction, or a hematologic disorder.

8. **Extremities.** Joint swelling or effusions may be signs of an underlying collagen-vascular disease. Finger clubbing suggests the presence of a chronic pulmonary disease (e.g., cystic fibrosis, bronchiectasis, pulmonary fibrosis, or cancer). Evaluate for findings suggestive of a deep venous thrombosis (palpable venous cord, localized warmth, tenderness, erythema, or swelling).

9. **Nervous System.** Carefully note the patient's mental status. Agitation may be a sign of hypoxia; lethargy may indicate hypercarbia and portend respiratory failure.

C. Monitoring

In the patient with moderate to severe hemoptysis, continuously monitor both oxygen saturation (SaO_2) and cardiac rhythm.

D. Laboratory Studies

1. *Routinely* obtain the following laboratory tests in patients with hemoptysis:

   a. Complete blood count (CBC), including platelets.

   b. Electrolyte panel, glucose, blood urea nitrogen, and creatinine levels.

    c. Prothrombin time (PT)/and partial thromboplastin time (PTT).

    d. Chest roentgenogram.

    e. Electrocardiogram.

    f. Urinalysis.

    g. Sputum (for Gram stain and culture; acid-fast stain and culture).

    h. Tuberculin skin test [PPD] (unless the patient has had a positive PPD documented in the past).

2. Further evaluation should be guided by the severity of the hemoptysis and its likely cause as determined by the history, physical examination, and laboratory results. Additional studies that *may* be appropriate, depending on the clinical situation, include one or more of the following:

    a. *Arterial blood gase* (ABG).

    b. *Type and cross match* for 4–6 units packed red blood cells (in the setting of massive hemoptysis).

    c. *Fiberoptic bronchoscopy* or *rigid bronchoscopy*

    d. *Spirometry* (may indicate air-flow obstruction of the small airways; flow-volume loops may be helpful in diagnosing upper-airway obstruction).

    e. *Ventilation–perfusion nuclear scan, lower-extremity duplex examination,* and/or *pulmonary angiogram* (to evaluate for deep venous thrombosis or pulmonary embolism).

    f. *Pulmonary angiography* (may also be useful in evaluating patients for suspected pulmonary arteriovenous malformations).

    g. *Chest computed tomography scan* (may reveal bronchiectasis, adenopathy, malignancy).

    h. *Echocardiogram* (to evaluate cardiac function and/or valvular dysfunction).

III. DIFFERENTIAL DIAGNOSIS

The differential diagnosis of hemoptysis includes the large number of potential causes outlined below:

A. **Infection.** Tracheobronchitis, bacterial or viral pneumonia, fungal infection (e.g., aspergilloma, coccidioidomycosis), lung abscess, bronchiectasis, tuberculosis, and pulmonary parasitic infections (e.g., paragonimiasis).

B. **Neoplasia.** Bronchogenic, tracheal, or metastatic carcinoma; bronchial adenoma.

C. **Cardiovascular Disease.** Congestive heart failure (CHF), mitral stenosis, pulmonary embolism or infarction, pulmonary arteriovenous malformation, Rasmussen's aneurysm (dilated artery in a tuberculous cavity), Eisenmenger's syndrome (ventricular septal defect with pulmonary hypertension resulting in right-to-left shunting and cyanosis).

D. **Collagen-Vascular Disease.** Pulmonary vasculitis (e.g., Wegener's granulomatosis), autoimmune disorders (e.g., Goodpasture's syndrome), systemic lupus erythematosus, progressive systemic sclerosis, ankylosing spondylitis.

E. **Trauma.** Penetrating lung injury, pulmonary contusion, foreign-body aspiration, rupture of pulmonary artery by pulmonary artery catheterization.

F. **Miscellaneous.** Cystic fibrosis, idiopathic pulmonary hemosiderosis, broncholithiasis, pulmonary sequestration, thrombocytopenia.

IV. TREATMENT

The goals of therapy are to prevent asphyxia, stop the bleeding, and treat the underlying cause of hemoptysis (Fig. 14–3).

A. General Measures

1. Secure and support airway, breathing, and circulation as appropriate (see Chapter 1).
   a. Obtain vital signs; continuously monitor cardiac rhythm and SaO_2.
   b. Administer supplemental oxygen as necessary.
   c. Establish intravenous (IV) access.
2. Initiate laboratory evaluation as outlined in II. D. 1, above.
3. Identify and treat any underlying coagulation disorder.

B. Non–Life-Threatening Hemoptysis

1. In patients with a suspected bronchitis and/or other bacterial pulmonary infection, empiric antibiotic treatment should be given. Possible antibiotic choices include any of the following:
   a. Amoxicillin 250–500 mg PO every 8 hours; *or*
   b. Trimethoprim/sulfamethoxazole (Septra DS) 1 PO every 12 hours; *or*
   c. Doxycyline 200 mg PO at once, then 100 mg PO every 12 hours; *or*
   d. Amoxicillin/clavulanate (Augmentin) 250–500 mg PO every 8 hours; *or*
   e. Cefuroxime (Ceftin) 250 mg PO every 12 hours; *or*
   f. Azithromycin 500 mg PO once on day 1, then 250 mg once daily on days 2–5 for a total dose of 1.5 g.
2. Follow-up in pulmonary clinic and consideration for elective bronchoscopy is mandatory in the patient with hemoptysis and *any* of the following:
   a. Abnormal chest roentgenogram.
   b. Cigarette use.
   c. Suspected foreign-body aspiration.
   d. Age $\geq$ 40 years.
   e. History of hemoptysis $\geq$ 1 week duration.

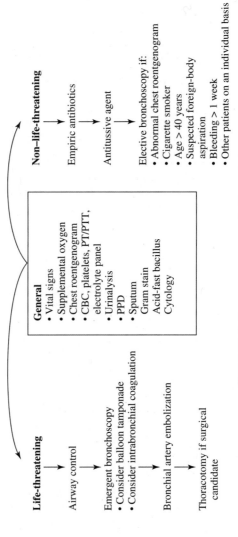

Figure 14–3. Emergency management of hemoptysis.

Life-threatening

Airway control

Emergent bronchoscopy
• Consider balloon tamponade
• Consider intrabronchial coagulation

Bronchial artery embolization

Thoracotomy if surgical
  candidate

General
• Vital signs
• Supplemental oxygen
• Chest roentgenogram
• CBC, platelets, PT/PTT,
  electrolyte panel
• Urinalysis
• PPD
• Sputum
  Gram stain
  Acid-fast bacillus
  Cytology

Non-life-threatening

Empiric antibiotics

Antitussive agent

Elective bronchoscopy if:
• Abnormal chest roentgenogram
• Cigarette smoker
• Age > 40 years
• Suspected foreign-body
  aspiration
  • Bleeding > 1 week
  • Other patients on an individual basis

3. Consider treatment with an antitussive agent (e.g., codeine 30 mg PO every 6 hours).

C. Life-Threatening Hemoptysis

1. Meticulously secure and support airway, breathing, oxygenation, and circulation.
   a. Administer humidified oxygen, establish large-bore IV access, and place the suspected bleeding lung in a dependent position. Administer crystalloid as necessary for pulse and blood pressure support.
   b. Endotracheal intubation and mechanical ventilation are indicated in patients who are unable to adequately maintain a patent airway, or in those with severe hypoxemia or ventilatory failure. Selective intubation of one mainstem bronchus, or placement of a double-lumen endotracheal tube, may be necessary to prevent asphyxiation in cases of massive hemoptysis with a known site of bleeding.

2. Emergently consult pulmonary, anesthesia, and thoracic surgery specialists. Many of the procedures discussed in III. C. 3, below, require special expertise and should only be performed by physicians skilled in their application. While awaiting arrival of the consultant for delivery of definitive care, arrange for ICU admission, continue to monitor the patient closely, and support oxygenation and vital signs as necessary.

3. Definitive care:
   a. Emergent bronchoscopy should be undertaken to localize the source of bleeding and aid in therapeutic intervention. Both rigid bronchoscopy (for airway control, suction capability, and application of balloon catheters or laser therapy) and flexible fiberoptic bronchoscopy (for extended visualization) should be available.
      i. Balloon tamponade can be accomplished by placing a Fogarty catheter into the bleeding subsegment via bronchoscopy.
      ii. Intrabronchial coagulation can be performed using fibrin, thrombin, and/or other coagulative agents applied to the bleeding site via a fiberoptic bronchoscope.
      iii. Endobronchial irradiation or brachytherapy may be helpful in arresting bleeding coming from an endobronchial tumor.
      iv. The YAG laser has also been used to induce coagulation and arrest bleeding in cases of hemoptysis arising from endobronchial lesions associated with bronchogenic carcinoma. Not all patients with endobronchial tumors are candidates for laser therapy, and treatment options must be tailored to meet the needs of individual patients.
   b. Bronchial artery embolization, by an experienced angiographer, has been successfully used to provide emergent hemostasis in patients with life-threatening hemoptysis.

This treatment may control bleeding and obviate the need for thoracotomy in a significant number of cases.

   c. Thoracotomy with surgical resection of the bleeding site is necessary in a small number of patients with life-threatening hemoptysis unresponsive to the other treatment modalities outlined above.

V. DISPOSITION

A. Discharge

Discharge from the ED should be considered if *all* of the following conditions are met:

1. The patient is clinically stable with satisfactory vital signs and laboratory data.
2. Appropriate follow-up care has been arranged.
3. The work-up in the ED is negative for any acute problem that would require immediate hospitalization (e.g., pulmonary thromboembolism, serious pneumonia, or CHF).
4. The episode of hemoptysis was not life-threatening.
5. The patient has been observed in the ED for at least several hours without experiencing further hemoptysis.

B. Admit

1. Patient with *any* of the following should be admitted:
   a. Suspected pulmonary embolism, active tuberculosis (*caution:* establish strict and appropriate respiratory isolation), or other disorders that require inpatient evaluation and management.
   b. Suspected pneumonia, CHF, mitral stenosis, cystic fibrosis, or other conditions that would benefit from inpatient management.
   c. Unreliable patients or patients with a poor social situation in need of bronchoscopy or significant further evaluation.
2. Patients with *any* of the following should be admitted to the ICU:
   a. Clinically unstable.
   b. Experienced massive, life-threatening hemoptysis, or recurrent significant hemoptysis.
   c. In acute respiratory failure or those with the potential for significant respiratory compromise if further hemoptysis occurs.
   d. Unable to adequately protect the airway.
   e. Have severe underlying cardiopulmonary disease.

VI. PEARLS AND PITFALLS

A. Ensure adequate airway, oxygenation, ventilation, and hemodynamic stability for all patients presenting with hemoptysis.

B. Appropriately rule-out oropharyngeal bleeding or hematemesis.

C. Remember the many potential causes of hemoptysis; thoroughly investigate all possible causes.

D. Obtain a chest roentgenogram on all patients with hemoptysis.

E. Give a trial of empiric antibiotics to patients with hemoptysis and suspected pulmonary infection.

Do not do any of the following:

A. Fail to establish respiratory isolation for patients suspected of having active tuberculosis.

B. Discharge patients from the ED unless adequate follow-up (preferably in a pulmonary clinic) has been arranged.

BIBLIOGRAPHY

Goldman JM: Hemoptysis: emergency assessment and management. Emerg Med Clin North Am 1989;7(2):325–338.

O'Neil KM, Lazarus AA: Hemoptysis. Indications for bronchoscopy. Arch Intern Med 1991; 151(1):171–174.

Thompson AB, Teschler H, Rennard SI: Pathogenesis, evaluation, and therapy for massive hemoptysis. Clin Chest Med 1992;13(1):69–82.

Wedzicha JA, Pearson MC: Management of massive hemoptysis. Respir Med 1990;84(1):9–12.

Winter SM, Ingbar DH: Massive hemoptysis: pathogenesis and management. J Intensive Care Med 1988;3:171.

DEEP VENOUS THROMBOSIS AND PULMONARY EMBOLISM

> *"The diagnosis of disease is often easy, often difficult, and often impossible."*
>
> PETER MERE LATHAM

I. ESSENTIAL FACTS

A. Definitions

1. *Deep venous thrombosis* (DVT) is the formation of a thrombus in a deep vein: usually the iliac, femoral, or popliteal veins of the lower extremities.

2. *Pulmonary embolism* (PE) is the obstruction of a portion of the pulmonary vascular bed by a displaced thrombus, air bubble, or other particulate matter. Its most common precipitant is DVT.

3. *Postphlebitic syndrome* may occur in 20–40% of patients after an episode of DVT. Destruction of the venous valves results in chronic pain, swelling, hyperpigmentation, and/or skin ulceration in the involved extremity. The risk of recurrent DVT is

increased, and the syndrome can be particularly disabling when an upper extremity is involved.

B. Important Statistics

1. Acute DVT is one of the most common diseases of the vascular system. Approximately 50% of documented DVTs will subsequently cause pulmonary embolism.
2. More than 600,000 PEs occur in the United States yearly. PE is the primary cause of death in 100,000 patients annually and a contributing cause of death in another 100,000 patients. Pulmonary thromboembolism is second only to hemorrhage as a leading cause of pregnancy-related mortality in the United States.
3. The mortality of undiagnosed and untreated PE is estimated to be 30%; 10% of deaths occur within 60 minutes of the event. Anticoagulation therapy reduces mortality to $\leq 8\%$.
4. Ninety percent of PEs occur in hospitalized patients.

C. Risk Factors

1. General risk factors include blood stasis, endothelial injury, and/or hypercoagulable states (e.g., antithrombin III deficiency, protein C deficiency, protein S deficiency, defective fibrinolysis, or abnormal levels of plasminogen and/or plasminogen activator).
2. Specific *clinical* risk factors are presented in Table 14–5.
3. The absence of risk factors as identified above does *not* rule out the presence of DVT and/or PE: $\geq 10\%$ of patients have *no* identifiable risk factors.

II. CLINICAL EVALUATION

A. History

Important elements of the history include patient's risk factors for thromboembolic disease (see Table 14–5), other significant health problems or medical conditions, and the presence/absence of symptoms of DVT and/or PE (see below).

B. Symptoms and Signs of DVT

1. Discoloration, including erythema.
2. Edema.
3. Extremity pain.
4. Extremity tenderness.
5. Palpable cord.
6. Homan's sign (pain behind the knee on forceful foot dorsiflexion).
7. Subcutaneous venous distention.

Table 14–5. SPECIFIC CLINICAL RISK FACTORS FOR DEEP VENOUS THROMBOSIS AND PULMONARY EMBOLISM

Age > 60 years
Antiphospholipid antibodies
Estrogen-containing oral contraceptive use
Heart disease (especially congestive heart failure)
Inherited hypercoagulable states (see C.1 in text)
Malignancy
Myeloproliferative disease (including polycythemia vera and thrombocytosis)
Nephrotic syndrome
Obesity

Paralysis, prolonged bed rest, and/or other immobilization
Paroxysmal nocturnal hemoglobinuria
Pregnancy
Previous history of thromboembolic disease
Trauma
Ulcerative colitis
Surgery (especially age > 40 years, duration of procedure > 30 min, lower-extremity orthopedic surgery, abdominal or pelvic surgery for malignant disease)

Adapted from McGlynn TJ Jr: In Kammerer WS, Gross RJ (eds): Medical Consultation. 2nd Ed. Baltimore, Williams & Wilkins 1990, pp. 97–106.

Unfortunately, ≥ 50% of DVTs are completely asymptomatic, and ≤ 50% of patients with clinical evidence of DVT are suffering from some other condition.

C. Symptoms and Signs of PE

Signs and symptoms of PE are nonspecific (Table 14–6).

D. Directed Physical Examination

This should include vital signs, skin, HEENT evaluation, neck, chest, heart, abdomen, extremities, and mental status.

E. Monitoring

Continuously monitor oxygen saturation (SaO_2) and cardiac rhythm.

F. Diagnostic Tests for DVT

1. **Contrast Venography.** Considered the "gold standard" for the diagnosis of DVT. Complications include induced thrombosis (≈ 3–4% of patients) and the postvenographic syndrome (leg pain, swelling, and tenderness; ≈ 5-10% of patients). Because it is invasive, requires a contrast injection, and has associated complications, contrast venography is generally used only when absolutely necessary (e.g., DVT is strongly suspected clinically and one or more of the noninvasive studies below is(are) nondiagnostic).

2. **Doppler Ultrasound.** A noninvasive, operator-dependent study. At many institutions, it is the initial diagnostic procedure of choice for the diagnosis of DVT. Proximal venous thrombi are detected with > 90% accuracy. The sensitivity of this test in detecting calf thrombi is only about 50%.

3. **Real-Time Ultrasound.** Also noninvasive and highly operator dependent. In skilled hands, it is accurate in the diagnosis of femoral and popliteal DVT's (mean sensitivity of 96%; mean specificity of 99%). It is also useful in the diagnosis of conditions that can mimic a DVT (e.g., Baker's cyst). Iliac vein DVTs may be missed, and it is inaccurate in the diagnosis of calf DVTs.

4. **Impedance Plethysmography.** The diagnostic procedure of choice at many institutions. Sensitivity and specificity are ≤ 87–95% for proximal vein DVTs. Nonocclusive thrombi may result in a falsely negative test, and it is only 50% sensitive for calf thrombi.

5. **Radioiodinated Fibrinogen.** Not commonly ordered in the ED because it takes 1–2 days to complete, but its diagnostic accuracy is ≤ 92% for DVTs in the thigh, popliteal, and calf area (it is not reliable, however, in detecting DVTs in the pelvic area).

6. **Radionuclide Venography.** Has good sensitivity, poor specificity, and is only marginally useful in detecting calf thrombi.

G. Diagnostic Tests for PE

1. Initial Studies

a. *Chest roentgenography* is useful in diagnosing other conditions that may mimic PE (e.g., pneumonia, congestive heart failure). The diagnosis of pulmonary embolism can never be made on the basis of a chest film alone.

b. Arterial blood gas (ABG) is routinely obtained, but ABG abnormalities have no specificity in the diagnosis of PE. "Normal" ABGs do not completely rule out PE (13% of patients with confirmed PE will have a $PaO_2 \geq 80$ mmHg). To correctly interpret the ABGs, look for the presence

Table 14–6. SYMPTOMS AND SIGNS OF PULMONARY EMBOLISM

SYMPTOMS	SIGNS
Apprehension	**Accentuated S2**
Chest pain (pleuritic and nonpleuritic)	Cyanosis
Cough	Diaphoresis
Dyspnea	Fever
Hemoptysis	Lower-extremity edema
Sweating	**Rales**
Syncope	S3 or S4 gallop
	Tachycardia (> 100 beats/min)
	Tachypnea (> 16/min)
	Thrombophlebitis

Bold-faced items above are the most commonly reported symptoms and signs.

Table 14–7. VENTILATION/PERFUSION LUNG SCANS: RISK OF PULMONARY EMBOLISM AND CLINICAL RELEVANCE

V/Q STUDY RESULT	PULMONARY EMBOLISM	CLINICAL RELEVANCE
Normal	1–2% of patients	PE ruled out.
Low probability	12% of patients	Nondiagnostic result; further evaluation is required unless clinical suspicion is low.
Intermediate probability	33% of patients	Nondiagnostic result; further evaluation is required.
High probability	88% of patients	If patient has no contraindications to anticoagulation, begin therapy. If anticoagulation is contraindicated, then further evaluation is required.

Adapted from PIOPED Investigators. JAMA 1990;263:2753–2759.

of a respiratory alkalosis (80% of patients with PE have a decreased PCO_2) and/or an abnormal A–a gradient:

$$A\text{–a gradient} = PAO_2 - PaO_2;$$
$$PAO_2 = FiO_2 \ (PB - 47) - PaCO_2/0.8$$

where FiO_2 is the inspired concentration of oxygen (0.21 for room air), PaO_2 is the blood gas oxygen level, $PaCO_2$ is the blood gas carbon dioxide level, and PB is the atmospheric pressure (760 mmHg at sea level). A normal PCO_2 *and* a normal A–a gradient make acute PE unlikely (but they do not absolutely rule-out PE if the clinical picture is highly suggestive for same). The A–a gradient increases with age; in the normal young person without pulmonary disease, the A–a gradient should be 5–10 mmHg.

   c. *Electrocardiography* (ECG) is mandatory in the patient with a suspected PE, but the results are again nonspecific. Sinus tachycardia is seen in approximately 75% of patients with a PE. Other findings may include right-sided strain, right-axis deviation, right bundle-branch block (RBBB), S1 Q3 T3 pattern, and/or atrial arrhythmias.

2. **Pulmonary Scintigraphy (Ventilation–Perfusion [V/Q] Scanning)** is usually the first "diagnostic" test to pursue in the evaluation of a patient suspected of PE. Typical V/Q scan results, the risk of PE with a given V/Q scan result, and the clinical relevance of that result are presented in Table 14–7.

3. **Lower-Extremity Noninvasive DVT Study** (see II. F, above). When the V/Q scan is nondiagnostic (e.g., low probability and/or intermediate probability study), demonstrating a DVT by noninvasive means obviates the need for pulmonary angiography because the treatment is generally the same: anticoagulation and risk factor modification. Approximately 70% of patients with PE will have a demonstrable coexisting thrombus in the deep veins of the thighs or pelvis.

4. **Pulmonary Angiography.** The "definitive" test in the diagnosis of pulmonary thromboembolism. Morbidity is low, and mortality is 0.25%. Angiography is indicated in the following situations:

a. The patient has a high-probability V/Q scan but anticoagulation is contraindicated.

b. The patient has failed anticoagulation therapy and surgery for PE is being considered.

c. The patient has a nondiagnostic V/Q scan, no evidence of lower-extremity DVT, and PE is strongly suspected clinically.

Note: recent data suggest that patients with a *non–high-probability* V/Q scan and repeatedly negative serial impedance plethysmography (IPG) studies ($\leq$ 5 IPGs over a 2-week time period) have a good prognosis without anticoagulant therapy; in these patients, pursuing pulmonary angiography may not be necessary.

H. Laboratory Studies

Routinely obtain the following blood studies in the patient clinically suspected of having either a DVT or PE:

1. Complete blood count (including platelets).
2. Electrolyte panel.
3. Glucose.
4. Blood urea nitrogen creatinine.
5. Prothrombin time (PT)/activated partial thromboplastin time (aPTT) (if thrombolytic therapy is indicated, also obtain a thrombin time (TT), bleeding time, and fibrinogen level).
6. Pregnancy test (in reproductive age females).
7. Urinalysis.

III. DIFFERENTIAL DIAGNOSIS

A. **Differential diagnosis of DVT** includes Baker's cyst (posterior knee swelling caused by membrane enclosed synovial fluid), cellulitis, knee injury, hematoma, lymphangitis, lymphatic obstruction, muscle strain, muscle tear, postphlebitic syndrome, and vasomotor changes in a paralyzed leg.

B. **Differential diagnosis of PE** includes acute myocardial infarction, angina, anxiety attack, asthma or chronic obstructive pulmonary disease exacerbation, congestive heart failure, costochondritis, herpes zoster infection, hyperventilation, lung cancer, musculoskeletal pain, pancreatitis, pericarditis, pleurisy, pneumonia, pneumothorax, rib fracture, and tuberculosis.

IV. THERAPY

Note: the diagnostic and therapeutic strategies for DVT and PE are presented in Figures 14–4 and 14–5, respectively.

A. Initial Therapy: Secure and support the airway, breathing, and circulation (also see Chapter 1).

1. If the patient is dyspneic and/or PE is a reasonable consideration, rapidly obtain an ABG and then administer supplemental *oxygen* and continuously *monitor* both SaO_2 and the cardiac rhythm.

2. Rapidly obtain vital signs, intravenous (IV) access, and an ECG, and perform a directed physical examination.

3. The hypotensive patient secondary to a massive PE should have blood pressure supported with crystalloid infusion and vasopressors (e.g., dopamine, begin at 5 µg/kg/min IV and titrate as necessary). Urgently consult pulmonary, cardiothoracic surgery, and interventional radiology specialists for rapid confirmation of the diagnosis and initiation of appropriate treatment in the hemodynamically unstable patient.

4. Obtain a chest roentgenogram and order relevent laboratory studies (see II. H.).

B. Anticoagulation: Heparin

1. Heparin is the initial anticoagulant of choice for most patients with DVT and for hemodynamically stable patients with PE. It prevents further propagation of the thrombus, but it *does not* enhance clot lysis. Consider initiating heparin in appropriate candidates while awaiting diagnostic confirmation of acute PE—especially in the unstable patient.

2. *Dosing:*
   a. Loading dose: 80 units/kg. In the setting of acute PE, some experts recommend a larger heparin loading dose (10,000–20,000 units IV) and waiting 2 hours before beginning the maintenance infusion.
   b. Maintenance infusion: begin with 18 units/kg/hr after the loading dose. Recheck PTT 6 hours after initiating therapy (generally this will be after admission) and adjust as necessary to maintain the aPTT 1.5–2.5 times control.

3. *Contraindications:*
   a. Absolute: active internal bleeding, intracranial bleeding, intracranial lesions predisposed to bleeding, and malignant hypertension.
   b. Relative: hemorrhagic diathesis, recent stroke, recent major surgery, severe hypertension, bacterial endocarditis, severe renal failure, severe hepatic failure, and diabetic retinopathy.

C. Thrombolytic Therapy

1. Thrombolytic therapy produces fairly rapid and complete clot lysis. Hemodynamically unstable patients with an acute PE improve more rapidly with thrombolytic therapy than with

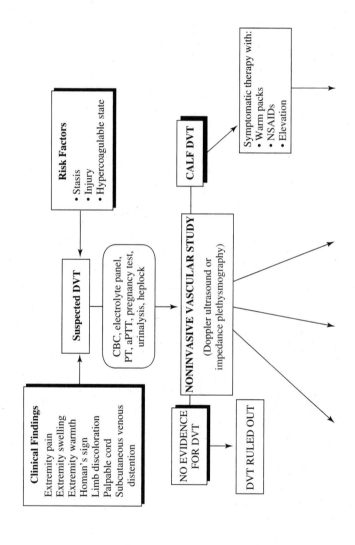

Clinical Findings

Extremity pain
Extremity swelling
Extremity warmth
Homan's sign
Limb discoloration
Palpable cord
Subcutaneous venous
distention

Risk Factors

• Stasis
• Injury
• Hypercoagulable state

Suspected DVT

CBC, electrolyte panel,
PT, aPTT, pregnancy test,
urinalysis, heplock

NONINVASIVE VASCULAR STUDY

(Doppler ultrasound or
impedance plethysmography)

**NO EVIDENCE
FOR DVT**

DVT RULED OUT

CALF DVT

Symptomatic therapy with:
• Warm packs
• NSAIDs
• Elevation

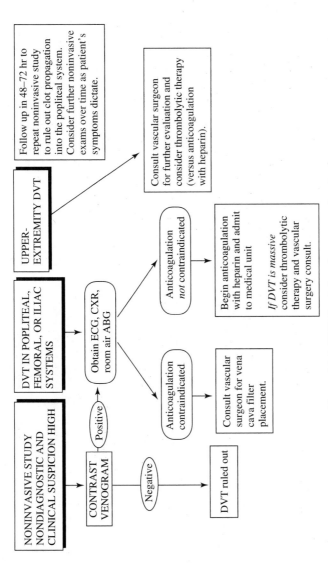

Figure 14–4. DVT diagnosis and management protocol.

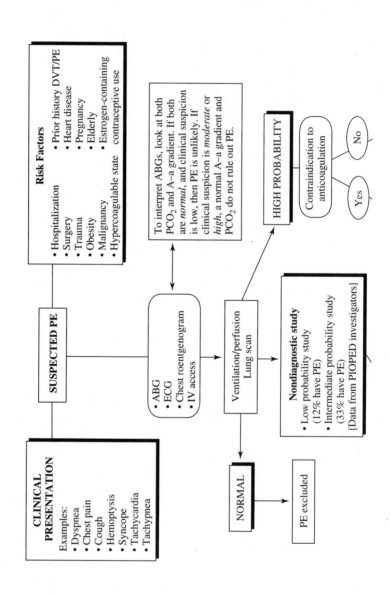

CLINICAL PRESENTATION

Examples:
- Dyspnea
- Chest pain
- Cough
- Hemoptysis
- Syncope
- Tachycardia
- Tachypnea

Risk Factors

- Hospitalization
- Surgery
- Trauma
- Obesity
- Malignancy
- Hypercoagulable state
- Prior history DVT/PE
- Heart disease
- Pregnancy
- Elderly
- Estrogen-containing contraceptive use

SUSPECTED PE

- ABG
- ECG
- Chest roentgenogram
- IV access

To interpret ABGs, look at both PCO_2 and A–a gradient. If both are *normal*, and clinical suspicion is low, then PE is unlikely. If clinical suspicion is *moderate* or *high*, a normal A–a gradient and PCO_2 do not rule out PE.

Ventilation/perfusion Lung scan

NORMAL

PE excluded

Nondiagnostic study
- Low probability study (12% have PE)
- Intermediate probability study (33% have PE)
[Data from PIOPED investigators]

HIGH PROBABILITY

Contraindication to anticoagulation

Yes   No

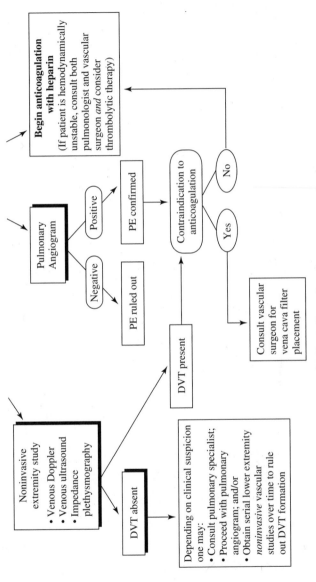

Figure 14-5. PE diagnosis and management protocol.

heparin, and it may reduce the risk of venous hypertension and the post-thrombotic syndrome in acute DVT.

2. **Indication.** Acute PE with hemodynamic instability.

3. **Controversial Indication.** Acute massive DVT (in either an upper or lower extremity).

4. **Dosing of Thrombolytic Agents.**

   a. Streptokinase 250,000 units IV over 30 minutes, followed by a maintenance infusion of 100,000 units/hr for 24 hours (or longer in massive PE with huge DVT—up to 72 hours infusion).

      Side effects include hemorrhage requiring transfusion (4% of patients), oozing from puncture wounds, fever (20% of patients), hypotension, and marked allergic reactions (6% of patients). Consider administering hydrocortisone 100 mg IV to minimize allergic phenomena.

   b. Urokinase 4400 units/kg IV load over 10 minutes, followed by a maintenance infusion of 4400 units/kg/hr IV for 12 hours.

      Side effects include hemorrhage in the same rate as that seen with streptokinase, but allergic reactions are rare.

   c. Tissue Plasminogen Activator (t-PA): 100 mg infused through a peripheral vein over 2 hours (50 mg/hr).

5. **Laboratory Monitoring and Heparin Use**

   a. With thrombolytic therapy, the bleeding time, TT, aPTT, PT, and fibrinogen level should be checked before the start of treatment. With streptokinase and urokinase, a TT should be checked 4 hours after the initial bolus to confirm an adequate lytic state.

   b. After thrombolytic therapy, a continuous heparin infusion should be started to achieve an aPTT of 1.5–2.0 times control.

      i. Streptokinase and urokinase: do *not* bolus with heparin. Begin the heparin infusion when the aPTT after thrombolytic administration is <100 sec (3–4 hours after the thrombolytic infusion has been stopped).

      ii. t-PA: bolus with 5000 units of heparin and begin the heparin infusion (1000 units/hr) immediately after the t-PA is given.

6. **Contraindications to Thrombolytic Therapy.** See Table 13–16.

D. Inferior Vena Cava Barriers

1. These mechanical barriers are placed by a vascular surgeon under fluoroscopic guidance via either an internal jugular or femoral vein cutdown approach. They are effective and may reduce the recurrence rate for PE to ≤ 5%. Rarely, actual

ligation of the inferior vena cava is sometimes utilized instead of a percutaneously placed venous filter.

2. **Indications for Venous Filter Placement**

   a. Patient has suffered an acute PE and/or DVT and antico-agulation therapy is contraindicated.
   b. Patient has suffered a recurrent DVT and/or PE even though appropriately anticoagulated.
   c. Patient has suffered a massive, life-threatening PE.

E. Surgical Embolectomy

This procedure carries a high mortality rate ($\geq 25\%$), and its current role in the treatment of PE is controversial. It should be considered in the patient with persistent, severe hypotension secondary to a massive and life-threatening PE when thrombolytic therapy is absolutely contraindicated or ineffective.

V. DISPOSITION

A. Discharge

If an isolated *calf* DVT is demonstrated, anticoagulation is probably not warranted (although the issue is controversial), and the patient may be discharged to home. Treatment should be initiated with an anti-inflammatory agent (e.g., aspirin) and warm compresses. Follow-up in 48-72 hours is mandatory. A repeat lower-extremity study (e.g., doppler ultrasound or IPG) should be done at the time of follow-up to rule out proximal propagation of the calf thrombus into the popliteal system. The risk of proximal propagation of a clot is about 15%; and a popliteal DVT *does* require admission and anticoagulation.

B. Admit

All patients with a popliteal or higher DVT, an upper-extremity DVT, or a PE must be admitted to the hospital for anticoagulation and monitoring of therapy. Patients with an acute PE should be admitted to a telemetry bed, and patients with hemodynamic instability should be admitted to the ICU.

VI. PEARLS AND PITFALLS

A. The possibility of PE should be considered in any patient presenting with chest pain, dyspnea, or syncope.

B. The possibility of DVT should be considered in any patient presenting with extremity pain or swelling.

C. The absence of risk factors does not rule out the possibility of venous thromboembolic disease.

D. "Normal" ABGs do not rule out the possibility of PE in a patient with a history strongly suggestive of same.

E. Upper-extremity DVT can cause PE, and the postphlebitic syndrome may be particularly disabling. These patients should receive a vascular surgery consult and be admitted for anticoagulation. An upper-extremity DVT is treated with thrombolytic therapy at some institutions.

F. Isolated calf thrombi mandate close outpatient follow-up and serial noninvasive vascular studies to rule out proximal clot propagation; a popliteal DVT mandates hospitalization and anticoagulation.

G. An acute PE that causes hemodynamic instability is an indication for thrombolytic therapy; pulmonary, cardiothoracic surgery, and interventional radiology specialists should be urgently consulted.

BIBLIOGRAPHY

Bolgiano EB, Foxwell MM, Browne BJ, Barish RA: Deep venous thrombosis of the upper extremity: Diagnosis and treatment. J Emerg Med 1990;8:85–91.

Carson JL, Kelley MA, Duff A, et al: The clinical course of pulmonary embolism. N Engl J Med 1992;326(19):1240–1245.

Hobson RW, Mintz BL, Jamil Z, et al: Diagnosis of acute deep venous thrombosis. Surg Clin N Am 1990;70:143–157.

Hull RD, Raskob GE, Coates G, et al. A new noninvasive management strategy for patients with suspected pulmonary embolism. Arch Intern Med 1989:149:2549–2555.

Landefeld CS, McGuire E, Cohen AM: Clinical findings associated with acute proximal deep vein thrombosis: A basis for quantifying clinical judgment. Am J Med 1990;88:382–388.

McGlynn TJ, Jr: Pulmonary embolism and venous thrombosis. Chapter 9. In Kammerer WS, RJ Gross (eds): Medical Consultation. 2nd Ed. Baltimore; Williams & Wilkins, 1990, pp. 97–106.

PIOPED Investigators: Value of the ventilation/perfusion scan in acute pulmonary embolism. JAMA 1990;263:2753–2759.

Valenzuela TD, Croghan MK: Pulmonary embolism. Chapter 299. In Harwood-Nuss A, Linden C, Luten RC, Sternbach G, and Wolfson AB (eds): The Clinical Practice of Emergency Medicine. Philadelphia, JB Lippincott, 1991, pp. 932–935.

SPONTANEOUS PNEUMOTHORAX

> *"...there is much gas within his thorax, resulting in panting and troubled breathing."*
>
> HUANG TI (THE YELLOW EMPEROR)

I. ESSENTIAL FACTS

A. Definition

Pneumothorax refers to the presence of air in the intrapleural space between the visceral and parietal pleural surfaces.

1. *Spontaneous pneumothoraces* occur without any preceding trauma or obvious cause, and are classified as primary or secondary.

   a. *Idiopathic* or *primary spontaneous pneumothoraces* occur in otherwise healthy individuals.

    b. *Secondary spontaneous pneumothoraces* occur in patients with underlying pulmonary disease.

2. *Traumatic pneumothoraces* occur as the result of direct or indirect trauma to the chest.

3. A *tension pneumothorax* (may be either spontaneous or traumatic) results when air accumulates in the pleural space because of a one-way valve effect. This trapped air may cause pressure sufficient to restrict ventilation and/or displace the mediastinum to the opposite side, impairing venous return to the right heart and compromising cardiac output. It is a life-threatening emergency demanding immediate intervention!

B. Epidemiology

Primary spontaneous pneumothoraces are approximately seven times more common in males than in females, and secondary spontaneous pneumothoraces are approximately three times more common in males than in females. The majority of patients with a spontaneous primary pneumothorax are less than 35 years old at the time of their initial pneumothorax. There are approximately 20,000 new cases of spontaneous pneumothorax in the United States each year.

The recurrence rate for primary and secondary spontaneous pneumothoraces is similar. Nearly 50% of patients with spontaneous pneumothorax, not treated with thoracotomy for their initial event, have an ipsilateral recurrence. After an initial relapse, the incidence of subsequent recurrence is even higher.

C. Etiology

1. Primary spontaneous pneumothoraces typically result from rupture of apical subpleural parenchymal blebs or cysts with leakage of air into the pleural space. The pathogenesis of these subpleural blebs is unclear but they have been postulated to result from congenital abnormalities or bronchiole inflammation.

    a. Primary spontaneous pneumothoraces occur most often in *tall, thin, young men.*

    b. Cases of *familial* spontaneous pneumothorax have been described and may be associated with the HLA haplotype A2,B40.

    c. *Cigarette smoking* has also been implicated as a risk factor.

2. Secondary spontaneous pneumothoraces have been associated with a variety of underlying lung diseases, as outlined in Table 14–8.

3. Traumatic pneumothoraces are usually associated with blunt or penetrating chest trauma, iatrogenic injury, or barotrauma during mechanical ventilation.

Table 14–8. PULMONARY DISEASES
ASSOCIATED WITH PNEUMOTHORAX

Obstructive

Chronic obstructive pulmonary disease
Bullous emphysema
Asthma
Cystic fibrosis

Interstitial

Sarcoidosis
Idiopathic pulmonary fibrosis
Histiocytosis X
Tuberous sclerosis
Lymphangiomyomatosis
Idiopathic pulmonary hemosiderosis
Pulmonary alveolar proteinosis
Berylliosis

Neoplastic

Primary bronchogenic carcinoma
Metastatic pleural disease

Infectious

Bacterial pneumonia
Lung abscess
Mycobacterium tuberculosis and *M. avium*
Pneumocystis carinii pneumonia
Nocardia
Echinococcosis (hydatid disease)

Miscellaneous

Adult respiratory distress syndrome
Infant respiratory distress syndrome
Collagen vascular disease (e.g., rheumatoid disease and scleroderma)
Connective tissue disease (e.g., Marfan's syndrome and Ehlers-Danlos syndrome)
Esophageal rupture
Endometriosis (catamenial pneumothorax)
Pulmonary infarction

II. CLINICAL EVALUATION

A. History

Pertinent historical information in a patient with a pneumothorax should include the following:

1. History of *underlying lung disease*. Patients with chronic obstructive pulmonary disease (COPD) who develop secondary spontaneous pneumothoraces tend to have severe air-flow obstruction and frequently have air-trapping and bullous lung disease.

2. History of recent *trauma.*

3. History of any *past episodes* of pneumothorax.

4. *Family history* of pneumothorax.

5. History of *cigarette smoking.*

B. Symptoms

1. Common symptoms associated with a *spontaneous pneumothorax* include pleuritic *chest pain* and *dyspnea.*

2. The clinical symptoms associated with *secondary spontaneous pneumothorax* tend to be more severe than those associated with primary spontaneous pneumothorax because of the underlying lung disease and reduced physiologic reserve.

3. Patients with tension pneumothorax typically appear quite distressed with labored breathing. Patients may also demonstrate an altered level of consciousness secondary to profound hypoxemia and reduced cardiac output.

C. Signs

1. The physical examination of patients with spontaneous pneumothorax may be normal (in cases where a small pneumothorax is present), or may reveal *tachypnea, tachycardia, accessory muscle use* for respiration, and diminished or *absent breath sounds* on auscultation of the affected side. Percussion of the affected side demonstrates *hyperresonant tones.*

2. The signs of pneumothorax may be less apparent in patients with COPD and secondary spontaneous pneumothorax because some of these patients have diminished breath sounds or hyperresonant percussion tones at their baseline.

3. In addition to the signs mentioned above, patients with a tension pneumothorax may also demonstrate *cyanosis, hypotension, distended neck veins, tracheal shift* toward the contralateral side, and hyperinflation of the side of the chest with the pneumothorax. In severe cases, *pulseless electrical activity (PEA)* and hemodynamic collapse may occur.

D. Laboratory Studies

1. Arterial blood gas analysis (ABG) in patients with a primary spontaneous pneumothorax may be normal or reveal respiratory alkalosis, hypoxemia, and a widened alveolar–arterial (A–a) oxygen gradient. Patients with severe underlying lung disease and secondary spontaneous pneumothorax may experience respiratory acidosis and profound hypoxemia.

2. The chest roentgenogram in a patient with a pneumothorax usually demonstrates a line of visceral pleura oriented in a convex position toward the lateral chest wall and beyond which no lung markings are evident. Chest roentgenograms taken during full expiration may demonstrate a pneumothorax that is too small to identify on a standard posterior-anterior film. Occasionally, a large bulla will mimic a pneumothorax on the chest film. Computed tomography of the chest can distinguish between a bulla and a pneumothorax in uncertain cases.

In addition to demonstrating air in the pleural space, the chest roentgenogram in a patient with a tension pneumothorax may show collapse of the ipsilateral lung and shift of the trachea, heart, and mediastinum to the contralateral side. (*Reminder:* a tension pneumothorax should be diagnosed and treated at the time of the primary survey—before a chest roentgenogram is obtained.)

III. DIFFERENTIAL DIAGNOSIS

A. The clinical presentation of pneumothorax may be mimicked by other conditions that cause dyspnea and chest pain. These include pulmonary thromboembolism, pneumonia, myocardial infarction, pleurisy, pericarditis, aortic dissection, and esophageal spasm.

B. The roentgenographic differential diagnosis of pneumothorax includes any condition that simulates the presence of air in the intrapleural space, such as an emphysematous bulla, cyst, pneumatocele, or lung abscess with an air-fluid level. Occasionally, a skin fold overlying the chest cavity may mimic the visceral pleural line characteristic of a pneumothorax. In cases of skin folds, however, lung markings can usually be detected on both sides of the line.

IV. TREATMENT (Fig. 14–6)

A. Initial Interventions

1. Administer supplemental oxygen and maintain hemoglobin saturation (SaO_2) $\geq 95\%$ (maintain at 90% in the COPD patient at risk for carbon dioxide retention with high-flow oxygen). Administration of high concentrations of oxygen significantly increases the net gradient for gas absorption from the pleural space.

2. Obtain vital signs and intravenous (IV) access; continuously monitor both the cardiac rhythm and SaO_2.

3. The patient with a clinically identified tension pneumothorax should have immediate needle decompression of the pneumothorax followed by chest tube thoracostomy.

4. Order a portable chest roentgenogram.

B. Therapy to Evacuate Air from the Pleural Space

1. *Simple aspiration* of a primary spontaneous pneumothorax may be accomplished, under local anesthesia, by insertion of a 16-gauge IV cannula through the chest wall at the second anterior intercostal space in the midclavicular line. Once the pleural space has been entered, the needle is removed and a 3-way stopcock and 60-mL syringe are attached to the catheter. Air is then manually aspirated from the pleural space and expelled through the third port of the stopcock. Simple

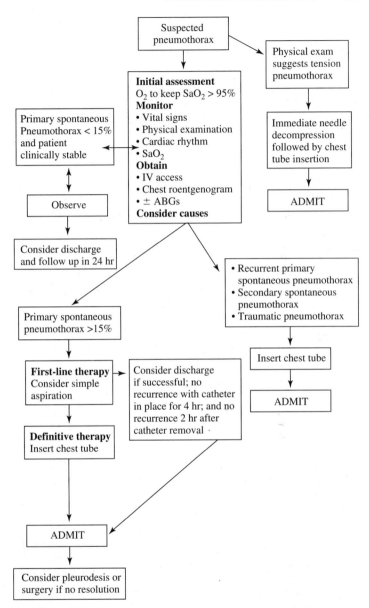

Figure 14–6. Emergency management of spontaneous pneumothorax.

aspiration is not generally recommended for patients with recurrence of a primary spontaneous pneumothorax or with a secondary spontaneous pneumothorax.

2. *Tube thoracostomy* should be performed in cases of recurrent or secondary spontaneous pneumothorax or when simple aspiration is ineffective. A small chest tube or "flutter valve" may be successful in managing patients with a primary spontaneous or iatrogenic pneumothorax. However, treatment of patients with a secondary spontaneous pneumothorax or a traumatic pneumothorax usually requires placement of a larger chest tube with a water-seal apparatus for drainage. The risk of re-expansion pulmonary edema may be higher when suction is applied to the chest tube, therefore suction should be applied only when the lung fails to expand after chest tube placement.

3. *Chemical pleurodesis:* various sclerosing agents, such as tetracycline, bleomycin, or talc can be introduced into the pleural space through a chest tube in order to induce an inflammatory response and prevent recurrence of the pneumothorax. In general, consider chemical pleurodesis in patients with recurrent primary spontaneous pneumothorax or secondary spontaneous pneumothorax.

4. *Open thoracotomy* may be necessary to oversew or remove pleural blebs in patients with recurrent primary spontaneous pneumothoraces despite treatment with tube thoracostomy and chemical pleurodesis. Some patients with recurrent secondary spontaneous pneumothoraces also require open thoracotomy to remove or oversew bullae in cases of persistent air leakage (bronchopleural fistula) following tube thoracostomy placement.

C. Special Circumstances

1. **Small Pneumothorax.** Clinically stable patients with spontaneous primary pneumothoraces that occupy less than 15% of the hemithorax may be observed without intervention if careful medical follow-up can be ensured. It is estimated that approximately 1.25% of the volume of the hemithorax is absorbed in 24 hours. Therefore, most small pneumothoraces take 2–4 weeks to completely resorb after the air leakage has stopped. Hospitalized patients may benefit from the administration of high concentrations of supplemental oxygen, which accelerates the rate of pleural air absorption.

2. **Traumatic Pneumothorax.** A pneumothorax resulting from blunt or penetrating chest trauma almost always requires chest tube insertion. The clinician should be alert for the possibility of an associated hemothorax in these cases, and the surgical team should be involved early in the course of the patient's management.

3. **Pneumothorax Associated With Mechanical Ventilation.** Patients who develop a pneumothorax while receiving positive-pressure mechanical ventilation are at high risk of developing a tension pneumothorax and should be managed with tube thoracostomy.

4. **Tension Pneumothorax.** In a critically ill patient with physical examination findings suggestive of a tension pneumothorax, time should not be wasted by obtaining a chest roentgenogram. These patients should be given high concentrations of supplemental oxygen and a large-bore needle should be inserted into the pleural space through the second anterior intercostal space at the mid-clavicular line to emergently decompress the tension pneumothorax, followed by chest tube thoracostomy.

V. DISPOSITION

A. Discharge

Patients with a primary, spontaneous pneumothorax may be discharged from the ED if *all* of the following conditions apply:

1. Room air SaO_2 is $\geq 95\%$.

2. The patient is relatively asymptomatic and otherwise healthy.

3. The patient is reliable and follow-up in 24 hours (including a repeat chest roentgenogram) is arranged.

4. The patient's spontaneous pneumothorax involved $\leq 15\%$ of the hemithorax, and there is no evidence that it is increasing in size while the patient is observed in the ED.

5. If the patient's spontaneous pneumothorax was treated with simple catheter aspiration, a repeat chest roentgenogram taken 4 hours after aspiration shows no pneumothorax while the catheter is still in place, and another chest roentgenogram taken 2 hours after catheter removal again shows no pneumothorax.

B. Admit

Patients with any of the following should be admitted:

1. Recurrent primary spontaneous pneumothorax.

2. Secondary spontaneous pneumothorax.

3. Traumatic pneumothorax.

4. Tension pneumothorax.

5. Unstable vital signs.

6. Hypoxemia.

7. Pneumothoraces $> 15\%$ of the hemithorax not reduced with simple aspiration.

8. Need for tube thoracostomy placement or chemical pleuro-desis.

VI. PEARLS AND PITFALLS

A. Mechanically remove intrapleural air in all unstable patients.

B. Consider causes of secondary spontaneous pneumothorax before labeling a pneumothorax as a primary or idiopathic spontaneous pneumothorax.

C. Administer high concentrations of oxygen to all hospitalized patients (except COPD patients at risk for severe carbon dioxide retention).

D. Provide follow-up in 24 hours for patients discharged from the ED.

E. Treat patients with suspected tension pneumothorax before obtaining a chest roentgenogram.

Do not do any of the following:

A. Perform simple needle aspiration in a traumatic pneumothorax—these patients require tube thoracostomy drainage.

B. Wait for a chest roentgenogram before treating an unstable patient with a suspected tension pneumothorax.

C. Discharge a patient home unless they have normal vital signs, an $SaO_2 \geq 95\%$, and are reliable.

BIBLIOGRAPHY

Beers MF, Sohn M, Swartz M: Recurrent pneumothorax in AIDS patients with Pneumocystis pneumonia. A clinicopathologic report of three cases and review of the literature. Chest 1990;98(2):266–270.

Conces DJ, Tarver RD, Gray WC, et al: Treatment of pneumothoraces utilizing small caliber chest tubes. Chest 1988;94:55–57.

Light RW: Pneumothorax. Chapter 77. In Murray JF, Nadel JA (eds): Textbook of Respiratory Medicine. Philadelphia, WB Saunders, 1988, pp. 1745–1759.

Vallee P, et al: Sequential treatment of a simple pneumothorax. Ann Emerg Med 1988;5:45–47.

Wait MA, Estrera A: Changing clinical spectrum of spontaneous pneumothorax. Am J Surg 1992;164(5):528–531.

15

Infectious Disease Emergencies

ACQUIRED IMMUNODEFICIENCY SYNDROME

"The terrors of disease are always with us."
THOMAS A. DOOLEY (1927–1961)

I. ESSENTIAL FACTS

A. Definition

Acquired immunodeficiency syndrome (AIDS) is caused by infection with the human immunodeficiency virus (HIV). The two known strains of the virus are HIV-1 and HIV-2; the vast majority of infection in the United States is due to HIV-1. Infection with HIV leads to depression of cell-mediated immunity and an increased susceptibility to opportunistic infection. *AIDS* is defined as the occurrence of a significant or life-threatening opportunistic infection and/or neoplastic process (e.g., Kaposi's sarcoma, primary central nervous system lymphoma) in the setting of HIV infection.

B. Classification

Table 15–1 presents a classification system for HIV infection.

C. Epidemiology

1. It is estimated that more than one million people are infected with HIV in the United States. Over 240,000 cases of AIDS have been reported since 1981; 60% of these patients have died.

2. High-risk groups for HIV infection include the following (with the percentage of diagnosed AIDS cases noted in parentheses):
   a. Homosexual/bisexual men (58% of AIDS cases).
   b. Injection drug users (23%).
   c. Homosexual injection drug users (6%).
   d. Transfusion recipients (2%) (with those who received blood products between 1978 and March 1985 at greatest risk).
   e. Sexual partners or children of high-risk mothers (6%).
   f. Hemophiliacs (1%).
   g. Four percent of patients with AIDS do not fit into one of the above categories.

Table 15–1. 1993 REVISED CLASSIFICATION SYSTEM FOR HIV INFECTION AND EXPANDED AIDS SURVEILLANCE CASE DEFINITIONS IN ADULTS

	CLINICAL CATEGORIES		
CD4 + T-CELL CATEGORIES	A ASYMPTOMATIC (ACUTE HIV INFECTION OR PGL)	B SYMPTOMATIC (PREVIOUSLY CLASS IV NON-AIDS)	C AIDS INDICATOR CONDITIONS
1. ≥ 500/mm³	A1	B1	C1[a]
2. 200–499/mm³	A2	B2	C2[a]
3. < 200/mm³ (AIDS indicator T-cell count)	A3[a]	B3[a]	C3[a]

Category B Conditions

Bacillary angiomatosis
Candidiasis, oropharyngeal (thrush)
Candidiasis, vulvovaginal; persistent, frequent, or poorly responsive to therapy
Cervical dysplasia (moderate or severe)/cervical carcinoma in situ
Constitutional symptoms, i.e., persistent fevers (> 38.5° C) or diarrhea (> 1 month's duration)
Hairy leukoplakia
Herpes zoster (two episodes or more than one dermatome)
Idiopathic thrombocytopenic purpura
Listeriosis
Pelvic inflammatory disease (particularly with tubo-ovarian abscess)
Peripheral neuropathy

Category C Conditions

Candidiasis of bronchi, trachea, or lungs
Candidiasis, esophageal
Cervical cancer, invasive[b]
Coccidioidomycosis, disseminated or extrapulmonary
Cryptococcus, extrapulmonary
Cryptosporidiosis, chronic intestinal (> 1 month's duration)
Cytomegalovirus disease (other than liver, spleen, or nodes)
Cytomagalovirus retinitis (with loss of vision)
Encephalopathy, HIV-related
Herpes simplex virus: chronic ulcer(s) (> 1 month's duration); or bronchitis, pneumonitis, or esophagitis
Histoplasmosis, disseminated or extrapulmonary
Isosporiasis, chronic intestinal (> 1 month's duration)
Kaposi's sarcoma
Lymphoma, Burkitt's (or equivalent term)
Lymphoma, immunoblastic (or equivalent term)
Lymphoma, primary, of brain
Mycobacterium avium complex or *M. kansasii,* disseminated or extrapulmonary
Mycobacterium tuberculosis, any site (pulmonary[b] or extrapulmonary)
Mycobacterium, other species or unidentified species, disseminated or extrapulmonary
Pneumocystis carinii pneumonia
Pneumonia, recurrent[b]
Progressive multifocal leukoencephalopathy
Salmonella septicemia, recurrent
Toxoplasmosis of brain
Wasting syndrome due to HIV

PGL, persistent generalized lymphadenopathy.
[a]AIDS surveillance case definition.
[b]Added in the 1993 expansion of the AIDS surveillance case definition.

D. Laboratory Diagnosis of HIV Infection

1. Serologic Tests for HIV

a. The *enzyme-linked immunosorbent assay* (ELISA) measures antibody against HIV envelope antigens. It is the initial screening serologic test for HIV infection. In high-risk groups, specificity is 99%. The specificity is much lower in low-risk individuals. A strongly positive ELISA in a low-risk population is more likely to be a true positive (87%) than is a weakly positive test (2%).

b. The Western Blot assay allows for detection of serum antibodies to several particular HIV antigens. It is more specific for HIV infection than the ELISA. It is used as a confirmatory test for all positive ELISA results.

2. T-Cell Subsets

a. In HIV disease, there is a marked decline in CD4 T-cell lymphocytes, with no change or a slight increase in CD8 T-cell lymphocytes (T8 or T-suppressor cells).

b. A CD4 count < $200/mm^3$ is associated with an increased risk of progression to AIDS. Most opportunistic infections occur when the CD4 count is < $200/mm^3$.

E. Therapy for HIV Infection

1. Zidovudine (AZT).
This drug was first demonstrated to have antiretroviral activity against HIV-1 in 1985. In symptomatic HIV-infected patients, its use has slowed progression to AIDS and prolonged survival. After the diagnosis of AIDS, its use has been associated with increased median survival from < 9 months to > 2 years.

a. *Indications.* Zidovudine is appropriate in HIV-infected patients whose CD4 count drops < $500/mm^3$.

b. *Dose.* 500–600 mg daily (100 mg PO five times per day or 200 mg PO every 8 hours). 300 mg daily may be used in patients intolerant of larger doses.

c. *Side Effects.* Headache, fatigue, malaise, myopathy, nausea, vomiting, confusion, anemia, neutropenia, and hepatitis. With continued use, in vitro resistance to the drug frequently occurs.

2. Didanosine (DDI).
Use of this drug can result in increased weight, improved cutaneous hypersensitivity reactions, and increased CD4 counts in patients with either AIDS or AIDS-related complex.

a. *Indications.* Patients with advanced HIV infection who are intolerant of zidovudine or in whom zidovudine has been unsuccessful. Sequential use of zidovudine followed by didanosine seems to delay clinical deterioration.

b. *Dose.* Patient weight ≥ 50 kg: 200 mg PO bid;
Patient weight 35-49 kg: 125 mg PO bid.

    c. **Side Effects.** Gastrointestinal disturbances, pancreatitis, painful peripheral neuropathy, and hepatic failure.

  3. **Zalcitabine** (dideoxycytidine, or DDC). Patients with advanced HIV disease experience increased CD4 counts and weight gain when this medication is used in combination with zidovudine or when used alone.

    a. **Indications.** Use in combination with zidovudine in patients with HIV infection and $\leq$ 300 CD4 cells/mm^3 who have either clinical or immunologic deterioration, or use alone in patients intolerant or resistant to zidovudine.

    b. **Dose.** 0.75 mg PO tid, given together with zidovudine (200 mg tid).

    c. **Side Effects.** Peripheral neuropathy, rash, fever, stomatitis, and esophageal ulceration.

  4. **Stavudine** (D4T). Use of this drug results in an increase in CD4 cell counts and decrease in P24 antigenemia.

    a. **Indications.** Patients intolerant of other antiretroviral agents (i.e., zidovudine, DDC, DDI).

    b. **Dose.** 0.5-1.0 mg/kg/day PO.

    c. **Side Effects.** Peripheral neuropathy, pancreatitis.

II. RESPIRATORY SYMPTOMS IN THE HIV-POSITIVE PATIENT

A. Potential Causes of Respiratory Symptoms

1. *Pneumocystis carinii* pneumonia (PCP)

2. Bacterial pneumonia (especially *Streptococcus pneumoniae* and *Hemophilus influenzae*)

3. *Coccidioides immitis*

4. *Cryptococcus neoformans*

5. Cytomegalovirus

6. *Histoplasma capsulatum*

7. *Mycobacteria avium-intracellulare*

8. *Mycobacterium tuberculosis*

9. Neoplasm (e.g., Kaposi's sarcoma [KS], lymphoma, bronchogenic carcinoma)

10. Pneumothorax

11. Pulmonary edema

12. Sinusitis

B. Symptoms

1. Productive cough suggests bacterial pneumonia or possibly sinusitis. A chronic, dry, nonproductive cough is seen with

PCP. Mycobacterial infection may also cause a chronic cough.

2. Dyspnea of recent onset (< 48 hours duration) should suggest bacterial pneumonia, pulmonary embolus, or spontaneous pneumothorax. Dyspnea of subacute onset (1–4 weeks) or chronic (>1 month duration) is most commonly a manifestation of PCP. Pulmonary KS or HIV-related cardiomyopathy with pulmonary edema may also cause subacute or chronic dyspnea.

3. Pleuritic chest pain is a common symptom and can be seen with bacterial pneumonias, spontaneous pneumothorax (associated with PCP), pleural tuberculosis, or pulmonary embolus (especially in debilitated and immobile patients).

C. Important Historical Questions

1. Previous travel history or residence:
   a. Southwestern United States: risk for coccidioidomycosis.
   b. Midwest/Ohio river valley: risk for histoplasmosis.
   c. Latin America/Africa/Southeast Asia: high risk for endemic tuberculosis; increased risk for parasitic infestation.

2. Use and compliance with PCP prophylaxis:
   a. Life-long PCP prophylaxis is recommended for HIV-infected patients with *any* of the following:
      i. CD4 count < 200/mm^3.
      ii. Constitutional symptoms (e.g., oral candidiasis or unexplained fever) for ≥ 2 weeks (regardless of CD4 count).
      iii. Prior documented episode of PCP.
   b. PCP prophylactic regimens include any of the following:
      i. Trimethoprim-sulfamethoxazole: one double-strength tablet (160 mg trimethoprim + 800 mg sulfamethoxazole) PO daily, 7 days a week. *Or*
      ii. Aerosolized pentamidine: administered by the Respirgard II regimen (300 mg once per month) or the Fisoneb nebulizer (initial loading regimen of five 60-mg doses over a 2-week period, followed by a 60-mg dose every 2 weeks). *Or*
      iii. Dapsone: 100 mg PO every day.
   c. The risk of PCP is much less in patients on prophylaxis. If aerosolized pentamidine is being used, then an atypical presentation of PCP may occur (e.g., upper-lobe infiltrates, extrapulmonary disease).

3. Past medical history.

4. Current medications and allergies.

5. Habits (e.g., cigarette, alcohol, illicit drug use; sexual practices).

6. Economic situation and social support system.

D. Use of the CD4 Count

Most HIV-infected patients who are receiving appropriate primary care have had a baseline CD4 count. This is crucial in assessing their risk for opportunistic infections. PCP is rare when the CD4 count is > 300/mm^3. Ninety-five percent of cases occur in patients with CD4 counts < 200/mm^3. Bacterial pneumonias and sinusitis may occur at any CD4 count. The presentation of tuberculosis is more "typical" (i.e., productive cough, upper-lobe infiltrates) when the CD4 count is high. When the count is < 200/mm^3, atypical pulmonary presentations are the rule (e.g., hilar/medias tinal adenopathy, lower-lobe infiltrates, miliary pattern).

E. Directed Physical Examination

1. **General.** Note the patient's overall appearance, degree of respiratory distress, and cachexia.

2. **Vital Signs.** Obtain pulse, blood pressure, respiratory rate, and temperature. A weight is appropriate if the patient's condition allows.

3. **Skin.** Note any lesions or rashes. The presence of multifocal KS (flat or nodular dark red to purple lesions) increases the likelihood of pulmonary involvement with KS. Flesh-colored or erythematous nodular skin lesions may suggest disseminated *Cryptococcus.*

4. **HEENT.** The presence of oral candidiasis is a marker of immunodeficiency and indicates an increased risk for opportunistic pulmonary infection. Hairy leukoplakias are whitish plaques on the sides of the tongue that cannot be dislodged with gentle scraping. Oral ulcers may be caused by herpes simplex virus (HSV), candidiasis, or medications. KS may also cause oral lesions. Carefully evaluate both fundi.

5. **Neck.** Note suppleness and adenopathy.

6. **Chest.** Consolidation on examination suggests bacterial pneumonia. A normal pulmonary examination is present in approximately 50% of patients with PCP.

7. **Heart.** Auscultate for heart sounds, murmurs, rubs, and/or gallops.

8. **Abdomen.** Look for distention, bowel sounds, masses, or findings of localized peritoneal irritation.

9. **Genitourinary Tract.** Note any evidence of infection (e.g., ulcers, perianal abscess, prostatitis, pelvic inflammatory disease, other sexually transmitted disease) or signs of pregnancy.

10. **Extremities.** Search for joint inflammation or infection.

11. **Neurologic Status.** Note any evidence of mental status deterioration and/or focal findings.

F. Laboratory Studies/Diagnostic Tests

1. *Routinely* obtain the following:
   a. Complete blood count (CBC) with differential count.
   b. Chest roentgenogram.
   c. Electrolyte panel.
   d. Glucose level.
   e. Blood urea nitrogen and creatinine levels.
   f. Sputum Gram stain, acid-fast bacillus (AFB) stain and culture.

2. Additional studies *may be required* depending on clinical circumstances:
   a. Arterial blood gas (ABG).
   b. Lactate dehydrogenase (LDH) level.
   c. Blood cultures (aerobic, fungal, and mycobacterial).
   d. Limited sinus computed tomography (CT).
   e. Urinalysis and culture.
   f. Cryptococcal capsular antigen (blood and/or cerebrospinal fluid [CSF]).
   g. *Histoplasma capsulatum* antigen (blood and/or urine).

3. Laboratory/diagnostic test results:
   a. CBC: anemia, leukopenia, and thrombocytopenia are relatively common.
   b. Chest roentgenogram (Table 15–2): a lobar infiltrate usually suggests bacterial pneumonia or *Cryptococcus* infection. Interstitial infiltrates are highly suggestive of PCP. Presence of a pneumothorax strongly suggests underlying PCP.

Table 15–2. ROENTGENOGRAPHIC PATTERNS AND COMMONLY ASSOCIATED DISORDERS IN THE HIV-INFECTED PATIENT

Interstitial Alveolar Infiltrates	***Pleural Effusion***
Pneumocystis carinii pneumonia	Kaposi's sarcoma
Kaposi's sarcoma	Tuberculosis
Cytomegalovirus pneumonia	Cryptococcal pneumonia
	Nocardiosis
Reticulonodular-Micronodular Infiltrates	***Intrathoracic Adenopathy***
Tuberculosis	Tuberculosis (late onset)
Histoplasmosis	Kaposi's sarcoma
Coccidioidomycosis	*Mycobacterium avium-intracellulare*
Lymphoid interstitial pneumonitis	
Focal Infiltrates	***Cavity/Pneumatocele***
Bacterial pneumonia	*P. carinii* pneumonia
P. carinii (upper lobes)	Tuberculosis
Tuberculosis	*Aspergillus* sp.
Cryptococcal pneumonia	Nocardiosis
	Rhodococcus equi
	S. aureus (septic emboli)

From White DA, Gold JWM (eds): Med Clin N Am 1992;76:1.

c. Sputum Gram stain: purulent sputum suggests a bacterial pneumonia. If the cough is nonproductive, attempt to obtain sputum (for Gram stain, culture, PCP stain, and AFB stain) after administering aerosolized saline. Bronchoscopy with bronchoalveolar lavage may ultimately be necessary.

d. ABGs: most patients with PCP have a widened alveolar–arterial oxygen gradient (A–a gradient) even if the chest roentgenogram is normal. It is essential to calculate the A–a gradient in all dyspneic patients:

$$A–a = PA(alveolar)O_2 - PaO_2 \text{ (from the blood gas).}$$
$$PAO_2 = FiO_2 \text{ (PB} - 47) - PaCO_2/R$$
where

FiO_2 = inspired concentration of oxygen (0.21 with room air), PB = atmostpheric pressure (760 mmHg at sea level), $PaCO_2$ = carbon dioxide measurement from the blood gas, and R = respiratory quotient (generally assumed to be 0.8).

In young patients without pulmonary disease, the normal A–a gradient is 5–10 mmHg.

e. LDH: this enzyme is significantly elevated in individuals with extensive PCP (it may also be elevated in the patient with lymphoma).

G. Therapy

Figure 15–1 presents the emergent therapy of pulmonary infections in HIV-infected patients.

1. **Initial Management**

   a. Place the patient on oxygen (2–4 L/min via nasal cannula) and continuously monitor the oxygen saturation (SaO_2) with a pulse oximeter. Supplement oxygenation as necessary to maintain $\geq 95\%$ SaO_2. Patients with PCP may have a rapid deterioration in oxygenation.

   b. Rapidly obtain vital signs and intravenous (IV) access, and perform a directed physical examination.

   c. The volume-depleted patient should be appropriately resuscitated with IV crystalloid (normal saline [NS] or lactated Ringer's solution [LR]).

   d. Obtain relevant laboratory studies (see II. F, above) and a chest roentgenogram.

2. **Antibiotic Therapy: Presumed Bacterial Pneumonia**

   a. Therapy should be directed by sputum Gram stain results. If unclear, empiric therapy should cover both *S. pneumoniae* and *H. influenzae*.

   b. Reasonable initial parenteral antibiotic choices include
      i. Ampicillin + sulbactam (Unasyn) 1.5–3.0 g IV every 6 hours; *or*

      ii. Cefuroxime 1.5 g IV every 8 hours; *or*

      iii. Ceftriaxone 1–2 g IV every 12–24 hours.

3. **Antibiotic Therapy: Presumed *P. carinii* Pneumonia**

  a. PCP is a likely diagnosis if *any* of the following conditions apply:

    i. CD4 count is $< 200/mm^3$.

    ii. Patient is not on PCP prophylaxis or is noncompliant with prophylaxis.

    iii. Diffuse infiltrates or pneumothorax are present on the chest roentgenogram.

  b. If PCP is clinically suspected, begin antibiotic therapy before confirmation of the diagnosis:

    i. Trimethoprim-sulfamethoxazole (first-choice agent) 20 mg/kg trimethoprim + 100 mg/kg sulfamethoxazole in four divided doses PO or IV for 21 days. *Or*

    ii. Pentamidine (alternative agent for severe disease) 4 mg/kg IV daily for 21 days. *Or*

    iii. Dapsone + trimethoprim 100 mg dapsone PO daily + 5 mg/kg trimethoprim PO qid for 21 days. *Or*

    iv. Atovaquone (alternative agent for mild to moderate disease only) 750 mg PO tid given with fatty foods to promote absorption.

  c. Corticosteroids may be used as adjunctive therapy. Prednisone, added to the above antibiotic regimens, reduces morbidity and mortality in the setting of PCP when the patient's oxygenation is compromised.

    Indication. Begin as soon as possible in the patient with PCP when either the PaO_2 on room air is ≤ 70 mmHg or the A–a gradient is ≥ 35 mmHg.

    Dose. 40 mg PO bid (days 1–5), 20 mg PO bid (days 6–10), 20 mg PO every day (days 11–21).

4. **Antiretroviral Agents.** In the long term, HIV-infected patients benefit from antiretroviral therapy; however, it should not be started while the patient is hospitalized for an acute infection. In patients with PCP, antibiotic therapy (e.g., trimethoprim + sulfamethoxazole) can increase the risk of neutropenia with zidovudine.

H. Disposition

1. *Discharge*

  Consider discharging the HIV-infected patient with mild pneumonia if *all* of the following conditions apply:

  a. The patient is not significantly ill.

  b. Oral intake is possible.

  c. Room-air PaO_2 is > 70 mmHg.

  d. The patient is reliable.

  e. The home situation is adequate.

  f. Follow-up has been arranged in 24–48 hours.

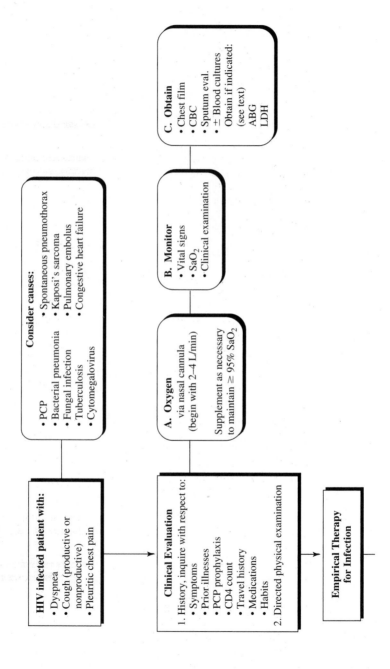

HIV infected patient with:
• Dyspnea
• Cough (productive or nonproductive)
• Pleuritic chest pain

Consider causes:
• PCP   • Spontaneous pneumothorax
• Bacterial pneumonia   • Kaposi's sarcoma
• Fungal infection   • Pulmonary embolus
• Tuberculosis   • Congestive heart failure
• Cytomegalovirus

Clinical Evaluation
1. History, inquire with respect to:
   • Symptoms
   • Prior illnesses
   • PCP prophylaxis
   • CD4 count
   • Travel history
   • Medications
   • Habits
2. Directed physical examination

A. Oxygen
via nasal cannula (begin with 2–4 L/min)

Supplement as necessary to maintain ≥ 95% SaO₂

B. Monitor
• Vital signs
• SaO₂
• Clinical examination

C. Obtain
• Chest film
• CBC
• Sputum eval.
• ± Blood cultures
  Obtain if indicated: (see text)
  ABG
  LDH

Empirical Therapy for Infection

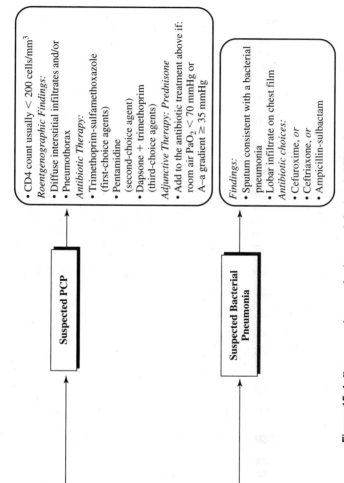

Suspected PCP

- CD4 count usually < 200 cells/mm^3

Roentgenographic Findings:
- Diffuse interstitial infiltrates and/or
- Pneumothorax

Antibiotic Therapy:
- Trimethoprim-sulfamethoxazole (first-choice agents)
- Pentamidine (second-choice agent)
- Dapsone + trimethoprim (third-choice agents)

Adjunctive Therapy: Prednisone
- Add to the antibiotic treatment above if: room air PaO$_2$ < 70 mmHg or A–a gradient ≥ 35 mmHg

Suspected Bacterial Pneumonia

Findings:
- Sputum consistent with a bacterial pneumonia
- Lobar infiltrate on chest film

Antibiotic choices:
- Cefuroxime, *or*
- Ceftriaxone, *or*
- Ampicillin–sulbactam

Figure 15–1. Emergency therapy of pulmonary infections in HIV-infected patients.

369

2. *Admit*

Patients who do not satisfy all of the above discharge criteria should be admitted to the hospital. In addition, patients requiring parenteral pentamidine must be monitored in the hospital (significant side effects may include hypoglycemia, hyperglycemia, prolonged orthostatic hypotension, hypomagnesemia, renal failure, pancreatitis, leukopenia, and cardiac arrhythmias).

III. NEW-ONSET CENTRAL NERVOUS SYSTEM SYMPTOMS OR SIGNS IN THE HIV-INFECTED PATIENT

A. Potential Causes of Central Nervous System (CNS) Symptoms and Signs

1. AIDS-related dementia (the most common neurologic disorder, eventually affecting 40–60% of patients)

2. *Cryptococcus neoformans*

3. Herpes simplex virus

4. Medications (zidovudine [AZT], dapsone, amphotericin, and acyclovir may all cause headaches; zidovudine may also cause confusion)

5. *M. tuberculosis*

6. Primary CNS lymphoma

7. Progressive multifocal leukoencephalopathy (a demyelinating process resulting from papovavirus infection)

8. *Toxoplasma gondii*

9. *Treponema pallidum* (syphilis)

B. Symptoms and Signs

One or more of the following may be present: altered mental status, cognitive decline, headache, seizures, meningismus, fever, focal neurologic abnormalities, and/or visual complaints.

C. Important Historical Questions

Knowledge of the most recent CD4 count is helpful. Opportunistic infection of the CNS is rare when the CD4 count is > 200 cells/mm^3. (See II. C and D, above.)

D. Physical Examination

Perform the physical examination as outlined in II. E, above. In addition, a detailed neurologic evaluation is mandatory:

1. **Mental Status.** Note the patient's level of consciousness, orientation, short- and long-term memory, speech, and basic

cognitive capabilities (e.g., spell "WORLD" backward, count backward by 3 from 20).

2. **Cranial Nerves.** Examine each specifically and include a thorough fundoscopic examination (retinal hemorrhage, edema, and/or fluffy white perivascular retinal lesions are seen with cytomegalovirus [CMV] retinitis).

3. **Musculoskeletal.** Evaluate muscle bulk, tone, joint range of motion, and the strength of major muscle groups. Deep tendon reflexes should also be noted.

4. **Sensory.** Evaluate several modalities (e.g., pain, light touch, and proprioception).

5. **Cerebellar.** General measures of coordination include rapid alternating movements, the finger-to-nose test, and the heel-to-shin test.

Caution: a normal neurologic examination does not exclude meningitis. In cryptococcal meningitis, nuchal rigidity is rare (22% of patients), as is photophobia (18%). A focal examination suggests a CNS mass lesion (e.g., toxoplasmosis, lymphoma, tuberculoma).

E. Laboratory Studies/Diagnostic Tests

1. *Routinely* obtain the following in the HIV-infected patient with new CNS symptoms:
   a. CBC with differential count.
   b. Electrolyte panel.
   c. Glucose level.
   d. Calcium, magnesium, and phosphate levels.
   e. BUN/creatinine levels.
   f. Head CT without and with contrast (or magnetic resonance imaging [MRI] depending on availability).
   g. Lumbar puncture (the CT scan should be done *prior* to the lumbar puncture in the HIV-infected patient: CNS mass lesions are an ever-present concern).
   Note: if the CD4 count is known to be < 300/mm^3, the patient should have an aggressive evaluation, including a CT scan and lumbar puncture with CSF analysis. If the CD4 count is > 300/mm^3 and a non-CNS cause for symptoms and signs is found, then the evaluation may be individualized.

2. Additional studies *may be required* depending on clinical circumstances:
   a. ABG.
   b. Blood cultures (aerobic, fungal, and mycobacterial).
   c. Urinalysis and culture.
   d. Cryptococcal capsular antigen (blood and/or CSF).
   e. *H. capsulatum* antigen (blood and urine).
   f. Serum anti-toxoplasma antibody.
   g. Serum or CSF VDRL test.

3. Laboratory/diagnostic test results:
   a. Imaging studies:
      i. CT scan: the most common finding is diffuse cortical atrophy associated with HIV encephalopathy. The presence of multiple (usually three or more) nodular contrast-enhancing lesions with surrounding edema suggests toxoplasmosis. Nonenhancing lesions are most commonly seen with progressive multifocal leukoencephalopathy. Herpes simplex virus encephalitis is suggested by enhanced cortical uptake on the contrast-enhanced scan.
      ii. MRI: this study is more sensitive than CT but probably less specific. Progressive multifocal leukoencephalopathy reveals characteristic white-matter abnormalities.
   b. CSF: obtain the following studies: cell count and differential, protein, glucose, Gram stain, india ink preparation, AFB stain and culture, cryptococcal antigen, VDRL test, bacterial culture, and fungal culture. *Note:* cell counts are frequently noninflammatory in AIDS patients with cryptococcal meningitis, but CSF cryptococcal antigen is positive in 90% of patients.
   c. Non-CSF cultures: 68% of patients with cryptococcal meningitis also have a positive culture from an extrameningeal source.
   d. Serum cryptococcal antigen: serum cryptococcal antigen is more sensitive (99%) than CSF cryptococcal antigen (90%) in AIDS patients with cryptococcal meningitis.
   e. Toxoplasma titers: 95% of patients with CNS toxoplasma infection have anti-toxoplasma IgG antibody in the serum.

F. Therapy

The therapy of CNS symptoms and signs in the HIV-infected patient is outlined in Figure 15–2.

1. Initial Management

Assess, secure, and support the airway, breathing, and circulation as indicated:

a. Guard the airway, and administer supplemental oxygen.
b. Obtain vital signs, establish IV access, and check the fingerstick glucose level. Order relevant laboratory tests.
c. Treat hypotension with crystalloid resuscitation. If clinical evidence of pulmonary edema (cardiogenic or noncardiogenic) contraindicates fluid administration, administer **dopamine** (2–20 µg/kg/min IV).
d. Administer **thiamine** (100 mg IV), **glucose** (25–50 g IV if the fingerstick glucose level is < 80 mg/dL), and **naloxone** (0.4–2 mg IV) as necessary for the patient with an altered level of consciousness.

2. **Seizure Control:** (also see Chapter 20)

   a. Benzodiazepines are the initial drugs of choice if the patient is actively seizing:
      i. Diazepam (5–10 mg IV, no faster than 2 mg/min; may be repeated in 5–10 minutes if necessary); *or*
      ii. Lorazepam (4 mg IV, no faster than 2 mg/min; may be repeated in 5–10 minutes if necessary).
   b. Additional drugs may include one or more of the following as necessary:
      i. Phenytoin (15–20 mg/kg IV load, no faster than 50 mg/min). Fluconazole and ketoconazole can decrease phenytoin metabolism. Monitor levels carefully. Zidovudine (AZT) can also alter phenytoin levels.
      ii. Phenobarbital (250 mg slowly IV, repeated in 6 hours if needed; in the setting of status epilepticus, give 10–20 mg/kg IV at the rate of 100 mg/min).
   c. Aggressively pursue the cause of new-onset seizures.

3. **Therapy of Specific Conditions**

   a. Toxoplasmosis
      i. Primary therapy: Pyramethamine (200 mg PO loading dose, followed by 1–1.5 mg/kg PO daily [50–100 mg daily]) and sulfadiazine (4-6 g PO daily) and folinic acid (10–50 mg PO daily).
      ii. Chronic maintenance therapy: Pyramethamine (25–50 mg PO daily) and folinic acid (5–20 mg PO daily) and sulfadiazine (500 mg–1 g PO every 6 hours) or clindamycin (300 mg PO qid, if the patient is intolerant of or allergic to sulfadiazine).
      iii. Drug interactions: Pyramethamine may increase bone marrow suppression in patients already taking AZT; anemia worsens when taken with trimethoprim-sulfamethoxazole; sulfadiazine will prolong prothrombin times (PTs) when patients are concomitantly taking warfarin.
   b. Cryptococcal Meningitis
      i. Primary therapy: Amphotericin B (0.3–0.6 mg/kg daily, until fever, headache, and nausea resolve [usually 2-week minimal course]). When amphotericin B is stopped, begin fluconazole at doses of 400 mg PO per day to complete an 8-week course.
      ii. Chronic suppressive therapy: Fluconazole 200 mg PO daily for the life of the patient.
   c. Neurosyphilis
      i. Aqueous penicillin G (2 million units IV every 4 hours for 10 days) or procaine penicillin (2.4 million units IM daily for 10 days).
      ii. Probenecid (500 mg PO bid) should be added to either of the above regimens for the 10 days of treatment.

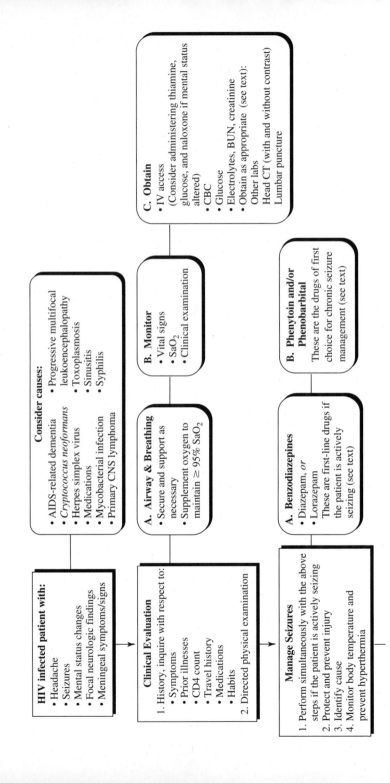

HIV infected patient with:
- Headache
- Seizures
- Mental status changes
- Focal neurologic findings
- Meningeal symptoms/signs

Consider causes:
- AIDS-related dementia
- *Cryptococcus neoformans*
- Herpes simplex virus
- Medications
- Mycobacterial infection
- Primary CNS lymphoma
- Progressive multifocal leukoencephalopathy
- Toxoplasmosis
- Sinusitis
- Syphilis

Clinical Evaluation
1. History, inquire with respect to:
   - Symptoms
   - Prior illnesses
   - CD4 count
   - Travel history
   - Medications
   - Habits
2. Directed physical examination

A. Airway & Breathing
- Secure and support as necessary
- Supplement oxygen to maintain ≥ 95% SaO$_2$

B. Monitor
- Vital signs
- SaO$_2$
- Clinical examination

C. Obtain
- IV access
  (Consider administering thiamine, glucose, and naloxone if mental status altered)
- CBC
- Glucose
- Electrolytes, BUN, creatinine
- Obtain as appropriate (see text):
  Other labs
  Head CT (with and without contrast)
  Lumbar puncture

Manage Seizures
1. Perform simultaneously with the above steps if the patient is actively seizing
2. Protect and prevent injury
3. Identify cause
4. Monitor body temperature and prevent hyperthermia

A. Benzodiazepines
- Diazepam, *or*
- Lorazepam
These are first-line drugs if the patient is actively seizing (see text)

B. Phenytoin and/or Phenobarbital
These are the drugs of first choice for chronic seizure management (see text)

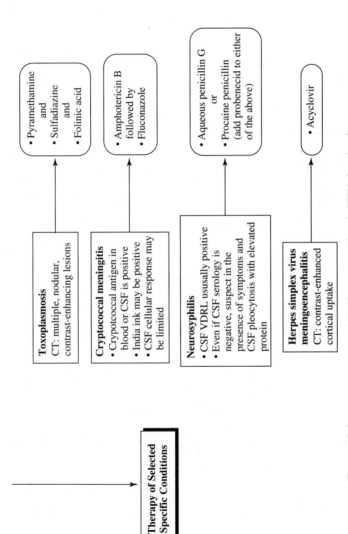

Figure 15–2. Emergency therapy of CNS symptoms/signs in HIV-infected patients.

375

    d. Herpes Simplex Virus Meningoencephalitis.
      i. Acyclovir (10-12 mg/kg IV every 8 hours).

G. Disposition

The patient with AIDS who presents with new or changed CNS symptoms or signs should be admitted to the hospital.

IV. GASTROINTESTINAL COMPLAINTS IN THE HIV-INFECTED PATIENT

A. Gastrointestinal symptoms, especially diarrhea, occur in as many as 50% of North American and European patients with AIDS and in almost 90% of patients in developing countries.

B. Symptoms and Their Causes

1. Painful Oral Lesions

Causes

a. Herpes simplex virus: ulcers are located on the hard palate and lips.
b. *Candida albicans*: erythematous shiny lesions (atrophic candidiasis), or inflammatory erosions, or superficial ulcers with an overlying whitish plaque (thrush). Candidal infection is common when the CD4 count is < $300/mm^3$.
c. Recurrent aphthous ulcers of undetermined cause.
d. Dideoxycytidine (DDC): may cause stomatitis.

2. Dysphagia and Odynophagia Secondary to Esophagitis

Causes

- *C. albicans* (may cause esophagitis even in the absence of oral lesions).
- Herpes simplex virus (HSV).
- Cytomegalovirus (CMV).

a. Dysphagia is more common with candidal infection; odynophagia is more common with CMV or HSV esophagitis.
b. All three diseases occur with CD4 counts < $200/mm^3$ and are rare with higher counts.

3. Abdominal Pain

Causes

a. Acalculous cholecystitis secondary to CMV or *Crytosporidium.* Symptoms may include right-upper-quadrant colicky pain with nausea and vomiting.
b. AIDS cholangiopathy. Symptoms include right-upper-quadrant pain with jaundice.
c. Pancreatitis secondary to medications (didanosine [DDI], pentamidine, dideoxycytidine [DDC], and trimethoprim-sulfamethoxazole). Symptoms may include midepigastric pain and left-upper-quadrant pain.

4. **Gastrointestinal Bleeding**

   a. Occult bleeding may be due to HSV, CMV, candidal esophagitis, or Kaposi's sarcoma of the gastrointestinal tract.

   b. Proctocolitis secondary to HSV, CMV, *Neisseria gonorrhoeae*, or *Entamoeba histolytica* may also cause bleeding.

   c. Massive bleeding is usually due to CMV, gastrointestinal KS, or gastrointestinal lymphoma.

5. **Diarrhea**

   a. Blood in the diarrhea suggests *Campylobacter, Shigella, E. histolitica,* or *Salmonella.*

   b. Watery diarrhea is suggestive of *Giardia, Cryptosporidium, M. avium-intracellulare,* or HIV enteropathy.

   c. Rectal symptoms, including tenesmus, suggest proctocolitis due to *N. gonorrhoeae,* HSV, syphilis, *Chlamydia,* or *Campylobacter.*

   d. Prior antibiotic use suggests *Clostridia difficile.*

C. Important Historical Questions

Review the CD4 count: this is crucial for all decision-making. CMV, *M. avium-intracellulare,* and severe HSV infections are all extremely rare with CD4 counts > $100/mm^3$. (See II. C and D, above.)

D. Physical Examination

Perform the physical examination as outlined in II. E, above.

E. Recommended Diagnostic Approach

1. The basic laboratory evaluation should include the following:
   a. CBC with differential count.
   b. Electrolyte panel.
   c. Glucose level.
   d. BUN and creatinine levels.

2. Further diagnostic testing depends on the patient's presenting complaint:
   a. **Dysphagia.** If oral thrush is present, treat the patient for presumed candidal esophagitis. If oral thrush is absent, consult a gastroenterologist for upper endoscopy.
   b. **Abdominal Pain**
      i. Obtain the following additional laboratory studies:
         • Amylase level.
         • Bilirubin level.
         • Liver function tests (SGOT, SGPT, alkaline phosphatase, PT).
         • Urinalysis.
         • Upright chest roentgenogram and supine and upright abdominal films.

      ii. Upper abdominal pain, or findings suggestive of biliary disease, should be pursued with abdominal ultrasound.

  c. **Gastrointestinal Bleeding**

      i. Check platelet count, PT, and partial thromboplastin time (PTT). Depending on the severity of hemorrhage, serial hematocrits and typed and crossmatched blood may be necessary.

      ii. Consult a gastroenterologist for endoscopy (esophago-gastroduodenoscopy and colonoscopy). At the time of endoscopy samples of luminal fluid and biopsies will be obtained. A radionuclide-tagged erythrocyte scan may assist in localization of the bleeding site(s).

  d. **Diarrhea**

      i. Routinely obtain the following studies:
- Serum magnesium level.
- Stool for fecal leukocytes.
- Culture for enteric pathogens, including *Campylobacter, Salmonella,* and *Shigella.* If the patient has taken antibiotics in the past several months, assay for *C. difficile* toxin.
- Stool for ova and parasites (may require several specimens over time), including *E. histolytica, Cryptosporidium,* and *Isospora belli.*

      ii. Obtain blood cultures in toxic or febrile patients. *Salmonella* may commonly cause bacteremia. If the CD4 count is $< 100/mm^3$ also culture the blood for *Mycobacteria.*

F. Therapy

The therapy of gastrointestinal symptoms in HIV-infected patients is given in Figure 15–3.

1. **Initial Management**

Secure and support the airway, breathing, and circulation as indicated.

a. Provide supplemental oxygen.

b. Supporting ED staff should obtain vital signs and establish IV access. Relevant laboratory tests should be ordered.

c. The HIV-infected patient with diarrhea or gastrointestinal bleeding may be severely volume depleted and may have profound electrolyte abnormalities. Resuscitate with NS or LR infusion; monitor pulmonary status and cardiac function closely.

2. **Treatment of Specific Infections**

a. *Candidiasis*

    i. Oral thrush:
- Clotrimazole troche (10 mg): one dissolved in mouth five times a day for 10–14 days; *or*

- Nystatin pastille (200,000 unit): one or two dissolved in mouth five times per day for 10–14 days; *or*
- Fluconazole (100 mg): one PO daily for 10–14 days (use in refractory or severe cases).

ii. Candidal esophagitis:
- *Fluconazole:* 200 mg PO loading dose, followed by 100 mg PO daily for 21 days; *or*
- *Amphotericin B:* 0.3 mg/kg IV daily for 7–10 days (use in cases refractory to fluconazole).

b. *Oral/Esophageal Herpes Simplex Virus Infections*
- Acyclovir: 200 mg PO five times per day for 7–10 days (exact duration of therapy is determined by clinical response). Severe cases may require intravenous acyclovir (5 mg/kg infused over 1 hour every 8 hours).

c. *Recurrent Aphthous Ulcers*
- Fluocinonide (0.05%, Lidex ointment) mixed with 50% Orabase gel and applied to lesions five times per day; *or*
- Decadron elixir: 0.5 mg/mL used as a mouth wash/rinse two or three times per day.

d. *Infectious Diarrhea*
i. *Salmonella, Shigella,* and/or *Campylobacter:*
- Ciprofloxacin: 500 mg PO bid for 7–10 days. Chronic suppressive therapy may be necessary for patients with *Salmonella* or *Shigella* infections.

ii. *C. difficile:*
- Metronidazole: 250 mg PO qid for 10 days (less expensive agent); *or*
- Vancomycin: 125 mg PO qid for 10 days.

iii. *Isospora belli:*
- Trimethoprim-sufamethoxazole DS (160 mg trimethoprim + 800 mg sulfamethoxazole): one PO qid for 10 days, then one PO bid for 21 days.

iv. *Cryptosporidium:*
- There is no effective antimicrobial treatment (octreotide: 50 μg SQ every 8 hours, with the dose increased to 500 μg SQ every 8 hours, can decrease diarrhea in up to 33% of patients).
- Paromomycin or high dose azithromycin may be beneficial. Consult an infectious disease specialist.

v. *Giardia lamblia:*
- Metronidazole: 250 mg PO tid for 5 days, *or*
- Quinacrine: 100 mg PO tid for 5 days.

vi. *E. histolytica:*
- Metronidazole: 750 mg PO tid for 10 days; then iodoquinol: 650 mg PO tid for 20 days.

vii. Cytomegalovirus:
- Ganciclovir: 5 mg/kg IV twice daily for 14–21 days; *or*
- Foscarnet: 60 mg/kg IV every 8 hours for 14–21 days, then 90–120 mg/kg/day maintenance therapy.

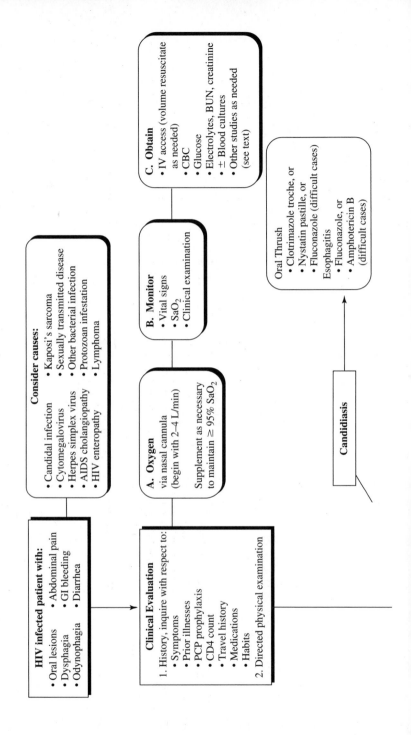

HIV infected patient with:
- Oral lesions
- Dysphagia
- Odynophagia
- Abdominal pain
- GI bleeding
- Diarrhea

Consider causes:
- Candidal infection
- Cytomegalovirus
- Herpes simplex virus
- AIDS cholangiopathy
- HIV enteropathy
- Kaposi's sarcoma
- Sexually transmitted disease
- Other bacterial infection
- Protozoan infestation
- Lymphoma

Clinical Evaluation
1. History, inquire with respect to:
   - Symptoms
   - Prior illnesses
   - PCP prophylaxis
   - CD4 count
   - Travel history
   - Medications
   - Habits
2. Directed physical examination

A. Oxygen
via nasal cannula
(begin with 2–4 L/min)

Supplement as necessary
to maintain ≥ 95% SaO$_2$

B. Monitor
- Vital signs
- SaO$_2$
- Clinical examination

C. Obtain
- IV access (volume resuscitate as needed)
- CBC
- Glucose
- Electrolytes, BUN, creatinine
- ± Blood cultures
- Other studies as needed (see text)

Candidiasis

Oral Thrush
- Clotrimazole troche, or
- Nystatin pastille, or
- Fluconazole (difficult cases)

Esophagitis
- Fluconazole, or
- Amphotericin B (difficult cases)

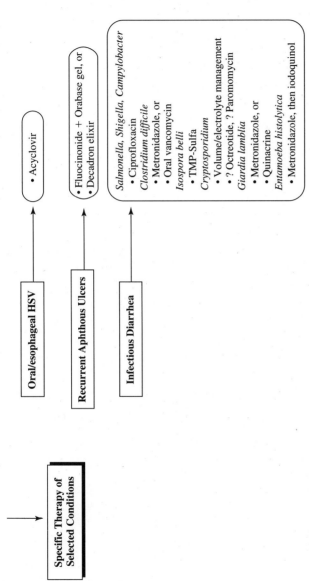

Figure 15–3. Emergency therapy of gastrointestinal symptoms in HIV-infected patients.

381

e. ***Antimotility Agents for Diarrhea.*** If the patient is not febrile and there is no blood or leukocytes in the stool, symptomatic therapy with antimotility agents is appropriate while awaiting further laboratory results (e.g., cultures, stool for ova and parasite examination).
- Loperamide (Imodium): 4 mg PO loading dose, then 2 mg after each stool; maximum dose is 16 mg per day; or
- Diphenoxylate/atropine (Lomotil): 2 tablets PO up to four times per day.

G. Disposition

1. *Discharge*

The HIV-infected patient with a simple or minor gastrointestinal complaint may be discharged from the ED if *all* of the following conditions apply:
a. No serious or life-threatening problem has been identified.
b. The patient's medical status is stable, and vital signs are normal.
c. Oral intake is possible and adequate.
d. The patient is able to care for him/herself, or patient's caretaker is capable of providing appropriate home care.
e. Follow-up or necessary referral has been arranged.

2. *Admit*

Admission is appropriate if *any* of the above conditions are not satisfied. In particular, the following patients must be admitted:
a. The patient with moderate to severe volume depletion, electrolyte abnormalities, or unstable vital signs.
b. The patient who cannot maintain adequate oral intake.
c. The patient with intractable diarrhea.
d. The patient with severe weakness.
e. The patient without adequate home care.

V. PEARLS AND PITFALLS

A. Pneumothorax in an AIDS patient indicates the presence of underlying *Pneumocystis* pneumonia.

B. The patient with HIV disease and oral thrush having a high CD4 count (> 300/mm^3) should be considered at higher risk for other opportunistic infections than would be predicted by the CD4 count alone.

C. Nonhealing ulcers in patients with HIV disease are most commonly due to herpes simplex virus (HSV) infection. Particularly large ulcers due to HSV occur most commonly when the CD4 count is < 100/mm^3.

D. Positive mycobacterial blood cultures can represent either *M. tuberculosis* or *M. avium* complex. Both are usually seen in the setting of CD4 counts < 100/mm^3. Empiric antituberculosis therapy should be started and continued until specific culture results are known.

E. Medications can be a cause of mucosal ulcers in patients with HIV disease. Foscarnet can cause penile ulceration (~5–10%); dideoxycytidine (DDC) can cause oral and esophageal ulceration (13%).

F. Remember to think of acute HIV infection in the patient who presents with fever, rash, lymphadenopathy, and pharyngitis.

BIBLIOGRAPHY

Cohn DL: Bacterial pneumonia in the HIV-infected patient. Infect Dis Clin N Am 1991; 5:485.

The National Institutes of Health—University of California Expert Panel for Corticosteroids as Adjunctive Therapy for *Pneumocystis* Pneumonia: Consensus statement on the use of corticosteroids as adjunctive therapy for *Pneumocystis* pneumonia in the acquired immunodeficiency syndrome. N Engl J Med 1990;323:1500.

Crowe SM, Carlin JB, Steward KI, et al: Predictive value of CD4 lymphocyte numbers for the development of opportunistic infections and malignancies in HIV-infected patients. J AIDS 1991;4:770.

Holtzman DM, Kaku DA, So YT: New onset seizures associated with human immuno-deficiency virus infection: causation and clinical features in 100 cases. Am J Med 1989;87:173.

Phair J, Munoz A, Detels, et al: The risk of *Pneumocystis carinii* pneumonia among men infected with human immunodeficiency virus type 1. N Engl J Med 1990;322:161.

Sande MA, Volberding PA (eds): Medical Management of AIDS. Philadelphia, WB Saunders, 1992.

Scully C, Laskaris G, Pindborg J, et al: Oral manifestations in HIV infection and their management. More common lesions. Oral Surg Oral Med Pathol 1991;71:158.

Smith PD, Quinn TC, Strober W, et al: Gastrointestinal infections in AIDS. Ann Intern Med 1992;116:63.

The Medical Letter Consultants: Drugs for AIDS and associated infections. Med Lett 35(Issue 904);1993:79–86.

White DA, Gold JWM (eds): Medical management of AIDS patients. Med Clin N Am 1992;76:1.

ANIMAL BITES

> *"Beware the Jabberwock, my son!*
> *The jaws that bite, the claws that catch!"*
>
> LEWIS CARROLL

I. ESSENTIAL FACTS

A. General Information

Human and other mammalian bites are important because they are common, may have a substantial risk for infection, and occasionally result in significant tissue injury. The risk of infection depends on the location of the wound, the biting animal, tissue damage incurred, patient characteristics, and time elapsed before treatment (Table 15–3). Unusual pathogens of note may include:

1. *Pasteurella multocida:* a small gram-negative coccobacillus that is commonly carried in the mouths of many animals, including dogs and cats. Wound infections develop within 24 hours of the bite and are characterized by an intense inflammatory response.

2. *Eikenella corrodens:* a fastidious gram-negative rod that is isolated from 30% of human bite wounds. The organism has a predilection to infect heart valves.

3. *Capnocytophaga canimorsus* (DF-2): a rare, slow growing, virulent, gram-negative bacterium that may cause a significant and life-threatening infection (25% mortality rate) after dog bites. Symptoms and signs may begin 3–10 days after the bite incident, and include fever (92% of patients), leukocytosis (65% of patients), dermatologic lesions (petechiae, maculo-papular rash, painful erythema, gangrene), disseminated intra-vascular coagulation (DIC), cellulitis, hypotension (25% of patients), and renal failure (25% of patients).

B. Epidemiology

Over one million mammalian and human bites occur annually in the United States; 80% of these result in only minor injury. Bite

Table 15–3. RISK FACTORS FOR BITE-WOUND INFECTIONS

	LOW RISK	HIGH RISK
Location	Face, scalp, ears, and mouth	Hand, wrist, or foot Scalp (in infants) Over a joint
Wound Type	Large clean lacerations	Puncture wound Nondebridable crush injury
Patient		Age >50 Asplenia Chronic alcoholism Altered immune status Diabetes mellitus Peripheral vascular disease Chronic corticosteroid therapy Prosthetic or diseased car- diac valve Prosthetic joint
Species	Rodents	Domestic cat Human (hand wounds) Primates Pigs

wounds account for 1% of all patient visits to the ED, and 1–2% necessitate hospitalization.

1. **Dog Bites**

   a. Eighty percent of mammalian bites are inflicted by dogs, with an overall infection rate of 15–20%.

   b. Infection is greatest for crush injuries, puncture wounds, and bites to the hand (the latter have an infection rate as high as 40%).

   c. Common infectious agents include *Staphylococcus aureus, P. multocida, Corynebacterium* sp., and alpha-hemolytic streptococci.

2. **Cat Bites**

   a. Three to fifteen percent of mammalian bites are inflicted by cats.

   b. The cat's needle-like teeth result in puncture wounds (frequently involving bone, joints, and deeper fascial layers) with a high incidence of infection ($\approx$ 50%).

   c. *P. multocida* is isolated from > 50% of these wounds.

3. **Human Bites**

   a. Human beings are the third most common cause of mammalian bites. Most of these are sustained in fights, but 15–20% are secondary to "love nips" (i.e., related to sexual activity).

   b. Human bites have traditionally been considered highly infection prone, but this is more a consequence of the bite's location (e.g., the hand) and delays in patient presentation and wound care than it is because of the organisms involved. In fact, human bites in locations other than the hand, if treated promptly, have no greater risk of infection than a dog bite.

   c. Common infectious agents include streptococci, *S. aureus, Corynebacterium* sp., *Bacteroides* sp., and *E. corrodens*. Fifty to eighty percent of wounds yield a mixture of both aerobic and anaerobic bacteria.

   d. A *closed-fist injury* ("fight bite") is a laceration over the metacarpophalangeal joint secondary to striking an opponent's tooth. There is frequently direct inoculation of organisms from the mouth into the bone or joint, leading to osteomyelitis or septic arthritis. In addition, when the fingers of the closed fist are extended, injured extensor tendons retract proximally, sealing off the tissues and setting the stage for a rapidly progressive infection of the tendon and adjacent tissue layers.

4. **Other Bites.** The true incidence of other mammalian bites is uncertain. The bacteriology in the bite wound generally approximates the mouth organisms of the biting animal (Table 15–4).

Table 15–4. UNUSUAL PATHOGENS ASSOCIATED WITH SPECIFIC ANIMAL BITES OR SCRATCHES

ANIMAL	PATHOGEN
Alligator	*Aeromonas hydrophila*[a]
	Citrobacter diversus
	Enterobacter agglomerans
	Pseudomonas
	Serratia
Coyote	*Francisella tularensis*
Cougar	*Pasteurella multocida*
Gerbil	*Streptobacillus moniliformis*
Hamster	*Acinetobacter anitratum*
Lion	*P. multocida*
	Staphylococcus aureus
	E. coli
Opossum	*P. multocida*
Panther	*P. multocida*
Piranha	*A. hydrophila*
Pig	*F. tularensis*
	P. multocida
	Streptococcus agalactiae
	Streptococcus milleri
	Streptococcus equisimilis
	Proteus sp.
	E. coli
	Bacteroides sp.
Polar bear	Unknown ("seal finger")
Rat	*S. moniliformis*[a]
	Spirillum minor[a]
	Leptospira interrogans
	P. multocida
	Coagulase-negative staphylococci
Rooster (peck)	*Streptococcus bovis*
	Clostridium tertium
	Aspergillus niger
Seal	Unknown ("seal finger")
Shark	*Vibrio carachariae*
Squirrel	*F. tularensis*
Tiger	*P. multocida*[a]
	Acinetobacter
	E. coli
	Streptococci
	Staphylococci
	Diphtheroids
Wolf	*P. multocida*

[a]Most commonly isolated pathogens.

5. **Complications.** In addition to tissue damage and local wound infections, complications of bite wounds include the following:
   a. Infectious tenosynovitis.
   b. Osteomyelitis.
   c. Septic arthritis.
   d. Sepsis.
   e. Rabies.
   f. Other systemic diseases: bubonic plague, cat-scratch dis-

ease, leptospirosis, rat-bite fever, tetanus, tularemia, and sporotrichosis.

II. CLINICAL EVALUATION

A. History

Determine the following:

1. Dominant hand and occupation of the patient.
2. Circumstances of the injury: area(s) of the body injured, type of animal, current location of the animal, provoked or unprovoked attack.
3. Time since the injury.
4. Specific complaints resulting from the bite.
5. Comorbid conditions, including significant vascular disease, diabetes mellitus, and other immunocompromising disorders and/or medications.
6. Medication allergies, including antibiotics, analgesics, and anesthetics.
7. Tetanus immunization status.

B. Directed Physical Examination

The physical examination should include the following (assuming that all life-threatening injuries have already been identified and appropriately treated):

1. Thorough inspection of the skin and soft tissues: note the presence/absence of lacerations, punctures, scratches, swelling, crush injury, and/or devitalized tissue.
2. A careful vascular examination: note relevant pulses, skin temperature, and capillary refill.
3. Assessment of the range of motion of all affected areas and careful evaluation of the functional status of potentially involved tendons.
4. Assessment of nerve function (both motor and sensory): sensory function in the hand is best evaluated and documented by noting two-point discrimination on the volar pads of the fingertips (should be ≤5 mm in the axis of the digit; compare with the uninjured side).
5. Evaluation for skeletal injury.
6. In the late-presenting patient, also a careful search for any evidence of local or systemic infection, including regional adenopathy.

C. Laboratory Studies

1. The *minimally injured* patient, presenting with an acute bite, will generally not require a laboratory evaluation. Consider the following studies as needed:
   a. Roentgenograms of the affected area should be obtained in the following circumstances:
      i. A fracture is suspected.

        ii. A potential foreign body is present (e.g., tooth fragment).

        iii. Bone, joint, and/or tendon has potentially been penetrated.

    b. In high-risk wounds (e.g., significant bite wounds to the hand) a Gram stain and culture should be obtained.

2. Consider the following in the *late-presenting* patient with a localized wound infection:

    a. Wound site Gram stain and culture: obtain both aerobic and anaerobic cultures after superficial decontamination (before debridement of devitalized tissues). Optimal cultures are acquired by percutaneous or deep wound aspiration.

    b. ± Complete blood count.

3. The *seriously ill* patient with a bite-wound infection requires a thorough laboratory evaluation that minimally should include the following:

    a. Complete blood count, including platelets.

    b. Electrolyte panel.

    c. Glucose level.

    d. Blood urea nitrogen (BUN) and creatinine levels.

    e. Prothrombin time/partial thromboplastin time (PT/PTT).

    f. Blood cultures (at least two).

    g. Wound-site Gram stain and cultures.

    h. Appropriate roentgenograms.

III. THERAPY

A. Analgesia

Patients in pain should have analgesia provided at the outset. Medication choices are numerous. Commonly used intramuscularly (IM) administered agents in adults include meperidine (1 mg/kg IM) ± hydroxyzine (25-50 mg IM); and/or ketorolac (30-60 mg IM).

B. Wound Cleansing

Thoroughly wash all bites and scratches with soap and water. A mild soap is important to remove the animal's saliva from the wound. At this stage, any grossly apparent particulate matter should also be removed. If the bite was caused by a wild animal (e.g., raccoon, skunk), the wound should subsequently be thoroughly irrigated with 1% benzalkonium chloride, which has been experimentally demonstrated capable of killing the rabies virus.

C. Local Anesthesia

The choice of agent depends on the patient's age, allergy history, and local wound characteristics. In most instances, 1% lidocaine (without epinephrine) is used. Infiltrate the wound edges slowly using a 25-gauge or smaller needle to minimize pain. The maximum dose of lidocaine for local infiltration is 4 mg/kg (0.4 mL/kg of a 1% solution). Lidocaine's tendency to cause tissue burning can be reduced by mixing the lidocaine with an 8.4% sodium bicarbonate solution (1 mL sodium bicarbonate for every 10 mL of lidocaine).

D. Wound Irrigation

Irrigate the wound with copious volumes (500–2000 mL or more, depending on the wound) of normal saline. A 1% povidone-iodine solution can be used in wounds clinically considered to be high risk for infection (Table 15–3). Other disinfectants (e.g., hydrogen peroxide or detergent-based scrubs) are toxic to tissues and should be avoided. The ideal irrigation pressure is 5–8 psi. This is achieved by forcefully pressing on the plunger of a 30-mL syringe equipped with an 18–20-gauge plastic catheter.

E. Debridement

Remove with care any eschar, devitalized tissue, and foreign material. Puncture wounds should have the wound margins excised (approximately a 1–2-mm rim) to allow for improved cleansing and better drainage.

F. Wound Closure

Closure of the wound is controversial in the setting of animal bites. Pertinent considerations include whether the wound will heal satisfactorily without closure, infection risks, and cosmetic considerations. If wound closure is deemed clinically appropriate, subcutaneous sutures should not be used.

1. Fresh (< 24 hours old) *facial bites* without evidence of inflammation may be closed after careful and thorough wound cleansing and preparation.
2. Bites to other areas in need of closure or bites > 24 hours old are best handled by delayed primary closure. *Technique*: thoroughly cleanse the wound, control all bleeding sites, debride as necessary, apply a layer of fine mesh gauze to the wound, pack open, dress, and follow closely; if there is no purulence or wound margin erythema at 3–5 days follow-up, closure may then be accomplished.
3. Infected wounds should be left open.

G. Antimicrobial Therapy

1. Antibiotic prophylaxis (Table 15–5) is recommended for 3–5 days in patients with fresh bite wounds with *any* of the following characteristics:
   a. Cat bites.
   b. Hand bites.

  c. Moderate to severe tissue damage (e.g., crush injury or edema).

  d. Occurring in patients with immunocompromising conditions (e.g., diabetes mellitus).

  e. Potentially involving a tendon, bone, or joint.

  f. Puncture wounds.

2. Infected wounds require empiric antibiotic therapy subsequently guided by aerobic and anaerobic culture results. Amoxicillin + clavulanate (500 mg PO tid for 10 days) is an excellent oral agent for the outpatient treatment of mild local wound infections secondary to dog, cat, pig, or human bites. If parenteral antibiotic therapy is necessary, reasonable initial

Table 15–5. ANIMAL BITE WOUNDS: ANTIMICROBIAL PROPHYLAXIS

SOURCE	DRUG	DOSE	COMMENTS
Cat bites or High-risk dog bites (e.g., hand, considerable tissue damage)	Amoxicillin + clavulanate (Augmentin)	500 mg/125 mg PO tid for 3–5 days	Moderately effective but expensive agent; 10% incidence of GI side effects.
	or		
	Cefuroxime (Ceftin)	250–500 mg PO bid for 3–5 days	Also expensive, but with fewer GI side effects than the above.
	or		
	Penicillin VK *and* Cephalexin or Dicloxacillin* (*addition of latter agents not necessary in cat bites)	500 mg PO qid for 3–5 days 500 mg PO qid for 3–5 days	Less expensive regimen than the above, but requires two antibiotics qid, which is inconvenient.
	or		
	Erythromycin (dogs)	500 mg PO qid for 3–5 days	Use erythromycin or tetracycline only if necessary because of penicillin *and* cephalosporin allergy. Treatment failures may occur.
	or		
	Tetracycline (cats) (or doxycycline)	500 mg PO qid for 3–5 days (100 mg PO bid for 3–5 days)	
Human bites	Amoxicillin + clavulanate (Augmentin)	500 mg/125 mg PO tid for 3–5 days	Probable oral drug of choice in this setting.

Important clinical points: 1. The most important aspect of infection prevention is thorough and meticulous wound care (cleansing, irrigation, and debridement), not antibiotic administration. 2. If antibiotic prophylaxis is deemed clinically appropriate the sooner it is given from the time of the bite, the better the efficacy. 3. In the setting of high-risk wounds (e.g., crush injuries; severe contamination; bone, tendon, or joint exposure) consider immediate administration of a parenteral agent. Possible choices include ceftriaxone (1–2 g IV), ampicillin-sulbactam [Unasyn] (1.5–3 g IV), or ticarcillin-clavulanate [Timentin] (3.1 g IV).

choices include ceftriaxone (1-2 g IV every 12–24 hours), ampicillin + sulbactam [Unasyn] (1.5-3 g IV every 6 hours), or ticarcillin-clavulanate [Timentin] (3.1 g IV every 4-6 hours). Obtain early infectious disease consultation if needed. Osteomyelitis or septic arthritis will require orthopedic consultation, usually an operative procedure, and 4–8 weeks of antimicrobial therapy.

H. Tetanus Immunization

Bite wounds should be considered tetanus-prone injuries. If a patient has already recieved a primary immunization series, but has not recieved a booster in the past 5 years, then an adult tetanus booster should be administered (see Tetanus Prophylaxis, later in this chapter).

I. Rabies Prophylaxis

1. Rabies encephalitis is uniformily fatal once acquired. Fortunately, successful vaccination programs in this country have significantly reduced the incidence of rabies in both domestic animals and humans.

2. About 85% of all cases of animal rabies in the United States now occurs in wildlife. Skunks, raccoons (especially in the mid-Atlantic and Southeastern regions), bats, foxes, coyotes, bobcats, and other carnivores may be afflicted and should be considered rabid unless proven otherwise.

3. The risk of rabies in rodents (e.g., chipmunks, mice, rats, squirrels) and lagomorphs (rabbits) is minute.

4. The likelihood that a domestic dog or cat is infected with rabies varies from region to region. Any questions regarding the need for postexposure prophylaxis should be referred to the local health department or an infectious disease specialist familiar with patterns of the disease in the local area.

5. Rabies prophylaxis recommendations are presented in Table 15–6.

J. Additional Care

1. Elevation of the injured area is essential for several days postinjury.

2. Immobilization for 3–5 days is recommended for all bites over joints. When splinting the wrist and hand, immobilization should be in the proper position: 20 degrees wrist extension, metacarpal-phalangeal joints flexed 70–90 degrees, and proximal interphalangeal and distal interphalangeal joints flexed 10 degrees.

3. Prescribe analgesic medications (e.g., nonsteroidal anti-inflammatory agents ± medium-potency oral opioids).

Table 15–6. SUMMARY OF RABIES PROPHYLAXIS RECOMMENDATIONS

Animal Species	Condition of Animal at Time of Attack	Treatment of Exposed Person[a]
Dog and cat	Healthy and available for 10 days of observation	None, unless animal develops rabies[b]
	Rabid or suspected rabid	RIG[c] and HDCV (or RVA)
	Unknown (escaped)	Consult local public health officials. If treatment is indicated, give RIG[c] and HDCV (or RVA)
Skunk, bat, fox, coyote, raccoon, bobcat, and other carnivores	Regard as rabid unless proven negative by laboratory tests[d]	RIG[c] and HDCV (or RVA)
Livestock, rodents, and lagomorphs (rabbits and hares)	Consider individually. Local and state public health officials should be consulted on questions about the need for rabies prophylaxis. Bites of squirrels, hamsters, guinea pigs, gerbils, chipmunks, rats, mice, other rodents, rabbits and hares almost never call for antirabies prophylaxis.	

[a]*All bites and other wounds should be thoroughly cleansed with soap and water,* followed by copious irrigation with 1% benzalkonium chloride (if available) and then normal saline. If postexposure rabies prophylaxis is indicated, both rabies immune globulin (RIG) and human diploid cell rabies vaccine (HDCV) [or rabies vaccine, adsorbed (RVA)] should be given as soon as possible. Give postexposure prophylaxis *regardless* of the time elapsed since exposure occurred. Pregnancy does not contraindicate rabies prophylaxis. Local reactions to vaccines are common, and they do not contraindicate continuing teatment. Discontinue vaccine if fluorescent-antibody tests for rabies of the sacrificed animal's neural tissue are negative. Dosing:
- RIG: 20 IU/kg. If anatomically possible, one-half the dose should be infiltrated around the wound and the other half given IM (gluteal muscle).
- HDCV: 1 mL IM in the deltoid region on days 0, 3, 7, 14, and 28 (if patient not previously vaccinated).
- RVA: 1 mL IM in the deltoid region on days 0, 3, 7, 14, 28 (if patient not previously vaccinated).
- Individuals previously vaccinated with either HDCV or RA should not receive RIG; they should, however, receive 1 mL IM "booster" doses of either HDCV or RVA on days 0 and 3.

[b]During the usual 10-day animal holding period, begin treatment with RIG and HDCV (or RVA) at the first sign of rabies in the dog or cat that has inflicted the bite. Symptomatic animals should be killed immediately and tested.

[c]If RIG is not available, use antirabies serum, equine (ARS). Do not use more than the recommended dosage in the package insert.

[d]The animal should be killed and tested as soon as possible. Holding for observation is not recommended.

IV. DISPOSITION

A. Discharge

Most bite wounds are minor injuries, and the patient can be discharged to home after thorough and meticulous wound management. Follow-up of all bite wounds within 48 hours is appropriate.

B. Admit

Patients with *any* of the following conditions should be admitted to the hospital for continued daily wound care and inpatient parenteral antibiotic therapy:

1. Systemic manifestations of infection.

2. Severe cellulitis.

3. Failure to respond to appropriate outpatient treatment within 48 hours.

4. Bite-wound infections that involve a bone, joint, tendon, or nerve.

5. Unreliable patients.

Remember to obtain early and necessary consultation as appropriate (e.g., infectious disease specialist, orthopedist, hand surgeon).

V. PEARLS AND PITFALLS

A. In any wound case, carefully assess for neurovascular, joint, tendon, and osseous injury.

B. Improper wound cleansing and failure to appropriately immobilize and elevate the bitten extremity are the most common reasons for subsequent infections.

C. Early orthopedic consultation for closed-fist injuries ("fight bites") is essential.

D. Document and update as necessary the patient's tetanus immunization status.

E. The decision to culture, suture, and/or give prophylactic antibiotics depends on the wound, patient factors, and the animal inflicting the bite.

BIBLIOGRAPHY

Berk WA, Welch RD, Bock BF: Clinical issues in clinical management of the simple wound. Ann Emerg Med 1992;21:72–80.
Chisholm CD: Wound evaluation and cleansing. Emerg Med Clin N Am 1992;10:665–672.
Fishbein DB, Robinson LE: Rabies. N Engl J Med 1993;329(22):1632–1638.
Goldstein EJ: Bite wounds and infection. Clin Infect Dis 1992:14;633–640.
Weber DJ, Hansen AR: Infections resulting from animal bites. Infect Dis Clin N Am 1991; 5:663–680.

BOTULISM

"What is food to one, is to other bitter poison."

LUCRETIUS (99–55 BC)

I. ESSENTIAL FACTS

A. Definition

Botulism is a descending paralysis caused by a neurotoxin elaborated by *Clostridium botulinum.* The toxin is the most potent poison known to affect humans. Of the five different toxins that cause disease in humans (A,B,E,F,G), type A has the highest associated mortality.

B. Epidemiology

Most outbreaks can be traced to home-canned vegetables, fruits, and meat products. The incubation period is usually 18–36 hours but ranges from 2 hours to 8 days.

C. Botulism in Infancy

The entity of *infant botulism* should be considered in "failure to thrive" or a "floppy" baby.

II. CLINICAL EVALUATION

A. History

Usually home-processed food has been ingested in the previous 36 hours. Multiple cases may be present.

B. Signs and Symptoms

A descending bilateral flaccid paralysis is the major feature of the disease. Death is the result of respiratory or bulbar paralysis.

1. Onset of symptoms may be gradual and subtle.

2. Fever is usually absent.

3. Diplopia, dysarthria, dysphagia, dry mouth, and dilated pupils (five Ds; usually at least three of these signs and symptoms are present). Lateral rectus muscle weakness is usually present.

4. Decreased vital capacity may be present.

5. Vomiting and abdominal pain commonly occur.

6. Descending bilaterial paralysis; mental status is usually normal and sensory deficits do not occur.

7. Urinary retention is common.

C. Laboratory Studies

1. Usual tests, including cerebrospinal fluid studies, are not helpful.

2. Detection of toxin in serum, stool, or leftover food requires special procedures. Prior to giving antitoxin, obtain 30 mL of blood and a stool specimen, if possible, for diagnostic testing.

3. Stool and/or food should be cultured for *C. botulinum.*

III. DIAGNOSIS

A. Presumptive diagnosis is clinical.

B. Definitive diagnosis is by identification of toxin in serum, stool, or leftover food.

C. Differential diagnosis includes Guillain-Barré syndrome (ascending paralysis), tick paralysis, cerebral vascular accidents, and myasthenia gravis (botulism patients do not respond to edrophonium [Tensilon]). Electromyography can be useful in differentiating confusing cases.

IV. THERAPY

A. The most common cause of death is respiratory paralysis.

B. Provide oxygen as required. Oxygen saturation (SaO_2) should be continuously monitored with pulse oximetry. Obtain frequent vital capacity readings to monitor the patient's course. Arterial blood gas measurements may be needed, especially for marginal SaO_2. Be prepared for emergency intubation.

C. Give two vials trivalent (ABE) antitoxin (made from horse serum). This can be obtained from most public health departments. Meticulously follow the package insert on sensitivity testing and autitoxin administration. One vial is given intramuscularly (IM) and one intravenously (IV). The IV dose is injected very slowly at a dilution of 1:10. Repeat with two more vials in 2–4 hours if symptoms persist. If the toxin is known, type-specific antitoxin may be used. Anaphylaxis occurs in 3–5% of patients, and hypersensitivity reactions in 20%. If the antitoxin cannot be obtained from the local public health department, it may be obtained from the Centers for Disease Control (M–F, 8 AM–4:30 PM (404) 639–3670; other times: (404) 639-2888).

Tests for skin and eye sensitivity should be performed before any injection.

1. The skin sensitivity test dose is 0.1 mL of a 1:100 saline dilution of the antitoxin given subcutaneously. The reaction is read in 5–30 minutes and is positive if a wheal with hyperemic areola appears. The size of the reaction correlates with the degree of sensitivity.

2. Eye sensitivity tests are performed by instilling a 1:10 dilution of antitoxin with saline in one eye and a control drop of saline instilled in the other. Lacrimation and conjunctivitis appearing in 10–30 minutes is considered an indicator of sensitivity.

D. Lavage the stomach if no respiratory impairment is present. Give an enema unless diarrhea is present.

E. Some authorities recommend a trial of oral quinidine hydrochloride (20–30 mg/kg daily) to enhance acetylcholine release. The patient's cardiac rhythm must be continuously monitored.

V. DISPOSITION

Patients should be hospitalized. Individuals with any degree of neurologic or respiratory impairment must be admitted to an ICU for close monitoring.

VI. PEARLS AND PITFALLS

A. Notify the local and/or state public health department immediately. Other persons may be at risk.

B. Think of wound botulism, though it is an extremely rare condition. The incubation period is longer (4–14 days). Signs and symptoms are the same as those of classic botulism except that there are no gastrointestinal symptoms. Wound botulism occurs in a setting of crush injury or major trauma.

C. Do not assume neurologic findings are symmetrical. They are bilateral but not always symmetrical.

BIBLIOGRAPHY

Arnon SS: Infant botulism. Annu Rev Med 1980;31:541.
Hughes JM, Blumenthal JR, Merson MH, et al: Clinical features of types A and B foodborne botulism. Ann Intern Med 1981;95:442.
MacDonald KL, Cohen ML, Blake PA. The changing epidemiology of adult botulism in the United States. Am J Epidemiol 1986;124:794–799.
Ruthman JC, Hendricksen DK, Bonefield R: Emergency department presentation of type A botulism. Am J Emerg Med 1985;3:203.

CELLULITIS

> *"Webster was much possessed by death
> And saw the skull beneath the skin."*
>
> THOMAS STEARNS ELIOT (1888–1965)

I. ESSENTIAL FACTS

A. Definitions

Cellulitis is a spreading infection of the skin characterized by cutaneous erythema, warmth, and edema. *Erysipelas* is a distinctive type of superficial cellulitis with prominent lymphatic involvement that leads to sharply demarcated raised borders.

B. Epidemiology

Risk factors for cellulitis include

1. Venous insufficiency.

2. Chronic edema.

3. Injection drug use.

4. Alcoholism.

5. Peripheral vascular disease.

6. Diabetes mellitus.

II. CLINICAL EVALUATION

A. History

Inquire about trauma (lacerations, bites, puncture wounds) resulting in a portal of entry. Trauma occurring in water may suggest specific organisms (salt water: *Vibrio* sp.; fresh water: *Aeromonas hydrophilia*). Animal bites (discussed earlier in this chapter) can lead to cellulitis with odd organisms. Pre-existing skin disease (superficial mycoses, vesiculobullous skin disorders, psoriasis, etc.) may also serve as a portal of entry for bacteria.

B. Symptoms and Signs

Local symptoms include tenderness, pain, and erythema at the site of cellulitis. Systemic symptoms may include malaise, fever, and chills. Fever, tachycardia, lymphangiitis, and regional lymphadenopathy may develop. Diffuse erythema, warmth, and edema are common. Bullae may be present.

C. Important Clinical Situations

1. **Periorbital Cellulitis.** Usually the result of eyelid trauma, conjunctivitis, or sinusitis. There is full mobility of the eye without pain.

2. **Orbital Cellulitis.** A suppurative process that involves the orbital structures. The portal of entry is usually an infected sinus or trauma. Eye movements are painful. Proptosis, ophthalmoplegia, and visual changes are important features. Complications of orbital cellulitis are cavernous sinus thrombosis, meningitis, and brain abscess.

3. **Cellulitis Following an Animal Bite.** See discussion earlier in this chapter.

4. **Cellulitis Following Water-Related Injury.** *Vibrio vulnificus* is a slender, curved gram-negative rod that causes cellulitis in the setting of salt water-contaminated wounds. Prominent bullae formation is typical. Cellulitis can also occur as part of a sepsis syndrome due to *V. vulnificus* in patients with liver disease who have ingested *Vibrio*-containing seafood.

   Aeromonas hydrophilia can cause cellulitis in wounds contaminated with fresh or brackish water.

5. **Cellulitis in the Injection Drug User.** *Staphylococcus aureus* is an extremely common cause of cellulitis in injection drug users. Involvement of deeper tissue layers can complicate cellulitis and lead to a surgical emergency in this patient

population. When fascial involvement occurs, anaerobic organisms are commonly implicated.

6. **Cellulitis Following Puncture Wounds.** Puncture wounds through shoes may lead to cellulitis/osteomyelitis due to gram-negative rods, particularly *Pseudomonas aeruginosa.*

D. Directed Physical Examination

The physical examination minimally should include the following:

1. **Vital Signs.** Temperature, pulse, blood pressure.

2. **Skin.** Evaluation of the lesion and its extent of spread. Presence of warmth associated with erythema. Presence of bullous lesions.

3. **Lymph Glands.** Regional or generalized lymphadenopathy.

4. **Heart.** Note whether a cardiac murmur is present.

E. Laboratory Studies

1. A complete blood count (CBC) is generally not needed in afebrile, nontoxic-appearing patients.

2. Blood cultures should be considered in the presence of systemic symptoms or fever and in the patient who will be hospitalized.

3. Wound cultures: culture the lesion if the wound is open. If bullae are present, culture/Gram stain of the bullae fluid is helpful.

4. Obtain a roentgenogram if an overlying ulcer is present or a necrotizing infection is suspected. This is especially important in diabetic patients.

III. DIFFERENTIAL DIAGNOSIS

Fixed drug eruptions, reactions to insect bites, reactions to immunizations, sunburn, superficial thrombophlebitis.

IV. THERAPY

The emergency medical therapy of cellulitis is presented in Figure 15–4.

A. Elevate the affected area if possible.

B. If the infection is in an extremity (e.g., hand), splinting is appropriate.

C. Heat or warm moist packs should be used every 4–6 hours.

D. Administer antibiotics. Most cases of cellulitis involve group A beta-hemolytic streptococci or *S. aureus.* Penicillinase-resistant

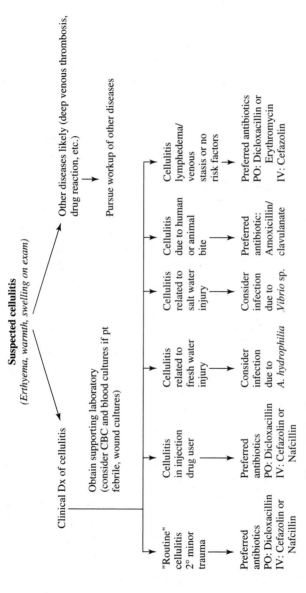

Figure 15-4. Emergency therapy of cellulitis (see Table 15-7 for medication dosing).

399

penicillin, cephalosporin, or erythromycin are usually adequate (Table 15–7). Empiric coverage for other causes of cellulitis should be considered in special situations. The penicillin-allergic patient with cellulitis can be given erythromycin, trimethoprim-sulfamethoxazole, or clindamycin. Oral antibiotics can be dosed at "skin dose" (i.e., dicloxacillin 250 mg qid, erythromycin 250 mg qid), unless cellulitis is severe or is accompanied by systemic symptoms.

E. Administer analgesia. Cellulitis is frequently exquisitely tender and appropriate pain medications (e.g., acetaminophen, acetaminophen with codeine, or oxycodone) should be prescribed.

V. DISPOSITION

A. Discharge

Many patients with cellulitis can be managed as outpatients. Reliable patients who are not systemically ill can be given a trial of outpatient therapy. The extent of the cellulitis should be marked on the skin. Close follow-up in 24 hours is needed to determine the response to antibiotics. Good candidates for outpatient therapy are young adults, patients without systemic symptoms/fever, and patients with a proven record of compliance. At the time of the follow-up visit, if the cellulitis is not improving, admission is appropriate.

B. Admit

The following situations necessitate admission:

1. Facial cellulitis.

2. Orbital/periorbital cellulitis.

3. Cellulitis due to *Vibrio* or *Aeromonas* spp.

4. Toxic on presentation, fever $\geq 38.5°C$.

5. Underlying diabetes mellitus.

6. Concern for noncompliance (alcoholism) or homelessness.

VI. PEARLS AND PITFALLS

A. Tetanus immunization status should be ascertained in all patients and updated if appropriate.

B. Clinical improvement is indicated by decreased pain, swelling, and erythema. Occasionally, erythema may initially worsen and does not necessarily indicate a treatment failure as long as pain and swelling are improved. It is usually due to the killing of organisms and release of bacterial enzymes.

C. In the patient with recurrent cellulitis, look for evidence of tinea pedis. Simple treatment of tinea may prevent recurrences of cellulitis by eradicating the portal of entry of the bacteria.

Table 15–7. ANTIBIOTIC THERAPY OF CELLULITIS

CLINICAL SITUATION	SUSPECTED ORGANISM	ANTIBIOTIC CHOICES
Lymphedema, venous stasis, minor trauma, lymphangitis present on examination	Beta-hemolytic streptococci	PO: Dicloxacillin 250–500 mg PO qid Erythromycin 250–500 mg PO qid IV: Cefazolin 1 g IV every 8 hours Nafcillin 1 g IV every 4–6 hours Incise and drain abscess if present.
Injection drug users, clinical evidence of abscess (no evidence of endocarditis—patient not systemically ill).	S. aureus	PO: Dicloxacillin 250–500 mg PO qid Erythromycin 250–500 mg PO qidIV: Cefazolin 1–2 g IV every 8 hours Nafcillin 1–2 g IV every 4–6 hours Vancomycin 1 g IV every 12 hours
Fresh- or brackish water-related injuries	A. hydrophilia	PO: Ciprofloxacin 500 mg PO bid Trimethoprim-sulfamethoxazole (160 mg/800 mg) PO bid IV: Ceftriaxone 1 g IV every 12 hours Ciprofloxacin 400 mg IV every 12 hours Imipenem 500 mg IV every 6 hours
Salt water-related injuries	Vibrio sp.	PO: Doxycycline 100 mg PO bid IV: Doxycycline 100 mg IV every 12 hours Choramphenicol 1 g IV every 6 hours
Cellulitis associated with bite wounds		
Dog/cat	S. aureus P. multocida Streptococcus spp. Capnocytophaga canimorsus (DF2)	PO: Amoxicillin/clavulanate (Augmentin) 250–500 mg PO every 8 hours Cefuroxime 250–500 mg PO every 12 hours IV: Ampicillin/sulbactam 1.5–3.0 g IV every 6 hours Ceftriaxone 2 g IV every 24 hours

Table continued on following page

Table 15–7. ANTIBIOTIC THERAPY OF CELLULITIS *Continued*

CLINICAL SITUATION	SUSPECTED ORGANISM	ANTIBIOTIC CHOICES
Human bite	*S. aureus* *S. viridans* Group A streptococci *Eikenella corrodens* Anerobes	PO: Amoxicillin/clavulanate 250–500 mg every 8 hours IV: Ampicillin/sulbactam 1.5–3.0 g IV every 6 hours
Cellulitis associated with diabetic foot ulcer	Group A streptococci *S. aureus* gram-negative rods Panaerobes	IV: Cefoxitin 2 g IV every 6–8 hours Cefotetan 1–2 g IV every 12 hours Ticarcillin-clavulanate 3.1 g IV every 4–6 hours Ciprofloxacin 400 mg IV every 12 hours + Clindamycin 600–900 mg IV every 8 hours

BIBLIOGRAPHY

Caputo GM, Cavanagh PR, Ulbrecht JS, et al: Assessment and management of foot disease in patients with diabetes. N Engl J Med 1994;331(13):854–860.

Hill MK, Sanders CV: Localized and systemic infection due to vibro species. Inf Dis Clin N Am 1987;3:687.

Leum DP: Skin and soft tissue infections in intravenous drug abusers. In Levine DP, Sobel JD (ed): Infections in Intravenous Drug Abusers. New York, Oxford University Press, 1991; pp. 183–206.

Steinberg DG, Stollerman GH: Dangerous pyogenic skin infections. Hosp Pract 1989;24:95.

INFECTIVE ENDOCARDITIS

"There is an awful warmth about my heart like a load of immortality."

JOHN KEATS (1818)

I. ESSENTIAL FACTS

A. Definition

Infective endocarditis (IE) is a microbial infection of the heart valves or, less commonly, the endocardium. Most infections are caused by bacteria and are associated with continuous bacteremia.

B. Epidemiology

1. Bacterial causes and underlying cardiac pathology in IE have changed markedly over the past several decades. This change is attributable to several factors:

   a. The advent of antimicrobial therapy.

      b. Decreasing frequency of rheumatic heart disease.

      c. Increasing frequency of injection drug use.

2. Risk factors include

      a. Underlying heart disease (valvular, rheumatic, congenital).

      b. Injection drug use.

      c. Prosthetic cardiac valves.

      d. Recent procedures (dental, urologic, gynecologic, or gastrointestinal manipulations).

C. Classification

1. **Native-Valve Endocarditis.** Approximately 70% of patients have an underlying structural abnormality: mitral valve prolapse (30%), degenerative lesions of the aorta and/or mitral valves (20%), congenital heart disease (13%), rheumatic heart disease (6%), and hypertrophic cardiomyopathy (5%) (Fig. 15–5).

2. **Injection Drug Use-Associated Endocarditis.** Approximately 70% of patients are without structural heart disease (Fig. 15–6).

3. **Prosthetic-Valve Endocarditis**

      a. Early prosthetic-valve endocarditis (within 2 months of replacement) is usually a consequence of operative contamination.

      b. Late prosthetic-valve endocarditis (> 2 months after replacement) is more commonly associated with incidental bacteremia (procedures, intravenous (IV) catheter infection, etc.)

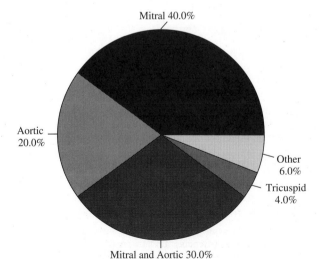

Figure 15–5. Valves affected in native-valve endocarditis.

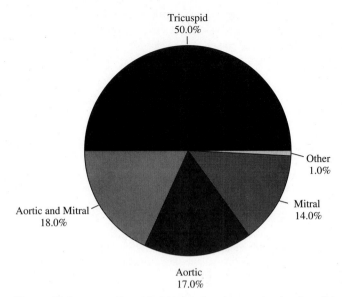

Figure 15–6. Valves affected in injection drug use-associated endocarditis.

4. **Indolent (Subacute) Endocarditis.** This is an episode of IE that involves less virulent organisms and is manifested by constitutional symptoms (malaise, arthralgias, anorexia). The patient is initially medically stable without any complications from the endocarditis (abscess, significant embolization, conduction abnormality, congestive heart failure [CHF]).

II. CLINICAL EVALUATION

The evaluation of IE is presented in Figure 15–7.

A. History

Determine any history of underlying heart disease; the presence of prosthetic valves; injection drug use; recent dental, urologic, gynecologic, or gastrointestinal procedures; history of rheumatic fever; and history of recent antibiotic usage.

B. Symptoms

The older classification of acute and subacute does not identify specific causes or give treatment for each type of endocarditis. Nonetheless, the following are generally true:

1. Infections with less virulent pathogens (e.g., *Streptococcus viridans,* enterococci) tend to be insidious and present with fatigue, malaise, arthralgias, weight loss, and anorexia.

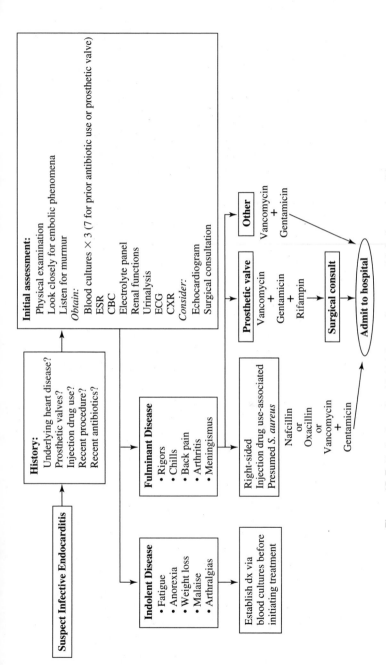

Figure 15–7. Evaluation of and initial therapy for suspected infective endocarditis.

2. Infections with virulent bacteria (e.g., *Staphylococcus aureus, Streptococcus pneumoniae*) more often present with rigors, chills, meningismus, back pain, and arthritis.

3. Relying on the presence of "classic" diagnostic criteria will result in most cases being missed.

4. Elderly patients have fewer symptoms and a diminished febrile response to IE.

C. Signs

More than 50% of patients with IE have fever, a heart murmur, and embolic phenomena. Fewer than 25% will have the "classic" signs (Osler's nodes, Janeway's lesions, Roth's spots), although approximately 50% have some skin findings. (Table 15–8; also see Infectious Causes of Arthritis in Chapter 22.)

D. Laboratory Studies

1. **Blood Cultures.** The principal diagnostic test for IE. Success of pathogen recovery depends primarily on the volume of blood cultured. Timing of cultures is not important because bacteremia is continuous. The most common reason for "culture-negative" endocarditis is prior antibiotic treatment.
   a. Three blood cultures should be obtained for suspected native-valve endocarditis.

Table 15–8. SYMPTOMS AND PHYSICAL FINDINGS OF INFECTIVE ENDOCARDITIS

SYMPTOMS	PERCENT (%)	PHYSICAL FINDINGS	PERCENT (%)
Fever	80	Fever	90
Chills	40	Heart murmur	85
Weakness	40	Changing murmur	5–10
Dyspnea	40	New murmur	3–5
Sweats	25	Embolic phenomena	> 50
Anorexia	25	Skin manifestations	50
Weight loss	25	Osler's nodes	10–23
Malaise	25	Splinter hemorrhages	15
Cough	25	Petechiae	20–40
Skin lesions	20	Janeway's lesions	< 10
Stroke	20	Splenomegaly	20–57
Nausea and vomiting	20	Septic complications (pneumonia,	20
Headache	15	meningitis, etc.)	
Myalgia and arthralgia	15	Mycotic aneurysms	20
Edema	15	Clubbing	12–52
Chest pain	15	Retinal lesion	5–10
Delirium and coma	10	Signs of renal failure	10–15
Hemoptysis	10		
Back pain	10		
Abdominal pain	10–15		

From Hook EW: Infective endocarditis. In Cummins RO, Eisenberg MS (eds): Blue Book of Medical Diagnosis. Philadelphia, WB Saunders, 1986, p. 307.

b. Seven blood cultures should be obtained over time for patients with subacute symptoms and those having had prior antibiotic treatment or valve replacement.

2. **Immune Mediators.** Most patients with IE will have anemia, and the majority will have an elevated erythrocyte sedimentation rate (mean: 57 mm/hr). Other mediators are less useful.

3. **Urinalysis.** Approximately 50% of all IE patients will have microscopic hematuria or erythrocyte casts.

4. **Electrocardiography.** The electrocardiogram (ECG) may be useful for detecting conduction abnormalities caused by myocardial abscess.

5. **Chest Roentgenography.** Useful to detect CHF, and it may help to identify a specific cause (e.g., multiple "cannonball" emboli in the lungs seen with *S. aureus* endocarditis of the tricuspid valve).

6. **Echocardiography.** Not necessary for the diagnosis. Positive predictive value is 70%, negative predictive value is 80%. If a vegetation is visualized, however, the prognosis may be worse.

E. Special Cases

1. **Right-Sided *S. aureus* Injection Drug Use-Associated Endocarditis.** Patients have an aggressive endocarditis, with fevers, chills, and chest pain. A systolic murmur is common, as are septic pulmonary emboli on chest films. Prognosis is favorable and surgical intervention is seldom needed.

2. **Endocarditis in the Elderly.** The elderly have fewer symptoms and diminished febrile response to IE. They are much more likely to acquire IE after invasive urologic, gastrointestinal, or vascular procedures. A specific cause, *Streptococcus bovis,* may be associated with lesions of the colon (such as carcinoma) in this group. Mortality for IE is higher in the elderly.

3. **Prosthetic-Valve Endocarditis.** These patients often present with cardiac decompensation manifested as CHF or progressive cardiac conduction abnormalities. Surgical intervention is often required. Mortality is high.

III. DIFFERENTIAL DIAGNOSIS

Includes acute rheumatic fever with carditis, collagen vascular disease (especially systemic lupus erythematosus), atrial myxoma, nonbacterial thrombotic endocarditis, paraneoplastic disease (especially hypernephroma), and *S. aureus* bacteremia without endocarditis.

Table 15–9. EMERGENCY MEDICAL THERAPY
OF INFECTIVE ENDOCARDITIS

DISEASE	DRUG	DOSAGE	COMMENTS
Indolent endocarditis	None emergently		Obtain serial blood cultures to confirm diagnosis
Fulminant endocarditis			
Presumed *S. aureus* in IDU-associated endocarditis			
Standard	Nafcillin or	2 g IV q 6 hr	Do not give antibiotics until blood cultures are obtained
	Oxacillin or	2 g IV q 4 hr	
	Vancomycin and	0.5 g IV q 6 hr	
	Gentamicin	1–1.5 mg/kg IV q 8 hr	
Potential for methicillin-resistant *S. aureus*	Vancomycin	0.5 IV q 6 hr	
Other IDU-associated or native-valve endocarditis	Vancomycin and	0.5 g IV q 6 hr	
	Gentamicin	1–1.5 mg/kg IV q 8 hr	
Prosthetic-valve endocarditis	Vancomycin and	0.5 g IV q 6 hr	Surgical consultation
	Gentamicin and	1–1.5 mg/kg IV q 8 hr	
	Rifampin	300–600 mg PO q 12 hr	

Fulminant Endocarditis with Complications

(CHF, perivalvular invasion, conduction abnormality, significant embolization)

Above *plus* surgical consultation

IDU, injection drug user.

IV. THERAPY

A. Initial Management

Assess, secure, and support the airway, breathing, and circulation as clinically necessary (see Chapter 1. II).

B. Antimicrobial Therapy

Begin empiric antibiotic therapy after obtaining blood cultures (Table 15–9). Ultimately, effective treatment requires identification of the causative agent.

C. Surgical Therapy

Debridement of infected perivalvular tissue and/or valve replacement may be necessary. Obtain surgical consultation as needed.

V. DISPOSITION

    A. Admission is mandatory in all cases of acute endocarditis.

    B. Injection drug users with a fever should be admitted until endocarditis can be ruled out.

VI. PEARLS AND PITFALLS

    A. Have a high index of suspicion, especially in patients with a history of weight loss, anorexia, low-grade fever, and malaise.

    B. Obtain early surgical consultation in prosthetic valve endocarditis or endocarditis associated with CHF, conduction abnormalities, perivalvular invasion, significant embolus, or echocardiographically demonstrable large or unstable vegetations.

    C. Inquire about antecedent dental, urologic, gynecologic, or gastrointestinal procedures.

    D. Obtain an ECG to look for conduction abnormalities.

    E. Obtain blood cultures prior to antibiotic treatment.

BIBLIOGRAPHY

Delaney KA: Endocarditis in the emergency department. Ann Emerg Med 1991;20:405–413.

Hecht SR, Berger M: Right-sided endocarditis in intravenous drug users. Ann Intern Med 1992; 117:560–566.

Terpening MS, Buggy BP, Kauffman CA: Infective endocarditis: clinical features in young and elderly patients. Am J Med 1987;83:626–634.

Threlkeld MG, Cobbs CG: Infectious disorders of prosthetic valves and intravascular devices. Chapter 62. In Mandell GL, Douglas RG, Bennett JE (eds): Principles and Practice of Infectious Disease. New York, Churchill Livingstone, 1994.

ADULT EPIGLOTTITIS

> *"It's as if the morbid condition was an evil creature which,*
> *when it found itself closely hunted,*
> *flew at the throat of its pursuer."*
>
> SIR ARTHUR CONAN DOYLE

I. ESSENTIAL FACTS

A. Definition

    Epiglottitis is an infection of the epiglottis and/or supraglottic structures. It can result in complete airway obstruction and death.

B. Epidemiology

    1. Epiglottitis has a bimodal age distribution. The classic description of the disease is in children (ages 3–7). In the last two decades, however, adult epiglottitis has been increasingly

recognized as an uncommon and occasionally lethal entity with a peak occurrence in patients aged 20–40 years.

2. *Hemophilus influenzae* is the most commonly identified bacterial pathogen in both children and adults. Other causative agents include *Staphylococcus aureus,* various streptococci, *Candida albicans,* and viruses. In many cases, there is no identifiable pathogen.

3. In the adult population, studies reveal overall mortality rates of 6–7% (usually from acute airway obstruction).

II. CLINICAL EVALUATION

A. History

In the pediatric patient, acute epiglottitis is characteristically of short duration (< 24 hours) and dramatic presentation. In the adult, the illness is more varied. Some patients present within 8 hours of symptom onset in marked distress with impending airway compromise. These fulminant cases are usually due to *H. influenzae.* Others present with a more gradual onset of mild to moderate symptoms and are probably at less risk for airway obstruction.

B. Symptoms and Signs

The two predominant symptoms are dysphagia and sore throat. Other symptoms may include odynophagia, a muffled "hot potato" voice, drooling (< 25% of adults), hoarseness, and/or respiratory distress. Patients commonly are febrile (~38°C) and may be tachycardic or tachypneic. The pharynx may appear benign. (*Note:* the "classic" pediatric patient with epiglottitis is toxic-appearing, sitting up, leaning forward, drooling, and with stridor.)

C. Physical Examination

1. **General.** Note the patient's overall toxicity and position of maximal comfort. Have a bag–valve oxygen mask, intubation and cricothyrotomy equipment, and suction set up at the bedside before proceeding with the examination. The examination should be done carefully and delicately. *Do not agitate the patient or cause discomfort in any way.*

2. **Vital Signs.** Check for fever, tachycardia, and tachypnea.

3. **HEENT and Neck.** Gently palpate for cervical adenopathy and laryngeal tenderness; visually inspect the mouth and pharynx for signs of pharyngitis. Do *not* manipulate the oropharynx or use a tongue blade to examine the posterior pharynx of moderately ill or toxic patients (pediatric or adult) as you may precipitate complete airway obstruction.

4. **Lungs.** Listen for wheezes, rales, and/or rhonchi. Note any

signs of increased respiratory effort (e.g., accessory muscle use and intercostal retractions).

5. **Extremities.** Evaluate for cyanosis and capillary refill.

D. Monitoring and Laboratory Studies

1. In the adult patient, obtain the following if possible:
   a. Complete blood count (CBC) and differential.
   b. Blood cultures.
   c. Intravenous (IV) access.
   d. Continuous oxygen saturation (SaO_2) monitoring.
2. Soft-tissue lateral neck roentgenograms may show evidence of epiglottic swelling (e.g., thumblike appearance of the epiglottis), ballooned hypopharynx, swollen aryepiglottic folds, and/or prevertebral soft tissue swelling. The sensitivity of neck films in adults is 75–95%. A normal lateral neck film, however, does *not* rule out epiglottitis. *Caution:* the ill patient with suspected epiglottitis must not leave the ED. Do not send the stable patient to radiology unless accompanied by a physician with necessary airway management equipment (oxygen, bag–valve mask, intubation tray, and cricothyrotomy equipment).
3. Endoscopy/indirect laryngoscopy performed by the consultant otolaryngologist definitively establishes the diagnosis of epiglottitis/supraglottitis. Findings may include a "classic" cherry-red and edematous epiglottis or supraglottic swelling. *Cautions:* the moderately ill or toxic patient with suspected epiglottitis should have laryngoscopy performed in the operating room suite with anesthesia, surgical staff, and all needed airway equipment available. Stable patients, without any evidence of airway compromise or respiratory distress (e.g., stridor, drooling or wheezing), who have normal soft tissue neck films, may undergo either indirect laryngoscopy or fiberoptic endoscopy in the ED by the otolaryngologist. Again, all necessary airway management equipment should be available.

III. DIFFERENTIAL DIAGNOSIS

A. Acute thyroiditis

B. Angioedema

C. Croup

D. Foreign body

E. Peritonsillar abscess

F. Pharyngitis

G. Retropharyngeal abscess

H. Tonsillitis

I. Traumatic conditions

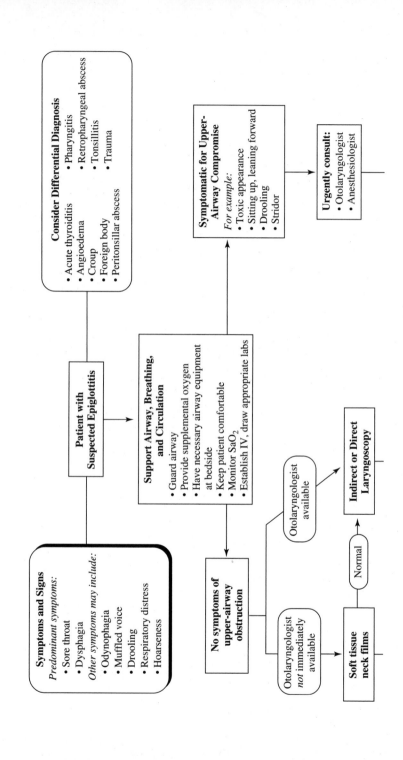

Symptoms and Signs
Predominant symptoms:
• Sore throat
• Dysphagia
Other symptoms may include:
• Odynophagia
• Muffled voice
• Drooling
• Respiratory distress
• Hoarseness

Patient with Suspected Epiglottitis

Consider Differential Diagnosis
• Acute thyroiditis
• Angioedema
• Croup
• Foreign body
• Peritonsillar abscess
• Pharyngitis
• Retropharyngeal abscess
• Tonsillitis
• Trauma

Support Airway, Breathing, and Circulation
• Guard airway
• Provide supplemental oxygen
• Have necessary airway equipment at bedside
• Keep patient comfortable
• Monitor SaO$_2$
• Establish IV, draw appropriate labs

Symptomatic for Upper-Airway Compromise
For example:
• Toxic appearance
• Sitting up, leaning forward
• Drooling
• Stridor

Urgently consult:
• Otolaryngologist
• Anesthesiologist

No symptoms of upper-airway obstruction

Otolaryngologist available

Otolaryngologist *not immediately available*

Indirect or Direct Laryngoscopy

Soft tissue neck films

Normal

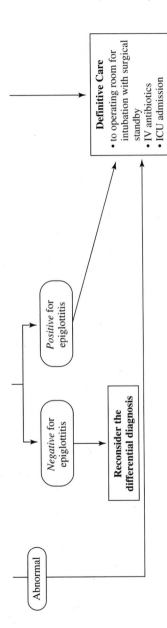

Figure 15—8. ED evaluation of and therapy for adult epiglottitis.

413

IV. THERAPY

Figure 15–8 presents the ED management of adult epiglottitis.

A. Initial Management

Support the airway, breathing, and circulation.

1. Guard the airway, have suction and necessary intubation/ cricothyrotomy equipment at the bedside, and provide supplemental oxygen.

2. Urgently consult necessary specialties (e.g., otolaryngology and anesthesiology).

3. *Airway management is the crucial treatment priority.* Pediatric patients are kept comfortable and subsequently intubated *in the operating room* by anesthesia with a surgical team present. The moderately ill or toxic adult patient with any suggestion of respiratory compromise should be treated in a similar fashion.

4. *Simultaneously* with the above, supporting ED staff should initiate continuous monitoring of SaO_2, obtain vital signs, establish IV access, and obtain needed blood work (do not distress the patient in any way).

5. *Caution:* do *not* attempt intubation in the ED unless the patient has a respiratory arrest; in that case, also stat page an anesthesiologist and otolaryngologist.

B. Antibiotics

Urgent empiric treatment with parenteral antibiotics is indicated; cultures will take several days and in many cases will be negative. Antibiotic choices for the adult include any of the following:

1. Cefotaxime 2 g IV every 6 hours.

2. Ceftriaxone 1-2 g IV every 12 hours.

3. Ceftizoxime 2 g IV every 8 hours.

4. Cefuroxime 1.5 g IV every 6 hours.

5. Ampicillin (2 g IV every 6 hours) *and* chloramphenicol (50-100 mg/kg/day in divided doses every 6 hours).

C. Corticosteroids

Corticosteroids have been used in many institutions, but there are no randomized controlled trials proving their benefit.

D. Post-ED Management

Arrange for ICU admission.

V. DISPOSITION

Any patient with proven epiglottitis should be admitted to the ICU.

VI. PEARLS AND PITFALLS

A. Consider epiglottitis in any patient with severe dysphagia or odynophagia, especially if the pharynx is benign or the patient is returning to the ED after a previous evaluation for sore throat/pharyngitis.

B. Airway management is the highest treatment priority. Adult patients who require intubation (in the operating room with an anesthesiologist and a surgical team available) include those with obstructive airway symptoms, difficulty with oral secretions or swallowing, significant supraglottic swelling, or otherwise significant toxicity (e.g., marked leukocytosis and/or high fever).

Do *not* do any of the following:

A. Manipulate the oropharynx or airway of any patient (child or adult) if he/she is toxic or has evidence of upper-airway compromise.

B. Leave suspected epiglottitis patients alone in either the ED or radiology suite.

BIBLIOGRAPHY

Baxter FJ, Dunn GL: Acute epiglottitis in adults. Can J Anaesth 1988;35(4):428.
Fontanarosa PB, Polsky SS, Goldman GE: Adult epiglottitis. J Emerg Med 1989;7:223.
Murrage KJ, Janzen VD, Ruby RR. Epiglottitis: adult and pediatric comparisons. J Otolaryngol 1988;17(4):194.
Rivron RP, Murray J: Adult epiglottitis: is there a consensus on diagnosis and treatment? Clin Otolaryngol 1991;16:338.

FOOD-BORNE DISEASE

"He that eats till he is sick must fast till he is well."

ENGLISH PROVERB

I. ESSENTIAL FACTS

A. Definition

Food-borne disease is a broad category of illnesses caused by bacteria, viruses, parasites, chemicals, heavy metals, and/or naturally occuring toxins; the unifying characteristic of these various syndromes is the utilization of foodstuffs for disease transmission. Gastrointestinal symptoms are the most common manifestations of food-borne disease.

B. Epidemiology

1. **Incidence**

    a. There are an estimated 6–81 million cases of food-borne disease in the United States each year. Most of these go unreported because the patient does not seek medical care or a specific cause is never determined.

    b. Some patients are at particularly increased risk of serious illness due to food-borne disease, including the very young, the elderly, diabetics, and the immunocompromised (including human immunodeficiency virus [HIV] infection).

2. **Pathogenesis**

The majority of food-borne illnesses are due to bacterial pathogens, which can cause diarrhea and/or other symptoms via the following mechanisms:

    a. *Enterotoxin production,* resulting in stimulation of adenylate cyclase and the production of a noninflammatory, secretory, watery diarrhea. Fecal leukocytes are uncommon.

        i. Enterotoxins may be either preformed in food or formed in vivo. Examples include diarrhea caused by *Vibrio cholera* and enterotoxin-producing *Escherichia coli.*

        ii. The most common food-borne disease in this country is caused by a protein enterotoxin produced by *Staphylococcus aureus.* Common implicated foodstuffs are meats and cream or custard-filled bakery items. The incubation period is usually 1–6 hours; classic symptoms include vomiting, crampy abdominal pain, and diarrhea (with vomiting more prominent than diarrhea).

    b. *Mucosal invasion,* resulting in an inflammatory diarrhea. Systemic symptoms may include fever and abdominal pain; fecal leukocytes are common. The stool may also contain blood and/or mucus. Examples include diarrhea caused by *Campylobacter, Shigella, Salmonella, Yersinia,* and some *E. coli.*

    c. *Systemic infection,* for example, enteric or typhoid fever caused by *Salmonella* (most commonly *S. typhi* and *S. paratyphi*).

II. CLINICAL EVALUATION

A. History

This is the most important step in identifying food-borne illnesses. Two or more people reporting a similar illness following a communal meal is strongly suggestive of a food-borne disease. A typical scenario is the sudden onset of gastrointestinal symptoms (e.g., nausea, vomiting, abdominal pain, and/or diarrhea) minutes to hours following food ingestion. Risk factors for various types of food-borne illness are foreign travel, daycare exposure, food prepared in metal containers, or ingestion of any of the following: raw (unpasteurized) milk, seafood, shellfish, raw or undercooked meat, poultry or eggs, mushrooms, or home-canned food. Ask the patient to list everything eaten in the last 72 hours. Be sure to inquire about any new foods recently consumed.

B. Symptoms

The different syndromes of food-borne disease may present with a wide variety of symptoms (Table 15–10); gastrointestinal complaints (e.g., abdominal pain or cramping, nausea, vomiting, and/or diarrhea) are the most common. Systemic complaints, depending on disease, may include fever, malaise, and/or headache. Unusual symptoms can include a metallic taste (e.g., in the setting of heavy-metal poisonings) or neurologic symptoms (e.g., in the setting of botulism or neurotoxic seafood poisoning).

C. Physical Examination

1. **Vital Signs.** Note tachycardia, postural vital signs, respiratory rate, and temperature.

2. **HEENT.** The oral mucosa and tongue may reveal evidence of significant dehydration; check the conjunctiva for jaundice.

3. **Chest.** Listen for wheezes, rales, and/or rhonchi.

4. **Heart.** Note degree of tachycardia and listen for murmurs, rubs, or gallops.

5. **Abdomen.** Evaluate for distention, bowel sounds, tenderness, localized peritoneal irritation, and masses. Check for heme in the stool.

6. **Neurologic.** Perform a screening neurologic examination.

D. Laboratory

1. Laboratory evaluation is generally unnecessary for most patients with only acute, mild gastrointestinal symptoms.

2. In the patient with significant toxicity, minimally obtain the following:

   a. Complete blood count (CBC).
   b. Electrolyte panel; blood urea nitrogen (BUN) and creatinine levels.
   c. Magnesium level (in the setting of significant diarrhea).

3. Obtain stool for fecal leukocytes and enteric pathogen culture if diarrhea has been present for > 24–48 hours or if it is accompanied by fever or blood or pus in the stool. Stool assay for *Clostridia difficile* toxin should also be obtained if the patient has been on antibiotics within the past 4–6 weeks.

4. Additional studies may be required, depending on clinical circumstances (e.g., stool for ova and parasite [O and P] examination in the patient with diarrhea after travel).

III. DIAGNOSIS

In most cases, the diagnosis of food-borne disease is made clinically (see Table 15–10).

Table 15–10. CAUSES OF FOOD-BORNE DISEASE

AGENT	ONSET	CLINICAL FEATURES N V D C F B	FECAL LEUKOCYTES	DURATION
Bacterial				
Bacillus cereus				
1. Emetic	1–6 hr	+ +	No	6–24 hr
2. Diarrheal	6–24 hr	+ – –	No	12–24 hr
Campylobacter	2–10 days	+ + + + + + May cause Guillian-Barré syndrome	Yes	7–14 days
Clostridium botulinum	12–72 hr	+ + Symmetrical descending motor paralysis, cranial nerve and respiratory paralysis, death	No	1 day–months
Clostridium perfringens	5–24 hr	+ – + + – –	No	1–2 days
E. coli				
1. Enterotoxin	8–48 hr	+ +	No	1–3 days
2. Invasive	6–48 hr	+ + + + + +	Yes	2–7 days
3. Hemorrhagic (e.g., 0157:H7)	1–8 days	+ + + + – + Hemolytic-uremic syndrome in children	Yes	5–8 days
Listeria	—	Spontaneous abortion, meningitis	No	3–4 weeks
Salmonella	6–72 hr	+ + + + + + Also causes enteric fever	Yes	2–7 days
Shigella	6 hr–7 days	+ + + + + +	Yes	4–7 days
S. aureus	1–6 hr	+ + + + – –	No	24–48 hr
Vibrio parahemolyticus	12–24 hr	+ + + + + –	Yes	1–7 days
Vibrio cholerae	1–5 days	+ + + – – –	No	3–5 days
Vibrio vulnificus	1–36 hours	– – – – + – Soft tissue infections, sepsis	No	May be fatal in 6 hr
Yersinia enterocolitica	1–11 days	+ + + + + – Pseudoappendicitis	Yes	5–14 days
Viruses				
Hepatitis A	15–45 days	+ + – – – –	No	2–4 weeks
Norwalk	1–3 days	+ + +	No	48–72 hr
Rotavirus	1–3 days	+ + + – + –	No	3–10 days

Pathophysiology	Food Source	Diagnosis	Therapy
Preformed enterotoxin	Fried rice	Clinical; culture food	Rehydration ± antiemetics for both syndromes
Enterotoxin	Custards, cereals, sauces, puddings, meatloaf	Clinical; culture food	
Mucosal invasion	Raw milk, meat products, poultry, water	Culture stool	Rehydration; quinolones or erythromycin for moderate to severe cases
Preformed neurotoxin	Improperly canned foods (low-pH vegetables, fruits; meats)	Culture or toxin assay from food, stool, or vomitus	Supportive care and polyvalent antitoxin
Enterotoxin formed in vivo	Meat, gravies, poultry	Culture stool or food source	Rehydration
Enterotoxin	Meats, cheese, seafood, water	—	Rehydration; antibiotics
Mucosal invasion	Cheese, water	—	Same
(Shigella-like toxin)	Raw or undercooked beef, salad, raw milk, water	Culture stool	(Antibiotics not indicated for O157:H7)
Unknown	Soft cheeses, dairy products	Blood culture, CSF culture	Ampicillin, TMP/SMX
Mucosal invasion	Eggs, poultry, meats, fruits, vegetables	Stool culture, blood culture	Rehydration; antibiotics usually not necessary except in severe cases or enteric fever
Mucosal invasion	Potato/egg salad, fecal-oral	Stool culture	Rehydration; quinolone or TMP/SMX
Preformed toxin	Meats, custards, cream fillings, potato/egg salad	Clinical	Rehydration; antiemetics
Unknown	Fish, shellfish	Stool culture, food source culture	Rehydration; supportive care
Enterotoxin	Water, fish, shellfish	Stool culture, food source culture	IV hydration, doxycycline
—	Raw seafood, oysters	Blood culture	Chloramphenicol, tetracycline
Mucosal invasion	Meats, milk	Stool culture	Antibiotics if invasive disease
Fecal-oral	Shellfish (oysters), fruits, salad, water	Serology	Supportive
Mucosal invasion		Radioimmunoassay for IgM antibodies	Supportive
Mucosal invasion	Fecal-oral	Viral antigen in stool	Supportive

Table continued on following page

Table 15–10. CAUSES OF FOOD-BORNE DISEASE *Continued*

AGENT	ONSET	CLINICAL FEATURES N V D C F B	FECAL LEUKOCYTES	DURATION
Protozoans				
Entamoeba histolytica	2 days–months	– – + + + +	Yes	
Cryptosporidium	2–14 days	– + + + + – Chronic diarrhea in HIV+ patients	No	10–14 days in healthy pts
Giardia	1–4 weeks	– – + + – –	No	6 wks–months
Trichinella	1–2 days	– – + – + –	No	GI sx last 2–3 days; later myositis, periorbital edema, fever
Seafood				
Ciguatoxin	1–6 hr	+ + + – – – Paresthesias, blurred vision	No	Days–months
Paralytic shellfish toxin	10 min–3 hr	Headache, dizziness, paresthesias, paralysis, ataxia	No	6 hr–7 days
Scombroid	1–6 hr	Histamine reaction (erythema, urticaria, pruritus, HA, dizziness)	No	3 hr–3 days
Mushrooms				
Muscarine	3 min–3 hr	+ + + + – –	No	—
Amatoxin	6–24 hr	+ + + + + + Hepatic failure, renal failure, death	—	—
Miscellaneous				
Heavy metals (cadmium, copper, iron, tin, zinc)	5 min–8 hr	+ + + Metallic taste to food	No	
Monosodium glutamate (MSG)	3–30 min	Burning sensation in chest, neck, extremities, lacrimation, diaphoresis	No	2 hr

Abbreviations: N, nausea; V, vomiting; D, diarrhea; C, abdominal cramps; F, fever; B, bloody diarrhea.

Adapted from Sack RB, Barker LR: In Principles of Ambulatory Medicine, Baltimore, Williams & Wilkins, 1991.

IV. THERAPY

Most food-borne diseases are self-limited and require only supportive care. Exceptions, however, include amatoxin-containing mushroom poisoning, botulism, cholera, and enteric fever.

A. Initial Management

Secure and support the airway, breathing, and circulation as clinically indicated.

Pathophysiology	Food Source	Diagnosis	Therapy
Mucosal invasion	Water, vegetables	Stool O & P	Metronidazole followed by iodoquinol
	Water, raw milk	Stool O & P	Paromomycin; or high-dose azithromycin
	Water, salad, fruits	Stool O & P	Metronidazole
Mucosal invasion	Undercooked pork, game	Serology	No satisfactory treatment; consult infectious disease
Dinoflagellate-produced toxin	Fish (snapper, barracuda)	Radioimmunoassay for toxin in fish	Supportive
Neurotoxin produced by dinoflagellates	Shellfish	Toxin assay in shellfish	Supportive
Toxin produced by bacteria in improperly stored fish	Fish (tuna, mackerel, bonito, skipjack mahi-mahi)	Histamine level in fish > 20 mg/dL	Supportive (may use antihistamines)
Toxin stimulates parasympathetic nerves	*Amanita muscaria*	Clinical	Atropine
Multisystem cytotoxic effects	*Amanita phalloides* and other *Amanita* spp.	Thin-layer chromatography of mushroom, vomitus, or stool	A B Cs; GI lavage + charcoal; supportive care; liver transplantation for hepatic failure
—	Lemonade, fruit punch, soft drinks (served in metal containers)	Clinical	Supportive
Idiopathic	Chinese restaurant food	Clinical	Supportive

1. Airway and respiratory compromise may be a life-threatening complication of botulism, ciguatoxin, and paralytic shellfish toxin. Provide appropriate airway control and respiratory support as clinically indicated.

2. Volume and electrolyte depletion may be significant. Replace volume losses with IV crystalloid (normal saline or lactated Ringer's solution); manage electrolyte abnormalities as indicated.

B. Adjunctive Therapy

One or more of the following may also be administered:

1. **Antibiotics.** Nonpregnant patients > 18 years old with an inflammatory diarrhea may be empirically started on a quinolone antibiotic (e.g., ofloxacin 300 mg PO bid for 3 days; also see Chapter 5). Antibiotic therapy, however, may prolong the carrier state when diarrhea is caused by *Salmonella*.

2. **Antidiarrheal Agents.** Examples include loperamide (4 mg initially, then 2 mg after each stool up to 16 mg/day) or diphenoxylate/atropine (Lomotil; 15-20 mg/day of diphenoxylate component in three to four divided doses).

   Do not use these drugs if there is clinical evidence of invasive disease (e.g., fever, abdominal pain, or blood in stool).

3. **Antiemetic Agents.** Examples include prochlorperazine (5-10 mg PO tid–qid or 25 mg PR bid), metoclopramide (10 mg PO 30 minutes before meals and at bedtime), or promethazine (12.5-25 mg PO every 4–6 hours).

   These agents can be helpful if the patient has primarily emetic symptoms (e.g., staphylococcal or *Bacillus cereus* food poisoning).

V. DISPOSITION

A. Discharge

Most patients with a clinical syndrome compatible with food-borne disease can be treated in the ED and discharged to home once symptoms have been controlled, volume depletion corrected, and oral intake is possible. Ready access to follow-up is mandatory if symptoms persist or the illness worsens.

B. Admit

Patients unable to take oral fluids and maintain adequate hydration, or those who have profound volume depletion or significant metabolic derangements (e.g., metabolic acidosis or hypokalemia), should be admitted to the hospital for continued IV fluid and electrolyte management and other therapy as indicated. Very young, elderly, or immunocompromised individuals should be evaluated carefully and considered for hospitalization. Patients with potentially life-threatening poisonings (e.g., amatoxin-containing mushroom poisoning, botulism) require ICU admission.

VI. PEARLS AND PITFALLS

A. Beware of the patient with neurologic symptoms. Airway compromise and/or respiratory insufficiency are life-threatening potential complications of botulism, ciguatoxin, and paralytic shellfish poisoning.

B. Volume and electrolyte deficits may be profound and life-threatening; correct volume depletion and electrolyte disorders as appropriate.

C. Consider the possibilities of upper-gastrointestinal hemorrhage and/or inflammatory bowel disease in any patient with bloody diarrhea. Endoscopy may be necessary for definitive diagnosis.

D. *Yersinia* and *Campylobacter* infections may mimic an acute appendicitis ("pseudoappendicitis").

E. Obtain an occupational history. Food-handlers with possible infectious diarrhea should have their stool cultured. Instruct such patients not to work until medical treatment is completed, symptoms have completely resolved, and they are medically cleared to return to work.

F. Discuss with the laboratory any special culture requests (e.g., culture for *E. coli* O157:H7, stool assay for *C. difficile* toxin or *Giardia* antigen).

G. Report to the public health department any notifiable disease. Examples include amebiasis, botulism, cholera; hepatitis A, B, and non-A, non-B; salmonellosis, shigellosis, trichinosis, and typhoid fever.

BIBLIOGRAPHY

Bean NH, Griffin PM, et al: Foodborne disease outbreaks, 5 year summary, 1983–1987. MMWR CDC Surveillance Summaries 1990;Mar 31(1):15.

Guerrant RL, Bobak DA: Bacterial and protozoal gastroenteritis. N Engl J Med 1991; 325(5):327.

Neil MA, Osterholm MT, Swerdlow DL: New threats from foodborne infections. Patient Care 1994;28(12):47.

Sack RB, Barker LR: Acute gastroenteritis and associated conditions. Chapter 26. In Barker LR, Burton JR, Zieve PD (eds): Principles of Ambulatory Medicine. 3rd Ed. Baltimore, Williams & Wilkins, 1991, pp. 281–290.

Sanders WE: Intoxications from the seas: ciguatera, scombroid, and paralytic shellfish poisoning. Infect Dis Clin N. Am 1987;1(3):665.

COMMON HAND INFECTIONS

> *Mercutio: Go villain, fetch a surgeon.*
> *Romeo: Courage, man. The hurt cannot be much.*
> *Mercutio: No, 'tis not so deep as a well, nor so wide as a church door; but 'tis enough, 'twill serve. Ask me tomorrow, and you shall find me a grave man.*

WILLIAM SHAKESPEARE (1564–1616)

I. PARONYCHIA AND EPONYCHIA

A. Definition

Paronychia is an inflammatory condition of the radial or ulnar lateral nail fold. *Eponychia* is the term used when the same condition exists under the basal nail fold (cuticle).

B. Pathogenesis and Etiology

Recurrent trauma, such as with manipulation of the cuticle, introduction of a foreign body, and moisture, predispose to invasion by pathogenic organisms, typically gram-positive cocci (especially *Staphylococcus aureus*), and also fungi and yeast.

C. Clinical Picture

The patient typically has tenderness, erythema, warmth and edema of the involved nail fold(s). Often a collection of pus is visible through the nail. Cellulitis of more proximal tissues is frequently encountered. Pain, caused by pressure from the accumulation of pus between the nail and nail fold, may be intense. Fever is uncommon in isolated paronychia/eponychia.

D. Management

1. Drainage of accumulated pus is the mainstay of therapy. A No. 11 scapel blade is introduced between the nail and nail fold and advanced until the abscess cavity is entered and pus drains (Fig. 15–9). Often anesthesia is not required for simple paronychia/eponychia. If inflammation and pain are particularly severe, or if the infection extends into the subungual space, then a digital nerve block using 1% lidocaine without epinephrine should be performed prior to abscess drainage. If a large amount of pus is drained, a small piece of packing gauze should be inserted to allow for continuous drainage. The patient should soak the digit in warm water for 20 minutes three to four times a day to prevent resealing of the involved nail fold.

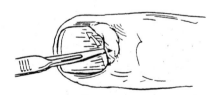

Figure 15–9. Technique for draining simple paronychia. Note that the No. 11 blade is brought between the nail and the eponychium parallel to the nail plate. This simple maneuver will drain the vast majority of paronychiae. (From Trott A: Wounds and Lacerations: Emergency Care and Closure. St. Louis, Mosby-Year Book, 1991.)

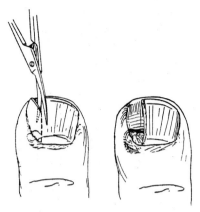

Figure 15–10. When a paronychia extends below the nail and insinuates between the nail bed and nail plate, partial nail removal must take place. Once the nail removal is accomplished, a small packing or drain is left in place for 5–7 days. (From Trott A: Wounds and Lacerations: Emergency Care and Closure. St. Louis, Mosby-Year Book, 1991.)

2. With subungual involvement, partial nail removal is recommended after a digital nerve block. For a lateral subungual abscess, a longitudinal cut in the nail all the way to the germinal matrix is made, and the segment of nail is removed (Fig. 15–10). For a subungual abscess with eponychia, horizontally incising the proximal nail, leaving the distal nail intact, will allow drainage and packing of the abscess and afford protection of the distal nailbed (Fig. 15–11). The lateral nail fold, or *eponychium*, is loosely packed for a few days, after which warm water soaks are applied as described above. Rechecking of the wound after 2–3 days is essential.

3. Systemic antibiotics are generally reserved for complex paronychiae (i.e., those with subungual involvement or more proximal cellulitis). An antistaphylococcal penicillin (e.g., dicloxacillin 250–500 mg PO qid for 7 days) or a first-generation cephalosporin (e.g., cephalexin 250–500 mg PO qid for 7 days) is generally adequate. Erythromycin (250–500 mg PO qid for 7 days) is an alternative for the patient with a history of serious beta-lactam antibiotic allergy. One should be suspicious of dermatophyte or *candidal* involvement when a patient's paronychia, particularly one that has been chronic, does not resolve with the above measures.

II. HERPETIC WHITLOW

A. Definition, Pathogenesis, and Clinical Picture

Herpetic whitlow is an infection caused by herpes simplex virus (HSV), type 1 or 2, affecting one or more fingers, particularly at

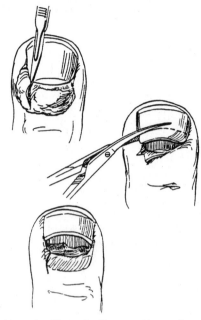

Figure 15–11. A complex "horseshoe" paronychia usually needs to be drained both by incising the paronychia directly and removing either a portion or all of the nail as illustrated. Note that a packing is left in place for 5–7 days to prevent adherence of the eponychium to the germinal matrix. (From Trott A: Wounds and Lacerations: Emergency Care and Closure. St. Louis, Mosby-Year Book, 1991.)

the tips. The virus is spread by direct contact. Occupational exposure (e.g., dental hygienists, cosmetologists) and autoinoculation during a primary outbreak of oral or genital herpes are important risk factors. Abrupt onset of edema, erythema, and localized tenderness, with painful vesicles or pustules, is common. Fever with regional lymphadenopathy also occurs. The clinical picture can be indistinguishable from that of pyogenic infection of the finger; herpetic whitlow may also become secondarily infected with bacteria. An important clue in distinguishing whitlow is the infection of more than one finger simultaneously. The pulp of the finger remains soft, distinguishing whitlow from felon (see below). HSV cultures are helpful (cultures may be negative once crusting of the lesion occurs).

B. Management

The infection is generally self-limited and requires neither surgical nor medical therapy. Acyclovir is reserved for especially severe infections or for immunocompromised patients. The dose

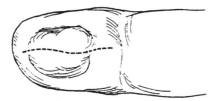

Figure 15–12. Technique for draining a felon. Note that the incision is made directly over the area of maximal tenderness and fluctuance. (From Trott A: Wounds and Lacerations: Emergency Care and Closure. St. Louis, Mosby-Year Book, 1991.)

is 400 mg PO tid for 10 days. Topical acyclovir has not been shown to be of benefit.

III. FELON

A. Definition, Pathogenesis, and Clinical Picture

A *felon* is a collection of pus in the pulp space of the fingertip. As with paronychiae, gram-positive cocci are the typical infecting organisms. Puncture wounds, often trivial, may predispose one to this infection. The pad of the fingertip is painful, swollen, and erythematous, and frequently the abscess is pointing toward the volar surface.

B. Management

The simplest procedure to drain a felon is to make a longitudinal midline incision directly over the abscess, stopping short of the distal flexor crease (Fig. 15–12). A digital nerve block is required beforehand. An alternative is the hockey-stick incision (Fig. 15–13). A nonadhesive wick is placed for the next 48 hours and removed at follow-up. Soaking three to four times a day is then prescribed. Antibiotics are recommended.

IV. PALMAR-SPACE INFECTIONS

A. Clinical Picture

Infection in the deep space of the palm usually occurs as a result of a puncture wound to the palm or as an extension of infection in adjacent flexor tendon sheaths. The infection is under pressure from the tension of the palmar fascia, and edema tends to spread dorsally, although maximal pain is in the midpalmar area.

B. Management

This infection is often complex and requires drainage by a hand surgeon. Consultation is mandatory.

V. SEPTIC TENOSYNOVITIS

A. Definition and Pathogenesis

Septic tenosynovitis is an infection of the flexor tendon sheaths. In general, this is the result of lacerations or puncture wounds over the joint creases allowing entry of pathogenic streptococci or staphylococci. The continuity of the tendon sheaths allow bacteria to spread quickly along the sheath's entire length, leading to a serious and potentially debilitating infection.

B. Clinical Picture

The patient often presents late (> 8 hours) after the injury has occurred. Elucidating the lacerating object (e.g., human or animal teeth, gravel surface, wood) is very important. In the event of no obvious trauma to the digit, consider hematogenous spread of bacteria, particularly *Neisseria gonorrheae* with disseminated gonococcal infection.

The four cardinal signs of flexor tendon infections are

1. Tenderness along the tendon.
2. A "sausage" digit.
3. Flexed posture of the digit.
4. Marked pain with passive extension.

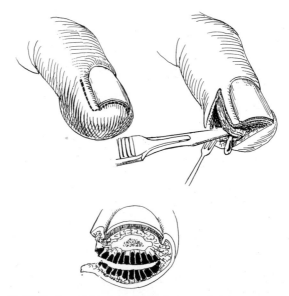

Figure 15–13. Hockey-stick incision for the drainage of a felon. *Note:* An incision on the ulnar side of the index, middle, and ring fingers is appropriate. The little finger is best incised on the radial side. The site of the incision on the thumb is also preferably on the radial side, but it may depend on the occupation of the patient. (From Chase RA: Atlas of Hand Surgery. Philadelphia, WB Saunders, 1973, p. 606.

C. Management

The severity and potential long-term disability related to the infection mandates orthopaedic consultation, hospital admission for parenteral antibiotics, and urgent surgical decompression.

VI. BITE WOUNDS TO THE HAND

Bite wounds are discussed in Animal Bites, earlier in this chapter.

VII. PEARLS AND PITFALLS

A. Ensure tetanus immune status is updated.

B. Trauma-related infections tend to involve a single gram-positive species (typically *S. aureus*); infections associated with bites, diabetes mellitus, or injection drug use tend to be polymicrobial.

C. Obtain a roentgenogram if glass or other foreign body is suspected.

D. A well-padded splint, keeping the hand immobile, is a very effective method of pain control for a hand infection.

BIBLIOGRAPHY

Hausman MR, Lisser SP: Hand infections. Orthop Clinics N Am 1992;23:171–178.
Simon RR, Koenigsknecht SJ: Emergency Orthopedics: The Extremities. 2nd Ed. East Norwalk, CT, Appleton & Lange, 1987, pp. 314–316.
Trott A: Wounds and Lacerations: Emergency Care and Closure. St. Louis, Mosby-Year Book, 1991, pp. 207–212.
Uehara DT (ed): The hand in emergency medicine. Emerg Med Clin N Am 1993; II(3).
Warden TM, Fourré MW: Incision and drainage of cutaneous abscesses and soft tissue infections. In Roberts JR, Hedges JR (eds): Clinical Procedures in Emergency Medicine. 2nd Ed. Philadelphia, WB Saunders, 1991, pp. 591–610.

VIRAL HEPATITIS

"Most men form an exaggerated estimate of the powers of medicine, founded on the common acceptance of the name, that medicine is the art of curing diseases. . . .
A far more just definition would be that medicine is the art of understanding diseases, and of curing or relieving them when possible."

JACOB BIGELOW (1786–1879)

I. ESSENTIAL FACTS

A. Definition

Viral hepatitis is an inflammatory condition of the liver secondary to a viral infection. Approximately 95% of cases are caused by one or more of the hepatotrophic viruses (i.e., hepatitis viruses A, B, C, D, or E).

B. The Hepatotrophic Viruses

1. **Hepatitis A Virus (HAV).** HAV is the most common form of viral hepatitis worldwide. It is most prevalent in areas with crowding and poor sanitation; even in some developed Western nations, antibodies to HAV can be found in the serum of 50–60% of the population > age 50.

   a. Mode of transmission: fecal–oral or water-borne infection (including infection from ingesting contaminated shellfish).

   b. Incubation period: 2–6 weeks (mean: 26 days). Peak infectivity occurs in the 2 weeks prior to the onset of jaundice and during early clinical illness. Many infections are subclinical and undiagnosed.

   c. Outcome of HAV infection: most cases resolve uneventfully. There is no carrier state, but 5–10% of infections will persist for months, with intermittent clinical relapse, before eventual resolution. Fewer than 1/1000 cases result in fulminant hepatitis (i.e., severe hepatitis culminating in liver failure and, in 60–70% of cases, death).

2. **Hepatitis B Virus (HBV).** Worldwide, the prevalence of HBV varies greatly. In the United States, < 10% of the adult population show evidence of prior HBV exposure, and only 0.2% of adults are chronic carriers of HBV.

   a. Mode of transmission: parenteral and sexual routes primarily (other body fluids that contain the virus and may be infectious include breast milk, seminal fluid, sweat, tears, vaginal secretions, and urine). Groups at particular risk for infection with HBV include

      i. Blood-product recipients: about 5% of transfusion-associated hepatitis is now due to HBV. Despite meticulous screening of blood products, transmission may still occur when those products contain HBV at a level below the sensitivity threshhold of the hepatitis B surface antigen (HBsAg) assay.

      ii. Health care workers, especially those with frequent contact with blood products, saliva, or other potentially contaminated body fluids, or who frequently treat patients who are likely to have acute or chronic HBV infection.

      iii. Hemodialysis patients.

      iv. Household or close physical contacts of infected individuals.

      v. Infants of infected mothers (these may acquire the virus by maternal–fetal transmission, especially during parturition).

      vi. Institutionalized individuals (e.g., mentally handicapped patients, prisoners).

      vii. Organ-transplant recipients.

      viii. Parenteral drug users.

      ix. Sexual contacts of infected individuals (unprotected

anal-receptive intercourse may put an individual at particular risk of infection).

Note: > 30% of patients with acute HBV give no history of recognized exposure and are not in one of the above-described high-risk groups.

b. Incubation period: 2–6 months (mean:11.8 weeks); the patient is infectious beginning very early in the incubation period. The size of the inoculum may determine the length of incubation.

c. Outcome of HBV infection: 90–95% of patients recover completely. Unfortunately, 5–10% become chronic carriers of the virus and 0.1–1.0% die from fulminant hepatitis. Chronic HBV carriers are at an increased risk for developing hepatocellular carcinoma.

3. **Hepatitis C Virus (HCV).** In this country, HCV causes 80–90% of hepatitis associated with blood transfusions. Anti-HCV antibody is present in 1% of volunteer blood donors.

a. Mode of transmission: similar to HBV and usually parenteral; 42% of cases occur in injection drug users, and 6% of cases are secondary to blood-product transfusion. Up to 50% of cases have no identifiable parenteral risk factor.

b. Incubation period: 6 weeks–6 months (may be as short as 2 weeks; mean:7.8 weeks). Seroconversion can take ≤ 12 months.

c. Outcome of HCV infection: the infection is frequently indolent, with ≤ 75% of post-transfusion cases anicteric and relatively asymptomatic. Unfortunately, ≤ 60% of post-transfusion HCV-infected patients become chronic carriers. The disease progresses to cirrhosis in 20% of chronically infected patients in 1.5–2 years. Hepatocellular carcinoma is a reported complication.

4. **Hepatitis D Virus (HDV, or the "delta" agent).** This is a "defective" virus whose replication is dependent on the presence of HBsAg synthesis. HDV may therefore only occur as a "coinfection" during an acute HBV infection or as a "superinfection" in chronic carriers of HBV. Concomitant infection with HDV should be suspected in any patient with fulminant HBV infection or in the chronic carrier of HBV who develops a sudden exacerbation of hepatitis.

a. Mode of transmission: similar to HBV and usually parenteral.

b. Incubation period: 4–8 weeks.

c. Outcome of HDV infection: while only about 5-10% of patients with coinfection develop chronic HDV infection, the majority of patients with superinfection become chronic carriers; ≤ 70% of chronic carriers develop chronic active hepatitis. Fulminant hepatitis occurs in as many as 17% of patients; it is more common when HDV is acquired as a superinfection rather than a coinfection.

5. **Hepatitis E Virus (HEV).** In developing nations, HEV has occurred in rural and urban epidemics, especially when floods have disrupted already poor sanitary conditions. Though imported cases have been recognized in the United States, secondary transmission or epidemic disease has not been seen.
   a. Mode of transmission: fecal–oral pattern similar to HAV.
   b. Incubation period: 2–9 weeks (mean:6 weeks).
   c. Outcome of HEV infection: this disease is more severe than HAV, with a mortality of 1–2% in the general population (and 10–20% in pregnant women). The disease appears to be self-limited, however, without an identified carrier state.

6. **Non-A-Non-B-Non-C Hepatitis.** About 5–10% of post-transfusion hepatitis cases and a number of sporadic community-acquired non-A-non-B hepatitis cases are not accounted for by current serologic tests. Probably one or more other hepatitis viruses are yet to be identified.

C. Other Nonviral Causes of Hepatitis

Other causes are numerous and include alcohol, medications, toxins, metabolic diseases, and miscellaneous disorders (see III, below).

II. CLINICAL EVALUATION

A. History

1. Inquire about risk factors for viral hepatitis as identified in Table 15–11.

2. Accurately identify any pre-existing medical problems (e.g.,

Table 15–11. RISK FACTORS FOR ACUTE VIRAL HEPATITIS

Ethnic background and birthplace (especially Asian, Oceanic, or North African; or close exposure to these individuals)

Exposure to poor sanitary conditions

Hemodialysis

History of organ transplantation

History of recent surgery

Illicit drug use (especially parenteral)

Known exposure to an infectious agent causing hepatitis (including health care workers with high-risk exposure)

Previous history of hepatitis, including type (if known)

Recent travel history

Sexual orientation and patterns of contact

Transfusions or administration of blood products

congestive heart failure, renal insufficiency, alcoholism, prior history of liver disease, pulmonary disease, cancer). *Gilbert's syndrome* is a benign inherited condition that results in mild, chronic unconjugated hyperbilirubinemia (usually bilirubin ≤ 3-4 mg/dL).

3. Obtain a thorough medication history, including prescription medications and over-the-counter preparations. Acute hepatitis can be caused by a number of agents (see III, below).

4. Consider the possibility of occupational exposure (e.g., heavy metals), toxin exposure, mushroom ingestion, and/or drug overdose (e.g., acetaminophen).

B. Symptoms and Signs

1. **Prodromal Phase** (Prior to the Onset of Jaundice): May be characterized by one or more of the following: anorexia, fatigue, fever, malaise, nausea and vomiting, right-upper-quadrant fullness and tenderness, and/or a serum sickness-like syndrome (urticarial rash and/or symmetrical arthropathy). Polyarteritis nodosum, glomerulonephritis, polymyalgia rheumatica, and essential mixed cryoglobulinemia may also be manifestations of HBV.

2. **Icteric Phase.** From the time of initial transaminase elevation, patients may show a progression from dark urine (bilirubinuria), to acholic stool, then jaundice. Anorexia, malaise, and fatigue are persistent. The liver is palpable in 70% of patients, and the liver edge is smooth and tender. Percussion of the lower right posterior ribs may produce a sickening sensation in the patient. In HAV, systemic symptoms begin to resolve when the patient becomes jaundiced.

Note: most cases of acute viral hepatitis are anicteric and relatively asymptomatic; this is especially so for HAV in young children and for HCV. Symptoms may be only mild and flu-like, and the diagnosis is only made if liver transaminases are checked and found to be elevated.

3. **Fulminant Hepatitis.** A relatively rare complication of hepatitis characterized by an overwhelming infection that destroys large numbers of hepatocytes and results in the rapid development of hepatic failure. Manifestations include profound jaundice, high initial transaminase levels, prolonged prothrombin time, hepatic encephalopathy, and ascites. Complications may include bleeding, coma, renal failure, cerebral edema, pneumonia, and sepsis. The mortality of fulminant hepatitis is 60–70%.

C. Physical Examination

Obtain vital signs and examine the skin, HEENT and neck, chest, heart, abdomen (include a rectal examination and stool heme test), and neurologic status.

D. Laboratory Studies

1. *Routinely* obtain the following studies in the patient suspected of acute viral hepatitis:
   a. Complete blood count.
   b. Bilirubin level.
   c. Glucose level.
   d. Prothrombin time (PT).
   e. Hepatic transaminases (AST [SGOT] and ALT [SGPT]): in viral hepatitis these are elevated 5–30 times above normal, with ALT > AST.
   Appropriate hepatitis serologies (begin with HAV and HBV serologies—see 4, below)

2. Additional studies *may be necessary,* depending on clinical circumstances (e.g., electrolyte panel, blood urea nitrogen (BUN), creatinine level, toxicologic screen).

3. Other viral serologies (in complicated cases, consider having the laboratory save acute serum for potential future studies) are sometimes helpful.

4. Hepatotrophic virus serologies:
   a. **Hepatitis A** (Fig. 15–14). Hepatitis A antibody (anti-HAV) is produced about the time that jaundice appears. This antibody is initially an IgM immunoglobulin; it remains detectable in the serum for several months. Following acute infection, IgG anti-HAV develops and probably lasts for life.
   b. **Hepatitis B** (Fig. 15–15)
      i. Hepatitis B surface antigen (HBsAg) is usually the first manifestation of infection with HBV. It typically appears within 1 month of exposure and 1–2 months

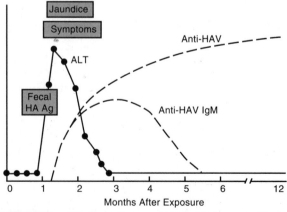

Figure 15–14. The clinical, serologic, and biochemical course of typical HAV infection. (Reproduction of "Clinical Chemistry Lewis Laboratory Guide to Thyroid Testing" has been granted with approval of Abbott Laboratories, all rights reserved by Abbott Laboratories.)

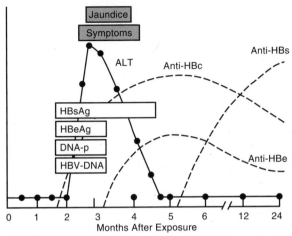

Figure 15–15. The clinical, serologic, and biochemical course of typical acute HBV infection.(Reproduction of "Clinical Chemistry Lewis Laboratory Guide to Thyroid Testing" has been granted with approval of Abbott Laboratories, all rights reserved by Abbott Laboratories.)

before the onset of clinical disease; it disappears with resolution of infection. Persistence of HBsAg beyond 6 months from symptom onset indicates a chronic carrier state (though this assay may be negative in the very low-level carrier).

ii. Hepatitis B surface antibody (anti-HBs) is indicative of recovery from HBV infection and confers immunity to reinfection. It is usually not seen for ≥ 1 month after HBsAg is cleared from the serum. In subclinical infections, anti-HBs appears early and HBsAg may never be detectable. Anti-HBs is the antibody induced by the hepatitis B vaccine.

iii. Hepatitis B core antibody (anti-HBc) appears generally just before clinical illness develops. After HBsAg disappears, and before anti-HBs appears, anti-HBc (of predominantly the IgM class) may be the only marker of acute HBV infection (the "core window"). Anti-HBc decreases after resolution of symptoms but typically persists for life. Anti-HBc of the IgG class may be the only marker of a very low-level carrier in the patient who is HBsAg and anti-HBs antibody negative.

iv. Hepatitis B e antigen (HBeAg) is found in acute infection and is indicative of high infectivity. It disappears in patients whose infections resolve, but 25–50% of chronic HBsAg carriers are positive for HBeAg for years.

v. Hepatitis Be antibody (anti-HBe) usually develops just as HBeAg disappears; this indicates that resolution of infection will occur. Anti-HBe generally disappears within 1–2 years after an acute infection.

See Table 15–12 for HBV serologic test interpretation.

c. **Hepatitis C.** Antibody to HCV (anti-HCV) becomes positive a mean of 15 weeks after the clinical onset of hepatitis (range: 4 weeks to >1 year). The anti-HCV assay, however, has had many difficulties. For example, up to 60% of positive screening tests in blood donors are falsely positive; the test is also insensitive in many patients, especially those who do not go on to develop chronic hepatitis. The newer second-generation enzyme-linked immunoassay (EIA) tests appear to be more sensitive and specific. A radioimmunoblot assay (RIBA) is now used to confirm positive blood screening tests. Detection of HCV-RNA using the polymerase chain reaction (PCR) detects ongoing viral replication and is extremely sensitive, but it is not yet commercially available.

d. **Hepatitis D.** A serologic test for antibody to HDV (anti-HDV) is available. *Remember:* patients simultaneously must have HBsAg in their serum to have hepatitis D.

e. **Hepatitis E.** Serologic testing for HEV (anti-HEV) may be obtained through the hepatitis branch of the Centers for Disease Control and Prevention (CDC). An assay should be commercially available soon.

III. DIFFERENTIAL DIAGNOSIS

The symptoms of acute viral hepatitis are nonspecific. Diagnosis depends on a high index of suspicion; relevant findings from the history and physical examination; and laboratory confirmation (including relevant viral serologies as outlined above). The differential includes the following:

A. The hepatotrophic viruses.

B. Other viruses: adenovirus, Coxsackie B, cytomegalovirus, Epstein-Barr, herpes simplex, mumps, rubella, rubeola, varicella-zoster, and yellow fever.

C. Nonviral infections: leptospirosis, liver abscess (amoebic or bacterial), malaria, Q fever, schistosomiasis, syphilis, and toxoplasmosis.

D. Toxins: acetaminophen poisoning, alcohol abuse, carbon tetrachloride exposure, *Amanita phalloides* mushroom ingestion, vitamin A or D abuse.

E. Medications:

1. Hepatocellular injury: alpha methyldopa, halothane, isoniazid, ketoconazole, niacin, nonsteroidal anti-inflammatory drugs, phenytoin, sulfonamides.

2. Cholestatic jaundice (characterized by an unusually high bilirubin): antithyroid agents, chlorpromazine (Thorazine), erythromycin estolate, estrogenic and androgenic steroids, oral hypoglycemics.

Table 15–12. INTERPRETATION OF HEPATITIS B SEROLOGIC TESTS

SEROLOGIC TEST			
HBsAg	Anti-HBs	Anti-HBc	Suggested Diagnoses and Follow-Up
+	−	−	Early hepatitis B infection: probably preclinical or early clinical illness. HBeAg/anti-HBe testing possibly indicated: If −/− ("e window") or −/+: resolution likely. If +/−: still highly infectious. HDV testing may be considered if epidemiologically indicated. Needs follow-up testing until anti-HBs is positive (i.e., acute infection has resolved).
+	−	+	Diagnostic of any of the following: 1. Acute HBV infection: has not developed anti-HBs yet. Positive IgM subclass of anti-HBc will confirm acute infection. Consider "e" antigen testing as outlined above. Needs follow-up testing for anti-HBs until positive. 2. Chronic HBV carrier (negative IgM anti-HBc). Consider HAV or HCV as cause of the acute hepatitis. 3. HDV may be present as coinfection or superinfection; consider testing for anti-HDV and IgM of anti-HBc if epidemiologically indicated.
+	+	+	Acute hepatitis B. Atypical pattern: usually HBsAg is gone by the time anti-HBs appears. Should resolve because anti-HBs is present, although occasionally this pattern can be seen with a second infection due to HBV of a different surface antigen serologic subtype.
−	+	+	Remote hepatitis B infection. Recovery is indicated by positive anti-HBs. Consider HAV, HCV, other virus, or other cause of acute hepatitis.
−	−	+	One of the following: 1. Remote HBV infection: anti-HBs now at undetectable level. A negative IgM anti-HBc assay can confirm that the infection is remote. In addition, HBeAg should be negative. Consider HAV, HCV, or other cause of acute hepatitis. 2. Acute or early resolving HBV infection: the "core window" after HBsAg disappears but before anti-HBs appears. A positive test for IgM anti-HBc suggests this diagnosis. While the patient may still be infectious at a low level (if HBeAg is still positive), resolution should occur because HBsAg has disappeared; follow-up is needed to be sure anti-HBs becomes positive. 3. Low-level carrier: HBsAg is too low to measure. IgM anti-HBc should be negative. If acute hepatitis is present, consider HAV, HCV, other virus, or other cause.

Table continued on following page

Table 15–12. INTERPRETATION OF HEPATITIS B SEROLOGIC TESTS
Continued

SEROLOGIC TEST			
HBsAg	Anti-HBs	Anti-HBc	Suggested Diagnoses and Follow-Up
−	+	−	Either of the following: 1. Remote HBV infection: anti-HBc now too low to detect. 2. Past immunization with hepatitis B vaccine: HBsAg is the only immunogenic antigen in the vaccine. If acute infection is present, consider HAV, HCV, other virus, or other cause of hepatitis.
−	−	−	No evidence of HBV infection. Consider HAV, HCV, other virus, or other cause of hepatitis.

From McMullen R: In Medical Diagnostics. Philadelphia, WB Saunders; 1992.

3. Fatty infiltration: amiodarone, tetracycline (high-dose parenteral), valproic acid.

F. Biliary tract disease.

G. "Benign postoperative jaundice": marked by elevation of bilirubin and alkaline phosphatase levels with normal or near-normal transaminase levels.

H. Shock.

I. Gilbert's syndrome.

J. Metabolic conditions: hemochromatosis, Wilson's disease.

K. Pregnancy-related jaundice (either of the following may complicate the third trimester):

1. Acute fatty liver: bilirubin and transaminase levels are high, PT prolonged; it is associated with a high mortality rate.

2. Cholestatic jaundice of pregnancy: characterized by only mild elevation of bilirubin and transaminase levels; it is a relatively benign condition.

IV. THERAPY

A. Supportive Care

1. Volume replacement: the patient with acute viral hepatitis may be volume depleted and/or may have significant electrolyte abnormalities. Initial ED care consists of necessary crystalloid replacement and electrolyte management. The vomiting patient should be treated with antiemetics (e.g., metoclopramide 10 mg IM or IV every 6 hours).

2. Diet: most patients are anorectic, and a low-fat, high-carbohydrate diet should be recommended. Clear liquids may

be the only oral intake initially tolerated. Malnourished or profoundly anorectic patients should be prescribed vitamin supplements. If the PT is elevated, vitamin K is appropriate (2.5–10 mg SQ or IM, may repeat once after 6–8 hours).

3. Activity: patients are usually profoundly fatigued and bed rest is reasonable. Activity may be slowly increased as tolerated, but never to the point that fatigue is exacerbated.

4. Corticosteroids and interferon are *not* of benefit in the management of acute viral hepatitis.

B. Patient Education

1. Prevent transmission:
   a. Hepatitis A: Patients should practice meticulous hygiene with appropriate hand-washing. Eating and drinking utensils should not be shared; the patient should use separate bathroom facilities in the household if possible. Once clinical illness develops, viral shedding decreases rapidly. The patient should not work in commercial food preparation until jaundice has completely resolved.
   b. Hepatitis B: transmission requires exposure to blood or bodily secretions. Needle and body-secretion precautions (including sexual abstinence) should be followed until HBsAb develops, indicating resolution. Nursing children, children ≤ age 5, and sexual partners are at the greatest risk for exposure.
   c. Hepatitis C: transmission is generally parenteral; needle and body-secretion precautions should be followed.

2. Eliminate hepatotoxins: unnecessary medications with hepatotoxic potential should be discontinued. Alcohol consumption must stop until all evidence of hepatic injury has disappeared.

C. Viral Hepatitis Prophylaxis to Contacts

Immunoprophylaxis is appropriate for family members and close personal contacts (see V, below). Although the appropriate prophylactic regimen will vary with the specific virus, gamma globulin (immune globulin [IG] 0.02 mL/kg IM) should be offered to household contacts while awaiting viral serologies.

D. Notification of the Public Health Department

Viral hepatitis is a reportable disease, and the appropriate public health department should be notified when the diagnosis is confirmed.

E. Post-ED Management

Arrange for appropriate disposition and follow-up (see VI, below).

V. VIRAL HEPATITIS PROPHYLAXIS

Patients, emergency personnel, and hospital staff frequently seek advice and request prophylaxis for possible exposure to hepatitis. Occasionally, public health department epidemiologic investigators may identify contacts of known hepatitis cases and suggest prophylaxis for them.

A. Hepatitis A Prophylaxis

Immune globulin (IG) is administered for HAV prophylaxis.

1. **Pre-exposure Prophylaxis.** Should be offered to travelers to areas endemic for HAV (e.g., the Middle East, Southeast Asia, Africa, South America, and Eastern Europe) before their trip.

   Dose of IG
   - Short stay (< 3 months) in high-risk area: 0.02 mL/kg IM.
   - Long stay (> 3 months) in high-risk area: 0.06 mL/kg IM every 5 months.

2. **Post-exposure Prophylaxis.** Should be given to persons living in the same household, sexual contacts, or other public health department-identified contacts of an individual with HAV. It protects against clinical illness in 80–90% of recipients for ≤ 3 months after administration. Administer IG as soon as possible after exposure; it probably is not effective if given > 2 weeks after exposure.

   Dose of IG
   - 0.02 mL/kg IM.

B. Hepatitis B Prophylaxis

Hepatitis B vaccine, ± hepatitis B immune globulin (HBIG) is (are) administered for HBV prophylaxis.

1. **Pre-exposure Prophylaxis.** Hepatitis B vaccine is the most effective way to prevent HBV. See Table 15–13 for dosing of the HBV vaccine. Vaccination is appropriate for
   a. All infants.
   b. High-risk adolescents (including injection drug users, patients with multiple sexual partners, and/or teenagers from communities where injection drug use, teenage pregnancy, and sexually transmitted diseases are common).
   c. High-risk adults (including health care workers, injection drug users, patients with multiple sexual partners or sexually transmitted diseases, homosexual and bisexual men, hemodialysis patients, individuals who it is anticipated will receive multiple blood-product infusions, sexual partners of HBV carriers, certain international travelers, patients and staff of institutions for the developmentally disabled, and inmates of long-term correctional facilities).
   d. Adoptees from countries where HBV is endemic.

Table 15–13. DOSING OF HBV VACCINE[a,b]

	RECOMBIVAX	ENGERIX-B
Birth to 10 years	2.5 μg (0.25 mL)	10 μg (0.5 mL)[c]
Infants born to HBsAG (+) mothers	5 μg (0.5 mL)	10 μg (0.5 mL)
Children and adolescents age 11–19 years	5 μg (0.5 mL)	20 μg (1.0 mL)
Adults ≥ 20 years	10 μg (1.0 mL)	20 μg (1.0 mL)
Immunocompromised patients (including dialysis patients)	40 μg (1.0 mL)[d,f]	40 μg (2.0 mL)[e,f]

[a]The vaccine is normally given in a three-dose series at 0, 1, and 6 months. There are no official recommendations for booster intervals.

[b]The IM injection must be given in the deltoid (anterolateral thigh in infants and young children).

[c]Engerix-B has been approved for a dosing schedule of 0, 1, and 2 months for neonates born to infected mothers and others requiring rapid vaccination such as departing travelers; a booster dose is required at 12 months.

[d]Special dialysis formulation, but schedule is 0, 1, and 6 months.

[e]Dosing schedule is 0, 1, 2, and 6 months.

[f]Need for booster dose (HBsAb level ≤ 10 mIU/mL) should be assessed shortly after the course, then annually.

    e. Alaskan Eskimos.
    f. All household contacts of HBV carriers.

  2. **Post-exposure Prophylaxis.** HBIG is indicated, *in addition to hepatitis B vaccine* as outlined in Table 15–13, in unvaccinated persons who have suffered exposure to HBV. Exposure is defined as birth to a HBsAg-positive mother; percutaneous, ocular, or mucous membrane contact to blood known or presumed to contain HBV; percutaneous bites by known or presumed HBsAg-positive individuals; or household or sexual contacts of individuals known or presumed to be HBsAg-positive.

    Dose of HBIG
- Infants born to HBsAG (+) mothers: 0.5 mL IM within 12 hours of birth; initiate HBV vaccine.
- Infants < 12 months old and acute hepatitis B in mother, father, or caretaker: 0.5 mL IM; initiate HBV vaccine.
- Unvaccinated exposed person: 0.06 mL/kg IM; initiate HBV vaccine.
- Previously vaccinated with (+) response but now with inadequate antibody level (i.e., anti-HBsAg titer < 10 mIU/mL): HBIG not necessary; administer HBV vaccine booster dose.
- Previously vaccinated and known vaccine *nonresponder:* two doses of HBIG (0.06 mL/kg per dose) or one dose of HBIG plus 1 dose of HBV vaccine.

Note: HBIG should be given IM as soon as possible after exposure (preferably within 24 hours; effectiveness after 14 days is uncertain). If hepatitis B vaccine is administered concomitantly, administer HBIG and the vaccine at separate sites.

C. Hepatitis C Prophylaxis

Prevention of hepatitis C is currently limited to screening blood for HCV antibody, and avoiding injection drug use (or at least avoiding any needle-sharing). The rate of sexual transmission remains unclear, but appears to be relatively low. Recommending barrier contraception for monogamous couples in which partners are discordant for anti-HCV remains controversial. There is no vaccine available. IG (see A, above) may be given for postexposure prophylaxis, but its effectiveness is equivocal.

D. Hepatitis D Prophylaxis

Because HDV requires infection with HBV, prevention of hepatitis B as outlined above will prevent hepatitis D.

E. Hepatitis E Prophylaxis

Prevention of HEV requires improved public sanitation. No vaccine is available. Passive protection by IG is of uncertain effectiveness (even if it is manufactured with plasma obtained in countries where the disease is endemic).

VI. DISPOSITION

A. Discharge

Most patients with viral hepatitis may be discharged to home after appropriate ED care. Discharge medications may include antiemetics and multivitamin supplements. The patient should avoid all potential hepatotoxins and follow-up should be arranged within 1 week.

B. Admit

In *any* of the following circumstances the patient should be hospitalized:

1. Diagnosis is uncertain.
2. Intractable vomiting.
3. Prothrombin time prolonged > 4 seconds above control.
4. Patient lives alone.
5. Evidence of fulminant hepatitis (e.g., encephalopathy, severe coagulopathy).

VII. PEARLS AND PITFALLS

A. The symptoms of acute viral hepatitis are nonspecific. Maintain a high index of suspicion for this disease, especially in patients with significant risk factors.

B. In patients with acute hepatic dysfunction, keep the differential diagnosis in mind. Jaundice has many causes besides acute viral hepatitis. Many of these disorders pose a greater threat to the patient's well-being than acute viral hepatitis.

C. Adequate care of the patient goes beyond making the diagnosis and includes fluid and electrolyte management, patient education, arranging appropriate follow-up, providing prophylaxis to high-risk contacts, and notifying the public health department.

BIBLIOGRAPHY

Centers for Disease Control: Hepatitis B virus: a comprehensive strategy for eliminating transmission in the United States through universal childhood immunization. Recommendation of the Immunizations Practices Advisory Committee (ACIP). MMWR 1991; 40(NO RR-13).

Frymoyer CL: Preventing the spread of viral hepatitis. Am Fam Phys 1993;8(8):1479–1486.

Kelen GD, Green GB, Purcell R, et al: Hepatitis B and hepatitis C in emergency department patients. N Engl J Med 1992;326:399–1404.

LaBrecque DR: Acute and chronic hepatitis. Chapter 57. In Stein JH (Editor-in-Chief): Internal Medicine. St. Louis, Mosby-Year Book, 1994, pp. 586–601.

McMullen R: Viral hepatitis. Chapter 98. In Dugdale DC, Eisenberg MS (eds): Medical Diagnostics. Philadelphia, WB Saunders, 1992, pp. 833–856.

LYME DISEASE

> *"Every man carries a parasite somewhere."*
> JAPANESE PROVERB

I. ESSENTIAL FACTS

A. Definition

Lyme disease is a tick-borne spirochetal infectious disease that typically occurs in stages and can involve multiple body systems, including the skin and the cardiac, neurologic, and musculoskeletal systems.

B. Causative Organism

Borrrelia burgdorferi, a spiral shaped spirochete.

C. Vector

Transmission occurs via *Ixodes* ticks. Two *Ixodes* species have been proven to transmit Lyme disease in the United States: *I. scapularis* in the Northeast and Minnesota/Wisconsin region; and *I. pacificus* in the West. It is most often the juvenile nymphal ticks, which are approximately the size of the head of a pin, that transmit Lyme disease. Because of the small size of these ticks, only ~ 50% of people with Lyme disease recall a tick bite. These ticks probably need to feed on humans for longer than 12 hours to transmit the spirochete.

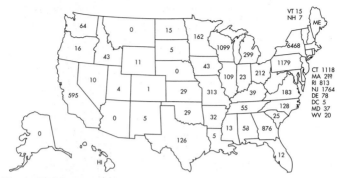

Figure 15–16. Reported Lyme disease cases—United States, 1989–1990. 1990 data are provisional. (From Lyme disease surveillance—United States. 1989–1990. MMWR 1991;40(25)417–421.

D. Epidemiology

1. Lyme disease is the most common vector-borne disease in the United States; more than 30,000 cases were reported between 1982 and 1990.

2. Forty-six states have reported cases of Lyme disease (Fig. 15–16). Highly endemic areas include the northeastern states, Minnesota, Wisconsin, and California. Lyme disease also occurs worldwide.

3. Most patients acquire infection during the months of May and August, the time period that corresponds to the active feeding period of the *Ixodes* nymphal ticks.

II. CLINICAL EVALUATION

A. History

1. Patients should be asked about outdoor activities and residence or travel to highly endemic regions.

2. A history of a tick bite may help in making a correct diagnosis.

B. Signs and Symptoms

Conceptually, one can view Lyme disease as occurring in three stages, with stage 1 and stage 2 equivalent to "early infection" and stage 3 equivalent to "late infection" (Table 15–14). Individual patients, however, can have highly variable presentations and disease progression.

1. *Early Infection*

a. **Erythema Migrans.** This cutaneous manifestation of Lyme disease, which occurs in ~ 70% of patients, develops at the site of the tick bite, typically 7–10 days after the bite. In

Table 15–14. MANIFESTATIONS OF LYME DISEASE BY STAGE[a]

| SYSTEM[b] | EARLY INFECTION | | LATE INFECTION |
	LOCALIZED (STAGE 1)	DISSEMINATED (STAGE 2)	PERSISTENT (STAGE 3)
Skin	Erythema migrans	Secondary annular lesions, malar rash, diffuse erythema or urticaria, evanescent lesions, lymphocytoma	Acrodermatitis chronica atrophicans, localized scleroderma-like lesions
Musculoskeletal system		Migratory pain in joints, tendons, bursae, muscle, bone; brief arthritis attacks; myositis[c]; osteomyelitis[c]; panniculitis[c]	Prolonged arthritis attacks, chronic arthritis, peripheral enthesopathy, periostitis or joint subluxations below lesions of acrodermatitis
Neurologic system		Meningitis, cranial neuritis, Bell's palsy, motor or sensory radioculoneuritis, subtle encephalitis, mononeuritis multiplex, myelitis[c], chorea[c], cerebellar ataxia[c]	Chronic encephalomyelitis, spastic parapareses, ataxic gait, subtle mental disorders, chronic axonal polyradiculopathy, dementia[c]
Lymphatic system	Regional lymphadenopathy	Regional or generalized lymphadenopathy, splenomegaly	
Heart		Atrioventricular nodal block, myopericarditis, pancarditis	
Eyes		Conjunctivitis, iritis[c], choroiditis[c], retinal hemorrhage or detachment[c], panophthalmitis[c]	Keratitis
Liver		Mild or recurrent hepatitis	
Respiratory system		Nonexudative sore throat, nonproductive cough, adult respiratory distress syndrome[c]	
Kidney		Microscopic hematuria or proteinuria	
Genitourinary system		Orchitis[c]	
Constitutional symptoms	Minor	Severe malaise and fatigue	Fatigue

[a]The classification by stages provides a guideline for the expected timing of the illness's manifestations, but may vary from case to case.
[b]Systems are based from the most to the least commonly affected.
[c]The inclusion of this manifesation is based on one or a few cases.
From Steere AC: Lyme disease. N Engl J Med 1989;321:586–596.

445

most patients, the rash presents with an erythematous annular border that gradually expands and frequently leaves a central clearing. In some patients, the central portion of the rash may develop necrotic or vesicular features. The median diameter of the rash is 15 cm. Untreated, the rash remains for 3–4 weeks. Approximately 30–40% of patients also develop multiple skin lesions. These lesions, which are smaller than the primary erythema migrans lesion, usually appear several weeks after the tick bite and represent dissemination of spirochetes.

b. **Flu-like Symptoms.** These symptoms often accompany the erythema migrans rash. Approximately 15% of patients may present with flu-like symptoms without evidence of erythema migrans.

c. **Musculoskeletal Symptoms.** Approximately 3–4 weeks after the tick bite, patients may develop migratory pains in joints, tendons, bursae, muscles, and bones. In general, one or two sites are affected at a time, but, on occasion, up to 10 sites can be involved. Patients often have concomitant malaise and fatigue. Approximately 6 months after the tick bite, brief attacks of arthritis occur in ~ 60% of patients. These attacks usually do not exceed several weeks in duration. Most often the arthritis is oligoarticular and involves large joints, especially the knee.

d. **Neurologic Symptoms.** Neurologic manifestations, which occur in 10–15% of untreated patients at this stage, typically begin 2–3 months after the tick bite and most commonly include acute meningitis, cranial nerve abnormalities (especially Bell's palsy), and peripheral neuropathy. For those patients with meningitis, cerebrospinal fluid (CSF) analysis typically shows a lymphocytic pleocytosis of ~ 100 cells/mm^3.

e. **Cardiac Symptoms.** Approximately 5–10% of patients with Lyme disease develop cardiac manifestations, most commonly some form of atrioventricular block. For the patient with first-degree heart block, progression to second- or third-degree heart block is more likely if the PR– interval is longer than 0.30 seconds. Although patients with severe heart block often require temporary cardiac pacing, the heart block almost always resolves within 1 week.

2. *Late Infection*

a. **Musculoskeletal Symptoms.** Chronic Lyme arthritis typically begins a year or more after the initial infection and attacks typically last months at a time. The arthritis is usually monoarticular or oligoarticular and, as with earlier stages of arthritis, the knees and shoulders are the joints most commonly involved. As each year passes, the number of patients who have recurrent attacks of arthritis decreases by 10–20%. Usually, attacks of arthritis resolve after several years. Patients who have HLA-DR4 more often have a lack of response to antibiotic therapy and develop chronic arthritis. In rare cases, permanent joint disability can result.

b. **Neurologic Symptoms.** Chronic nervous system involvement usually begins a year or more after initial infection and most often manifests as encephalopathy, polyneuropathy, or leukoencephalitis. Subacute encephalopathy is the most common of these manifestations and is characterized by disturbances in mood, memory, and sleep. Lymphocytic pleocytosis is rare at this stage. Chronic Lyme neurologic disease, unlike chronic Lyme arthritis, may persist for longer than 10 years.

c. **Cutaneous Symptoms.** Years after the tick bite, patients may develop a chronic skin disorder known as acrodermatitis chronica atrophicans. This late cutaneous manifestation of Lyme disease is rarely seen in the United States, but occurs in approximately 10% of European patients with the disease. The lesion initially presents as an erythematous to violaceous cutaneous plaque or nodule but later is characterized by thinning of the skin and subcutaneous tissues. Acrodermatitis chronica atrophicans typically involves the extensor surfaces of the extremities, particularly in regions around joints.

C. Laboratory Studies

1. **Cultures.** Although *B. burgdorferi* has been isolated from blood, skin, CSF, and synovial fluid, routine culturing for the purposes of clinical diagnosis is not recommended, mainly because of the low-yield, high cost, and long delay for positive cultures to develop.

2. **Skin Biopsy.** Warthin-Starry staining of skin biopsy specimens can identify spirochetes in approximately 50% of patients, but it is not recommended on a routine basis.

3. **Serology.** The only practical laboratory method for diagnosing Lyme disease is serologic testing. For screening, the enzyme-linked immunosorbent assay (ELISA) has supplanted the less sensitive and specific immunofluorescence assay (IFA). If tested several months after the initial tick bite, most patients will have a positive ELISA test. Western blot testing has also been employed, but criteria for a "positive" Western blot for Lyme disease remain controversial. The Western blot should be viewed as providing supplemental information, not as a definitive confirmatory test. In general, one should diagnose Lyme disease on the basis of clinical findings with serologic testing used as supporting evidence. Because false-negative serologic tests occur primarily in the first 6 weeks of infection, serologic tests are more reliable with late Lyme disease. In neurologic Lyme disease, CSF usually shows an elevated concentration of specific antibodies to *B. burgdorferi*.

4. **False-Negative and -Positive Results.** Several problems with the currently available serologic tests exist:

 a. False-negative results are common when patients are tested within the first several weeks after having a tick bite.
 b. Patients who receive antibiotics for early illness may not develop a positive antibody response when tested at a later point.
 c. False-positive results can occur with syphilis, relapsing fever, Rocky Mountain spotted fever, and mononucleosis.
 d. No standardization of testing exists and several studies have demonstrated marked interlaboratory variability.

III. DIFFERENTIAL DIAGNOSIS

A. Early Infection

Includes localized reactions to spider bites, ringworm, idiopathic Bell's palsy, viral meningitis, parvovirus, rubella, and influenza.

B. Late Infection

Includes systemic lupus erythematosus, rheumatoid arthritis, multiple sclerosis, localized scleroderma, and chronic fatigue syndrome.

IV. THERAPY

A. Early Disease

Antimicrobial therapy is indicated in early disease to relieve symptoms and to prevent later sequelae of Lyme disease (Table 15-15).

1. **Erythema Migrans, Acute Flu-like Symptoms.** Oral doxycycline is the drug of choice, but should not be administered to children < 9 years of age or to pregnant women. Amoxicillin is considered the second choice drug and is often combined with probenecid. Recent studies of oral regimens demonstrated equal efficacy with doxycycline, amoxicillin plus probenecid, cefuroxime, and azithromycin. The erythema migrans lesions typically resolve in 3–4 days with treatment; untreated, this lesion persists a median of 28 days. Failures occur in < 10% of patients. A self-limited intensification in symptoms with the onset of antimicrobial therapy (Jarisch-Herxheimer reaction) occurs in approximately 15% of patients.

2. **Neurologic Symptoms.** For those patients with neurologic involvement limited to Bell's palsy, oral regimens (doxycycline or amoxicillin) are recommended. Antimicrobial therapy decreases the duration of the Bell's palsy. Patients with radiculitis or meningitis should be treated intravenously with either ceftriaxone or penicillin G.

Table 15–15. TREATMENT OF LYME DISEASE[a]

		DRUG	ADULT DOSAGE	PEDIATRIC DOSAGE[b]
Erythema Migrans		Doxycycline[c] (*Vibramycin*, and others)	100 mg PO bid	
	OR	Amoxicillin (*Amoxil*, and others)	250–500 mg PO tid	25–50 mg/kg/day divided tid
Alternative:		Cefuroxime axetil (*Ceftin*)	500 mg bid	250 mg bid
Neurologic disease				
Bell's palsy		Doxycycline[c]	100 mg PO bid	
	OR	Amoxicillin	250–500 mg PO tid	25–50 mg/kg/day divided tid
More serious		Ceftriaxone (*Rocephin*)	2 g/day IV	75–100 mg/kg/day IV
CNS disease[d]	OR	Penicillin G	20–24 million units/day IV	300,000 units/kg/day IV
Cardiac Disease				
Mild		Doxycycline[c]	100 mg PO bid	
	OR	Amoxicillin	250–500 mg PO tid	25–50 mg/kg/day divided tid
More serious[e]		Ceftriaxone	2 grams/day IV	75–100 mg/kg/day IV
	OR	Penicillin G	20–24 million units/day IV	300,000 units/kg/day IV
Arthritis[d]				
Oral		Doxycycline[c]	100 mg PO bid	
	OR	Amoxicillin	500 mg PO tid	50 mg/kg/day divided tid
Parenteral		Ceftriaxone	2 g/day IV	75–100 mg/kg/day IV
	OR	Penicillin G	20–24 million units/day IV	300,000 units/kg/day IV

[a]Recommendations are based on limited data and should be considered tentative. The duration of treatment is not well established for any indication; it is usually based on severity of disease and rapidity of response. Clinicians generally recommend 10–30 days for oral drugs and 14–21 days for intravenous treatment.

[b]Should not exceed adult dosage.

[c]Or tetracycline HCl (*Achromycin,* and others) 250–500 mg qid. Neither doxycycline nor any other tetracycline should be used for children < 9 years old or for pregnant or lactating women.

[d]In late disease, the response to treatment may be delayed for several weeks or months.

[e]A temporary pacemaker may be necessary.

From Treatment of Lyme disease. Med Let 1992;34:95–97.

3. **Arthritis.** For early arthritis, oral and intravenous regimens are accepted. Recommended regimens include oral doxycycline, amoxicillin, intravenous ceftriaxone, or intravenous penicillin G. Approximately 50% of patients have complete resolution of arthritis within several weeks of completing therapy. Antimi-

crobial therapy is less effective in those who have received intra-articular steroids.

4. **Cardiac Symptoms.** Mild involvement with first-degree atrioventricular block < 0.30 seconds can be treated with oral doxycycline, but all other cardiac involvement should be treated with intravenous ceftriaxone or intravenous penicillin G. Temporary pacemakers may be needed.

B. Late Disease

Positive antibody responses frequently remain after effective therapy and resolution of clinical symptoms; this should not be interpreted to mean that infection remains and that patients need to be retreated.

1. **Arthritis.** For late arthritis, differences in efficacy between oral and intravenous regimens have not been demonstrated. Therapy may be either oral (doxycycline or amoxicillin) or intravenous (ceftriaxone or penicillin G), but, many physicians prefer treating with intravenous antimicrobials at this stage.

2. **Neurologic Symptoms.** Chronic neurologic involvement should be treated with intravenous regimens (ceftriaxone or penicillin G). Approximately 60% of patients have significant improvement after antimicrobial treatment, but resolution of symptoms may take months. There is no evidence that multiple courses of antimicrobial agents are indicated in those patients who have persistent symptoms after one course of intravenous therapy.

3. **Cutaneous Symptoms.** Suggested oral regimens include doxycycline or amoxicillin. Residual scarring and hyperpigmentation may remain after therapy.

C. Experimental Malaria Therapy

Blood infected with malaria has been administered to several patients, but this therapy has no proven benefit and is potentially extremely dangerous.

D. Therapy for the Pregnant Patient

For pregnant patients who receive treatment for Lyme disease, adverse outcomes with the fetus are uncommon. If oral antimicrobials are used, doxycycline should not be given.

E. Prophylactic Therapy for Tick Bites

Administering oral antimicrobial agents to patients who are bitten by a tick is controversial. A recent study, which performed a cost-effective analysis, concluded that patients living in highly endemic areas for Lyme disease should receive prophylactic antimicrobials for tick bites if the patient identified the tick as an *Ixodes* species. *The Medical Letter,* however, does not recommend prophylactic treatment of tick bites. Regardless of whether patients receive prophylactic antimicrobials, they should be educated about the signs and symptoms of Lyme disease and advised to seek medical care promptly should these signs or symptoms develop.

V. DISPOSITION

A. Discharge

Patients with Lyme disease rarely require hospital admission. Before discharging the patient from the ED, one should provide education about the signs and symptoms that may develop with Lyme disease, and advise the patient to seek medical care promptly should these signs or symptoms develop.

B. Admit

Patients with cardiac involvement who have high-grade atrioventricular block (or a first-degree block with a PR– interval ≥ 0.30 seconds) should be admitted to the hospital for cardiac monitoring. Patients with acute meningitis will also require admission.

VI. PEARLS AND PITFALLS

A. Inquire about outdoor exposure, recent travel to a region highly endemic for Lyme disease, and recollection of a tick bite.

B. Look carefully for an erythema migrans rash.

C. Perform a careful neurologic examination on all patients suspected of having Lyme disease.

D. Remember that very early in the illness patients often have negative serologic tests.

Do *not* do any of the following:

A. Overdiagnose Lyme disease in patients with chronic, nonspecific complaints.

B. Repeatedly administer intravenous antimicrobial regimens to patients who do not immediately respond to therapy.

C. Administer intravenous antimicrobial regimens to patients because they have persistently positive serologic tests after antimicrobial therapy.

D. Administer doxycycline to pregnant women or to children < 9 years of age.

BIBLIOGRAPHY

Logigian EL, Kaplan RF, Steere AC: Chronic neurologic manifestations of Lyme disease. N Engl J Med 1990;323:1438–1444.

Lyme disease surveillance—United States, 1989–1990. MMWR 1991;40:417–421.

Magid D, Schwartz B, Craft J, Schwartz JS: Prevention of Lyme disease after tick bites. N Engl J Med 1992;327:534–541.

Malane MS, Grant-Kels JM, Feder HM, Luger SW: Diagnosis of Lyme disease based on dermatologic manifestations. Ann Intern Med 1991;114:472–481.

Massarotti EM, Luger SW, Rahn DW, et al: Treatment of early Lyme disease. Am J Med 1992;92:396–403.

Spach DH, Liles WC, Campbell GL, et al: Tick-borne diseases in the United States. N Engl J Med 1993;329(13):936–947.

Treatment of Lyme disease. Med Lett 1992;34:95–97.

MENINGITIS AND ENCEPHALITIS

> *"MIND, n. A mysterious form of matter secreted by the brain.*
> *Its chief activity consists in the endeavor to ascertain its own nature,*
> *the futility of the attempt being due to the fact that*
> *it has nothing but itself to know itself with."*
>
> AMBROSE BIERCE (1842–1914)

I. ESSENTIAL FACTS: MENINGITIS

A. Definition

Meningitis is inflammation of the meninges. It may be caused by infectious agents (bacteria, viruses, or fungi), neoplasia, or other inflammatory conditions (e.g., sarcoidosis, vasculitis).

B. Etiology

1. **Bacterial Meningitis**

   a. *Streptococcus pneumoniae* is the most common cause of bacterial meningitis in adults, and it is responsible for 30–50% of meningitis cases in children. It may occur concomitantly with pneumococcal pneumonia, pneumococcal endocarditis, otitis media, sinusitis, or mastoiditis. Risk factors include recent head injury (e.g., skull fracture), sickle cell anemia, alcoholism, immunoglobulin deficiency, and splenectomy.

   b. *Neisseria meningitidis* is responsible for 10–30% of bacterial meningitis cases in adults and 30–40% of childhood cases. It is rare in infants. A rash (petechial or purpuric) may be noted in ≤ 50% of meningococcal infections. Peak disease incidence is in winter and spring.

   c. *Hemophilus influenzae,* type B, is responsible for 1–3% of bacterial meningitis cases in adults. Before the introduction of vaccines against *H. influenzae* type b, it was the most common cause of bacterial meningitis in young children. It usually occurs following upper-respiratory-tract infections (otitis media 66%, pharyngitis 50%). Children who are close contacts with the infected patient should receive rifampin prophylaxis.

d. *Listeria monocytogenes* may cause meningitis in neonatal patients, the elderly, renal transplant recipients who are receiving immunosuppressive therapy (corticosteroids or cytotoxic agents), alcoholic patients, and lymphoma or leukemia patients.

e. *Staphylococcus aureus* causes meningitis primarily in post-operative neurosurgical patients and injection drug users.

f. *Staphylococcus epidermidis* is a major pathogen in patients with infected ventricular shunts.

g. Group B streptococci are a major pathogen in neonates but a rare cause of meningitis in adults.

h. Gram-negative bacilli *(Escherichia coli, Klebsiella, Entero-bacter, Proteus, Citrobacter, Pseudomonas)* are seen in infants, postoperative neurosurgical patients, and head-injury patients (especially those with a cerebrospinal fluid leak).

2. **Viral Meningitis**

a. Meningitis may be caused by a variety of viral agents, including picornaviruses (especially enteroviruses [e.g., coxsackieviruses, echovirus], which are responsible for 70% of viral meningitis), paramyxoviruses (mumps), herpesviruses, and lymphocytic choriomeningitis.

b. Most patients with viral meningitis are < age 40.

c. Enteroviral infections occur predominantly in summer.

d. Mumps meningitis is seen in winter and late spring, with a predominance in males.

e. Herpes simplex meningitis is usually associated with episodes of primary genital or oral herpes infection (though it also may occur with recurrent herpes infections).

f. Lymphocytic choriomeningitis occurs throughout the year. Often there is a history of animal exposure (especially hamsters).

II. ESSENTIAL FACTS: ENCEPHALITIS

A. Definition

Encephalitis is inflammation of brain tissue: cerebrum, cerebellum, and/or brainstem.

B. Etiology

1. In the United States, herpesviruses are the major cause of acute nonepidemic viral encephalitis.

2. Additional viruses known to cause encephalitis include togaviruses, bunyaviruses, and picornaviruses (summer and early fall); varicella zoster, Epstein-Barr virus, rubella, and

paramyxoviruses (winter epidemics); California and western equine encephalitis (usually seen in younger patients; vectors are mosquitoes); Eastern equine encephalitis; Japanese encephalitis; St. Louis encephalitis, human immunodeficiency virus (HIV)-induced encephalitis, and rabies.

3. Examples of nonviral causes of encephalitis include vasculitis, fungal infection, Lyme disease, malaria, Rocky Mountain spotted fever, syphilis, toxoplasmosis, and tuberculosis.

III. CLINICAL EVALUATION: BACTERIAL MENINGITIS

A. History, Signs, and Symptoms

1. There are three patterns of onset of clinical illness:
   a. Meningitis that develops over 1–7 days and is commonly associated with respiratory symptoms (50% of cases).
   b. Meningitis that develops suddenly with the rapid onset of headache, confusion, lethargy, and loss of consciousness, leading to hospitalization within 24 hours (30% of cases). Respiratory symptoms are uncommon.
   c. Meningitis that develops subacutely, with the onset occurring after 1–3 weeks of respiratory symptoms (20% of cases).

2. Principal symptoms and signs in adults include
   a. Fever (present commonly, but not invariably).
   b. Headache (very common).
   c. Seizures (a poor prognostic sign).
   d. Vomiting.
   e. Altered consciousness or confusion (an altered mental status or confusion is usual; < 5% of cases present with the patient completely awake and alert).
   f. Stiff neck or back. This sign is present in 80% of patients, but it may be a late finding.
      i. Kernig's sign. Pain with passive extension of the knee when the hips are flexed.
      ii. Brudzinski's sign: Flexion of hips and knees produced by passive neck flexion.
   g. Petechiae. Two-thirds of patients with meningococcal meningitis have petechiae. Petechiae may also be seen in viral meningitis (caused by coxsackievirus or echovirus) and with other causes of bacterial meningitis. Meningococcal meningitis may also be associated with purpura or vasculitic lesions.

B. Laboratory Studies

The following are appropriate considerations in the patient with suspected meningitis or encephalitis.

1. *Routinely* obtain the following:
   a. Complete blood count (CBC).
   b. Blood cultures.

    c. Electrolyte panel.
    d. Blood urea nitrogen (BUN) and creatinine levels.
    e. Glucose level.
    f. Urinalysis.

2. Lumbar puncture and head computed tomography (CT) scan: cerebrospinal fluid (CSF) must be obtained from patients suspected of having meningitis or encephalitis. A head CT should be obtained before the lumbar puncture if the patient has papilledema, depressed level of consciousness, focal neurologic examination, and/or known or suspected HIV infection.

3. Additional studies *may be necessary,* depending on the clinical circumstances (e.g., arterial blood gas, chest roentgenogram, serologic studies).

C. Lumbar Puncture

1. CSF count is elevated (usually > 500 cells/mm^3) in patients with bacterial meningitis, and there is typically a neutrophilic predominance. *Any neutrophils in the CSF are abnormal, even if the total cell count is not elevated (i.e., < 5 cells/mm^3).* Monocytic cells may be seen in bacterial meningitis caused by *L. monocytogenes,* in partially treated or resolving meningitis, and in tuberculous or fungal meningitis.

2. CSF pressure is typically elevated (> 18 cm H_2O).

3. CSF protein is usually elevated (> 100 mg/dL).

4. CSF glucose is generally decreased (< 40 mg/dL or $< 40\%$ of the simultaneous blood glucose concentration, provided the blood glucose concentration is < 250 mg/dL).

5. Gram stain of CSF may permit a rapid presumptive diagnosis. Approximately 80% of untreated bacterial meningitis cases can be diagnosed on Gram stain.

6. CSF cultures are positive in 70–80% of cases of bacterial meningitis. Anaerobic cultures of CSF should be performed when anaerobic organisms are a possibility (as with brain abscess, middle-ear infection, mastoiditis, sinus infections, malignancies, shunt infections, or head trauma).

7. Counterimmunoelectrophoresis (CIE) of CSF can be used to detect the presence of capsular polysaccharide from *H. influenzae, S. pneumoniae,* and *N. meningitidis.* CIE is particularly useful in the setting of partially treated meningitis or in patients with equivocal Gram stain results. The false-negative rate of CIE is about 10% compared with cultures.

8. India ink and acid-fast preparations should be obtained in the setting of suspected fungal or tuberculous meningitis, respectively. Negative results, however, do not rule out significant CSF infection with either fungi or acid-fast organisms.

IV. CLINICAL EVALUATION: VIRAL MENINGITIS

A. History, Signs, and Symptoms

1. Prodromal symptoms usually occur over several days and typically include
   a. Headache (usually frontal or retro-orbital).
   b. Malaise, nausea, vomiting, listlessness, and photophobia.
   c. Fever (usually, but not always).
   d. Neurologic symptoms. Mental status is usually normal, but ~ 10% of patients with viral meningitis have seizures, coma, or motor or sensory impairments.

2. Physical examination findings may suggest specific causative agents, such as
   a. Parotitis caused by mumps.
   b. Rash caused by echovirus or coxsackievirus.
   c. Pleurodynia caused by coxsackievirus.
   d. Genital herpes caused by herpesvirus.

B. Lumbar Puncture Results

1. CSF cell count in viral meningitis is usually 10–150 cells/mm^3 but may be as high as 1000 cells/mm^3. Cells are typically lymphocytic; but in 30% of patients there may be early polymorphonuclear leukocyte predominance, usually followed in 6–24 hours by lymphocytic predominance.

2. CSF glucose is usually normal, but it is occasionally low in patients with herpes or mumps.

3. CSF protein is usually normal or only slightly elevated.

4. CSF viral cultures are often negative; cultures of stool, urine, or throat, or serologic tests may yield diagnostic information.

V. CLINICAL EVALUATION: ENCEPHALITIS

A. History, Signs, and Symptoms

1. Patients with viral encephalitis usually have signs of meningeal irritation (headache, nausea, vomiting, or nuchal rigidity) plus alterations in consciousness (mild lethargy to drowsiness, stupor, or coma).

2. Focal neurologic findings and seizures are common.

3. In herpes simplex encephalitis, temporal lobe manifestations, such as bizarre behavior or hallucinations, may be noted.

4. Fever is usually present.

B. Lumbar Puncture Results

1. Erythrocytes and/or xanthochromic fluid may be found in herpes simplex encephalitis.

2. CSF leukocyte count is usually 50–500 cells/mm^3. A lymphocytic pleocytosis is typical.

3. CSF glucose is usually normal.

4. CSF protein is usually mildly elevated.

5. Opening pressure is normal or slightly elevated.

VI. DIFFERENTIAL DIAGNOSIS

Meningitis is a consideration in any patient with a fever and a headache, fever and altered level of consciousness, fever and meningeal irritation (e.g., "stiff" neck), or headache and meningeal irritation (even if the patient is afebrile). Other diagnoses to be considered include encephalitis, brain abscess, sepsis (from any source), vascular headaches, subarachnoid hemorrhage, seizure disorder or postictal state, severe electrolyte disorder, hypoxia, respiratory acidosis, head or neck trauma, toxin exposure (including intentional drug ingestion), drug withdrawal (e.g., alcohol), or behavioral disorder.

VII. THERAPY

Figure 15–17 presents the emergency therapy of acute meningitis and encephalitis.

A. Initial Management

Assess, secure, and support the airway, breathing, and circulation as indicated. (See Chapter 1. II.)

1. Administer supplemental oxygen, and protect the airway as necessary.

2. Obtain vital signs, establish intravenous (IV) access, and check the fingerstick glucose level if mental status is altered. Monitor both cardiac rhythm and oxygen saturation (SaO_2) in seriously ill patients.

3. Treat hypotension with IV crystalloid. If the clinical examination indicates pulmonary vascular congestion, support the blood pressure as necessary with dopamine.

4. Consider parenteral thiamine, glucose, and naloxone if the patient's mental status is altered.

B. Evaluation for Suspected Meningitis/Encephalitis

1. Complete a rapid but thorough physical examination.

2. Perform a lumbar puncture. Obtain a head CT scan *before* the lumbar puncture if indicated (see III. B. 2). A head CT is mandatory in the patient with suspected encephalitis.

C. Antibiotic Therapy

1. Therapy for suspected bacterial meningitis should be initiated in the ED as rapidly as possible, and within 30 minutes of the

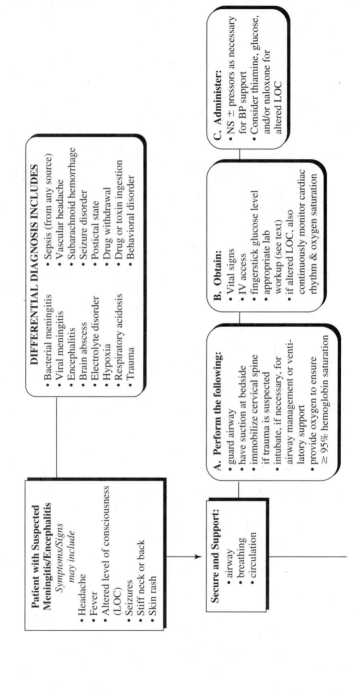

Patient with Suspected Meningitis/Encephalitis

Symptoms/Signs may include

- Headache
- Fever
- Altered level of consciousness (LOC)
- Seizures
- Stiff neck or back
- Skin rash

DIFFERENTIAL DIAGNOSIS INCLUDES

- Bacterial meningitis
- Viral meningitis
- Encephalitis
- Brain abscess
- Electrolyte disorder
- Hypoxia
- Respiratory acidosis
- Trauma
- Sepsis (from any source)
- Vascular headache
- Subarachnoid hemorrhage
- Seizure disorder
- Postictal state
- Drug withdrawal
- Drug or toxin ingestion
- Behavioral disorder

Secure and Support:
- airway
- breathing
- circulation

A. Perform the following:
- guard airway
- have suction at bedside
- immobilize cervical spine if trauma is suspected
- intubate, if necessary, for airway management or ventilatory support
- provide oxygen to ensure ≥ 95% hemoglobin saturation

B. Obtain:
- Vital signs
- IV access
- fingerstick glucose level
- appropriate lab workup (see text)
- if altered LOC, also continuously monitor cardiac rhythm & oxygen saturation

C. Administer:
- NS ± pressors as necessary for BP support
- Consider thiamine, glucose, and/or naloxone for altered LOC

458

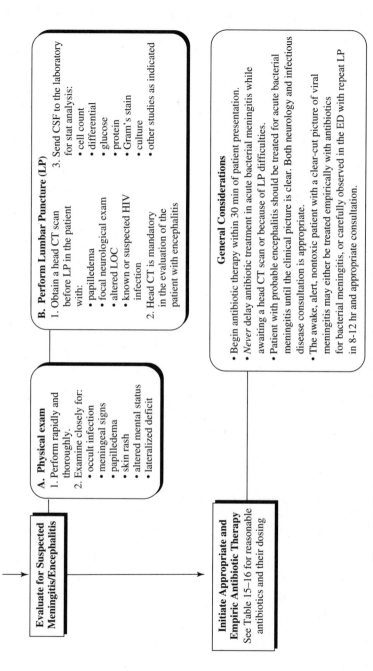

Evaluate for Suspected Meningitis/Encephalitis

A. Physical exam
1. Perform rapidly and thoroughly.
2. Examine closely for:
   • occult infection
   • meningeal signs
   • papilledema
   • skin rash
   • altered mental status
   • lateralized deficit

B. Perform Lumbar Puncture (LP)
1. Obtain a head CT scan before LP in the patient with:
   • papilledema
   • focal neurological exam
   • altered LOC
   • known or suspected HIV infection
2. Head CT is mandatory in the evaluation of the patient with encephalitis
3. Send CSF to the laboratory for stat analysis:
   • cell count
   • differential
   • glucose
   • protein
   • Gram's stain
   • culture
   • other studies as indicated

Initiate Appropriate and Empiric Antibiotic Therapy
See Table 15–16 for reasonable antibiotics and their dosing

General Considerations
• Begin antibiotic therapy within 30 min of patient presentation.
• *Never* delay antibiotic treatment in acute bacterial meningitis while awaiting a head CT scan or because of LP difficulties.
• Patient with probable encephalitis should be treated for acute bacterial meningitis until the clinical picture is clear. Both neurology and infectious disease consultation is appropriate.
• The awake, alert, nontoxic patient with a clear-cut picture of viral meningitis may either be treated empirically with antibiotics for bacterial meningitis, or carefully observed in the ED with repeat LP in 8–12 hr and appropriate consultation.

Figure 15–17. Emergency therapy of the patient with acute meningitis or encephalitis.

patient's presentation. In the setting of suspected bacterial meningitis, antibiotics should *not* be withheld while awaiting a head CT scan (before the lumbar puncture) or if the clinician is unable to perform the lumbar puncture because of anatomic difficulties. Under those circumstances, obtain blood cultures rapidly and initiate antibiotic therapy prior to performing head CT and/or lumbar puncture.

2. Antibiotic choices:
   a. Table 15–16 presents appropriate empiric antibiotic therapy for the ED patient with suspected bacterial meningitis.
   b. Subsequent therapy should be guided by identification of the organism on Gram stain and eventual culture results.

Table 15–16. EMPIRIC ANTIBIOTIC THERAPY FOR ADULT BACTERIAL MENINGITIS IN THE ED

PATIENT CHARACTERISTICS	MOST LIKELY PATHOGENS	ANTIBIOTICS OF CHOICE
Otherwise healthy, ≤ 50 years	*S. pneumoniae, N. meningitidis, H. influenzae*	Ceftriaxone (100 mg/kg/day, up to 4 g/day, divided into 2 doses q 12 hr) *or* Cefotaxime (2 g IV q 4 hr) *or* Ceftizoxime (3 g IV q 8 hr)
> 50 yrs, immunocompromised and/or alcoholic	Same as above, but *L. monocytogenes* and/or enteric gram-negative rods also possible	Same as no. 1 above, but add Ampicillin (2 g IV q 4 hr)
Injection drug user	*S. pneumoniae, N. meningitidis,* enteric gram-negative rods, *H. influenzae, S. aureus*	Same as no. 1 above. Also add either Vancomycin (1 g IV q 12 hr) OR Nafcillin (50 mg/kg IV q 6 hr)
Status post head trauma or intracranial surgery	*S. pneumoniae, H. influenzae,* staphylococci, enteric gram-negative rods including *Pseudomonas* sp.	May subsitute Ceftazidime (2 g IV q 8 hr) for any of the third-generation cephalosporins listed in no. 1 above and add either Vancomycin *or* Nafcillin
Neutropenic	*S. pneumoniae, H. influenzae,* enteric gram-negative rods including *Pseudomonas* sp., staphylococci, *L. monocytogenes*	Ceftazidime, Ampicillin, and Vancomycin or Nafcillin
Shunt-associated meningitis	Coag-negative staphylococci, *S. aureus, Proprionibacterium acnes,* gram-negative enteric rods, and enterococci	Ceftazidime (or other third-generation cephalosporin listed under no. 1 above) and Vancomycin ± Rifampin (600 mg IV/day)

3. In the setting of an alert and oriented, nontoxic patient clinically suspected of having viral meningitis, the ED physician may decide to empirically treat for bacterial meningitis until the clinical situation is absolutely clear and CSF cultures are negative, or to closely observe the patient and withhold antibiotics pending a repeat lumbar puncture in 8–12 hours (the repeat lumbar puncture should demonstrate a lymphocyte predominance). There is no specific antibiotic therapy for viral meningitis (except in the setting of herpes simplex meningoencephalitis, where IV acyclovir should be utilized [*dose:* 10 mg/kg IV every 8 hours]).

4. Encephalitis should be treated empirically as bacterial meningitis by the ED physician until the cause of the encephalitis is clear. Both neurology and infectious disease consultations are appropriate.

VIII. DISPOSITION

A. Discharge

The patient with clear-cut viral (not herpetic) meningitis on the basis of presentation and lumbar puncture results may be discharged from the ED if all of the following conditions hold: patient is reliable, awake, alert, and nontoxic; has normal vital signs; has a reliable third party who can observe the patient; and follow-up is possible within 12–24 hours. It is prudent and appropriate to also obtain internal medicine, neurology, or infectious disease consultation on these patients prior to ED discharge, or to admit them for observation and repeat lumbar puncture.

B. Admit

All patients with suspected bacterial meningitis or encephalitis should be admitted. The patient with altered mental status or vital-sign instability should be admitted to the ICU for close monitoring.

C. Chemoprophylaxis

1. Meningococcal prophylaxis should be reserved for close contacts (family, roommates, mouth-to-mouth resuscitators):
   a. Rifampin (drug of choice) 600 mg PO bid for 2 days (10 mg/kg/day bid PO for 2 days for children).
   b. Minocycline (2 mg/kg/d PO every 12 hours for 5 days) is an alternative drug to rifampin, but it is not favored because of the high frequency of vestibular toxicity.
   c. Prophylaxis may *also* be possible with one dose of ciprofloxacin 750 mg PO (*not* FDA approved, can *not* be used in pregnant patients, nursing women, or patients < age 18).

2. Chemoprophylaxis is also appropriate for close contacts of patients with *H. influenzae* meningitis. The drug of choice is

rifampin, one dose of 20 mg/kg (not to exceed 600 mg per dose) PO per day for 4 days.

IX. PEARLS AND PITFALLS

A. Suspect meningitis (and pursue diagnosis with a lumbar puncture) in any patient with a fever and mental status changes (even if another infectious source is apparent), fever and meningeal signs, fever and a moderate to severe headache, or headache and meningeal signs.

B. A head CT is *not* mandatory before lumbar puncture in all cases, but do obtain a head CT first in the setting of papilledema, altered mental status, focal neurologic examination, or known/suspected HIV infection.

C. Do not delay antibiotic therapy because of delays in obtaining a head CT or a lumbar puncture. For typical cases, treatment should begin within 30 minutes of the patient's ED arrival.

D. It is difficult to distinguish bacterial from viral meningitis on the basis of CSF laboratory studies alone, owing to the large overlap in findings. If in doubt, treat for bacterial meningitis until culture results are negative.

BIBLIOGRAPHY

Durand ML, Calderwood SB, Wever DJ, et al: Acute bacterial meningitis in adults: a review of 493 episodes. N Engl J Med 1993;328:21–28.

Quagliarello V, Scheld WM: Bacterial meningitis: Pathogenesis, pathophysiology, and progress. N Engl J Med 1992;327:864–872.

Tunkel AR, Wispelwey B, Scheld WM: Bacterial meningitis: Recent advances in pathophysiology and treatment. Ann Intern Med. 1990;112:610–623.

Walsh-Kelly C, Nelson DB, Smith DS, et al: Clinical predictors of bacterial versus aseptic meningitis in childhood. Ann Emerg Med 1992;21:910–914.

INFECTIOUS MONONUCLEOSIS

"The fact that your patient gets well does not prove that your diagnosis was correct."

SAMUEL J. METIZER (1851–1921)

I. ESSENTIAL FACTS

A. Definition

Infectious mononucleosis (IM) is a clinical syndrome characterized by fever, malaise, pharyngitis, and lymphadenopathy. Laboratory findings include lymphocytosis with atypical lymphocytes and positive tests for heterophil antibodies. Ninety percent of cases are caused by Epstein-Barr virus (EBV).

B. Epidemiology

1. EBV is worldwide in distribution. The clinical manifestations vary with age, and the typical IM syndrome is most common in developed countries. In the United States, the highest incidence of primary infection is in persons 15–19 years of age.

2. Transmission is usually by salivary exchange, but blood-borne infection is also possible. The communicability of EBV is low to moderate and the source of infection is usually not found. Ninety percent of patients shed virus in saliva during the first week of illness and for weeks to months afterward. In addition, most asymptomatic persons who are EBV-seropositive have intermittent viral shedding in their saliva.

II. CLINICAL EVALUATION

A. History and Symptoms

1. IM should be suspected when a patient complaining of sore throat has prominent malaise, fever, and lymphadenopathy.

2. In a typical case, a 3–5-day prodrome of fatigue, myalgia, and malaise is followed by a 1–3-week period in which the major symptoms are sore throat, fever, headache, and fatigue. Of febrile cases, 90% have fever for > 1 week; 50% have fever for > 2 weeks. The total duration of illness is usually < 4 weeks, but 3% of cases last longer.

3. The rare complication of splenic rupture (0.1–0.2%) is suggested by left-upper-quadrant abdominal pain radiating to the left shoulder. Splenic rupture occurs between days 4 and 28 of illness and is usually spontaneous.

B. Signs and Physical Examination Findings

1. Most common signs include lymphadenopathy (90% of cases), fever > 38.3°C (75%), splenomegaly (50%), exudative pharyngitis (40%), and petechiae on the hard palate (27%). Lymphadenopathy, pharyngitis, and splenomegaly are significantly less common in elderly patients with primary EBV infection than in adolescents and young adults.

2. Other signs include hepatomegaly (20% of cases; but 42% in patients > age 40), neurologic abnormalities (2%; may include aseptic meningitis, encephalitis, cranial nerve palsies, transverse myelitis, or Guillain-Barré syndrome), pulmonary consolidation and pleural effusions (< 1% of cases), myocarditis and pericarditis (< 1% of cases).

3. Urticarial or morbilliform rashes occur in 4% of cases. Patients inadvertently treated with ampicillin will develop a rash 90% of the time. This generally does not represent an ampicillin allergy.

4. A rare but potentially life-threatening complication of IM is

airway obstruction due to pharyngeal lymphoid tissue hyperplasia.

C. Laboratory Evaluation

1. **Hematologic Tests.** An absolute (lymphocyte count > 4000/mm^3) and relative (lymphocytes account for > 50% of total leukocytes) lymphocytosis are each seen in > 90% of patients with IM. Also, in > 90% of patients, atypical lymphocytes account for > 10% of the total leukocytes. These hematologic findings may be only intermittently present through the course of the illness. Hemolytic anemia with anti-I antibody and significant thrombocytopenia occur occasionally.

2. **Serologic Tests**

   a. The Monospot and other card or slide tests are usually used to detect the heterophil antibody that is characteristic of EBV infection (Fig. 15–18). A positive test means the titer is ≥ 1:80. Positive and negative predictive values are both 95% in young adult populations. False-negative results are usually positive when repeated 1–2 weeks later: 50% of patients have a positive heterophil test after 1 week of illness; the fraction rises to 90% by the end of the third week. Heterophil-negative IM is more common in children and the elderly.

   b. Specific anti-EBV antibodies are the "gold standard" for diagnosing EBV infection but are normally out of the scope of emergency medicine practice. The presence of antibodies to viral capsid antigen (VCA) and the absence of antibody to EB nuclear antigen (EBNA) indicate current or recent IM.

3. **Biochemical Tests.** Mild elevations of the transaminase or alkaline phosphatase levels occur in 90% of IM cases, with peak values by the second to third week of illness. These tests should not be routinely ordered, however.

4. **Imaging Studies.** These generally have no place in the diagnosis or management of IM. If splenic rupture is suspected, an abdominal computed tomography (CT) scan is the test of choice; surgical consultation should be obtained in this setting.

III. DIFFERENTIAL DIAGNOSIS

A. Pharyngitis. IM causes < 2% of cases of pharyngitis. The main differential point is to distinguish patients requiring antibiotics (primarily due to group A streptococci or gonococci) from other causes (see Pharyngitis, later in this chapter).

B. Prolonged malaise, fever, and lymphadenopathy.

   1. Cytomegalovirus (CMV) infection may cause fever, spleno-

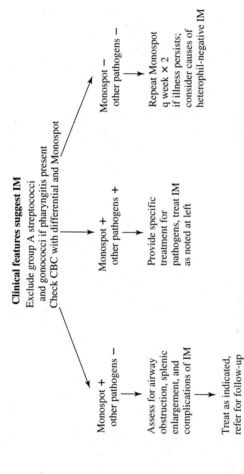

Figure 15-18 Flow diagram for diagnosis and management of IM.

Clinical features suggest IM

Exclude group A streptococci
and gonococci if pharyngitis present
Check CBC with differential and Monospot

Monospot +
other pathogens −

Assess for airway
obstruction, splenic
enlargement, and
complications of IM

Treat as indicated,
refer for follow-up

Monospot +
other pathogens +

Provide specific
treatment for
pathogens, treat IM
as noted at left

Monospot −
other pathogens −

Repeat Monospot
q week × 2
if illness persists;
consider causes of
heterophil-negative IM

465

Table 15–17. MISCELLANEOUS CAUSES OF HETEROPHIL-NEGATIVE INFECTIOUS MONONUCLEOSIS

Viruses	Hepatitis (A, B, C), mumps, adenovirus, HIV
Bacteria	Listeriosis, subacute bacterial endocarditis, brucellosis, chronic meningococcemia, syphilis, cat-scratch disease
Parasites	Toxoplasmosis, trichinosis
Noninfectious	Serum sickness, systemic lupus erythematosus, polyarteritis nodosa, drug reactions (isoniazid, para-aminosalicylic acid, sulfasalazine, phenytoin, and rubella vaccine)

Table 15–18. MEDICATIONS FOR INFECTIOUS MONONUCLEOSIS

For symptomatic relief of fever and pharyngitis:
1. Acetaminophen 650 mg PO q 4 hr
2. Viscous lidocaine 5 mL diluted with water to 10 mL, swish and spit q 2–4 hr

For relief of mild airway compromise associated with pharyngeal swelling in outpatients:
Prednisone 40 mg PO bid for 5 days, then tapered over 1 week

For relief of airway compromise associated with pharyngeal swelling in inpatients:
Methylprednisolone 40 mg IV q 6 hr

megaly, hepatitis, and atypical lymphocytosis. Pharyngitis and cervical adenopathy are unusual signs of CMV infection.

2. Toxoplasmosis may cause fever, splenomegaly, generalized lymphadenopathy, and atypical lymphocytosis; pharyngitis is uncommon.

3. Rubella may mimic IM but is associated with a rash that affects the face. When it occurs, the rash of IM spares the face.

4. Hematologic malignancy, such as leukemia or lymphoma, may require lymph node or bone marrow biopsy for diagnosis.

5. *Heterophil-negative* IM is the term applied to patients with the typical signs and symptoms of IM but a negative heterophil test. Half of these cases are due to EBV, one-third to CMV, and the remainder to other causes (Table 15–17).

IV. MANAGEMENT

Figure 15–18 and Table 15–18 present the management of IM.

A. The therapy of uncomplicated IM is supportive and should include activity limitations. Patients with significant pharyngitis or fever may benefit from topical anesthetics (viscous lidocaine) or acetaminophen; these patients should also have a throat culture obtained to exclude concomitant group A beta-hemolytic streptococcal infection. Care must be taken to avoid volume depletion.

B. Corticosteroids are useful in preventing airway obstruction and the need for emergency surgery (tonsillectomy or tracheostomy). Patients with stridor in the supine position or severe odynophagia should be admitted to the hospital and receive intravenous corticosteroids. Patients with dyspnea or more severe stridor may require urgent surgical intervention.

C. Although most splenic ruptures in patients with IM are nontraumatic, activity restriction is prudent. Physical training should be deferred for 1 month, vigorous athletics for 2 months, and strenuous contact sports for 3–6 months. If the patient is a competitive athlete involved in strenuous contact sports, splenic imaging to exclude nonpalpable splenomegaly should be considered prior to giving clearance for full-contact activity. Patients with suspected splenic rupture at the time of presentation need urgent surgical evaluation.

V. DISPOSITION

A. Discharge

Patients with uncomplicated IM may be discharged to home care. Patients with splenomegaly should have a follow-up outpatient clinical evaluation.

B. Admit

Patients who are debilitated, volume depleted, or suffering from complications of IM (moderate to severe airway compromise, splenic rupture, severe hepatitis, hemolytic anemia, myocarditis, or neurologic compromise) should be admitted to the hospital for observation and therapy.

VI. PEARLS AND PITFALLS

A. Consider and exclude bacterial causes of pharyngitis (such as group A streptococci and gonococci) in patients with pharyngitis.

B. Instruct the patient to avoid activities that exchange saliva with other persons.

C. Treat patients with severe odynophagia and pharyngeal swelling with intravenous corticosteroids and consider hospital admission.

D. Restrict activities and arrange follow-up for patients with splenomegaly discharged from the ED.

E. Do not overlook abdominal complaints in a patient with IM.

F. Avoid excessive palpation of the spleen in a patient with IM.

G. Do not administer ampicillin to a patient with IM.

BIBLIOGRAPHY

Axelrod P, Finestone AJ: Infectious mononucleosis in older adults. Am Fam Phys 1990;42:1599–1606.
Cheeseman SH: Infectious mononucleosis. Semin Hematol 1988;25:261–268.
Chetham MM, Roberts KB: Infectious mononucleosis in adolescents. Pediatr Ann 1991;20:206–213.
Konvolinka CW, Wyatt DB: Splenic rupture and infectious mononucleosis. J Emerg Med 1988;7:471–475.

OTITIS MEDIA AND OTITIS EXTERNA

". . . my ears hum . . ."
SAPPHO (612 BC)

I. ESSENTIAL FACTS

A. Definitions

Acute *otitis media* is a suppurative infection of the middle ear. *Otitis externa* is infection of the external auditory canal. *Serous otitis media* occurs when the middle ear space is filled with a noninfectious fluid, often in the setting of a viral upper-respiratory-tract infection.

B. Causative Organisms

1. **Otitis Media.** *Streptococcus pneumoniae* and nontypable *Hemophilus influenzae* are the most likely causes in children and adults. Beta-lactamase-producing organisms are an increasing problem. Viral agents (influenza, respiratory syncytial virus, adenovirus) may play a primary or secondary role. Mycoplasma is rarely found in middle-ear isolates from patients with otitis media but has been associated with bullous myringitis. *Pneumococcus* and *H. influenzae,* however, probably cause most cases of bullous myringitis, especially in young children.

2. **Otitis Externa.** *Pseudomonas aeruginosa* is the most common cause of otitis externa in children and adults. Other causes include *Staphylococcus aureus, S. pyogenes,* fungi (*Aspergillus* and *Candida*), other gram-negative bacteria (*Proteus, Escherichia coli*), and viruses (herpes zoster). Trauma or exposure to chlorinated water is the usual predisposing cause.

II. CLINICAL EVALUATION

A. Symptoms

1. **Otitis Media.** Pain in the ear and fever are common symptoms (in 40–60% of cases). Nausea, vomiting, vertigo, and hearing loss are seen less frequently. Predisposing conditions include

viral infections, allergy, and prior ear infections. Tympanocentesis provides the only accurate method for obtaining culture material, but it is not usually necessary. Antibiotic selection should be based on knowledge of the likely bacteria.

2. **Otitis Externa.** Pain in the affected ear and pruritus are common, but fever is rare. Otoscopic examination reveals erythema, serosanguineous or purulent discharge, and granulation tissue in the external canal. Swimming and frequent use of cotton-tipped swabs may be predisposing factors. Culture of material from the external canal can be useful. Elderly, diabetic patients are at risk of developing invasive ("malignant") otitis externa. These patients are ill, febrile, and with frequent deep tissue involvement. Severe neurologic complications may develop in patients with invasive otitis externa; this group of patients requires admission, otolaryngology consultation, and parenteral antibiotic treatment.

3. **Serous Otitis Media.** Serous otitis media is painless and the patient notes decreased hearing in the affected ear.

B. Signs

The diagnosis of otitis media and otitis externa is usually made on the basis of clinical findings, including otoscopic examination of the color, contour, translucence, and mobility of the tympanic membrane. Cultures obtained via myringotomy are rarely indicated but may be useful in the following situations:

1. Severe systemic toxicity.

2. Immunosuppressed patients.

3. Patients not responding to prior antibiotic therapy.

4. Signs of infection beyond the middle ear (mastoiditis or temporal bone osteomyelitis).

Roentgenography and computed tomography may occasionally be useful in complicated cases.

III. THERAPY

Figure 15–19 and Table 15–19 present the therapy of otitis media and otitis externa.

A. For otitis media in adults, give amoxicillin or trimethoprim-sulfamethoxazole. Some authors recommend the routine use of amoxicillin with clavulanic acid (Augmentin), though most would reserve this for patients who do not respond to less expensive therapy. Other possible drugs include cefaclor and cefuroxime.

B. For otitis externa, gently cleanse the ear canal of any debris. Topical therapy is then usually effective for uncomplicated otitis externa. Acetic acid 2% (five drops qid) or otic solutions

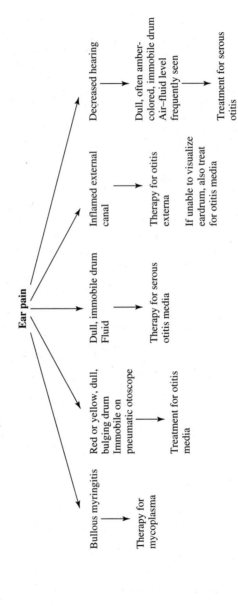

Figure 15–19. Symptoms, findings, and treatment of ear pain.

Table 15–19. THERAPY FOR OTITIS MEDIA AND OTITIS EXTERNA IN ADULTS

Otitis Media	
Uncomplicated	Amoxicillin 500 mg tid for 10 days *or* Trimethoprim-sulfamethoxazole DS bid for 10 days
Infection not responding to therapy for uncomplicated infection	Amoxicillin/clavulanate (Augmentin) 500 mg tid for 10 days *or* Cefaclor (Ceclor) 500 mg PO tid for 10 days *or* Cefuroxime (Ceftin) 250–500 mg PO bid for 10 days
Serous Otitis Media	Phenylephrine nasal spray (0.25–0.50%) 2 puffs each nostril bid–qid × 3 days
Otitis Externa	
Uncomplicated[a]	Acetic acid 2% 5 drops tid–qid *or* Polymyxin drops *or* Neomycin drops
Extensive swelling or exudate	Acetic acid 2% with 1% hydrocortisone 5 drops tid–qid *Consider adding* Ciprofloxacin 500 mg PO bid × 7–10 days

[a]For prominent exudate or swelling, place a cotton wick in the external canal and leave in place for 1–2 days. Drops should be used to moisten the wick, which serves to keep the medicine in contact with the canal.

containing antibiotics and hydrocortisone (Cortisporin-otic) are effective also. If there is extensive swelling and/or exudate, 2% acetic acid drops with 1% hydrocortisone may be useful. A cotton wick, moistened with otic drops and placed in the external canal, should be considered for the first 24–48 hours in patients with prominent edema and exudate.

C. If the tympanic membrane cannot be well visualized in the presence of otitis externa, it is reasonable to treat the patient with systemic antibiotics for otitis media in addition to treatment for externa. Patients with invasive external otitis due to *P. aeruginosa* should be hospitalized, seen by an otolaryngologist, and treated with intravenous antibiotics for an extended period of time.

D. For serous otitis media, decongestants are indicated.

E. Bullous myringitis often indicates mycoplasma; treat with erythromycin 250–500 mg qid for 10 days.

F. Adjunctive therapy includes pain medications. Decongestants may be of empiric benefit.

IV. PEARLS AND PITFALLS

A. Consider placing a cotton wick in the external canal for patients with otitis externa and extensive swelling or exudate.

B. Treat for otitis media if the tympanic membrane cannot be well visualized in the patient with otitis externa.

C. Ruptured tympanic membranes should be treated as for otitis media.

D. Cultures are generally not necessary for uncomplicated infections.

BIBLIOGRAPHY

Celin SE, Bluestone CD, Stephenson J, et al: Bacteriology of acute otitis media in adults. JAMA 1991;299:2249–2252.

Evans P, Hofmann L: Malignant external otitis: a case report and review. Am Fam Phys 1994; 49(2):427–431.

Kligman EW: Treatment of otitis media. Am Fam Phys 1992;45(1):242–250.

Schwartz LE, Brown RB: Purulent otitis media in adults. Arch Intern Med 1992; 152:2301–2304.

PEDICULOSIS AND SCABIES

> *"It is easy to stand a pain, but difficult to stand an itch."*
>
> CHANG CH'AO

Pediculosis

I. ESSENTIAL FACTS

A. Definitions

Pediculosis is infestation by sucking lice. Three species infest humans: crab or pubic louse *(Phthirus pubis),* head louse *(Pediculus humanus capitis),* and body louse *(Pediculus humanus corporis).*

B. Transmission

1. Pubic lice (also called crab lice or crabs) are transmitted most commonly by sexual contact. Sharing a bed with an infested individual is the usual nonsexual route. Fomite transmission (clothing, towels, toilet seats) is possible but rare.

2. Head lice are transmitted by direct contact or contact with personal objects (hat, comb or brush).

3. Body lice feed upon the skin and reside in the seams of clothing, where the eggs are usually deposited. Transmission occurs with sharing of clothing; infestation is uncommon except in crowded living conditions (e.g., emergency shelters) and when hygiene is poor.

II. CLINICAL EVALUATION

A. Symptoms and Signs

Pruritis is the prominent symptom. Patients often see the lice or nits (cemented eggs on hair shafts), though the latter may be mistaken for dandruff. Small erythematous punctae are a manifestation of the bites. Intense scratching results in excoriations and bloody crusts. Secondary eczematization or infection (impetigo, cellulitis) with regional adenopathy may obscure the diagnosis. Urticaria may occur as an acquired sensitivity. Postinflammatory hyperpigmentation occurs only in protracted cases.

Head lice commonly infect the scalp around the ears and the occipital hairline. Lesions from body lice usually occur at points where clothing comes into close contact with skin (e.g., under collars, at waistlines). Pubic lice may be also found in the axilla, beard, eyelashes, and eyebrows.

B. Physical Examination

Careful observation with a hand lens will reveal pubic and head lice and their nits; the nits are usually found on the proximal hair shaft close to the skin. Confirmation of body lice infestation may require inspection of the seams of the patient's clothing.

III. DIFFERENTIAL DIAGNOSIS

The differential diagnosis includes other causes of eczema, dandruff, skin infection, and urticaria.

IV. THERAPY

A. Medications

Table 15–20 presents dosing and application of medications for treating pediculosis.

1. Permethrin 1% is ovicidal and safe in infants and during pregnancy and lactation. It is the drug of choice.

2. Pyrethrins with piperonyl butoxide are not as effective as permethrin, but are less expensive. Both pyrethrins and permethrin are available over-the-counter.

3. Malathion 0.5% is effective, safe, and the main treatment used in the United Kingdom.

4. Lindane 1% has been used commonly in the past. It is potentially toxic to the central nervous system (especially if used frequently), and it cannot be used on infants or on pregnant or nursing women. A repeat application 2 weeks after the first treatment is frequently necessary.

Table 15–20. MEDICAL THERAPY FOR PEDICULOSIS AND SCABIES

Drug	Application	Dispense	Comments
Pediculocides			
Permethrin 1% (Nix) Cream Rinse	Apply to unwetted affected area and leave on for 10 min before rinsing.	2 fluid ounces each for scalp or body.	Dispense enough for infested family members.
Pyrethrins with piperonyl butoxide (Rid, R & C shampoo, A-200 shampoo)	Apply to unwetted affected area and leave on for 10 min before rinsing.	2 fluid ounces each for scalp or body; and enough for a repeat treatment.	A repeat dose in 7–10 days is recommended if symptoms continue.
Malathion 0.5%	Apply to unwetted affected areas and leave on for 12 hr before rinsing.	As above.	As above.
Lindane 1% (Kwell) shampoo	Shampoo hair first and then dry thoroughly. Then apply Lindane to scalp and/or pubic hair. Work into a lather and leave on hair for 4 min before rinsing.	1–2 fluid ounces per application.	As above.
Scabicides			
Permethrin 5% (Elimite)	Rub into the skin from the neck down (including the soles of the feet) and leave on for 8–12 hr before showering.	Dispense 30 g for the average adult.	
Lindane 1% (Kwell) lotion or cream	Apply to the skin before bathing. Leave on for 8–12 hr before rinsing off.	30–60 g will treat the average adult.	A second application may be necessary in 7 days; but warn the patient about repeated use. This medication should *not* be used in pregnant patients, nursing mothers, or children < 10 years old.
Crotamiton 10% (Eurax)	After showering or bathing rub cream or lotion from the chin down and leave on for 24 hr, then reapply a second dose and leave on for another 24 hr. Then wash off.	60-g tube or bottle (sufficient for two applications in an adult).	Retreatment is frequently necessary. This is the preferred drug in young children/infants, pregnant patients, and nursing mothers.

B. General Measures

Pediculosis is a household and community illness. Treatment needs to be directed toward the patient, his personal effects (including clothing, bed linen), his contacts, and his living environment.

1. Machine-washing and hot-cycle drying cloth items is effective. Dry-cleaning and sealing in a plastic bag for 10 days are alternatives. Dry heat alone has been found to be effective for body lice. This may be more practical in an emergency shelter setting.

2. Vacuuming furniture, mattresses, and rugs will eliminate some environmental lice.

3. All sexual contacts and nonsexual close contacts should be treated simultaneously to avoid reinfestation.

4. After treatment, a tweezers or nit comb, often included with the medication, should be used to remove as many nits as possible.

5. Eyelid nits and lice can be treated with an occlusive ointment (e.g., white petrolatum) applied two to five times daily for 10 days. Do not use pediculocides on the eyelids.

Scabies

I. ESSENTIAL FACTS

A. Definitions

1. *Scabies* is infestation with the mite *Sarcoptes scabiei,* an obligate parasite of the epidermis of humans. Much smaller than a louse, the mite is usually invisible to the naked eye.

2. Norwegian scabies is a clinical variant of the infestation characterized by crusted, psoriasiform lesions containing thousands of mites. This form tends to occur in debilitated patients and patients with immune compromise (including the acquired immunodeficiency syndrome). It is quite contagious and is curiously relatively asymptomatic.

B. Transmission

Scabies is transmitted by close contact with infected individuals, their bedding, or articles of clothing. Symptoms are caused by an acquired sensitivity to the mite, noted 2–4 weeks after primary infection, or within 2 weeks of recurrent infections.

II. CLINICAL EVALUATION

A. Symptoms and Signs

1. Intense pruritus, often nocturnal, is characteristic. It is initially localized to the sites of burrows, but subsequently becomes generalized. In infants this may manifest as irritability.

2. The linear burrows (1–10 mm long) are pathognomonic but may be obscured by excoriations and secondary infection.

3. Skin lesions typically consist of erythematous papules, vesicles, or pustules at the sites of burrows. Impetiginization, eczema, and/or urticaria may also occur.

4. The mites have a predilection for the interdigital webs of hands, flexor surfaces of wrists, elbows, and axillary regions, nipples (in women), belt line, groin, buttocks, and penis. Adolescents

and adults are spared their faces and heads; infants frequently have involvement in these areas.

5. Erythematous indurated nodules may occur on the glans penis and buttocks as a result of sensitization and may persist for months following adequate treatment.

6. Pruritic eruption among several members of a family suggests scabies.

B. Diagnosis

1. Diagnosis is definitive if the mite, eggs, or feces are seen microscopically. A No. 15 scalpel blade, dipped in immersion oil, is used to scrape the end of one or more burrows. The contents are placed on a slide to which a drop of immersion oil is added. A coverslip is added and the slide is observed under the microscope at $10 \times$ magnification. Fingerwebs and intertriginous areas are especially good sites for finding mites.

2. Burrows can be demonstrated using dark ink applied to suspicious lesions and then wiped off with alcohol. The burrow with take up the ink and will be apparent after wiping. The same can be done with topical tetracycline and the use of a fluorescent lamp; the burrows will illuminate yellow-green under a Wood's lamp.

3. Late in the course of the infestation, the mites or eggs may not be demonstrable. In this situation, the clinical manifestation of intense pruritus and lesions with secondary excoriations is enough to suggest the diagnosis.

III. DIFFERENTIAL DIAGNOSIS

The differential diagnosis includes dermatitis herpetiformis, atopic eczema, contact dermatitis, xerosis, and pruritis associated with a systemic disease.

IV. THERAPY

A. Medications

Table 15–20 presents medications for treatment of scabies.

1. Permethrin 5% cream (prescription needed) applied from the neck down is the treatment of choice.

2. Lindane 1% and crotamiton 10% are alternatives, but are more toxic and less effective, respectively. Crotamiton is the drug of choice, however, in the pregnant patient, nursing mothers, and children < 10 years old.

3. Norwegian scabies may require repeated treatment to effect a cure.

B. General Measures

1. Itching may persist for weeks and is usually caused by hypersensitivity rather than persistent infestation. Antipruritics (e.g., benadryl or hydroxyzine 25-50 mg PO every 6 hours as needed) are usually required.

2. Antibiotics may be necessary for secondary bacterial infections (e.g., dicloxicillin, cephalexin, or erythromycin 250-500 mg PO every 6 hours for 7-10 days).

3. Treat sexual and close nonsexual contacts.

4. Clothing or bed linen not used in the previous 2 days need not be treated. Otherwise treat as described under Pediculosis.

V. PEARLS AND PITFALLS

A. A second sexually transmitted disease is present in 30% of those infested with pubic lice. A thorough sexual history and examination are essential.

B. Topical corticosteroids can be used for local control of pruritus or an eczematous response. Do not use while lindane is on the skin. Start with the application of triamcinolone cream (0.025%) to involved sites (excluding the face and genital areas).

C. There is no evidence to support routine environmental cleaning with a pediculocide. The only exceptions are cleansing the toilet seat (in the case of a patient with pediculosis) and cleansing wigs, hairbrushes, and combs (in the case of a patient with head lice).

D. Excessive use of lindane by patients in an attempt to control pruritus is common. Central nervous system side effects may result from excessive cutaneous absorption. An irritant dermatitis may result from repeated applications of gamma benzene hexachloride. Resultant pruritus will create unwarranted patient concern for persistence of infestation.

BIBLIOGRAPHY

Blondell RD: Parasites of the skin and hair. Prim Care 1991;18:167–83.
Burns DA: The treatment of human ectoparasite infection. Br J Dermatol 1991;125: 89–93.
Centers for Disease Control and Prevention. 1993 Sexually transmitted diseases treatment guidelines. MMWR 1993;42(No. RR-14).

PHARYNGITIS

"To blow and swallow at the same time is not easy."
TITUS MACCIUS PLAUTUS

I. ESSENTIAL FACTS

A. Definition

Pharyngitis is an infection of the oropharynx caused by a variety of viruses and bacteria. Most infections are self-limited; complications may include otitis media, sinusitis, cervical adenitis, peritonsillar abscess, retropharyngeal abscess, and nonsuppurative sequelae of *Streptococcus pyogenes* infection (e.g., rheumatic fever, glomerulonephritis).

B. Etiology

1. Viruses cause most cases of pharyngitis.
2. Bacteria may cause as many as 30% of cases in epidemic settings (Table 15–21).
   a. *S. pyogenes* infections occur most frequently in school-age children.
   b. *Mycoplasma* may cause pharyngitis in individuals 10–30 years old.
3. Distribution of causative agents depends on the patient's age and clinical setting.
   a. Pharyngitis in young children is commonly caused by several different viruses, including: respiratory syncytial virus, adenovirus, rhinovirus, parainfluenza virus, and enteroviruses.
   b. In adults, parainfluenza virus, influenza virus, adenovirus, enteroviruses, Epstein-Barr virus, and herpes simplex virus also cause pharyngitis.

II. CLINICAL EVALUATION

A. History

Sore throat usually develops acutely. Accompanying symptoms often include generalized malaise, myalgia, fever, coryza, cough, and laryngitis. Although symptoms and physical findings do not provide a specific diagnosis, there are suggestive findings.

B. Physical Examination

1. Tender cervical lymphadenopathy, in association with an exudative pharyngitis and fever suggest streptococcal infection, but only a minority of patients with streptococcal pharyngitis will have all of these.
2. Exudative pharyngitis alone is not a specific finding for streptococcal infection. It can be seen with Epstein-Barr virus, adenovirus, herpes simplex virus, and other viral infections.
3. Scarlet fever is suggested by a bright erythematous rash with a sandpaper quality involving the trunk, face, and skin folds (Pastia's lines). There is circumoral pallor. The rash usually

Table 15–21. MICROBIAL CAUSES OF ACUTE PHARYNGITIS

	SYNDROME/DISEASE	ESTIMATED IMPORTANCE[a]
Viral		
Rhinovirus (89 types and 1 subtype)	Common cold	20
Coronavirus (4 or more types)	Common cold	≥ 5
Adenovirus (types 3, 4, 7, 14, 21)	Pharyngoconjunctival fever, ARDs	5
Herpes simplex virus (types 1 and 2)	Gingivitis, stomatitis, pharyngitis	4
Parainfluenza virus (types 1–4)	Common cold, croup	2
Influenza virus (types A and B)	Influenza	2
Coxsackievirus A (types 2, 4–6, 8, 10)	Herpangina	< 1
Epstein-Barr virus	Infectious mononucleosis	< 1
Cytomegalovirus	Infectious mononucleosis	< 1
Human immunodeficiency virus	Primary HIV infection	< 1
Bacterial		
Streptococcus pyogenes (group A beta-hemolytic streptococcus)	Pharyngitis/tonsillitis, scarlet fever	15–30
Mixed anaerobic infection	Gingivitis, pharyngitis (Vincent's angina)	< 1
	Peritonsillitis/peritonsillar abscess (quinsy)	< 1
Neisseria gonorrhoeae	Pharyngitis	< 1
Corynebacterium diphtheriae	Diphtheria	≥ 1
Corynebacterium ulcerans	Pharyngitis, diphtheria	< 1
Corynebacterium hemolyticum (*Arcanobacterium hemolyticum*)	Pharyngitis, scarlatiniform rash	< 1
Yersinia enterocolitica	Pharyngitis, enterocolitis	< 1
Treponema pallidum	Secondary syphilis	< 1
Chlamydial		
Chlamydia psittaci	ARDs, pneumonia	Unknown
Mycoplasmal		
Mycoplasma pneumoniae	Pneumonia/bronchitis/pharyngitis	< 1
M hominis (type 1)	Pharyngitis in volunteers	Unknown
Unknown		40

[a]Estimated percentage of cases of pharyngitis due to indicated organism in civilians of all ages.

ARDs, adult respiratory distress syndrome; HIV, human immunodeficiency virus.

From Mandell GL, Douglas RG Jr, Bennett JE: Principles and Practice of Infectious Diseases, 3rd ed. New York, Churchill Livingstone, 1990, p. 494.

spares the palms and soles and desquamates in the resolving phase. A "strawberry" tongue may be present.

III. DIFFERENTIAL DIAGNOSIS

A. *Diphtheria* is suggested by an adherent gray-black membrane with edema of the tonsillar fauces.

B. *Peritonsillar abscess* (quinsy) most commonly occurs at the superior pole of the tonsil. It often produces dysphagia and physical findings of impaired palatal motion and a fluctuant mass with a laterally displaced uvula.

C. *Retropharyngeal abscess* typically causes referred pain to the back of the neck. Symptoms include fever, neck pain, sore throat, dysphagia, and drooling. Dyspnea may be present. Examination may reveal erythema and bulging of the posterior wall of the pharynx.

D. *Epiglottitis* is suggested by sore throat, fever, cervical adenopathy, and severe dysphagia. The severity of the sore throat is frequently out of proportion to physical examination findings.

E. *Neisseria gonorrhoeae* can cause an acute exudative pharyngitis or tonsillitis in the setting of orogenital contact (although 90% of cases are asymptomatic).

IV. DIAGNOSIS

A. Clinical Diagnostic/Treatment Strategy

"Predictive" markers used clinically in the diagnosis of streptococcal pharyngitis include fever > 38° C, exudative tonsillitis, anterior cervical adenopathy, and lack of cough. If three or four of these clinical findings are present, empiric therapy (without culture) is a cost-effective decision. If two of these findings are present, empiric therapy or culture is reasonable. If only one finding is present, culture only is reasonable (Fig. 15–20).

B. Laboratory Studies

1. Throat cultures are considered the "gold standard" for the diagnosis of group A streptococcal pharyngitis. In general, cultures should be performed for streptococcal isolation only ("rule out" beta-hemolytic streptococcus) unless the clinical setting also suggests the possibility of *N. gonorrhoeae*.

2. Antibody studies such as antistreptolysin-O (ASO) titer and streptozyme titers are useful only for retrospective diagnosis (e.g., in the setting of rheumatic fever or glomerulonephritis).

3. Pharyngeal Gram staining is useful in identifying patients with a high likelihood of streptococcus. It is reliable only when performed by experienced personnel.

4. Rapid (10-minute) "strep" tests are available to diagnose streptococcal infection. Sensitivity (60–95%), and specificity (95–100%) approach that of standard culture. A positive test is justification for treatment, but a negative test should be followed by a culture. The best clinical strategy for laboratory diagnosis of streptococcus is controversial, and it varies from one ED to another.

V. THERAPY

Figure 15–20 presents the treatment protocol for pharyngitis.

A. Streptococcal pharyngitis can be treated effectively with intra-muscular (IM) benzathine penicillin (1.2 million units IM in a single dose for adults), or with oral (PO) penicillin VK (250 mg PO qid, or 500 mg PO bid, for 10 days in adults). Ten days of oral antibiotic therapy is necessary to prevent a relapse; the recidivistic rates of streptococcal infection are unacceptably high. Oral penicillin is preferred in reliable patients, as the risk of life-threatening anaphylaxis is less.

B. Erythromycin (250 mg PO qid for 10 days) is an effective alternative for penicillin-allergic patients.

C. The objectives of therapy are to prevent suppurative complications, to prevent rheumatic fever, to eliminate streptococci from the pharynx, to decrease disease transmission, and to relieve symptoms. Antibiotics may ameliorate symptoms if they are given in the first 24 hours of streptococcal infection; otherwise, symptomatic benefit is difficult to demonstrate.

D. No specific treatment is available for viral pharyngitis except amantadine for influenza A infections and acyclovir for herpes virus infections.

E. Treatment of contacts (e.g., household, sexual) is controversial. Empiric treatment of symptomatic contacts is indicated, especially if there is culture documentation of the index case.

F. Adjunctive therapy:

1. Acetaminophen (650 mg PO every 4 hours) for fever.

2. Salt-water gargles ($\frac{1}{2}$ teaspoon salt in $\frac{1}{2}$ glass of water, gargle and spit, every 4-6 hours)

3. Pain medications (e.g., acetaminophen with codeine or oxy-codone PO every 4–6 hours for moderately severe pain).

4. Recent data suggest that dexamethasone (10 mg IM) may significantly improve pain relief in patients with acute exudative pharyngitis. Empiric antibiotic therapy for strep-tococcal pharyngitis should be prescribed concomitantly. Dexamethasone should not be used in the setting of known acquired immunodeficiency syndrome, pregnancy, sus-pected peritonsillar abscess, thrush, or ulcerative pharyn-gitis.

VI. DISPOSITION

Outpatient therapy is indicated for simple pharyngitis. Occasion-ally, moderately ill or dehydrated patients with streptococcal phar-yngitis require admission.

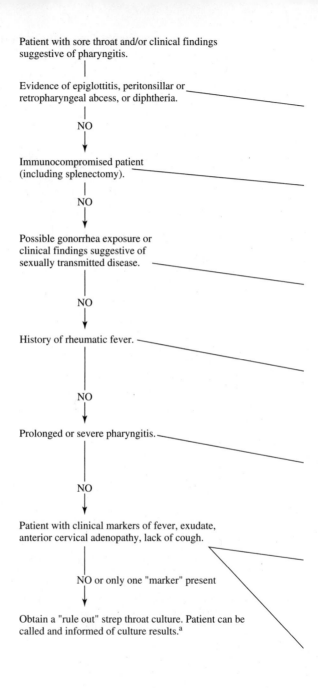

Patient with sore throat and/or clinical findings suggestive of pharyngitis.

Evidence of epiglottitis, peritonsillar or retropharyngeal abcess, or diphtheria.

NO

Immunocompromised patient (including splenectomy).

NO

Possible gonorrhea exposure or clinical findings suggestive of sexually transmitted disease.

NO

History of rheumatic fever.

NO

Prolonged or severe pharyngitis.

NO

Patient with clinical markers of fever, exudate, anterior cervical adenopathy, lack of cough.

NO or only one "marker" present

Obtain a "rule out" strep throat culture. Patient can be called and informed of culture results.[a]

[a] *Some clinicians begin the patient on penicillin PO and contact the patient to cancel the treatment if the culture is negative.*

482   **Figure 15–20.** Pharyngitis treatment protocol.

YES

Evaluate for potential airway compromise.
CBC, IV access, and otolaryngology consult mandatory.

YES

Gram stain, throat culture, and CBC.
Treat as appropriate for suspected cause.
Close follow-up mandatory, and admission
reasonable. (Splenectomized patients with
pharyngitis can develop fulminant sepsis.)

YES

Obtain GC cultures, give ceftriaxone 250 mg IM.
Obtain RPR, and consider concomitant
chlamydia treatment. Follow-up and proof of
cure mandatory.

YES

Obtain throat culture and, in the non-penicillin-
allergic patient, treat with penicillin PO or
benzathine penicillin IM. (Use erythromycin in
the penicillin-allergic patient.)

YES

Consider the possibilities of *Yersinia,*
C. diphtheriae, C. hemolyticum, and
mononucleosis. Throat culture mandatory,
monospot test reasonable. Close follow-up mandatory.

YES: three or four "markers" present

Empiric treatment:
In the non-penicillin-allergic patient, give
penicillin PO or benzathine penicillin IM. Use
erythromycin in the penicillin-allergic patient.

YES: only two "markers" present

Obtain a "rule out strep" culture or treat empirically.

VII. PEARLS AND PITFALLS

A. There are several clinical approaches to the management of acute pharyngitis. The diagnostic approach (e.g., use of cultures versus rapid "strep" test versus Gram stain), and therapy (e.g., empiric therapy, oral penicillin, intramuscular penicillin, treat initially and stop, or continue pending cultures), is dependent on local ED practice, resources, and patient population.

B. Oral versus intramuscular penicillin involves trade-offs between lower compliance with oral penicillin versus increased pain and higher risk of life-threatening anaphylaxis with intramuscular benzathine penicillin therapy.

C. When the discomfort of the patient is out of proportion to physical examination findings, suspect epiglottitis.

BIBLIOGRAPHY

Bisno AL: Group A streptococcal infections and acute rheumatic fever. N Engl J Med 1991;325:783–793.

Kiselica D: Group A beta-hemolytic streptococcal pharyngitis: current clinical concepts. Am Fam Phys 1994;49(5):1147–1154.

Lieu TA, Fleisher GR, Schwartz JS: Cost-effectiveness of rapid latex agglutination testing and throat culture for streptococcal pharyngitis. Pediatrics 1990;85:246–256.

O'Brien JF, JL Falk, JL Meade: Dexamethasone as adjuvant therapy for severe acute pharyngitis. Ann Emerg Med 1993;22:212–213.

PNEUMONIA

> "In the mortality bills, pneumonia is
> . . . 'the Captain of the men of death.' "
>
> SIR WILLIAM OSLER

I. ESSENTIAL FACTS

A. Definition

1. *Pneumonia* is an inflammatory process of the lung parenchyma; its prevalence in adults with an acute respiratory illness is 3–10%.

2. *Community-acquired pneumonia* is a pulmonary infection contracted outside of the hospital setting.

3. *"Typical pneumonia"* is a community-acquired pneumonia caused by a bacterial pathogen; the patient "typically" presents with a sudden high fever, toxicity, purulent sputum, and ± pleuritic chest pain (Table 15–22).

4. *"Atypical pneumonia"* is a community-acquired pneumonia caused by a nonpyogenic organism. The term is frequently applied to any pneumonia that presents with diffuse constitutional symptoms and a nonproductive cough (Table 15–22).

Table 15–22. ETIOLOGY OF ACUTE PNEUMONIA BASED UPON DIFFERENCES IN PRESENTATION

	"TYPICAL" PRESENTATION	"ATYPICAL" PRESENTATION
Age	Any age	Usually young
Symptoms and Signs	Sudden onset Fever > 103° F common Shaking chills Pleuritic chest pain Tachycardia/tachypnea Consolidation on auscultation	Gradual-onset High fever less common Chills uncommon Pleuritic pain uncommon Pulse and respirations often in normal range Rales without consolidation
Sputum		
Gram Stain	Many PMNs Single predominant organism	Variable numbers of PMNs or mononuclear cells No predominant organism
Volume and character	Purulent sputum	Scant or absent sputum
Chest Roentgenogram	Lobar or segmental consolidation; may be patchy bronchopneumonia Effusion may occur (usually large)	Interstitial, patchy infiltrates Effusion uncommon (usually small)
Leukocyte Count	Usually 15,000–25,000 with left shift	Usually normal
Leading Causes		
Common	*Streptococcus pneumoniae* *Hemophilus influenzae* *Branhamella catarrhalis* *Legionella pneumophila*	*Mycoplasma pneumoniae* *Chlamydia pneumoniae* (TWAR) Influenza A and B *Legionella pneumophila*
Uncommon	*Klebsiella pneumoniae* *Staphylococcus aureus* Gram-negative bacilli Mixed anaerobic bacteria *Mycobacterium tuberculosis*	Adenovirus Measles *Chlamydia psittici* *Coxiella burnetii* (Q fever)

PMNs, polymorphonuclear leukocytes.

5. *Aspiration pneumonia* is a pulmonary infection caused by the aspiration of oropharyngeal contents, usually in patients with an altered level of consciousness or impaired swallowing. Aspiration of gastric contents may also cause a chemical pneumonitis.
6. *Nosocomial pneumonia* is a pulmonary infection acquired in the hospital setting.
7. *Human immunodeficiency virus (HIV)-associated pulmonary infections* are presented in Acquired Immunodeficiency Syndrome (AIDS), earlier in this chapter.

B. Mortality

Pneumonia is the sixth most common cause of death in the United States and the most common cause of infection-related death. The exact mortality rate varies greatly depending on patient characteristics and the causative agent; in bacteremic patients with aerobic gram-negative pneumonia it is as high as 50%.

C. Etiology

Tables 15–23 and 15–24 present the etiology of acute pneumonia.

Table 15–23. PREVALENCE OF MICROORGANISMS CAUSING COMMUNITY-ACQUIRED PNEUMONIA

PATHOGEN	ESTIMATED %
Streptococcus pneumoniae	15–40
Hemophilus influenzae	4–15
Mycoplasma pneumoniae	3–14
Staphylococcus aureus	2–10
Chlamydia pneumoniae	2–10
Legionella sp.	1–22
Viruses (esp. influenza A)	1–10
Pneumocystis carinii	1–6
Other gram-negative bacilli	2–8
Other (fungi, mycobacteria)	< 1
Mouth anaerobes	unknown
No pathogen identified	3–40

Table 15–24. CAUSATIVE AGENTS OF ACUTE PNEUMONIA IN ADULTS

Bacterial

Streptococcus pneumoniae
Staphylococcus aureus
Hemophilus influenzae
Mixed anaerobic bacteria
Escherichia coli
Klebsiella pneumoniae
Enterobacter cloacae
Serratia marcescens
Pseudomonas aeruginosa
Legionella pneumophila

Mycobacterial

Mycobacterium tuberculosis

Bacteria-like agents

Mycoplasma pneumoniae
Chlamydia pneumoniae (TWAR)
Chlamydia psittaci

Rickettsia

Coxiella burnetii

Parasites

Pneumocystis carinii

Viruses

Influenza A virus
Influenza B virus
Adenovirus types
Cytomegalovirus
Varicella
Measles

Fungi

Aspergillus spp.
Candida spp.
Coccidioides immitis
Cryptococcus neoformans
Histoplasma capsulatum

II. CLINICAL EVALUATION

A. General

1. The diagnosis of pneumonia is based primarily upon the history, physical examination, and chest roentgenogram. With the exception of HIV-positive and immunocompromised patients, an infiltrate on the chest film is a key element of the diagnosis.

2. Clinical features of the most common community-acquired pneumonias are outlined in Table 15–25.

3. Even with an aggressive investigation, the specific cause of a given pneumonia can be established in only 50–60% of patients.

B. History

1. A detailed history is crucial; certain patient characteristics may increase their risk for particular pathogens (Table 15–26).

2. *Cough* is almost always a prominent complaint, although the elderly or immunocompromised patient may lack this symptom.

3. Bacterial pneumonias are usually associated with *purulent* (yellow, rust-colored, or bloody) *sputum.* Patients with atypical pneumonias (e.g., pneumonia caused by *Pneumocystis carinii* or viral pathogens) frequently have nonproductive coughs.

4. *Chest pain* is frequent and is usually pleuritic in nature.

5. *Extrapulmonary symptoms* may include ear pain, sinus discomfort, sore throat, headache, abdominal pain, diarrhea, and confusion. These complaints are especially common with the atypical pneumonias.

C. Physical Examination

1. *Fever* is common. Elderly or debilitated patients with overwhelming infection, however, may be afebrile. Patients self-medicating with antipyretic agents may also be afebrile at the time of presentation.

2. *Tachycardia* is a natural response to fever. A pulse–temperature deficit (relative bradycardia for the degree of fever) has been reported with influenza virus, *Legionella,* or *Chlamydia psittaci.*

3. *Tachypnea* is common.

4. *Chest examination:*
   a. Decreased breath sounds may be the only finding early in pneumonia, with rales becoming prominent as the infection progresses.
   b. Evidence of consolidation (including dullness to percussion, bronchial breath sounds, egophony [E to A changes],

Table 15–25. SPECIFIC COMMON PATHOGENS

	STREPTOCOCCUS PNEUMONIAE	HEMOPHILUS INFLUENZAE	MYCOPLASMA PNEUMONIAE
History	The most common cause of pneumonia; frequently seen in previously healthy adults Abrupt onset with single shaking chill (80% of cases)	Often associated with debilitating conditions (alcoholism, cancer, immunosuppression) or recent hospitalization Usually sudden onset	The most common cause of pneumonia in young adults Highest incidence in fall and winter Onset insidious in 70% Presenting symptoms: cough 95%, malaise 75%, headache 72%, sore throat 51%, pleuritic chest pain 30%, rhinorrhea 32%, earache 24%, nausea 29%, diarrhea 13%
Physical Examination	Ill-appearing and febrile Tachycardia and tachypnea Signs of consolidation	Ill-appearing and febrile Tachycardia and tachypnea Signs of consolidation	Usually not ill-appearing Pulmonary signs: fever 80%, rales 80% Extrapulmonary signs: pharyngitis 41%, lymphadenopathy 21%, rash (maculopapular, vesicular, erythema multiforme) 20%, bullous myringitis 12%, myocarditis 4%
Roentgenography	Lobar or sublobar consolidation classic Pleural effusions in 20%	Bronchopneumonia is the most common pattern Lobar consolidation can occur	Variable Patchy bronchopneumonia (40%)—insidious onset and nonspecific symptoms Lobar or segmental consolidation (40%)—acute onset suggestive of bacterial pneumonia Interstitial (20%)—longer duration of symptoms with less fever and more dyspnea Pleural effusions are seen in 20% of patients

PMNs, polymorphonuclear leukocytes; WBC, white cell (leukocyte) count.

Table 15–25. SPECIFIC COMMON PATHOGENS *Continued*

	CHLAMYDIA PNEUMONIAE (TWAR)	LEGIONELLA PNEUMOPHILA
History	Implicated in pneumonia outbreaks in military recruits and civilian populations May be insidious or abrupt in onset Presenting symptoms: pharyngitis, hoarseness, headache, fever; respiratory-tract symptoms may not appear for days to weeks "*Mycoplasma*-like"	Infection follows inhalation of organism from contaminated drinking water May be insidious or abrupt in onset Presenting symptoms: anorexia, malaise 100%, fever 95%, cough (usually minor) 90%, mental confusion, abdominal pain, diarrhea
Physical Examination	Temperature elevation sometimes present Pharyngeal erythema (nonexudative) common Sinus tenderness present in 33% Rales on chest auscultation almost always present	Nonremitting fever > 39°C, relative bradycardia, tachypnea Signs of consolidation
Roentgenography	Nonspecific unilateral interstitial lower-lobe infiltrate	Initially patchy infiltrate with progression to lobar consolidation Lower lobes most often affected Pleural effusions 50% Macroscopic abscesses 25%
Laboratory Studies		
Hematology	Normal or ↑ WBC	↑ WBC—left shift
Sputum	Few leukocytes No organisms	Moderate PMNs Faintly staining gram-negative rods (rarely) Direct fluorescent antibody (DFA) stain, 30–80% sensitivity
Cultures		Blood cultures positive in 20–38% Sputum culture positive in 70%
Serology	A four-fold rise in fluorescent antibody titers in acute and convalescent sera (2–3 weeks apart) confirms a clinical diagnosis. A single IgG titer of 1:512 on acute sera is considered presumptive evidence of infection	

Table continued on following page

Table 15–25. SPECIFIC COMMON PATHOGENS *Continued*

	STAPHYLOCOCCUS AUREUS	MIXED ANAEROBIC (ASPIRATION)	INFLUENZA VIRUS
History	Infection occurs in immunocompromised hosts and in healthy adults as a complication of influenza A Abrupt onset, with hectic fevers, multiple chills, productive cough, and pleuritic chest pain In hematogenously spread pneumonia (e.g., injection drug users) symptoms may be less dramatic	Associated with an altered level of consciousness (seizures, alcoholism, elderly) Associated with airway compromise (neuromuscular disease, vomiting, esophageal disease)	Peak incidence is in winter Usually gradual onset, but occasionally may be acute and fulminant Presenting symptoms: malaise, rhinorrhea, headache, sore throat, then progressive cough
Physical Examination	Ill-appearing, tachycardia, temperature > 40° C Lung findings variable ranging from clear to consolidated	Variable, depending on amount of aspirated material (mild fever to respiratory failure)	Temperature elevation to 39° C. Rales present but no consolidation.
Roentgenography	Lower-lobe bronchopneumonia typical Abscesses, pleural effusions, and empyema common complications The radiographic appearance of single or multiple small round infiltrates characteristic of hematogenously acquired *S. aureus* pneumonia	Lower lobes usually (often superior segment)	Perihilar infiltrates
Laboratory Studies			
Hematology	↑ WBC—left shift	WBC variable	Normal or ↑ WBC
Sputum	Many PMNs Large gram-positive cocci in clusters	Many PMNs Mixed oral flora Fetid odor	Few leukocytes No organisms
Cultures	Blood cultures positive in 20%	Blood cultures usually negative Sputum culture— mixed flora and/or *Bacteroides* and/or anaerobic streptococci	Tissue culture (nasopharyngeal swabs, sputum, lung aspirates or lung biopsy) 60% sensitivity

PMNs, polymorphonuclear leukocytes; WBC, white cell (leukocyte) count.

Table 15–25. SPECIFIC COMMON PATHOGENS *Continued*

	STREPTOCOCCUS PNEUMONIAE	HEMOPHILUS INFLUENZAE	MYCOPLASMA PNEUMONIAE
Laboratory Studies			
Hematology	↑ WBC—left shift	↑ WBC—left shift	WBC usually normal
Sputum	Many PMNs Gram-positive diplo-cocci often intracel-lular	Many PMNs Small pleomorphic gram-negative coc-cobacilli	Few PMNs Normal flora
Cultures	Blood cultures posi-tive in 25%	Blood cultures posi-tive in 33%	
Serology			A four-fold rise in complement fixation titers in acute and convalescent sera (2–3 weeks apart) confirms a clinical diagnosis. A single titer of 1:64 on acute sera is considered presumptive evi-dence of infection.
Other			Cold agglutinins present in 50% DNA probe (spu-tum) 90% sensitive but expensive
Complications	Parapneumonic effusion in 20–40% Empyema rare	Bacteremia, empy-ema, abscess—common (type B only)	Pleural effusions—20% (usually small) Hemolytic anemia, arthritis, myocardi-tis, aseptic meningi-tis, Guillain-Barré syndrome (all un-common)
Usual Course	Crisis (deferves-cence in 24–48 hr) or lysis (7–10 days)	Usually slow re-covery Mortality higher with type B	Gradual resolution over 1–3 weeks

Table continued on following page

and/or tactile fremitus) is highly suggestive of a bacterial process; dullness to percussion may also signify a pleural effusion.

c. Patients with *C. pneumoniae, C. psittaci, Coxiella burnetii* (Q fever), influenza virus, and *Mycoplasma pneumoniae* usually have an unremarkable chest examination despite impressive infiltrates on the chest film.

5. *Extrapulmonary signs,* suggesting an atypical pathogen, in-clude skin rashes, nonexudative pharyngitis, and/or bullous myringitis.

Table 15–25. SPECIFIC COMMON PATHOGENS *Continued*

	Chlamydia Pneumoniae (TWAR)	Legionella Pneumophila
Other		DNA probe 70% sensitivity and expensive Urinary antigen 75–90% sensitivity, inexpensive, not positive early in infection ↓ phosphate, hyponatremia hematuria
Complications	Probably few	Multisystem failure, respiratory failure very common
Usual Course	Gradual resolution over 1–3 weeks	Mortality is high; often rapid progression to multilobar disease Recovery is usually difficult and slow

PMNs, polymorphonuclear leukocytes; WBC, white cell (leukocyte) count.

6. A *splenectomy scar* suggests the possibility of infection with encapsulated organisms (including *Streptococcus pneumoniae* and *Hemophilus influenzae*).

7. *Mental status changes* may result from hypoxia, hypercarbia, electrolyte abnormalities, and/or concurrent meningitis. Altered mentation may be the only sign of infection in elderly patients.

D. Radiographic Evaluation

1. Any of the following mandate chest roentgenography:
   a. Symptoms:
      i. Acute dyspnea.
      ii. Pleuritic chest pain.
      iii. Fever for > 3 days.
      iv. Cough for > 7 days.
   b. Signs:
      i. Respiratory rate > 25 breaths/min.
      ii. Pulse > 100 beats/min.
      iii. Cyanosis.
      iv. Splinting.
      v. Focal pulmonary findings (rales, wheezes, egophony).

2. The following radiographic abnormalities may be noted:
   a. Lobar consolidation suggests a bacterial pneumonia; it is routinely present with infection caused by *S. pneumoniae* or *Klebsiella pneumoniae.*
   b. Cavitation with pneumatocele formation suggests infection with *S. aureus,* gram-negative bacilli, or *M. tuberculosis.*

Table 15–25. SPECIFIC COMMON PATHOGENS Continued

	STAPHYLOCOCCUS AUREUS	MIXED ANAEROBIC (ASPIRATION)	INFLUENZA VIRUS
Serology			
Other			
Complications	Respiratory failure common Lung abscess, empyema occasional Endocarditis, osteomyelitis uncommon	Lung abscess, empyema occasional	Bacterial superinfection complicates 1% of influenza A pneumonias *(S. pneumoniae, S. aureus, H. influenzae)* Respiratory failure uncommon
Usual Course	High mortality Slow recovery	Depends on underlying condition Slow recovery	Variable

    c. Bilateral diffuse infiltrates suggest infection with *P. carinii* or a viral pathogen.

    d. A perihilar distribution of infiltrates is frequently noted in early *M. pneumoniae* or influenza infection.

    e. *M. tuberculosis* and *K. pneumoniae* have a predilection for upper-lobe involvement; *K. pneumoniae* is classically associated with bulging or sagging of the major fissure.

    f. Infiltrates in the superior or basilar segments of the lower lobes or posterior segments of the upper lobes suggest aspiration.

E. Laboratory Studies

1. **Complete Blood Count (CBC).** The leukocyte count is usually elevated and a left shift is frequently present. The leukocyte count may be normal in the atypical pneumonias. Leukopenia in the presence of a bacterial pneumonia is a poor prognostic sign.

2. **Arterial Blood Gas (ABG).** Reasonable in patients with respiratory distress or who are otherwise seriously ill.

3. **Tuberculin Skin Test (PPD).** Should be placed on any pneumonia patient with concomitant risk factors for tuberculosis (Table 15–26). A positive test indicates that infection has occurred, but it does not prove the presence of active disease; false-negative PPD tests occur in 20% of patients with tuberculosis. Control skin tests (e.g., measles, mumps, *Candida*) should be placed in debilitated patients.

Table 15–26. PNEUMONIA: EPIDEMIOLOGIC CATEGORIES AND EMPIRIC THERAPY

CATEGORY	MOST COMMON ORGANISMS	SUGGESTED ANTIBIOTIC		ADDITIONAL NOTES
		PRIMARY	SECONDARY	
Age 5–40 years "healthy"	*S. pneumoniae* *Mycoplasma pneumoniae* *Chlamydia pneumoniae* Influenza virus *H. influenzae*	PO: Erythromycin or azithromycin or clarithromycin	Doxycycline or tetracycline	Gram stain may allow specific diagnosis: if *S. pneumoniae*—Pen G or VK or amoxicillin; if *H. influenzae*—AM/CL or cephalosporin (second or third generation). No clarithromycin, azithromycin, or tetracyclines in pregnant women.
Age > 40 years "healthy"	*S. pneumoniae* *H. influenzae* *M. pneumoniae* (uncommon)	PO: Cefuroxime or cefixime or AM/CL IV: Cefuroxime or TC/CL or 3 Ceph AP or AM/SB	PO: TMP-SMX	
Age > 40 years underlying disease: diabetes, congestive heart failure, alcoholism	As above plus... *Klebsiella pneumoniae* *Legionella* Other gramnegative bacilli *M. tuberculosis*	As above plus... PO or IV: Erythromycin	As above plus... PO or IV: Erythromycin	In the subgroup of patients who are at risk for *M. tuberculosis* (HIV-positive, homeless, immigrants, alcoholics, history of neoplasia, nursing home residents), consider placing PPD and obtaining sputum samples. Isolate until active *M. tuberculosis* is ruled out (see Tuberculosis, later in this chapter).
Aspiration: CVA, alcoholism, sedation	*Streptococcus pneumoniae* Oral anaerobes Gram-negative bacilli	IV: Clindamycin or cefoxitin or AM/SB or TC/CL	IV: Clindamycin + APAG or IMP	
Chronic obstructive pulmonary disease	*H. influenzae* *S. pneumoniae* *Branhamella catarrhalis* *Legionella*	PO: TMP-SMX or amoxicillin or cefuroxime or cefixime IV: Cefuroxime or 3 Ceph AP	PO: Doxycycline	Consider adding erythromycin in areas where *Legionella* is endemic or if the patient fails to respond to initial therapy in 48 hr.
Cystic fibrosis	*Pseudomonas aeruginosa* *S. aureus*	IV: APAG + AP Pen or 3 Ceph AP	PO: CIP IV: CIP or IMP	Do not use CIP in children < 18 years of age or in nursing or pregnant women.

AM/SB, ampicillin-sulbactam; AM/CL, amoxicillin-clavulanate; APAG, antipseudomonal aminoglycoside (tobramycin, gentamicin, amikacin); AP Pen, antipseudomonal penicillin (piperacillin, ticarcillin); CIP, ciprofloxacin; IMP, imipenem-cilastatin; MRSA, methicillin-resistant *S. aureus*; TC/CL, ticarcillin-clavulanate; TMP-SMX, trimethoprim-sulfamethoxazole; 3 Ceph AP, third-generation antipseudomonal cephalosporin (ceftizoxime, cefoperazone, ceftazidime).

From Sandford JP: Guide to Antimicrobial Therapy. Dallas, Antimicrobial Therapy, Inc., 1993, p. 21.

Table 15–26. PNEUMONIA: EPIDEMIOLOGIC CATEGORIES AND EMPIRIC THERAPY *Continued*

CATEGORY	MOST COMMON ORGANISMS	SUGGESTED ANTIBIOTIC		ADDITIONAL NOTES
		PRIMARY	*SECONDARY*	
HIV-positive patient	*Pneumocystis carinii* *S. pneumoniae* *H. influenzae* *M. tuberculosis*	See Acquired Immunodeficiency Syndrome earlier in this chapter.		
Intravenous drug use	As for "Age > 40 years" plus *S. aureus* (septic emboli)	IV: AM/SB or TC/CL or 3 Ceph AP	IV: IMP or vancomycin	
Nosocomial pneumonia	Gram-negative bacilli *S. aureus* *Legionella*	IV: IMP or (AP Pen + APAG) or (TC/ CL + APAG) or Ceph 3 AP + APAG)	IV: CIP + ampicillin Aztreonam for APAG	These agents do not cover MRSA; if prevalent in your hospital add vancomycin
Nursing home patient	*S. pneumoniae* *K. pneumoniae* *H. influenzae* *S. aureus* *M. tuberculosis* Influenza virus	IV: AM/SB or TC/CL or Ceph 3 AP	IV: IMP	See notes on *M. tuberculosis,* above. Influenza A should be treated with either amantadine or rimantadine (must be started within 48 hr of illness onset).
Post-influenzal pneumoniae	*S. pneumoniae* *H. influenzae* *S. aureus*	IV: AM/SB or TC/CL or 3 Ceph AP	IV: IMP or vancomycin	

4. **Sputum.** Evaluation of properly collected *sputum* is important; it leads to a presumptive microbiologic diagnosis in > 60% of cases.
   a. Appearance:
      i. *Color:* yellow-green sputum indicates purulence and is the most common sputum color in patients with bacterial pneumonia. Blood-colored sputum is seen in one-third of patients with *Legionella.* "Rusty" sputum is commonly (although not solely) associated with *S. pneumoniae.* "Currant jelly" sputum is found in *K. pneumoniae* infections. Watery sputum suggests *M. pneumoniae.*
      ii. *Amount:* most bacterial pneumonias result in copious sputum production. Dehydration and atypical pneumonias result in scant amounts of sputum.
      iii. *Odor:* fetid sputum suggests anaerobic organisms.
   b. Microscopic evaluation:
      i. *Gram stain:*
         • To ensure minimal oropharyngeal contamination, strict criteria should be applied to the evaluation of the sputum Gram stain. An adequate sample has ≥ 25

neutrophils and ≤ 10 epithelial cells per low-power field (100×).

- Physician evaluation of Gram stains is most reliable for the diagnosis of *S. pneumoniae* (gram-positive, lancet-shaped diplococci), and less reliable for the diagnosis of *H. influenzae* (small gram-negative coccobacilli). *S. aureus* appears as tetrads or grape-like clusters of gram-positive cocci. Gram-negative cocci suggest *Branhamella catarrhalis.*
- The presence of leukocytes without bacteria suggests *C. pneumoniae, Legionella, Mycoplasma,* or viral infection.

ii. Giemsa or Gomori methenamine silver stain detects *P. carinii.* The sensitivity for induced sputum samples is 50–80%. This test should be routinely employed in HIV-positive patients with suspected pneumonia.

iii. Direct fluorescent antibody stain is a rapid (2–4 hour) test for detecting *Legionella* when this organism is suspected. Its sensitivity ranges from 20–80%; specificity is 99%.

iv. Acid-fast stain is used to detect *M. tuberculosis.* Active pulmonary disease can usually be confirmed by sputum evaluation. Ideally, three morning sputum samples should be obtained. Broncoscopy is occasionally required.

5. **Cultures**
   a. Sputum:
      i. Sputum cultures are less useful clinically than the Gram stain in making a causative diagnosis, especially for the ED physician. Cultures are not routinely necessary in patients with community-acquired pneumonia.
      ii. Cultures are negative in 45–50% of patients with bacteremic pneumococcal and *H. influenzae* pneumonias.
      iii. Sputum cultures are essential in the following clinical settings:
         - Suspected *Legionella* infection. Culture requires special techniques with charcoal yeast extract agar. Sensitivity is 80–100%; specificity is 100%.
         - Suspected *M. tuberculosis.* The patient with active pulmonary tuberculosis may have negative acid-fast stains but positive sputum cultures. Unfortunately, cultures may require 4 to 6 weeks.
   b. Blood cultures have a low sensitivity (10–33%), but are diagnostic when positive. They should be obtained on any pneumonia patient ill enough to require hospitalization.

6. **Serologic Studies.** A variety of serologic tests are sometimes of use in confirming a diagnosis. These may be requested by the medicine or infectious disease consultant when one or more

of the following organisms are suspected: *Legionella* sp., *M. pneumoniae, Chlamydia* sp., and/or *Coxiella burnetii.*

7. **Urinary Antigen Assay.** Detects *Legionella* antigen. Although its sensitivity is 75–90%, antigenuria does not occur early in the infection, which limits its diagnostic usefulness.

I. DIFFERENTIAL DIAGNOSIS

Many of the symptoms, signs, and roentgenographic findings of lower-respiratory-tract infections can be mimicked by noninfectious conditions, including the following:

A. Atelectasis.

B. Aspiration of gastric acid or toxins.

C. Collagen-vascular diseases.

D. Congestive heart failure.

E. Drug toxicity.

F. Foreign-body aspiration.

G. Goodpasture's syndrome.

H. Inhalation injury.

I. Neoplasm.

J. Pulmonary contusion.

K. Pulmonary embolism.

L. Sarcoidosis.

M. Wegener's granulomatosis.

II. THERAPY

A. Initial Management

Assess, secure, and support the airway, breathing, and circulation as indicated. (See Chapter 1. II.)

B. Antibiotic Therapy

1. After addressing immediately life-threatening considerations and supporting oxygenation and vital signs as required, complete the directed history and a more thorough physical examination. A chest roentgenogram and sputum sample should be obtained.
2. On the basis of the information above, the patient should be assigned an epidemiologic category and empiric antibiotic therapy initiated (see Table 15–26 for appropriate initial antibiotic choices and Table 15–27 for antibiotic dosing).

Table 15–27. ANTIBIOTIC THERAPY FOR PNEUMONIAE[a]

DRUG	DOSE	COMMENT/DURATION OF THERAPY (OUTPATIENT ONLY)
Erythromycin	PO: 250–500 mg qid	10 days: *S. pneumoniae, C. pneumoniae* 10–14 days: *M. pneumoniae* 21 days: *L. pneumophila* High dose: *L. pneumophila*
Azithromycin *(Zithromax)*	PO: 500 mg (2 tablets) on day 1, then 250 mg (1 tablet) day 2–5	5 days
Clarithromycin *(Biaxin)*	PO: 250–500 mg bid	10–14 days
Doxycycline *(Doryx, Vibramycin)*	PO: 100 mg bid	10–14 days: *C. pneumoniae* 10–14 days: *M. pneumoniae*
Tetracycline	PO: 500 mg qid	10–14 days: *C. pneumoniae* 10–14 days: *M. pneumoniae*
Penicillin (VK) (G)	PO: 500 mg qid IV: 1.2–2.4 million units/24 hours	7–10 days: Initial inpatient treatment for *S. pneumoniae*
Amoxicillin	PO: 500 mg tid	7–10 days
Ampicillin	IV: 4–12 g/24 hours	
Amoxicillin-clavulanate *(Augmentin)*	PO: 500 mg tid	7–10 days
Ampicillin-sulbactam *(Unasyn)*	IV: 1.5–3 g q 6 hr	
Ticarcillin-clavulanate *(Timentin)*	IV: 3.1 g q 6 hr	
Ticarcillin *(Ticar)*	IV: 200–300 mg/kg/day in four divided doses	
Piperacillin *(Pipracil)*	IV: 200–300 mg/kg/day in four divided doses	
Cefuroxine axetil *(Ceftin)*	PO: 250–500 mg bid	7–10 days
Cefuroxime sodium *(Zinacef)*	IV: 1.5 g q 8 hr	
Cefixime *(Suprax)*	PO: 400 mg daily	7–10 days
Cefoxitin *(Mefoxin)*	IV: 1–2 g q 6 hr	
Ceftriaxone *(Rocephin)*	IV or IM: 2–4 g daily	
Ceftazidime *(Tazidime)*	IV or IM: 1 g q 8–12 hr	
Trimethoprim-sulfamethoxizole DS *(Bactrim DS, Septra DS)*	PO: 1 pill bid	7–10 days

[a]Refer to Table 15–26 for specific antibiotic choice.

Table 15–27. ANTIBIOTIC THERAPY FOR PNEUMONIAE[a] *Continued*

DRUG	DOSE	COMMENT/DURATION OF THERAPY (OUTPATIENT ONLY)
Ciprofloxacin *(Cipro)*	PO: 500 mg bid IV: 400 mg bid	10–14 days Contraindicated in pregnancy, nursing mothers, or age < 18 yrs
Clindamycin *(Cleocin)*	IV: 0.6–1.8 g/day in four divided doses	
Gentamicin	IV: 1 mg/kg q 8 hr	1–2 mg/kg loading dose
Tobramycin	IV: 1 mg/kg q 8 hr	1–2 mg/kg loading dose
Amikacin	IV: 5 mg/kg q 8 hr	5–10 mg/kg loading dose
Imipenem *(Premaxin)*	IV: 500 mg q 6 hr	
Vancomycin *(Vancocin)*	IV: 500 mg q 6 hr	

From Sandford, JP: Guide to Antimicrobial Therapy. Dallas: Antimicrobial Therapy, Inc. 1993, p. 21.

C. Supportive Care

1. **Pulmonary Toilet.** Encourage coughing. Suction, ± postural drainage, may be necessary if the patient's own efforts fail to adequately clear secretions.

2. **Ventilation.** Ventilatory status is reflected by PCO_2. Normal or slightly low values ($PCO_2 \leq 40$ mmHg) are to be expected. Higher levels of PCO_2 with declining serum pH suggest impending ventilatory failure. Continue to support respiratory status as required by optimizing oxygenation, pulmonary toilet, and hydration status. Intubation and mechanical ventilation may be necessary in the patient with progressive respiratory failure (see Chapters 11 and 14).

3. **Bronchodilator Therapy (Nebulized Beta Agonists).** Appropriate in the patient with known asthma or chronic obstructive pulmonary disease, or who is otherwise wheezing on pulmonary examination (see Chapter 14).

4. **Isolation**

   a. Patients at high risk for *M. tuberculosis* infection should be kept in respiratory isolation until active disease is ruled out (see Tuberculosis, later in this chapter.)

   b. Patients with methicillin-resistant *S. aureus* (MRSA) as identified by sputum culture need respiratory isolation for the duration of their antibiotic therapy.

V. DISPOSITION

A. Discharge

1. Reliable, otherwise healthy, nontoxic and nonelderly patients

(< age 65) with a reasonable home situation can generally be treated as outpatients.

2. Follow-up with the patient's primary care physician should be arranged within 1 week.

3. The duration of antibiotic therapy depends on the causative agent and clinical setting. For most community pneumonias, a 10-day course of antibiotics is appropriate. Patients with suspected *C. pneumoniae* or *M. pneumoniae* infection may benefit from longer treatment (2–3 weeks).

4. A follow-up chest roentgenogram is recommended in 6 weeks (to ensure clearance of the infiltrate).

B. Admit

Patients with pneumonia and *any* of the following should be hospitalized:

1. High-morbidity pneumonias (aspiration, cavitary process, gram-negative organisms, multilobar involvement, nosocomial pneumonia, suspected *S. aureus*).

2. Hypoxemia (PO_2 < 65 mmHg on room air) or risk for ventilatory compromise (rising PCO_2);

3. Significant co-morbid condition (≥ age 65, AIDS, alcoholism, underlying severe cardiopulmonary disease, concurrent corticosteroid use, diabetes mellitus, injection drug use, homelessness, malnutrition, pregnancy, primary or secondary B- or T-cell disorder, recent hospitalization or intubation).

4. Significantly ill patient (altered mentation, marked dyspnea, dehydration, high fever, nausea/vomiting, toxic appearance).

5. Suspected complicated effusion or empyema.

6. Unreliable or inadequate home situation.

VI. PEARLS AND PITFALLS

A. Patient characteristics, appearance of the infiltrate on the chest roentgenogram, and sputum Gram stain are the key elements in determining the causative agent of the patient's pneumonia.

B. An infiltrate must be present on the chest film to make the diagnosis of pneumonia (exceptions: dehydrated, elderly, or immunocompromised patient).

C. Always consider the possibility of tuberculosis, *P. carinii* pneumonia, empyema, pulmonary embolus with infarction, congestive heart failure, and/or a neoplastic process when evaluating the patient with an infiltrate on chest film.

D. If the patient does not require hospitalization, close follow-up is mandatory.

BIBLIOGRAPHY

Ashbourne J, Downey P, Westfall M: Pneumonia. In Rosen (ed): Emergency Medicine: Concepts and Clinical Practice. 3rd Ed. St. Louis, CV Mosby, 1992; pp. 1162–1177.

Heckerling PS, Tape TG, Wigton RS, et al: Clinical prediction rule for pulmonary infiltrates. Ann Intern Med 1990;113(9):664–670.

Johnson DH, Cunha BA: Atypical pneumonias. Postgrad Med 1993;93:69.

Mansel JK, Rosenow EG, et al: *Mycoplasma pneumoniae* pneumonia. Chest 1989;95:639–646.

Musher DM: Infections caused by *Streptococcus pneumoniae:* clinical spectrum, pathogenesis, immunity, and treatment. Clin Infect Dis 1992;14(4):801–807.

Nguyen MH, Stout JE, Yu VL: Legionellosis. Infect Dis Clin N Am 1991;5:561.

Torres A, Serra-Batlles J, Ferrer A, et al: Severe community-acquired pneumonia: epidemiology and prognostic factors. Am Rev Respir Dis 1991;144(2):312–318.

SEXUALLY TRANSMITTED DISEASES

> *"For your physicians have expressly charg'd,*
> *In peril to incur your former malady,*
> *That I should yet absent me from your bed."*
>
> WILLIAM SHAKESPEARE (1564–1616)

Gonorrhea and Chlamydia

Neisseria gonorrhoeae and *Chlamydia trachomatis* cause a variety of clinical syndromes in both men and women. Because of their significant rate of coinfection and the similarity in presentation of many of their syndromes, they are discussed together. Pelvic inflammatory disease is discussed in Chapter 18.

I. ESSENTIAL FACTS

A. Gonorrhea is a major cause of morbidity worldwide, with an estimated 2.5 million cases reported annually in the United States.

B. *Chlamydia trachomatis* is an obligate intracellular pathogen that requires cell culture for in vitro growth. It is the most prevalent sexually transmitted bacterial pathogen in the United States.

C. Many patients infected with gonorrhea or chlamydia are asymptomatic and thus maintain a large reservoir of infection in the community.

D. Serious complications of these infections include acute pelvic inflammatory disease, female infertility, and ectopic pregnancy.

II. GENITAL GONOCOCCAL AND NONGONOCOCCAL SYNDROMES

A. Mucopurulent cervicitis

1. **Presentation.** Gonorrhea, chlamydia, and herpes simplex virus (HSV) are the major agents in mucopurulent cervicitis (MPC).

Patients are often asymptomatic, though they may present with vaginal discharge, bleeding, or lower-abdominal pain. Chlamydial infection generally is associated with longer incubation (5–21 days versus 2–7 days with gonorrhea) and milder symptoms than infections caused by *N. gonorrhoeae*. Cervical discharge tends to be mucoid or mucopurulent and scant to moderate in amount. Asymptomatic infection may persist for extended periods of time.

2. **Diagnosis.** A presumptive diagnosis is made by the presence of purulent or mucopurulent endocervical discharge (appearing yellow or green on the swab) and a Gram stain showing > 20 polymorphonuclear leukocytes (PMN's) per high-power field with or without intracellular gram-negative diplococci present. The specimen should not be heavily contaminated with vaginal squamous epithelial cells; it should not be interpreted if the patient is menstruating. The definitive diagnosis is established by a positive culture. False-negative cultures also occur. Rapid monoclonal immunofluorescent antibody tests to detect chlamydial antigen are available and are about 75% sensitive.

3. **Differential Diagnosis.** Consider HSV as an alternative cause of cervicitis. Also consider primary vaginal pathogens (e.g., trichomonads) in the differential of vaginal discharge. Cervical neoplasia is a possibility when encountering a friable and exudative cervix on speculum examination.

4. **Therapy.** Therapy for uncomplicated MPC is discussed below (see II. C).

B. Urethritis in Males

1. **Presentation.** Gonococcal urethritis typically causes a copious penile discharge often associated with dysuria 2–7 days following exposure. Nongonococcal urethritis (NGU), caused by chlamydia (30–50% of NGU) and *Ureaplasma urealyticum* (10–40%), is more common than gonococcal urethritis (GU). NGU often causes milder symptoms, and is more often asymptomatic than gonococcal disease. The incubation period for NGU is 1–5 weeks.

2. **Diagnosis.** Presumptive diagnosis of GU is made by a urethral Gram stain showing PMNs with intracellular gram-negative diplococci. Seeing > 4 PMNs per high-power field without gonococci in three different areas on the urethral smear makes the presumptive diagnosis of NGU. Cultures for both gonococci and chlamydia should be sent.

3. **Therapy.** Therapy for GU and NGU is discussed below (see II. C). Patients with epididymitis should be treated for a longer duration than those with uncomplicated urethritis.

C. Treatment of Uncomplicated Endocervical or Urethral Gonorrhea and Chlamydia

Table 15–28 presents a summary of gonorrhea and chlamydia treatment.

1. Simultaneous treatment of gonorrhea and chlamydia is recommended because their coinfection rate is as high as 50%. Ceftriaxone 125–250 mg IM once for gonorrhea plus doxycycline 100 mg PO bid (or tetracycline 500 mg PO qid) for 7 days for chlamydia is the regimen of choice.

2. Alternatives for ceftriaxone include cefixime (400 mg PO once), ciprofloxacin (500 mg PO once), ofloxacin (400 mg PO once), and spectinomycin (2 g IM once).

3. Alternative regimens to the tetracyclines include erythromycin base or stearate (500 mg PO qid for 7 days [recommended for a pregnant patient]), azithromycin (1 g PO once), ofloxacin (300 mg PO bid for 7 days [if the patient is not pregnant]), sulfisoxazole (500 mg PO qid for 10 days [avoid in the third trimester of pregnancy]), and amoxicillin (500 mg PO tid for 10 days [a reasonable choice for pregnant patients who do not tolerate erythromycin]). Ten days of chlamydia therapy are recommended for epididymitis.

Table 15–28. TREATMENT FOR GONORRHEA AND CHLAMYDIA IN ADULTS

INFECTION SITE/ DIAGNOSIS	DRUG OF CHOICE/DOSE	ALTERNATIVE(S) (SEE TEXT)
Gonorrhea		
Cervical,[a] urethral,[a] rectal,[a] pharyngeal	Ceftriaxone 125–250 mg IM once	Cefixime, ciprofloxacin, ofloxacin, spectinomycin[b]
Conjunctivitis	Ceftriaxone 1 g IM once and irrigation	
Pelvic inflammatory disease (PID) (outpatient)[a]	Ceftriaxone 250 mg IM	Cefoxitin 2 g IM plus probenicid 1 g PO
Disseminated gonococcal infection (see text)[a]	Ceftriaxone 1 g IV for 7–10 days, or ~ 3 days followed by oral therapy with cefixime or ciprofloxacin to complete a 10-day course.	Ceftizoxime, cefotaxime, spectinomycin
Chlamydia		
Cervical, urethral, rectal, conjunctival, PID	Doxycycline 100 mg PO for 7 days (14 days for PID; 10 days for epididymitis)	Erythromycin (during pregnancy), azithromycin, ofloxacin, sulfisoxazole, or amoxicillin

[a]Requires treatment for chlamydial coinfection.
[b]Ineffective for pharyngeal gonorrhea.

III. EXTRAGENITAL GONOCOCCAL SYNDROMES

A. Pharyngitis

1. **Presentation.** Acquired by orogenital contact (predominantly fellatio) with an infected person. Cunnilingus is less risky than fellatio, and pharynx-to-pharynx transmission is rare. It is occasionally manifested as acute exudative pharyngitis or tonsillitis but > 90% of cases are asymptomatic. The pharynx is the sole site of infection in < 5% of patients; thus presumptive diagnosis is often made at other sites.

2. **Diagnosis.** A Gram-stained smear of the pharynx is unreliable. Definitive diagnosis is by positive culture.

3. **Therapy.** Ceftriaxone (125-250 mg IM once) and cefixime (400 mg PO once) are the drugs of choice. Avoid spectinomycin, amoxicillin, or ampicillin, as these drugs tend to be ineffective for gonococcal pharyngitis, even with susceptible organisms in vitro.

B. Conjunctivitis

1. **Presentation.** In adults, this is most frequently acquired by autoinculation in a patient with anal or genital gonorrhea. The infection tends to be very purulent and may spread rapidly to cause preseptal cellulitis, orbital cellulitis, and panophthalmitis, with potential eye loss if not treated promptly. Neonatal infection is prevented in most countries by use of postpartum prophylactic ophthalmologic preparations (silver nitrate, erythromycin, or tetracycline). Copiously purulent conjunctivitis should lead one to suspect gonorrhea, particularly in a sexually active patient.

2. **Diagnosis.** A Gram stain showing intra-PMN gram-negative diplococci gives a presumptive diagnosis; culture gives the definitive diagnosis. Cultures of the cervix and rectum in females, the urethra (and rectum if receptive anal intercourse is reported) in males, and, if indicated, the pharynx in both sexes must be collected.

3. **Therapy.** Single-dose ceftriaxone 1 g IM in the adult is the regimen of choice. Eye irrigation with normal saline and ophthalmologic consultation for any suspicion of deeper infection are also indicated. *C. trachomatis* infection should be considered in the patient who does not respond promptly to therapy.

C. Disseminated Gonococcal Infection and Gonococcal Arthritis

See Infectious Causes of Arthritis in Chapter 22.

IV. EXTRAGENITAL CHLAMYDIA INFECTION

A. Fitz-Hugh-Curtis Syndrome

1. **Presentation.** Fitz-Hugh-Curtis syndrome, or perihepatitis, may occur in women. Most cases are associated with chlamydial salpingitis, in contrast with the association with gonococcal pelvic inflammatory disease (PID) in the past. There is pleuritic upper (usually right-sided) abdominal pain, often accompanied by symptoms and signs of PID. Occasionally, a hepatic friction rub is heard. Symptoms of perihepatitis occur in 3–10% of women with acute PID. This is one of the most common causes of upper-quadrant pain in young sexually active women.

2. **Diagnosis.** A presumptive diagnosis of Fitz-Hugh-Curtis syndrome is based on clinical criteria in a sexually active woman. Cervical culture is often positive. Definitive diagnosis is by direct visualization of the liver capsule and culture of peritoneal fluid for *N. gonorrhoeae* and *C. trachomatis.* Early in its course, laparoscopy will show edema of the liver capsule. Delayed presentation or therapy will allow frank exudate and "violin strings" fibrinous adhesions to occur. Liver function tests will be normal. The differential diagnosis includes acute cholecystitis, other intraabdominal processes, pneumonia, pleurisy, and pyelonephritis.

3. **Therapy.** Therapy for Fitz-Hugh-Curtis syndrome is the same as that for PID (see Chapter 18).

B. Other Extragenital Syndromes

Other extragenital syndromes caused by *C. trachomatis* but not discussed in this book include lymphogranuloma venereum, ocular trachoma, neonatal inclusion conjunctivitis, and neonatal pneumonia. See Chapter 22 for a discussion of Reiter's syndrome.

V. DISPOSITION AND FOLLOW-UP OF PATIENTS WITH GONORRHEA OR CHLAMYDIA

A. Most patients with these infections may be treated and discharged from the ED.

B. Patients with a disseminated gonococcal infection, including gonococcal arthritis, should be hospitalized.

C. Indications for hospitalization of patients with suspected perihepatitis are similar to those for patients with acute PID: unlikely outpatient compliance, pregnancy, peritonitis, suspected pelvic abscess, failure to respond to outpatient therapy within 72 hours, adolescents, and uncertain diagnosis.

D. Treatment failures using combined ceftriaxone/doxycycline (or erythromycin) therapy are rare. Routine follow-up cultures in the nonpregnant patient are not essential. If symptoms persist or recur after completion of therapy, follow-up cultures are recommended.

E. Patients with a sexually transmitted disease (STD) should also have a serologic test for syphilis (e.g., RPR or VDRL) checked and be referred for human immunodeficiency virus counseling and antibody testing.

VI. PEARLS AND PITFALLS

A. All sex partners of the patient in the past 30 days should be examined, cultured, and treated with a regimen effective against gonorrhea and chlamydia.

B. The patient should be advised to refrain from sexual activity until he or she and partners have completed treatment.

C. Gonorrhea and chlamydia in pregnancy: Avoid flouroquinolones and tetracyclines. Follow-up endocervical and rectal cultures 4–7 days following completion of therapy are recommended.

D. All cases of chlamydia and gonorrhea should be reported to the local public health department.

BIBLIOGRAPHY

Bowie WR: Urethritis in males. In Holmes KK, Mardh P-A (eds): Sexually Transmitted Diseases. 2nd Ed. New York, McGraw-Hill, 1990, pp. 627–640.

Centers for Disease Control and Prevention: 1993 Sexually transmitted diseases treatment guidelines. MMWR 1993;42(No. RR-14).

Drugs for sexually transmitted diseases. Med Lett Drugs Ther 1991;33:119.

Handsfield HH, McCormack WM, et al: A comparison of single-dose cefixime with ceftriaxone as treatment for uncomplicated gonorrhea. N Engl J Med 1991;325 (19):1337.

Martin DH, et al: A controlled trial of a single dose of azithromycin for the treatment of chlamydial urethritis and cervicitis. N Engl J Med 1992;327:921.

Genital Herpes

I. ESSENTIAL FACTS

Genital herpes is caused by herpes simplex virus, type 2 (HSV-2), and, less commonly, type 1 (HSV-1). It is one of the most common STDs, and it accounts for 5% of STD clinic visits.

II. CLINICAL EVALUATION

A. Symptoms and Signs

1. **Initial Infection**

   a. Herpetic lesions are painful, multiple vesicles. The vesicles tend to coalesce, pustulate, and form superficial ulcers that heal without scarring. Lesions appear 2–20 days after exposure (mean: 6 days), and symptoms last 12 days on average.

b. Accompanying symptoms frequently include fever, malaise, anorexia, dysuria, and vaginal or urethral discharge.

c. Tender regional lymphadenopathy develops toward the end of the first week of illness.

d. Transient aseptic meningitis, myelitis, or lumbosacral myeloradiculitis occasionally occurs with initial infections.

e. Initial episodes are asymptomatic in up to 60% of cases. Patients who have had a prior HSV-1 infection often have milder initial episodes of genital herpes (type 1 or 2).

2. **Recurrent Disease**

a. Itching or burning locally often precedes the outbreak of vesicles.

b. Lesions progress through the same stages as primary lesions, crusting over 4–5 days after appearance.

c. Systemic symptoms are uncommon.

B. Diagnosis

1. A presumptive diagnosis is clinical (presence of typical genital lesions) and is often all that is required.

2. The Tzanck preparation has limited utility (sensitivity only 40-50%).

3. Definitive diagnosis is made by viral culture.

4. Serologies generally do not play a role in the management of genital herpes in the ED.

III. DIFFERENTIAL DIAGNOSIS

The differential diagnosis includes syphilis, chancroid, and traumatic ulcers. Patients with genital ulcers not typical for HSV should have a VDRL (or RPR) and darkfield microscopy done.

IV. THERAPY

A. Systemic Therapy

Table 15–29 presents the medical therapy of HSV infection. Systemic therapy is indicated for initial episodes (unless spontaneously healing), severe recurrences, and for suppression of frequent recurrences.

1. Acyclovir is the treatment of choice.
   a. *Oral Dose:* either 400 mg PO tid or 200 mg PO five times each day for 7-10 days. (Herpes proctitis requires a higher dose of acyclovir: 800 mg PO tid or 400 mg PO five times each day for 7–10 days).
   b. *Intravenous Dose:* 5 mg/kg IV every 8 hours for 7 days, or in the case of neurologic involvement, 10-12.4 mg/kg IV

Table 15–29. MEDICAL THERAPY OF GENITAL HERPES SIMPLEX INFECTIONS

CONDITION	DRUG	DOSE/ROUTE/DURATION
Initial Mucocutaneous Outbreak	Acyclovir	400 mg PO tid or 200 mg PO five times daily for 7–10 days
Proctitis	Acyclovir	800 mg PO tid or 400 mg PO five times daily for 7–10 days
Initial outbreak, immuno-compromised patient	Acyclovir	5 mg/kg IV q 8 hr for 7 days or 400 mg PO five times daily for 7 days, then suppressive therapy (below)
Acyclovir resistance	Foscarnet	40–60 mg/kg IV q 8 hr for 21 days, then suppressive therapy (below)
Recurrent (and Severe) Episodes	Acyclovir	400 mg PO tid or 200 mg PO five times daily for 7–10 days
Suppressive Therapy (for frequent episodes or immunocompromised)	Acyclovir	400 mg PO bid
Acyclovir resistance	Foscarnet	50 mg/kg IV daily, 5–7 days per week for up to 15 weeks

every 8 hours for 10 days. Intravenous acyclovir may be used if symptoms are severe, neurologic complications are present, or if the patient is immunocompromised.

   c. Topical acyclovir is generally not recommended because of its limited efficacy and need for frequent application.

2. Suppressive therapy: in patients with more than six recurrences per year acyclovir 400 mg PO bid reduces the frequency of symptomatic episodes. Limited and infrequent recurrent episodes, however, do not benefit from acyclovir therapy.

3. Foscarnet is indicated for the treatment of severe genital herpes in immunocompromised patients in the setting of viral *acyclovir resistance. Dose* 40–60 mg/kg IV every 8 hours for 21 days, followed by suppressive therapy of 50 mg/kg/day IV given once per day 5–7 days per week for up to 15 weeks.

B. Local and Supportive Care

1. Advise the patient to keep the area involved clean and dry.

2. Sexual abstinence should be practiced until all lesions have healed. Condoms are recommended for 6 months following an initial infection because of high rates of viral shedding.

V. DISPOSITION

A. Discharge

Most patients with genital herpes infection may be discharged from the ED with appropriate treatment and education initiated.

B. Admit

Patients with severe systemic manifestations (e.g., volume depletion, protracted nausea and vomiting), immunocompromised patients with systemic symptoms, and patients with neurologic manifestations requiring intravenous therapy should be admitted.

VI. PEARLS AND PITFALLS

A. Patients with lesions should be advised to avoid sexual contact.

B. Asymptomatic patients may still shed the virus and transmit the infection; many experts advise wearing a condom to prevent any potential exposure. Condoms are probably protective if all exposed skin is covered.

C. The patient's sexual partner(s) should be educated about signs and symptoms of HSV infection and should seek STD evaluation if symptoms occur.

D. HSV infection in patients with acquired immunodeficiency syndrome commonly manifests with atypical and chronic anogenital or oral ulcers. Suppressive therapy is often used to reduce frequent or severe recurrences. Acyclovir resistance does occur and should be considered in culture-confirmed ulcers that fail to respond.

BIBLIOGRAPHY

Centers for Disease Control and Prevention. 1993 Sexually transmitted diseases treatment guidelines. MMWR 1993;42(No. RR-14):22–26.
Hook EW 3rd, Cannon RO, et al: Herpes simplex virus infection as a risk factor for human immunodeficiency virus infection in homosexuals. J Infect Dis 1992;165:251.
Koutsky LA, Stevens CE, et al: Underdiagnosis of genital herpes by current clinical and viral-isolation procedures. N Engl J Med 1992;326:1533.
Whitley RJ, Gnann JW: Drug therapy: acyclovir: a decade later. N Engl J Med 1992;327:782.

Syphilis

I. ESSENTIAL FACTS

A. Definition

Syphilis is a chronic infection, highlighted by clinically apparent stages (primary, secondary, and tertiary [or late]), caused by the spirochete *Treponema pallidum*. This discussion emphasizes aspects of primary and secondary syphilis, as later stages are rarely encountered in the ED.

B. Epidemiology

1. More than 50,000 cases of primary and secondary syphilis were reported to the Centers for Disease Control (CDC) in 1990; the incidence has been increasing since 1986.

2. Most of this increase has involved ethnic and racial minorities.

3. In contrast to the early 1980s, rates of this disease have dropped dramatically in the gay community.

C. Routes of Exposure

1. Most infections are acquired during sexual contact with an infected individual in the primary (chancre) stage of disease.

2. Transplacental transmission is a secondary route of exposure, leading to congenital syphilis.

II. CLINICAL PRESENTATION

A. Signs and Symptoms

1. **Primary.** The classic syphilitic chancre is a genital ulcer several millimeters to 2 cm in size, indurated, painless, and solitary. However, atypical and multiple lesions are common, and extragenital lesions (oral, anal, rectal in homosexual men, cervical lesions in women) are seen. Regional painless adenopathy usually is present.

2. **Secondary.** Manifests 2–10 weeks after the appearance of the primary chancre as systemic symptoms (malaise, fever, arthralgias) and a generalized nonpruritic macular and papular rash. Palm and sole involvement is highly suggestive. Condylomata lata may be confused with mucosal condylomata acuminata (warts). Patchy alopecia and mucous patches are other common mucocutaneous findings. Generalized adenopathy usually is present. The primary chancre may still be present when secondary lesions first appear.

B. Laboratory Studies

Diagnosis of primary and secondary syphilis is by positive darkfield examination of suspicious lesions or a positive serologic test and a suggestive presentation.

1. Darkfield examination is a definitive test for early syphilis. Perform darkfield microscopy on any genital, oral, or anal ulcer not typical of genital herpes. The results should be interpreted only by experienced personnel. Darkfield examination of oral and rectal lesions must be interpreted cautiously because of the presence of commensal spirochetes.

2. A VDRL or RPR test is used for screening; a fluorescent treponemal antibody absorption test (FTA-ABS) or microhemagglutination *T. pallidum* (MHA-TP) test more specifically confirms the presence of treponemes. If RPR results are positive, perform a VDRL test to determine the baseline titer against which the response to therapy may be gauged. The RPR or VDRL test is positive in only 50–70% of patients with primary syphilis, but sensitivity increases with the duration of

untreated disease. Therefore, if primary syphilis is suspected, the patient should return in several weeks for a repeat serologic test. The RPR (or VDRL) test is positive in 99–100% of patients with secondary syphilis. Both nonspecific and specific treponemal serologies may be falsely negative in HIV-positive patients with clinical evidence of syphilis.

III. DIFFERENTIAL DIAGNOSIS

A. The differential diagnosis for primary syphilis includes other causes of genital ulcer disease: chancroid, genital herpes, traumatic ulcer, fixed drug eruption, and squamous cell carcinoma.

B. Secondary syphilis may be confused with drug rash, pityriasis rosea, viral exanthemata, superficial dermatophyte infection, and mucosal warts.

IV. THERAPY

For primary and secondary, as well as early latent syphilis (known to be < 1 year's duration):

A. The drug of choice is benzathine penicillin G (2.4 million units IM, as a single dose). More intensive therapy (the above injection given weekly for up to three doses) has been recommended, especially for human immunodeficiency virus (HIV)-positive patients, to erradicate cerebrospinal fluid (CSF) treponemes.

B. In penicillin-allergic patients:

1. Doxycycline 100 mg PO bid (or tetracycline 500 mg PO qid) for 2 weeks.

2. If tetracyclines are contraindicated (as in pregnancy), or not tolerated, erythromycin 500 mg PO four times daily for 15 days.

It is extremely important that the patient be counseled about strict adherence to these oral regimens. If compliance cannot be ensured with an oral regimen, the CDC recommends skin testing for penicillin allergy and desensitization if necessary.

C. Another potentially effective option is ceftriaxone 250 mg IM daily for 10 days, if there is no history of anaphylaxis with penicillin. Again, compliance and follow-up must be ensured.

D. Always counsel patients about the possibility of the Jarisch-Herxheimer reaction—fever, chills, malaise, arthralgias, myalgia, headache, or appearance or exacerbation of rash—which can occur after any therapy for syphilis. It is treated with bedrest and aspirin and resolves within 24 hours.

V. FOLLOW-UP

A. A VDRL test needs to be repeated at 3, 6, and 12 months to make sure that the titer declines to a nonreactive or low level. For HIV-positive patients, repeat serologies are recommended at more frequent intervals (1, 2, 3, 6, 9, and 12 months).

B. All patients diagnosed with early syphilis should undergo a thorough STD examination. Likewise, all should be counseled regarding HIV risks and encouraged to be tested for HIV.

C. Persons exposed to syphilis should undergo a thorough STD examination and serologic testing. Treat those exposed within the preceding 3 months as for early syphilis, regardless of serology results.

D. Routine CSF examination is not required for HIV-negative adults with early syphilis. Controversy exists over routine lumbar puncture for early syphilis in those who are HIV-positive. Many authors recommend this.

E. Perform lumbar puncture for neurologic involvement, including meningeal or cranial, optic, or auditory nerve symptoms or signs.

F. Report all cases to the local public health department.

VI. PEARLS AND PITFALLS

A. Consider primary syphilis in any patient with a genital ulcer, even painful or atypical-appearing ones.

B. A negative RPR or VDRL test does not rule out primary syphilis.

C. Perform an RPR or VDRL test with any rash that could be consistent with secondary syphilis.

BIBLIOGRAPHY

Centers for Disease Control: Primary and secondary syphilis—United States, 1985–1990. MMWR 1991;40:314.
Centers for Disease Control and Prevention: 1993 Sexually transmitted diseases treatment guidelines. MMWR 1993;42(No. RR-14):27–46.
Musher DM, Hamill RJ, Baughn RE: Effect of human immunodeficiency virus (HIV) infection on the course of syphilis and on the response to treatment. Ann Intern Med 1990;113:872.

SINUSITIS

"Sit down now and pray forsooth that the mucus in your nose may not run. Nay, rather wipe your nose and do not blame God!"

EPICTETUS (60?–120?)

I. ESSENTIAL FACTS

A. Definition

Sinusitis is an inflammation of one or more of the paranasal sinuses. It is categorized as acute or chronic based upon the duration of a patient's symptoms: in *acute sinusitis* symptoms are present for ≤ 4 weeks; in *chronic sinusitis* symptoms have been present for ≥ 3 months. Patients with symptom duration between these two parameters are generally evaluated and treated for acute sinusitis. The distinction is important because symptoms, signs, and diagnostic/treatment modalities differ between the two entities.

B. Epidemiology

1. Acute and chronic sinusitis cause 16 million physician visits annually, and chronic sinusitis affects ≈ 31 million people in the United States.

2. Sinusitis occurs most commonly in the fall, winter, and spring; it complicates 0.5% of common upper-respiratory-tract infections.

C. Pathophysiology

Sinusitis can result from an alteration in ostial size, mucociliary transport, oxygen exchange, or mucosal blood flow. Of these, the most important is ostial obstruction. The *microbiology* of sinusitis differs depending on the risk factors present and the chronicity of the disease (Table 15–30).

II. CLINICAL EVALUATION

A. History

1. **Acute Sinusitis.** This entity can often be diagnosed by history alone. *The symptoms most constant and predictive of sinusitis include*
   a. Facial pain; which varies depending on which sinus(es) is/are affected.
      i. Maxillary: pain is felt over the cheeks, maxillary molars, and hard palate. It is worse in the upright position.
      ii. Ethmoid: pain is felt in the retro-orbital area and upper lateral aspect of the nose. It is worse in the supine position.
      iii. Frontal: pain is over the lower forehead. It is worse in the supine position.
      iv. Sphenoid: pain may be referred to multiple locations, including the retro-orbital, frontal, facial, or postauricular areas. It is worse in the supine position.
   b. Pain that fails to improve with decongestant use.

Table 15–30. RISK FACTORS AND MOST LIKELY ORGANISMS IN ACUTE SINUSITIS

RISK FACTORS	PREDOMINANT ORGANISMS
Obstruction of Sinus Ostia Upper-respiratory-tract infection Allergic rhinitis Deviated nasal septum Hypertrophied adenoids Nasal polyps or tumors Nasal foreign bodies Topical decongestant overuse	*Streptococcus pneumoniae* (55%) *Hemophilus influenzae* (20%) Respiratory viruses (15%) Anaerobes (9%) *Branhamella catarrhalis* Streptococci (group A beta-hemolytic and alpha-hemolytic)
Environmental Situations Swimming/diving Barotrauma Cold weather	Same as above
Dental Infection	Gram-negative bacilli Anaerobes Streptococci
Impaired Ciliary Motility Cystic fibrosis Immotile cilia syndrome Kartagener's syndrome	*Pseudomonas aeruginosa* *Staphylococcus aureus*
Nosocomial Infection Nasopharyngeal tubes Nasotracheal tubes Nasal packing Nasal and cranial fractures	*Escherichia coli* *P. aeruginosa* *Serratia* sp. Polymicrobial organisms
Immunocompromised Patients Systemic illness Diabetes mellitus Corticosteroid therapy	*H. influenzae* *S. pneumoniae* Fungi (aspergillus species; fungal species causing mucormycosis; *Candida albicans*)
Acquired Immunodeficiency Syndrome	*H. influenzae* *S. pneumoniae* *P. aeruginosa* *Pseudallescheria boydii* *Legionella pneumophila* *Acanthamoeba castellani*

From Herr RD: Acute sinusitis: diagnosis and treatment update. Am Fam Phys 1991; 44(6):2055–2062.

    c. Maxillary toothache (maxillary sinusitis).
    d. Purulent nasal discharge.

        Less predictive but frequently encountered symptoms include
    e. Fever and malaise.
    f. Nasal congestion.
    g. Preceding upper-respiratory-tract infection.
    h. Headache.

     i. Sore throat.

     j. Cough.

2. **Chronic Sinusitis.** The symptoms of chronic sinusitis are similar to, but more protracted ($\geq$ 3 months) and subtle than, those of acute sinusitis. Fever and purulent nasal discharge are rarely present. The history is usually not sufficient to make the diagnosis, and an imaging study (sinus computed tomography [CT]) is frequently necessary. A patient may complain of one or more of the following:

     a. Pain: location is identical to above acute sinusitis descriptions, but less severe. Patients will often describe pain as a chronic daily headache.

     b. Nasal congestion.

     c. Postnasal drip.

     d. Otalgia.

     e. Minor nosebleeds.

     f. Eye pain.

     g. Intermittent facial swelling.

     h. Halitosis.

     i. Chronic cough.

     j. Fatigue and lightheadedness.

B. Physical Examination

The directed examination should focus on the patient's vital signs, head/neck, and pulmonary system. Possible findings include the following:

1. **Acute Sinusitis**

     a. Temperature > 38°C (20% of patients).

     b. Purulent nasal discharge (50% of patients): most commonly emanates from behind the middle turbinate.

     c. Nasal mucosal edema.

     d. Facial tenderness (50% of patients).

     e. Abnormal transillumination (60% of patients). Transillumination is a useful test for diagnosing maxillary or frontal sinus disease, but it requires training and experience to interpret the findings adequately. A completely opaque sinus correlates with active infection. (*Technique:* the test is performed in a darkened room. A bright light source is placed over the midpoint of the inferior orbital rim. With the patient's mouth open, the physician assesses transmission of light through the maxilla and, if possible, the hard palate. To transilluminate the frontal sinus, the light source must be placed inferior to the medial border of the supraorbital ridge. The symmetry of the blush can be evaluated bilaterally).

2. **Chronic Sinusitis.** A thorough head and neck examination are required as above, however, the findings are frequently subtle. Transillumination is not useful in chronic disease because of

the diffuse swelling of all sinus mucosa and the rarity of sinus fluid collections.

C. Diagnostic Studies

1. **Laboratory Testing.** No test is of diagnostic utility. A complete blood count (CBC) may reveal a leukocytosis but this finding is neither sensitive nor specific.

2. **Cultures.** Nasal cultures are not useful. Sinus aspirates, obtained by an otolaryngology consultant through sinus puncture, should be reserved for those patients with severe disease, disease unresponsive to appropriate antibiotics, and/or those who are markedly immunosupressed (e.g., human immunodeficiency virus-infected patients with low CD4 counts with a suspected unusual pathogen).

3. **Imaging Studies.** These need not be obtained in patients with convincing acute signs and symptoms.
   a. *Plain radiographs (sinus series):* Data are scarce regarding their sensitivity and specificity for sinusitis. The Water's view is the most helpful (an air-fluid level, opacification, or mucosal thickening > 6 mm has a sensitivity of 70% for maxillary disease). The ethmoid sinuses are visualized poorly.
   b. *Limited sinus CT* is the most sensitive imaging technique available and is useful in the evaluation of patients with atypical acute presentations or suspected ethmoid and sphenoid disease, and all those with possible chronic sinusitis. Findings must always be clinically correlated (16% false-positive rate). In many centers, the cost is comparable to plain radiography.

4. **Nasal Endoscopy.** This technique permits extensive examination of the entire nasal cavity, including the ostiomeatal complex. It is an office otolaryngologic procedure employed in the evaluation of patients with severe or chronic symptoms.

III. DIFFERENTIAL DIAGNOSIS

The differential diagnosis includes simple upper-respiratory-tract infections, allergic or vasomotor rhinitis, polyps, sinus tumors, sinus retention cysts, nasal foreign body, dental infections, and vasculitis.

IV. COMPLICATIONS

In the antibiotic era, complications are rare, but can be life-threatening.

A. *Osteomyelitis* may result from frontal sinusitis eroding into the frontal bones. Patients present with headache, fever, and a characteristic doughy edema over the affected bone known as "Pott's puffy tumor."

B. *Orbital cellulitis* is most commonly a complication of ethmoid sinusitis. It usually begins with edema of the eyelids and rapidly progresses to ptosis, proptosis, chemosis, and diminished extraocular movements. Patients are febrile and acutely ill.

C. *Cavernous sinus thrombophlebitis* can result from retrograde extension of infection along venous channels from the orbit, ethmoid, or frontal sinuses. These patients are febrile and "toxic" appearing. Lid edema; proptosis; chemosis; third, fourth, and sixth cranial nerve palsies; fixed and dilated pupils; and venous engorgement may all be present.

D. *Intracranial extension* directly through bone or via venous channels can lead to a variety of syndromes, including brain abscess, empyema, and meningitis.

V. THERAPY

Table 15–31 presents the medical treatment of sinusitis.

A. **Acute Sinusitis.** The components of therapy for acute sinusitis include antibiotics, decongestants, and occasionally antihistamines.

B. **Recurrent or Chronic Sinusitis.** Therapy for patients with recurrent or prolonged symptoms is similar to that for acute sinusitis, with the following adaptations:

1. *Antibiotics:* an empiric, prolonged trial (3–4 weeks) of antimicrobial therapy is recommended. Because patients in this category are more likely to have unusual or resistant organisms, the antibiotic chosen should be effective against *Staphylococcus aureus,* anaerobes, and beta-lactamase-producing *Hemophilus influenzae* and *Bramhamella catarrhalis.*

2. *Decongestants and antihistamines:* oral decongestants and antihistamines (if indicated for suspected allergic symptoms) should be continued for 3–4 weeks.

3. *Corticosteroids:* nasally inhaled steroids may be used in patients who have not adequately responded to antihistamines. Because they may theoretically potentiate infection, patients should be monitored closely for signs of worsening infection.

4. *Otolaryngology consultation/referral:* patients with suspected chronic disease should be referred to an otolaryngologist. Needle aspiration of the maxillary sinus and/or surgery is sometimes necessary if maximal medical therapy fails to improve or resolve symptoms.

Table 15–31. OUTPATIENT MEDICAL TREATMENT OF ACUTE OR CHRONIC SINUSITIS

DRUG	DOSE	COMMENT
Antibiotics		Choose an agent effective against the most likely organisms.
Initial Treatment		Except where noted, *continue therapy for 14 days* for patients with acute sinusitis. Penetration into infected sinuses is low.
Amoxicillin	250–500 mg PO q 8 hr	
Trimethoprim-sulfamethoxazole[a] (Bactrim DS, Septra DS)	1 tab PO q 12 hr	
Alternative Agents		
Amoxicillin-Clavulanate[a] (Augmentin)	250–500 mg PO q 8 hr	
Cefuroxime axetil[a] (Ceftin)	250 mg PO q 12 hr	
Cefalor[a] (Ceclor)	250–500 mg PO q 8 hr	
Clarithromycin[a] (Biaxin)	250–500 mg PO bid	
Azithromycin[a]	500 mg PO on day one, then 250 mg PO on days 2–7	
Dental Infections		
Penicillin VK	250–500 mg PO q 6 hr	
Impaired ciliary motility		
Ciprofloxacin	500 mg PO q 12 hr	
Decongestants		The use of decongestants is essential to decrease mucosal edema and allow drainage of sinus secretions. A combination of both topical and systemic agents should be employed.
Topical		
Phenylephrine hydrochloride (Neosynephrine)	One spray each nostril, then repeat after 1 min. Use q 4 hr during first four days of treatment.	Topical formulations should be limited to 4 days to avoid the phenomenon of rebound hyperemia (rhinitis medicamentosa).
Oxymetazoline hydrochloride (Afrin)	Two–three drops or two sprays each nostril twice daily	Use decongestants with caution in patients with hypertension. Phenylpropanolamine is the best choice in this setting.
Systemic		
Pseudoephedrine hydrochloride (Sudafed)	30–60 mg PO qid	
Phenylpropanolamine hydrochloride	75 mg PO q 12 hr (maximum dose)	

[a]Patients with unresolved, recurrent or chronic symptoms should have a *3–4 week course* of an antibiotic which covers: *S. aureus,* anaerobes, and beta-lactamase producing *H. influenzae* and *B. catarrhalis.*

Table 15–31. OUTPATIENT MEDICAL TREATMENT OF ACUTE OR CHRONIC SINUSITIS *Continued*

DRUG	DOSE	COMMENT
Antihistamines		Antihistamines may provide additional decongestion if there is an allergic component to the problem, but because they thicken secretions, their use should be limited to those patients with suspected allergy.
Diphenhydramine *(Benedryl)*	25–50 mg PO q 6 hr	
Terphenadine *(Seldane)*	60 mg PO q 12 hr	Many antihistamines are available. Three in common use are listed here. Clinically they differ in the amount of sedation they produce: Seldane (none); Chlor-Trimeton (little); Benadryl (marked). *Caution:* seldane must be taken only as prescribed; beware of drug interactions; improper dosing or drug interaction (e.g., with erythromycin) have caused prolonged QT intervals and sudden death in some patients.
Chlorpheniramine *(Chlor-Trimeton)*	4 mg PO q 6 hr	
Steroids		Nasally inhaled steroids may be employed in patients who have an *allergic component to their chronic symptoms,* in whom antihistamines have failed. The potentiation of infection is a stated concern of many authors, but remains unproven.
Nasal inhalers		
Beclomethasone dipropionate *(Beconase, Vancenase)*	2–4 puffs q 6 hr	
Flunisolide *(Nasalide)*	2–4 puffs q 12 hr	
Triamcinolone acetonide *(Nasocort)*	2–3 puffs q 6 hr	

VI. DISPOSITION

A. Discharge

Most patients with acute, uncomplicated sinusitis may have treatment initiated in the ED and then be discharged to home. Prior to discharge, the patient should be informed of the complications of sinusitis listed above. Follow-up in 2–3 days is strongly recommended to ensure improvement in signs and symptoms.

B. Admit

Patients with *any* of the following should be admitted to the hospital for thorough otolaryngologic evaluation and parenteral antibiotic therapy:

1. Severely ill or "toxic" appearance with high fever and/or rigors.

2. Severe pain requiring parenteral opioids.

3. Failure to improve after 2–3 days of outpatient therapy.

4. Debilitated or immunocompromised patient (consult otolaryngology urgently and evaluate for mucormycosis or invasive aspergillosis).

     5. Suspected complication from sinusitis (e.g., osteomyelitis, orbital cellulitis).

VII. PEARLS AND PITFALLS

A. The diagnosis of acute sinusitis can usually be made by the history and physical examination alone. A laboratory evaluation and/or imaging studies are not necessary in most otherwise healthy patients.

B. The most sensitive test revealing sinus inflammation, when imaging is deemed necessary, is a limited sinus CT.

C. Effective therapy of sinusitis requires antibiotics *and* nasal/oral decongestants. In addition, antihistamines should be added if allergic symptoms are a component of the disease.

D. Chronic sinusitis often presents with vague and confusing symptoms. Empiric, prolonged antibiotic/decongestant therapy and otolaryngologic referral are appropriate.

E. Follow-up is necessary for all patients with acute sinusitis to document improvement of signs/symptoms.

F. Consider the possibility of a serious invasive fungal infection in the debilitated or immunocompromised patient with signs/symptoms of sinusitis: urgent otolaryngologic consultation and admission are required.

BIBLIOGRAPHY

Bolger WE, Kennedy DW: Changing concepts in chronic sinusitis. Hosp Pract September 1992; 20–28.

Godley FA. Chronic sinusitis: An update. Am Fam Phys 1992;45:2190–2199.

Lanza DC, Kennedy DW: Current concepts in the surgical management of chronic and recurrent acute sinusitis. J Allergy Clin Immunol 1992;90(3)Part 2:505–511.

Wald ER: Sinusitis in children. N Engl J Med 1992;326(5)319–323.

Williams W Jr., Simel DL, Roberts L, Samsa, G: Clinical evaluation for sinusitis. Ann Intern Med 1992;117(9)705–710.

TETANUS PROPHYLAXIS

> *"H' had got a hurt*
> *D'th' inside of a deadlier sort."*
>
> SAMUEL BUTLER (1612–1680)

I. ESSENTIAL FACTS

In the United States between 1982 and 1989, 95% of tetanus cases occurred in patients $\geq$ 20 years of age; 59% of cases occurred in individuals $\geq$ 60 years old.

II. PROPHYLAXIS

A. Any wound may be contaminated and potentially infected by tetanus organisms. Tetanus prophylaxis must be considered in all wounds. This includes chronic ulcers, bites and scratches, burns, frostbite, corneal abrasions, foreign bodies in eyes, friction abrasions, and illicit needle use, especially skin popping. The first step is prompt, adequate surgical care: excision of dead tissue, removal of foreign material, and mechanical cleansing, including irrigation.

B. Adsorbed tetanus and diphtheria toxoids (Td) is the preferred preparation for active tetanus immunization (for patients ≥ 7 years old). This is to enhance diphtheria protection, as a large proportion of adults are susceptible. The dose is 0.5 mL IM. The patient ≥ 7 years old who did not receive primary immunization to tetanus as a young child should receive two doses of Td 4–8 weeks apart, followed by a third dose 6–12 months later. Booster doses should then follow every 10 years, or as directed in the flow diagram (Fig. 15–21).

C. Tetanus immune globulin (TIG) is indicated for the patient with any wound other than a clean minor one *and* who has never received or is uncertain of having received a primary series. Those who served in the military can be assumed to have received a primary series. The dose of TIG is 250 units IM.

D. When Td and TIG are given at the same time, use different syringes, needles, and sites. When uncertain about immunization history, risk, or wound, err on the side of overimmunization. A patient with tetanus must receive full immunization after recovery, as the disease does not confer immunity.

BIBLIOGRAPHY

Immunization Practices Advisory Committee (ACIP): Diphtheria, tetanus, and pertussis: recommendations for vaccine use and other preventive measures. MMWR 1991; 40(RR-10):1-28.

Update on adult immunization: recommendations of the Immunization Practices Advisory Committee (ACIP). MMWR 1991;40(RR-12):16–19, 49, 70.

TUBERCULOSIS

> "In its beginning the malady [tuberculosis] is easier to cure but difficult to detect, but later it becomes easy to detect but difficult to cure."
>
> NICCOLO MACHIAVELLI (1469–1527)

I. ESSENTIAL FACTS

A. Definition

Tuberculosis (TB) is an infection caused by the organism *Mycobacterium tuberculosis,* a slow-growing, aerobic bacillus

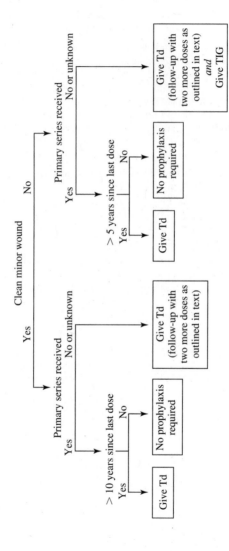

Figure 15-21. Tetanus prophylaxis summary.

that cannot be decolorized with acid alcohol after staining (acid fast). Though pulmonary infection is most common, TB can involve any organ system. Patients with human immunodeficiency virus (HIV) infection frequently have extrapulmonary involvement (~ 24-45% extrapulmonary infection in HIV-infected patients; > 70% in patients with acquired immunodeficiency syndrome [AIDS]).

B. Mode of Transmission

Almost all infections result from inhalation of air-borne particles known as *droplet nuclei*. These particles are very small (1–5 μm) and are generated when persons with pulmonary or laryngeal tuberculosis cough, sneeze, speak, or sing.

C. Pathogenesis

Infection begins when a person inhales droplet nuclei that contain *M. tuberculosis.* These organisms first become established in the alveoli of the lungs and then spread throughout the body. Newly infected immunocompetent persons usually contain the infection ("dormant" or latent infection), but ~ 1.0% will develop an acute clinical illness (*primary disease* [Fig. 15–22]). Months, years, or decades later, ~ 5-10% of patients with dormant infection will develop clinically apparent tuberculosis (*reactivation disease*). The risk of developing reactivation disease is highest during the first several years after the person was infected. In HIV-infected patients, ~ 30% will develop primary disease; of the patients who have dormant infection, ~ 30% will develop reactivation disease (Fig. 15–23).

D. Epidemiology

1. **Incidence.** In recent years, the incidence of TB has increased, mainly because of the HIV epidemic. Approximately 25,000 cases of tuberculosis are reported annually, and 10–15 million persons in the United States have latent *M. tuberculosis* infection.

2. **Risk Factors**

   a. Major risk factors include
      i. HIV infection.
      ii. Injection drug use.
      iii. Close contacts of smear-positive patients.
      iv. Homelessness.
      v. Prior residence in an endemic country (Southeast Asia, Africa, Caribbean, Mexico, and Central America).
      vi. Institutionalization (e.g., prison).
   b. Minor risk factors include
      i. Diabetes mellitus.
      ii. Previous gastrectomy.
      iii. History of silicosis.

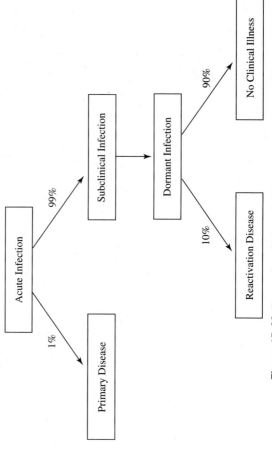

Figure 15–22. Progression of tuberculosis in immunocompetent patients.

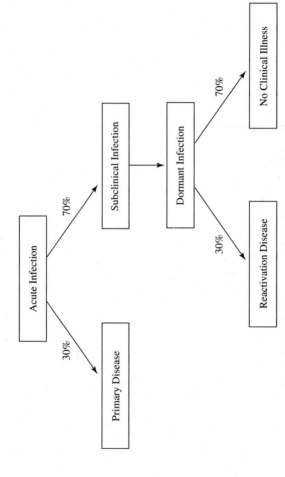

Figure 15–23. Progression of tuberculosis in patients with HIV infection.

3. **Multidrug-Resistant Tuberculosis.** In recent years, several large outbreaks of multidrug-resistant TB have occurred. These have predominantly been in the eastern United States in patients in institutional settings, especially HIV-infected individuals.

E. Key Fact

Lifetime risk of reactivation in immunocompetent patients with a positive purified protein derivative (PPD) test is ~ 10%. The *yearly* risk of reactivation of TB in an HIV-infected individual with a positive PPD test is 8%.

II. CLINICAL EVALUATION

A. History

Determine the patient's risk factors for TB (see above). Prior PPD reactor status should be documented if known.

B. Symptoms

Classic symptoms of tuberculosis include fever, night sweats, weight loss, cough with sputum production, dyspnea, and hemoptysis. In individuals with AIDS, or in the elderly, these classic symptoms may be absent or replaced by more vague symptoms related to extrapulmonary TB, including anorexia, malaise, weakness, pleuritic chest pain (secondary to tuberculous effusions), nausea, headache, and back or bone pain.

C. Signs

Pulmonary signs are nonspecific and include dullness to percussion and decreased fremitus when pleural effusion or thickening is present. With more extensive disease, signs of consolidation (tubular breath sounds) may occur. Erythema nodosum may occasionally be seen with primary infection.

D. Directed Physical Examination

1. **Vital Signs.** Note fever, tachycardia, and/or tachypnea.

2. **Skin:** Look for erythema nodosum (a rare finding of primary TB), and/or findings suggestive of HIV infection (e.g., Kaposi's sarcoma).

3. **Lymph Nodes.** Adenopathy may be present as part of localized or disseminated TB, or as a sign of co-existent HIV infection.

4. **Pulmonary Examination.** Note dullness to percussion (pleural effusion/thickening), rales, and/or signs of consolidation.

5. **Neurologic Examination.** Central nervous system abnormalities or significant mental status changes may occur. Meningeal signs may or may not be present.

E. Routine Tests

1. **Chest Roentgenography.** This is the key test and often suggests the diagnosis of TB even when the disease was not initially suspected.
   a. Classic chest film manifestations of primary TB include
      i. Hilar adenopathy.
      ii. Pleural effusions.
      iii. Miliary pattern (multiple "millet seed"-sized infiltrates throughout lungs).
   b. Classic chest film manifestations of reactivation TB include
      i. Upper-lobe infiltrates.
      ii. Cavitation.
      iii. Pleural effusions.
   c. Chest film patterns frequently seen in patients with *early* HIV infection (well-preserved immune function) are similar to those of reactivation TB in immunocompetent hosts (see above).
   d. Chest film patterns frequently seen in patients with late HIV infection or AIDS (severely immunosuppressed) are similar to those of primary TB in immunocompetent hosts (see above).
   e. Chest film patterns frequently seen in HIV-infected patients with multidrug-resistant TB include
      i. Alveolar infiltrates.
      ii. Reticular interstitial infiltrates.
      iii. Cavitation.

2. **PPD Testing.** The major role of PPD testing is in patient screening. It may also be helpful in occasional cases where TB is suspected, but the clinical presentation is atypical. In general, skin test sensitivity develops 2–10 weeks after primary infection with *M. tuberculosis.* Criteria for positive PPD testing are given in V. A. below. *Cautions:* if infiltrates are present, obtain sputum for acid-fast bacilli (AFB) (do not start with PPD testing); do not repeat PPD testing in patients with the history of a positive PPD test.

3. **Sputum for AFB.** The definitive diagnosis of TB is made by identifying *M. tuberculosis* in a sputum culture. Three sets of sputum for smear and culture should be obtained (ideally morning specimens from three separate days). Smear positivity is present in 50–80% of patients with pulmonary TB and increases to 98% in patients with cavitary disease. The yield is lower in HIV-infected patients, presumably because of the lower frequency of cavitary pulmonary disease among HIV-infected individuals. Antimicrobial susceptibility testing should be performed on all positive isolates.

4. **Urinalysis.** Sterile pyuria may suggest renal TB.

5. **Liver Function Tests.** Alanine aminotransferase, aspartate aminotransferase, and alkaline phosphatase levels may be

elevated if the liver is involved. Baseline values must be obtained before a patient is placed on isoniazid therapy.

III. THERAPY

Table 15–32 presents the medical therapy of tuberculosis.

A. General Treatment Principles

1. Before effective antituberculosis therapy became available, approximately 50% of patients with active pulmonary TB died. With current recommended regimens, tuberculosis can effectively be treated in most cases (although the specter of multidrug-resistant disease is worrisome).

2. Simultaneous administration of multiple drugs is appropriate in an attempt to prevent drug resistance. Therapy should be initiated with *four drugs* (i.e., isoniazid, rifampin, pyrazinamide, and ethambutol) until susceptibility to isoniazid and rifampin is demonstrated (if the organism is sensitive to isoniazid and rifampin, ethambutol may then be discontinued).

3. During recent years, shorter courses of therapy have been shown as effective as longer, traditional regimens. In immunocompetent patients, therapy can be completed in 6 months; in HIV-infected patients, therapy should be continued for 9 months (Table 15–32). After 2 months of therapy, the pyrazinamide can be stopped (assuming isoniazid and rifampin sensitivity); the isoniazid and rifampin should be continued for the duration of the remaining treatment course. This regimen is also highly effective for extrapulmonary TB. When a strain of multidrug-resistant *M. tuberculosis* is isolated or suspected, consultation with an infectious disease expert (or TB specialist) should occur in order to optimize therapy.

4. If noncompliance with recommended treatment is a concern, providers should contact their local public health departments for advice and assistance in providing directly observed therapy.

Table 15–32. TREATMENT OF TUBERCULOSIS IN ADULTS

DRUG	DAILY DOSE	MAXIMUM DAILY DOSE	DURATION
Isoniazid	5 mg/kg	300 mg	6 months[a]
Rifampin	10 mg/kg	600 mg	6 months[a]
Pyrazinamide	15–30 mg/kg	2 g	Initial 2 months
Ethambutol[b]	15–25 mg/kg	2.5 g	

[a]Therapy should be extended to 9 months in HIV-infected patients.
[b]Ethambutol is used in initial therapy *until* susceptibility to INH and rifampin is demonstrated.

B. Medications

1. Isoniazid (INH) is an inexpensive bactericidal agent that remains the cornerstone of TB therapy. This drug's two major side effects are hepatotoxicity (1-2%) and peripheral neuritis (1-2%). The incidence of hepatoxicity increases with older patients and with alcohol ingestion. Peripheral neuritis occurs more commonly in patients with diabetes, alcoholism, uremia, pregnancy, seizure disorders, and malnutrition. It can be prevented by the concomitant administration of pyridoxine (10-25 mg/day). INH reduces serum levels of the antifungal drugs ketoconazole and fluconazole, thereby making them ineffective in some patients; it also may increase serum phenytoin levels. Patients taking disulfiram (Antabuse) may suffer behavioral abnormalities while also taking INH.

2. Rifampin is bactericidal for *M. tuberculosis* and is a relatively safe and easily administered drug. Its major side effects are gastrointestinal upset, skin eruptions, hepatitis, and rarely, thrombocytopenia. In addition, rifampin accelerates the clearance of drugs metabolized by the liver and may render them inactive. Patients taking rifampin should be advised that their body fluids, such as tears, urine, and sweat, will become orange colored; soft contact lenses may become permanently discolored.

3. Pyrazinamide is a bactericidal agent in an acid environment. Adverse reactions associated with pyrazinamide include liver toxicity and hyperuricemia. Clinically relevant adverse reactions are rarely seen, especially when the pyrazinamide is discontinued after the first 2 months of therapy.

4. Ethambutol is bacteriostatic against *M. tuberculosis*. The most common adverse reaction to ethambutol is optic neuritis, manifesting as blurred vision, central scotoma, and red-green color blindness. This side effect occurs in < 1% of persons who take ethambutol at a daily dose of 15 mg/kg.

C. Multidrug-Resistant TB

Therapy for multidrug-resistant TB depends on the results of antimicrobial susceptibility testing. Drugs that are used include INH, rifampin, pyrazinamide, ethambutol, streptomycin, ciprofloxacin, ethionamide, cycloserine, and clofazimine. Despite aggressive treatment with multiple agents, patients generally have persistently positive (or intermittently positive) sputum cultures and high mortality rates.

IV. INFECTION CONTROL

Patients with confirmed or suspected TB who come into the ED should be placed in a room that is adequately ventilated (ideally an isolation room). Patients with a productive cough, pulmonary cavitation on chest roentgenography, and a positive AFB sputum smear are the most contagious. Appropriate high-filtration masks should be worn by health care workers to decrease their likelihood of becoming infected. The patient should also wear a mask. The best protective masks are disposable, valveless, particulate respirators.

V. PREVENTION: TUBERCULIN (PPD) TEST

A. Testing

Initial preventative screening should be performed with the intradermal administration of 5 tuberculin units of PPD and two additional antigens as controls (mumps, candida, or tetanus toxoid). Tests should be read between 48 and 72 hours after PPD administration. A positive test should be based on the presence of induration, not erythema; the diameter of induration should be measured transversely to the long axis of the forearm. The significance of induration (i.e., whether the test should be interpreted as positive) depends on the patient group tested.

B. Interpretation of PPD Testing.

Table 15–33 presents the interpretation of the PPD test.

Table 15–33. INTERPRETATION OF PPD TESTING

INDURATION (INDICATING A POSITIVE REACTION)	APPROPRIATE GROUP	PREVENTIVE THERAPY (INH)
≥ 5 mm	Close contacts of smear-positive patients	All
	HIV-infected patients or persons with risk factors for HIV infection who have an unknown HIV status	All
	Persons who have chest films consistent with old healed tuberculosis	All
≥ 10 mm	Injection drug users	All
	Patients with diseases that increase the risk of TB (silicosis, diabetes, Hodgkin's disease, end-stage renal disease)	All
	Persons from countries wth a high prevalence of TB	< 35 years old, or recent converter[a]
	Nursing home and prison residents	< 35 years old, or recent converter
	Homeless patients	< 35 years old, or recent converter
	Health care workers	< 35 years old, or recent converter
≥ 15 mm	No identifiable risk factors for TB	< 35 years old, or recent converter

[a]A person who has developed a positive PPD test within the past 2 years.

C. Treatment Following a "Positive" PPD Test

1. The PPD test provides information on whether a person has been infected with *M. tuberculosis* at some time, but it cannot determine whether the disease is active or dormant. Therefore, *all persons with a positive PPD test should have a chest roentgenogram.*

2. All persons < 35 years of age with a positive PPD test should receive preventive therapy. In addition, all recent converters (within 2 years) should receive preventive therapy.

3. The standard treatment regimen is isoniazid 10 mg/kg daily for children and 300 mg daily for adults. Treatment should be continued for 6 months (except for HIV-infected patients, who should receive 12 months of therapy). INH therapy is highly effective in preventing reactivation of *M. tuberculosis.*

4. *Cautions:* severe and sometimes fatal hepatitis may develop in patients on INH, even after only a few months of therapy. Risk is increased by alcohol consumption and increasing age. Patients should be instructed to abstain from alcohol while taking INH. Liver function tests should be checked before initiating therapy and periodically throughout therapy. Patients should be clinically evaluated *every month* while on therapy, and they must be instructed to stop INH immediately and seek medical attention for any symptoms suggestive of hepatitis (e.g., malaise, anorexia, nausea/vomiting, right-upper-quadrant discomfort, jaundice).

VI. DISPOSITION

A. Discharge

The patient with known or suspected active tuberculosis may be discharged to home if *all* of the following conditions apply:

1. The patient is not seriously ill.

2. No worrisome comorbid conditions are present.

3. No extrapulmonary disease is evident.

4. The patient is reliable.

5. Close outpatient follow-up is ensured.

In most cases, only a suspicion for tuberculosis will be generated in the ED, with further outpatient work-up and confirmation of the diagnosis necessary. The patient must be made aware of the contagious nature of his/her disease. Until the patient has been on multidrug therapy for *at least 2 weeks,* he/she should wear an appropriate mask, avoid intimate contact with others, and cough into a tissue (the tissue should subsequently be incinerated). Any patient with a presumptive or confirmed diagnosis of tuberculosis should be reported to the public health department.

B. Admit

The patient with known or suspected tuberculosis should be admitted to an appropriate isolation room in the hospital if *any* of the following conditions apply:

1. The patient is unreliable.

2. The patient has moderate to severe disease (e.g., cavitary disease, marked wasting, malnutrition).

3. The patient has extrapulmonary disease.

4. The patient has another significant comorbid condition.

VII. PEARLS AND PITFALLS

A. Maintain a high index of suspicion for tuberculosis, especially in the patient with known or suspected HIV infection, weight loss, night sweats, chronic cough, persistent fever, or hemoptysis.

B. The patient with a positive PPD test must have a chest film obtained.

C. The patient begun on isoniazid (INH) prophylaxis should be educated with respect to concomitant risk of liver toxicity. The patient must refrain from alcohol use while on INH and must have close (monthly) outpatient follow-up.

D. Patients must have liver function tests checked before INH therapy is started, and the liver function tests should be periodically rechecked throughout treatment.

E. Pyridoxine should be prescribed with INH to prevent peripheral neuropathy in pregnant women, malnourished adults, or patients with other medical illnesses.

F. The patient with tuberculosis should be offered HIV counseling and antibody testing.

G. The patient with suspected or known tuberculosis must be reported to the public health department.

BIBLIOGRAPHY

American Thoracic Society and Centers for Disease Control. Diagnostic standards and classification of tuberculosis. Am Rev Respir Dis 1990;142:725–735.

Barnes PF, Bloch AB, Davidson PT, Snider DE: Tuberculosis in patients with human immunodeficiency virus infection. N Engl J Med 1991;324:1644–1650.

Centers for Disease Control: Screening for tuberculosis in high-risk populations, and the use of preventative therapy for tuberculosis infection in the United States: Recommendations of the Advisory Committee for the Elimination of Tuberculosis. MMWR 1990;39:1–12(No. RR-8).

Centers for Disease Control and Prevention: Initial therapy for tuberculosis in the era of multidrug resistance: Recommendations of the Advisory Council for the Elimination of Tuberculosis. MMWR 1993;42(No. RR-7):1–8.

Davidson PT: Treating tuberculosis: what drugs, for how long? Ann Intern Med 1990;112:393–395.

Dooley SW, Castro KG, Hutton MD, et al: Guidelines for preventing the transmission of tuberculosis in health-care settings, with special focus on HIV-related issues. MMWR 1990;39:1–29(No. RR-17).

Fischl MA, Daikos GL, Uttamchandani RB, et al. Clinical presentation and outcome of patients with HIV infection and tuberculosis caused by multiple-drug-resistant bacilli. Ann Intern Med 1992;117:184–190.

Small PM, Schecter GF, Goodman PC, et al: Treatment of tuberculosis in patients with advanced human immunodeficiency virus infection. N Engl J Med 1991;324:289–294.

URINARY TRACT INFECTIONS

"One must agree with Hippocrates, Galen, and many others, ancient and modern, that there is no surer way to determine the temperaments and constitutions of people of either sex than to look at the urine."

DAVACH DE LA RIVIERE (18TH CENTURY)

I. ESSENTIAL FACTS

A. Definition

The term *urinary tract infection* (UTI) is nonspecific and refers to a number of different conditions:

1. *Acute cystitis:* bacterial infection of the bladder.

2. *Urethritis:* infection confined to the urethra.

3. *Pyelonephritis:* bacterial infection of the kidney.

B. Epidemiology

An estimated 6 million cases of acute cystitis and 250,000 cases of pyelonephritis occur annually in the United States. Twenty percent of women will have a urinary tract infection during their lifetime, and 3% experience recurrent infections. Cystitis and pyelonephritis are 50-fold more common in young adults and middle-aged women than in men. In the elderly the ratio is 1:1.

C. Etiology

1. **Cystitis.** A majority of cases are due to *Escherichia coli* (80%), with other enteric gram-negative organisms occurring occasionally. *Staphylococcus saprophyticus* causes 10–15% of cystitis cases in sexually active young females.

2. **Pyelonephritis**

   a. Uncomplicated: > 90% *E. coli, Klebsiella.*
   b. Recurrent: mostly *E. coli* with increased antibiotic resistance, *Proteus, Enterobacter, Klebsiella.*
   c. Associated with calculi: *Proteus, Klebsiella,* enterococci, *Staphylococcus aureus.*
   d. Associated with urologic manipulation, obstruction, or

urinary catheters: *E. coli, Pseudomonas, Proteus, Klebsiella, Enterobacter, Serratia, S. aureus.*

3. **Urethritis.** Gonorrhea and chlamydia are the most common causes. Herpes simplex virus, type 2, and *Ureaplasma urealyticum* can occasionally cause urethritis. In males ≤ 35 years of age dysuria is more likely a manifestation of a sexually transmitted disease (STD) than a urinary tract infection.

II. CLINICAL EVALUATION

A. History/Symptoms

1. **Cystitis.** A past history of cystitis is common. Diaphragm use is a common predisposing condition. Hematuria, dysuria, frequency, voiding small volumes of urine, and lower-abdominal (suprapubic) discomfort are often present.

2. **Pyelonephritis.** Symptoms may include fever, chills, nausea, vomiting, flank or abdominal pain, and malaise. Irritative voiding symptoms due to a concomitant cystitis may or may not be present.

3. **Urethritis.** A history of a new sexual partner is common. Internal dysuria (pain felt within the urethra or at the meatus) and urethral discharge are the most common symptoms.

B. Signs

1. **Cystitis.** Temperature is normal; suprapubic tenderness may be present.

2. **Pyelonephritis.** Fever, tachycardia, and flank pain are usually present.

3. **Urethritis.** Urethral discharge (males); females may have co-existent cervicitis.

C. Physical Examination

1. **Vital Signs.** Presence of fever makes pyelonephritis the more likely diagnosis.

2. **Abdominal Examination.** Examine for suprapubic tenderness (specific for cystitis), costovertebral angle tenderness with percussion (pyelonephritis).

3. **Pelvic Examination.** Should be performed in any patient with a new sexual partner, vaginal symptoms, or risks for STDs. The symptoms of pelvic inflammatory disease (PID) may be similar to those of pyelonephritis.

4. **Rectal Examination.** In males who present with signs/

symptoms of a UTI a prostate examination should be carefully performed to evaluate for prostatitis.

D. Laboratory Studies

1. **Suspected Cystitis (Simple).** In the setting of symptoms consistent with a UTI any of the following findings on urinalysis is sufficient to confirm the diagnosis:
   a. Microscopic hematuria.
   b. Microscopic bacteriuria (any organism per oil immersion field of *unspun* clean-catch Gram-stained urine).
   c. Pyuria (> 8 leukocytes/mL unspun urine as seen using the hemocytometer). In men 1–2 leukocytes/mL is considered abnormal; > 1–2 epithelial cells/mL suggests contamination.

2. **Suspected Cystitis.** When faced with potential complication by pregnancy, diabetes, old age, recent UTI, or recent instrumentation, perform the following:
   a. Urinalysis.
   b. Urine Gram stain.
   c. Urine culture.

3. **Suspected Pyelonephritis**

   a. Urinalysis.
   b. Urine Gram stain.
   c. Urine culture and sensitivities.
   d. Complete blood count (CBC).

4. **Suspected Urethritis**

   a. Gonorrheal culture/Gram stain (males: urethral culture; females: cervical culture).
   b. Chlamydial culture.
   c. Urinalysis: In men obtain urethral culture before collecting urine.

III. DIFFERENTIAL DIAGNOSIS

Urethritis, cystitis, pyelonephritis, prostatitis, and vaginitis should be considered in the differential diagnosis.

IV. THERAPY

Table 15–34 outlines UTI therapy.

V. DISPOSITION

A. Discharge

1. Patients with cystitis.

2. Patients with urethritis.

Table 15–34. THERAPY OF URINARY TRACT INFECTIONS

CONDITION	SYMPTOMS	LABORATORY	TREATMENT
Acute "Uncomplicated Cystitis"	One or more of the following: Dysuria Increased frequency Urgency Suprapubic discomfort	Urinalysis: Positive leukocyte esterase on dipstick, or microscopic pyuria, hematuria, or bacteriruia	Three days treatment with one of the following: TMP-sulfa DS PO bid Norfloxacin 400 mg PO bid Ciprofloxacin 250 mg PO bid Ofloxacin 200 mg PO bid Trimethoprim 100 mg PO bid
Cystitis or Asymptomatic Bacteriuria in the Pregnant Patient Treatment of asymptomatic bacteriuria is also appropriate in the setting of persistent bacteriuria posturologic procedures, post indwelling catheter removal, prior to prosthesis placement, or ± diabetes mellitus	Symptoms as per uncomplicated cystitis above; may also be asymptomatic (i.e., asymptomatic bacteriuria)	Urinalysis: results as per above, or asymptomatic bacteriuria. Urine culture is mandatory (even with asymptomatic bacteriuria). Urine culture results showing ≥ 100 colony-forming units (cfu)/mL with symptoms, or ≥ 100,000 cfu/mL without symptoms or pyuria, is significant and mandates completion of antibiotic therapy course	Seven to ten days of treatment with one of the following regimens: Cefadroxil 500 mg PO bid Cephalexin 250–500 mg PO qid Cephradine 250–500 mg PO qid Nitrofurantoin 100 mg PO qid Amoxicillin 250–500 mg PO tid Ampicillin 250–500 mg PO qid
Acute "Complicated Cystitis" (cystitis in patients with any of the following characteristics): Age > 50 Diabetes mellitus History of recurrent infections Immunocompromised Known urinary tract anatomic abnormality Male gender Recent hospitalization Recent urinary tract catheterization Symptoms ≥ 6 days	Symptoms as per uncomplicated cystitis above	Urinalysis: results as per above Urine culture is mandatory; culture results with ≥ 100 cfu/mL are significant in the presence of symptoms	Seven-day antibiotic regimen with one of the agents listed for uncomplicated cystitis above Young healthy men with the *isolated cystitis syndrome* usually respond to 7 days of antibiotics; those who do respond generally do not benefit from a urologic evaluation for an anatomical abnormality. In other males, consider the possibility of bacterial prostatitis, prostatic enlargement, impaired bladder-emptying, or stones (any of which may require prolonged antibiotic therapy for 2–6 weeks and urologic evaluation).

TMP-sulfa, trimethoprim-sulfamethoxazole; PMNs, polymorphonuclear leukocytes.

Table 15–34. THERAPY OF URINARY TRACT INFECTIONS *Continued*

CONDITION	SYMPTOMS	LABORATORY	TREATMENT
Urethritis	Symptoms may include one or more of the following: Dysuria (gradual onset, mild symptoms) History of a new sexual partner Lower abdominal pain Dysuria in males ≤ age 35 Urethral discharge Vaginal symptoms	Pelvic examination in females, including: cervical Gram stain, cervical gonorrhea and chlamydia cultures, KOH and normal saline preparations of vaginal secretions, urinalysis (may show leukocytes without any organisms) In males: Urethral swabs for Gram stain (nongonoccual urethritis is indicated by ≥ 5 PMNs per oil immersion field), and gonorrhea and chlamydia cultures Obtain these specimens prior to obtaining a urine specimen for urinalysis	Treat for both gonorrhea and chlamydia simultaneously: Gonorrhea treatment (one of the following): Cefixime 400 mg PO once Ceftriaxone 125 mg IM once Ciprofloxacin 500 mg PO once Ofloxacin 400 mg PO once Spectinomycin 2 g IM once Chlamydia treatment (one of the folowing): Doxycyline 100 mg PO bid for 7 days Azithromycin 1 g PO once Ofloxacin 300 mg PO bid for 7 days Erythromycin 500 mg PO qid for 7 days
Acute Pyelonephritis in Young Otherwise Healthy Nonpregnant Women (mild illness)	One or more of the following: Fever Flank pain Back pain (costovertebral angle tenderness) Cystitis symptoms frequently also accompany the above	Urinalysis (pyuria almost always present and usually accompanied by bacteriuria) Obtain CBC and pregnancy test. Urine culture is mandatory. Followp in the ED in 48 hr is recommended to make sure patient is improving and tolerating outpatient therapy. Follow-up urine cultures should be obtained 2 weeks after completing antibiotic therapy.	Reliable patients who can take oral medications and who have mild illness can be treated as an outpatient with 14 days of one of the following agents (treatment should subsequently be guided by urine culture when results are available): TMP/sulfa DS PO bid Norfloxacin 400 mg PO bid Ciprofloxacin 500 mg PO bid Ofloxacin 200–300 mg PO bid

Table continued on following page

3. Reliable nonelderly patients with uncomplicated pyonephritis who are not pregnant, not vomiting (can tolerate oral medication), and not toxic.
4. Patients with pyelonephritis sent home should have close follow-up within 24–48 hours.

B. Admit

1. Patients with pyelonephritis in whom compliance is a concern.

2. Patients with uncomplicated pyelonephritis who cannot tolerate oral medication or who require parenteral analgesia.

3. Patients with complicated pyelonephritis (diabetics, pregnant

Table 15–34. THERAPY OF URINARY TRACT INFECTIONS *Continued*

CONDITION	SYMPTOMS	LABORATORY	TREATMENT
Acute Pyelonephritis (moderate to severe illness requiring hospitalization, including the following): Diabetes mellitus Immunocompromised History of complicated infections or multiply resistant organisms in the past Known or suspected anatomic abnormality, including obstruction or nephrolithiasis Inadequate home situation Males Nausea and vomiting Older age Pain requiring parenteral analgesia Persistently abnormal or unstable vital signs Pregnant patients Renal insufficiency Unreliable patients	Symptoms of increased severity as compared to the above, patient with nausea and vomiting or otherwise systemically ill	Urinalysis as per above. At the minimum also obtain the following: CBC, pregnancy test (in reproductive age females), electrolyte panel, blood cultures, and urine culture. A urinary tract imaging procedure (e.g., renal ultrasound) should be performed in patients clinically suspected of an anatomic abnormality or obstruction (e.g., history of complicated infections or nephrolithiasis, severe flank pain, or unstable vital signs). Also obtain a urology consult in those settings. Follow-up urine cultures should be obtained 2 weeks after completing antibiotic therapy.	Administer one of the following parenteral regimens and hospitalize the patient: Ceftriaxone 1–2 g IV q 12 hr (or other appropriate third-generation cephalosporin) TMP/sulfa 160/800 mg IV q 12 hr Ciprofloxacin 200–400 mg IV q 12 hr Ofloxacin 200–400 mg IV q 12 hr Gentamicin 2 mg/kg IV load followed by 1–1.5 mg/kg IV q 8 hr (do not use in renal insufficiency; follow levels carefully) Ticarcillin-clavulanate 3.1 g IV q 8 hr Aztreonam 1 g IV q 8–12 hr Total treatment course (IV + PO after hospital discharge) should be 14 days In the pregnant patient, appropriate agents include ceftriaxone (or other third-generation cephalosporin), TMP-sulfa, gentamicin, or aztreonam (do *not* use the fluoroquinolones) If enterococci are suspected, initiate treatment with one of the following: Ampicillin + gentamicin, *or* Vancomycin + gentamicin

TMP-sulfa, trimethoprim-sulfamethoxazole; PMNs, polymorphonuclear leukocytes.

patients, elderly patients, individuals with urinary tract obstruction, individuals with infected renal calculi).

4. Patients with persistently abnormal vital signs (e.g., tachycardia) should be admitted.

5. Patients with an obstructed and infected urinary tract have a true urologic emergency; consult a urologist immediately.

VI. PEARLS AND PITFALLS

A. Some patients with pyelonephritis complain of flu-like symptoms—nausea, vomiting, and fever—with no symptoms referable to the urinary tract. Consider a urinalysis as part of your workup in patients with "the flu."

B. Women complaining of "external" dysuria (labia are uncomfortable with urination) are more likely to have vaginitis or an STD. A pelvic examination and necessary cultures should be part of their evaluation.

C. Trimethoprim-sulfamethoxazole and the fluoroquinolones offer the advantage of causing less candidal vaginitis, as they have less anaerobic activity than most antibiotics.

D. Men with symptoms of cystitis should always have their urine cultured. Many authorities suggest referral of men with UTI to urologists.

E. Do not use fluoroquinolones in women who are nursing or pregnant (may cause cartilage damage in the fetus); they are also *not* recommended in patients < age 18.

F. Diabetics, the elderly, and males do not qualify for short-course therapy for cystitis.

G. Injection drug users who present with pyelonephritis may have seeded the kidney from bacteremia secondary to endocarditis. *S. aureus* is a common pathogen in this setting.

BIBLIOGRAPHY

Blum RN, Wright RA: Detection of pyuria and bacteriuria in symptomatic ambulatory women. J Gen Intern Med 1992;7:140.

Kiningham RB: Asymptomatic bacteriuria in pregnancy. Am Fam Phys 1993;47(5): 1232–1238.

Stamm WE, Hooton TM: Management of urinary tract infections in adults. N Engl J Med 1993; 329(18):1328–1334.

16

Gastrointestinal Emergencies

APPENDICITIS

*"It's this damned belly that gives
a man his worst troubles."*

HOMER

I. ESSENTIAL FACTS

A. Definition

Appendicitis is an acute inflammation of the appendix. Its most common precipitant is obstruction of the appendiceal lumen, resulting in the following: rising intraluminal pressure, appendiceal edema, ischemia, bacterial tissue invasion, and eventual gangrene with perforation. The latter typically occurs within 24–36 hours of symptom onset. The cause of the obstruction may be a fecalith, dietary material, lymphoid hyperplasia, barium, a tumor, granulomatous disease, a parasite, or an anatomic variation (e.g., extra-appendiceal bands).

1. Appendicitis is the most common cause of the acute abdomen.

2. Failure to make an accurate diagnosis early in the course of appendicitis remains the primary cause of morbidity and mortality from this disease and a frequent cause of litigation against ED physicians.

B. Epidemiology

1. The incidence of appendicitis is one to two cases per 1000 persons per year. The incidence is highest in the second and third decades of life.

2. Appendicitis is slightly more common in males and nearly twice as common in whites as blacks. More cases occur in the summer and winter months than at other times of the year.

3. The mortality of correctly diagnosed and treated *unperforated* appendicitis is 0.1%. Mortality rates increase greatly *with perforation* and are as follows: 2–6% in the general population, 15% in the elderly patient, 19.4% in the pregnant patient, and 20% in children < 2 years old.

II. CLINICAL EVALUATION

A. History (Table 16–1)

Abdominal pain is the most prominent complaint in patients with appendicitis. At its onset, the pain is characteristically dull, constant, and visceral in nature. Sixty percent of cases will present with the following classic symptoms: initially vague and poorly localized abdominal discomfort (epigastric or periumbilical) that gradually begins to localize in the right lower quadrant. Prominent accompanying symptoms include anorexia (90% of patients), malaise, and nausea and vomiting (75% of patients). Nausea and vomiting usually occur *after* the onset of abdominal pain. Early vomiting may signal immediate danger of perforation.

Caution: appendicitis may present very atypically, especially in very young patients, pregnant patients, and the elderly.

B. Physical Examination (Table 16–1)

1. Obtain vital signs and evaluate the HEENT (look for scleral icterus), neck, chest, and heart.

2. Carefully evaluate the abdomen, including the genitourinary tract and rectum.
   a. Localized abdominal tenderness in the right iliac fossa, alone or in conjunction with tenderness in other areas of the abdomen, is the most sensitive sign in appendicitis (seen in 96–100% of patients), but specificity is low. Localized muscle rigidity, guarding, and cutaneous hyperesthesia are sometimes also seen.
   b. Symptoms and signs with perforation typically include generalized, severe abdominal pain; high or spiking fever;

Table 16–1. THE USEFULNESS OF SELECTED SYMPTOMS, SIGNS, AND LABORATORY RESULTS IN ACUTE APPENDICITIS

SIGNS/SYMPTOMS	SENSITIVITY	SPECIFICITY	POSITIVE PREDICTIVE VALUE	NEGATIVE PREDICTIVE VALUE
Tenderness	1.00	.12	.83	1.00
Anorexia	.61	.72	.91	.29
Pain migration	.69	.84	.95	.37
Rebound	.55	.78	.92	.27
Elevated temperature	.73	.50	.87	.29
Nausea/vomiting	.74	.36	.84	.23
Elevated leukocyte count	.93	.38	.87	.53
Left shift	.71	.68	.91	.29

Adapted from Alvarado A, A practical score for the early diagnosis of acute appendicitis. Ann Emerg Med 1986;15:557–561.

chills; tachycardia; rapid, shallow respirations; abdominal guarding; rebound tenderness; and "board-like" rigidity of the abdomen. The patient tends to lie supine and motionless with knees and hips flexed.

  c. Patients with appendicitis in the third trimester of pregnancy generally present with *right-upper*-quadrant pain and tenderness.

C. Laboratory Studies

  1. Laboratory evaluation should *minimally* include the following:

    a. Complete blood count (CBC; the leukocyte count is > 10,000/μL in ~ 90% of patients with appendicitis).

    b. Serum pregnancy test (obtain on females of reproductive age).

    c. Urinalysis.

  2. Additional studies that are sometimes useful and *may* be occasionally indicated include one or more of the following:

    a. Electrolyte panel, blood urea nitrogen, and creatinine levels.

    b. Amylase and bilirubin levels.

    c. Electrocardiogram (mandatory in all patients ≥ 40 years old or with ischemic heart disease risk factors).

    d. Prothrombin time (PT)/partial thromboplastin time (PTT).

    e. Upright chest roentgenogram and supine and upright abdominal roentgenograms.

    f. Other imaging studies (e.g., abdominal/pelvic ultrasound, barium enema, or, rarely, computed tomography examination). Criteria for appendicitis on ultrasound include any of the following: complex mass suggestive of an abscess, visualized appendix > 6 mm in diameter, or appendiceal muscular wall thickness ≥ 3 mm. Sensitivities ≤ 96% and specificities ≤ 94% have been reported. In expert hands, ultrasound can be helpful in excluding nonsurgical disease (e.g., nephrolithiasis, mesenteric adenitis, ileitis) and in diagnosing surgical disease other than appendicitis (e.g., ectopic pregnancy, cholecystitis in the pregnant patient with right-upper-quadrant pain).

III. DIFFERENTIAL DIAGNOSIS

  A. The differential diagnosis of appendicitis depends on the patient's age, sex, symptoms, and signs.

  B. The most commonly encountered conditions that mimic an acute appendicitis and result in a "negative" laparotomy are presented in Table 16–2.

Table 16–2. THE ETIOLOGY OF A NEGATIVE LAPAROTOMY IN PATIENTS SUSPECTED OF ACUTE APPENDICITIS

ALL ADULTS	ADULT FEMALES	CHILDREN
Abdominal pain of unknown cause	Pelvic inflammatory disease	Abdominal pain of unknown cause
Diverticulitis	Ovarian cysts	Mesenteric adenitis
Ileitis	Endometriosis	Ileocolitis
Cholelithiasis	Ectopic pregnancy	Meckel's diverticulum
Pancreatitis	Abdominal pain of unknown cause	Testicular torsion
Bowel obstruction		Urinary tract infection
Gastroenteritis		Henoch–Schönlein purpura
		Pancreatitis
		Gastroenteritis

IV. THERAPY

A. Initial Therapy and Assessment

1. Obtain vital signs, keep the patient NPO, establish intravenous (IV) access, and initiate crystalloid infusion as necessary (1–2 L normal saline or lactated Ringer's solution IV in the otherwise healthy adult patient).

2. Obtain a directed history, perform a physical examination and order relevant laboratory tests as outlined in II, above.

3. The patient with nausea and vomiting should have a nasogastric tube placed to provide low intermittent suction. Administration of parenteral antiemetics is appropriate (e.g., prochlorperazine 5–10 mg slowly IV or metoclopramide 10 mg slowly IV).

B. Definitive Therapy

1. Obtain a general surgery consult.

2. In consultation with the surgeon:
   a. Administer preoperative antibiotics (e.g., cefotetan or cefoxitin 2 g IV). Preoperative antibiotics reduce the incidence of postoperative wound infections and postoperative abscess formation if perforation has occurred.
   b. Administer appropriate analgesia (e.g., meperidine initially 12.5–25 mg IV, titrated to pain as necessary).

3. Prompt surgical intervention (appendectomy via laparotomy or laparoscopy) is required for definitive treatment. Delay is the most common cause of complications.

544 / GASTROINTESTINAL EMERGENCIES

V. DISPOSITION

A. The patient strongly suspected of acute appendicitis must be admitted to the hospital and undergo immediate laparotomy to minimize the risk of perforation. Additional diagnostic testing should not be pursued if it will delay laparotomy when the clinical suspicion of appendicitis is high. If the suspicion is lower, and there is no clear-cut indication for immediate surgery, ultrasound may be helpful in further clarifying the diagnosis.

B. The reliable patient with a low, but still possible, likelihood of early appendicitis may be discharged from the ED with mandatory follow-up in 6–8 hours. The patient should be kept NPO over this time period and informed of the symptoms and signs suggestive of disease progression. It is appropriate to involve a consulting surgeon in disposition-planning.

VI. PEARLS AND PITFALLS

A. Abdominal pain is the most common complaint in patients suffering from appendicitis, and pain usually precedes other symptoms.

B. Delays in diagnosis and early definitive operative therapy increase the risk of perforation; morbidity and mortality rise significantly with perforation.

C. The young patient, the pregnant patient, and the elderly patient may present very atypically. The most common location of pain in the third-trimester pregnant patient is the right upper quadrant.

D. Signs and symptoms vary with the anatomic location of the appendix. A retroileal appendix may irritate the ureter, causing referred pain to the testicles. A pelvic appendix can lie adjacent to the pelvic wall, rectum, or bladder, leading to symptoms of diarrhea, dysuria, hematuria, or suprapubic pain. A high retrocecal appendix may cause right-upper-quadrant pain. The abdominal examination may be nontender in the patient with a pelvic appendix; tenderness may be illicited with a rectal or vaginal digital examination.

E. Most patients (but not all!) with an acute appendicitis will have a leukocyte count $> 10,000/\mu L$.

F. Most patients (but not all!) will be anorectic.

G. Preoperative antibiotics decrease the incidence of postoperative wound infection and decrease the incidence of postoperative abscess formation if the appendix has perforated.

Do not do any of the following:

A. Delay obtaining early surgical consultation in suspected acute appendicitis.

B. Dismiss the diagnosis of appendicitis due to the presence of cervical motion tenderness (30% of female patients with appendicitis will have concomitant cervical motion tenderness).

BIBLIOGRAPHY

Alvarado A: A practical score for the early diagnosis of acute appendicitis. Ann Emerg Med 1986;15:557–564.

Hockberger RS, Henneman PL, Boniface K: Disorders of the small intestine: Appendicitis. Chapter 81. In Rosen P, Barkin RM, et al (eds): Emergency Medicine: Concepts and Clinical Practice. 3rd Ed. St. Louis, Mosby-Year Book, 1992, pp. 1627–1633.

Maxwell JM, Ragland JJ: Appendicitis—improvements in diagnosis and treatment. Am Surg 1991;57:282–285.

Puylaert J, et al: A prospective study of ultrasonography in the diagnosis of appendicitis. N Engl J Med 1987;317(11):666–669.

Silen Z: Cope's Early Diagnosis of the Acute Abdomen. 18th Ed. New York, Oxford Univ. Press, 1991.

GALLBLADDER DISEASE

"The longer I live, the more I am convinced that . . . half the unhappiness in the world proceeds from little stoppages, from a duct choked up, . . ."

SYDNEY SMITH (1771-1845)

I. ESSENTIAL FACTS

A. Definitions

An estimated 35 million people (15% of the population of the United States) have gallstones, and 20% of these individuals will eventually develop symptoms. Gallstone-induced diseases include biliary colic, cholecystitis, cholangitis, and gallstone pancreatitis.

1. *Biliary colic* is characterized by moderate to severe abdominal pain (usually in the epigastrium or right upper quadrant) of relatively sudden onset secondary to one or more stones obstructing the cystic duct. After 1–4 hours the pain usually resolves. Unlike cholecystitis, biliary colic is not accompanied by either fever or leukocytosis.

2. *Cholecystitis* is acute inflammation of the gallbladder, usually following obstruction of the cystic duct by a gallstone (95% of cases). A bacterial contribution to inflammation is present in 50–85% of cases. In 5% of patients with cholecystitis, cystic duct obstruction occurs in the absence of gallstones (acalculous cholecystitis). Acalculous cholecystitis most frequently occurs in severely ill individuals in the setting of extensive burns, immobility, prolonged fasting, postoperative states, human immunodeficiency virus disease, and/or trauma.

3. *Choledocholithiasis* is the occurrence of stones in the common bile duct.

4. *Cholangitis* is inflammation of a bile duct, usually in the setting of a common bile duct stone. It is the most life-threatening complication of cholelithiasis. Complete or partial obstruction of the common bile duct results in increased intraluminal pressure and eventual bacterial infection. The prevalence of bacteremia is 25–40%, and the presence of gram-negative sepsis increases mortality.

5. *Gallstone pancreatitis* is pancreatic inflammation secondary to impaction of either a gallstone or biliary sludge in the common channel of the biliary and pancreatic ducts.

B. Biliary Tract Stones

1. Gallstones are classified as cholesterol stones (85–90% of gallstones in the United States) and pigment stones (further subdivided as "black" and "brown" stones).

2. Risk factors for cholesterol stones include American Indian heritage, high triglyceride and low HDL-cholesterol levels, medications (e.g., clofibrate, estrogens, and gemfibrozil), female gender (women have twice the risk of men), obesity, older age, parity (increasing risk with a history of two or more children), primary biliary cirrhosis, rapid weight loss, and spinal cord injury.

3. Risk factors for pigment stones include advanced acquired immunodeficiency syndrome, alcoholic cirrhosis, biliary infection (e.g., *Escherichia coli, Ascaris lumbricoides, Clonorchis sinensis*), biliary stasis, chronic hemolysis, chronic hypercalcemia, ileal dysfunction, older age, and total parenteral nutrition.

C. Complications of Cholecystitis

1. Cholecystoenteric fistula.

2. Emphysematous cholecystitis, or "gas gangrene" of the gallbladder (seen in males three times more often than in females, is more common in diabetics, and acalculous in 28% of cases; the estimated mortality is 10%).

3. Free perforation into the abdominal cavity (this is the most serious complication of cholecystitis and is associated with a 30% mortality).

4. Gallstone ileus (obstruction of the small bowel by a large gallstone that has gained access to the bowel via a cholecystoenteric fistula).

5. Localized perforation and abscess formation.

II. CLINICAL EVALUATION

A. History

1. Abdominal pain is the most prominent feature of symptomatic gallstone disease. It is usually of sudden onset, visceral in

nature, constant (not colicky, despite the term "biliary colic"), and is usually located in the epigastrium or right upper quadrant (less frequently in the left upper quadrant). The pain may radiate to the right scapula. On careful questioning, many patients have a prior history of similar pain that spontaneously resolved. Accompanying symptoms may include anorexia, bloating, nausea, and vomiting.

2. Cholecystitis begins as typical biliary colic pain, but the discomfort does *not* resolve. As inflammation progresses, pain increases in intensity and localizes more to the right upper quadrant. (*Caution:* pain may be minimal or absent in the aged, patients receiving steroids, or those with diabetes mellitus.) A low-grade fever is common and may be the only clinical sign of cholecystitis in the elderly.

3. Cholangitis patients generally present with abdominal pain, fever, chills, nausea, and vomiting. The pain of biliary colic accompanied by high spiking fevers and jaundice (Charcot's triad) is present in 50–70% of patients. In some individuals, altered mentation and shock also occur (Reynold's pentad).

4. Gallstone pancreatitis is indistinguishable from acute pancreatitis of another cause (see Pancreatitis, later in this chapter).

B. Physical Examination

1. Obtain vital signs and evaluate the HEENT (look for scleral icterus), neck, chest, and heart. The presence of high fever, rigors, or hemodynamic compromise suggests cholangitis, gallbladder perforation, or empyema and necessitates immediate vital sign support, crystalloid resuscitation, and general surgical consultation.

2. Carefully evaluate the abdomen, including the genitourinary tract and rectum. Right-upper-quadrant or midepigastric tenderness is frequently present and may be accompanied by guarding and local peritoneal signs. Murphy's sign (pain and transient inspiratory arrest with palpation in the right upper quadrant) may be present but is not specific.

C. Laboratory Studies

1. *Minimally* obtain the following:
   a. Complete blood count with platelet count. Acute cholecystitis usually is accompanied by a mild to moderate leukocytosis (10,000–15,000/μL). The leukocyte count in cholangitis may be of the same range or markedly higher.
   b. Electrolyte panel, glucose, blood urea nitrogen, and creatinine levels.
   c. Amylase, bilirubin, and alkaline phosphatase levels. A mildly elevated bilirubin level (< 5 mg/dL) occurs in about 25% of patients with cholecystitis. Alkaline phosphatase and serum transaminase levels may be 2–4 times normal. A

markedly elevated bilirubin or alkaline phosphatase level may be seen in cholangitis. Amylase can be elevated secondary to the passage of a stone, severe vomiting, or associated pancreatitis.

   d. Urinalysis.

   e. Electrocardiogram (ECG) (mandatory in patients ≥ 40 years old, or in those with a history of ischemic heart disease, coronary artery disease risk factors, or unstable vital signs).

   f. Serum or urine pregnancy test (mandatory in female patients of reproductive age).

2. Additional studies may also be appropriate depending on clinical circumstances (e.g., blood cultures, liver function tests, prothrombin time/partial thromboplastin time).

D. Imaging Procedures

1. **Acute Abdominal Series** (upright chest roentgenogram; supine and upright abdominal roentgenograms). Though only 15–20% of gallstones are visible on plain x-ray films, an acute abdominal series is reasonable and may be helpful in ruling out alternative diagnoses.

2. **Abdominal Ultrasound.** This is the imaging study of choice in evaluating the patient with suspected gallbladder disease. The identification of gallstones by ultrasound is nearly 100% accurate but does not prove the stones are the cause of the patient's abdominal complaints. The presence of a thickened gallbladder wall, fluid collections around the gallbladder, "sludge" in the gallbladder, and/or pain over the gallbladder when pressed with the transducer greatly improves the diagnostic accuracy of the study in the setting of suspected cholecystitis. Adjacent structures such as the liver, common bile duct, kidney, ureter, and pancreas can also be visualized. A dilated common bile duct may be seen in cholangitis (but cholangitis can also occur without ductal dilatation).

3. **Hepatobiliary Scintigraphy (HIDA Scan).** This is the most sensitive study to confirm the diagnosis of cholecystitis but is seldom obtained in the ED because it requires a fasting state and may require several hours to complete. In the setting of cholecystitis, radiolabeled material is present in the common bile duct but not the gallbladder. It is the imaging study of choice when acalculous cholecystitis is suspected.

4. **Other Imaging Modalities.** Abdominal *computed tomography* may be more accurate at detecting common bile duct stones and is useful when a pancreatic process, such as pancreatitis or malignancy, is suspected. In the setting of choledocholithiasis, *endoscopic retrograde cholangiopancreatography* (ERCP) is the definitive diagnostic test and may also be therapeutic.

III. DIFFERENTIAL DIAGNOSIS

Depending on the patient's presentation, the following disease processes should be considered:

A. Acute appendicitis (may cause right-upper-quadrant pain early in its course, in the third trimester of pregnancy, or in the setting of a retrocecal appendix or a malpositioned cecum).

B. Acute myocardial infarction.

C. Acute viral hepatitis.

D. Alcoholic or other drug-related hepatitis.

E. Bile duct stricture.

F. Cancer (including bile duct, gallbladder, gastric, hepatic, metastatic, and pancreatic).

G. Hepatic abscess.

H. Hepatobiliary parasitosis.

 I. Pancreatitis.

 J. Peptic ulcer disease.

K. Perihepatitis (secondary to gonorrhea or *Chlamydia* infection in the setting of pelvic inflammatory disease).

L. Pyelonephritis.

M. Pneumonia.

N. Renal colic.

O. Sclerosing cholangitis.

IV. THERAPY

Figure 16–1 presents the therapy of gallbladder disease in the ED.

A. Initial Therapy and Assessment

1. Obtain vital signs, keep the patient NPO, establish intravenous (IV) access, and initiate crystalloid infusion.

2. Support oxygenation and vital signs as necessary.

3. Obtain a directed history, perform a physical examination, and order relevant laboratory tests as outlined in II, above.

4. The patient with nausea and vomiting should have a nasogastric tube placed to provide low intermittent suction; even in the absence of emesis, a nasogastric tube is appropriate in the setting of cholecystitis or cholangitis. Administration of parenteral antiemetics is also reasonable (e.g., prochlorperazine 5–10 mg slowly IV; or metoclopramide 10 mg slowly IV).

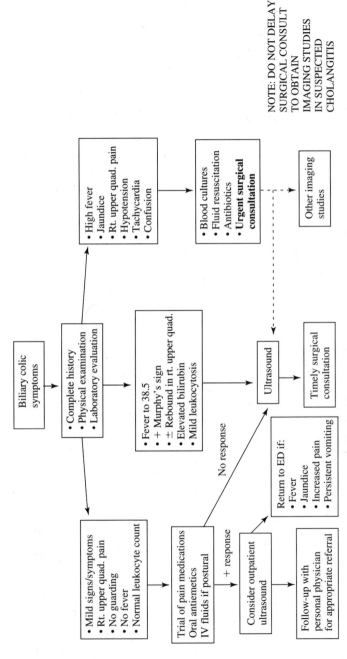

Figure 16-1. ED management of gallbladder disease.

Biliary colic symptoms

- Complete history
- Physical examination
- Laboratory evaluation

- High fever
- Jaundice
- Rt. upper quad. pain
- Hypotension
- Tachycardia
- Confusion

- Blood cultures
- Fluid resuscitation
- Antibiotics
- **Urgent surgical consultation**

Other imaging studies

- Fever to 38.5
- + Murphy's sign
- ± Rebound in rt. upper quad.
- Elevated bilirubin
- Mild leukocytosis

Ultrasound

Timely surgical consultation

No response

- Mild signs/symptoms
- Rt. upper quad. pain
- No guarding
- No fever
- Normal leukocyte count

Trial of pain medications
Oral antiemetics
IV fluids if postural

+ response

Return to ED if:
- Fever
- Jaundice
- Increased pain
- Persistent vomiting

Consider outpatient ultrasound

Follow-up with personal physician for appropriate referral

NOTE: DO NOT DELAY SURGICAL CONSULT TO OBTAIN IMAGING STUDIES IN SUSPECTED CHOLANGITIS

B. Obtain a General Surgery Consult

Note: urgent surgical consultation is not necessary in isolated biliary colic, although outpatient referral is appropriate.

C. Provide Analgesia

1. Opioid agents for adequate pain relief are usually required, but ideally they should *not* be administered until after the surgical consultant has had the opportunity to examine the patient. If consultation is not readily available, or will be delayed, proceed with reasonable pain control.

2. Medication choices: meperidine is classically preferred over morphine because it causes less spasm of the spincter of Oddi:
   a. Meperidine 12.5–25 mg given slowly IV, repeat every 15–60 minutes as required. Titrate carefully to avoid vital sign compromise. May also be given intramuscularly (IM) (1 mg/kg IM every 3–4 hours). *Or*
   b. Morphine 1–3 mg IV every 5 minutes initially, titrated carefully to avoid vital sign compromise.

D. Administer Antibiotics

Obtain two blood cultures and then begin antibiotic therapy in the setting of either acute cholecystitis or cholangitis. Antibiotic choices may include any of the following:
   a. Mezlocillin (3–4 g IV every 4–6 hours) and metronidazole (15 mg/kg IV over 1 hour to start, followed by 7.5 mg/kg IV every 6 hours; do not exceed 4 g in 24-hour period). *Or*
   b. Cefotetan (1–2 g IV every 12 hours) and gentamicin (2 mg/kg IV load, then 1–1.5 mg/kg IV every 8 hours, with subsequent dosing dependent on serum levels). *Or*
   c. Ampicillin (2 g IV every 6 hours) and gentamicin (see dose above) and metronidazole (see dose above). *Or*
   d. Imipenem (500 mg IV every 6 hours). *Or*
   e. Ticarcillin/clavulanate (Timentin 3.1 g IV over 30 minutes every 4–6 hours). *Or*
   f. Ampicillin/sulbactam (Unasyn 1.5–3.0 g IM or IV every 6 hours).

E. Arrange for Definitive Care

1. Biliary colic (symptomatic gallstones without inflammatory complications):
   a. Patients may electively be scheduled for cholecystectomy in the near future.
   b. A minority of patients may be candidates for extracorporeal shock-wave lithotripsy (candidates should have a history of biliary colic, no evidence of inflammation, no more than three radiolucent stones that are all ≤ 30 mm in diameter, and a functioning gallbladder). It is an expensive procedure, and long-term maintenance therapy with oral bile acids is probably required.

2. Cholecystitis: early surgical intervention is appropriate, though the procedure performed and its timing are the decision of the surgeon.

   a. Prompt laparoscopic cholecystectomy is currently the favored procedure.

   b. Open cholecystectomy is necessary, however, in patients with marked clotting disorders, peritonitis, portal hypertension, or severe associated pancreatitis, and in those in the third trimester of pregnancy or in septic shock. The mortality of either laparoscopic or open cholecystectomy is usually $\leq 1\%$ (mortality is higher in elderly individuals).

   c. Patients deemed too ill to tolerate either of the above should be considered for cholecystostomy (extraction of gallstones followed by drainage of the biliary tree through a catheter left in the gallbladder). Elective cholecystectomy may then be considered at a later date when the patient's clinical situation has improved.

3. Cholangitis: biliary decompression should be urgently achieved by ERCP and endoscopic sphincterotomy. Cholecystectomy may then be performed in several days after stabilization in suitable operative candidates.

V. DISPOSITION

A. Discharge

Patients with isolated biliary colic may be discharged to home if *all* of the following conditions are met:

1. Vital signs are normal.

2. Adequate pain control has been achieved, and the acute symptomatic episode is resolving.

3. There is absolutely no evidence of associated inflammation or infection.

4. No other associated condition mandating hospitalization has been found.

5. Follow-up has been arranged for definitive care of symptomatic cholelithiasis.

B. Admit

Patients with cholecystitis, cholangitis, or gallstone pancreatitis require hospitalization. ICU admission is appropriate in the setting of vital sign instability or suspected sepsis.

VI. PEARLS AND PITFALLS

A. Inquire with respect to prior episodes of symptomatic biliary disease.

B. Fever, without abdominal pain, may be the only manifestation of cholecystitis in the elderly, the diabetic patient, or those taking corticosteroids.

C. Initiate antibiotics and fluid resuscitation early in the hemodynamically unstable patient with biliary tract disease.

D. Use vasopressors to support hemodynamic status in the patient unresponsive to appropriate crystalloid resuscitation.

E. Initiate nasogastric suction in the patient with persistent nausea and vomiting.

F. Remember that cholecystitis can occur in the absence of gallstones, and that cholangitis can occur after cholecystectomy.

G. Acute myocardial infarction may mimic biliary tract disease! An ECG is an appropriate component of the initial evaluation of the patient with suspected gallbladder symptoms who is ≥ 40 years old or who has any risk factors for coronary artery disease.

BIBLIOGRAPHY

Apstein MD, Carey MC: Biliary tract stones and associated diseases. Chapter 65. In Internal Medicine. 4th Ed. Stein JH (ed). St. Louis, Mosby-Year Book, 1994, pp. 646–662.

Cox GR, Browne, BJ: Acute cholecystitis in the emergency department. J Emerg Med 1989; 7:501–511.

Johnston DE, Kaplan MM: Pathogenesis and treatment of gallstones. N Engl J Med 1993; 328(6):412–421.

Marshall JB: Current options in gallstone management. Postgrad Med 1994;95:115–128.

Young M: Acute diseases of the pancreas and biliary tract: Management in the emergency department. Emerg Med Clin N Am 1989;7(3):555–573.

GASTROINTESTINAL HEMORRHAGE

"I'll empty all these veins,
And shed my dear blood drop by drop."

WILLIAM SHAKESPEARE

I. ESSENTIAL FACTS

A. Definitions

Gastrointestinal (GI) hemorrhage is categorized as "upper" or "lower" depending on its source:

1. *Upper-GI-tract Bleeding* occurs proximal to the ligament of Treitz. Major causes include duodenal ulcer, gastric ulcer, gastric erosions, varices, Mallory–Weiss tear, esophagitis, and duodenitis. *Hematemesis* (red blood or dark, coffee ground material) defines upper-tract bleeding, while *melena* implies an upper source.

2. *Lower-GI-tract Bleeding* occurs distal to the ligament of Treitz. Major causes include diverticulosis, angiodysplasia, polyps, cancer, anorectal disorders (e.g., hemorrhoids, fissures), bacterial dysentery, and inflammatory bowel disease. Hematochezia (red blood or dark, mahogany-colored stool) with a negative nasogastric aspirate implies lower-tract bleeding.

B. Epidemiology

1. In the United States, 85,000 patients are admitted annually for GI bleeding, representing 2% of all medical and surgical hospital admissions. Ten to 20% of these patients ultimately require surgery to control hemorrhage.

2. Significant upper-tract bleeding is three to four times more common than major lower-tract bleeding.

3. The overall mortality rate is 8%, which has been constant over the last 40 years despite improved diagnostic and management techniques.

II. CLINICAL EVALUATION

A. History

Inquire with respect to the following:

1. Gastrointestinal symptoms: pain, nausea, vomiting, anorexia, diarrhea, prior history of GI disease (including hemorrhage), and liver disease.
   a. Epigastric pain suggests peptic ulcer disease.
   b. Anorexia, weight loss, and chronic anemia suggest cancer.
   c. Severe retching prior to bleeding suggests a Mallory-Weiss tear.
   Caution: in the patient with a prior history of GI hemorrhage, there is a significant chance that bleeding is now from a *different* source. For example, in individuals with known varices there is a 50% chance that the current hemorrhage is secondary to a different cause; only one-half of patients with Mallory–Weiss tears give a history of vomiting prior to the onset of hemorrhage.

2. Quantity and color of vomitus and stool.

3. Symptoms associated with hypovolemia and/or anemia: dizziness, fatigue, dyspnea, syncope, and angina.

4. Other active medical and surgical problems, including a known history of a bleeding disorder.

5. Past medical and surgical history.

6. Alcohol use, including history of related complications.

7. Cigarette use: smoking is a known risk factor for peptic ulcer disease.

8. Medications, especially those that may predispose to GI bleeding (aspirin, NSAIDs, prednisone, or anticoagulants).

9. Allergy history.

B. Physical Examination

1. Obtain vital signs, evaluate the skin, HEENT (look for scleral icterus), neck, chest, heart, abdomen, and genitalia, and perform a rectal examination (test stool for heme).

2. Stigmata of liver disease may include palmar erythema, spider angiomas, and Dupuytren's contractures.

3. Hematomas, ecchymoses, or petechiae may suggest a bleeding disorder.

C. Laboratory Studies

1. Obtain the following studies:
   a. Complete blood count (CBC) with differential and platelet count. *Caution:* an initially normal hematocrit does not rule out an acute life-threatening hemorrhage. Equilibration takes time, although it occurs faster with vigorous crystalloid resuscitation. The decision to transfuse a patient with an acute GI bleed should be made on the basis of vital signs, clinical status, and response to intravenous (IV) fluid replacement rather than on the basis of isolated laboratory findings (see IV, below).
   b. Electrolyte panel; glucose, blood urea nitrogen (BUN), and creatinine levels. BUN may be elevated from volume loss (prerenal azotemia), the GI protein load secondary to hemorrhage, or renal insufficiency.
   c. Prothrombin time (PT)/partial thromboplastin time (PTT).
   d. Blood type and crossmatch. Patients at risk for imminent cardiac arrest due to profound hypovolemic shock should receive low-titer O-negative blood at the outset of the resuscitation (see IV, below). Otherwise, type-specific red cells (requires 15 minutes of laboratory time at the blood bank) or complete cross-matched red cells (45–60 minutes of laboratory time) are used as available and as required. Whole blood should be used preferentially over packed red cells for the patient who requires both volume and hemoglobin replacement.
   e. Electrocardiogram (mandatory in patients ≥ 40 years old, and those with a history of or known risk factors for coronary artery disease, anemia, or abnormal vital signs).
   f. Urinalysis.

2. Depending on clinical circumstances, one or more of the following may also be appropriate:
   a. Abdominal series (upright posterior–anterior chest, supine and upright abdominal films). Obtain if viscus perforation is suspected.
   b. Chest roentgenogram.

    c. Ethanol level.

    d. Liver function tests.

    e. Pregnancy test (mandatory in females of reproductive age).

    f. Serum calcium, magnesium, and phosphate levels.

D. Gastric Aspirate

1. A nasogastric or orogastric tube should be placed, at least temporarily, in all patients with an acute GI hemorrhage. The purpose of the tube is to
   a. Attempt to identify an acute upper-tract hemorrhage (although a negative tube aspirate and lavage does not rule out an upper-tract bleed that has stopped or a duodenal hemorrhage occurring distal to a closed pylorus);
   b. Monitor the rate of bleeding if hemorrhage is found;
   c. Decompress the stomach; and
   d. Evacuate the stomach in preparation for endoscopy.

2. Theoretically, gastric decompression may assist with hemostasis by stimulating contraction of gastric musculature, but there is no clinical evidence that the course of GI hemorrhage is favorably influenced by this procedure. Iced saline lavage should *not* be used.

3. There is *no* conclusive evidence that insertion of a nasogastric or orogastric tube increases the risk of variceal hemorrhage.

4. Nasogastric or orogastric tubes are uncomfortable, may induce nasal hemorrhage or mucosal injury, and predispose to gastroesophageal reflux and aspiration. Discontinue the tube as soon as possible after reasonable placement and lavage.

III. DIFFERENTIAL DIAGNOSIS

A. Upper-Gastrointestinal-Tract Hemorrhage

1. Nongastrointestinal hemorrhage:
   a. Hemoptysis.
   b. Nasal bleeding.
   c. Pharyngeal bleeding.

2. Esophagus:
   a. Cancer.
   b. Esophagitis.
   c. Esophagogastric mucosal tear (Mallory–Weiss tear).
   d. Rupture (Boerhaave's syndrome [very rare]).
   e. Varices.

3. Stomach (gastric):
   a. Mucosal vascular ectasia.
   b. Neoplasms (carcinoma, lymphoma, polyps).
   c. Peptic ulcer disease.
   d. Varices.

4. Duodenum:
   a. Duodenitis.
   b. Peptic ulcer disease (duodenal ulcer is more common than gastric ulcer).
   c. Submucosal neoplasms (e.g., leiomyoma).
   d. Vascular–enteric fistula (from an aortic aneurysm or graft).

B. Lower-Gastrointestinal-Tract Hemorrhage

1. Upper-gastrointestinal-tract hemorrhage (see above).
2. Small and large bowel:
   a. Amyloidosis.
   b. Angiodysplasia.
   c. Antibiotic-related colitis.
   d. Diverticulosis.
   e. Infectious enterocolitis.
   f. Inflammatory bowel disease.
   g. Ischemia.
   h. Meckel's diverticulum.
   i. Neoplasia (carcinoma, lymphoma).
   j. Polyps.
   k. Radiation.
   l. Vascular–enteric fistula.
3. Rectum:
   a. Anal fissure.
   b. Hemorrhoids.
   c. Neoplasia.
   d. Polyps.
   e. Proctitis.

IV. THERAPY

The treatment goals of the ED physician in managing a patient with an acute GI hemorrhage are to ensure adequate oxygenation and ventilation, stabilize hemodynamic parameters, institute early and appropriate consultation, and arrange for reasonable disposition and definitive care. Fortunately, in 85% of patients GI bleeding stops spontaneously.

A. Initial Management

Secure and support the patient's airway, breathing, and circulation as necessary (also see Chapters 1, 11, and 12).

1. Place the patient on oxygen (2–5 L/min minimum via nasal cannula) and continuously monitor the oxygen saturation (SaO_2) and cardiac rhythm.
2. Rapidly obtain vital signs, large-bore IV access (at least two 14–16-gauge IV lines are recommended), and order necessary laboratory studies, including an emergent blood type and crossmatch. Consider serial hematocrits.

3. Begin crystalloid resuscitation with warm normal saline or lactated Ringer's solution.

 a. The adult patient with significant volume loss, as evidenced by abnormal vital signs, poor skin perfusion, low urine output, *or* altered mentation, should receive 1–2 L warmed crystalloid as rapidly as possible. In the critically ill patient in extremis, low-titer O-negative whole blood should be started emergently at the outset of the resuscitation (see Blood Component Therapy, Chapter 21).

 b. If the clinical status has not stabilized after 2-L rapid crystalloid infusion, begin type-specific blood transfusion as well. Maintain the patient's platelet count > 50,000/μL by transfusing platelets if necessary. If coagulation studies (PT/PTT) are abnormal, correct any pre-existing coagulopathy with 2 units fresh frozen plasma.

 c. Monitor cardiopulmonary systems carefully and avoid inducing congestive heart failure or pulmonary edema. A central venous catheter and central venous pressure (CVP) monitoring may assist in managing fluid resuscitation (consider a Swan-Ganz catheter in the patient with significant cardiopulmonary disease or renal insufficiency).

4. *Simultaneously* with the above, obtain a directed history and perform a physical examination. Place a nasogastric (or orogastric tube) to evaluate for and monitor upper-tract hemorrhage. In the patient with a moderate or worse bleed, a Foley catheter is appropriate to monitor urine output.

B. Consultations

Continued management of the patient with acute GI hemorrhage generally requires a team of physicians. Who is consulted depends on the patient's clinical condition (e.g., severity of bleeding), whether hemorrhage is from the upper or lower tract, and the capabilities of the institution. *Most patients needing admission will require urgent consultation from a gastroenterologist, the admitting medicine service, and a general surgeon.*

1. **Gastroenterology.** Consultation is appropriate in the patient with either an acute upper or lower-tract hemorrhage.

 a. Upper-tract endoscopy is sensitive in identifying the exact source of the bleed, which may influence subsequent therapy. Endoscopy may also be used for therapeutic interventions (e.g., injection sclerotherapy or ligation for variceal hemorrhage; laser therapy, injection therapy, or electrocoagulation for acutely bleeding ulcers).

 b. Proctosigmoidoscopy is the initial diagnostic procedure of choice for most patients with an acute lower-tract bleed. Colonoscopy may ultimately become necessary.

2. **Admitting Medical Service.** Whether the patient is admitted to the ICU or ward depends on patient characteristics (see Disposition, below). Notify the admitting service early.

3. **General Surgery.** The patient with an acute and significant GI bleed should have a general surgery consult. Both upper- and lower-tract bleeding that persists (> 5-unit blood transfusion) despite aggressive medical management may require acute surgical intervention.

4. **Interventional Radiology.** Arteriography may occasionally be used to define the site of persistent bleeding as well as treat the bleed (via selective arterial vasopressin infusion or arterial embolization with autologous clot or Gelfoam). Angiography is the procedure of choice to evaluate persistent and significant lower-tract hemorrhage. Hemorrhage must be ≥ 0.5 mL/min to visualize the bleeding site.

5. **Nuclear Medicine.** In patients with intermittent GI bleeding from an undetermined site, radionuclide scanning (using radiolabeled red cells or sulfur colloid) can be used to identify the approximate area of hemorrhage, even with a very low rate of blood loss (0.1–0.5 mL/min). Radionuclide scanning, however, is not as specific as angiography.

C. Medications

1. **Histamine H_2 Blockers.** These are beneficial in the overall treatment of peptic ulcer disease and in the prevention of stress ulceration. They have not been demonstrated effective, however, in stopping acute upper-tract hemorrhage. Despite this, their use is reasonable and common in this setting. Medication choices include the following:
   a. Ranitidine 50 mg IM or IV every 6–8 hours; *or*
   b. Cimetidine 150 mg IV load, followed by continuous infusion of 37.5 mg/hr; alternatively, 300 mg IM or IV every 6–8 hours.

2. **Vasopressin (Pitressin).** Vasopressin causes vascular bed constriction. It is indicated in the temporary control of significant or persistent esophageal variceal hemorrhage.
   Dose: begin with 0.2–0.4 units/min IV and titrate the dose carefully. Maximum dose is 0.9 unit/min IV.
   Caution: vasopressin may exacerbate cardiac ischemia, congestive heart failure, peripheral vascular disease, hypertension, and/or fluid overload. Use with great caution in patients with known cardiac disease or vascular disease. Concomitant administration of IV nitroglycerin (begin at 10 μg/min IV and titrate as necessary, do not allow systolic blood pressure to fall below 95-100 mmHg) may reduce unwanted side effects and enhance overall drug efficacy.

D. Adjunctive Therapy for Esophageal Variceal Hemorrhage

1. **Endoscopic Therapy.** This is usually the first-line definitive therapy in patients with confirmed variceal hemorrhage.

Treatment modalities include sclerotherapy and variceal ligation. Though effective in acute hemorrhage control, improvement in overall patient survival has not been demonstrated to date.

2. **Pitressin.** See C. 2, above.

3. **Balloon Tamponade.** This is indicated in the patient with severe variceal hemorrhage uncontrolled by other measures. The Sengstaken–Blakemore tube (a triple-lumen rubber tube with a gastric balloon, esophageal balloon, and a lumen for nasogastric suction), Linton–Nachlas tube (a triple-lumen rubber tube with a large-volume gastric balloon, gastric suction lumen, and esophageal suction lumen), and the Minnesota tube (a modified Sengstaken–Blakemore tube with esophageal suction capability proximal to the esophageal balloon) are capable of stopping acute hemorrhage in up to 90% of patients. Rebleeding rates are high, however, and complication rates of 30% have been reported. Prior to placement, most authorities recommend endotracheal intubation for airway protection. These devices should only be placed by experienced personnel in the ICU.

4. **Transjugular Intrahepatic Portosystemic Shunt (TIPS).** In this procedure, angiographic catheters are used to place an expandable metal-mesh stent between the hepatic vein and a branch of the portal vein. The stent results in immediate reduction in portal hypertension and variceal hemorrhage control in the majority of patients (88% in one study).

5. **Other Treatment Modalities.** These may include angiography with selective arterial vasopressin infusion or embolization, shunt surgery, and liver transplantation.

V. DISPOSITION

A. Discharge

A patient with a history of minor GI bleeding and no evidence of significant blood loss may be discharged to home if *all* of the following conditions are met:

1. Patient is reliable;

2. Vital signs are normal (including orthostatic vital signs);

3. History, physical examination, nasogastric aspiration (no frank blood or coffee ground material), and stool examination (± heme positive, but no frank blood, maroon stools, or melena) indicate there is no significant ongoing blood loss;

4. Hematocrit is normal and stable;

5. No significant comorbid condition mandating hospitalization is found; and

6. Follow-up in 24 hours is assured to recheck vital signs and

hematocrit. The patient should be instructed to return immediately in the event of orthostatic symptoms, hematemesis, hematochezia, or melenotic stools.

B. Admit

Patients with a significant GI hemorrhage require hospitalization. ICU admission is appropriate in the patient with hypotension (at any time), unstable vital signs, persistent bleeding, significant anemia or decrease in hematocrit over the course of ED stay, age > 75 years, or other worrisome comorbid condition(s).

VI. PEARLS AND PITFALLS

A. Ensure adequate oxygenation, ventilation, and volume resuscitation.

B. Obtain blood for type and crossmatch early.

C. Obtain a nasogastric aspirate in all patients. Remember, however, that the aspirate may be negative in upper-tract hemorrhage if bleeding is intermittent or duodenal contents are not sampled.

D. A normal hematocrit does *not* exclude a significant hemorrhage or the need for blood transfusion.

E. Obtain early consultation (gastroenterology, admitting medicine service, and general surgery) on any patient with significant GI hemorrhage.

F. Maintain platelet count > 50,000/μL in the patient with active bleeding; correct an identified coagulopathy with fresh frozen plasma.

BIBLIOGRAPHY

Garden OJ, Carter DC: Balloon tamponade and vasoactive drugs in the control of acute variceal hemorrhage. *Baillieres Clin Gastroenterol* 1992;6(3):451–463.

Gogel HK, Tandberg D: Emergency management of gastrointestinal hemorrhage. Am J Emerg Med 1986;4(2):150–162.

Laine L, Peterson WL: Bleeding peptic ulcer. N Engl J Med 1994;331(11):717–727.

Sarin SK, Lahoti D: Management of gastric varices. Baillieres Clin Gastroenterol 1992; 6(3):527–548.

Steffes C, Fromm D: Current diagnosis and management of upper gastrointestinal bleeding. Adv Surg 1992;25:331–361.

HEPATIC FAILURE

"It was at one time considered the seat of life; hence its name—liver, the thing we live with."

AMBROSE BIERCE (1842-1914?)

I. ESSENTIAL FACTS

A. Definitions

Cirrhosis occurs when a chronic and progressive disease of the liver (e.g., continued alcohol-induced injury, chronic viral hepatitis) results in disruption of the normal microscopic hepatic lobular architecture, with resultant fibrosis and nodular regeneration. *Hepatic failure,* which may be either acute or chronic, occurs when hepatic injury is so severe that the liver's vital functions are compromised. It may manifest as one or more of the following entities:

1. *Hepatic encephalopathy* is a neuropsychiatric syndrome characterized by mental status changes and altered neuromuscular activity.
   a. Worsening encephalopathy in the patient with known liver failure may occur secondary to azotemia, gastrointestinal hemorrhage, hypokalemic metabolic alkalosis, hypoxia, increased dietary protein, infection, medications (e.g., analgesics, sedative-hypnotics), and/or serious electrolyte derangements.
   b. Hepatic encephalopathy is staged as follows:
      i. **Stage 1.** Depression, disordered sleep, and cognitive dysfunction.
      ii. **Stage 2.** Asterixis (irregular flexion of the extremities, best seen in the fingers when the patient's arms are horizontal and the hands dorsiflexed at the wrists), confusion, disorientation, and lethargy.
      iii. **Stage 3.** Barely responsive patient, with confused speech and profound somnolence (asterixis may now be absent).
      iv. **Stage 4.** Coma.
   c. In the setting of *acute* liver injury, development of encephalopathy within 1 or more weeks of the onset of jaundice defines *fulminant hepatic failure;* urgent transfer to a medical center skilled in liver transplantation is appropriate.

2. *Portal hypertension* is elevation of portal vein pressure. Its manifestations may include ascites, splenomegaly, and/or collateral vein development. Collateral vessels can include prominent abdominal wall veins (caput medusae), esophageal and gastric varices, and/or small intestinal, colonic, and rectal (hemorrhoidal) varices. Significant gastrointestinal hemorrhage is a life-threatening complication. Splenomegaly may cause thrombocytopenia (pancytopenia in severe cases).

3. *Ascites* is the abnormal accumulation of fluid in the peritoneal cavity. Most patients with ascites in the United States have cirrhosis.

4. *Spontaneous bacterial peritonitis* (SBP) is infection of ascitic fluid via a presumed hematogenous route. Classic findings

include fever, abdominal pain, and/or worsened encephalopathy, but clinical manifestations may be subtle. Diagnostic paracentesis is appropriate in any patient with new ascites or ascites and clinical deterioration, even in the absence of fever or abdominal complaints. The mortality of SBP is 40–60% even with therapy.

5. *Hepatorenal syndrome* is unexplained progressive renal failure in the patient with severe hepatic failure.

6. *Miscellaneous* manifestations may include
   a. Coagulopathy secondary to compromised synthetic function of vitamin K-dependent coagulation factors (with a prolonged prothrombin time [PT]).
   b. Impaired drug clearance of hepatically metabolized or excreted drugs.
   c. Abnormal blood glucose, including serious hypoglycemia.
   d. Impaired oxygenation and ventilation secondary to ascites and right to left shunting (a PaO_2 of 60–70 mmHg is not infrequent).
   e. Endocrine abnormalities, including hypogonadism and increased aldosterone.

B. Mortality

1. In 1990, over 27,000 people died of liver failure in the United States.

2. Hepatic cirrhosis is the fourth most common cause of death in 25–45-year-old individuals living in urban areas of the United States.

3. Patients with chronic liver disease and ascites have a 50% mortality within 2 years.

4. The cirrhotic patient's risk of developing hepatocellular carcinoma is 15–25%.

5. Approximately 2000 causes of *acute* liver failure occur annually in the United States, with a mortality of nearly 80%.

II. CLINICAL EVALUATION

A. History

1. Question the patient carefully about his/her presenting complaints.

2. In patients with known chronic liver disease, inquire with respect to
   a. The cause of liver disease.
   b. Prior complications and hospitalizations for hepatic failure.
   c. Current use and prior history of ethanol consumption.
   d. Other drug use.
   e. Symptoms/signs of ascites (e.g., abdominal pain, change in abdominal girth, change in weight, fever).

    f. Symptoms/signs of encephalopathy (may need to discuss with another family member).

    g. Symptoms/signs of gastrointestinal hemorrhage.

    h. Current medication use and drug allergies.

3. In patients with acute-onset liver disease, inquire with respect to
   a. Risk factors for viral hepatitis (see Hepatitis in Chapter 15), drug-induced hepatitis, and other potential causes of liver disease.
   b. Current use and prior history of ethanol consumption.
   c. Other drug use.
   d. Current medication use and drug allergies.

4. Always consider the possibility of toxin exposure (e.g., alcohol, heavy metals, occupational chemical use), mushroom ingestion, and/or drug overdose (e.g., acetaminophen).

5. Accurately identify any pre-existing significant other medical problems (e.g., alcoholism, cancer, congestive heart failure, pulmonary disease, renal insufficiency).

B. Symptoms and Signs

1. Nonspecific symptoms of hepatic failure may include anorexia, fatigue, malaise, nausea, and right-upper-quadrant tenderness. Jaundice may not be present initially, but eventually develops.

2. Worsened disease is usually characterized by increasing jaundice, pruritis, anorexia, and vomiting.

3. Asterixis is characteristic of mild to moderate encephalopathy. *Fetor hepaticus* is a sweet to musty pungent breath odor reminiscent of damp rodents.

4. Other manifestations may include abdominal pain, coagulopathy, fever/infection, gastrointestinal hemorrhage, hepatic encephalopathy, hypogonadism, new or worsened ascites, peripheral edema, and/or renal dysfunction.

C. Physical Examination

Obtain vital signs and evaluate the skin, HEENT (look for scleral icterus), neck, chest, heart, abdomen (include a rectal examination and stool heme test), extremities, and neurologic system. In the stable patient, comparing current with prior body weights is helpful.

1. Findings characteristic of hepatic insufficiency may include ascites, prominent abdominal-wall veins, spider angiomata (spider-like, fiery red vascular skin lesions that blanch with pressure and then refill from the center outward), palmar erythema (blotchy, purplish-red discoloration of the hypothenar area), gynecomastia, Dupuytren's contracture (a thickened plaque of the ring and sometimes little fingers resulting in a thick, fibrotic cord and the development of an eventual

flexion contracture of the involved finger[s]), testicular atrophy, and/or decreased body hair in males.

2. Carefully palpate the liver and spleen for size and tenderness. The cirrhotic liver is initially large, but as the disease progresses it becomes small and shrunken.

3. Increased muscle tone, mid-sized and sluggishly reactive pupils, and hyperventilation are early clinical signs of increasing intracranial pressure.

D. Laboratory Evaluation

1. *Routinely* obtain the following studies:
   a. Complete blood count (including platelets).
   b. Electrolyte panel.
   c. Glucose, blood urea nitrogen, and creatinine levels.
   d. Bilirubin level.
   e. Prothrombin time (PT). This test is immediately available, has important prognostic implications, and is a useful measure of hepatic synthetic function.
   f. Electrocardiogram.
   g. Chest roentgenogram.
   h. Urinalysis.

2. In the patient with *hepatic encephalopathy,* include the following in addition to the studies listed in D.1, above:
   a. Albumin.
   b. Arterial blood gas.
   c. Blood cultures.
   d. Calcium, magnesium, and phosphate levels.
   e. Toxicologic screen.
   f. Arterial ammonia level. The blood ammonia level is elevated in approximately 90% of encephalopathic patients, but it correlates poorly with the degree of mental status alteration. Cerebrospinal fluid glutamine (which reflects brain ammonia metabolism) is usually increased and is a more stable parameter than blood ammonia, but requires a lumbar puncture.

3. In the patient with an *acute gastrointestinal hemorrhage,* include the following in addition to the studies in D.1, above:
   a. Serial hematocrits.
   b. Partial thromboplastin time.
   c. Emergent blood type and crossmatch.

4. In the patient with suspected *spontaneous bacterial peritonitis,* include the following in addition to the studies in D.1, above:
   a. Albumin level.
   b. Blood cultures.
   c. Urine culture.
   d. Diagnostic paracentesis (obtain at least 50 mL of ascitic fluid). *Note:* if the physical examination does not clearly demonstrate ascites, paracentesis should be done under

ultrasound guidance. A concomitant coagulopathy does *not* contraindicate paracentesis unless the patient is suffering from disseminated intravascular coagulation or primary fibrinolysis.

   i. Routinely order the following tests on the obtained ascitic fluid: cell count, albumin, Gram stain, culture, and total protein. Optimal culture yields occur when ascitic fluid is directly inoculated into blood culture bottles at the bedside (10 mL of ascitic fluid per bottle for aerobic, anaerobic, and microaerophilic cultures). A polymorphonuclear cell count $\geq 250/mm^3$ is a reasonable laboratory diagnostic criterion for SBP. The serum–ascites albumin gradient correlates directly with portal pressure (patients with gradients ≥ 1.1 g/dL have portal hypertension).

   ii. Additional studies that should *not* be routinely ordered, but may be appropriate in certain circumstances, include glucose, lactate dehydrogenase, and amylase levels; tuberculosis smear and culture; and/or cytologic evaluation.

5. Additional studies may be necessary *depending on clinical circumstances* (e.g., hepatitis serologies, acetaminophen level, amylase, ceruloplasmin, iron studies, head computed tomography).

III. DIFFERENTIAL DIAGNOSIS

A. *Chronic liver failure* may be secondary to any of the following (the most common causes are *alcoholic cirrhosis* and *chronic viral hepatitis*):

1. Alcoholic cirrhosis.

2. Autoimmune hepatitis (may be seen in young girls and postmenopausal women).

3. Cardiac cirrhosis (liver injury in the setting of chronic right-sided heart failure).

4. Chronic viral hepatitis.

5. Drug-induced chronic hepatitis (the most common responsible agents include alpha-methyldopa, dantrolene sodium, isoniazid, nitrofurantoin, and nonsteroidal anti-inflammatory drugs; hepatic failure may be prevented if the offending drug is stopped in time).

6. Metabolic diseases (including Wilson's disease, alpha-1 antitrypsin deficiency, and hemochromatosis).

7. Postjejunoileal bypass.

8. Primary biliary cirrhosis.

9. Sarcoidosis (cirrhosis is a rare complication of this disease).

10. Schistosomiasis (a very unusual cause of cirrhosis in the United States).

11. Sclerosing cholangitis.

12. Toxin exposure (including chronic exposure to arsenic, methotrexate, or excessive amounts of vitamin A).

B. *Acute liver failure* may be secondary to any of the following (the most common causes are *viral hepatitis* and *drug-induced liver injury*):

1. Acetaminophen poisoning.

2. Acute fatty liver of pregnancy.

3. Heatstroke.

4. Hepatotrophic viruses (including hepatitis viruses A, B, C, D, E and non-A non-B non-C).

5. Idiosyncratic drug reactions (e.g., amiodarone, dapsone, disulfiram, halothane, isoniazid, phenytoin, propylthiouracil, sulfonamides, and valproate).

6. Ischemia.

7. Malignant infiltration.

8. Other viruses (e.g., cytomegalovirus, herpes simplex virus).

9. Reye's syndrome.

10. Toxin exposure (e.g., *Amanita phalloides* mushrooms, carbon tetrachloride, phosphorus).

11. Veno-occlusive disease.

12. Wilson's disease.

C. *Ascites* may be caused by any of the following:

1. Acute hepatic failure.

2. Alcoholic hepatitis.

3. Biliary ascites.

4. Bowel obstruction.

5. Bowel infarction.

6. Budd-Chiari syndrome (hepatic vein thrombosis).

7. Cancer (e.g., liver metastases, peritoneal carcinomatosis).

8. Chronic hepatic failure.

9. Congestive heart failure.

10. Fatty liver of pregnancy.

11. Myxedema.

12. Nephrotic syndrome.

13. Pancreatic disease.

14. Portal vein thrombosis.

15. Serositis.

16. Tuberculosis.

17. Veno-occlusive disease.

IV. THERAPY

The patient in hepatic failure may be critically ill from a compromised airway, cerebral edema, hypoxia, hypoventilation, hypovolemia, gastrointestinal hemorrhage, life-threatening infection, and/or a major electrolyte disorder. The priorities of the ED physician are to (1) support the patient's airway and vital signs, (2) rapidly initiate a diagnostic evaluation, (3) identify and initiate therapy for the specific manifestations of hepatic failure, and (4) expedite appropriate consultation and a reasonable disposition.

A. Initial Management

Assess, secure, and support airway, breathing, circulation, and neurologic status as indicated (see Chapter 1. II).

1. Administer supplemental oxygen, and protect the airway as necessary. Endotracheal intubation may be necessary for definitive airway management or to allow for hyperventilation in the setting of increased intracranial pressure.

2. Obtain vital signs, establish intravenous (IV) access, check the fingerstick glucose level if the mental status is altered, and order appropriate laboratory studies (see II, above). Monitor both cardiac rhythm and oxygen saturation (SaO_2) in seriously ill patients.

3. Treat hypotension with IV crystalloid. If the clinical examination indicates pulmonary vascular congestion, support blood pressure as necessary with dopamine.

4. Consider parenteral thiamine, glucose, and naloxone if mental status is altered.

5. Consider potential toxin exposure (e.g., acetaminophen poisoning, toxic mushroom ingestion) and manage as required (see Chapter 23).

6. Provide general supportive care as necessary (e.g., Foley catheter, nasogastric tube [place orally instead of nasally in the patient with a significant coagulopathy]) and protect the comatose patient's eyes from desiccation and injury. Do not leave the patient with severe encephalopathy in the ED room alone. Keep the guardrails up on the patient's stretcher; soft restraints are appropriate to prevent self-harm.

B. Specific Therapy for Hepatic Failure

1. Hepatic Encephalopathy

a. Secure and support airway, breathing, circulation, and deficits as outlined under IV. A, above.

b. Identify and treat any precipitating factors (e.g., azotemia, gastrointestinal hemorrhage, hypokalemic metabolic alkalosis, hypoxia, increased dietary protein, infection, medications, and/or electrolyte derangements). Even mild hyponatremia, hypoglycemia, and/or volume depletion may worsen encephalopathy and must be corrected.

c. Meticulously review the patient's medication use, and withhold all potentially central nervous system depressant drugs.

d. Restrict or eliminate dietary protein until the clinical condition improves. Adequate caloric intake (25–30 kcal/ kg) should still be provided either enterally or parenterally. Remember to administer thiamine prior to glucose-containing solutions; multivitamin supplementation is also appropriate.

e. Administer specific medications for hepatic encephalopathy: Lactulose is the drug of first choice. Combined lactulose + neomycin therapy is reasonable in the patient who is unresponsive to either agent alone. Metronidazole may be considered in patients unresponsive to lactulose and/or neomycin.

   i. **Lactulose.**
      Dose: begin with 30 mL (20 g) PO tid–qid (may be administered via a nasogastric tube in obtunded patients). In severe cases (e.g., those associated with concomitant gastrointestinal hemorrhage), 30 mL may be given every hour until catharsis is achieved, but avoid volume depletion secondary to medication-induced diarrhea. Maintenance dosing should be adjusted to produce one to two soft stools per day without frank diarrhea. Lactulose may also be given as an enema (300 mL of lactulose in 700 mL tap water). *And/or*

   ii. **Neomycin.**
      Dose: 1 g PO (or via a nasogastric tube) every 6 hours. (Enema dose is 1–2 g in 100–200 mL normal saline bid–qid; enema is less effective than PO administration). *Caution:* ototoxicity and/or renal injury have been reported. Do not use in patients with renal insufficiency; avoid prolonged use. *Or*

   iii. **Metronidazole.**
      Dose: 250 mg PO qid. Avoid prolonged use.

f. Consider flumazenil (0.5 mg IV over 30 seconds, repeated every 1 minute up to a maximum cumulative dose of 5 mg): this benzodiazepine antagonist has been reported to produce temporary improvement in hepatic encephalopathy. It is expensive (approximately $22 per 0.5-mg dose).

g. Patients with evidence of cerebral edema should be managed by elevating the head of the bed (to 20 degrees) and administering IV mannitol (0.3–0.4 g/kg of a 20% solution given rapidly IV; dose may be repeated at least once after several hours). Consider intubation and hyperventilation.

2. Acute Variceal Hemorrhage

a. Secure and support airway, breathing, and circulation as outlined under IV. A, above.
b. See Acute Gastrointestinal Hemorrhage, earlier in this chapter, for specific therapeutic recommendations.

3. Ascites

a. Secure and support airway, breathing, and circulation as outlined under IV. A, above.
b. Diagnostic paracentesis is appropriate in the patient with new-onset ascites or suspected spontaneous bacterial peritonitis (see II. D. 4, above).
c. Begin dietary sodium restriction ($\leq$ 2 g/day).
d. Recommend bed rest with frequent position changes (to avoid decubitus ulcers); gradual resumption of activity may occur once diuresis has been initiated.
e. Diuretic therapy: reasonable goals are a weight loss secondary to diuresis of 0.5 kg/day in patients without edema and 1 kg/day in those with edema.

   Combination Therapy. Spironolactone and furosemide. Begin with 100 mg of spironolactone and 40 mg of furosemide PO every AM. If the patient does not respond to the above in 2–3 days (as evidenced by a decrease in body weight and an increase in urinary sodium excretion to > 10 mEq/L), increase the dose of spironolactone to 200 mg and furosemide to 80 mg PO every AM. Maximum doses of these medications in this setting are 400 mg of spironolactone and 160 mg of furosemide q day. Amiloride may be substituted for spironolactone in the above combination diuretic regimen. The starting dose is 10 mg PO every AM, and the maximum daily dose is 40 mg. Amiloride's advantage over spironolactone is its faster onset of action and the absence of painful gynecomastia as a side effect.

   Caution: carefully warn the patient to *not* consume potassium-rich foods or potassium supplements while taking either spironolactone or amiloride. Daily weights should be measured. Unreliable patients, those unable to maintain close (e.g., every 24–48 hours initially) outpatient monitoring of electrolyte levels and renal function, or individuals with renal insufficiency should be admitted prior to initiating the above combination regimen.
f. In patients with severe ascites or those unresponsive to diuretic therapy as outlined above, consider large-volume

paracentesis combined with albumin infusion (25 g albumin IV for every 2 L ascites removed). This therapeutic modality has been shown to shorten the hospital stay and decrease complications in patients with significant ascites uncontrolled by maintenance diuretics. It may be repeated one to three times per month if required.

g. In patients whose ascites is unresponsive to the above-described interventions, treatment options may include peritoneovenous shunting (unfortunately associated with significant complications, including coagulopathy, disseminated intravascular coagulation, shunt failure, and infection/sepsis); transjugular intrahepatic portosystemic stent shunts; and liver transplantation in suitable candidates.

4. Spontaneous Bacterial Peritonitis

a. Secure and support airway, breathing, and circulation as outlined under IV. A, above.

b. Obtain blood cultures and diagnostic paracentesis as outlined under II. D. 4, above.

c. Initiate antibiotic therapy: reasonable initial choices include cefotaxime (2 g IV every 6 hours), ceftriaxone (1 g IV every 12 hours), or ampicillin-sulbactam (3 g IV every 6 hours) for 5–10 days. Repeat paracentesis should be performed in 48–72 hours to ensure appropriateness of inpatient antibiotic therapy.

d. The risk of recurrence of SBP may be reduced with long-term norfloxacin prophylaxis (400 mg PO daily).

5. Hepatorenal Syndrome

a. Stop all diuretics and potentially nephrotoxic medications (including aspirin or other nonsteroidal anti-inflammatory drugs).

b. Rule out occult blood loss or any other cause of prerenal azotemia. A saline challenge and/or invasive central venous monitoring are appropriate to assist in accurate assessment of volume status.

c. Consult nephrology.

d. Hospitalize the patient for continued therapy of the underlying liver disease and appropriate diagnostic and supportive care.

6. Miscellaneous

a. Patients with coagulopathy (prolonged PT) should be given vitamin K (5–10 mg PO or 10 mg SQ daily for several days).

b. Meticulously dose all medications, and avoid drugs that are hepatotoxic or hepatically metabolized and/or excreted.

c. Routinely prescribe multivitamins and folic acid (1 mg/day).

C. Expedite Appropriate Consultation

1. The patient in hepatic failure may benefit from a variety of consultants (e.g., gastroenterology, internal medicine, nephrology, critical care, and/or transplant specialist) depending on the patient's presentation. Obtain consultant involvement early as required.

2. Liver transplantation has significantly improved survival and prognosis for most forms of end-stage liver disease. Patients with acute liver failure should be considered for urgent transplantation, as 1-year survival with a transplant is > 60%. Early consultation with transplant specialists and transfer to a center capable of this procedure are appropriate.

V. DISPOSITION

A. Discharge

The patient with *chronic liver failure of known cause* may be managed as an outpatient if *all* of the following conditions apply:

1. Vital signs are stable and normal.

2. Encephalopathy, if present, is grade 1 only and the patient does not live alone.

3. There is no evidence of gastrointestinal hemorrhage.

4. There is no evidence of a significant infection (including spontaneous bacterial peritonitis).

5. Ascites, if present, is not severe.

6. No other condition mandating hospitalization is present.

7. The patient is reliable.

8. Expeditious outpatient follow-up has been arranged.

B. Admit

Patients with hepatic failure who do not meet all of the above criteria for ED discharge should be hospitalized. Hospitalization is especially appropriate in patients with *any* of the following:

1. Acute-onset liver failure.

2. Hepatic encephalopathy of grade 2 or worse.

3. Gastrointestinal hemorrhage.

4. Significant ascites.

5. Ascites unresponsive to outpatient management.

6. Need for large-volume paracentesis to manage refractory ascites.

7. Suspected or confirmed spontaneous bacterial peritonitis.

8. Other significant infection.

9. Renal insufficiency or suspected hepatorenal syndrome.

10. Inadequate home situation.

VI. PEARLS AND PITFALLS

A. Secure and support the patient's airway, oxygenation, ventilation, and vital signs. Beware of occult blood loss, cerebral edema, trauma, life-threatening electrolyte disorder, and/or infection.

B. Routinely administer thiamine, glucose, and naloxone to the patient presenting with altered mentation.

C. Remember, mental status changes may not be secondary to hepatic encephalopathy; consider the possibilities of drug overdose, electrolyte disorder, meningitis, subdural hematoma, and/or toxin ingestion (see Chapter 20 on Coma for a more extensive differential diagnosis).

D. Acute hepatic failure may be secondary to an idiosyncratic drug reaction or toxin exposure. Urgently evaluate all patients with recent-onset hepatic failure for potential reversible causes and/or the need for appropriate antidote administration.

E. The initial therapy of mild to moderate ascites in the setting of cirrhosis is dietary sodium restriction and diuretic therapy. The combination of spironolactone and furosemide is more effective than either agent used individually. Carefully instruct the patient prescribed a potassium-sparing diuretic (e.g., spironolactone or amiloride) to avoid potassium-rich foods and potassium supplements.

F. The patient with ascites who is treated with large-volume therapeutic paracentesis should have an albumin infusion and be temporarily admitted for observation to ensure the procedure is well tolerated.

G. The symptoms and signs of SBP may be subtle. Diagnostic paracentesis is appropriate whenever the diagnosis of SBP is even remotely possible or ascites is a new clinical finding for the patient.

H. Transfer to a center experienced in liver transplantation should be considered expeditiously in any patient with acute-onset liver failure or who is otherwise an appropriate transplant candidate.

BIBLIOGRAPHY

Arroyo et al: Treatment of ascites in cirrhosis. Diuresis, peritoneovenous shunt, and large-volume paracentesis. Gastroenterol Clin N Am 1992; March 21(1):237–256.

Groover J: Alcoholic liver disease. Emerg Med Clin N Am 1990;8(4):887–903.

Lee WM: Acute liver failure. N Engl J Med 1993;329(25):1862–1872.

Runyon BA: Care of patients with ascities. N Engl J Med 1994;330(5):337–342.

Tito L et al: Total paracentesis associated with IV albumin management of patients with cirrhosis and ascites. Gastroenterology 1990;98(1):146–151.

PANCREATITIS

"A physician is obligated to consider more than a diseased organ, more even than the whole man—he must view the man in his world."

HARVEY CUSHING (1869-1939)

I. ESSENTIAL FACTS

A. Definition

Pancreatitis is an inflammatory condition of the pancreas associated with at least some autodigestion of the organ by its own enzymes. It may be either an acute or a chronic illness; the latter is characterized by persistent or recurrent bouts of abdominal pain and evidence of insufficient pancreatic function (e.g., diabetes, steatorrhea).

B. Epidemiology

1. The annual incidence of acute pancreatitis is estimated to be 10–30 per 100,000 people.
2. The causes of acute pancreatitis include
   a. Gallstones (45% of cases).
   b. Alcohol (35% of cases).
   c. Miscellaneous (10% of cases; including toxins, drugs, trauma, hypertriglyceridemia, hypercalcemia, inherited conditions, infections, vascular abnormalities, peptic ulcer disease, Crohn's disease, cystic fibrosis, Reye's syndrome, and hypothermia).
   d. Idiopathic (10% of cases).
3. Most acute episodes are mild and self-limited; 25% of attacks are severe, with a mortality rate approaching 9%.
4. The overall mortality rate from pancreatitis has decreased from 25% to 5% over the past 25 years, due largely to the improved identification, treatment, and monitoring of patients at risk for complications.
5. Most cases (75%) of *chronic pancreatitis* in the United States are due to chronic alcohol abuse.

II. CLINICAL EVALUATION

A. History

1. Abdominal pain is a prominent complaint (90% of patients). It is generally epigastric, sharp, penetrating, and continuous, and in 50% of patients it radiates to the back. The degree of pain, however, has a poor correlation with the extent of pancreatic inflammation.
2. Associated symptoms may include nausea and vomiting (60–90% of cases), anorexia, and occasionally dyspnea or fever.

3. A careful history regarding medication use, toxin exposure, trauma, alcohol ingestion, and history of other medical/surgical problems must be obtained.

   a. *Medications* associated with acute pancreatitis include acetaminophen, azathioprine, cimetidine, didanosine, erythromycin, estrogens, furosemide, mercaptopurine, methyldopa, metronidazole, pentamidine, ranitidine, salicylates, sulfonamides, and sulindac.

   b. *Toxins* associated with acute pancreatitis include ethanol, methanol, organophosphorous insecticides, and scorpion venom.

B. Physical Examination

Obtain vital signs and evaluate the skin, HEENT, neck, chest, heart, abdomen (include a rectal examination and stool heme test), extremities, and neurologic system. In the stable patient, also obtain orthostatic vital signs.

   a. A temperature > 38.0° C suggests severe inflammation or sepsis. Trousseau's sign (spasmodic muscular contractions of the upper extremity secondary to pressure on the involved nerves) may be elicited while taking the blood pressure if the patient is significantly hypocalcemic. Hypotension suggests retroperitoneal hemorrhage, volume depletion, sepsis, or fluid sequestration secondary to a massive inflammatory response. Tachypnea may be due to pain, hypoxia, pulmonary infiltrates, and/or pleural effusion.

   b. Tenderness in the epigastric and periumbilical region is found in 98% of cases and peritoneal signs are found in 30–40% of cases. A palpable epigastric mass suggests an abscess, pseudocyst, or carcinoma. Hypoactive or absent bowel sounds and distention are consistent with ileus.

C. Laboratory Studies

1. *Minimally* obtain the following:

   a. Complete blood count (CBC) with platelet count. Mild leukocytosis is common; a markedly elevated leukocyte count suggests severe inflammation or infection.

   b. Electrolyte panel, glucose, blood urea nitrogen [BUN], and creatinine levels.

   c. Amylase and bilirubin levels. Ten percent of patients with acute pancreatitis have a *normal* serum amylase level. Even if initially elevated, amylase levels return to normal in 2–3 days after symptom onset and do *not* correlate with resolution of disease. Urine amylase may be elevated even if the serum amylase is normal. Pancreatic isoenzymes (i.e., salivary and pancreatic) should be obtained to confirm that an elevated amylase level is pancreatic in origin. Gallstone pancreatitis tends to result in higher serum amylase levels (> 1000 units/L in 89% of patients with gallstone pancreatitis in one study) than alcoholic pancreatitis.

    d. Serum lipase. Serum lipase is more specific but less sensitive than serum amylase. The lipase level remains elevated for 7–10 days after onset of symptoms.

    e. Urinalysis.

    f. Electrocardiogram (ECG) (mandatory in patients ≥ 40 years old and in those with a history of ischemic heart disease, coronary artery disease risk factors, or unstable vital signs).

    g. Serum or urine pregnancy test. Mandatory in female patients of reproductive age.

2. *One or more* of the following *may* also be appropriate depending on clinical circumstances:

    a. Arterial blood gas.

    b. Blood cultures.

    c. Calcium, magnesium, and phosphate levels.

    d. Ethanol level.

    e. Liver function tests. Liver function tests should be ordered if gallstone pancreatitis or alcoholic liver disease is suspected.

    f. Serum triglyceride level.

    a. Toxicologic screen.

D. Imaging Procedures

1. **Acute Abdominal Series** (upright chest roentgenogram; supine and upright abdominal roentgenograms). These films are appropriate in the patient clinically suspected of pancreatitis and may be helpful in ruling out alternative diagnoses.

    a. Subdiaphragmatic air on the chest film or upright abdominal film indicates visceral perforation.

    b. Chest-film findings consistent with acute pancreatitis include pleural effusion, atelectasis, and/or diffuse infiltrates.

    c. Abdominal films in pancreatitis may reveal a jejunal ileus ("sentinel loop"), generalized ileus, and/or a radiolucency around the kidney ("renal halo") caused by perirenal fat medially and by inflammatory changes laterally.

    d. Ninety percent of patients with chronic pancreatitis have pancreatic calcifications.

1. **Abdominal Ultrasound.** Ultrasound is not routinely necessary in patients with pancreatitis unless biliary tract disease is suspected, and it is often difficult to obtain a high-quality study because of overlying intestinal gas. A pancreatic abscess or pseudocyst may occasionally be seen. A normal study does not exclude the diagnosis of pancreatitis.

2. **Contrast-Enhanced Abdominal Computed Tomography (CT) Scan.** This is the modality of choice when pancreatic imaging is clinically necessary (e.g., when the diagnosis is in doubt, when the patient fails to improve with medical therapy, when a pseudocyst or pancreatic phlegmon is suspected, or in

the patient with life-threatening disease). In addition, a normal CT examination excludes the diagnosis of severe pancreatitis.

E. Assessing the Severity of Acute Pancreatitis

The Ranson criteria and the modified Glasgow criteria have been used to predict the severity of disease and to assess mortality risk. An assessment must be made initially and within 48 hours of patient presentation. See Table 16–3.

Table 16–3. ADVERSE PROGNOSTIC FACTORS IN SEVERE ACUTE PANCREATITIS[a]

Ranson's Criteria

Pancreatitis not due to gallstones
  On admission
    Age > 55 years
    White-cell count > 16,000/mm^3
    Glucose > 200 mg/dL
    Lactate dehydrogenase > 350 units/L
    Aspartate aminotransferase > 250 units/L
  Within 48 hours of hospitalization
    Decrease in hematocrit > 10 points
    Increase in BUN > 5 mg/dL
    Calcium < 8 mg/dL
    PaO$_2$ < 60 mmHg
    Base deficit > 4 mmol/L
    Fluid deficit > 6 L

Gallstone-induced pancreatitis
  On admission
    Age > 70 years
    White-cell count > 18,000/mm^3
    Glucose > 220 mg/dL
    Lactate dehydrogenase > 400 units/L
    Aspartate aminotransferase > 250 units/L
  Within 48 hours of hospitalization
    Decrease in hematocrit > 10 points
    Increase in BUN > 2 mg/dL
    Serum calcium < 8 mg/dL
    Base deficit > 5 mmol/L
    Fluid deficit > 4 L

Modified Glasgow Criteria

  Within 48 hours of hospitalization
    Age > 55 years
    White-cell count > 15,000/mm^3
    Glucose > 180 mg/dL
    BUN > 45 mg/dL
    Lactate dehydrogenase > 600 units/L
    Albumin < 3.3 g/dL
    Calcium < 8 mg/dL
    PaO$_2$ < 60 mmHg

[a]The presence of three or more risk factors at the times indicated is associated with increased morbidity and mortality. To convert values for glucose to millimoles per liter, multiply by 0.05551. To convert values for BUN to millimoles per liter, multiply by 0.357. To convert values for calcium to millimoles per liter, multiply by 0.250.

Modified from Steinberg W, Tenner S, adverse pronostic factors in severe acute pancreatitis. N Engl J Med 1994;330:1198–1210.

III. DIFFERENTIAL DIAGNOSIS

The differential diagnosis of pancreatitis includes the following:

A. Acute appendicitis.*

B. Acute myocardial infarction.

C. Bowel infarction.*

D. Bowel obstruction.*

E. Cholelithiasis and cholecystitis.

F. Diabetic ketoacidosis.*

G. Dissecting abdominal aortic aneurysm.*

H. Ectopic pregnancy.*

I. Gastritis.

J. Hepatitis.

K. Methanol poisoning.

L. Peptic ulcer disease.

M. Perforated duodenal ulcer.

N. Peritonitis.*

O. Pneumonia.

P. Pulmonary embolus.

Q. Renal colic.

Note: conditions with an asterisk above may present with an elevated serum amylase level.

IV. THERAPY

The management of the patient with pancreatitis in the ED involves supportive care appropriate for the severity of disease. *Some patients with acute pancreatitis are critically ill and will require aggressive resuscitation and ICU admission.*

A. Initial Management

Assess, secure, and support the airway, breathing, and circulation as indicated (see Chapter 1. II).

1. Administer supplemental oxygen, establish intravenous (IV) access, keep the patient NPO, obtain vital signs, and check the fingerstick glucose level. Monitor both cardiac rhythm and oxygen saturation (SaO_2) in seriously ill patients.

2. Treat hypotension with intravenous crystalloid. If clinical examination indicates pulmonary vascular congestion, support blood pressure as necessary with dopamine.

3. Obtain a directed history, perform a physical examination, and order relevant laboratory tests as outlined in II, above.

4. The patient with nausea and vomiting or ileus should have a nasogastric tube placed and also should receive parenteral antiemetics (e.g., *prochlorperazine* 5–10 mg slowly IV; or *metoclopramide* 10 mg slowly IV).

B. Provide Analgesia

1. Analgesia with opioid agents is usually required.

2. Medication choices: *meperidine* is preferred over *morphine* because it causes less spasm of the spincter of Oddi:
   i. Meperidine 12.5–25 mg given slowly IV; repeat every 15–60 minutes as required. Titrate carefully to avoid vital sign compromise. May also be given IM (1 mg/kg IM every 4 hours). *Or*
   ii. Morphine 1–3 mg IV every 5 minutes initially, titrated carefully to avoid vital sign compromise.

C. Adjunctive Therapy

1. *Correct electrolyte abnormalities* (e.g., hypokalemia, hypomagnesemia, and/or hypocalcemia) as necessary.

2. *Antibiotics* are indicated if concomitant bililary tract obstruction is present or a pancreatic abscess is demonstrated on the CT scan. Choices include

   a. Imipenem (500 mg IV every 6 hours). *Note:* a recent study found that imipenem reduced the incidence of pancreatic sepsis (from 30% to 12%) in patients with necrotizing pancreatitis, although mortality was not affected. *Or*
   b. Mezlocillin (4 g IV every 6 hours) and metronidazole (15 mg/kg IV over 1 hour to start, followed by 7.5 mg/kg IV every 6 hours; do not exceed 4 g in a 24-hour period). *Or*
   c. Ticarcillin/clavulanate (Timentin: 3.1 g IV over 30 minutes every 4–6 hours). *Or*
   d. Ampicillin/sulbactam (Unasyn: 1.5–3.0 g IM or IV every 6 hours).

3. *Endoscopic therapy:* in patients with gallstone pancreatitis, the removal of impacted gallstones via endoscopic retrograde cholangiopancreatography (ERCP) and endoscopic sphincterotomy within 24 hours of admission appears to decrease morbidity and may reduce mortality. Consult a gastroenterologist early.

4. *Surgery:* indications for general surgery include an uncertain diagnosis, cholangitis, pancreatic abscess, and/or a pseudocyst that fails to respond to 4–6 weeks of conservative medical therapy. Consult a general surgeon early.

5. *Peritoneal lavage* (daily for 7 days) is controversial, but may be beneficial in patients with severe pancreatitis (> 5 Ranson

580 / GASTROINTESTINAL EMERGENCIES

criteria risk factors; see Table 16–3). Consult a general surgeon early.

V. DISPOSITION

A. Discharge

Consider discharging the patient with *mild* pancreatitis from the ED to home if *all* of the following conditions are met:

1. Vital signs are normal.
2. Pain is mild and can be controlled with oral analgesic agents.
3. The patient is able to take clear liquids PO in the ED.
4. The patient is reliable.
5. There is no evidence of biliary tract disease.
6. There is no evidence of a systemic complication.

Discharge the patient with an oral analgesic (e.g., meperidine tablets 50–150 mg PO every 4 hours), recommend a clear liquid diet and no ethanol intake, and ensure follow-up within several days.

B. Admit

Patients who do not meet the above criteria for discharge will require hospitalization to the medicine service. If hemorrhagic or necrotizing pancreatitis is suspected, ICU admission is appropriate.

VI. PEARLS AND PITFALLS

A. The patient with acute pancreatitis may be critically ill. Assess and manage the airway, breathing, and circulation immediately. Resuscitate as necessary.

B. Always remember the differential diagnosis. Abdominal catastrophes that may elevate the serum amylase level, in addition to acute pancreatitis, include acute appendicitis, dissecting abdominal aortic aneurysm, perforated duodenal ulcer, bowel obstruction, bowel infarction, ruptured ectopic pregnancy, and generalized peritonitis of any cause. Obtain surgical consultation early as clinically appropriate.

C. Evaluate the patient carefully for complications, including respiratory compromise, adult respiratory distress syndrome, shock, acute renal failure, hypocalcemia, hemorrhage, cholangitis, concomitant cholecystitis, pseudocyst, phlegmon, and/or pancreatic abscess.

D. Check and manage glucose and electrolyte abnormalities as required.

E. Administer antiemetics and place a nasogastric tube in the patient with significant vomiting.

F. Provide adequate analgesia.

   Do not do any of the following:

A. Dismiss the diagnosis of pancreatitis based on a normal amylase level.

B. Use vasopressors to support blood pressure until fluid resuscitation has been maximized.

BIBLIOGRAPHY

Marshall JB: Acute pancreatitis: A review with an emphasis on new developments. Arch Intern Med 1993;153:1185–1198.

Moulton JS: The radiologic assessment of acute pancreatitis and its complications. Pancreas 1991;6(1):S13–S22.

Ranson JH: Acute pancreatitis: Pathogenesis, outcome and treatment. Clin Gastroenterol 1984; 13:843–863.

Steinberg WM: Predictors of severity of acute pancreatitis. Gastroenterol Clin N Am 1990; 19(4):849–861.

Steinberg W, Tenner S: Acute pancreatitis. N Engl J Med 1994;330:1198–1210.

17

Renal Emergencies

ACID–BASE DISORDERS

> *"In all things you shall find everywhere the Acid and the Alcaly."*
>
> OTTO TACHENIUS (d. 1670)

I. ESSENTIAL FACTS

A. Introduction

The human body is remarkably capable of maintaining its concentration of free hydrogen ions within an extremely narrow range. It does this despite the daily production of a comparatively large amount of acid. This homeostasis may be disturbed in a wide variety of disease states when acid synthesis or excretion is altered or buffering capacity is compromised. The accurate analysis of acid–base disturbances can aid in making a correct initial clinical diagnosis and assessing its severity; indeed, it may provide critical clues to unsuspected problems or impending catastrophe.

1. The addition of inorganic and certain organic acids would quickly alter systemic pH were it not for buffers present in the

intra- and extracellular fluid. Bicarbonate is the most important of these. It binds protons to form carbonic acid, which is subsequently dehydrated and released from the lungs as carbon dioxide:

$$H^+ + HCO_3^- = H_2CO_3 = H_2O + CO_2$$

The lungs must maintain a rate of carbon dioxide excretion that keeps pace with carbonic acid production.

2. The kidney is responsible for regenerating bicarbonate as well as excreting some acids directly.

3. The *Henderson–Hasselbach equation* is useful in understanding the interrelationship of these components. It may be modified slightly to reflect the fact that PCO_2 is proportional to the less easily measured H_2CO_3:

$$pH = 6.1 + \log \frac{[HCO_3^-]}{0.0301 \times PCO_2}$$

or

$$[H^+] \text{ (in nEq/L)} = 24 \times \frac{PCO_2 \text{ (mmHg)}}{[HCO_3^-] \text{ (mEq/L)}}$$

At a pH of 7.40, H^+ is 40 nEq/L.

B. Definitions

The first step in acid–base analysis is to identify the deviation of pH and HCO_3^- or PCO_2 from normal (normal HCO_3^- is 23–28 mEq/L and normal PCO_2 is 35–45 mmHg) and characterize the primary disturbance according to the following four categories:

1. *Metabolic acidosis:* decreases plasma bicarbonate concentration. It may result from addition of acid (endogenous or exogenous) or enhanced bicarbonate excretion.

2. *Metabolic alkalosis:* increases plasma bicarbonate concentration. It may result from ingestion of bicarbonate or enhanced proton excretion, such as HCl loss through vomiting or aldosterone-mediated renal tubular H^+ secretion.

3. *Respiratory acidosis:* elevates PCO_2 as the result of hypoventilation relative to CO_2 production. Ventilatory disorders may arise as a result of intrinsic pulmonary diseases or central nervous system processes that alter respiratory "drive."

4. *Respiratory alkalosis:* decreases PCO_2 as a result of increased ventilation relative to PCO_2 production.

Note: interpretation of acid–base status becomes more challenging when more than one of the above disorders is present simultaneously. For example, patients may present with metabolic alkalosis, respiratory acidosis, and metabolic acidosis concomitantly.

C. The Anion Gap

1. Calculation of the anion gap is a prerequisite to proper analysis of acid–base disturbances. The anion gap approximates the difference in concentration of routinely measured serum anions and cations and is calculated as follows:

$$\text{Anion gap} = [Na^+] - ([Cl^-] + [HCO_3^-])$$

The normal anion gap is 10–12 mEq/L.

2. Normally, the anion gap represents primarily albumin and phosphate. Metabolic acidosis with a *normal* anion gap occurs when hyperchloremia offsets bicarbonate loss or when the added acid is HCl.

3. In the setting of metabolic acidosis, a "widened" (increased) anion gap implies the addition of a nonmeasured proton donor such as lactate, acetoacetate, or beta hydroxybutyrate. *Note:* the many causes of an elevated anion gap include the following:
   a. Alcohol.
   b. Toluene.
   c. Methanol.
   d. Uremia.
   e. Diabetic ketoacidosis.
   f. Paraldehyde.
   g. Iron, isoniazid.
   h. Lactic acid.
   i. Ethylene glycol.
   j. Strychnine, salicylates.

   Note: the first letters of these causes spell the mnemonic AT MUD PILES.

D. Compensation for a Primary Acid–Base Disturbance

1. **Underlying Principles.** Acid–base derangements develop when a toxin or illness compromises the ability of the kidneys or lungs to maintain homeostasis or when their capacity to adapt is overwhelmed by increased acid or base release. When one organ system falters, the other will attempt to diminish the net alteration in hydrogen ion concentration through certain well-described and predictable compensatory mechanisms. Examples include the following:
   a. When a respiratory acidosis develops (increased PCO_2), the kidney responds by increasing reclamation of HCO_3^-.
   b. When a respiratory alkalosis develops (decreased PCO_2), the kidney decreases HCO_3^- reabsorption.
   c. In the setting of metabolic acidosis (decreased serum HCO_3^-), ventilation is increased to lower PCO_2 and return systemic pH toward normal.
   d. Metabolic alkalosis (increased HCO_3^-) induces a mild compensatory hypoventilation that increases PCO_2.

2. **Primary and Compensatory Changes.** When confronted

with a patient with an acid–base disturbance, determine what is the *primary* or initiating abnormality and what is the compensation for that abnormality. To do this, simply check the variation of the systemic pH from normal and decide whether the alteration in HCO_3^- or PCO_2 would produce that shift; that alteration is considered the primary disorder. Remember, also, the following principles:

a. Appropriate compensatory changes will not overcorrect or even normalize the pH; compensation acts only to *ameliorate* the primary acid–base disorder.

b. Ventilatory changes occur *within minutes* to compensate for primary metabolic disturbances.

c. Renal responses to respiratory disturbances, however, take time. In the setting of a primary respiratory alkalosis, compensatory renal bicarbonate loss occurs after 24–48 hours. In the setting of a primary respiratory acidosis, the maximal bicarbonate concentration is achieved by the kidneys after about 3–5 days. It is helpful to think of respiratory derangements as acute or chronic when judging the adequacy of the renal response. Failure of the kidney to respond appropriately indicates a concomitant metabolic abnormality.

d. There are limits to the compensatory mechanisms. For example, hypoventilation will increase PCO_2 in response to severe metabolic alkalosis but generally not to the extent that hypoxia develops.

e. The formulas in Table 17–1 are useful in approximately predicting the expected compensatory changes. The greater the severity of the acid–base disturbance, the less accurate the predictions become. *Compensation that "overshoots" or falls far short of the prediction indicates concomitant derangement of the compensating organ system.* This is discussed further in III. E, below.

II. CLINICAL EVALUATION

Laboratory data (blood chemistries, arterial blood gas, and anion gap) will reveal which acid–base disorder(s) is(are) present. It may be more difficult, however, to pinpoint the exact cause of the disorder(s). A thorough history and physical examination, with special attention to the following factors, will help the clinician determine the precise nature of the disorder and its necessary treatment.

A. History

1. Inquire about factors that affect intravascular volume and electrolytes, including the following: vomiting, diarrhea, anorexia, and blood loss. Volume-depleted patients may complain of thirst and note a diminution in urine output.

2. Accurately identify pre-existing medical problems (e.g., dia-

Table 17–1. GUIDELINES FOR PREDICTING METABOLIC AND RESPIRATORY COMPENSATION FOR ACID–BASE DISTURBANCES

PRIMARY DISORDER	INITIATING DISTURBANCE	COMPENSATORY RESPONSE	LIMITS OF COMPENSATION
Metabolic	*Changes in $[HCO_3^-]$*	*Change in PCO_2*	
Acidosis	$\downarrow\downarrow\downarrow$ $[HCO_3^-]$	$\downarrow\downarrow$ PCO_2	$PCO_2 = 1.5x$ $[HCO_3^-]+8 \pm 2.$
Alkalosis	$\uparrow\uparrow\uparrow$ $[HCO_3^-]$	$\uparrow\uparrow$ PCO_2	PCO_2 increases 6 mmHg per 10-mEq/L increase in $[HCO_3^-]$
Respiratory	*Change in PCO_2*	*Change in $[HCO_3^-]$*	
Acidosis			
acute (hours)	$\uparrow\uparrow\uparrow$ PCO_2	$\uparrow$ $[HCO_3^-]$	$[HCO_3^-]$ increases 1 mEq/L for each 10-mmHg increment in PCO_2
chronic (days)	$\uparrow\uparrow\uparrow$ PCO_2	$\uparrow\uparrow$ $[HCO_3^-]$	$[HCO_3^-]$ increases 3–3.5 mEq/L for each 10-mmHg increment in PCO_2
Alkalosis			
acute (hours)	$\downarrow\downarrow\downarrow$ PCO_2	$\downarrow$ $[HCO_3^-]$	$[HCO_3^-]$ drops 2.5 mEq/L for each 10-mmHg decrement in PCO_2
chronic (days)	$\downarrow\downarrow\downarrow$ PCO_2	$\downarrow\downarrow$ $[HCO_3^-]$	$[HCO_3^-]$ drops 5.0 mEq/L for each 10-mmHg decrement in PCO_2

Adapted from Narins RG: Clinical disorders of fluid and electrolyte metabolism, 4th ed. New York: McGraw-Hill, 1987, p. 59.

betes, congestive heart failure, renal insufficiency, alcoholism, hepatic compromise, and pulmonary disease).

3. Obtain a thorough medication history. Many drugs can affect volume and acid–base status (e.g., acetazolamide, antacids, diuretics, insulin, iron, isoniazid, paraldehyde, salicylates).

4. Consider the possibility of exposure to toxins, including carbon monoxide, cyanide, ethanol, ethylene glycol, methanol, toluene, and strychnine.

B. Physical Examination

Obtain vital signs and evaluate the skin, HEENT, neck, chest, heart, abdomen (include a rectal examination and stool heme test), extremities, and nervous system. In the stable patient, obtain orthostatic vital signs and compare current to baseline body weight.

1. The mucosa of the tongue may reveal evidence of dehydration (a dry, longitudinally furrowed tongue indicates marked dehydration). Note the breath for the smell of acetone or the fruity odor of ketones. Fundoscopic changes may be seen in methanol poisoning, diabetes mellitus, or hypertensive crises.

2. Rapid and deep respirations may be a compensation for metabolic acidosis.

3. Cold, clammy limbs indicate hypoperfusion and vasoconstriction, which causes lactic acidosis. Peripheral edema may indicate right-sided congestive heart failure, hepatic disease, or hypoalbuminemia.

4. The patient's mental status may be altered by infection, severe dehydration, hypo- or hyperglycemia, marked electrolyte abnormalities (including significant acid–base disturbances), traumatic injury, primary central nervous system (CNS) disease, or drug/toxin ingestion.

C. Laboratory Studies

1. The following are the *minimal* studies necessary to adequately evaluate a patient with an acid–base disorder:

   a. Arterial blood gas (ABGs).
   b. Electrolyte panel.
   c. Glucose, blood urea nitrogen (BUN), and creatinine levels.
   d. Anion gap (calculated from the serum electrolytes).

2. Additional studies that are frequently useful, depending on clinical circumstances, may include one or more of the following:

   a. Urinalysis (including pH, specific gravity, and crystal examination).
   b. Blood ethanol level.
   c. Serum osmolarity.
   d. Serum ketones.
   e. Serum lactate level.
   f. Urinary electrolytes.
   g. Serum and/or urine toxicologic screen.

III. SPECIFIC ACID–BASE DISORDERS

A. Metabolic Acidosis

1. Causes of a *normal anion gap* metabolic acidosis include

   a. Enteric losses:
      i. Diarrhea: excess bicarbonate loss occurs in the stool. The ensuing volume contraction stimulates the renin–angiotensin system with resultant renal NaCl reabsorption and hyperchloremia.
      ii. Small bowel or pancreatic fistulas: may also cause significant gastrointestinal bicarbonate loss.

    iii. Ureteroenterostomies: surgical diversion of urine from the ureters to the sigmoid colon stimulates exchange of luminal chloride for blood bicarbonate and causes a hyperchloremic metabolic acidosis.

  b. Renal tubular acidoses (RTAs): disorders of the urinary acidification mechanism. They occur in a variety of disease states, including tubulointerstitial diseases (e.g., interstitial nephritis), autoimmune diseases (e.g., lupus nephritis), and diabetes mellitus. Mild RTAs may not become manifest until the kidney is stressed acutely by an added acid load.

    i. Type I (distal) RTA: characterized by a hyperchloremic, hypokalemic metabolic acidosis with a urinary pH > 5.5.

    ii. Type II (proximal) RTA: characterized by a hyperchloremic, hypokalemic metabolic acidosis with a urinary pH < 5.5 (though, initially, urine pH may be > 5.5 until serum bicarbonate concentration falls to 15–18 mEq/L).

    iii. Type IV (distal, hyperkalemic) RTA: usually occurs in the setting of renal insufficiency and is characterized by a hyperchloremic metabolic acidosis and hyperkalemia.

  c. Miscellaneous causes of a non-anion gap metabolic acidosis include vigorous volume resuscitation with normal saline, use of carbonic anhydrase inhibitors (e.g., acetazolamide), and adrenal insufficiency.

2. Causes of an *increased anion gap* metabolic acidosis include

  a. Exogenous acid: always consider the possibility of an ingested drug or toxin in the patient with a widened anion gap acidosis. Possible agents include salicylate, ethylene glycol, methanol, and paraldehyde.

    i. Salicylates act directly on the CNS, stimulating ventilation and promoting oxygen consumption and carbon dioxide production; they also inhibit oxidative phosphorylation. A mixed acid–base disorder (respiratory alkalosis and anion gap metabolic acidosis [lactate]) may result.

    ii. Ethylene glycol, the primary constituent of antifreeze, is metabolized to glycolic and oxalic acids. Renal and cardiopulmonary failure are life-threatening complications of poisoning. Laboratory clues to ethylene glycol ingestion are an increased osmolal gap, an anion gap metabolic acidosis, and the presence of "envelope" or needle-shaped calcium oxalate crystals in the urine.

    iii. Methanol is widely available as a solvent, a solid burning alcohol (Sterno), and as an additive to many substances (e.g., windshield wiper fluid, fuel substitutes, gasoline antifreeze). Methanol is metabolized to formic acid; like ethylene glycol, it causes an increased osmolal gap and an anion gap metabolic acidosis. Poisoning results in CNS dysfunction, abdominal pain, visual disturbances, and fundoscopic changes. Complications include blindness, renal failure, and death.

b. Endogenous acid: another source of unmeasured anions are those generated intrinsically. The added acid may accumulate rapidly and overwhelm buffering and compensatory mechanisms to the point of life-threatening acidosis.

    i. Lactic acidosis: occurs when lactic acid production is not matched by the metabolism of lactate back to pyruvate.

- Type A lactic acidosis occurs secondary to tissue hypoxia (e.g., shock, respiratory failure, severe anemia, carbon monoxide or cyanide poisoning, and local vascular compromise).

- Type B lactic acidosis occurs with apparently normal tissue perfusion and oxygenation. It may result from organ failure (e.g., liver disease, renal disease, sepsis, neoplasia), a drug or toxin (e.g., ethanol, ethylene glycol, methanol, phenformin, salicylates), or congenital errors of metabolism.

    An unusual cause of lactic acidosis can occur in patients with short-bowel syndromes. Intestinal overgrowth of lactobacilli may result in accumulation of the D-isomer of lactate. Because routine laboratory testing detects only L-lactate, this derangement may be missed unless specifically looked for.

    ii. Ketoacids are synthesized when glucose is unavailable because of starvation, insulin-deficient states (e.g., diabetic ketoacidosis), or when poor oral glucose intake is combined with absent hepatic glycogen stores (e.g., alcoholic ketoacidosis). Serum ketones are detected through the nitroprusside reaction; this test is quite sensitive for acetoacetate, weakly positive for acetone, but negative for the predominant ketoacid, beta hydroxybutyrate. Therefore, a negative serum ketone test does not rule out ketoacidosis.

    iii. In advanced chronic renal insufficiency, the accumulation of phosphate, sulfate, and other organic anions may cause an increased anion gap acidosis.

c. Pseudometabolic acidosis: may occur secondary to underfilling of Vacutainer tubes at the time of blood drawing. Serum bicarbonate declines and the anion gap increases when excess air is present in the blood tube (secondary to carbon dioxide diffusing out of the blood and into the air in the tube). To avoid this problem, completely fill vacutainer tubes.

B. Metabolic Alkalosis

1. *Gastrointestinal tract acid loss:* severe vomiting or prolonged nasogastric suction causes alkalosis because of HCl loss and volume depletion.

2. *Enhanced renal bicarbonate reclamation:* occurs in response to decreased renal perfusion and activation of the renin–angiotensin system. Renal hypoperfusion may occur secondary to intravascular volume depletion, diuretic use, poor oral intake, congestive heart failure with poor forward output, and decreased plasma oncotic pressure (e.g., in cirrhosis, nephrotic syndrome, or malnutrition). As the kidney attempts to maintain intravascular volume through sodium reabsorption, it retrieves its associated anions chloride and bicarbonate.

3. *Increased urinary acid secretion:* primary hyperaldosteronism and states of mineralocorticoid excess are associated with increased sodium reabsorption and enhanced urinary potassium and acid losses causing hypertension, hypokalemia, and metabolic alkalosis.

4. *Excessive bicarbonate intake:* the bicarbonate-secreting capacity of the kidney is readily overwhelmed by exogenous bicarbonate intake (bicarbonate-containing antacids, milk-alkali syndrome) or excess oral or parenteral alkali supplementation.

C. Respiratory Acidosis (increased PCO$_2$)

1. *Acute causes* of respiratory acidosis include
   a. CNS depression from ingested toxins, drugs (e.g., general anesthetics, opioids, sedative-hypnotics), head injury, infection, or acute cerebrovascular accidents.
   b. Neuromuscular abnormalities, which may compromise ventilation and include cervical spinal cord injury, specific neuromuscular diseases (e.g., Guillain-Barré syndrome), toxins (e.g., botulism), or drugs.
   c. Airway or pulmonary function impairment may result from airway obstruction (e.g., foreign-body aspiration, epiglottitis, laryngeal edema), severe bronchospastic disease, or pulmonary parenchymal disease (e.g., pneumonia, hemorrhage, adult respiratory distress syndrome).
   d. Hemodynamic compromise, which may result from severe cardiac dysfunction or massive pulmonary embolism.

2. *Chronic causes* of respiratory acidosis include
   a. CNS depression from brain stem neoplasms, prolonged use of sedatives or opioids, severe endocrine dysfunction, or obesity associated with chronic hypercapnia.
   b. Neuromuscular abnormalities secondary to amyotrophic lateral sclerosis, multiple sclerosis, polio, or muscular dystrophies.
   c. Airway and pulmonary diseases, including chronic obstructive pulmonary disease (COPD), structural limitations to ventilation (e.g., scoliosis, kyphosis, obesity), or severe long-standing parenchymal diseases.

D. Respiratory Alkalosis

Respiratory alkalosis may also develop acutely or be sustained for a prolonged interval. Enhanced bicarbonate excretion by the kidneys begins almost immediately but is rapidly diminished as bicarbonate concentrations are lowered. Approximately half of the compensation occurs within the first 24 hours and the remaining excretion requires 2–3 days. Causes include the following:

1. *CNS-mediated causes,* including infection, vascular accident, trauma, or drugs (e.g., salicylates). These may centrally stimulate hyperventilation. Other causes include intermittent panic attacks or the anxiety associated with arterial puncture.

2. *Pulmonary parenchymal diseases:* pulmonary edema, embolism, pneumonia, or fibrosis. These may cause hypocapnia through stimulation of nociceptive receptors within the lung.

3. *Hypoxemia* for any reason (e.g., hemodynamic collapse, high altitude, severe anemia) may augment respiration.

4. *Miscellaneous causes* of hypocapnia, including pregnancy (normal PCO_2 in the third trimester is 30 mmHg), hepatic disease, heat exposure, or excessive ventilation from mechanical ventilators.

E. Mixed Acid–Base Disorders

In a wide variety of clinical situations, the acid–base disturbance will be more complex than a single primary disorder and secondary compensation. It is important to identify other concomitant disorders; they will provide clues to the presence and severity of underlying diseases and influence therapy.

1. Combined Metabolic Derangements

a. Because bicarbonate is the primary buffer for added acids, a consistent stoichiometric relationship exists between the anion gap and the bicarbonate concentration. The addition of an organic or inorganic acid (other than HCl) produces an increase in the anion gap, which should equal the decrement in serum bicarbonate. Expressed another way:

$$\Delta AG \text{ (change in anion gap)} = \Delta HCO_3^- \text{ (change in bicarbonate).}$$

Calculation and comparison of the ΔAG and ΔHCO_3^- will determine whether more than one metabolic derangement is present simultaneously.

i. For example, in a simple lactic acidosis from physical exertion, the addition of lactic acid might cause the bicarbonate to decrease by 10 mEq/L (with a measured serum bicarbonate of 24 [normal serum bicarbonate] − 10 = *15 mEq/L*). The lactate is an unmeasured anion and the anion gap should also increase by 10 mEq/L (with the resultant anion gap being 12 [normal anion gap] + 10 = *22 mEq/L*). The *decrement* in the bicarbonate is equal to the *increment* in the anion gap; this is a simple anion gap metabolic acidosis.

ii. Sometimes, the ΔAG may *exceed* the ΔHCO_3^-. In this case, the original blood HCO_3^- concentration, prior to the addition of acid, was elevated (i.e., a metabolic alkalosis was present before the addition of a metabolic acidosis). Such a derangement might develop in a diabetic with intractable vomiting (metabolic alkalosis) who then develops ketoacidosis (anion gap metabolic acidosis).

iii. Sometimes, the ΔHCO_3^- may *exceed* the ΔAG. In this circumstance, the source of the added acids is both measured (i.e., HCl) and unmeasured anions. In other words, a normal and elevated anion gap acidosis coexist. Such a derangement might develop in a patient with severe diarrhea from cholera (non-anion gap metabolic acidosis) who secondarily develops profound volume depletion and lactic acidosis (anion gap metabolic acidosis).

b. *Remember:* occasionally a patient with combined metabolic alkalosis and normal anion gap acidosis will have *normal* concentrations of HCO_3^- and PCO_2. For example, a patient with concomitant diarrhea (non-anion gap metabolic acidosis) and vomiting (metabolic alkalosis) may present with a normal serum pH, PCO_2, and serum bicarbonate, yet still suffer from an acid–base disturbance. In this instance, the decrement in serum bicarbonate (from the diarrhea) is exactly offset by the loss of protons (in the vomitus); other than the history, the clue to the presence of this disorder is coexistent hypokalemia.

2. **Combined Respiratory and Metabolic Derangements.** Primary disorders of both types may coexist. These combinations may have the same effect on systemic pH and be additive, or they may offset each other and be counterbalancing. The key to identification of these mixed disturbances is evaluating the degree to which secondary compensation has taken place. Using the formulas listed in Table 17–1, it is possible to approximately predict the expected compensation. If the compensation differs significantly (overcorrection or undercorrection) from its predicted value, then a disturbance exists in that compensating organ system as well.

a. *Example:* a patient chronically on diuretics (with a resultant metabolic alkalosis) may then begin to retain carbon dioxide over and above compensation secondary to worsening COPD. While some degree of carbon dioxide retention to offset the alkalosis is normal, compensatory mechanisms always correct toward, but not to, normal. If the pH is normalized, then the degree of carbon dioxide retention is abnormal and a concomitant respiratory acidosis and metabolic alkalosis are present.

     b. *Example:* a patient on diuretics with a chronic metabolic alkalosis has a measured serum bicarbonate of 35 mEq/L. Using Table 17–1, one would predict a mild compensatory respiratory acidosis and a resultant PCO_2 of approximately 46 mmHg. If the measured PCO_2 from the ABG is actually 38 mmHg, then the patient has inadequately compensated for the metabolic alkalosis and has a mild respiratory alkalosis as well.

IV. THERAPY

A. *The cornerstone of therapy for an acid–base disorder is identification and treatment of the underlying disease process.* It is futile and potentially dangerous to attempt to ameliorate the chemical derangements without directing care toward the initiating insult. In fact, most acid–base disturbances are corrected by endogenous mechanisms given proper patient care (such as airway and breathing management, volume resuscitation, antibiotics, insulin, and nutritional repletion) and time.

B. *The primary therapy for severe, uncompensated metabolic acidosis should be proper ventilatory management* (e.g., hyperventilation to a PCO_2 of 25 mmHg, if necessary). Sodium bicarbonate therapy, after appropriate use of hyperventilation, is currently controversial. Potential complications of bicarbonate therapy include paradoxical cerebrospinal fluid and intracellular acidosis, impaired tissue oxygen delivery, hypokalemia, hypernatremia, hyperosmolality, volume overload, "overshoot" alkalosis, and/or hypocalcemia. On the other hand, profound metabolic acidosis compromises myocardial function and lowers the threshold for ventricular fibrillation. Consider sodium bicarbonate therapy in the following situations: (after first maximizing ventilatory management):

1. In *diabetic ketoacidosis* if the pH is < 7.00 or the measured serum HCO_3^- is < 6 mEq/L.

2. In *alcoholic ketoacidosis* if the pH is < 7.10.

3. In *lactic acidosis or other causes of metabolic acidosis* if the pH is < 7.2.

The goal of sodium bicarbonate is to keep the measured pH higher than the referenced thresholds above; the goal is *not* to normalize the pH. If intravenous sodium bicarbonate therapy is selected, it should be given slowly, the patient must be monitored carefully for evidence of volume overload; and arterial pH and blood chemistries must be checked frequently to avoid overcorrection, hypokalemia, and/or hypernatremia.

V. PEARLS AND PITFALLS

A. The proper identification of an acid–base disorder requires a thorough history and physical examination and a directed laboratory evaluation that minimally should include a serum electrolyte panel, ABG, and anion gap.

B. A normal blood pH, PCO_2 and serum bicarbonate does not rule out the presence of an acid–base disorder! One must also consider the anion gap and the clinical setting.

C. Compensatory mechanisms act to ameliorate, but not normalize, the pH change.

D. Clues to the presence of a mixed acid–base disturbance come from the history, electrolytes (e.g., hypokalemia in the setting of combined diarrhea and vomiting), the anion gap (e.g., when $\Delta AG \neq \Delta HCO_3^-$ from normal), and/or when the actual compensatory change is different from that predicted (see Table 17–1).

E. The possibility of toxin exposure should be considered in any patient with an anion gap metabolic acidosis.

F. The primary treatment of an acid–base disorder is appropriate therapy of the underlying condition responsible for the disorder.

G. Hyperventilation (to a PCO_2 of 25 mmHg, if necessary) is the treatment of choice for an uncompensated and severe metabolic acidosis.

BIBLIOGRAPHY

Narins RG: Acid–base disorders: definitions and introductory concepts. In Maxwell MH, Kleeman CR, Narins RG, (eds): Clinical Disorders of Fluid and Electrolyte Metabolism. 4th Ed. New York. McGraw-Hill, 1987.

ACUTE RENAL FAILURE

> *"Bones can break, muscles can atrophy,*
> *glands can loaf, even the brain can*
> *go to sleep without immediately endangering*
> *survival; but should the kidneys fail . . . neither bone,*
> *muscle, gland, nor brain could carry on."*
>
> HOMER W. SMITH

I. ESSENTIAL FACTS

A. Definition

Acute renal failure (ARF) is an abrupt decrease in renal function that results in nitrogenous waste retention. Serum blood urea nitrogen (BUN) and creatinine increase; volume, electrolyte, and acid–base disturbances may also occur. It is a true medical emergency associated with high morbidity and mortality.

1. An increased serum *creatinine* is generally a reliable marker of an impaired glomerular filtration rate (GFR) and compromised

renal function. Under steady-state conditions, a decrease in the GFR by 50% results in a doubling of the creatinine. The creatinine increases by 1.0–1.5 mg/dL per day in the complete absence of kidney function; daily increments are even greater in the setting of muscle injury (e.g., trauma, rhabomyolysis).

Note: acetoacetate (in ketoacidosis) and some commonly used medications (e.g., trimethoprim, cefoxitin, cimetidine) may spuriously elevate creatinine despite normal kidney filtration.

2. The *BUN* also increases in ARF (usually by 10–20 mg/dL per day), but it is not as reliable a marker of declining renal function as serum creatinine. Exogenous or endogenous protein loads may increase BUN independently of renal activity. Examples of the former include a high-protein diet and gastrointestinal hemorrhage; examples of the latter include burns, sepsis, and trauma. In the setting of low urine flow (e.g., dehydration, congestive heart failure, obstructive uropathy), BUN may also be elevated despite initially normal renal function.

3. *Oliguria* (< 30 mL/hr in the adult patient) may or may not occur in ARF; 30–50% of patients with ARF are nonoliguric.

B. Causes

ARF is classically divided into three broad diagnostic categories: prerenal, renal, and postrenal.

1. *Prerenal ARF* results from hypoperfusion of the kidney. If renal blood flow were normal, renal function would be normal because the kidneys are, at least initially, intact. As hypoperfusion persists, however, acute tubular necrosis (ATN; a type of intrinsic "renal" ARF) may result.

    a. Prerenal insults are responsible for 50–70% of all cases of ARF.
    b. Prerenal ARF may result from hypovolemia, impaired cardiac output, or hemodynamically mediated hypoperfusion at the microvascular level (e.g., renal prostaglandin inhibition secondary to nonsteroidal anti-inflammatory drugs [NSAIDs] or decreased glomerular efferent arteriolar tone secondary to angiotensin converting-enzyme inhibition). See III for a more extensive listing of prerenal causes.
    c. Clinical clues to the diagnosis may include
        i. A reasonable clinical scenario, including a history of volume loss, hypotension, congestive heart failure, shock, liver failure, NSAID or angiotensin converting enzyme (ACE) inhibitor use.
        ii. Elevated BUN/creatinine ratio (> 20:1).
        iii. Oliguria (< 500 mL/24 hr).
        iv. Normal or nearly normal urinary sediment (hyaline casts or rare granular casts may sometimes be seen).

v. Compatible urine indices (see Table 17–2):
- High urine specific gravity.
- High urine osmolality (> 500 mOsm/L).
- Low urinary sodium (≤ 20 mEq/L).
- Low fractional excretion of filtered sodium (FE Na < 1%).

Caution: none of the above clues is absolute. For example, recent diuretic use will elevate the urine sodium; glucosuria will elevate the urine sodium and osmolality. Patients with postrenal and renal ARF may, not infrequently, also have low urinary sodium.

2. *Postrenal ARF* occurs secondary to urinary tract obstruction and may be intrarenal or extrarenal. To adversely affect renal function (as measured by a rising serum creatinine), obstruction is bilateral, or the patient had renal insufficiency prior to the obstruction, or the patient has a solitary obstructed kidney.

   a. Postrenal insults account for only 1–10% of cases of ARF.
   b. Postrenal ARF may result from renal tubular obstruction (e.g., uric acid crystals, myeloma protein, methotrexate crystals), ureteral obstruction, or urethral obstruction (see III, below).
   c. Clinical clues to the diagnosis include one or more of the following:
      i. A reasonable clinical scenario, including males with suspected benign prostatic hypertrophy; individuals with known or suspected retroperitoneal carcinoma or sarcoma; patients with accelerated cellular turnover (e.g., high uric acid levels secondary to the treatment of

Table 17–2. INTERPRETING URINARY INDICES IN ARF

URINARY INDICES	PRERENAL ARF	ATN	POSTRENAL ARF
Osmolality	> 500 mOsm/L	< 350 mOsm/L	Initially > 500 mOsm/L, but decreases
Specific gravity	> 1.010	< 1.010	Variable
BUN/Creat (plasma)	> 20/1	10/1	> 20/1
U creat/P creat	≥ 20	≤ 10	Variable
U Na	≤ 20	≥ 40	> 100 in the postobstructive diuretic phase
FE Na	< 1%	> 2%	Variable

Notes: 1. In postrenal ARF most urinary indices are variable and depend on the completeness of obstruction and/or whether obstruction is superimposed on an interstitial process. 2. FE Na = (U Na/P Na) × (P creat/U creat); U-urine; p-plasma.

Adapted from Bursten S: Acute renal failure. Chapter 29. In Dugdale DC, Eisenberg MS (eds): Medical Diagnostics. Philadelphia, WB Saunders, 1992, p. 242.

acute leukemia or lymphoma); individuals receiving methotrexate therapy.

ii. Acute anuria indicates obstruction 90% of the time. Bladder catheterization is immediately indicated.

iii. Elevated BUN/creatinine ratio (> 20:1).

iv. Abdominal ultrasound or computed tomography (CT) scan showing hydronephrosis.

Note: early in extrarenal obstruction, a sonogram may be negative (in some cases hydronephrosis may take 24–72 hours to develop after the onset of obstruction).

v. Abnormal urine sediment (hematuria, pyuria, and/or crystals); the urine sediment may also be normal.

Urine indices are variable and generally nondiagnostic in postrenal ARF (see Table 17–2).

3. *Renal ARF* results from intrinsic disease of the renal parenchyma.

a. It is responsible for 20–30% of cases of ARF.

b. Renal ARF may result from damage to the renal tubules (ATN), interstitium (interstitial nephritis), glomeruli (glomerulonephritis), and/or blood vessels (vasculitis, thrombosis). In hospitalized patients, ATN is the most common cause of ARF and may be secondary to prolonged prerenal ischemia, nephrotoxins (e.g., aminoglycosides, radiographic contrast agents), or pigmenturia (e.g., intravascular hemolysis, rhabdomyolysis). Renal cortical necrosis is the most severe form of ATN; it may occur in conjunction with abruptio placenta, septic abortion, trauma, burns, sepsis, toxins, or hemorrhagic pancreatitis.

c. Clinical clues to the diagnosis include the following:

i. A reasonable clinical scenario, including a history of prolonged prerenal insult with subsequent ARF unresponsive to volume replacement; nephrotoxin exposure followed by a rising creatinine; renal failure after an episode of either intravascular hemolysis or rhabdomyolysis.

ii. Prerenal and postrenal ARF have been appropriately excluded (see B. 1 and 2, above).

iii. Abnormal urine sediment (e.g., erythrocytes, leukocytes, proteinuria, pigmented granular casts, erythrocyte casts, leukocyte casts, or eosinophiluria [using Hansel's stain; eosinophiluria indicates interstitial nephritis]).

iv. Urine indices (see Table 17–2): these are frequently helpful in differentiating ATN from prerenal ARF. In ATN, the following are commonly seen:

• Urine specific gravity < 1.010.

• Urine osmolality < 350 mOsm/L.

• Urinary sodium ≥ 40mEq/L.

• FE Na > 2%.

C. Epidemiology

1. Five percent of all hospitalized patients and $\leq 20\%$ of ICU patients develop some form of ARF.

2. Mortality varies depending on the underlying cause of the renal dysfunction: it is 30–35% if the cause is medical and $\geq 50\%$ if the cause is surgical. Nonoliguric ARF has a lower mortality rate than oliguric ARF (20–26% versus 40–65%, respectively). In most cases, the high mortality rate of ARF is related to the primary disease process and its associated complications (e.g., infection, cardiovascular disease, hemorrhage, other organ system failure).

3. Risk factors for ARF include
   a. Alcohol or other drug abuse.
   b. Cardiovascular disease (including ischemic heart disease and chronic congestive heart failure).
   c. Chronic liver disease.
   d. Chronic renal insufficiency.
   e. Diabetes mellitus.
   f. Elderly patients.
   g. Hypercalcemia.
   h. Hypertension.
   i. Hyperuricosuria.
   j. Infection (including hepatitis, infection with *Escherichia coli* 0157:H7, human immunodeficiency virus [HIV] infection, sepsis).
   k. Malignancy.
   l. Prostate disease.
   m. Systemic collagen vascular diseases (e.g., systemic lupus erythematosus [SLE]).
   n. Toxin exposure (including prescribed medications with nephrotoxic potential).
   o. Volume depletion.

II. CLINICAL EVALUATION

The history, physical examination, and laboratory findings are crucial in making the diagnosis of ARF. Every effort should be made to uncover the underlying cause since therapy varies with the cause of the syndrome.

A. History

1. Inquire about factors that affect intravascular volume, including vomiting, diarrhea, blood loss, and oral intake. Volume-depleted patients may complain of thirst and note a diminution in urine output. Bloody diarrhea may be associated with *E. coli* 0157:H7 infection and the hemolytic uremic syndrome (HUS). A history of a recently acquired and/or treated infectious disease raises the possibility of a rapidly progressive glomer-

ulonephritis. Hemoptysis is common with pulmonary–renal syndromes (e.g., SLE, Wegener's granulomatosis, Goodpasture's syndrome).

2. Ask about urinary tract symptoms, including flank pain, urgency, frequency, dysuria, hematuria, hesitancy, adequacy of the urinary stream, incontinence, and urine volume.

3. Accurately identify pre-existing medical problems (e.g., diabetes mellitus, congestive heart failure, prior renal insufficiency, alcoholism, hepatic compromise, rheumatologic disease, prostate disease, malignancy).

4. Obtain a thorough medication history. Many drugs can affect both volume status and intrinsic renal function.

5. Consider the possibility of exposure to toxins, including severe acetaminophen overdose, carbon tetrachloride, ethylene glycol, heavy metals, methanol, paraquat, and/or *Amanita phalloides* mushroom ingestion.

B. Physical Examination

Obtain vital signs and evaluate the skin, HEENT, neck, chest, heart, abdomen (include a rectal examination and stool heme test), extremities, and nervous system. In the stable patient, obtain orthostatic vital signs and compare current to baseline body weight.

1. Note skin turgor (as a reflection of dehydration). A rash or purpura may represent an underlying collagen vascular disease, thrombotic thrombocytopenic purpura (TTP), the HUS, or significant infection.

2. The mucosa of the tongue may also reveal evidence of dehydration. Note the breath for the smell of acetone or the fruity odor of ketones. Fundoscopic changes may be seen in methanol poisoning, diabetes mellitus, or hypertensive crises.

3. Carefully evaluate for costovertebral angle tenderness, renal artery bruits, suprapubic tenderness, palpable kidneys, and bladder distention.

4. Evaluate for uterine and ovarian masses in females. In males, note the urethral meatus for size and patency, examine scrotal contents, and assess the prostate for size, tenderness, and nodules.

5. Peripheral edema may indicate right-sided congestive heart failure, hepatic disease, or hypoalbuminemia. Also evaluate the joints for tenderness and/or inflammatory abnormalities.

C. Laboratory Studies

1. The following are the *minimal* studies necessary to initially evaluate a patient with ARF:

   a. Creatinine and BUN levels (compare with prior values if available).

   b. Electrolyte panel, glucose level.

    c. Anion gap (calculated from the serum electrolytes).

    d. Urinalysis (including microscopic examination of the sediment for erythocyte casts [glomerulonephritis], leukocyte casts [interstitial nephritis, pyelonephritis], tubular or "muddy brown casts" [ATN], dysmorphic erythrocytes [origin in the upper urinary tract] and/or normal erythrocytes [origin in the lower urinary tract]).

    e. Urine sodium and determination of the FE Na (see Table 17–2).

    f. Complete blood count.

    g. Calcium, magnesium, phosphate, and uric acid levels.

    h. Electrocardiogram (ECG).

    i. Chest roentgenogram.

    j. Serum or urine pregnancy test (in sexually active females of reproductive age).

2. Additional studies that are frequently useful to the ED physician, depending on clinical circumstances, may include *one or more* of the following:

    a. Renal ultrasound (to evaluate for obstruction and renal size, and to verify the presence of two kidneys).

    b. Arterial blood gas (ABG).

    c. Appropriate cultures (e.g., blood, urine, stool).

    d. Blood ethanol level.

    e. Creatinine kinase level (CK; elevated in rhabdomyolysis).

    f. Liver function tests.

    g. Serum osmolality.

    h. Toxicologic studies.

    i. Urine and serum eosinophils (may be positive in interstitial nephritis).

3. Other studies may be requested by the medicine or nephrology consultant, depending on clinical circumstances (e.g., anti-glomerular basement membrane [GBM] antibody [Goodpasture's disease, anti-GBM disease], antineutrophilic cytoplasmic antibody [positive in Wegener's granulomatosis], antinuclear antibodies [in SLE], antistreptolysin O titer [in poststreptococcal glomerulonephritis], erythrocyte sedimentation rate, hepatitis virus antibodies [hepatitis A, B, and/or C], serum complement, serum and urine protein electrophoresis [SPEP and UPEP, respectively; abnormal in multiple myeloma and Bence-Jones proteinuria]).

III. DIFFERENTIAL DIAGNOSIS

The many causes of ARF are outlined in detail below:

A. Prerenal Acute Renal Failure

1. **Decreased Intravascular and Extravascular Volume**

    a. Burns

    b. Dehydration (diaphoresis or other skin losses, excessive

    renal losses [diuretics, osmotic diuresis], poor oral intake, respiratory losses).

  c. Gastrointestinal losses (diarrhea, nasogastric suctioning, vomiting).

  d. Hemorrhage.

2. **Decreased Intravascular Volume/Renal Perfusion with Increased Extravascular Volume**

  a. Anaphylaxis.

  b. Cirrhosis.

  c. Congestive heart failure.

  d. Nephrotic syndrome.

  e. Sepsis.

  f. Third-spacing (including crush injury, pancreatitis, postsurgery).

3. **Medications (Microvascular Hemodynamically Mediated Changes)**

  a. ACE inhibitors (e.g., captopril, enalapril).

  b. NSAIDs.

4. **Other**

  a. Hepatorenal syndrome.

  b. Overtreatment of chronic severe hypertension.

  c. Renal artery stenosis.

B. Renal Acute Renal Failure

1. **Acute Tubular Necrosis**

  a. Drugs (acyclovir, aminoglycosides, amphotericin, cisplatin, cyclosporine, pentamidine, radiographic contrast agents).

  b. Hypercalcemia.

  c. Ischemia (hypotension, hypoxia, prolonged prerenal insult, sepsis, shock, trauma).

  d. Obstetrical complications (abruptio placentae, septic abortion).

  e. Pigmenturia (hemoglobinuria, myoglobinuria).

  f. Poisoning (acetaminophen overdose, carbon tetrachloride, ethylene glycol, heavy metals, methanol, paraquat, *A. phalloides* mushroom ingestion).

2. **Glomerular Diseases**

  a. Primary renal disease (acute poststreptococcal glomerulonephritis, antiglomerular basement membrane disease, idiopathic rapidly progressive glomerulonephritis, IgA nephritis, membranoproliferative glomerulonephritis).

  b. Systemic diseases (cryoglobulinemia, Goodpasture's syndrome, HUS, Henoch-Schönlein purpura, SLE, TTP).

  c. Systemic infection (bacterial endocarditis, hepatitis B infection, HIV-associated nephropathy, ventriculoatrial shunt infection, visceral abscesses).

    d. Vasculitis (hypersensitivity vasculitis, polyarteritis nodosa, Wegener's granulomatosis).

3. **Interstitial Nephritis**

    a. Antibiotics (including cephalosporins, penicillins, quinolones, rifampin, sulfonamides, tetracycline, vancomycin).

    b. Diuretics.

    c. NSAIDs.

    d. Other medications (allopurinol, aspirin, azathioprine, captopril, carbamazepine, cimetidine, phenobarbital, phenytoin).

    e. Systemic infections (including *Legionella,* leptospirosis, mononucleosis, *Mycoplasma,* Rocky Mountain spotted fever, *Streptococcus,* syphilis, *Toxoplasma*).

4. **Vascular Diseases**

    a. Atheroembolic disease (including bacterial endocarditis, multiple cholesterol emboli syndrome).

    b. Systemic disease (acute vasculitis, malignant hypertension, nephrosclerosis, scleroderma).

C. Postrenal Acute Renal Failure

1. **Intrarenal Obstruction.** Methotrexate crystals, uric acid crystals.

2. **Extrarenal Obstruction**

    a. Ureteral obstruction (blood clot; calculi; fungus ball; necrotic papillae; retroperitoneal carcinoma, fibrosis, or sarcoma).

    b. Urethral obstruction (bladder dysfunction, bladder tumor, blood clot, calculi, cervical carcinoma, prostatic disease, phimosis, stricture).

IV. THERAPY

A. Management of Immediately Life-Threatening Conditions

The patient in acute renal failure may be critically ill from either a concomitant medical/surgical disorder or the ARF itself. The highest initial priorities of the ED physician are evaluating for, and *simultaneously* treating as necessary, hypoxia, hypoventilation, hypovolemia, hemodynamic instability, cardiac dysfunction, life-threatening electrolyte disturbances (especially hyperkalemia), and significant toxin exposure.

1. *Assess, secure, and support* the *airway and breathing* as required.

2. *Simultaneously* with the above, supporting ED staff should initiate continuous monitoring of the cardiac rhythm and oxygen saturation. Obtain vital signs and intravenous (IV)

access, and perform the necessary physical examination, appropriate laboratory studies, and a 12-lead ECG. Closely scrutinize the ECG for evidence of myocardial ischemia and hyperkalemia.

3. *Hypovolemia and/or hypotension* should be treated with crystalloid infusion. Normal saline (NS) is the initial fluid of choice. Do *not* use lactated Ringer's solution (LR) in the setting of ARF; LR contains potassium (4 mEq/L) and may exacerbate hyperkalemia. If hemorrhage is the cause of hemodynamic instability, consider appropriate blood products as indicated.

   a. Use pressors in *nonhemorrhagic shock* if findings on cardiopulmonary examination contraindicate further normal saline administration. In most instances, dopamine will be the drug of choice (*dose:* begin with 2–5 µg/kg/min IV infusion and adjust as necessary to maintain a systolic blood pressure [BP] of approximately 95–100 mmHg).

   b. Volume management is critical in patients with ARF. If the patient is hemodynamically stable, a fluid challenge is reasonable to rule out at a prerenal cause of ARF (see IV. B, below). Do not, however, excessively volume overload the patient; pulmonary edema should always be avoided.

4. *Maximize cardiac function.* Impaired cardiac output may be caused by congestive heart failure, myocardial ischemia, hypertensive crisis, constrictive pericarditis, significant valvular heart disease, massive pulmonary embolus, or cardiac tamponade. Therapy should be directed at maximizing oxygenation, optimizing fluid management, and treating the specific condition(s) as indicated. See the appropriate sections in this manual pertaining to the relevant cardiopulmonary condition in need of therapy.

5. *Manage life-threatening hyperkalemia.* Emergently institute therapy for the clinical and ECG manifestations of hyperkalemia, which occur when the serum potassium is > 6.0–6.5 mEq/L. Hyperkalemic ECG changes begin with peaked T waves and progress to a prolonged PR-interval, widened QRS complex, eventual loss of the P wave, final widening of the QRS complex into a sine-wave configuration, and, ultimately, ventricular fibrillation. The following medications may be life-saving (also see the discussion of hyperkalemia in Electrolyte Disorders later in this chapter):

   a. Calcium chloride: 5–10 mL of a 10% solution (13.6 mEq/10 mL) IV over 2–5 minutes. The dose may be repeated in 5 minutes if no response is seen. Calcium is the initial drug of choice in the symptomatic hyperkalemic patient. Its effects occur immediately and last approximately 60 minutes.

   b. Sodium bicarbonate: 50 mEq IV over 5 minutes. The dose may be repeated in 10–15 minutes if ECG changes persist. Onset of action occurs in 5–10 minutes and effects may last 1–2 hours.

   c. Glucose: 25 g (50 mL of 50% dextrose in water) given IV over 5 minutes, *and*
      Insulin: 8–10 units regular insulin IV given concomitantly.
         Glucose and insulin shift potassium from the extracellular fluid (ECF) into cells. A response is seen in 30 minutes and effects last ≤ 4–6 hours.
   d. Sodium polystyrene sulfonate (Kayexalate):
      i. Oral (PO): 15–30 g in 50–100 mL of 20% sorbitol orally, may repeat every 3–4 hours, up to 4–5 doses per day, *or*
      ii. Rectal (PR): 50 g in 200 mL of 20% sorbitol (or 20% dextrose in water if sorbitol not available) given as a retention enema (the patient should retain the enema for 30–60 minutes). The dose may be repeated every 4–6 hours, up to four doses per day.
   e. Dialysis is indicated for severe hyperkalemia when the above therapy is not adequate and/or there are other indications for dialysis (see IV. D, below).

6. *Identify and manage toxin exposures.* The patient's ARF may be due to poisoning, and management should proceed as outlined in detail in Chapter 23.

B. Identification and Treatment of Postrenal and Prerenal Causes of ARF

   After imminently life-threatening conditions have been identified and managed, the next priority is to accurately diagnose and treat postrenal and other prerenal causes of ARF.

1. **Postrenal ARF Management.** Anuria or fluctuating urine output suggests obstruction.
   a. A Foley catheter should always be placed in the patient with ARF to rule out bladder outlet obstruction. The indwelling catheter can be used to closely monitor urine output.
   b. Ureteral obstruction, as revealed by renal ultrasound examination, mandates urologic consultation. Percutaneous nephrostomy may be necessary depending on the cause of obstruction.
   c. With relief of severe obstruction, a postobstructive diuresis may ensue: manage fluid and electrolytes closely as guided by vital signs, clinical examination, urine output, and serum/urine electrolyte measurements.

2. **Prerenal ARF Management.** Accurate therapy depends on the specific cause. If there is any possibility of hypovolemia, fluid challenge is appropriate. Normal saline is the crystalloid of choice; 500–1000 mL or more should be infused over 30–60 minutes as clinically indicated. Blood products should be considered as needed if hemorrhage is a contributing cause. Vital signs, cardiopulmonary status, and urine output must be monitored carefully. Do not worsen the patient's clinical status

by excessive volume replacement and resultant pulmonary edema.

C. Conversion of Oliguric ARF into Nonoliguric ARF

Nonoliguric ARF is easier to manage and has a lower mortality rate than oliguric ARF. If the patient remains oliguric despite ruling out postrenal causes and after appropriate fluid challenge, attempt to establish increased urine output with pharmacologic manipulation.

One or more of the following agents may be tried. Also consult a nephrologist.

1. Furosemide (Lasix)

   Dose: 40–80 mg given slowly IV. If there is no response in 30–60 minutes the dose may be doubled. Continuous furosemide infusions (2–4 mg/min till the desired dose is administered) decrease ototoxicity and require lower total doses.

   Caution: administration of furosemide to the patient with ARF is associated with a significant risk of hearing loss. To minimize this risk, the drug should be given slowly, and doses > 200 mg should probably not be used.

2. Metolazone: this medication may facilitate diuresis when administered with IV furosemide.

   Dose: 5–10 mg PO given concomitantly with IV furosemide.

3. Mannitol

   Dose: 12.5–25 g of 25% mannitol given IV over 5–10 minutes. In the setting of rhabdomyolysis, this initial mannitol dose may be followed by a combined mannitol and bicarbonate infusion (25 g of mannitol and 100 mEq of sodium bicarbonate added to 800 mL of 5% dextrose in water; infuse at 200 mL/hr for 5 hours [1 L total]).

   Caution: mannitol may exacerbate volume overload and pulmonary edema. If the patient does not initiate diuresis with the above 12.5–25-g dose, repeat doses should not be given.

4. Dopamine: at low doses dopamine dilates renal vessels. Clear-cut efficacy in the setting of ARF, however, has not been demonstrated.

   Dose: 1–3 µg/kg/min IV.

D. Hemodialysis

Hemodialysis utilizes a semipermeable membrane to remove certain substances from the blood by virtue of differences in their rates of diffusion from the blood, across that membrane, and into a dialysate solution. Prompt consultation with a nephrologist is mandatory; the patient will require proper venous access (i.e., dialysis catheter placement). Any of the following are reasonable indications for dialysis in the patient with ARF if the described abnormalities are not correctable by more conservative measures:

1. Hyperkalemia: ECG changes and/or a potassium level > 6.5 mEq/L.

2. Severe hyponatremia (serum sodium < 120 mEq/L) in the setting of hypervolemia, ARF, and/or significant mental status changes.

3. Hypervolemia: severe congestive heart failure unmanageable with diuretics and other appropriate therapy.

4. Uremia: BUN > 100 mg/dL, creatinine >10 mg/dL, changed mental status and/or other uremic symptoms/signs, uremic pericarditis, or bleeding.

5. Acidosis: pH < 7.2 and ongoing acid production not correctable by other means (e.g., hyperventilation and/or parenteral sodium bicarbonate).

6. Poisoning:
   a. Acute acetaminophen ingestion if the 4-hour postingestion blood level is >300 μg/mL.
   b. *A. phalloides* mushroom ingestion.
   c. Ethylene glycol; *any* of the following are indications for hemodialysis: symptomatic poisoning, significant metabolic acidosis, significant renal dysfunction, pulmonary edema, or serum level > 25 mg/dL.
   d. Lithium; *any* of the following are indications for hemodialysis: moderate or severe central nervous system symptoms, cardiac arrhythmias, serum levels ≥ 3.5 mEq/L, or patients with renal insufficiency and levels ≥ 2.0 mEq/L.
   e. Methanol; *any* of the following are indications for hemodialysis: metabolic acidosis, visual symptoms, renal dysfunction, blood methanol level > 20–25 mg/dL, or a history of ingestion ≥ 40 mL by an adult.
   f. Severe parathion overdose.
   g. Salicylates; *any* of the following are indications for hemodialysis: severe toxicity as predicted by the Done nomogram (e.g., salicylate level > 120 mg/dL at 6 hours post-acute ingestion), ARF, pulmonary edema (cardiogenic or noncardiogenic), coma, severe acid–base and/or electrolyte abnormalities despite appropriate therapy, hepatic compromise, or coagulopathy.

V. DISPOSITION

A. Discharge

Patients with new-onset *mild* renal insufficiency may be discharged to home if *all* of the following conditions apply:

1. Prerenal and postrenal causes of azotemia have been identified and corrected.

2. All potential nephrotoxic drugs have been discontinued.

3. The patient has been instructed to avoid potassium-containing products and to restrict potassium in the diet.

4. Vital signs are normal.

5. No other condition or serious problem has been identified that mandates admission (e.g., patient is *not* hyperkalemic, acidotic, or in significant congestive heart failure).

6. Follow-up is arranged within several days.

7. The patient is reliable.

B. Admit

All patients with frank ARF require hospitalization for further evaluation and treatment and continued management of potential complications. The admitting service will vary with the specific cause of the ARF. Consultation with a nephrologist is always appropriate.

VI. PEARLS AND PITFALLS

A. The highest initial treatment priorities for the ED physician caring for the patient in ARF are the ABCs (airway, breathing, and circulation), appropriate fluid management, therapy for cardiac disease, correction of hyperkalemia, and necessary treatment of any toxin exposure.

B. Any prerenal contributions to ARF must be accurately identified and corrected; prolonged prerenal insults will ultimately cause ATN.

C. Place a Foley catheter to rule out bladder outlet obstruction and to closely monitor urine output.

D. Renal ultrasound should always be considered to rule out ureteral obstruction and to evaluate renal size, position, and number.

E. Discontinue all unnecessary medications and stop all potential nephrotoxins (e.g., radiographic contrast agents, aminoglycosides, NSAIDs, ACE inhibitors).

F. Carefully dose all medications in the patient with altered renal function. Many drugs require reduced dosing or prolonged intervals between doses. Review with a pharmacist as required before prescribing any new medication.

G. Look at a freshly spun urine specimen yourself (most laboratories underreport urine findings, especially casts).

H. Consider the possibility of toxin exposure; evaluate and treat as required.

I. Consider the possibility of a spuriously elevated BUN and/or creatinine:

1. BUN may be increased by any of the following despite normal renal function:
   a. High-protein diet.
   b. Gastrointestinal hemorrhage.
   c. Large hematomas.
   d. Tetracylines.
   e. Steroids.
   f. High tumor burden (lymphoma).
   g. Total parenteral nutrition.

2. Creatinine may be increased by any of the following despite normal renal function:
   a. Ketoacidosis.
   b. Cimetidine, trimethoprim (these block tubular secretion of creatinine).
   c. Cefoxitin (interferes with the serum creatinine assay).

J. Bleeding associated with uremia may benefit from desmopressin acetate (DDAVP; 0.3 µg/kg in 50 mL NS IV over 15–30 minutes).

K. Uric acid nephropathy may be prevented in the setting of cytotoxic therapy for hematologic malignancies by optimizing hydration, alkaline diuresis, and by pretreatment with allopurinol (600 mg PO initially, followed by 100–300 mg PO daily).

Do *not* do any of the following:

A. Iatrogenically volume overload the oliguric patient.

B. Administer potassium-containing medications or IV fluids (e.g., LR) to the patient with anuria, oliguria, or borderline elevated serum potassium, or the patient with frank ARF.

C. Administer IV furosemide rapidly or in doses in excess of 200 mg to the patient with ARF.

D. Prescribe any magnesium-containing compounds (e.g., antacids, sucralfate) to the patient with ARF.

E. Administer radiographic contrast agents to the patient with renal insufficiency.

BIBLIOGRAPHY

Adcox M, Collins B, Zager R: The differential diagnosis of acute renal failure, in Narins R, Stein J (eds): Diagnostic Techniques in Renal Disease. Contemporary Issues in Nephrology. New York, Churchill Livingstone, 1992, pp. 73–117.

Anderson RJ (ed): Acute renal failure, in The Principles and Practice of Nephrology. Philadelphia, BC Becker, 1991, pp. 626–666.

Anderson RJ: Prevention and management of acute renal failure. Hosp Pract 1993;15:61–75.

Jennette JC, Falk RJ: Diagnosis and management of glomerulonephritis and vasculitis presenting as acute renal failure. Med Clin N. Am 1990;74(4):893–907.

Martinez-Maldonado M, Kumjian D: Acute renal failure due to urinary tract obstruction. Med Clin N Am 1990;74(4):919–923.

ELECTROLYTE DISORDERS

> "...I will venture to predict that what the knowledge of anatomy at present is to the surgeon . . .
> so will chemistry be to the physician in directing him generally, what to do and what to shun;
> and, in short, enabling him to wield his remedies with a certainty and precision."
>
> WILLIAM PROUT (1785–1850)

Calcium

The normal total serum calcium is 8.7–10.6 mg/dL. Approximately 40–50% of this total is bound to protein (primarily albumin); 10–15% is complexed to a variety of anions (e.g., bicarbonate, citrate, and phosphate); and 45–50% is in a freely ionized state. The freely ionized portion is metabolically important and is responsible for the signs and symptoms of calcium disorders.

Changes in serum albumin result in proportional changes in total serum calcium: total serum calcium falls by 0.8 mg/dL for every 1.0-g/dL decrease in serum albumin. This is an important consideration in several clinical settings (e.g., the chronically ill or protein-malnourished patient). The metabolically active ionized serum calcium is not affected, however, by changes in the serum albumin. Many laboratories can measure the ionized portion, and this is the test of choice when an abnormal albumin concentration is suspected.

The patient's acid–base status also affects the ionized portion of serum calcium: acidemia increases and alkalemia decreases the ionized calcium.

I. HYPERCALCEMIA

A. Definition

Hypercalcemia is a serum level > 10.6 mg/dL. Minimally elevated values (10.7–11.5 mg/dL) warrant retesting on an outpatient basis multiple times to determine the mean serum calcium level. Signs and symptoms of hypercalcemia usually do not become manifest until the total serum calcium is >11.5 mg/dL.

B. Etiology

1. Hyperparathyroidism.
2. Malignancy (e.g., breast, head and neck, kidney, lung, multiple myeloma or other hematologic malignancies).
3. Nonparathyroid endocrine disorders:
   a. Acromegaly.
   b. Adrenal insufficiency.
   c. Hyperthyroidism.
   d. Pheochromocytoma.

      e. Vasoactive intestinal polypeptide hormone-producing tumors.

  4. Granulomatous diseases:
      a. Coccidioidomycosis.
      b. Histoplasmosis.
      c. Leprosy.
      d. Sarcoidosis.
      e. Tuberculosis.

  5. Medications:
      a. Estrogens and antiestrogens.
      b. Lithium.
      c. Thiazide diuretics.
      d. Vitamin A or D intoxication.

  6. Miscellaneous:
      a. Acute or chronic renal insufficiency.
      b. Familial hypocalciuric hypercalcemia.
      c. Iatrogenic (including parenteral nutrition).
      d. Milk-alkali syndrome (excessive, prolonged ingestion of large quantities of both alkali and milk or calcium salts).
      e. Paget's disease.
      f. Prolonged immobilization.
      g. Spurious hypercalcemia (from either laboratory error or prolonged application of a tourniquet prior to obtaining the blood sample).

C. Signs and Symptoms

These may include one or more of the following when the serum calcium level exceeds 11.5 mg/dL:

1. *Central nervous system:* difficulty concentrating, fatigue, headaches, memory loss, mental status changes, psychosis, stupor and coma.

2. *Gastrointestinal:* abdominal pain, anorexia, constipation, nausea and vomiting, pancreatitis, peptic ulcer disease, weight loss.

3. *Renal:* acute renal failure, loss of renal concentrating ability, nephrocalcinosis (calcium phosphate deposition in the renal tubules resulting in renal insufficiency), nephrolithiasis (renal calculi), polydipsia and polyuria.

4. *Cardiovascular:* arrhythmias, exacerbation of digitalis toxicity, hypertension, shortened QT-interval.

5. *Miscellaneous:* bone aches, conjunctivitis, difficulty focusing, pruritis, pseudogout, weakness.

D. Diagnosis

In addition to a confirmed elevated total serum calcium level, patient evaluation should include a careful history and physical examination (keeping in mind the disorders listed under I. B, above) and further laboratory workup (including a complete blood count [CBC]; serum electrolyte panel; blood urea nitrogen [BUN]; creatinine, glucose, phosphate, and magnesium levels; urinalysis; and electrocardiogram [ECG]). Depending on clinical circumstances, additional studies may be indicated (e.g., chest roentgenogram, serum parathyroid hormone assay, thyroid screen).

E. Therapy

The aggressiveness of therapy is determined by both the serum calcium level and the patient's symptoms.

1. Asymptomatic patients should have an elevated serum calcium level rechecked; if the elevated level is confirmed, a thorough diagnostic evaluation is indicated as outlined above. Under these circumstances, treatment of mild hypercalcemia in the asymptomatic patient depends on its cause and will generally be managed by the outpatient referral physician.

2. Patients with hypercalcemia accompanied by mild or worse symptoms should be treated with volume expansion ± furosemide.
   a. Administer 0.9% normal saline (NS) to expand the extracellular fluid volume: 1–2 L intravenously (IV) over 2–4 hours, followed by 200–300 mL/hr as the patient's clinical condition allows.
   b. Once volume expansion has been accomplished, administer furosemide (begin with 20–40 mg given slowly IV) to enhance renal calcium excretion.
   c. Maintain urine output at 200–300 mL/hr.
   d. *Caution:* closely monitor fluid and electrolyte status (especially serum potassium); do not allow the patient to become volume depleted.

3. Patients with significant hypercalcemia accompanied by moderate to severe symptoms frequently require *additional therapy* with one or more of the following agents as appropriate to the cause of hypercalcemia. Obtain specialist consultation (e.g., internal medicine, oncology, nephrology) and arrange for hospitalization.

   a. **Calcitonin**
      Caution: calcitonin is a foreign protein derived from salmon. Before administration, give a 1 unit test intradermal dose. A wheal and flare reaction contraindicates further administration.
      i. *Indications:* hypercalcemia secondary to enhanced bone resorption (e.g., hyperparathyroidism, malignancy-associated hypercalcemia, vitamin A intoxication, Paget's disease).
      ii. *Dose:* 4 units/kg subcutaneously (SQ) or intramuscularly (IM) every 12 hours. May increase to maximum dose of 8 units/kg every 6 hours if necessary.

    iii. *Comments:* onset of action occurs within 1–2 hours; the nadir in serum calcium is reached in 12–24 hours. Unfortunately, calcitonin is a relatively weak agent, and tachyphylaxis develops in several days. Side effects may include flushing, nausea, and vomiting. It is contraindicated in the setting of hypersensitivity to salmon protein or the gelatin diluent. If hypercalcemia is severe, calcitonin may be used with mithramycin (see E. 3. e., below) awaiting the onset of the latter. Concomitant glucocorticoid therapy may prolong the hypocalcemic effect.

b. **Glucocorticoids**

    i. *Indication:* hypercalcemia secondary to granulomatous diseases, vitamin D intoxication, calcium hyperabsorption (e.g., the milk-alkali syndrome), myeloma or other hematologic malignancies.

    ii. *Dose:* **hydrocortisone** (50–100 mg IV every 6 hours) or **prednisone** (20–50 mg orally [PO] bid).

    iii. *Comments:* time of onset is generally 2–3 days or longer. The usual and many glucocorticoid side effects may be encountered with continued use.

c. **Oral Phosphate**

    i. *Indication:* may be used to gradually lower mild hypercalcemia in the setting of concomitant hypophosphatemia.

    ii. *Dose:* 0.5–1.0 g elemental phosphorus PO tid.

    iii. *Comments:* do not administer phosphate if the renal function is abnormal, serum phosphate is elevated, or the product of serum calcium and phosphorus (measured in mg/dL) is $\geq$ 60. Side effects may include soft tissue calcification, nausea, and/or diarrhea. Oral phosphate is unlikely to be of much help in the setting of severe hypercalcemia. Intravenous phosphate should *not* be administered to treat hypercalcemia.

d. **Dialysis** (using a calcium-free dialysis fluid)

    i. *Indication:* significant symptomatic hypercalcemia in patients with severe congestive heart failure or renal failure.

    ii. *Comments:* serum levels are usually only lowered temporarily.

e. **Miscellaneous agents for the treatment of moderate to severe hypercalcemia.** One of the following agents is generally appropriate if significant and symptomatic hypercalcemia is unresponsive to NS volume expansion and furosemide. The underlying cause of hypercalcemia under these circumstances is frequently a malignancy.

    i. Mithramycin (plicamycin): 25 µg/kg in 500 mL 5% dextrose in water (D5W) infused IV over 4–6 hours (use one-half this dose in the setting of hepatic or renal dysfunction). The dose may be repeated if necessary in 24–48 hours. Side effects are significant and may include thrombocytopenia, nephrotoxicity, and hepato-toxicity. Mithramycin is contraindicated in patients with bleeding diatheses, bone marrow function impairment, coagulation disorders, pregnancy, or thrombocytopenia. Onset of action usually occurs within 24 hours and the nadir in serum calcium occurs in 2–4 days. Duration of action may be a few days to several weeks.

   ii. Pamidronate: if serum calcium is 12–13 mg/dL administer 60–90 mg in 1 L NS IV over 24 hours; do not repeat the dose within 7 days. If serum calcium is >13.5 mg/dL, use the 90-mg dose; do not repeat the dose within 7 days. This agent is potentially nephrotoxic. Serum calcium will begin to decrease in approximately 2 days; the nadir occurs within 7 days.

   iii. Etidronate: 7.5 mg/kg in 250 mL NS IV over 4 hours daily for 3–7 days. Potentially nephrotoxic; do not use if the serum creatinine is > 2.5 mg/dL. Serum calcium will begin to decrease in 2 days; the nadir occurs within 7 days.

   iv. Gallium nitrite: 200 mg/m2 in 1 L D5W or NS IV over 24 hours daily for 5 days. Maintain a saline diuresis throughout therapy. This drug is contraindicated in patients with a serum creatinine > 2.5 mg/dL. Experience with this agent is limited. A decrease in serum calcium occurs slowly; the nadir may occur as late as 8 days after the start of the infusion.

F. Disposition

1. Patients with mild and asymptomatic hypercalcemia (serum calcium < 11.5–12 mg/dL) may be discharged to home with appropriate outpatient follow-up for further diagnosis and therapy.

2. Individuals with serum calcium levels ≥ 12 mg/dL or more than just mild symptoms of hypercalcemia, and those requiring saline volume expansion ± furosemide treatment in the ED should be hospitalized.

II. HYPOCALCEMIA

A. Definition

1. Hypocalcemia is a serum calcium level < 8.6 mg/dL; symptoms may develop rapidly when hypocalcemia is significant (< 6.5 mg/dL). True hypocalcemia, however, implies that the metabolically active *ionized calcium* is abnormally low.

2. *Remember:* total serum calcium varies with changes in serum albumin without affecting the metabolically important ionized portion.

3. Acid–base status affects the ionized portion: alkalemia worsens symptomatic hypocalcemia.

B. Etiology

1. Situational:
   a. Alkalemia.
   b. Hypoalbuminemia.
   c. Increased concentrations of free fatty acids.

2. Hypoparathyroidism:
   a. Surgical removal.
   b. Infiltrative disease (e.g., amyloidosis, hemochromatosis, metastatic cancer, thalessemia, Wilson's disease).
   c. Idiopathic parathyroid gland hypofunction.
   d. Significant hyper- or hypomagnesemia.
   e. Ionizing radiation or chemotherapy.
   f. Congenital disorders (e.g., DiGeorge's syndrome).
   g. Pseudohypoparathyroidism (a hereditary condition clinically resembling hypoparathyroidism caused by a failure to respond to appropriate levels of parathyroid hormone).

3. Vitamin D disorders:
   a. Diminished absorption (including nutritional deficiency and fat malabsorption).
   b. Enhanced loss (e.g., chronic renal disease, liver disease).
   c. Vitamin D-resistant rickets.
   d. Renal failure.
   e. Rickets (the clinical condition caused by vitamin D deficiency in infancy and childhood resulting in abnormal ossification).

4. Miscellaneous conditions (resulting in rapid removal of ionized calcium):
   a. Acute pancreatitis.
   b. Blood transfusion (citrate binding of calcium).
   c. Osteoblastic metastases.
   d. Phosphate administration (including IV phosphate or phosphate enemas).
   e. Poisoning (e.g., ethylene glycol, hydrofluoric acid).
   f. Postparathyroidectomy ('hungry bone" syndrome).
   g. Release of cellular phosphate (e.g., chemotherapy, rapid tumor lysis, rhabdomyolysis).
   h. Sodium EDTA administration.
   i. Toxic shock syndrome.

C. Signs and Symptoms

These depend on both the actual degree of hypocalcemia and the rapidity of its onset. They may include one or more of the following: arrhythmias (heart block, ventricular arrhythmias), carpopedal spasm, Chvostek's sign (spasm of the facial muscles in response to tapping the facial nerve just anterior to the ear), prolonged QT-interval, mental status changes, muscle abnormalities (including tremor, twitching, tetany, or potentially life-threatening laryngospasm), paresthesias, seizures, and/or Trousseau's sign (carpopedal spasm produced by an upper-arm blood pressure cuff inflated to just above systolic blood pressure for 2–3 minutes).

D. Diagnosis

Laboratory evaluation should minimally include total serum calcium and serum albumin levels (or, preferably, a serum ionized calcium level), and phosphate, magnesium, serum electrolytes, BUN, creatinine, and glucose levels. Additional studies, depending on clinical circumstances and severity of hypocalcemia, may be indicated (e.g., arterial blood gas (ABG), CBC, ECG, and parathyroid hormone level).

E. Therapy

Treatment of hypocalcemia in the ED is indicated when symptomatic.

1. Calcium gluconate 10% (90 mg of elemental calcium per 10-mL ampule) is the emergency treatment of choice:

    Dose: 10–30 mL IV over 15–20 minutes. If symptoms are refractory, a continuous calcium infusion may be started at 3 mg of elemental calcium/kg per hour. Calcium gluconate is preferred over calcium chloride in this setting (calcium chloride can cause phlebitis; tissue necrosis may also occur with extravasation). The goal of IV calcium therapy is to control symptoms; do not attempt to normalize the serum calcium. *Caution:* if hyperphosphatemia is present, and the product of serum calcium and serum phosphate (measured in mg/dL) is ≥ 60, correct the hyperphosphatemia *before* administering IV calcium to avoid the risks of ectopic calcification. Calcium administration also worsens digoxin toxicity.

    Note: if the patient is *hypomagnesemic,* IV magnesium sulfate replacement (e.g., 2 g IV over 20–30 minutes) should occur simultaneously with the above. Depending on the degree of hypomagnesemia, additional doses may be necessary, or a continuous magnesium sulfate infusion may be initiated (≤ 10 g IV over 24 hours depending on degree of magnesium depletion). Magnesium sulfate is contraindicated in the patient with heart block or significant renal dysfunction.

2. Long-term management of hypocalcemia depends on its underlying cause (see II. B, above). Obtain appropriate specialist consultation as necessary (e.g., internal medicine, nephrology).

F. Disposition

1. Patients with asymptomatic hypocalcemia can generally be discharged from the ED. Outpatient follow-up is required for further evaluation and treatment of the cause of hypocalcemia.

2. Patients with symptomatic hypocalcemia requiring IV calcium therapy should be hospitalized.

Sodium

Note: an abnormal serum sodium level actually represents a disorder in water metabolism.

III. HYPERNATREMIA

A. Definition

Hypernatremia is a serum sodium concentration > 145 mEq/L. Hypernatremia is significant when the serum sodium concentration is > 150–155 mEq/L; it is severe if ≥ 160 mEq/L. *Remember:* hypernatremia indicates free-water depletion; it does not indicate the patient's saline or volume status. By definition, hypernatremia is a hyperosmolar, hypertonic state, but it may occur in the setting of total-body volume depletion, euvolemia, or volume expansion.

B. Etiology

1. Excessive water loss.
   a. Renal losses:
      i. Diabetes insipidus (central or nephrogenic, including drug induced [e.g., demeclocycline, lithium]).
      ii. Diuretics.
      iii. Glycosuria.
      iv. Partial renal obstruction or postobstructive diuresis.
      v. Renal failure.
      vi. Urea diuresis.
   b. Nonrenal losses:
      i. Gastrointestinal tract (diarrhea, fistulas, vomiting).
      ii. Respiratory tract.
      iii. Skin (burns, excess sweating, protracted fever, other skin conditions).
2. Inadequate water intake.
   a. Disordered thirst perception.
   b. Inability to obtain water (abnormal environment; altered mentation, including coma; infants; nonambulatory or immobile individuals, including nursing home or intubated patients).
   c. Hypodipsia.
3. Sodium intake in excess of water intake.
   a. Acute salt poisoning (ingestion of hypertonic saline, salt tablets, seawater).
   b. Iatrogenic (hypertonic dialysis baths, sodium bicarbonate administration, hypertonic saline infusions).
4. Mineralocorticoid excess.
   a. Congenital adrenal hyperplasia.

   b. Cushing's syndrome.
   c. Exogenous mineralocorticoid administration.
   d. Primary hyperaldosteronism.

C. Signs and Symptoms

   Signs and symptoms depend on the severity of hypernatremia and its rapidity of onset. The cardinal symptom is thirst if the patient is able to both sense and communicate this sensation. Other early symptoms may include irritability, lethargy, tremulousness, and weakness. If hypernatremia becomes severe, twitching, seizures, altered mentation, and eventual coma and death will occur. Depending on the cause of hypernatremia, concomitant signs of volume depletion may be present (e.g., tachycardia, depressed skin turgor, flat neck veins).

D. Diagnosis

   Minimal evaluation should include a serum electrolyte panel; BUN, creatinine, and glucose levels; serum osmolality; and urinalysis. Remember to correct the serum sodium for hyperglycemia (add 1.6 mEq/L to the serum sodium for every 100 mg/dL increase in the serum glucose over 100 mg/dL). Additional studies are frequently indicated as dictated by the clinical condition (e.g., ABG, CBC, chest roentgenogram, head computed tomography [CT], and endocrinologic evaluation).

E. Therapy

1. *Assess, secure, and support the airway, breathing, circulation, and neurologic status* as clinically indicated (see Chapter 1). These patients frequently have altered mentation; administer supplemental oxygen and protect the airway as necessary (see Chapter 11).

2. *Correct an abnormal volume status* if present. *Remember:* hypernatremia may occur in the setting of volume depletion, euvolemia, or volume overload.
   a. If volume depletion is present, correct hypovolemia by administering IV normal saline until a euvolemic state is established (the rate of administration will be determined by the patient's vital signs, overall clinical status, and urine output).
   b. If the patient is euvolemic, maintain euvolemia while correcting hypernatremia as outlined below.
   c. If the patient is volume overloaded, diuretic therapy is indicated (or dialysis in the setting of concomitant renal failure) while simultaneously correcting hypernatremia.

3. *Gradually correct hypernatremia. Caution:* do not correct hypernatremia too rapidly or cerebral edema may occur. The usual recommendation is to correct hypernatremia no faster than 1–2 mEq/L per hour, and correct only one-half of the free water deficit in the first 24 hours. The remainder of the deficit

should then be replaced in the subsequent 24–48 hours. Frequent measurements of serum sodium and appropriate adjustments in IV crystalloid replacement are indicated.

a. If hypernatremia is mild to moderate (serum sodium < 150–155 mEq/L) and the patient is conscious, he/she usually can respond to thirst by drinking free water. Alternatively, gradual correction of hypernatremia can be accomplished by administering 5% dextrose in 0.45% saline at the appropriate rate.

b. If hypernatremia is more severe (≥ 155 mEq/L), calculate the free-water deficit as outlined below and replace slowly.

$$\text{Free water deficit} = \text{normal total body water}$$
$$(\text{TBW}) - \text{abnormal TBW, where normal}$$
$$\text{TBW} = 0.6 \times (\text{weight in kg}).$$
Note: in cachectic patients use normal TBW = $0.5 \times$ (weight in kg).

$$\text{Abnormal TBW} = (\text{normal Na}^+) \times \frac{(\text{normal TBW})}{\text{observed Na}^+}$$

For example, in a 60-kg patient with a serum sodium concentration of 160 mEq/L, the appropriate calculation is as follows:

$$\text{normal TBW} = (0.6) \times (60 \text{ kg}) = 36 \text{ L}$$
$$\text{abnormal TBW} = [(140) \times (36)] / 160 = 31.5 \text{ L}$$
$$\text{Free water deficit} = 36 \text{ L} - 31.5 \text{ L} = 4.5 \text{ L}$$

As noted above, only one-half of the free-water deficit (2.25 L of free water in the above example) should be replaced in the first 24 hours. The remainder of the deficit should be replaced in the subsequent 24–48 hours. *Remember:* free-water replacement is in addition to the patient's maintenance fluid and electrolyte requirements.

4. *Evaluate for the cause of hypernatremia* (see I. B, above) *and treat as appropriate.* Obtain specialty consultation as necessary.

F. Disposition

1. Patients with mild hypernatremia (serum sodium ≤ 150 mEq/L) can generally be discharged to home with close outpatient follow-up provided serum sodium is gradually decreasing with ED management and the patient can take oral liquids without difficulty.

2. Patients with more significant hypernatremia (serum sodium > 150–155mEq/L) should be hospitalized for careful monitoring and gradual correction of their hypernatremia as outlined above.

IV. HYPONATREMIA

A. Definition

1. *Hyponatremia* is a serum sodium concentration < 136 mEq/L. It is the commonest fluid–electrolyte abnormality. Symptoms do not usually develop unless the serum sodium is ≤ 125 mEq/L; hyponatremia is severe if < 120 mEq/L.

2. *Remember:* hyponatremia indicates free-water excess; it does not indicate the patient's saline or volume status. Hyponatremia may occur in the setting of total-body volume depletion, euvolemia, or volume expansion.

B. Etiology

1. Isotonic hyponatremia (including pseudohyponatremia; serum osmolality 280-285 mOsm/kg serum H_2O).
   a. Hyperlipidemia.
   b. Hyperproteinemia.
   c. Laboratory or blood drawing error (e.g., blood draw proximal to a hypotonic intravenous infusion).

2. Hypertonic hyponatremia (serum osmolality > 285 mOsm/kg serum water).
   a. Hyperglycemia.
   b. Hypertonic infusions of glucose, mannitol, or glycine.

3. Hypotonic hyponatremia (serum osmolality < 280 mOsm/kg serum water).
   a. Hypovolemic hyponatremia (sodium deficit in excess of water deficit):
      i. Adrenal insufficiency.
      ii. Extrarenal losses (e.g., skin, lung, gastrointestinal tract; under these circumstances the urine sodium is usually < 10 mEq/L).
      iii. Renal losses (e.g., diuresis, renal insufficiency, partial urinary tract obstruction; under these circumstances the urine sodium is usually > 20 mEq/L).
      iv. Third spacing.
   b. Euvolemic hyponatremia (excess total-body water):
      i. Drugs (including clofibrate, cyclophosphamide, desmopressin, hypoglycemic agents [phenformin, sulfonylureas], indomethacin, opiates, oxytocin, thiazide diuretics, tricyclic compounds [amitriptyline, carbamazepine, thioridazine], and vincristine).
      ii. Adrenal glucocorticoid deficiency.
      iii. Hypothyroidism.
      iv. Potassium loss.
      v. Renal failure.
      vi. Reset osmostat.
      vii. SIADH (syndrome of inappropriate anti-diuretic hormone secretion; causes may include central nervous

system disorders, pulmonary disorders, and malignancies).

    viii. Water intoxication (including psychogenic polydipsia).

  c. Hypervolemic hyponatremia (excess total-body sodium and larger excess of total-body water):

    i. Congestive heart failure.

    ii. Liver failure.

    iii. Nephrotic syndrome.

    iv. Renal failure.

C. Signs and Symptoms

Signs and symptoms depend not only on the severity of hyponatremia but also on its rapidity of onset. Early complaints of anorexia, nausea, malaise, and apathy may progress to headache, mental status changes, and eventual seizures and/or coma as the hyponatremia becomes more severe. Miscellaneous findings may include depressed or abnormal deep-tendon reflexes, Cheyne-Stokes respirations, abnormal sensorium, or pseudobulbar palsy (weakness of the muscles innervated by the cranial nerves). Concomitant symptoms and signs of either volume depletion or volume overload may be present depending on the cause of the hyponatremia.

D. Diagnosis

1. Minimal evaluation should include a serum electrolyte panel; BUN, creatinine, and glucose levels; serum osmolality; and urinalysis. Remember to correct the serum sodium for hyperglycemia (add 1.6 mEq/L to the serum sodium for every 100-mg/dL increase in the serum glucose over 100 mg/dL). Additional studies are frequently indicated as dictated by the clinical condition (e.g., CBC, chest roentgenogram, head CT, urine sodium, endocrinologic evaluation [e.g., thyroid stimulating hormone level, serum cortisol level]).

2. Diagnosis of SIADH requires the following: hyponatremia; euvolemia; patient is not taking any diuretics; there is no evidence for cardiac, liver, or renal dysfunction; and adrenal and thyroid function are normal.

E. Therapy

1. *Assess, secure, and support the airway, breathing, circulation, and neurologic status* as clinically indicated (see Chapter 1). The hyponatremic patient may have profoundly altered mentation; administer supplemental oxygen and protect the airway as necessary (see Chapter 11). If the patient is actively seizing, initiate appropriate therapy to control seizure activity (see Chapter 20) while simultaneously treating severe hyponatremia as outlined below.

2. *Correct an abnormal volume status if present. Remember:*

hyponatremia may occur in the setting of volume depletion, euvolemia, or volume overload. Management of the patient's volume abnormality is crucial.

a. If volume depletion is present, treat for hypovolemia with normal saline as appropriate to the clinical condition. Also identify and treat the cause of volume depletion.

b. If the patient is euvolemic, maintain euvolemia while correcting hyponatremia as outlined below.

c. If the patient is volume overloaded, treat the underlying condition responsible for volume overload (e.g., congestive heart failure, renal failure or nephrotic syndrome, liver failure) while employing free-water restriction to correct the hyponatremia.

3. *Gradually correct hyponatremia. Caution:* the appropriate rate of correction of hyponatremia remains controversial and depends on the severity of hyponatremia, its duration, and accompanying symptoms. In general, do not allow the serum sodium concentration to increase faster than 0.5 mEq/L per hour, and do not increase the serum sodium concentration to > 125 mEq/L in the first 24–36 hours of therapy. Too rapid correction of hyponatremia may cause central pontine myelinolysis, which is associated with significant morbidity and may be fatal.

a. Under most circumstances, hyponatremia will respond to appropriate therapy of the patient's volume status, treatment of the underlying condition responsible for the volume abnormality and/or hyponatremia, and free water restriction (generally to 1000 mL/day).

b. Severe hyponatremia (serum sodium < 120 mEq/L) in euvolemic patients should be treated with NS administration combined with furosemide (begin with 0.5-1 mg/kg IV). Concomitant administration of furosemide (or other loop diuretic) is crucial to impair renal concentrating ability (resulting in a lower urine osmolality) so that net free-water excretion occurs. (*Note:* administration of NS alone in this setting, without furosemide, may actually worsen hyponatremia!).

c. When markedly severe hyponatremia is *accompanied by seizures or coma,* consider 3% saline administration (100–200 mL IV at the rate of 75–100 mL/hr) and furosemide. In this setting, furosemide causes loss of both salt and water in the urine, and the sodium loss (remember to measure the urine sodium) is replaced with the hypertonic saline to maintain euvolemia. The serum sodium should be increased by about 1 mEq/L per hour until life-threatening symptoms are controlled or for 4 hours. Then proceed with continued, slower, very gradual correction of hyponatremia as outlined above.

4. *Maintain serum potassium in the normal range.*

5. *Obtain specialist consultation as appropriate* (e.g., internal medicine, nephrology).

F. Disposition

1. Patients with asymptomatic, mild hyponatremia (serum sodium > 125 mEq/L) can frequently be discharged to home if they are euvolemic and no other condition mandating hospitalization has been identified. Mild free-water restriction (1000 mL/day) should be recommended and follow-up with the patient's primary care physician provided within 24–48 hours to recheck the serum sodium. In consultation with the patient's primary care physician, consider discontinuing any medication that may be contributing to the hyponatremia (see IV. B. 3. b, above).

2. Patients with symptomatic hyponatremia, or a serum sodium ≤ 125 mEq/L, should be hospitalized.

Potassium

The normal serum potassium level varies slightly between institutions, but is generally reported as 3.5–5.2 mEq/L. Total-body content of potassium varies depending on the patient's sex, muscle mass, and tissue wasting (if present); in a muscular male it may be as large as 50 mEq/kg body weight. Over 95% of the body's potassium is located within cells (potassium is the most prevalent intracellular cation). The differential concentration between intracellular and extracellular potassium is crucial in the maintenance of the transmembrane potential of excitable tissues.

Serum pH alters the serum potassium level: acidemia causes the movement of potassium from the intracellular to the extracellular fluid and increases the serum potassium level (in general, a decrease in serum pH of 0.1 raises serum potassium by 0.5 mEq/L); alkalemia has the opposite effect.

I. HYPERKALEMIA

A. Definition

1. *Hyperkalemia* is a serum potassium level > 5.2 mEq/L. It is the most life-threatening electrolyte abnormality. Serum levels > 6.0 mEq/L, or levels accompanied by ECG changes, require urgent intervention. The cardiotoxicity of hyperkalemia is worsened in the setting of acidemia, hypocalcemia, or hyponatremia.

2. Spurious hyperkalemia may occur as a consequence of hemolysis within the blood sample, profound thrombocytosis (platelet counts > 1 million/µL), profound leukocytosis (leukocyte count > 100,000/µL), prolonged application of the tourniquet prior to obtaining a blood sample, or excessive fist-clenching when obtaining the blood sample from a forearm vein (secondary to potassium release from muscle cells).

B. Etiology

1. Intracellular to extracellular potassium shifts.
   a. Acidemia.
   b. Cellular injury (including burns, crush injury, hemolysis, rhabdomyolysis, tumor lysis).
   c. Hyperkalemic periodic paralysis.
   d. Hypertonicity (e.g., secondary to hypertonic sodium, glucose, or mannitol infusions).
   e. Insulin deficiency.
   f. Medications (e.g., beta blockers, calcium channel blockers, succinylcholine).
   g. Poisoning with digoxin or fluoride.
2. Increased potassium intake.
   a. Oral (salt substitutes, potassium supplements).
   b. Parenteral (hyperalimentation, IV solutions, potassium salts of antibiotics [e.g., high-dose penicillin]).
3. Decreased renal excretion.
   a. Acute or chronic renal failure.
   b. Hypoaldosteronism (including Addison's disease or medication-induced [e.g., angiotensin-converting enzyme (ACE) inhibitors, cyclosporine, heparin]).
   c. Hyporeninemic hypoaldosteronism (secondary to acquired immunodeficiency syndrome, chronic interstitial nephritis, diabetes mellitus, nonsteroidal anti-inflammatory drugs [NSAIDs], obstructive uropathy, sickle cell nephropathy, systemic lupus erythematosus).
   d. Inadequate delivery of fluid and sodium to the distal nephron.
   e. Potassium-sparing diuretics (e.g., amiloride, spironolactone, triamterene).
   f. Renal tubular secretory defects (e.g., post-renal transplantation, tubulointerstitial renal diseases, type 4 renal tubular acidosis).

C. Symptoms and Signs

1. *Caution:* patients may be asymptomatic even if life-threatening hyperkalemia is present, and ECG manifestations are not consistent (abrupt pulseless electrical activity [PEA], ventricular tachycardia, ventricular fibrillation, or asystole may occur).
2. The classic ECG changes of hyperkalemia begin with peaked T waves (usually present when the serum potassium is > 6.5 mEq/L) and progress to a prolonged PR-interval, widened QRS complex, eventual loss of the P wave, final widening of the QRS complex into a sine-wave configuration, and, ultimately, ventricular fibrillation (or sometimes asystole). Various heart blocks and other arrhythmias may also occur.
3. Neuromuscular complaints, if present, may include altered muscle tone (increased or decreased), paresthesias, weakness, or paralysis.

D. Diagnosis

Minimal evaluation should include a serum electrolyte panel; ECG; glucose, BUN, and creatinine levels; CBC (including platelets); calcium and magnesium levels, and an ABG. In the asymptomatic patient with a normal ECG, consider the possibility of spurious hyperkalemia and recheck the laboratory result if indicated.

E. Therapy

Urgent therapy should be instituted if the serum potassium level is > 6.0–6.5 mEq/L, ECG changes are present, or the patient is otherwise symptomatic. Monitor the cardiac rhythm continuously. Following the acute treatment of hyperkalemia as outlined below, the cause of hyperkalemia must be identified and corrected.

1. **Membrane Stabilization: Calcium.** Calcium temporarily antagonizes the cardiac and neuromuscular manifestations of hyperkalemia; its effects occur immediately and last approximately 60 minutes. It is the initial drug of choice in the presence of ECG changes or otherwise severe hyperkalemia.

   Dose:
   - Calcium gluconate: 10–20 mL of a 10% solution (4.6 mEq/10 mL) IV over 2–5 minutes. The dose may be repeated in 5 minutes if no response is seen. *Or*
   - Calcium chloride: 5–10 mL of a 10% solution (13.6 mEq/10 mL) IV over 2–5 minutes. The dose may be repeated in 5 minutes if no response is seen.

   Simultaneously with the above, consider a *continuous* calcium infusion (start with 5–10 mEq/hr) and titrate as necessary to prevent recurrence of ECG manifestations.

   Caution: do not mix calcium with sodium bicarbonate or calcium carbonate will precipitate. Do not use IV calcium to treat hyperkalemia associated with digoxin toxicity: digoxin poisoning is exacerbated by hypercalcemia. Hyperkalemia (serum potassium > 5.5 mEq/L) secondary to acute digoxin toxicity is an immediate indication for dig-antibody therapy (see Chapter 23).

2. **Extracellular to Intracellular Shift of Potassium**

   a. Sodium bicarbonate shifts potassium intracellularly; it is especially effective and appropriate in the acidotic patient with hyperkalemia. The onset of action occurs in 5–10 minutes and effects may last 1–2 hours.

      Dose: 50 mEq IV over 5 minutes. The dose may be repeated in 10–15 minutes if ECG changes persist or further treatment of metabolic acidosis is required.

      Caution: hypervolemia, hypernatremia, and alkalemia are potential complications of sodium bicarbonate therapy; monitor volume status, electrolytes, and acid-base status carefully.

b. Glucose and insulin should also be given acutely to shift potassium from the extracellular fluid into cells. A response is seen in 30 minutes and effects last up to 4–6 hours.
   Dose:
   - Glucose: 25 g (50 mL of 50% dextrose in water [D50W]) given over 5 minutes, repeated if necessary to avoid hypoglycemia; *and*
   - Insulin: 8–10 units regular insulin IV.

   Caution: IV insulin has prolonged activity in the patient with renal failure. Monitor blood glucose closely after administering IV insulin; do not allow the patient to become hypoglycemic.

c. Albuterol (inhaled). Experience is limited, but beta-2 agonists have been used in the treatment of familial hyperkalemic periodic paralysis and hyperkalemia in the setting of renal failure. Onset of action occurs in 30 minutes; the duration of activity is 1–2 hours.
   Dose: optimal dose uncertain, consider 10 mg nebulized.

3. **Removal of Potassium from the Body**

   a. Cation-exchange resins are used to remove potassium from the body by binding it (in exchange for sodium) in the gastrointestinal tract. Benefit occurs within 30–60 minutes. Rectal administration works faster than oral administration, but the oral route is generally preferred. One gram of resin will bind 1 mEq of potassium.
      Dose: sodium polystyrene sulfonate (Kayexalate):
      - Oral (PO): 15–30 g in 50–100 mL of 20% sorbitol orally, may repeat every 3–4 hours up to 4–5 doses/day, *or*
      - Rectal (PR): 50 g in 200 mL of 20% sorbitol (or 20% dextrose in water if sorbitol is not available) given as a retention enema (the patient should retain the enema for 30–60 minutes). The dose may be repeated in 4–6 hours up to four doses/day.

      Caution: sodium polystyrene sulfonate exchanges 1.5 mEq of sodium for each 1 mEq of potassium removed. Use with care in the patient with moderate to severe hypertension or congestive heart failure.

   b. In the setting of normal renal function, loop diuretics may be used to promote increased urine production and potassium loss.
      Dose:
      - Furosemide: 40–80 mg IV; *or*
      - Bumetanide: 1-2 mg IV.

      Caution: maintain the patient's volume status as appropriate.

   c. Hemodialysis is indicated for severe hyperkalemia in the setting of renal failure or when the above therapy is otherwise not adequate. The onset of action is immediate.

F. Disposition

1. Patients with mild hyperkalemia (serum potassium < 6.0 mEq/L) may be discharged to home if all of the following conditions apply: hyperkalemia is asymptomatic, no ECG abnormalities are present, potassium has been removed from the body with appropriate ED therapy (e.g., loop diuretic therapy and/or sodium polystyrene sulfonate) and serum potassium is now in the normal range, the patient is reliable, the cause of hyperkalemia has been identified and corrected, and follow-up within 24 hours is possible.

2. Patients who have a serum potassium level $\geq$ 6.0 mEq/L, individuals with symptomatic hyperkalemia (including ECG changes), or those who do not meet the discharge criteria outlined in 1. above, require hospitalization to a monitored bed.

II. HYPOKALEMIA

A. Definition

1. *Hypokalemia* is a serum potassium level < 3.5 mEq/L. In the absence of transcellular potassium shifts (e.g., alkalemia), a decline in the serum potassium of 1 mEq/L reflects a total-body potassium deficit $\leq$ 200–400 mEq.

2. Hypokalemia should be considered in ED patients with alcohol abuse, cardiac complaints (including arrhythmias), diabetes mellitus, gastrointestinal disease (e.g., diarrhea or vomiting), hypertension, or neuromuscular complaints, and in individuals taking digoxin or diuretics.

3. Hypokalemia usually does not become symptomatic until the serum potassium level is < 3.0 mEq/L.

B. Etiology

1. Extracellular to intracellular potassium shifts.
    a. Acute glucose loads.
    b. Alkalemia.
    c. Anabolic states.
    d. Barium poisoning.
    e. Beta agonists.
    f. Delerium tremens.
    g. Hematologic causes (leukemia, treatment of megaloblastic anemia).
    h. Hypokalemic periodic paralysis.
    i. Insulin excess.
    j. Theophylline toxicity.
2. Inadequate intake (< 10-20 mEq/day).
    a. Dietary deficiency (including alcoholism, eating disorders, starvation).

    b. Iatrogenic (deficient potassium replacement in maintenance hydration fluids or hyperalimentation).

    c. Impaired absorption (including malabsorption, short-bowel syndrome).

3. Increased extrarenal losses (urine potassium usually < 15 mEq/L).

    a. Skin (burns, sweating).

    b. Gastrointestinal (diarrhea, gastric fluid loss, laxative abuse, villous adenoma, other).

4. Increased renal losses (urine potassium > 30 mEq/L despite body potassium depletion; these conditions may occur simultaneously with extrarenal losses as outlined above).

    a. Normal anion gap metabolic acidosis:

       i. Amphotericin.

       ii. Carbonic anhydrase inhibitors (e.g., acetazolamide).

       iii. Intestinal or biliary fistulas.

       iv. Laxative abuse.

       v. Renal tubular acidosis (type 1 and type 2).

       vi. Ureterosigmoidostomy.

    b. Increased anion gap metabolic acidosis:

       i. Diabetic ketoacidosis.

       ii. Alcoholic ketoacidosis.

       iii. Poisoning with ethylene glycol, methanol, or toluene.

    c. Metabolic alkalosis with low urinary chloride (< 20 mEq/L):

       i. Chloride losing diarrhea.

       ii. Previous diuretic use.

       iii. Gastrointestinal losses (vomiting, nasogastric drainage).

    d. Metabolic alkalosis with increased urinary chloride (> 20 mEq/L):

       i. Hypertensive patient (e.g., glucocorticoid excess, primary hyperaldosteronism).

       ii. Nonhypertensive patient (e.g., Bartter's syndrome [a syndrome of uncertain cause characterized by muscle weakness, renal potassium wasting, hypomagnesemia, metabolic alkalosis, hyperreninemia, hyperaldosteronism, and normotension], current diuretic therapy, magnesium deficiency).

C. Signs and Symptoms

If hypokalemia is significant, one or more of the following may be present:

1. Cardiovascular: cardiac arrhythmias, exacerbation of digitalis toxicity, ECG changes (progressing as follows: flattened T wave, prominent U wave, depressed ST segment).

2. Neuromuscular: cramps, hyporeflexia, muscle fatigue, myalgias, "restless" legs, weakness, and, if severe, paralysis.

3. Renal: metabolic alkalosis, impaired renal concentrating ability, polyuria.

4. Miscellaneous: gastric distention, ileus, polydipsia, rhabdomyolysis (if hypokalemia is severe), urinary retention, worsened hepatic encephalopathy.

D. Diagnosis

Minimal evaluation should include a serum electrolyte panel; and BUN, creatinine, glucose, and magnesium levels. Additional studies may be necessary depending on clinical circumstances and the severity of hypokalemia (e.g., ABG, ECG, urinary potassium, urinary chloride).

E. Therapy

The treatment of hypokalemia should include gradual replacement therapy and identification/treatment of the cause of hypokalemia. Magnesium replacement is also important if hypomagnesemia is concomitantly present. Usually hypokalemia is not an emergency, and it can be corrected safely and gradually using oral potassium supplements. In the absence of conditions causing transcellular potassium shifts, a nonacute decline in serum potassium of 0.5 mEq/L indicates a total-body potassium deficit as large as 100–200 mEq. *Caution:* always replace potassium cautiously and monitor potassium levels closely during replacement therapy; do not overtreat the patient and cause hyperkalemia! Overtreatment is especially likely when hypokalemia is not secondary to total-body depletion but is a consequence of intracellular shifts. Patients with the following are also at considerable risk for hyperkalemia in the setting of potassium replacement: diabetes mellitus, older age, renal insufficiency, certain medications (e.g., ACE inhibitors, cyclosporine, heparin, NSAIDs). *Remember:* the total extracellular potassium pool in an average-sized adult is only about 70 mEq. If replacement is excessive in quantity, or too rapid given the time needed for the body to appropriately modulate extracellular and intracellular levels, life-threatening hyperkalemia may result.

1. **Oral Replacement**
   a. This is the replacement route of choice in the asymptomatic, mildly to moderately hypokalemic patient who is capable of oral intake.
   b. Potassium chloride formulations:
      i. Liquid (10% = 20 mEq potassium per 15 mL; 20% = 40 mEq potassium per 15 mL).
      ii. Powder (15, 20, or 25 mEq potassium per package).
      iii. Tablets (multiple sizes available, slow-release 10 mEq or 20 mEq potassium per tablet most common).

      Note: potassium citrate or potassium gluconate are the potassium salts of choice when hyperchloremic metabolic acidosis accompanies hypokalemia (e.g., in type 1 [distal] renal tubular acidosis or severe diarrhea).

    c. *Dose:* depends on the severity of potassium depletion. Under most circumstances, 20–40 mEq PO every 12 hours is sufficient to gradually correct the deficit over time. Oral replacement should not exceed 40 mEq every 6–8 hours for more than two doses without re-evaluating serum potassium (the serum level can be rechecked 4–6 hours after an oral dose as necessary).

  2. **Intravenous Replacement**

    a. This route is appropriate in the hypokalemic patient incapable of oral intake, the symptomatic hypokalemic patient, the patient with profound hypokalemia (< 2.5 mEq/L) even if asymptomatic, or the patient on a digitalis preparation whose serum potassium is ≤ 3.0 mEq/L.

    b. *Dose:* IV replacement usually should not exceed 10 mEq/hr. The duration of therapy depends on the degree of hypokalemia, but do not administer > 40 mEq (at the rate of 10 mEq/hr) without rechecking the serum level. If hypokalemia is immediately life-threatening (e.g., serious cardiac arrhythmia, paralysis) a temporary infusion as rapid as 20–40 mEq/hr for 1 hour may be necessary, but should not be repeated without rechecking a serum level.

    c. Additional cautions:

      i. An infusion pump should be used.

      ii. The cardiac rhythm should be continuously monitored if the IV infusion rate is >10 mEq/hr.

      iii. Always monitor serum potassium levels frequently with replacement therapy.

      iv. The concentration of potassium in the fluid administered through a peripheral IV line should be ≤ 40 mEq/L. Local vein irritation and phlebitis are potential complications of potassium chloride administration.

F. Disposition

  1. The patient with mild to moderate hypokalemia (serum potassium 2.5–3.5 mEq/L) without significant symptoms can generally be managed with oral replacement therapy as an outpatient. Follow-up in 48–72 hours is recommended to recheck the potassium level.

  2. Patients with significant symptoms and/or a serum potassium level < 2.5 mEq/L should be admitted to a monitored hospital bed.

BIBLIOGRAPHY

Bilezikian JP: Management of acute hypercalcemia. N Engl J Med 1992;326(18):1196–1203.

Sterns RH, Narins RG: Disorders of potassium balance. Chapter 352. In Stein JH (ed): Internal Medicine, 4th Ed. St. Louis, Mosby-Year Book, 1994; pp. 2681–2693.

Wolfson AB (ed): Contemporary Issues in Emergency Medicine: Endocrine and Metabolic Emergencies. Harwood-Nuss A (series editor). New York, Churchill Livingstone, 1990.

NEPHROLITHIASIS

"So great was the extremity of his pain and anguish, that he did not only sigh but roar."

MATTHEW HENRY

I. ESSENTIAL FACTS

A. Definition

Nephrolithiasis is the formation of solid crystalline masses anywhere within the kidney or urinary tract.

B. Classification

The major renal calculi include calcium oxalate, calcium phosphate or apatite, uric acid, cystine, and struvite stones. Calcium-containing stones are radiopaque, but they must be at least 2 mm in diameter before they are visible on plain radiographs.

1. Calcium oxalate crystals are octahedral with a central cross. At least 60% of renal calculi are made of calcium oxalate. Causes include inherited disorders (rare, autosomal recessive), increased absorption of oxalate from the gastrointestinal tract (e.g., jejunal–ileal bypass, inflammatory bowel disease, small-bowel resection), and vitamin C ingestion; other cases are idiopathic.

2. Calcium phosphate and calcium apatite are amorphous crystals; they are responsible for 20% of renal calculi. Causes include primary hyperparathyroidism, sarcoidosis, thyrotoxicosis, other causes of hypercalcemia, vitamin A or D intoxication, and distal renal tubular acidosis (RTA). Fifty percent of cases are idiopathic.

3. Uric acid crystals are radiolucent, and are oval or diamond shaped; they are responsible for 7–10% of stones. Causes include low urinary pH, gout, myeloproliferative disease, malignancy, glycogen storage diseases, and diarrheal syndromes such as ulcerative colitis or regional enteritis. Hyperuricosuria may result in calcium oxalate stones by serving as a nidus for crystal formation or by reducing the activity of inhibitors of calcium oxalate crystal growth.

4. Struvite crystals are "coffin lid"-shaped, formed from magnesium, ammonium, and phosphate, and are responsible for 7–10% of stones. They are associated with infections caused by urea-splitting organisms (e.g., *Proteus, Pseudomonas, Klebsiella*) and an alkalotic urine. Large stones that assume the shape of the renal pelvis and calyces are termed *staghorn calculi*.

5. Cystine crystals are hexagonal and are responsible for only 2–3% of stones, which are radiopaque. They are caused by an autosomal recessive disorder associated with cystinuria and abnormal renal handling and transport of the dicarboxylic amino acids cystine, ornithine, lysine, and arginine (COLA).

C. Epidemiology

1. Nephrolithiasis has an annual incidence of 1% in white males, with a lifetime risk of 20%, a 5-year recurrence rate of 50%, and an 8-year recurrence rate of 63%. White females have a lifetime risk of 5–10%, with an 8-year recurrence rate of 18%. Blacks have a very low lifetime risk of 5–6% but a higher incidence of infection-associated stones.

2. Risk factors include
   a. Acidic or alkalotic urine (depending on the type of stone).
   b. Decreased urine volume.
   c. Diarrheal syndromes.
   d. Hyperparathyroidism.
   e. Medications (acetazolamide, triamterene, or sulfadiazine administration).
   f. Positive family history.
   g. Renal tubular acidosis (RTA).
   h. Thyrotoxicosis.
   i. Small-bowel disease.
   j. Vitamin A, D, and C intoxication.
   k. Volume depletion.

3. Approximately 20% of cases are associated with complications (e.g., infection, obstruction) requiring urologic intervention.

II. CLINICAL EVALUATION

A. History

Patients usually present with the sudden onset of severe pain in the costovertebral angle, flank, and/or lateral abdomen. Pain may be constant or colicky; the patient typically cannot find a comfortable position. The discomfort may be referred to the genitalia.

1. Associated symptoms frequently include nausea, vomiting, diaphoresis, and restlessness.

2. The patient may report a history of gross hematuria, prior stone formation, poor fluid intake, and/or dietary excess (e.g., meats, alcohol, purine or oxalate-containing foods).

3. Inquire about medication use, allergies (including prior reaction to intravenous [IV] contrast agents), history of renal insufficiency, pregnancy risk, fluid intake and loss, and other systemic diseases.

B. Physical Examination

Obtain vital signs and evaluate the skin, HEENT, neck, chest, heart, abdomen (include rectal examination and stool heme test), and genitalia.

1. Fever suggests concomitant infection. Hypotension with fever is indicative of urosepsis.

2. Auscultate the lungs carefully: a lower-lobe pneumonia may present with flank pain.

3. Anterior abdominal signs (e.g., pain with palpation, rebound tenderness, and/or guarding) should not be present in the setting of renal colic and suggest a more serious intra-abdominal process.

4. Carefully palpate the aorta for tenderness or enlargement suggestive of an aneurysm.

5. Evaluate the genitalia for any pathology (e.g., testicular masses, epididymitis, or torsion); consider concomitant obstetrical/gynecological emergencies (e.g., ectopic pregnancy, ovarian cyst, pelvic inflammatory disease).

C. Laboratory Evaluation

1. *Routinely* obtain the following values:
   a. Complete blood count (leukocyte count > 15,000/μL suggests concomitant infection).
   b. Glucose level
   c. Electrolyte panel; BUN and creatinine levels.
   d. Pregnancy test (obtain in women of reproductive age).
   e. Electrocardiogram (ECG; obtain in patients ≥ 40 years old or who otherwise have risk factors for ischemic heart disease).
   f. Urinalysis (microscopic hematuria is present in ≥ 80% of patients with renal colic; urine pH should be measured with an electrode for accuracy).
   g. Urine culture.

2. Imaging studies should include the following:
   a. A flat plate of the abdomen or a kidney ureter bladder (KUB) roentgenogram: this study should be routinely obtained in nonpregnant patients presenting with renal colic. Ninety percent of stones are radiopaque. Abdominal films may also suggest other diagnoses (e.g., acute intestinal obstruction or perforated viscus).
   b. An excretory urogram (EU) or an intravenous pyelogram (IVP) is the diagnostic study of choice in the patient with acute renal colic. In 96% of cases it establishes the diagnosis; it also demonstrates the severity of obstruction. The optimal time to obtain the IVP depends on the capabilities of the institution and the patient. In the stable patient

with classic renal colic, readily achieved pain control, and no evidence of infection, the study may be delayed till daylight hours when optimal radiology staff are available. Contraindications to an IVP include renal insufficiency, prior history of contrast agent allergy, or pregnancy.

   c. Ultrasound may be used to diagnose hydronephrosis suggestive of obstruction. It is not as sensitive as IVP, and it cannot visualize stones < 5 mm in diameter. Ultrasound is the imaging procedure of choice, however, in any of the following: pregnant patients, those with renal insufficiency or a history of prior contrast reactions, and individuals at high risk for contrast-induced renal injury (e.g., multiple myeloma, diabetic nephropathy, or severe volume depletion).

3. Additional laboratory tests may include

   a. Serum calcium, phosphate, and uric acid levels: these are appropriate, once the diagnosis is confirmed, to assess for possible causes of nephrolithiasis.

   b. Twenty-four-hour urine evaluation (for creatinine clearance, calcium, phosphate, citrate, oxalate, and cystine): this should *not* be ordered by the ED care provider. The referral physician may request this in patients who are multiple stone formers, are < age 21, or who had a complicated first-stone episode (e.g., required surgery). It should only be obtained after the patient has passed the stone and reached a steady-state metabolic condition.

   c. Stone evaluation: the referral physician may request this in patients with complicated first-stone episodes, patients < age 21, individuals with a positive family history, and those who have formed multiple stones.

III. DIFFERENTIAL DIAGNOSIS

A. Urologic disease, including pyelonephritis, renal abscess, renal cancer, trauma, tuberculosis, noncalculous causes of ureteral obstruction (e.g., tumor, blood clot, sloughed renal papilla from papillary necrosis, stricture), testicular torsion, and epididymitis.

B. Vascular disease, including aortic dissection, abdominal aortic aneurysm, and superior mesenteric artery occlusion.

C. Intra-abdominal disease, including intestinal ischemia, appendicitis, cholecystitis, other causes of peritonitis, gastroenteritis, diverticulitis, and intestinal obstruction.

D. Gynecologic disease, including ectopic pregnancy, ovarian torsion, ruptured ovarian cyst, pelvic inflammatory disease, endometriosis, and cancer.

E. Miscellaneous causes, including musculoskeletal disease; lower-lobe pneumonia; retroperitoneal bleed, fibrosis, or tumor; pancreatitis.

IV. THERAPY

Figure 17–1 presents the therapy of nephrolithiases.

A. First-Line Therapy: Hydration, Analgesia, and Antiemetics

1. Initiate IV crystalloid infusion. In the nonelderly patient with no history of cardiac dysfunction, begin with 1 L normal saline (NS) IV infused over 30–60 minutes followed by 200–250 mL/hr. Volume-depleted patients should be bolused with 500-mL increments till repleted. At the time of discharge, patients should be encouraged to maintain a urine output of > 2L/day to minimize recurrences.

2. Analgesia: the patient is frequently in severe pain and acute distress; early administration of analgesia is appropriate unless the diagnosis is in doubt. The following medications are helpful (the IV route of administration is preferable):
   a. Meperidine (Demerol): 25 mg IV, repeated every 15 minutes as necessary until adequate pain control is achieved; or 50–100 mg intramuscularly (IM) every 3–4 hours. *Caution:* multiple doses over time may lead to the accumulation of a toxic metabolite that can cause seizures. Meperidine should not be given to patients with acute or chronic renal failure. It is also contraindicated in patients taking monoamine oxidase inhibitors. *Or*
   b. Morphine sulfate: 1–3 mg IV, repeated every 5 minutes as necessary till adequate pain control is achieved; or 5–10 mg IM every 4–6 hours. *Or*
   c. Hydromorphone 0.5–1 mg IV, repeated in 15–30 minutes if necessary till adequate pain control is achieved.
   d. Parenteral ketorolac (Toradol) may be added to one of the above agents to further augment analgesia. *Dose:* 30–60 mg IM initially, followed by 15–30 mg IM every 6 hours. The smaller doses should be used in elderly patients. Do *not* use in patients with a history of peptic ulcer disease, individuals intolerant of nonsteroidal anti-inflammatory drugs (NSAIDs), or those with renal insufficiency.

3. Antemetics: these are frequently necessary and may be added to the above administered opioids. Choices include
   a. Prochlorperazine (Compazine): 5–10 mg given slowly IV, or 5–10 mg IM every 6 hours (maximum dose 40 mg/day), or 25 mg per rectum (PR) bid, or 5–10 mg orally (PO) tid–qid. *Or*
   b. Promethazine (Phenergan): 25 mg IV or IM every 4 hours, or 12.5–25 mg PR or PO every 4–6 hours. *Or*
   c. Hydroxyzine hydrochloride (Vistaril): 25–50 mg IM (*not* IV!) every 4–6 hours. *Or*

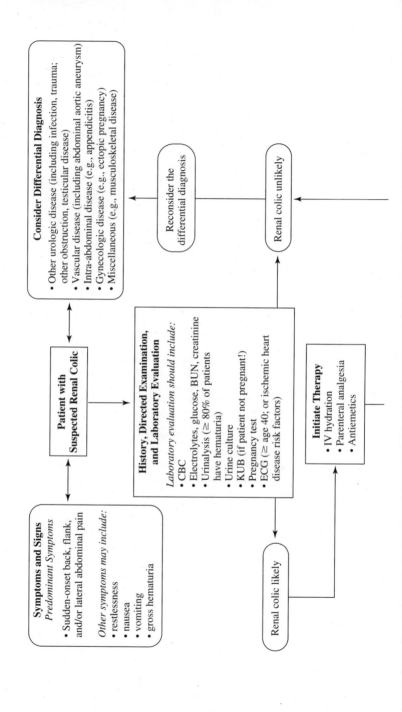

Patient with Suspected Renal Colic

Symptoms and Signs
Predominant Symptoms
- Sudden-onset back, flank, and/or lateral abdominal pain

Other symptoms may include:
- restlessness
- nausea
- vomiting
- gross hematuria

Consider Differential Diagnosis
- Other urologic disease (including infection, trauma: other obstruction, testicular disease)
- Vascular disease (including abdominal aortic aneurysm)
- Intra-abdominal disease (e.g., appendicitis)
- Gynecologic disease (e.g., ectopic pregnancy)
- Miscellaneous (e.g., musculoskeletal disease)

History, Directed Examination, and Laboratory Evaluation
Laboratory evaluation should include:
- CBC
- Electrolytes, glucose, BUN, creatinine
- Urinalysis (≥ 80% of patients have hematuria)
- Urine culture
- KUB (if patient not pregnant!)
- Pregnancy test
- ECG (≥ age 40; or ischemic heart disease risk factors)

Reconsider the differential diagnosis

Renal colic unlikely

Renal colic likely

Initiate Therapy
- IV hydration
- Parenteral analgesia
- Antiemetics

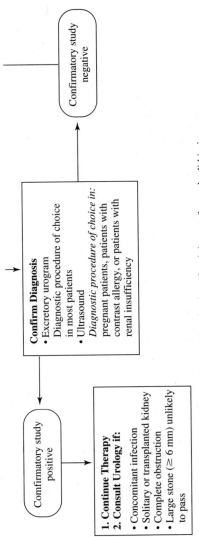

Figure 17–1. ED evaluation of and therapy for nephrolithiasis.

Confirm Diagnosis
• Excretory urogram
  Diagnostic procedure of choice
  in most patients
• Ultrasound
  Diagnostic procedure of choice in:
  pregnant patients, patients with
  contrast allergy, or patients with
  renal insufficiency

Confirmatory study
negative

Comfirmatory study
positive

1. Continue Therapy
2. Consult Urology if:
• Concomitant infection
• Solitary or transplanted kidney
• Complete obstruction
• Large stone (≥ 6 mm) unlikely
  to pass

     d. Trimethobenzamide (Tigan): 200 mg PR or 250 mg PO tid–qid.

B. Urologic Consultation/Surgical Intervention

1. Emergent urologic consultation is appropriate for patients with any of the following:
   a. Obstruction and concomitant urinary tract infection (this is a true urologic emergency!).
   b. Solitary or transplanted kidney with symptomatic nephrolithiasis.
   c. Complete obstruction.
   d. Large stones (> 6 mm) unlikely to pass spontaneously. *Remember:* the radiographic image is magnified; the actual stone is 80% of the size measured on the film.

2. Surgical interventions may include:
   a. Percutaneous nephrostomy tubes for hydronephrosis or obstruction with infection.
   b. Extracorporeal shock wave lithotripsy (ESWL) for large stones or staghorn calculi.
   c. Ureteroscopy and basket retrieval for large stones in the ureters.
   d. Open surgery for complications.

V. DISPOSITION

A. Discharge

1. Consider discharging a patient to home if *all* of the following conditions apply:
   a. Vital signs are normal.
   b. There is no evidence of concomitant urinary tract infection.
   c. Adequate pain relief has been established and parenteral opioids are no longer necessary.
   d. The patient is able to take fluids by mouth and can maintain hydration status.
   e. Patient is reliable with an adequate home situation.
   f. Patient has appropriate outpatient follow-up arranged.
   g. Renal function is normal.

2. Discharge medications may include
   a. Oral opioids for analgesia (e.g., oxycodone 5 mg PO every 4–6 hours).
   b. Anti-emetic agents (either PO or rectal suppositories).
   c. NSAIDs, but do not use in patients with renal insufficiency.

3. At the time of discharge, the patient should be instructed to maintain good oral intake and a urine output of at least 2 L/day. A urine strainer should be provided. When the stone is passed, it should be saved for possible future stone analysis.

B. Admit

Patients with nephrolithiasis should be admitted under *any* of the following circumstances:

1. Concomitant urinary tract infection, especially if there is suspicion of an ascending infection from the site of obstruction.

2. Unrelenting pain.

3. Severe volume depletion.

4. Inability to maintain oral intake.

5. Stone in a single kidney.

6. Stone in a transplanted kidney.

VI. PEARLS AND PITFALLS

A. Patients presenting with acute and severe flank or back pain may have a life-threatening condition (e.g., leaking abdominal aortic aneurysm, ectopic pregnancy). Remember the differential diagnosis of renal colic.

B. Urinary tract infection combined with ureteral obstruction is a true urologic emergency that mandates rapid confirmation of the diagnosis and immediate urinary tract decompression.

C. Always send the urine for culture in patients with symptomatic nephrolithiasis.

D. Approximately 90% of the time the patient will pass the stone spontaneously. Treatment consists of IV hydration, analgesia, and antiemetics.

E. Encourage discharged patients to drink plenty of fluids and to void frequently.

Do *not* do any of the following:

A. Administer IV contrast to the patient with contrast allergy, renal insufficiency, or pregnancy.

B. Discharge the patient unless he/she has adequate pain control, good urine output, is reliable, and has follow-up arranged.

BIBLIOGRAPHY

Mohammed AJS, Goldfarb S: Diagnostic approach to the patient with nephrolithiasis. Adv Nephrol 1991; Chapter 8, pp. 239–267.

Preminger GM: Renal calculi: pathogenesis, diagnosis and medical therapy. Semin Nephrol 1992;12(2):200–216.

Segura JW: Surgical management of urinary calculi. Semin Nephrol 1990;10(1):53–63.

Stewart C: Nephrolithiasis. Emerg Med Clin N Am 1988;6(3):617–630.

18

Gynecologic Emergencies

ABNORMAL VAGINAL BLEEDING

> *A careful physician . . ., before he attempts to administer a remedy to his patient, must investigate not only the malady of the [woman] he wishes to cure, but also [her] habits when in health, and [her] physical constitution."*
>
> CICERO

I. ESSENTIAL FACTS

Vaginal bleeding is a symptom, not a disease. It may represent the patient's normal menses or a life-threatening condition. Abnormal vaginal bleeding may occur in the nonpregnant, pregnant, or postmenopausal female. The responsibility of the ED physician is to determine the cause of the bleeding and to treat that cause as indicated.

A. Definitions

1. *Normal menstrual bleeding* occurs every 28 days (normal range, 21–35 days), with an average flow duration of 4.5 days (normal range 2–7 days), and a normal blood loss of approximately 35 mL (normal range 20–80 mL). In the United States, menarche usually occurs between ages 11 and 16 years (12.77 years mean); menopause occurs between the ages of 35 and 55 years (average age, 51 years).

2. *Abnormal vaginal bleeding* is bleeding that is different from the patient's usual menstrual bleeding. As such, abnormal vaginal bleeding is defined by the patient. Commonly used terms include the following:
   a. *Menorrhagia:* excessive bleeding in both amount and duration (with normal cycle length).
   b. *Metrorrhagia:* normal amounts of bleeding, but at irregular intervals.
   c. *Menometrorrhagia:* excessive bleeding at irregular intervals.
   d. *Oligomenorrhea:* regular bleeding at intervals > 35 days.
   e. *Polymenorrhea:* regular bleeding at intervals < 21 days.

B. Epidemiology

1. Abnormal vaginal bleeding occurs in 20% of women at some time in their life. It is responsible for ≤ 15% of outpatient visits and 25% of gynecologic surgeries.

2. In females < 10 years old, the most common causes are precocious puberty and vaginal foreign bodies.

3. In adolescents and women of reproductive age, abnormal genital bleeding is usually secondary to pregnancy, hormonal causes, or benign uterine conditions.

4. In postmenopausal patients, malignancy is the cause of bleeding 20% of the time. With increasing age the risk of malignancy increases.

II. CLINICAL EVALUATION

A. History

1. Determine the following: overall health, sexual history (e.g., new partner, number of partners, history of sexually transmitted diseases, vaginal complaints), method of birth control, prior pregnancy history (G P Ab status), prior gynecologic history (including last Pap smear), history of trauma, medication use, drug and alcohol use, and drug allergies.

2. Inquire with respect to the patient's normal menstrual cycle (interval, flow duration, and approximate amount of usual blood loss). It is difficult for both physician and patient to quantitate blood loss, but a fully soaked pad or tampon will absorb 20–30 mL of blood. Ask the patient when her last normal menstrual period (LMP) was and how current bleeding differs from usual menstrual flow. Normal menstrual blood does not clot; clotting may indicate more rapid vaginal bleeding than usual. Some patients will be able to identify the passage of tissue (possible products of conception) with blood.

3. Question the patient with respect to symptoms of blood loss or anemia (orthostatic dizziness, fatigue, dyspnea), history of bleeding tendency, pregnancy (missed menses, morning sickness, breast complaints), and abdominal complaints (pain, swelling, anorexia, nausea/vomiting).

B. Physical Examination

Obtain vital signs and evaluate the skin, HEENT, neck, chest, heart, and abdomen, and perform a pelvic examination. (*Caution:* do not perform a pelvic examination in the vaginally bleeding pregnant patient ≥ 20 weeks gestation.) If supine vital signs are normal, check for orthostatic changes.

1. Carefully evaluate for abdominal distention, bowel sounds, tenderness, localized peritoneal irritation, masses, and abdominal evidence of pregnancy. In the pregnant patient, note uterine tone, fundal height (palpable at the symphysis pubis at 12 weeks gestation, at the umbilicus by 16–20 weeks gestation), fetal movement, and fetal heart tones

(FHT; audible by Doppler at 10–12 weeks; normal 120–160 beats/min).

2. Have the patient empty her bladder before the pelvic examination.
   a. Evaluate the external genitalia for lesions, trauma, or evidence of infection.
   b. Speculum examination:
      i. Note vaginal discharge, lesions, bleeding, and/or abnormal tissue in the cervical os or vaginal canal.
      ii. Remove all blood from the vagina with large cotton-tipped swabs, gauze pads, or bedside suction if necessary. Save any tissue (other than blood clots) in a sterile container for subsequent evaluation by pathology.
      iii. Evaluate the cervix for friability or lacerations; determine if the origin of bleeding is the cervical os. Check for an open internal os by *carefully and gently* attempting passage of a sterile ring forceps through the os (the internal os is approximately 1.5 cm deep to the external os). If the ring forceps do not easily pass, then the internal os is closed. Do not insert them farther than 3 cm. It is normal for the external os to be open in a parous patient.
      iv. Obtain a Gram stain and gonorrhea/chlamydia cultures from the endocervix. Using a cotton-tipped swab, obtain fluid from the vaginal pool for wet mount (normal saline) and KOH preparations.
   c. Perform a bimanual examination: note any abnormal cervical motion tenderness and fundal size (the uterus is the size of an orange at 6–8 weeks gestation); evaluate the uterus and adnexa for pain and/or masses. An adnexal mass is palpable in only 50% of ectopic pregnancies.
   d. Perform a rectovaginal examination: change the glove on your examining hand and again, palpate for pain and/or masses.

C. Laboratory Studies

1. Initial laboratory evaluation should *minimally* include the following:
   a. Complete blood count (CBC), including platelet count. If the patient has significant vaginal bleeding, abdominal pain, or unstable vital signs, serial hematocrits (every 20–30 minutes) should be obtained.
   b. Serum or urine pregnancy test (in reproductive-age women). Modern qualitative pregnancy tests detect the beta subunit of human chorionic gonadotropin (hCG) in either urine or serum. The current beta-hCG threshold for these tests varies, but is as low as 10–50 mIU/mL (serum test more sensitive than urine); modern tests are capable of detecting pregnancy as early as 8–9 days postconception.
   c. Urinalysis.

2. Additional studies *may be indicated,* depending on clinical circumstances:
   a. Electrolyte panel, glucose, blood urea nitrogen (BUN), and creatinine levels.
   b. Electrocardiogram (mandatory in all patients with a history of coronary artery disease, or ≥ 40 years old with unstable vital signs or significant abdominal pain).
   c. Prothrombin time/partial thromboplastin time (PT/PTT).
   d. Blood type and cross match. Obtain type-specific blood emergently in the patient with significant vaginal bleeding, unstable vital signs, falling hematocrit, or an acute surgical abdomen.

3. *If the pregnancy test is positive,* also obtain the following:
   a. Blood type and Rh-factor status. Rh (−) pregnant patients with active vaginal bleeding or a spontaneous abortion will require an intramuscular injection of Rh immune globulin (RhoGAM).
   b. Quantitative beta-hCG level. This test is valuable in the stable patient with first trimester vaginal bleeding and will be especially helpful to the follow-up referral physician. During the first 8 weeks of a normal pregnancy, the beta-hCG doubles every 1.8–3 days. Failure of the beta-hCG to double in this manner indicates an abnormal pregnancy, including a possible ectopic pregnancy. The quantitative beta-hCG also is helpful in determining the optimal time for ultrasound examination. Transvaginal ultrasound will not be able to visualize an intrauterine pregnancy until the beta-hCG is > 1800 mIU/mL (International Reference Preparation units, IRP). Transabdominal ultrasound will not be capable of demonstrating an intrauterine gestational sac until the beta-hCG is ≥ 6000–6500 mIU/mL.
   c. Serum progesterone level. Like the beta-hCG test above, the serum progesterone level is helpful in estimating pregnancy viability during the first trimester in the stable patient. Its advantage over beta-hCG is that serial measurements are unnecessary (serum progesterone changes little in the first 8–10 weeks of pregnancy). A serum progesterone < 5 ng/mL is nearly 100% indicative of a nonviable pregnancy (but does not indicate its location). A serum progesterone > 25 ng/mL excludes ectopic pregnancy with 97.5% sensitivity. Progesterone values of 5–25 ng/mL are nondiagnostic.

III. DIFFERENTIAL DIAGNOSIS

A. Pregnancy-Related

1. Early (< 20 weeks gestation)
   a. Threatened abortion (uterine bleeding during the first half of pregnancy without cervical dilatation)
   b. Incomplete abortion (all or part of the placenta is retained in the uterus with continued bleeding)

      c. Inevitable abortion (gross rupture of membranes and cervical dilatation)

      d. Missed abortion (retention of dead products of conception for ≥ 4 weeks during the first half of pregnancy)

      e. Complete abortion (complete passage of uterine contents with subsequent closure of the cervix, with resolution of cramping and little persistent bleeding)

      f. Septic abortion (intrauterine infection in the setting of abortion, spontaneous or "therapeutic")

      g. Ectopic pregnancy

      h. Gestational trophoblastic disease

  2. Late (> 20 weeks gestation)

      a. Abruptio placenta

      b. Placenta previa

  3. Postpartum hemorrhage

B. Inflammation

  1. Cervicitis

  2. Endometritis

  3. Intrauterine device (IUD)-related infection

  4. Pelvic inflammatory disease (PID)

  5. Vaginitis

  6. Vulvitis

C. Trauma

  1. Direct trauma (abrasions, lacerations)

  2. Foreign body

  3. Sexual assault

D. Anatomic Abnormalities

  1. Benign lesions

      a. Cervical polyp

      b. Endometrial hyperplasia

      c. Endometrial polyp

      d. Uterine leiomyoma

  2. Malignant lesions

      a. Vulvar

      b. Vaginal

      c. Cervical

      d. Endometrial

      e. Tubal

      f. Ovarian

E. Hormonal

  1. Anovulation

  2. Estrogen breakthrough bleeding

3. Prolactin-secreting tumors

4. Thyroid dysfunction (hypo- and hyperthyroidism)

F. Systemic Diseases

1. Acquired coagulopathy (e.g., vitamin K deficiency)

2. Hepatic dysfunction

3. Leukemia

4. Renal failure

5. Thrombocytopenia

6. von Willebrand's disease

IV. DIAGNOSIS AND THERAPY

A. Initial Management

Assess, secure, and support the airway, breathing, and circulation as indicated (see Chapter 1. II).

1. Obtain vital signs, keep the patient NPO, establish intravenous (IV) access, and obtain necessary blood work.

2. *If vital signs are unstable,* administer oxygen, monitor both cardiac rhythm and oxygen saturation (SaO_2), and initiate crystalloid resuscitation. Treat for hypovolemic shock (see Chapter 12). Send blood for stat CBC, PT/PTT, beta-hCG level, and Rh typing, and order emergent type-specific blood (4–6 units minimum). If the patient is > 20 weeks gestation, also evaluate for disseminated intravascular coagulation (DIC) with a thrombin time, fibrinogen level, and measurement of fibrinogen degradation products. Emergent consultation with an obstetrician/gynecologist is appropriate in this setting.

3. Simultaneously with the above, obtain a directed history and perform a physical examination.

4. *If vital signs are stable,* be prepared for a sudden deterioration in the patient, and proceed as outlined below.

5. Continually reassess the patient's hemodynamic status throughout her ED stay.

B. Pregnancy Test Positive; < 20 Weeks Gestation

1. **Ectopic Pregnancy**

   a. **Diagnosis.** Abnormal menses or amenorrhea (15% of patients, however, deny a missed menses), vaginal bleeding (50–80% of patients), and variable degrees of abdominal/pelvic pain (may be referred to the back or shoulder). On examination, there is usually uterine and/or adnexal tenderness (an adnexal mass is palpable in 50% of patients). The uterus may be enlarged, but is smaller than expected for dates; the cervix is closed.

b. **Treatment**

    i. Secure and support the airway, breathing, and circulation as outlined in IV. A, above, and emergently consult an obstetrician/gynecologist if the patient is unstable. See Ectopic Pregnancy, later in this chapter, for further details.

    ii. Stable patients with normal vital signs, a stable hematocrit, and a benign physical examination with minimal vaginal bleeding have either a threatened abortion (see below) or an early unruptured ectopic pregnancy.

- Management will vary with the institution, and may include transvaginal ultrasound, gynecology consultation, culdocentesis, or expectant management.
- Expectant management of the stable and reliable patient with normal vital signs, a normal hematocrit, and an unremarkable pelvic examination except for mild vaginal bleeding is as follows: obtain quantitative beta-hCG and serum progesterone. Discharge the patient to home with the following instructions: rest, no sexual intercourse, return immediately for occurrence of abdominal pain or increased bleeding. Follow-up in 48 hours with an obstetrician/gynecologist for repeat quantitative beta-hCG and evaluation of progesterone determination (see II. C, above). If initial or follow-up beta-hCG is > 1800 mIU/mL, schedule the patient for a transvaginal ultrasound; further management will depend on the results of the ultrasound.

    iii. Rh (−) women should be administered rhoGAM (50 μg IM if < 12 weeks gestational age).

2. **Threatened Abortion (Miscarriage).** Approximately 20–25% of clinically pregnant patients experience some vaginal bleeding, and an estimated 50% of these go on to miscarry.

a. **Diagnosis.** Determine the approximate gestational age based on the LMP. There should be minimal or no uterine tenderness, no adnexal abnormalities, mild cramping with minimal bleeding, an enlarged uterus appropriate for gestational age, and a closed internal cervical os.

b. **Treatment**

    i. Obtain quantitative beta-HCG and serum progesterone levels (remember, early ectopic pregnancy is also a diagnostic possibility—see above), discharge the reliable and stable patient to home with bedrest, pelvic rest, and close follow-up with her obstetrician or family physician (see expectant management outlined under IV. B. 1. b. ii, above).

    ii. Rh (−) women should be administered rhoGAM (50 μg IM if < 12 weeks gestational age; 300 μg IM if ≥ 12 weeks gestational age).

3. **Inevitable and/or Incomplete Abortion**

a. **Diagnosis.** Vaginal bleeding, cramping, enlarged uterus appropriate for dates, an open internal os, and normal adnexa. If bleeding is persistent and tissue is present in the os or the vagina, the abortion is considered incomplete.

b. **Treatment**

i. Secure and support the airway, breathing, and circulation as outlined under IV. A, above.

ii. If the gestational age is < 6 weeks or > 14 weeks, the patient may completely empty the uterus without surgical intervention.

iii. Gently remove any fetal tissue seen at the os with ring forceps. Patients with persistent bleeding and cramping may need a surgical procedure (curettage) to empty the uterus; consult the obstetrician/gynecologist. Consider medical treatment of profuse bleeding in consultation with the obstetrician/gynecologist prior to curettage: add 20 units of oxytocin (Pitocin) to a liter bag of lactated Ringer's solution (LR) or normal saline (NS), begin infusion at 20mU/min, and titrate accordingly. Oxytocin will contract the uterus and decrease the rate of bleeding.

iv. Provide compassion and emotional support; arrange for social worker consultation for the grieving process if available.

v. The patient may be discharged with methergine (0.2 mg PO every 6 hours for 48 hours) after curettage to further contract the uterus and decrease bleeding.

vi. Rh (−) women should be administered rhoGAM as outlined previously.

4. **Complete Abortion**

a. **Diagnosis.** Contents of uterus were completely emptied, vaginal bleeding is minimal, cramping has resolved, the cervical os is only slightly dilated or is now closed, and the uterus is firm.

b. **Treatment**

i. Observe in ED. Discharge to home if vaginal bleeding is clearly decreased and vital signs and hematocrit are stable. Close outpatient follow-up is appropriate.

ii. Rh (−) women should be administered rhoGAM as outlined previously.

5. **Missed Abortion**

a. **Diagnosis.** Defined as the retention of the dead products of conception for ≥ 4 weeks. The uterus is smaller than expected for gestational age and is irregularly softened, the cervix is closed (there may be a brownish vaginal discharge), and adnexa are normal. If the ultrasound shows an intrauterine pregnancy, no fetal heart motion will be visible.

b. **Treatment**

    i. Most cases of fetal demise result in spontaneous abortion within 5 weeks of demise and can therefore be managed conservatively. Close follow-up with an obstetrician/gynecologist should be arranged.

    ii. If the missed abortion occurs in the second trimester, the patient is at increased risk for a coagulation disorder. If platelets are decreased and/or PT/PTT are increased, or infection is suspected, evaluate the patient for DIC. Secure and support the airway, breathing, and circulation as outlined under IV. A, above, consult an obstetrician/gynecologist urgently, and arrange for hospitalization.

    iii. Rh (−) women should be administered rhoGAM as outlined previously.

6. **Septic Abortion.** If any of the above-described spontaneous abortions are complicated by fever (T ≥ 38°C) the patient may have a septic abortion. Septic abortion is associated with prolonged rupture of membranes, a foreign body (e.g., IUD), or instrumentation in an attempt to induce abortion.

a. **Diagnosis.** Signs of infection (fever, leukocytosis), vaginal bleeding (may be accompanied by a foul-smelling discharge), cramping, abdominal pain (with or without peritoneal signs), uterine tenderness, and adnexal tenderness.

b. **Treatment**

    i. Secure and support the airway, breathing, and circulation as outlined under IV. A, above.

    ii. Obtain blood cultures and uterine discharge culture, and evaluate for DIC. Consult an obstetrician/gynecologist emergently and arrange for urgent evacuation of the uterine contents.

    iii. Begin antibiotics: for example, clindamycin (600 mg IV every 6 hours) and gentamicin or tobramycin (2 mg/kg IV load followed by 1.5 mg/kg IV every 8 hours).

    iv. Rh (−) women should be administered rhoGAM as outlined previously.

    v. Hospitalize the patient.

7. **Hydatidiform Mole.** This is a disorder of the trophoblast.

a. **Diagnosis.** Patients with this uncommon problem (1:2000 pregnancies) may have lower-abdominal pain, severe nausea and vomiting, heavy vaginal bleeding, and an enlarged uterus for dates. Blood pressure may be elevated (pregnancy-induced hypertension) and fetal heart tones are absent. Bilateral adnexal enlargement may occur secondary to theca-lutein cysts; the passage of grape-like hydatid vesicles from the cervix is diagnostic.

b. **Treatment.** Consult an obstetrician/gynecologist, obtain a quantitative beta-hCG level (values > 100,000 mIU/mL are suggestive of trophoblastic disease), order a pelvic ultrasound (which will reveal characteristic hydropic vesicles within the uterus), and arrange for hospitalization. Rh (−) women should be administered rhoGAM as previously outlined.

C. Pregnancy Test Positive; ≥ 20 Weeks Gestation

Note: fundal height at 20 weeks gestation should be at the level of the umbilicus.

1. **Placenta Previa.** This is defined as implantation of the placenta in the lower uterine segment within the zone of dilatation and effacement of the cervix. It is responsible for 20% of bleeding episodes in the second half of pregnancy, and it occurs in about 1 in 200 births.
   a. **Diagnosis.** Placenta previa classically presents as painless hemorrhage, usually after 28 weeks. Bleeding may be sudden and profuse. The uterus is soft and nontender.
   b. **Treatment**
      i. Secure and support the patient's airway, breathing, and circulation as outlined under IV. A, above.
      ii. Do *not* perform a speculum or bimanual examination! Digital or mechanical manipulation may precipitate catastrophic hemorrhage! (Pelvic examination should only be performed by the obstetrician *in the delivery suite* with a double set-up for both vaginal delivery and emergent cesarean section).
      iii. Consult an obstetrician/gynecologist emergently; attach an external fetal monitor.
      iv. Arrange for ultrasound to confirm placenta previa.
      v. Hospitalize the patient to the obstetrics unit.

2. **Abruptio Placenta.** This is defined as the separation of the placenta from its site of implantation in the uterus prior to delivery of the fetus. A partial separation may occur in as many as 1 in 85 deliveries. Abruptio placenta is responsible for 30% of bleeding episodes in the second half of pregnancy. Perinatal mortality may be as high as 20–35%.
   a. **Diagnosis.** Classic findings include the passage of dark blood and uterine pain/irritability. External bleeding may be minimal despite extensive maternal blood loss (concealed hemorrhage); the uterus is tender, firm, and contracted. With significant separation there is fetal distress, DIC, and maternal shock.
   b. **Treatment**
      i. Secure and support the airway, breathing, and circulation as outlined under IV. A, above.
      ii. Do *not* perform a speculum or bimanual examination!
      iii. Consult an obstetrician/gynecologist emergently; attach an external fetal monitor.
      iv. Evaluate for DIC.

  v. Rh (−) women should be administered rhoGAM (300 μg IM).
  vi. Hospitalize the patient to the obstetrics unit.

D. Postpartum Hemorrhage

1. **Early Postpartum Hemorrhage** (> 500 mL blood loss during the first 24 hours after delivery)

   a. **Causes.** Lacerations of the uterus and cervix; abnormal separation of the placenta; coagulopathy; and uterine atony (the most common cause). In the latter case, the uterus will be enlarged and boggy.

   b. **Treatment**
      i. Secure and support the airway, breathing, and circulation as outlined under IV. A, above.
      ii. Uterine atony should be treated with uterine massage, methergine (0.2 mg IM), and oxytocin infusion (20–30 units in 1 L of IV fluid, titrated as necessary). Consult an obstetrician/gynecologist.
      iii. If the uterus is firm upon presentation, then carefully examine the episiotomy site, vagina, and cervix for lacerations. Repair as indicated.
      iv. Treat coagulopathy as outlined in Chapter 21.

2. **Late Postpartum Hemorrhage** (> 24 hours after delivery)

   a. **Causes.** Retained placenta or infection.

   b. **Treatment.** Secure the airway, breathing, and circulation; consult an obstetrician for suction curettage. Administer antibiotics as indicated for infection.

E. Vaginal Bleeding in Nonpregnant Women

Note: profuse, persistent bleeding from a cervical, vaginal, or vulvar lesion should be treated with appropriate vital sign support, a vaginal pack or external pressure on the bleeding site, and emergent gynecologic consultation.

1. **Benign Lesions**

   a. **Uterine Leiomyoma ("Fibroids").** These benign uterine tumors occur most often in the 4th and 5th decades of life and are responsible for 30% of cases of nonpregnancy-related abnormal vaginal bleeding. Tumors of the submucosal type cause hemorrhage. Bimanual examination may reveal an enlarged or abnormally shaped uterus. Any patient with an abnormal uterus should be referred to a gynecologist for further diagnosis and definitive care.

   b. **Cervical Polyps.** These small pedunculated structures prolapse in the cervical os and may be visualized upon speculum examination. They are usually solitary, painless, red, and friable. They are an infrequent cause of bleeding; gynecologic referral for further diagnosis and definitive care is appropriate.

2. **Malignant Lesions**

   a. **Endometrial Carcinoma.** This is the most frequent genital malignancy responsible for abnormal vaginal bleeding. Risk factors include late menopause, nulliparity, obesity, hypertension, and diabetes mellitus. All patients with postmenopausal bleeding require an endometrial biopsy and should be referred to a gynecologist for further diagnosis and definitive care.

   b. **Cervical Carcinoma.** This tumor may cause vaginal bleeding in its invasive later stages. The peak incidence is in the 4th decade of life. A lesion responsible for bleeding will be red, raised, solid, and friable. Any tissue removed with ring forceps should be placed in formalin and sent for pathologic examination. Patients need urgent referral to a gynecologist for further diagnosis and definitive care.

   c. **Vulvar or Vaginal Carcinoma.** These tumors are uncommon causes of bleeding. Any solid tumor identified on the external genitalia or by speculum or bimanual examination in the vagina must be assumed malignant and the patient should be urgently referred to a gynecologist.

3. **Systemic Medical Diseases.** Thyroid dysfunction, renal disease, liver disease, or clotting abnormalities such as thrombocytopenia, von Willebrand's disease, or an acquired clotting disorder may all cause abnormal menses or significant vaginal bleeding. A careful history, physical examination, and review of systems will reveal other complaints that may point to a particular illness. Therapy is aimed at appropriate vital sign support, necessary consultation, and treatment of the underlying disease process.

4. **Miscellaneous Causes**

   a. **Intrauterine Device.** This foreign body may cause increased bleeding. In this setting, the IUD should be removed in the ED if the string is visible. The patient must be counseled to use another form of birth control.

   b. **Infection.** Some patients with vulvitis, vaginitis, cervicitis, or PID will present complaining of abnormal vaginal bleeding. See the relevant chapters elsewhere in this manual for pertinent recommended therapy of these disorders.

   c. **Trauma.** Evidence of trauma as a cause of abnormal vaginal bleeding should always be sought at the time of the pelvic examination. Some traumatic injuries may be secondary to a sexual assault that the patient is reluctant to report. It is the responsibility of the ED physician to identify such cases and follow appropriate ED protocols in gathering forensic evidence and caring for the patient. Large perineal, vaginal, or cervical lacerations should be managed by a gynecologist. Simultaneously evaluate for associated rectal trauma. Peritoneal symptoms and signs are suggestive of visceral perforation.

5. **Hormonal Causes**

   a. **"Breakthrough" Bleeding on Oral Contraceptives.** Some patients will experience "breakthrough" or mid-cycle bleeding while using oral contraceptives (most often "low-dose" pills, in which the estrogen content is inadequate to maintain the endometrium). Bleeding late in the cycle may be due to inadequate progesterone activity. Breakthrough bleeding is generally benign, although it may cause patient distress. Referral to the patient's primary care provider is appropriate. If necessary, the oral contraceptive may be changed to a formulation containing a higher dose of estrogen.

   b. **Anovulatory Dysfunctional Uterine Bleeding**

      i. Anovulation is the most common reason for dysfunctional uterine bleeding: unopposed estrogen results in a hyperplastic and unstable endometrium. The patient may have amenorrhea for < 6 months and then note frequent episodes of heavy bleeding or a single episode of profuse bleeding. Anovulatory bleeding is seen most often at the extremes of reproductive age, with most cases occurring in adolescents.

      ii. Treatment
         • Secure and support the airway, breathing, and circulation as indicated.
         • Always rule out pregnancy in this setting.
         • If the patient is hemodynamically unstable or suffering from severe anemia, hospitalization is appropriate. Patients with profuse or persistent bleeding may need urgent suction curettage.
         • Most patients will not have hemodynamic compromise and can be managed as outpatients. Bleeding can be controlled, if necessary, with oral contraceptives: use a 50-µg estrogen–progesterone combination pill (e.g., Ovral, Ortho-Novum 1/50), and begin with one pill PO every 6 hours until bleeding stops (24–48 hours), followed by one pill tid for 2 days, then one pill bid for 2 days, then one pill PO every AM till the 28-day cycle is completed. Concomitant administration of an antiemetic (e.g., prochlorperazine, 10 mg PO every 6 hours as needed) is reasonable. Warn the patient that she will have appropriate withdrawal bleeding after finishing the cycle. The patient should be referred to her primary care physician and continued on oral contraceptives for 3–6 months.

V. PEARLS AND PITFALLS

A. The highest treatment priorities in patients with abnormal vaginal bleeding are support of the patient's airway, breathing, and circulation.

B. A pregnancy test is mandatory on every female of reproductive age who presents with vaginal bleeding, unless a hysterectomy has been documented.

C. Assess the Rh status of every pregnant woman who is suffering from vaginal bleeding. RhoGAM is appropriate if the mother is Rh(−) unless the father is also known to be Rh(−).

D. A postmenopausal female with vaginal bleeding has endometrial cancer until proven otherwise. Refer the patient to her gynecologist for an endometrial biopsy.

E. Patients whose reproductive preventative health care measures (e.g., Pap smears) have been neglected should be informed of this and referred to a primary care provider as part of their ED discharge instructions.

F. *Do not* perform a speculum or bimanual examination in the ED on a pregnant patient with vaginal bleeding who is ≥ 20 weeks gestation. Either manipulation may induce massive hemorrhage if the patient has placenta previa.

BIBLIOGRAPHY

Cowan BD, Morrison JC: Management of abnormal genital bleeding in girls and women. N Engl J Med 1991;324(24):1710–1715.

Galle PC, McRae MA: Abnormal uterine bleeding. Postgrad Med 1993; 93(2):73–76, 80–81.

Hertweck SP: Dysfunctional uterine bleeding. Obstet Gyne Clin N Am March 1992; 19(1):129–149.

Hochbaum SR: Vaginal bleeding. Emerg Med Clin N Am 1987;5(3):429–441.

Turner LM: Vaginal bleeding during pregnancy. Emerg Med Clin N Am 1994;12(1): 45–54.

ECTOPIC PREGNANCY

> *"To learn how to treat disease, one must learn how to recognize it. The diagnosis is the best trump in the scheme of treatment."*
>
> JEAN MARTIN CHARCOT (1825–1893)

I. ESSENTIAL FACTS

A. Definition

Ectopic pregnancy results when a fertilized ovum implants at a site other than the endometrial lining of the uterus.

1. Most ectopic pregnancies occur in the fallopian tube; other sites include the cornua, ovary, cervix, or abdominal cavity.

2. The possibility of ectopic pregnancy should be considered in *any* reproductive-age female with abdominal pain, vaginal bleeding, back pain, syncope, or abnormal vital signs.

B. Epidemiology

1. The incidence of ectopic pregnancy has *increased* dramatically in the past two decades. In 1987, approximately 88,000 women were hospitalized with ectopic pregnancy (a four-fold increase since 1970).

2. The rise in reported cases is a result of several factors, including increased risk factor prevalence, known tendency for ectopic recurrence, increased awareness of the disease, and earlier diagnosis due to improved technology.

3. Identified *risk factors* include
   a. Prior ectopic pregnancy (the recurrence rate is approximately 15%).
   b. History of pelvic infection, especially pelvic inflammatory disease (PID).
   c. Current intrauterine device (IUD) use.
   d. Prior tubal surgery, including infertility surgery or any tubal sterilization procedure.

4. Fortunately, the case fatality rate has substantially *decreased* in the last two decades, from 35.5 deaths per 10,000 ectopic pregnancies in 1970 to 3.4 deaths per 10,000 ectopic pregnancies in 1987. Despite this, *ectopic pregnancy remains the leading cause of maternal mortality in the first 20 weeks of pregnancy, and many deaths occur as a result of a delay in diagnosis.*

II. CLINICAL EVALUATION

A. History

Obtain and document the patient's prior reproductive history, character and timing of last menstrual period, birth control method, prior ectopic history, gynecologic history (including history of PID and/or tubal surgery), other health problems, medication use, and drug allergies.

B. Signs and Symptoms

1. *Abdominal pain* is the most common complaint (reported in > 97% of patients with an ectopic pregnancy). The pain may be localized or diffuse; it may radiate to the back or shoulder.

2. *Vaginal bleeding* is the second most common complaint.

3. *Amenorrhea* is reported by approximately two-thirds of patients. If menses did occur, they were often delayed or atypical in flow or duration.

4. *Syncope* occasionally is the presenting complaint and occurs secondary to hypovolemia from intra-abdominal hemorrhage.

5. *Symptoms suggestive of pregnancy* (e.g., morning sickness, breast tenderness, urinary frequency) are present in only a *minority* of cases.

C. Physical Examination

Obtain vital signs and evaluate the skin, HEENT, neck, chest, heart, and abdomen. If supine vital signs are normal, check for orthostatic changes. Carefully perform a pelvic examination:

1. Evaluate the external genitalia for lesions or evidence of infection.

2. With a speculum examination note vaginal discharge, lesions, bleeding, and/or abnormal tissue in the cervical os or vaginal canal. Determine whether the internal cervical os is open or closed. Obtain a Gram stain and gonorrhea/chlamydia cultures from the endocervix. Obtain a sample of any vaginal secretions for normal saline and KOH preparations.

3. With a bimanual examination, note any abnormal cervical motion tenderness, and evaluate the uterus and adnexa for pain and/or masses. An adnexal mass is palpable in only 50% of ectopic pregnancies.

4. Change examination gloves and perform a rectovaginal examination: again, palpate for pain and/or masses.

D. Laboratory Studies

1. Initial laboratory evaluation should *minimally* include the following:
   a. Complete blood count (CBC). If the patient has significant vaginal bleeding, abdominal pain, or unstable vital signs, serial hematocrits (every 20–30 minutes) should be obtained.
   b. Serum or urine pregnancy test. Modern qualitative pregnancy tests detect the beta subunit of human chorionic gonadotropin (hCG) in either urine or serum. The current beta-hCG threshold for these tests varies, but is as low as 10-50 mIU/mL (serum test more sensitive than urine); modern tests are capable of detecting pregnancy as early as 8–9 days postconception. Over 95% of patients with ectopic pregnancy will have a positive result with these sensitive assays.
   c. Urinalysis

2. Additional studies *may be indicated,* depending on clinical circumstances:
   a. Electrolyte, blood urea nitrogen, glucose, and creatinine levels.
   b. Electrocardiogram (mandatory in all patients with a history of coronary artery disease, or ≥ 40 years old with unstable vital signs or significant abdominal pain).
   c. Prothrombin time/partial thromboplastin time (PT/PTT)
   d. Blood type and cross match. Obtain type-specific blood emergently in the patient with significant vaginal bleeding, unstable vital signs, falling hematocrit, or an acute surgical abdomen.

3. *If the pregnancy test is positive,* also obtain the following:

a. Blood type and Rh factor status. Rh(−) pregnant patients with active vaginal bleeding or a spontaneous abortion will require an intramuscular injection of Rh immune globulin [RhoGAM].

b. Quantitative beta-hCG. This test is valuable in the stable patient with first-trimester vaginal bleeding and will be especially helpful to the follow-up referral physician. During the first 8 weeks of a normal pregnancy, the beta-hCG doubles every 1.8–3 days. Failure of the beta-hCG to double indicates an abnormal pregnancy, including a possible ectopic. The quantitative beta-hCG also is helpful in determining the optimal time for ultrasound examination. Transvaginal ultrasound will not be able to visualize an intrauterine pregnancy until the beta-hCG is >1800 mIU/mL (International Reference Preparation units, IRP). Transabdominal ultrasound will not be capable of demonstrating an intrauterine gestational sac until the beta-hCG is ≥ 6000–6500 mIU/mL.

c. Serum progesterone level. Like the beta-hCG above, serum progesterone is helpful in estimating pregnancy viability in the stable patient. Its advantage over the beta-hCG is that serial measurements are unnecessary (serum progesterone changes little in the first 8–10 weeks of pregnancy). A serum progesterone < 5 ng/mL is nearly 100% indicative of a nonviable pregnancy (but does not indicate its location). A serum progesterone > 25 ng/mL excludes ectopic pregnancy with 97.5% sensitivity. Progesterone values of 5–25 ng/mL are nondiagnostic.

E. Diagnostic Adjuncts

1. Ultrasound

a. Transvaginal ultrasound is capable of visualizing an intrauterine gestational sac as early as 3 weeks postconception (5 weeks gestational age). Transabdominal ultrasound can first visualize an intrauterine pregnancy about 1 week later (6 weeks gestational age).

b. Demonstrating an intrauterine pregnancy by ultrasound essentially rules out an ectopic pregnancy (the risk of a combined ectopic pregnancy and intrauterine pregnancy is exceedingly rare) *except* in infertility patients. Infertility patients who have undergone pregnancy stimulation or in-vitro fertilization have a risk of heterotopic (simultaneous intrauterine and ectopic) pregnancy that approaches 1%.

c. Sonographic findings nondiagnostic for ectopic pregnancy, but suggestive of same, include complex or cystic adnexal masses and/or free peritoneal fluid. Demonstrating extrauterine fetal heart motion is absolutely diagnostic of ectopic pregnancy, but this finding is seen in <10–15% of confirmed ectopics.

Table 18–1. INTERPRETATION OF CULDOCENTESIS FLUID

CULDOCENTESIS FLUID	DIAGNOSIS
Nonclotting blood (> 0.5 mL)	Ectopic pregnancy
Red, clotting blood (> 0.5 mL)	Ectopic pregnancy (acutely ruptured), or Ruptured corpus luteum cyst
Pus	Pelvic inflammatory disease, or Ruptured abscess (e.g., appendiceal or diverticular abscess)
Clear or straw colored	Indeterminate or ruptured ovarian cyst
No fluid	Nondiagnostic

      d. *Caution:* ectopic pregnancy is *not* excluded if the ultrasound fails to demonstrate an intrauterine pregnancy or any other significant finding; in that circumstance, the study is simply nondiagnostic.

  2. Culdocentesis

      a. *Culdocentesis* is the aspiration of fluid from the rectouterine cul-de-sac via needle puncture of the posterior vaginal wall. It is used less frequently now than in the past because of improved sonographic techniques.

      b. Culdocentesis is a moderately accurate but uncomfortable procedure. It is positive in 85–90% of patients with ruptured ectopic pregnancies. Even in the stable patient prior to frank ectopic rupture, culdocentesis is positive in 65–70% of cases.

      c. Indications include the following:

         i. Unstable patients with suspected ectopic pregnancy who require rapid confirmation of intraperitoneal bleeding prior to operative intervention.

        ii. Ultrasound is unavailable and urgent diagnosis is necessary.

       iii. Ultrasound is nondiagnostic and urgent diagnosis is otherwise necessary.

      d. Fluid obtained from culdocentesis may be indicative of a variety of conditions (Table 18–1).

      e. Culdocentesis is contraindicated in a patient with a fixed pelvic mass, an enlarged retroverted uterus, or a coagulopathy.

III. DIFFERENTIAL DIAGNOSIS

    The differential diagnosis of ectopic pregnancy includes the following conditions:

A. Appendicitis.

B. Dysfunctional uterine bleeding.

   C. Endometriosis.

   D. Follicular or corpus luteum cyst.

   E. Ovarian torsion.

   F. Pelvic inflammatory disease.

   G. Renal colic.

   H. Urinary tract infection.

   I. Uterine fibroid.

   J. Threatened or incomplete abortion.

IV. THERAPY

The emergency medical therapy of the patient with an ectopic pregnancy is presented in Figure 18–1.

A. Initial Management

Assess, secure, and support the airway, breathing, and circulation as indicated (see Chapter 1. II).

1. Obtain vital signs, keep the patient NPO, establish intravenous (IV) access, and obtain necessary blood work.

2. *If vital signs are unstable,* administer oxygen, monitor both cardiac rhythm and oxygen saturation, (SaO_2), and initiate crystalloid resuscitation. Treat for hypovolemic shock (see Chapter 12). Send blood for stat CBC, PT/PTT, beta-hCG, and Rh typing, and order emergent type-specific blood (4–6 units minimum). Emergent consultation with an obstetrician/gynecologist is appropriate in this setting.

3. Simultaneously with the above, obtain a directed history and perform a physical examination.

4. *If vital signs are stable,* be prepared for a sudden deterioration in the patient, and proceed as outlined below.

5. Continually reassess the patient's hemodynamic status throughout her ED stay.

B. Definitive Care

Assuming the patient's qualitative pregnancy test is positive, definitive care is as follows:

1. *Initially unstable patient* (see stabilization therapy, above):
   a. If the patient's vital signs *do not* normalize with aggressive resuscitation, the patient requires emergent laparotomy. The gynecology consultant may elect to perform a culdocentesis to confirm intraperitoneal bleeding while the operating room is preparing for the case.

    b. If the patient's vital signs *do* normalize with aggressive IV resuscitation, then either transvaginal ultrasound or culdocentesis is a reasonable option.

        i. Culdocentesis: if positive, operative management is appropriate.

        ii. Ultrasound: if an intrauterine pregnancy is found, then ectopic pregnancy is essentially ruled out and other diagnoses should be considered. The only exception to this rule is the infertility patient who is now pregnant (see II, above). If ultrasound findings are diagnostic of an ectopic pregnancy, then operative management is indicated. If the ultrasound is nondiagnostic, then culdocentesis should be performed with further definitive therapy dependent on the results of this procedure.

2. *Initially stable patient, but with physical findings indicative of an acute abdomen or abnormal pelvic examination consistent with ectopic pregnancy:* manage as outlined in IV. B. 1. b, above. Definitive management of a nonbleeding, unruptured ectopic pregnancy in the *stable* patient depends on the gynecology consultant; get the consultant involved early.

3. *A stable patient with normal vital signs, a normal hematocrit, and a benign physical examination, but who is pregnant with minimal vaginal bleeding, has either a threatened abortion or an unruptured ectopic pregnancy.*

    a. Management will vary with the institution, and may include transvaginal ultrasound, gynecology consultation, culdocentesis, or expectant management.

    b. Expectant management of the reliable patient with normal vital signs, normal hematocrit, and an unremarkable pelvic examination except for vaginal bleeding is as follows:

        i. Obtain quantitative beta-hCG and serum progesterone levels.

        ii. Discharge the patient to home with the following instructions: rest; no sexual intercourse; and return immediately for occurrence of abdominal pain, worsened bleeding, or orthostatic symptoms.

        iii. Follow-up in 48 hours with an obstetrician/gynecologist for repeat quantitative beta-hCG and evaluation of progesterone determination (see II, above).

        iv. If the initial or follow-up beta-hCG is ≥1 800 mIU/mL, schedule the patient for a transvaginal ultrasound.

C. Rh Immune Globulin

Rh(−) patients who are pregnant should be given Rh immune globulin (RhoGAM; dose: 50 μg IM if <12 weeks gestation; 300 μg IM if ≥ 12 weeks gestation) if any of the following conditions apply:

1. Ectopic pregnancy.

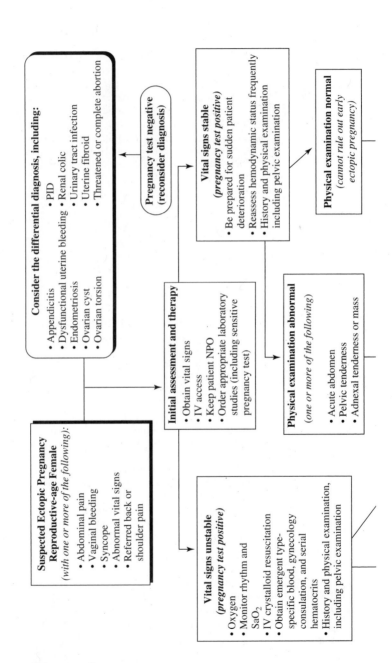

Suspected Ectopic Pregnancy Reproductive-age Female
(with one or more of the following):
- Abdominal pain
- Vaginal bleeding
- Syncope
- Abnormal vital signs
- Referred back or shoulder pain

Initial assessment and therapy
- Obtain vital signs
- IV access
- Keep patient NPO
- Order appropriate laboratory studies (including sensitive pregnancy test)

Consider the differential diagnosis, including:
- Appendicitis
- Dysfunctional uterine bleeding
- Endometriosis
- Ovarian cyst
- Ovarian torsion
- PID
- Renal colic
- Urinary tract infection
- Uterine fibroid
- Threatened or complete abortion

Pregnancy test negative (reconsider diagnosis)

Vital signs unstable *(pregnancy test positive)*
- Oxygen
- Monitor rhythm and SaO_2
- IV crystalloid resuscitation
- Obtain emergent type-specific blood, gynecology consultation, and serial hematocrits
- History and physical examination, including pelvic examination

Vital signs stable *(pregnancy test positive)*
- Be prepared for sudden patient deterioration
- Reassess hemodynamic status frequently
- History and physical examination including pelvic examination

Physical examination abnormal *(one or more of the following)*
- Acute abdomen
- Pelvic tenderness
- Adnexal tenderness or mass

Physical examination normal *(cannot rule out early ectopic pregnancy)*

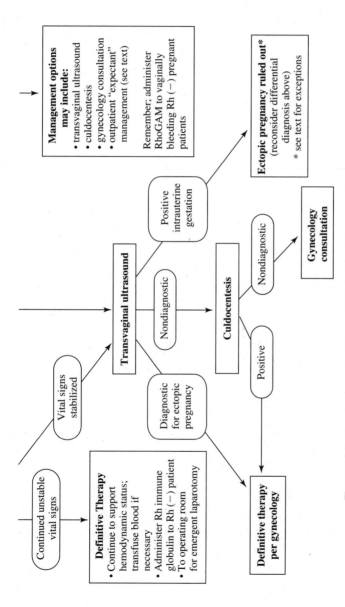

Figure 18–1. Emergency medical therapy of the patient with an ectopic pregnancy.

659

2. First-trimester vaginal bleeding (threatened abortion).

3. Completed abortion (spontaneous or induced).

V. DISPOSITION

Most patients with an established diagnosis of ectopic pregnancy require hospital admission for definitive medical or surgical treatment. In patients with a very early ectopic pregnancy, it is frequently impossible to make a definitive diagnosis at the initial ED visit. The reliable patient with normal vital signs, normal hematocrit, and insignificant findings on physical examination may be managed as outlined under IV. B. 3. b, above. If there is any doubt about the appropriateness of outpatient management of the stable patient, obtain a gynecology/obstetrics consultation.

VI. PEARLS AND PITFALLS

A. Obtain a stat pregnancy test on any female of reproductive age who presents with abdominal pain, vaginal bleeding, unstable vital signs, or amenorrhea.

B. Patients who have had a tubal sterilization procedure may rarely become pregnant; if pregnant, they are at significant risk for an ectopic pregnancy.

C. PID in pregnancy is rare; ectopic pregnancy must be ruled out.

D. A normal ultrasound examination (normal uterus, normal adnexa, no intrauterine gestation) does not rule out ectopic pregnancy; it is nondiagnostic in that instance.

E. Infertility patients who are pregnant after in vitro fertilization or pregnancy stimulation procedures can have a combined intrauterine and ectopic pregnancy.

F. Evaluate the Rh status of any pregnant patient with vaginal bleeding, and administer RhoGAM to Rh(−) mothers as indicated.

G. Patients who are not current with their preventative reproductive health care (e.g., Pap smears) should be referred to an appropriate primary care provider—and this information should be included in their ED discharge instructions.

BIBLIOGRAPHY

Abott JT, Emman LS, Lowenstein SR: Ectopic pregnancy: ten common pitfalls in diagnosis. Am J Emerg Med 1990;8(60):515–522.

Carson SA, Buster JE: Ectopic pregnancy. N Engl J Med 1993;329(16):1174–1181.

Diamond MP, DeCherney A (ed): Ectopic pregnancy. Obstet Gynecol Clin N Am 1991; 18(1):1–163.

Ectopic Pregnancy Surveillance, United States 1970–1987. MMWR 1990;39(SS-4):9–17.

Ory SJ: New options for diagnosis and treatment of ectopic pregnancy. JAMA 1992; 267(4):534–537.

VandoKrol L, Abbott JT: The current role of culdocentesis. Am J Emerg Med 1992; 10(4):354–359.

PELVIC INFLAMMATORY DISEASE

*"Variability is the law of life, and as no two faces are the same,
so no two bodies are alike, and no two individuals react alike and behave
alike under the abnormal conditions which we know as disease."*

SIR WILLIAM OSLER

I. ESSENTIAL FACTS

A. Definition

Pelvic inflammatory disease (PID) is a clinical syndrome caused by infection of one or more of the following: cervix, endometrium, myometrium, fallopian tubes, and/or other contiguous structures (e.g., peritoneum). The organisms involved are most commonly sexually transmitted agents (*Neisseria gonorrhoeae* and *Chlamydia trachomatis* together account for 80% of PID cases).

B. Risk Factors

Risk factors for PID include frequent sexual activity, multiple sexual partners, intrauterine device (IUD) use, prior history of PID, prior history of a sexually transmitted disease, recent menses, concurrent bacterial vaginosis, vaginal douching, intrauterine instrumentation (e.g., abortion), and age < 25 years.

C. Complications of PID

Complications of PID include perihepatitis (Fitz-Hugh–Curtis syndrome), tubo-ovarian abscess (7–16% of patients with PID), ectopic pregnancy (as much as a 10-fold increased risk after PID), recurrent infections, infertility (12% after one episode of PID, 25% after two episodes, 50% after three episodes), and/or chronic abdominal pain.

II. CLINICAL EVALUATION

A. History

Determine the patient's risk factors for PID (see I. B, above), duration and severity of symptoms, last menstrual period, pregnancy status, sexual history, and other health problems.

B. Symptoms and Signs

1. Symptoms may include lower-abdominal pain (patient's usual chief complaint), vaginal discharge, abnormal vaginal bleeding, nausea/vomiting, urinary tract symptoms, and/or fever.

2. Signs may include elevated temperature (T > 38°C in 30% of patients), abdominal tenderness (usually both lower quadrants), right-upper-quadrant abdominal tenderness (perihepa-

titis, present in 5% of PID cases), vaginal discharge, cervical inflammation, cervical motion tenderness, uterine tenderness, and adnexal tenderness and/or mass.

C. Directed Physical Examination

The physical examination should minimally include vital signs; evaluation of the patient's lungs, heart, and abdomen; and a carefully performed pelvic examination. At the time of the pelvic examination, a Gram stain, chlamydia culture, and gonorrhea culture should be obtained from the endocervix; a sample of vaginal pool fluid should be obtained for normal saline and 10% KOH slide preparations.

D. Laboratory Studies

1. *Minimal* laboratory evaluation should include
   a. Complete blood count (CBC) (leukocyte count frequently > 10 500/µL).
   b. Serum pregnancy test (a positive pregnancy test in a woman with abdominal pain suggests ectopic pregnancy; PID may also uncommonly occur in the first trimester of pregnancy).
   c. Urinalysis (to rule out urinary tract infections as a cause of lower-abdominal discomfort).
   d. Endocervical Gram stain (> 5 leukocytes/oil immersion field is indicative of infection).
   e. Vaginal pool normal saline and 10% KOH preparations (looking for trichomonads, clue cells, and/or yeast suggestive of concomitant vaginitis).
   f. Endocervical gonorrhea culture.
   g. Endocervical chlamydia culture.

2. Additional studies that are sometimes useful include
   a. Erthrocyte sedimentation rate (ESR) and/or C-reactive protein.
   b. Ultrasound examination (helpful in evaluating adnexal "fullness" suggestive of a tubo-ovarian abscess).
   c. Culdocentesis (may reveal purulent material in the setting of PID).
   d. Laparoscopy (performed in the operating room by the gynecology consultant; should be considered in the following patient situations: presence of an undiagnosed pelvic mass, PID that fails to respond to appropriate therapy, or when the diagnosis remains unclear [e.g., appendicitis can not be excluded]).

E. Diagnosing PID

1. All three of the following minimal criteria should be present:
   a. Lower-abdominal tenderness.
   b. Adnexal tenderness (usually bilateral).
   c. Cervical motion tenderness.

Note: The ED patient with all of the above should be empirically treated for PID.

2. One or more of the following, in addition to the above, increases the specificity of the diagnosis:
   a. Oral temperature > 38.3°C.
   b. Abnormal cervical or vaginal discharge.
   c. Elevated ESR (> 15 mm/hr) or C-reactive protein.
   d. Endocervical Gram stain revealing gram-negative intracellular diplococci or endocervical cultures positive for either *N. gonorrhoeae* or *C. trachomatis.*

3. "Elaborate" criteria for the diagnosis of PID may include endometritis on endometrial biopsy, tubo-ovarian abscess seen via ultrasound or other imaging procedure, or findings consistent with PID at laparoscopy.

4. *Cautions:* no single historical, physical, or laboratory finding is both sensitive and specific for PID. Many women complain of subtle, vague, or mild symptoms. Signs and symptoms may also be less pronounced in the immunocompromised or human immunodeficiency virus (HIV)-infected patient.

III. DIFFERENTIAL DIAGNOSIS

A. Appendicitis

B. Corpus luteum bleeding

C. Ectopic pregnancy

D. Endometriosis

E. Irritable bowel syndrome

F. Miscarriage

G. Ovarian cyst

H. Ovarian torsion

I. Ovarian tumors

J. Pelvic pain from prior PID episodes

K. Urinary tract infection

IV. THERAPY

A. Antibiotics

Antibiotics should be empirically instituted to minimize the potential sequelae of delayed or untreated infection. Table 18–2 outlines the Centers for Disease Control's antibiotic recommendations.

B. Analgesia

Nonsteroidal anti-inflammatory medication (e.g., ibuprofen 600 mg PO every 6–8 hours) and/or mild- to moderate-potency oral

Table 18–2. ANTIBIOTIC THERAPY FOR PELVIC INFLAMMATORY DISEASE

DRUG	DOSE	COMMENT
Outpatient Regimen		
Regimen A		
Ceftriaxone (Rocephin) or	250 mg IM single dose	Other cephalosporins that provide adequate gonococ-
Cefoxitin (Mefoxin) plus	2 g IM single dose	cal, gram-negative, and an-
Probenecid (Benemid)	1 g PO single dose	aerobic coverage may be used in appropriate doses.
to this add		
Doxycycline (Doryx, Vibramycin)	100 mg PO BID for 14 days	Do not administer tetracy- clines to pregnant patients.
Regimen B		
Ofloxacin	500 mg PO bid for 14 days	Do not administer fluoro- quiolones to pregnant pa- tients or patients <18 years
to this add		
Clindamycin or	450 mg PO qid for 14 days	
Metronidazole	500 mg PO bid for 14 days	
Inpatient Regimen		
Regimen A		
Cefoxitin sodium or	2 g IV every 6 hours	Continue this regimen for at least 48 hours after clinical
Cefotetan disodium (Cefotan)	2 g IV every 12 hours	improvement. After dis- charge, the patient should continue doxycycline 100 mg PO bid for 14 days.
to this add		
Doxycycline	100 mg IV every 12 hours	
Regimen B		
Clindamycin phosphate (Cleocin)	900 mg IV every 8 hours	Continue this regimen for at least 48 hours after clinical improvement. After dis-
to this add		charge, the patient should take doxycycline 100 mg PO
Gentamicin sulfate (Garamycin)	load: 2 mg/kg IV or IM maintenance: 1.5 mg/kg every 8 hours	bid, or clindamycin 450 mg PO qid, for 14 days.

opioids (e.g., oxycodone 5 mg PO every 4-6 hours) are beneficial and appropriate.

C. Counseling

Patients must be educated about the risk of reinfection by an untreated partner. Advise against sexual relations until both parties have completed a full course of therapy. Referral for HIV counseling and testing is appropriate in any patient who has acquired a sexually transmitted disease (STD). A serologic test for syphilis (e.g., RPR or VDRL) should also be obtained in any patient with a confirmed STD.

V. DISPOSITION

A. Discharge

Discharge to home is reasonable in the reliable patient with only mild disease. Follow-up in 48-72 hours is important to ensure response to therapy has occurred.

B. Admit

Admit to the hospital, with gynecologic consultation, patients suspected of PID who meet *any* of the following criteria:

1. Adolescent patient.
2. Diagnosis is uncertain.
3. Fails to respond to an appropriate outpatient regimen at time of follow-up.
4. Generalized peritoneal findings.
5. Immunocompromised patient (including HIV infection).
6. Intrauterine device is present.
7. Pregnant.
8. Severe pain requiring parenteral analgesia.
9. Suspected pelvic mass or tubo-ovarian abscess.
10. Toxic appearing.
11. Unable to take oral medications.
12. Unreliable.

VI. PEARLS AND PITFALLS

A. Obtain a serum pregnancy test in the workup of the patient suspected of PID, irrespective of the sexual or menstrual history reported by the patient.

B. Establishing the diagnosis of PID is difficult: in the ED setting, it is best to err on the side of overtreatment.

C. Obtain endocervical Gram stain and gonorrhea and chlamydia cultures in all women suspected of having PID.

D. Follow-up at 48-72 hours is mandatory in patients with PID.

E. Counseling to prevent future episodes of sexually transmitted diseases, evaluation and treatment of the partner, and referral for HIV counseling and testing is appropriate in any patient with a sexually transmitted disease.

F. If the patient is overdue for preventative Pap smear cervical cancer screening, include this information in her ED discharge instructions.

BIBLIOGRAPHY

Centers for Disease Control and Prevention: 1993 Sexually transmitted diseases treatment guidelines. MMWR 1993;42(No. RR-14):75–81.

McCormack WM: Pelvic inflammatory disease. N Engl J Med 1994;330(2):115–118.

Peterson HB, Galaid EI, Cates W: Pelvic inflammatory disease. Med Clin N Am 1990;74: 1603–1615.

Peterson HB, Galaid EI, Zenilman JM: Pelvic inflammatory disease: Review of treatment options. Rev Infec Dis 1990;12 (suppl.):656–664.

Washington AE, Cates W, Wasserheit JN: Preventing pelvic inflammatory disease. JAMA 1991;266:2574–2580.

VAGINITIS

"Nothing hinders a cure so much as frequent change of medicine . . ."

SENECA

I. ESSENTIAL FACTS

A. Definition

Vaginitis refers to a group of unrelated disorders that cause similar symptoms, including abnormal vaginal discharge, malodor, pruritis, spotting, and/or pain.

B. Etiology

Table 18–3 lists the many potential causes of vaginitis, the most common of which are bacterial vaginosis, candidiasis, and trichomoniasis.

1. *Bacterial vaginosis (BV).* This is a disturbance of the vaginal

Table 18–3. CAUSES OF VAGINITIS SYMPTOMS

Bacterial vaginosis (40–50%)
Vulvovaginal candidiasis (20–25%)
Trichomoniasis (15–20%)

Miscellaneous
  Atrophic vaginitis
  Puerperal atrophic vaginitis
  Foreign body
  Allergic vaginitis
  Chemical vaginitis
  Ulcerative vaginitis-associated *Staphylococcus aureus* and toxic shock syndrome
  Collagen vascular disease, Behcet's syndrome
  Herpes simplex virus—type II

Table 18–4. RISK FACTORS FOR CANDIDAL VAGINITIS

Pregnancy
Uncontrolled diabetes mellitus
High-estrogen oral contraceptives
Corticosteroid therapy
Tight-fitting, synthetic underclothing
Antimicrobial therapy
Intrauterine device

microbial ecosystem rather than a true infection; it is the most prevalent cause of vaginitis in women of reproductive age. BV is characterized by the overgrowth of *Gardnerella vaginalis, Mobiluncus* sp., genital *Mycoplasma,* and/or several species of facultative anaerobic bacteria.

2. *Vulvovaginal candidiasis (VVC).* This is the second most common cause of vaginitis among American women. Specific risk factors for VVC have been identified and are outlined in Table 18–4. *Candida albicans* is responsible for 90% of cases; other less frequent etiologic agents include *Torulopsis glabrata* and *Candida tropicalis.* These latter organisms may be more difficult to treat.

3. *Trichomoniasis. Trichomonas vaginalis* is a protozoan parasite that specifically infects genitourinary sites in men and women. Unlike BV and VVC, *T. vaginalis* is sexually transmitted. Its prevalence correlates with sexual activity and is highest among women with multiple sexual partners. The incubation period is 3–38 days. Most female partners of infected men, and 30–80% of male partners of infected women, are infected with this parasite.

II. CLINICAL EVALUATION

Table 18–5 presents the diagnostic features of vaginitis.

A. History

1. Symptoms related to vaginitis include vaginal discharge, pruritis, local discomfort, "external" dysuria (i.e., labial irritation with urination), and dyspareunia. Malodor is prominent with BV and trichomoniasis.

2. Determine and document the patient's last menstrual period, sexual and reproductive history, prior history of sexually transmitted diseases and vaginal infections, and pregnancy status.

B. Physical Examination

A careful and thorough pelvic examination is mandatory.

1. Inspect the vulvar area: note labial/perineal irritation, erosions, and any abnormal lesions.

2. Speculum examination: vaginal mucosa should be assessed for erythema, petechiae, ulceration, edema, atrophy, and adherent discharge. The color, consistency, pH, and volume of pooled vaginal secretions should be noted and a sample taken for normal saline and KOH slide preparations. Examine the cervix for exudate, ulcerations, other lesions, and bleeding. Obtain gonorrhea/chlamydia cultures and a Gram stain from the endocervix, ± a Pap smear (depending on the patient's health maintenance status and the "Pap smear policy" of the ED).

3. Bimanual examination: note any cervical and uterine tenderness, the uterine size, and the presence of uterine and/or adnexal masses.

4. Change gloves and complete the pelvic examination with a rectovaginal examination.

C. Diagnostic Studies

1. **Saline Wet Mount.** Add a drop of normal saline to a fresh slide of smeared vaginal secretions. Note the presence of any of the following:

   a. Clue cells: vaginal epithelial cells with obscured cell borders secondary to bacterial stippling; clue cells are indicative of BV (especially if the vaginal pH is $\geq$ 4.5).

   b. Trichomonads: twitching, motile protozoa the size of polymorphonuclear neutrophils.

   c. Yeast pseudohyphae: indicative of VVC.

   d. Polymorphonuclear neutrophils (PMNs): a ratio of PMNs to epithelial cells > 1 suggests an inflammatory process (e.g., trichomoniasis, other sexually transmitted disease).

   e. Morphology of epithelial cells: the presence of small round nucleated basal cells suggests estrogen deficiency.

Table 18–5. DIAGNOSTIC FEATURES OF VAGINITIS

	NORMAL	VULVOVAGINAL CANDIDIASIS	BACTERIAL VAGINOSIS	TRICHOMONIASIS
Symptoms	None or physiologic leukorrhea	Moderate pruritus, soreness	Malodorous discharge	Profuse discharge, and severely pruritic
Discharge	Variable—none to moderate	Scant to moderate; white, thick, and sometimes clumpy	Scant to moderate; white/gray; thin and homogenous	Profuse; gray to yellow; thin and homogenous
Amine (fishy odor) when 10% KOH is added to discharge	Negative	Negative	Positive	Sometimes positive
pH	$\leq$ 4.5 (5.0 during menses)	$\leq$ 4.5	5–6	5–7
Microscopy: normal saline and 10% KOH preparations		Fungal elements: budding yeast or pseudohyphae	Clue cells	Motile trichomonads and PMNs

2. **KOH Wet Mount.** Add a drop of 10% KOH to a fresh slide of smeared vaginal secretions.
   a. Note any odor produced (the "whiff" test): in BV (and occasionally trichomoniasis) the amines released will emit a "fishy" smell.
   b. Examine for yeast (either conidial forms or budding spores [oval shapes one-fourth the size of a PMN] and/or pseudohyphae).

3. **Vaginal pH.** Normal pH is < 4.5; pH ≥ 4.5 suggests BV or trichomoniasis.

4. **Gram Stain of the Endocervix.** > 5 leukocytes/oil-immersion field is indicative of infection/cervicitis; gram-negative intra-cellular diplococci suggest gonorrhea.

5. **Cultures.** Endocervical cultures are imperative for the diagnosis of cervicitis (e.g., gonorrhea, Chlamydia).

III. DIFFERENTIAL DIAGNOSIS

A. Vaginal Causes

Causes of vaginitis are listed in Table 18–3.

1. **Atrophic Vaginitis.** Reduced endogenous estrogen leads to gradual mucosal thinning, decreased glycogen, increased pH, and altered flora. Symptoms, when present, include vaginal soreness, dyspareunia, and occasional spotting or discharge. The saline wet mount shows small, round epithelial cells (immature squames that have not been exposed to sufficient estrogen).

2. **Vaginal Foreign Body.**

3. **Allergic Vulvovaginitis.** Presents as vulvar pruritus and burning. It is usually misdiagnosed as VVC. The causes include topical medications, douches, spermatozoa, and *Candida sp.*

4. **Chemical Vaginitis.** Is uncommon, but may be caused by disinfectants, deodorants, spermatocides, and cosmetics.

5. **Pinworm.** Vaginal itching (especially severe at night) unresponsive to usual therapies rarely may be caused by the pinworm *(Enterobius vermicularis)*. Cellophane tape pressed to the perianal or vulvar regions and then applied to a glass slide will reveal the worms.

B. Other

1. **Cervicitis.** Can present as a vaginal discharge. See Sexually Transmitted Diseases in Chapter 15.

2. **Herpes Simplex Virus.** Usually presents with a prodrome of tingling or discomfort in the genital region, followed by a

painful vesicular eruption. A primary infection is often accompanied by systemic symptoms such as fever and malaise. Lesions located along the vaginal vault or cervix may go unnoticed except for vaginal discharge. See Chapter 15.

3. **Urinary Tract Infection.** May cause dysuria (though usually "internal" [i.e., urethral discomfort] instead of "external" dysuria. Other symptoms may include suprapubic pain, urgency, frequency, and/or flank tenderness. Obtain a urinalysis, and culture if clinically indicated. See Chapter 15.

IV. THERAPY

Emergency medical therapy of vaginitis is presented in Table 18–6.

A. Bacterial Vaginosis

1. **Metronidazole (oral).** The immediate clinical cure rate of both multiple-day and single-dose regimens is 90%, but single-dose therapy has a 10–15% recurrence rate at 4 weeks. The most common side effects include a metallic taste; nausea (10%); transient neutropenia (7.5%), and a disulfiram reaction with alcohol. The most serious, but rare, side effects involve the central nervous system (seizures, peripheral neuropathy). This drug is contraindicated during the first trimester of pregnancy.

2. **Metronidazole (Topical).** Has similar efficacy to the oral preparation, and side effects are few. Minimal systemic absorption does occur; safety in the first trimester of pregnancy has *not* yet been determined.

3. **Clindamycin (Oral or Topical).** Has excellent activity against anaerobes and moderate activity against *G. vaginalis* and *Mycoplasma hominis.* This medication is the first effective alternative to metronidazole for BV. It has fewer adverse reactions and is safe to use during pregnancy. The mineral oil base of the topical preparation will weaken condoms and contraceptive diaphragms; use of these contraceptive devices should be avoided because of unreliability for 72 hours after using clindamycin cream.

4. **Amoxicillin (Oral).** Is a less effective alternative to metronidazole, but it is safe to use in pregnancy. Amoxicillin with clavulanic acid (Augmentin) is probably more effective than amoxicillin alone but is considerably more expensive and has a 10% rate of significant gastrointestinal side effects (especially diarrhea).

B. Vulvovaginal Candidiasis

1. **Azole and Polyene Antimycotics (Topical).** Are variously packaged as creams, lotions, vaginal tablets, suppositories, and coated tampons. Formulation does not effect clinical efficacy. The azoles are slightly more efficacious than the polyenes. Side

Table 18–6. EMERGENCY MEDICAL THERAPY FOR VAGINITIS

CAUSE	DRUG	DOSE	COMMENTS
Bacterial Vaginosis	Metronidazole (PO) (Flagyl, Metryl, Protostat)	500 mg bid for 7 days or 2 g initially	Side effects: see text
	Metronidazole (topical) (Metrogel-vaginal 0.75%)	5 g (one applicator) intravaginally bid for 5 days	Minimal systemic absorption.
	Clindamycin (topical) (Cleocin HCl)	2% cream applied intravaginally daily for 7 days	Equal efficacy to metronidazole Safe in pregnancy; see text.
	(Clindamycin [PO])	300 mg bid for 7 days	Safe in pregnancy.
Vulvovaginal Candidiasis	*Imidazoles* (topical)		Burning on initial application. Use 7 day treatment course in pregnancy.
	Clotrimazole (Gyne-lotrimin, Mycelex)	500-mg vaginal tablet (Mycelex), single dose or 1% vaginal cream (Gyne-Lotrimin, Mycelex-G) one applicatorful in vagina nightly for 7–14 nights or 200-mg vaginal tablet nightly for 3 nights	
	Miconazole (Monistat)	2% cream (Monistat 7), one applicatorful in vagina nightly for 7 nights or 200 mg vaginal suppository (Monistat 3) nightly for 3 nights or 100 mg vaginal tablet (Monistat) nightly for 7 nights	
	Butoconazole 2% (Femstat)	5 g (one applicator) cream intravaginally nightly for 3 days	
	Imidazoles (PO)		Consider for resistant or recurrent cases. Do not use in pregnant women.
	Fluconazole (Difulcan)	100–150 mg single dose	
	Ketoconazole (Nizoral)	200 mg bid for 5–14 days	
	Itraconazole (Sporanox)	200 mg/day for 3 days	
Trichomoniasis	Metronidazole (PO) (Flagyl, Metryl, Protostat)	2 g single dose for patient and for partner or 500 mg bid for 7 days	Side effects: see text. Treat sexual partner simultaneously.
Atrophic Vaginitis	Estrogen cream	One-half applicatorful intravaginally daily for 1–2 weeks, then one-half applicatorful twice weekly for 1–2 weeks.	

effects are minimal; burning upon initial application is reported.

2. **Azole Antimycotics (Oral).** These medications should be considered in resistant or recurrent cases; the risk of side effects is greater than with topical therapy. Patients treated with ketoconazole may experience the following: gastrointestinal upset (10%), anaphylaxis (rare), and hepatotoxicity (idiosyncratic, rare). Other agents have less adverse reactions.

3. **Recurrent and Chronic Vulvovaginal Candidiasis.** Proceed as follows:
   a. Confirm the diagnosis (consider culture documentation),
   b. If possible, correct any underlying causes (see Table 18–4), and
   c. Prescribe a long-term suppresive dose of an antifungal drug and/or refer the patient to a primary care provider. Daily low-dose oral ketoconazole (100 mg/day for 6 months) is the best-studied regimen.

C. Trichomoniasis

1. **Metronidazole.** Oral therapy is recommended because infection of the urethra and periurethral glands provides sources for endogenous reinfection. Standard therapy consists of 500 mg po bid for 7 days (cure rate of 95%). Many clinicians recommend a single dose of 2 g (cure rate of 82–88%; increases to > 90% when sexual partners are also treated). Side effects are as outlined above. Metronidazole is contraindicated during the first trimester of pregnancy.

2. **Clotrimazole Intravaginal Cream.** A reasonable alternative to metronidazole in the treatment of trichomoniasis during the first trimester of pregnancy.

3. **Vinegar Douche.** May provide symptomatic relief to women in the first trimester of pregnancy with trichomoniasis.

D. Atrophic Vaginitis

Treat with a topical estrogen cream.

V. PEARLS AND PITFALLS

A. Always consider the possibility of pregnancy in the female patient of reproductive age.

B. Consider the possibility of a concomitant sexually transmitted disease (e.g., gonorrhea, *Chlamydia*) in any patient with vaginal complaints; culture and treat as appropriate.

C. Patients with a recurrence of symptoms need a complete re-evaluation. Concurrent infections are common, and initial therapy may have eliminated only one of the pathogens.

D. Warn patients of possible medication side effects and the need to abstain from alcohol for at least 24 hours after completing a treatment course of metronidazole.

E. If a Pap smear was done at the time of the pelvic examination, ensure meticulous ED follow-up and patient notification of the Pap smear results. If a Pap smear was not done, but the patient is due for one (on the basis of health maintenance schedules), recommend this to the patient at the time of ED discharge and document this recommendation in the patient's chart.

BIBLIOGRAPHY

Centers for Disease Control and Prevention: 1993 Sexually transmitted diseases treatment guidelines. MMWR 1993;42 (No. RR-14):67–75.

Sobel JD: Vaginitis in adult women. Obstet Gynecol Clin N Am 1990;17(4):851-79.

Reed BD, Eyler A: Vaginal infections: Diagnosis and management. Am Fam Phys 1993;47(8): 1805–1816.

19

Endocrine Emergencies

ADRENAL CRISIS

"We have on our hands a sick man—a very sick man."

NICHOLAS I OF RUSSIA

I. ESSENTIAL FACTS

A. Definition

The acute loss of adrenal steroids is referred to as *adrenal crisis;* it constitutes a medical emergency and may present as vascular collapse, prominent abdominal symptoms, and significant electrolyte disturbances. Adrenal crisis is typically precipitated by trauma, surgery, labor and delivery, or a stressful intercurrent illness. It must be considered both in the differential diagnosis of shock and in illnesses accompanied by sustained hypotension refractory to ordinary volume repletion and supportive care.

B. Epidemiology

1. Complete *primary adrenal insufficiency* (destruction of the adrenal cortex) is a rare and potentially fatal disorder.

      a. It results in the complete loss of both glucocorticoid and mineralocorticoid production by the adrenal glands.

      b. Autoimmune and granulomatous diseases account for the majority of cases.

      c. Other causes include gram-negative bacterial infections, fungal infections, metastatic malignancy, sarcoidosis, and intra-adrenal hemorrhage associated with a bleeding disorder or anticoagulant use.

      d. Drugs that may precipitate adrenal crisis include ketoconazole, etomidate, levothyroxine, and rifampin.

      e. Partial primary adrenal insufficiency has been recognized with increasing frequency in patients with the acquired immunodeficiency syndrome (AIDS).

2. *Secondary adrenal insufficiency* is due to failure of normal pituitary ACTH production.

      a. It results in selective glucocorticoid deficiency with preservation of mineralocorticoid secretion.

      b. Long-term exogenous glucocorticoid administration (e.g., prednisone) is its most common cause. Any patient who has received supraphysiologic doses of a glucocorticoid for > 2 weeks is at risk for developing secondary adrenal insufficiency for a period of up to 9 months.

      c. Clinical manifestations in patients with this disorder are usually mild in comparison to the fulminant presentation of primary adrenal insufficiency.

II. CLINICAL EVALUATION

A. History

Inquire about the presence of other endocrine deficiencies, history of tuberculosis or systemic infection, history of malignancy, human immunodeficiency virus (HIV) status, glucocorticoid use within the past year, anticoagulant use, and symptoms of an illness or stressful event that may have precipitated the adrenal crisis. A family history that reveals endocrine deficiencies or other autoimmune phenomena may clarify the patient's diagnosis.

B. Symptoms

The patient with adrenal crisis will often complain of antecedent weakness, fatigue, weight loss, anorexia, orthostatic dizziness, or salt craving. Nausea, vomiting, and abdominal pain occurring at the time of presentation may mimic a surgical abdomen.

C. Signs

Tachycardia, orthostatic blood pressure changes or hypotension, and mild fever are common. Skin turgor is decreased; and in primary adrenal failure (not secondary) hyperpigmentation of the extensor surfaces, palmar creases, scars, and mucosal membranes may be seen. Other skin changes may include vitiligo, loss of adrenal androgen-dependent axillary and pubic hair in females, and atrophy or ecchymoses suggesting prior use of high-dose glucocorticoids or anticoagulants. Findings indicating previous glucocorticoid use include moon facies, a "buffalo hump," and central obesity. Abdominal examination typically reveals diffuse tenderness without localizing signs. Mental status changes include disorientation, confusion, lethargy, or unconsciousness.

D. Physical Examination

Obtain vital signs and examine the skin, HEENT and neck, chest, heart, abdomen (include rectal examination and stool heme test), genitourinary system, extremities, and neurologic status.

1. Note skin turgor (as a reflection of dehydration), and examine closely for infection, signs of chronic steroid use, and/or the hyperpigmentation changes of primary adrenal failure.

2. The abdomen is typically tender in adrenal crisis; but look for distention, bowel sounds, masses, or findings of localized peritoneal irritation. Localized findings suggest a surgical abdomen that has precipitated the adrenal crisis.

3. Mental status may be altered because of the adrenal failure, infection, severe dehydration, hypo- or hyperglycemia, marked electrolyte abnormality, traumatic injury, or drug ingestion/ withdrawal. A lateralized deficit suggests an acute cerebrovascular accident.

E. Laboratory Studies

1. *Routinely* obtain the following:
   a. Complete blood count (CBC) with platelet count.
   b. Glucose level.
   c. Electrolyte panel.
   d. Blood urea nitrogen (BUN) and creatinine levels.
   e. Blood cultures.
   f. Calcium, magnesium, and phosphate levels.
   g. Electrocardiogram (ECG).
   h. Chest roentgenogram.
   i. Urinalysis and culture.
   j. Pregnancy test (in reproductive-age females).

2. *Adrenal function studies* are mandatory (the results will not be available while the patient is in the ED):
   a. Cortisol (random serum).
   b. ACTH (place this sample on ice immediately and send it to the laboratory).

3. Additional studies *may be required,* depending on clinical circumstances (arterial blood gas, amylase, and bilirubin levels; abdominal films, etc.).

4. *Common laboratory results* include the following:
   a. **Electrolytes.** Hyponatremia, hyperkalemia, and hyperchloremic metabolic acidosis are the classic electrolyte

patterns seen in primary adrenal insufficiency. Hyperkalemia may not be present, however, because of decreased oral intake or gastrointestinal losses. In secondary adrenal insufficiency, the serum potassium is typically normal because mineralocorticoid function is preserved.

b. **CBC.** Neutropenia, lymphocytosis, and eosinophilia may occur.

c. **Glucose.** Hypoglycemia is seen most often in secondary adrenal insufficiency.

d. **BUN and Creatinine.** Azotemia is common.

e. **Calcium.** Hypercalemia occasionally occurs.

f. **Chest Film.** May reveal evidence of a malignancy or infection.

g. **Abdominal Films.** May show suprarenal calcifications consistent with tuberculous involvement of the adrenal glands.

h. **Abdominal Computed Tomography.** May reveal evidence of metastatic disease involving the adrenals, or bilaterally enlarged adrenals with hyperdense areas suggestive of hemorrhage.

i. **Adrenal Function Tests.** In adrenal insufficiency, the random serum cortisol obtained at the time of the patient's presentation will usually be less than 20 µg/dL, and further adrenal function tests will be necessary (see E. 5, below). If the cortisol level exceeds 20 µg/dL, a diagnosis of acute adrenal insufficiency is generally excluded. In primary adrenal insufficiency, the ACTH level drawn at the time of admission will be high, and in secondary adrenal insufficiency it will be low.

5. *A rapid ACTH stimulation test* should be performed during the patient's hospitalization if the random serum cortisol drawn at the time of presentation is < 20 µg/dL and adrenal insufficiency is clinically suspected.

a. *Caution:* both prednisone and hydrocortisone are measured in the cortisol assay and will interfere with the results of this test. Dexamethasone will *not* interfere with the cortisol assay.

b. Obtain a baseline serum cortisol determination at time "0."

c. Administer intravenously (IV) 250 µg of synthetic ACTH (cosyntropin).

d. Obtain serum cortisol levels at 30 minutes and 60 minutes after ACTH administration.

e. *Interpretation:* normal adrenal function is indicated by a rise in the cortisol level to 20 µg/dL or greater by 60 minutes. A rise in cortisol to less than 20 µg/dL by 60 minutes is consistent with either primary or secondary adrenal insufficiency. The latter two diagnoses may be further distinguished either by the ACTH level from the presenting blood specimen or by the cortisol response to three consecutive daily 8-hour IV infusions of 250 µg of synthetic ACTH in normal saline. An elevated baseline

ACTH level, or failure of the cortisol level to increase to
≥ 20 µg/dL in response to prolonged ACTH stimulation, is
indicative of primary adrenal insufficiency.

III. DIFFERENTIAL DIAGNOSIS

The typical hypotensive presentation of adrenal crisis evokes the
broad differential diagnosis of shock. Hypovolemic, cardiogenic,
distributive, and obstructive causes of shock must all be considered.
The fever that frequently accompanies glucocorticoid deficiency
mandates the exclusion of sepsis. Prominent gastrointestinal symptoms, along with hyperkalemia, necessitate consideration of an
intra-abdominal emergency. Diagnostic efforts other than laparotomy
should be employed, since surgery in the setting of unrecognized and
untreated adrenal crisis may have a fatal outcome. The hypoglycemia
that is often associated with secondary adrenal insufficiency raises the
possibility of alcohol abuse, insulinoma, overdose of a sulfonylurea
or insulin, or hepatic dysfunction.

IV. THERAPY

Emergency therapy of adrenal crisis is presented in Figure 19–1.

A. Initial Management

Assess, secure, and support airway, breathing, and circulation
as indicated (see Chapter 1. II).

1. Guard the airway, administer supplemental oxygen, establish
   IV access, monitor both cardiac rhythm and oxygen saturation
   (SaO_2), obtain vital signs, and check the fingerstick glucose
   level.

2. Use D5 normal saline (D5NS) as necessary for blood pressure
   support. Two to four liters are usually required in the first
   12–24 hours of the patient's care. D5NS is recommended over
   plain NS because hypoglycemia is so common and is a major
   source of morbidity in the patient in adrenal crisis.

3. Obtain a directed history, perform a physical examination, and
   obtain appropriate laboratory studies as outlined in II, above.

B. Adrenal Hormone Replacement

Steroid replacement therapy should be started immediately
without waiting for results of the baseline cortisol determination.

1. **Hydrocortisone.** This is considered the drug of choice in the
   setting of suspected adrenal insufficiency because it provides
   both glucocorticoid and mineralocorticoid replacement.
   Dose: 100 mg IV every 6 hours for the first 24 hours. After
   24 hours the hydrocortisone dose can usually be lowered to 50
   mg IV every 6 hours.
   If ACTH testing is to be performed, the patient should be

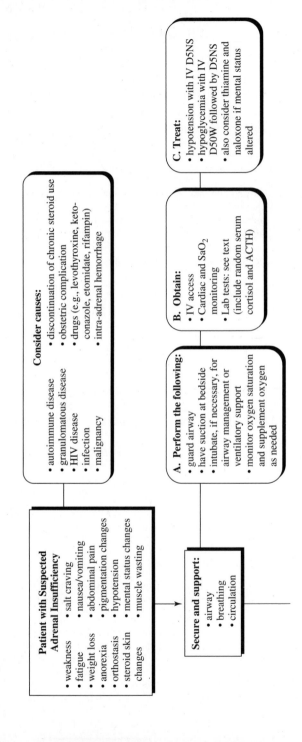

Patient with Suspected Adrenal Insufficiency

- weakness
- fatigue
- weight loss
- anorexia
- orthostasis
- steroid skin changes
- salt craving
- nausea/vomiting
- abdominal pain
- pigmentation changes
- hypotension
- mental status changes
- muscle wasting

Consider causes:

- autoimmune disease
- granulomatous disease
- HIV disease
- infection
- malignancy
- discontinuation of chronic steroid use
- obstetric complication
- drugs (e.g., levothyroxine, keto-conazole, etomidate, rifampin)
- intra-adrenal hemorrhage

Secure and support:

- airway
- breathing
- circulation

A. Perform the following:

- guard airway
- have suction at bedside
- intubate, if necessary, for airway management or ventilatory support
- monitor oxygen saturation and supplement oxygen as needed

B. Obtain:

- IV access
- Cardiac and SaO$_2$ monitoring
- Lab tests: see text (include random serum cortisol and ACTH)

C. Treat:

- hypotension with IV D5NS
- hypoglycemia with IV D50W followed by D5NS
- also consider thiamine and naloxone if mental status altered

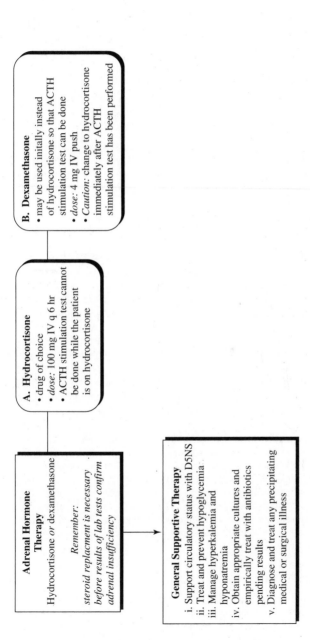

Adrenal Hormone Therapy
Hydrocortisone *or* dexamethasone

Remember:
steroid replacement is necessary before results of lab tests confirm adrenal insufficiency

A. Hydrocortisone
- drug of choice
- *dose:* 100 mg IV q 6 hr
- ACTH stimulation test cannot be done while the patient is on hydrocortisone

B. Dexamethasone
- may be used initially instead of hydrocortisone so that ACTH stimulation test can be done
- *dose:* 4 mg IV push
- *Caution:* change to hydrocortisone immediately after ACTH stimulation test has been performed

General Supportive Therapy
i. Support circulatory status with D5NS
ii. Treat and prevent hypoglycemia
iii. Manage hyperkalemia and hyponatremia
iv. Obtain appropriate cultures and empirically treat with antibiotics pending results
v. Diagnose and treat any precipitating medical or surgical illness

Figure 19–1. Emergency therapy of adrenal crisis.

stabilized on the hydrocortisone during hospitalization, then changed from hydrocortisone to dexamethasone, and ACTH testing performed 1 day later. (*Remember:* hydrocortisone will be measured in the cortisol assay during the ACTH stimulation test, and will falsely elevate the results.)

2. **Dexamethasone.** Some authors recommend starting treatment with dexamethasone, a pure glucocorticoid, to allow for ACTH testing *immediately.* Dexamethasone does not provide mineralocorticoid activity.

   Dose: 4 mg IV push.

   After the ACTH stimulation test, the patient *should* subsequently be treated with hydrocortisone (to provide mineralocorticoid effect) until the test results are available.

3. Improvement in the patient's blood pressure is generally noted within 6 hours of starting IV fluid and steroid replacement. Oral hydration and steroid replacement may be started when the patient's nausea and abdominal symptoms have resolved after several days in the hospital.

C. General Supportive Therapy

1. Support vital signs with D5NS as necessary.
2. Continuously monitor cardiac rhythm.
3. Treat and prevent hypoglycemia.
4. Manage electrolytes (sodium and potassium).
5. Obtain appropriate cultures (blood, urine, sputum, cerebrospinal fluid, etc.) and treat with empiric antibiotics pending culture results.
6. Vigorously diagnose and treat any major medical or surgical illness that precipitated the patient's decompensation.

D. Chronic Management

Maintenance therapy of adrenal insufficiency in the unstressed patient is generally provided with oral hydrocortisone or cortisone acetate (*dose:* 20–25 mg PO every morning and 10–12.5 mg PO every night). In primary adrenal failure, the addition of a more potent mineralocorticoid such as fludrocortisone (*dose:* 0.05–0.1 mg PO daily) is often needed to prevent hypotension and hyperkalemia. Patients should be instructed to wear a medical identification bracelet and to double or triple their maintenance steroid dose during periods of unusual stress or illness. A parenteral glucocorticoid preparation should also be provided for self-administration in case nausea and vomiting preclude the use of oral medication.

V. DISPOSITION

Adrenal crisis requires hospital admission for adequate volume replacement, initiation of steroid therapy, diagnosis and treatment of a precipitating illness, and definitive testing of the pituitary/adrenal axis. Patient's with hypotension, shock, or a life-threatening precipitating illness should be admitted to the ICU. In the absence of a major intercurrent illness, the patient usually recovers sufficiently for discharge on maintenance steroid therapy within 4–5 days. Results of the baseline ACTH determination, or 3-day ACTH stimulation test, must often be collated and interpreted on an outpatient basis.

VI. PEARLS AND PITFALLS

A. Start IV fluid resuscitation and steroid replacement therapy before laboratory confirmation of hypoadrenalism is available if there is a reasonable clinical suspicion of adrenal crisis.

B. Recognize that fever and abdominal pain, although seen in uncomplicated adrenal insufficiency, may indicate the presence of a serious infection or abdominal emergency.

C. Consider adrenal insufficiency as a frequent contributing cause of asthenia and hypotension in AIDS patients.

D. Expect the patient to have a major intercurrent illness requiring aggressive diagnostic and therapeutic efforts.

E. Advise patients on maintenance therapy for adrenal insufficiency to increase their glucocorticoid dose during periods of unusual stress or illness.

Do *not* do any of the following:

A. Assume that a normal potassium level excludes the diagnosis of adrenal crisis.

B. Send a patient who may have adrenal insufficiency to emergency surgery until fluid resuscitation and steroid replacement are well underway.

BIBLIOGRAPHY

Chin R: Adrenal crisis. Crit Care Clin 1991;7:23–42.
Frederick R, Brown C, Renusch J, Turner L: Addisonian crisis: emergency presentation of primary adrenal insufficiency. Ann Emerg Med 1991;20:802–806.
Guerra I, Kimmel PL: Hypokalemic adrenal crisis in a patient with AIDS. South Med J 1991; 84:1265–1267.
Khosla S, Wolfson JS, Demerjian Z, Godine JE. Adrenal crisis in the setting of high-dose ketoconazole therapy. Arch Intern Med 1989;149:802–804.

HYPERGLYCEMIA WITHOUT SIGNIFICANT KETOSIS

"They are as sick that surfeit with too much as they that starve with nothing."

WILLIAM SHAKESPEARE

I. ESSENTIAL FACTS

A. Definitions

1. *Hyperglycemia* is an abnormally elevated blood glucose level.

2. *Diabetes mellitus* is a metabolic disorder characterized by abnormal glucose utilization with an associated elevation of the blood glucose concentration. Diagnostic criteria for diabetes mellitus include an unequivocally increased random plasma glucose level (> 200 mg/dL) with classic symptoms of diabetes mellitus, or an abnormally elevated fasting plasma glucose level (> 140 mg/dL) on two occasions, or an elevated plasma glucose level (> 200 mg/dL at 2 hours and at least one other measurement) after an oral glucose tolerance test on two occasions.

B. In the ED, a diabetic patient with hyperglycemia, without significant ketoacidosis, is more common than a patient with either diabetic ketoacidosis or hyperglycemic hyperosmolar coma.

1. In a patient without a prior diagnosis of diabetes, hyperglycemia may be noted for the first time as part of a routine laboratory evaluation. This is not surprising since approximately 50% of all patients with type II diabetes mellitus are undiagnosed.

2. In a patient with a known history of diabetes (either type I or II), marked hyperglycemia may be present when the patient presents with a medical condition that affects glycemic control (e.g., myocardial infarction, infection).

II. CLINICAL EVALUATION

A. History

1. *Patient without known diabetes:* inquire about weight change, polyuria, polydipsia, change in energy level, visual complaints, orthostatic symptoms, dysuria and vaginal complaints, neurologic symptoms (e.g., lower-extremity hypoesthesia), recurrent skin infections, and a family history of diabetes.

2. *Patient with known diabetes:* the above historical questions are also important. In addition, inquire about the patient's use (and results of) home blood glucose monitoring, overall degree of glycemic control, prior glycosylated hemoglobin results, and compliance with diet and medical therapy.

B. Physical Examination

Obtain vital signs and examine the skin, HEENT and neck, chest, heart, abdomen (include a rectal examination and stool heme test), genitourinary system, extremities, and neurologic status.

1. Carefully evaluate the patient's tympanic membranes, sinuses,

and dentition/oropharynx for infection. Perform a fundoscopic examination searching for evidence of diabetic retinopathy (e.g., microaneurysms, retinal hemorrhages, hard exudates [glistening yellow or white lipid deposits], soft exudates ["cotton wool" spots], and/or vascular proliferation).

2. Check the patient's feet for ulcers and/or secondarily infected lesions.

3. Evaluate for evidence of a peripheral neuropathy (e.g., "stocking glove" hypoesthesia).

C. Laboratory Studies

1. *Routinely* obtain the following:
   a. Glucose level.
   b. Electrolyte panel.
   c. Blood urea nitrogen (BUN) and creatinine levels.
   d. Urinalysis.
   e. Anion gap.
   f. Complete blood count (CBC).

2. Additional studies *may be required,* depending on clinical circumstances (e.g., electrocardiogram, pregnancy test, chest roentgenogram).

III. THERAPY

Figure 19–2 presents the emergency therapy of hyperglycemia without ketoacidosis.

A. Fluid Therapy

Volume depletion should be treated with normal saline (NS) (300–1000 mL/hr, depending on the degree of patient volume depletion and comorbid conditions) until the patient has no orthostatic symptoms and is appropriately intravascularly repleted. Fluid replacement by itself will usually result in a reduction in the blood glucose level.

B. Insulin Therapy

Significant hyperglycemia (blood glucose > 300 mg/dL) will frequently require insulin treatment in addition to fluid therapy. Any patient with ketonuria will also require insulin therapy.

1. If the blood glucose is > 300 mg/dL, 5–10 units regular insulin subcutaneously (SQ) may be given. (Regular insulin given SQ will have an onset of action in 20 minutes and a peak effect at 2-4 hours, total duration of action is 4-6 hours.)

2. Newly diagnosed diabetic patients will need formal teaching about diabetes, home blood glucose monitoring, and the use of insulin. Most EDs are not equipped to initiate this teaching, so urgent referral to a diabetes education program and a physician skilled in diabetes care is appropriate.

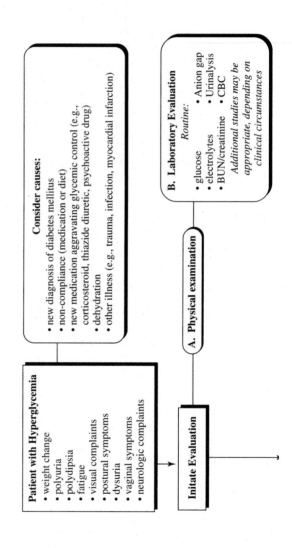

Patient with Hyperglycemia
- weight change
- polyuria
- polydipsia
- fatigue
- visual complaints
- postural symptoms
- dysuria
- vaginal symptoms
- neurologic complaints

Initate Evaluation

Consider causes:
- new diagnosis of diabetes mellitus
- non-compliance (medication or diet)
- new medication aggravating glycemic control (e.g., corticosteroid, thiazide diuretic, psychoactive drug)
- dehydration
- other illness (e.g., trauma, infection, myocardial infarction)

A. Physical examination

B. Laboratory Evaluation
Routine:
- glucose
- electrolytes
- BUN/creatinine
- Anion gap
- Urinalysis
- CBC

Additional studies may be appropriate, depending on clinical circumstances

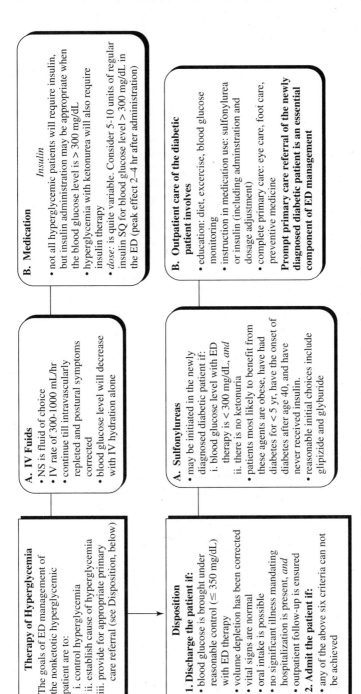

Figure 19-2. Emergency therapy of hyperglycemia without ketosis.

Therapy of Hyperglycemia

The goals of ED management of the nonketotic hyperglycemic patient are to:
- i. control hyperglycemia
- ii. establish cause of hyperglycemia
- iii. provide for appropriate primary care referral (see Disposition, below)

A. IV Fluids
- NS is fluid of choice
- IV rate of 300–1000 mL/hr
- continue till intravascularly repleted and postural symptoms corrected
- blood glucose level will decrease with IV hydration alone

B. Medication

Insulin
- not all hyperglycemic patients will require insulin, but insulin administration may be appropriate when the blood glucose level is > 300 mg/dL
- hyperglycemia with ketonurea will also require insulin therapy
- *dose:* is quite variable. Consider 5-10 units of regular insulin SQ for blood glucose level > 300 mg/dL in the ED (peak effect 2–4 hr after administration)

Disposition

1. Discharge the patient if:
- blood glucose is brought under reasonable control (≤ 350 mg/dL) with ED therapy
- volume depletion has been corrected
- vital signs are normal
- oral intake is possible
- no significant illness mandating hospitalization is present, *and*
- outpatient follow-up is ensured

2. Admit the patient if:
- any of the above six criteria can not be achieved

A. Sulfonylureas
- may be initiated in the newly diagnosed diabetic patient if:
  - i. blood glucose level with ED therapy is < 300 mg/dL, *and*
  - ii. there is no ketonuria
- patients most likely to benefit from these agents are obese, have had diabetes for < 5 yr, have the onset of diabetes after age 40, and have never received insulin.
- reasonable initial choices include glipizide and glyburide

B. Outpatient care of the diabetic patient involves
- education: diet, excercise, blood glucose monitoring
- instruction in medication use: sulfonylurea or insulin (including adminstration and dosage adjustment)
- complete primary care: eye care, foot care, preventive medicine

Prompt primary care referral of the newly diagnosed diabetic patient is an essential component of ED management

C. Sulfonylurea Therapy

1. Sulfonylureas may be initiated in the newly diagnosed diabetic in the ED *if* the blood glucose is *not* > 300 mg/dL *and* the urinalysis reveals *no* ketonuria. Sulfonylureas are most effective, however, with the institution of appropriate diabetic diet recommendations. Many patients initially started on these agents will not achieve improvement in their blood glucose levels ("primary sulfonylurea failure").

2. Multiple agents are available. Reasonable initial choices are
   a. Glyburide: starting dose 2.5–5.0 mg/day, *or*
   b. Glipizide: starting dose 5.0 mg/day.

D. General Therapeutic Interventions

1. Diabetes mellitus is a chronic disease that traditionally is difficult to initially manage thoroughly in the ED. Patients require education with respect to diet, medication, home blood glucose monitoring, exercise, eye care, foot care, and thorough primary medical care.

2. The ED physician should temporize any metabolic problems, identify exacerbating conditions needing urgent management, and make the appropriate referral for the delivery of primary diabetic care.

IV. DISPOSITION

A. Discharge

The patient with hyperglycemia without ketosis may be discharged home from the ED if the following *six* conditions are all applicable:

1. Blood glucose has been brought under reasonable control (< 300–350 mg/dL) in the ED with hydration and, if necessary, SQ regular insulin.

2. Volume depletion has been corrected.

3. Vital signs are normal.

4. Oral intake is possible.

5. No significant medical illness mandating hospitalization has been identified.

6. The patient is reliable and outpatient follow-up has been arranged (follow-up for repeat AM glucose check is recommended in 48–72 hours).

B. Admit

Patients who do not meet the above criteria are appropriate for admission to the medicine service for hydration, glucose control, treatment of any underlying medical illness in addition to diabetes, and the initiation of diabetes care teaching.

V. PEARLS AND PITFALLS

A. Search diligently for the cause of poor glucose control when the known diabetic patient presents with marked hyperglycemia (e.g., infection, occult myocardial infarction, diet or medication non-compliance).

B. The newly diagnosed diabetic patient with ketonuria will require insulin therapy (i.e., sulfonylureas are inappropriate in this setting).

C. Patients with marked elevations of their blood glucose level (> 300 mg/dL) are also unlikely to have their diabetes controlled with sulfonylureas alone.

D. All patients with diabetes should have their care referred to a primary care physician skilled in the management of patients with this disease or to a diabetologist.

DIABETIC KETOACIDOSIS

"The only way to successfully treat DKA is to handcuff the intern to the bed."

ANONYMOUS

I. ESSENTIAL FACTS

A. Definition

Diabetic ketoacidosis (DKA) is a metabolic acidosis that occurs in a state of deficient insulin secretion and excessive counterregulatory hormone secretion. These derangements result in hyperglycemia, ketosis, volume depletion, and other electrolyte abnormalities. DKA and diabetic hyperglycemic hyperosmolar coma (HHC) represent a continuum, with DKA generally occurring abruptly in younger patients with moderate hyperglycemia. Any patient presenting in DKA *and* coma will almost always be suffering from hyperosmolar coma.

B. Epidemiology

1. DKA occurs at an annual incidence of 14/100,000 general population: 20% are new cases of type I (insulin-dependent) diabetes.

2. Mortality from DKA ranges from 5% to 10%.

3. Precipitating factors include
   a. Infection (27–56% of all cases).
   b. Myocardial infarction.
   c. Cerebral vascular accident.
   d. Drugs (steroids, adrenergic agonists, pentamadine).

    e. Newly diagnosed type I diabetes.

    f. Accidental or purposeful noncompliance with insulin.

    g. Insulin occlusion in the tubing of insulin pumps.

    h. Abdominal disease (bleeding, infection, pancreatitis).

    i. Hyperthyroidism.

    j. Other stress.

II. CLINICAL EVALUATION

A. History

Look for the precipitating factors noted above. Patients with gastroenteritis and vomiting often incorrectly omit or decrease their insulin dose. If the initial history does not yield an obvious cause, search for an occult infection. In young women with recurrent DKA, consider the possibility of an eating disorder and purposeful omission of insulin.

B. Symptoms

Symptoms include nausea and vomiting, polydipsia, polyuria, weakness, anorexia, abdominal pain, and weight loss. Symptoms may also suggest a likely precipitating factor.

C. Signs

Signs include evidence of volume depletion (tachycardia, hypotension, poor skin turgor, dry mucous membranes); continuous, deep respirations (Kussmaul respirations); mental status changes (mild confusion to frank coma); and "fruity breath." Hypothermia without coexisting sepsis has been described.

D. Physical Examination

Obtain vital signs and examine the skin, HEENT and neck, chest, heart, abdomen (include a rectal examination and stool heme test), genitourinary system, extremities, and neurologic status.

1. The patient's eyes and tongue may reveal evidence of significant dehydration (e.g., a dry and longitudinally furrowed tongue). Carefully evaluate the patient's tympanic membranes, sinuses, and dentition/oropharynx for infection.

2. Rapid and deep respirations are a compensation for metabolic acidosis. Look for evidence of pneumonia or congestive heart failure.

3. Acute cholecystitis, cholangitis, pancreatitis, pyelonephritis, and an acute surgical abdomen may all precipitate DKA. DKA by itself may also cause marked abdominal pain, especially in the younger patient.

4. Carefully evaluate the extremities for ulcers or infections.

E. Laboratory Studies

1. *Routinely* obtain the following:
   a. Glucose level.
   b. Electrolyte panel.
   c. Complete blood count (CBC).
   d. Arterial blood gas (ABG).
   e. Electrocardiogram (ECG).
   f. Urinalysis.
   g. Anion gap.
   h. Blood urea nitrogen (BUN) and creatinine levels.
   i. Calcium, magnesium, phosphate levels.
   j. Chest roentgenogram.

2. Additional studies *may be required,* depending on clinical circumstances (blood cultures, urine culture, pregnancy test, etc.).

3. *Common laboratory results* include the following:
   a. Hyperglycemia: blood glucose level is usually > 300 mg/dL but may range from 200 mg/dL to 1500 mg/dL.
   b. Metabolic acidosis: pH < 7.25, HCO_3^-< 15 mEq/L. An anion gap variety of acidosis is usually present. Anion gap is calculated as

   $$Anion\ gap = (Na^+) - (Cl^- + HCO_3^-).$$
   Normal anion gap is 12 ± 2 mEq/L.

   With severe vomiting or diuretic therapy, a mixed acid–base disturbance may be present.
   c. Ketonuria and ketonemia.
   d. Hyper- or hyponatremia: measured serum sodium should be corrected for hyperglycemia (add 1.6 mEq/L of sodium to the measured sodium for every 100-mg/dL increase in glucose above normal). Approximately 50% of patients present with hypernatremia, indicating water deficits in excess of sodium; about 20% of patients present with hyponatremia. For these latter patients, total-body sodium deficits are severe. During treatment of DKA, the plasma sodium concentration will rise in all patients as glucose and water move into cells.
   e. Hyperkalemia: 80% of patients will present with normal or elevated potassium levels despite marked total-body potassium deficits. An *approximate* correction for the acidosis-induced elevation in measured serum potassium can be made by subtracting 0.6 mEq/L from the laboratory potassium for every 0.1-unit decrease from 7.4 in the pH on the ABG.
   f. Elevated serum osmolarity: if elevated markedly, obtundation may result. Coma will not occur until *effective* serum osmolarity (tonicity) is > 340 mOsm/L. Therefore, if a patient with DKA presents in coma with an effective serum osmolarity of 310 mOsm/L, another cause for the

coma should be sought. The formula for *effective osmolarity* is:

$$\text{Effective osmolarity} = 2(Na + K) + Glucose/18.$$

(In this setting, urea is not included in the calculation.)

g. Elevated leukocyte count: levels $\leq 30,000/\mu L$ are common, even in the absence of infection. A high percentage of bands *is* suggestive of infection.

h. Elevated amylase: concentrations are frequently high and cannot be used to diagnose pancreatitis.

i. Elevated creatinine: may be falsely elevated secondary to the interference of acetoacetate with the automated assay for creatinine.

III. DIFFERENTIAL DIAGNOSIS

A. *Patients with known diabetes:* if mental status is altered, quickly rule out hypoglycemia. If bedside blood glucose determination shows hyperglycemia, confirmation of DKA will usually require further laboratory evaluation as documented above.

B. *Conditions that mimic DKA* include acute appendicitis, pancreatitis, gastroenteritis, pyelonephritis, myocardial infarction, stroke, and drug overdose (including ethanol).

C. *Other causes of an anion-gap metabolic acidosis* include alcoholic ketoacidosis, methanol ingestion, uremia, paraldehyde ingestion, iron or isoniazid overdose, starvation ketosis, lactic acidosis, ethylene glycol ingestion, and salicylate overdose.

IV. THERAPY

Figure 19–3 presents the emergency therapy of diabetic ketoacidosis. Successful treatment of DKA is dependent on proper diagnosis, reversal of the metabolic abnormality, identification and treatment of any precipitating factors, and careful attention to clinical changes. Structured protocols should only serve as general guidelines. Decisions regarding admission to an ICU should be made on an individual basis since it has been shown that many patients do well on a general ward *if there is proper attention to clinical detail.*

A. Initial Management

Assess, secure, and support airway, breathing, and circulation as indicated. (See Chapter 1. II.)

1. Guard the airway, administer supplemental oxygen, establish intravenous (IV) access, monitor both cardiac rhythm and oxygen saturation (SaO_2), obtain vital signs, and check the fingerstick glucose level.

2. Initiate crystalloid volume resuscitation as outlined under B, below.

3. Simultaneously with the above, obtain a directed history, perform a physical examination, and obtain appropriate laboratory studies as outlined in II, above.

B. Fluid Therapy

Fluid therapy is of paramount importance in the treatment of a patient in DKA. In the adult, the average fluid deficit is 5-6 L.

1. Fluid administration alone will reduce both hyperglycemia and acidosis. Insulin should be withheld initially until appropriate fluid resuscitation has been started.

2. In most patients, normal saline (NS) is the initial fluid of choice.
   a. *For the hypotensive patient:* average replacement will be 1–2 L of NS over the first 1 hour, followed by 500 mL to 1 L/hr for the next 2–5 hours as vital signs and clinical parameters dictate. If hypotension persists despite aggressive and appropriate volume resuscitation, other causes of shock should be considered. When intravascular volume has been restored (i.e., patient neither hypovolemic or orthostatic), the IV hydration fluid may be changed to 0.45% saline at the rate of 150–300 mL/hr.
   b. *For the normotensive patient:* initiate fluids with NS at the rate of 500 mL–1L/hr for the first hour, followed by 500 mL/hr until the patient is no longer orthostatic; then change to 0.45% saline at the rate of 150–300 mL/hr.
   c. *Cautions:*
      i. In the patient with abnormal cardiac or renal function, pulmonary status must be closely followed. Invasive hemodynamic monitoring may be necessary.
      ii. Monitor both glucose and serum sodium frequently (hourly initially) and *avoid* sudden large shifts in either. Cerebral edema as a complication of the therapy of DKA has a significant mortality.

C. Insulin Therapy

1. Do *not* begin insulin until hypokalemia, as determined by the electrolyte panel, has been corrected.

2. Aggressive and appropriate IV hydration should be started *before* insulin therapy is initiated.

3. *Initial bolus of regular insulin:* 0.1 units/kg (should not exceed 10 units total) IV.

4. *Continuous IV regular insulin* (insulin drip): follow the initial insulin bolus with a continuous infusion. Mix 50 units of regular insulin in 500 mL of normal saline (0.1 unit/mL). Flush the tubing with 50 mL prior to patient administration.
   a. *Begin IV insulin drip* at 0.1 units/kg/hr. The goal is to decrease glucose levels by about 10%/hr. If blood glucose does not improve after 1 or 2 hours with this dose, the initial

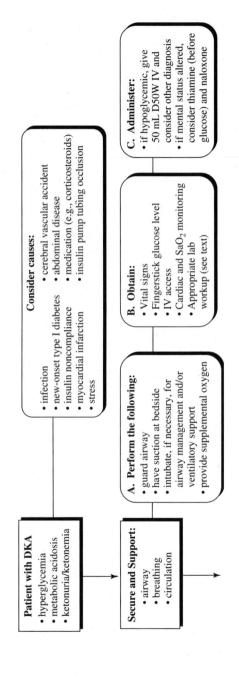

Patient with DKA
- hyperglycemia
- metabolic acidosis
- ketonuria/ketonemia

Consider causes:
- infection
- new-onset type I diabetes
- insulin noncompliance
- myocardial infarction
- stress
- cerebral vascular accident
- abdominal disease
- medication (e.g., corticosteroids)
- insulin pump tubing occlusion

Secure and Support:
- airway
- breathing
- circulation

A. Perform the following:
- guard airway
- have suction at bedside
- intubate, if necessary, for airway management and/or ventilatory support
- provide supplemental oxygen

B. Obtain:
- Vital signs
- Fingerstick glucose level
- IV access
- Cardiac and SaO_2 monitoring
- Appropriate lab workup (see text)

C. Administer:
- if hypoglycemic, give 50 mL D50W IV and consider other diagnosis
- if mental status altered, consider thiamine (before glucose) and naloxone

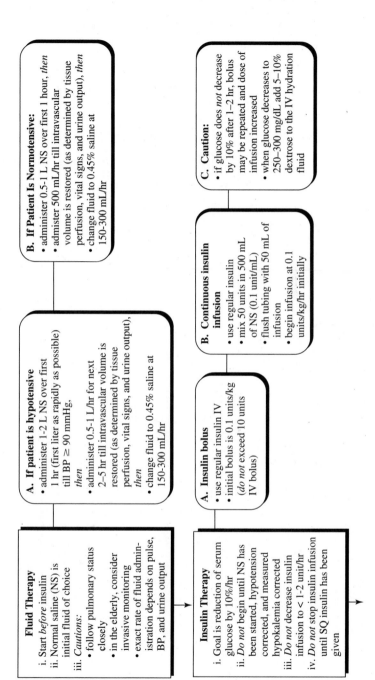

Fluid Therapy
i. Start *before* insulin
ii. Normal saline (NS) is initial fluid of choice
iii. *Cautions:*
  • follow pulmonary status closely
  • in the elderly, consider invasive monitoring
  • exact rate of fluid administration depends on pulse, BP, and urine output

A. If patient is hypotensive
  • administer 1-2 L NS over first 1 hr (first liter as rapidly as possible) till BP ≥ 90 mmHg, *then*
  • administer 0.5-1 L/hr for next 2–5 hr till intravascular volume is restored (as determined by tissue perfusion, vital signs, and urine output), *then*
  • change fluid to 0.45% saline at 150-300 mL/hr

B. If Patient Is Normotensive:
  • administer 0.5-1 L NS over first 1 hour, *then*
  • administer 500 mL/hr till intravascular volume is restored (as determined by tissue perfusion, vital signs, and urine output), *then*
  • change fluid to 0.45% saline at 150-300 mL/hr

Insulin Therapy
i. Goal is reduction of serum glucose by 10%/hr
ii. *Do not* begin until NS has been started, hypotension corrected, and measured hypokalemia corrected
iii. *Do not* decrease insulin infusion to < 1-2 unit/hr
iv. *Do not* stop insulin infusion until SQ insulin has been given

A. Insulin bolus
  • use regular insulin IV
  • initial bolus is 0.1 units/kg (*do not* exceed 10 units IV bolus)

B. Continuous insulin infusion
  • use regular insulin
  • mix 50 units in 500 mL of NS (0.1 unit/mL)
  • flush tubing with 50 mL of infusion
  • begin infusion at 0.1 units/kg/hr initially

C. Caution:
  • if glucose does *not* decrease by 10% after 1–2 hr, bolus may be repeated and dose of infusion increased
  • when glucose decreases to 250–300 mg/dL, add 5–10% dextrose to the IV hydration fluid

Figure 19–3. Emergency therapy of diabetic ketoacidosis.

Illustration continued on following page.

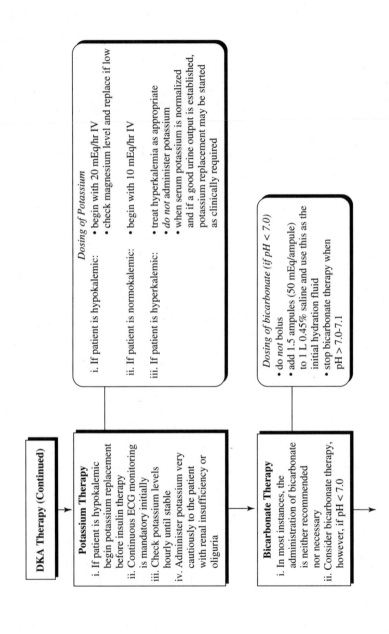

DKA Therapy (Continued)

Potassium Therapy

i. If patient is hypokalemic begin potassium replacement before insulin therapy

ii. Continuous ECG monitoring is mandatory initially

iii. Check potassium levels hourly until stable

iv. Administer potassium very cautiously to the patient with renal insufficiency or oliguria

Dosing of Potassium

i. If patient is hypokalemic:
  • begin with 20 mEq/hr IV
  • check magnesium level and replace if low

ii. If patient is normokalemic:
  • begin with 10 mEq/hr IV

iii. If patient is hyperkalemic:
  • treat hyperkalemia as appropriate
  • *do not* administer potassium
  • when serum potassium is normalized and if a good urine output is established, potassium replacement may be started as clinically required

Bicarbonate Therapy

i. In most instances, the administration of bicarbonate is neither recommended nor necessary

ii. Consider bicarbonate therapy, however, if pH < 7.0

Dosing of bicarbonate (if pH < 7.0)

• do *not* bolus
• add 1.5 ampules (50 mEq/ampule) to 1 L 0.45% saline and use this as the initial hydration fluid
• stop bicarbonate therapy when pH > 7.0-7.1

Phosphate Therapy

i. In most instances phosphate replacement will *not* be necessary while patient is in ED

ii. Consider replacement if serum phosphate is < 1.0 mg/dL

Dosing of phosphate

- do *not* bolus
- follow calcium and magnesium levels concomitantly
- if patient is *not* hyperkalemic, add 2-4 mL potassium phosphate solution (4 mEq potassium and 3 mmol phosphate per mL solution) to 1L of IV fluid and administer *no* faster than 3 mmol phosphate per hour

Figure 19-3. Continued

bolus may be repeated and the continuous infusion rate increased; but severe hypovolemia or other causes of insulin resistance (e.g., sepsis, Cushing's syndrome) should be considered.

b. Five to ten percent dextrose should be added to the hydration fluid when the blood glucose level has fallen to 250-300 mg/dL.

c. *Cautions:*
   i. The insulin infusion should not be decreased below 1-2 units/hr.
   ii. *The insulin infusion should never be stopped unless subcutaneous insulin has also been given.* In general, subcutaneous insulin is best administered when the patient is ready to eat.

D. Potassium Therapy

1. Most patients are suffering from profound potassium depletion, even if the measured serum potassium is normal or high.

2. *Cautions:*
   a. Potassium should be administered very carefully to all patients, especially those with either renal insufficiency or low urinary output.
   b. Check potassium levels hourly until stable. Do not cause hyperkalemia!
   c. Rate of potassium replacement depends on potassium levels as therapy proceeds (see below). Adjust replacement rates as clinically appropriate.

3. *In the hypokalemic patient:*
   a. Continuous ECG monitoring is mandatory.
   b. Withhold insulin therapy until potassium replacement has been initiated.
   c. Begin replacement with 20 mEq/hr IV (even higher replacement rates are sometimes necessary).

4. *In the normokalemic patient:* initiate potassium replacement at 10 mEq/hr IV.

5. *In the hyperkalemic patient:*
   a. Continuous ECG monitoring is mandatory.
   b. Check potassium levels at least hourly.
   c. *Withhold potassium* replacement until therapy of DKA results in normalization of potassium and a good urine output; then begin replacement as clinically indicated.

E. Bicarbonate Therapy

1. *Caution:* bicarbonate is *not* indicated in the treatment of DKA unless profound acidemia is present (pH < 7.0). Even for severe acidemia, many experts do not recommend the use of bicarbonate.

2. If bicarbonate is to be used for pH < 7.0, do *not* bolus the patient with bicarbonate. Instead, add 1.5 ampules of sodium

bicarbonate (50 mEq/ampule) to 1 L of 0.45% saline and use this as the initial IV hydration fluid over the first hour of therapy. Discontinue bicarbonate when the pH rises to > 7.0–7.1.

F. Phosphate Therapy

1. Though most patients in DKA are total-body phosphate depleted, phosphate replacement remains an unresolved issue.

2. *Consider* phosphate repletion *if* the measured serum phosphate is < 1.0–1.5 mg/dL.

3. If phosphate is to be replaced, also closely monitor serum calcium and magnesium levels.

4. If replacement is deemed necessary and the patient is not hyperkalemic, phosphate may be replaced as potassium phosphate (4 mEq potassium and 3 mmole of phosphate per 1 mL). Add 2–4 mL to 1 L of IV infusion and replace no faster than 3 mmol phosphate per hour.

V. DISPOSITION

A. Discharge

Occasionally patients with *mild ketoacidosis* may be treated in the ED and discharged to home. Discharge to home is reasonable only if *all* of the following nine conditions hold:

1. Patient is reliable.

2. Precipitating factor can be treated as an outpatient.

3. Patient can take oral fluids.

4. Vital signs have normalized.

5. pH and anion gap have normalized.

6. Serum potassium level is normal.

7. Glucose is reasonably controlled.

8. Serum bicarbonate level is > 15 mEq/L.

9. Close outpatient follow-up is available.

B. Admit

Most patients with DKA will require hospitalization, and many will need initial care in the ICU. The need for ICU admission versus admission to a general medical floor should be carefully considered. In the initial care of the patient with DKA, hourly clinical reassessment and electrolyte/glucose checks will be necessary until the patient's condition has truly stabilized. ICU admission is appropriate if *any* of the following condition(s) is(are) present in the patient:

1. Serious precipitating factor for DKA (e.g., myocardial infarction, sepsis).

2. Altered mental status.

3. Impaired renal or cardiac function.

4. Severe acidosis.

5. Hypo- or hyperkalemia or other significant electrolyte abnormality.

6. Other significant comorbid condition.

VI. PEARLS AND PITFALLS

A. Identify and treat any precipitating factor(s) that may have contributed to the cause of DKA.

B. Keep accurate flow charts to closely monitor vital signs, laboratory results, urine output, glucose levels, insulin therapy, electrolytes (e.g., sodium, potassium, bicarbonate, phosphate), and fluid administration.

C. Be aggressive with fluid replacement, especially if hypotension is present.

D. Admit to the ICU (or at least a telemetry bed) any patient with hypo- or hyperkalemia on presentation.

E. Measure sodium, potassium, and glucose levels hourly until stable.

F. Consider a nasogastric tube in the vomiting patient.

G. Begin subcutaneous insulin when the patient can tolerate food. Continue the IV insulin until the SQ insulin has a chance to reach peak effect (i.e., about 2 hours after administration).

Do *not* do any of the following:

A. Measure ABGs frequently. Most patients may be managed with only one ABG determination at presentation. Thereafter, serum potassium, bicarbonate, and blood glucose levels are adequate to dictate the course of therapy.

B. Dismiss the diagnosis of DKA if urinary ketones are not strongly positive. Some patients with DKA have a high ratio of beta-hydroxybutyrate to acetoacetate and the former does not react with commercially available strips or tablets for ketones.

C. Administer insulin prior to IV fluids.

D. Administer insulin until measured hypokalemia has been corrected.

E. Administer insulin to anuric patients.

F. Be misled by high amylase concentrations. However, acute pancreatitis may be a cause or a consequence of DKA. Lipase levels can also be elevated with DKA.

G. Give an IV bolus of sodium bicarbonate or phosphate.

H. Stop the insulin drip because of decreasing blood glucose levels. (*Comment:* the intravenous insulin has a half-life of about 4 minutes in patients with normal renal function, and continuous insulin is required to prevent recurrent ketogenesis. Decreasing blood glucose levels should be managed with increased glucose administration).

I. Administer "sliding scale insulin" after discontinuing the insulin drip. (*Comment:* insulin should be given in a physiologic regimen, with long- or intermediate-acting insulin combined with regular insulin to provide anticipatory needs based on caloric intake. Most patients with type I diabetes require 0.4–0.9 units insulin/kg/day).

BIBLIOGRAPHY

DeFronzo RA, Matsuda M, Barrett EJ: Diabetic ketoacidosis—a combined metabolic-nephrologic approach to therapy. *Diab Rev* 1994;2(2):209–238.

Hirsch IB, Herter CD: Intensive insulin therapy: Part II. Multicomponent insulin regimens. Am Fam Phys 1992;45:2141–2147.

Lipsky MS: Management of diabetic ketoacidosis. Am Fam Phys 1994;49(7):1607–1612.

Siperstein MD: Diabetic ketoacidosis and hyperosmolar coma. Endocrin Metab Clin N Am 21:415–432, 1992.

Walker M, Marshall SM, Alberti KGMM: Clinical aspects of diabetic ketoacidosis. Diab Metab Rev 5:651–663, 1989.

HYPERGLYCEMIC HYPEROSMOLAR COMA

"Man may be the captain of his fate,
but he is also the victim of his blood sugar."

WILFRID G. OAKLEY

I. ESSENTIAL FACTS

A. Definition

Hyperglycemic hyperosmolar coma (HHC) is a syndrome in which patients suffer from marked hyperglycemia, dehydration, hyperosmolarity, and profoundly altered mental status. Unlike diabetic ketoacidosis (DKA), significant ketoacidemia is not present.

B. Epidemiology

1. HHC occurs much less frequently than DKA. Patients are typically > age 60 and have type II diabetes. Twenty to 40% of patients have no previous history of diabetes.

2. Mortality rates range from 14% to 60%.

3. Precipitating factors include
   a. Poor access to water (especially common in nursing home patients);
   b. Major illness: chronic renal insufficiency, gram-negative

pneumonia, gastrointestinal hemorrhage, gram-negative sepsis, myocardial infarction, pancreatitis, subdural hematoma, burns, trauma, and stroke;

c. Drugs, including steroids, chlorpromazine, cimetidine, diuretics, phenytoin, and propranolol;

d. Surgery (especially cardiac surgery).

II. CLINICAL EVALUATION

A. History

Both HHC and hypoglycemia should be considered in any diabetic patient with altered mental status. Because of profound mental status changes in the patient, historical questions will often need to be directed to family members or nursing home personnel.

B. Symptoms

Symptoms typically develop over a period of days to weeks. The presentation of HHC can be variable depending on the degree of hyperosmolarity and dehydration. Although polyuria is a common early symptom, thirst is often impaired in the presence of hyperosmolarity. Oliguria may develop as volume depletion ensues. Symptoms of dehydration (e.g., dry mouth, dizziness, and weakness) and a variety of neurologic symptoms (both focal and nonfocal) may prompt medical attention.

C. Signs

Signs of dehydration are prominent: dry skin, poor skin turgor, sunken eyes, furrowed tongue, orthostatic hypotension, and/or shock. An altered mental status is the most common neurologic sign, and focal changes can occur. Nuchal rigidity, tremor, fasciculations, myoclonus, visual hallucinations, nystagmus, hyper- or hypo-reflexia, and focal or generalized seizures may also occur. Fever or hypothermia is not uncommon.

D. Physical Examination

Obtain vital signs and examine the skin, HEENT and neck, chest, heart, abdomen (include a rectal examination and stool heme test), genitourinary system, and extremities. Perform a careful neurologic examination.

E. Laboratory Studies

1. *Routinely* obtain the following:
   a. Complete blood count (CBC).
   b. Glucose level.
   c. Electrolyte panel.
   d. Arterial blood gas (ABG).
   e. Electrocardiogram (ECG).

f. Chest roentgenogram.
g. Urinalysis and urine cultures.
h. Anion gap.
i. Blood urea nitrogen (BUN)/creatinine levels.
j. Calcium, magnesium, phosphate levels.
k. Calculate "effective" serum osmolarity (see below).
l. Blood cultures.

2. Additional studies *may be required* (e.g., head computed tomography [CT], lumbar puncture).

3. *Common laboratory results* include the following:
   a. *Hyperglycemia:* blood glucose levels are usually > 600 mg/dL; mean blood glucose levels in most large series of HHC are > 1000 mg/dL.
   b. *Elevated serum osmolarity:* coma from hyperosmolarity does not occur until *effective* osmolarity (tonicity) exceeds 340 mOsm/L.

      "Effective" serum osmolarity = $2 (Na + K) + Glucose/18$

      The *syndrome* of HHC requires the presence of a calculated serum osmolarity ≥ 340 mOsm/L. If ketoacidosis is also present, the patient is classified as having DKA *with* hyperosmolar coma. If hyperglycemia and coma are present, but serum osmolarity does not exceed 340 mOsm/L, another cause for the mental status change should be aggressively sought.
   c. *Hypernatremia:* usually high–normal or high due to excessive loss of water. Serum sodium levels must be corrected for the hyperglycemia (for every 100 mg/dL elevation in the plasma glucose above 180 mg/dL, add 1.6 mEq/L to the measured serum sodium).
   d. Hyperkalemia: variable at presentation, the potassium level is usually normal or slightly elevated.
   e. *Elevated BUN:* usually quite high due to volume depletion. The BUN to creatinine ratio is consistent with prerenal azotemia.
   f. *Acidemia:* if there is an acidemia in the absence of ketosis, the most likely cause is a lactic acidosis, but other causes of an anion-gap acidosis should be considered.
   g. *Elevated leukocyte count:* Leukocytosis is common, even in the absence of infection.

III. DIFFERENTIAL DIAGNOSIS

Rule out hypoxia and hypoglycemia immediately. *Remember:* elderly patients may have hyperglycemia and neurologic dysfunction due to causes other than HHC (e.g., stroke, subdural hematoma, and meningitis). Metabolic causes that may mimic HHC include hypo- or hyperglycemia, hypo- or hypernatremia, other electrolyte abnormalities, thiamine deficiency, and drug overdose. Infection must always be considered.

IV. THERAPY

Figure 19–4 presents the emergency therapy of HHC.

Successful treatment is dependent on proper diagnosis, reversal of the metabolic abnormality, treatment of precipitating factors, and attention to clinical changes.

A. Initial Management

Assess, secure, and support airway, breathing, and circulation as indicated. (See Chapter 1. II.)

1. Guard the airway, administer supplemental oxygen, establish intravenous (IV) access, monitor both cardiac rhythm and oxygen saturation (SaO_2), obtain vital signs, and check the fingerstick glucose level.

2. Initiate crystalloid volume resuscitation as outlined under B, below.

3. Simultaneously with the above, obtain a directed history, perform a physical examination, and obtain appropriate laboratory studies as outlined in II, above.

B. Fluid Therapy

1. Fluid replacement is the main therapy of HHC. Typical fluid deficits are at the minimum 20–30% of total body water.

2. *Normal saline (NS) is the initial fluid of choice.*
   a. Replacement should be 1–2 L of NS over the first 1 hour (exact rate of replacement will be determined by the patient's vital signs [e.g., hypotension] and urine output), followed by 500–1000 mL/hr *until* intravascular volume is restored.
   b. After restoration of intravascular volume, *change replacement fluid to 0.45% saline* at 300–500 mL/hr to begin replacing the extensive free-water losses that occur in HHC.

3. *Cautions:*
   a. Because patients in HHC are usually elderly with significant comorbid conditions (e.g., cardiac and renal disease), invasive hemodynamic monitoring with either a central venous pressure (CVP) line or Swan–Ganz catheter is prudent as therapy proceeds.
   b. Monitor both glucose and serum sodium levels frequently and *avoid* sudden large shifts in either. The goal in fluid therapy is to replace one-half of the free-water deficit in the first 12–24 hours, and the remaining deficit in the next 24 hours.

C. Insulin Therapy

Insulin therapy does not need to be initiated early in the treatment of HHC; blood glucose will decrease 25% with fluid replacement alone.

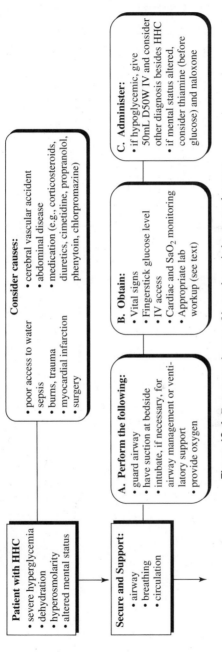

Figure 19–4. Emergency therapy of hyperglycemic hyperosmolar coma.

Illustration continued on following page.

Patient with HHC:
• severe hyperglycemia
• dehydration
• hyperosmolarity
• altered mental status

Consider causes:
• poor access to water
• sepsis
• burns, trauma
• myocardial infarction
• surgery
• cerebral vascular accident
• abdominal disease
• medication (e.g., corticosteroids, diuretics, cimetidine, propranolol, phenytoin, chlorpromazine)

Secure and Support:
• airway
• breathing
• circulation

A. Perform the following:
• guard airway
• have suction at bedside
• intubate, if necessary, for airway management or ventilatory support
• provide oxygen

B. Obtain:
• Vital signs
• Fingerstick glucose level
• IV access
• Cardiac and SaO_2 monitoring
• Appropriate lab workup (see text)

C. Administer:
• if hypoglycemic, give 50mL D50W IV and consider other diagnosis besides HHC
• if mental status altered, consider thiamine (before glucose) and naloxone

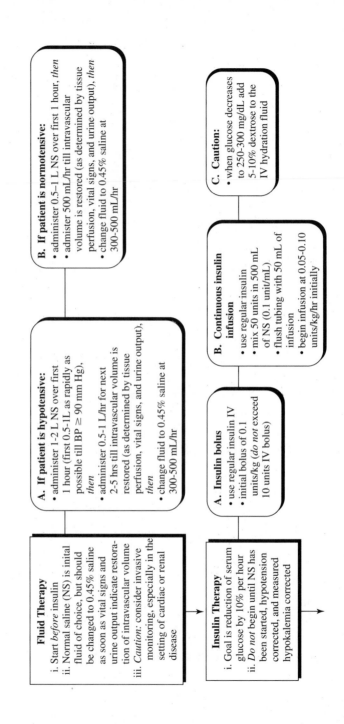

Fluid Therapy

i. Start *before* insulin
ii. Normal saline (NS) is initial fluid of choice, but should be changed to 0.45% saline as soon as vital signs and urine output indicate restoration of intravascular volume
iii. *Caution:* consider invasive monitoring, especially in the setting of cardiac or renal disease

A. If patient is hypotensive:
- administer 1-2 L NS over first 1 hour (first 0.5-1L as rapidly as possible till BP ≥ 90 mm Hg), *then*
- administer 0.5-1 L/hr for next 2-5 hrs till intravascular volume is restored (as determined by tissue perfusion, vital signs, and urine output), *then*
- change fluid to 0.45% saline at 300-500 mL/hr

B. If patient is normotensive:
- administer 0.5-1 L NS over first 1 hour, *then*
- administer 500 mL/hr till intravascular volume is restored (as determined by tissue perfusion, vital signs, and urine output), *then*
- change fluid to 0.45% saline at 300-500 mL/hr

Insulin Therapy

i. Goal is reduction of serum glucose by 10% per hour
ii. *Do not* begin until NS has been started, hypotension corrected, and measured hypokalemia corrected

A. Insulin bolus
- use regular insulin IV
- initial bolus of 0.1 units/kg (*do not* exceed 10 units IV bolus)

B. Continuous insulin infusion
- use regular insulin
- mix 50 units in 500 mL of NS (0.1 unit/mL)
- flush tubing with 50 mL of infusion
- begin infusion at 0.05-0.10 units/kg/hr initially

C. Caution:
- when glucose decreases to 250-300 mg/dL add 5-10% dextrose to the IV hydration fluid

Dosing of Potassium

i. If patient is hypokalemic: administer 10 mEq/hr IV (also check and replace serum magnesium if low)

ii. If patient is normokalemic: administer 5-10 mEq/hr IV

iii. If patient is hyperkalemic or anuric: *do not* administer potassium until clinical situation changes

Potassium Therapy

i. Continuous ECG monitoring is mandatory

ii. If patient is hypokalemic, begin potassium replacement before insulin therapy

iii. Check potassium levels hourly until stable

iv. Administer potassium very cautiously to the patient with renal insufficiency or oliguria

Figure 19–4. Continued.

1. Do *not* start insulin until hypotension and hypokalemia have been corrected.

2. *Initial bolus of regular insulin:* should not exceed 10 units IV.

3. *Continuous IV regular insulin* (drip): the initial insulin bolus should be followed with a continuous infusion. Mix 50 units of regular insulin in 500 mL of NS (0.1 unit/mL). Flush tubing with 50 mL prior to patient administration.
   a. *Begin IV insulin drip* at 0.05–0.1 units/kg/hr. *Smaller doses may be used if desired,* as some of these patients are very sensitive to insulin.
   b. When blood glucose has fallen to 250-300 mg/dL, 5–10% dextrose should be added to the hydration fluid.

4. *Caution:* follow glucose levels closely, and carefully dose insulin; avoid sudden dramatic changes in glucose.

D. Potassium Therapy

All patients with HHC have total-body potassium deficits. However, the possibility of *hyperkalemia* from overtreatment is more of a possibility with HHC than DKA because of the greater prevalence of pre-existing renal insufficiency with this population.

1. Continuous ECG monitoring should be considered for all patients with HHC.

2. If the patient is *not* hyperkalemic or anuric, begin replacement with 5–10 mEq/hr.

3. Potassium concentrations should be monitored hourly, and rates of potassium infusion should be dictated by laboratory levels. Patients with HHC generally do well receiving less potassium than patients with DKA.

V. DISPOSITION

ICU admission is mandatory for all patients with HHC.

VI. PEARLS AND PITFALLS

A. Assess and secure airway, breathing, and circulation immediately.

B. Monitor cardiac rhythm continuously.

C. Insert two large-bore IV lines and a Foley catheter.

D. Consider the use of a central line and/or Swan-Ganz catheter as treatment proceeds, especially in patients with pre-existing heart or renal disease.

E. Identify and treat any precipitating factor(s).

F. Keep accurate flow charts with vital signs, laboratory results, glucose levels, urine output, fluid therapy, insulin therapy, and electrolyte measurements (sodium and potassium).

G. Be aggressive with fluid replacement, especially if hypotension is present.

H. Admit the patient from the ED to the ICU.

I. Measure potassium, sodium, and glucose levels hourly until stable.

J. Consider toxicologic screening, CT scanning, and a lumbar puncture to further evaluate the patient's altered mental status.

Do not do any of the following:

A. Initiate insulin therapy prior to fluid therapy or even during fluid therapy if hypotension is present with extremely high blood glucose levels (> 600 mg/dL).

B. Use phenytoin to treat seizures in the setting of HHC.

C. Assume that any acidemia is secondary to DKA.

D. Routinely use furosemide for the treatment of oliguria. The only circumstance this drug would be appropriate is after adequate fluid replacement in the setting of hyperkalemia.

E. Administer "sliding scale insulin" after discontinuing the insulin infusion.

BIBLIOGRAPHY

Daugirdas JT, Kronfol NO, Tzamaloukas AH, Ing TS: Hyperosmolar coma: Cellular dehydration and the serum sodium concentration. Ann Intern Med 1989;119:855–857.

Khardori R, Soler NG: Hyperosmolar hyperglycemic nonketotic syndrome: Report of 22 cases and brief review. Am J Med 1984;77:899–904.

Pope DW, Dansky D: Hyperosmolar hyperglycemic nonketotic coma. Emerg Med Clin N Am 1989;7:849–857.

Siperstein MD: Diabetic ketoacidosis and hyperosmolar coma. Endocrin Metab Clin N Am 1992;21:415–432.

HYPOGLYCEMIA

"To a man with an empty stomach, food is God."

MAHATMA GANDHI

I. ESSENTIAL FACTS

A. Definition

Hypoglycemia is clinically present when the patient has "low" blood glucose, symptoms secondary to the "low" blood glucose, and improvement in symptoms with administration of glucose. Defining hypoglycemia with a "number" (e.g., < 65 mg/dL) is misleading because patients with diabetes can suffer symptoms of hypoglycemia at glucose levels higher or lower than those that produce symptoms in nondiabetic persons. The development of symptoms is also dependent on the rapidity of the fall of blood glucose. *Severe hypoglycemia* is defined as an event with symptoms consistent with hypoglycemia *requiring the assistance of another person* to treat the low blood glucose concentration. Patients with seizure or coma from hypoglycemia have severe hypoglycemia.

B. Epidemiology

1. Patients with insulin-dependent diabetes mellitus may average as many as 50–100 symptomatic hypoglycemic episodes per year.

2. The frequency of unrecognized hypoglycemia in insulin-dependent diabetics is unknown, although an incidence of asymptomatic nocturnal hypoglycemia (blood glucose < 53 mg/dL) of 29% *per night* has been documented.

3. Severe hypoglycemia occurs more commonly during sleep.

4. Approximately 30% of patients with insulin-dependent diabetes experience hypoglycemic coma at some time during their treatment.

5. The frequency of severe hypoglycemia is uncertain in patients with type II diabetes being treated with oral hypoglycemic agents.

6. Mortality from severe hypoglycemia in diabetic patients ranges from 3% to 5% in most series.

C. Etiology

1. Treatment of diabetes mellitus: patients receiving either insulin or sulfonylureas make up the majority of hypoglycemia cases.

2. Other drugs: alcohol, aspirin, colchicine, haloperidol, pentamadine, and quinine.

3. Chronic illnesses: chronic renal failure, hepatic insufficiency, and anorexia nervosa.

4. Neoplasms: hepatoma, sarcoma, insulinoma, and mesothelioma.

5. Endocrine causes: panhypopituitarism; or isolated deficiencies in cortisol, ACTH, and/or growth hormone.

6. Miscellaneous: sepsis, abrupt cessation of total parenteral nutrition (TPN), or inappropriate self-administered insulin.

II. CLINICAL EVALUATION

A. History

In the case of any patient presenting to the ED with altered mental status, medical information should be obtained from any possible source (e.g., family members, friends, Medic-Alert tags, driver's licence). If the patient presents comatose, a history of earlier inappropriate behavior or a seizure is common.

B. Symptoms

1. *Neurogenic symptoms:* diaphoresis, palpitations, tremors, nervousness, irritability, and hunger.

2. *Neuroglycopenic symptoms* (these usually follow the neurogenic symptoms above): confusion, weakness, blurry vision, focal neurologic deficits, seizures, and coma.

3. In general, neuroglycopenic symptoms do not develop until blood glucose levels decline to < 40 mg/dL. There is a wide variation in the blood glucose concentration at which neurogenic symptoms occur.

4. *Remember:* diabetic patients with normal or near-normal glycemic control have an increased risk of severe hypoglycemia. These patients often have no warning (neurogenic symptoms) of their hypoglycemia because of a deficient epinephrine response and thus present with neuroglycopenia.

C. Signs

Signs include tachycardia, diaphoresis, pallor, altered mental status, focal neurologic changes, and hypothermia.

D. Physical Examination

Rapidly assess (and secure) airway, breathing, and ventilation, vital signs, circulatory status, and neurologic status (pupillary response, level of consciousness, and any lateralized weakness). A more complete and detailed examination may follow once the primary survey and necessary immediate interventions have been completed.

E. Laboratory Studies

1. *Minimal workup* must include a bedside fingerstick glucose level, pulse oximetry oxygen saturation (SaO_2), and blood sent to the laboratory for glucose and electrolyte measurements.

2. Additional studies *may be necessary,* depending on clinical circumstances (e.g., alcohol level in the patient who appears intoxicated) and the patient's initial response to emergent therapy. In any patient presenting with altered mental status, a blood glucose level should be drawn prior to administering any glucose.

III. DIFFERENTIAL DIAGNOSIS

A presumptive diagnosis is clinical, especially if the patient is known to have diabetes or if there is a prompt response to treatment with intravenous (IV) glucose. A definitive diagnosis is made by laboratory testing. An immediate diagnosis may be established by bedside capillary blood glucose measurement. The differential diagnosis includes all causes of altered mental status.

IV. THERAPY

Figure 19–5 presents the emergency therapy of hypoglycemia.

A. Initial Management

Assess, secure, and support airway, breathing, and circulation as indicated. (See Chapter II). Guard the airway, administer supplemental oxygen, establish IV access, monitor both cardiac rhythm and SaO_2, obtain vital signs, and check the fingerstick glucose level. Administer glucose for hypoglycemia (i.e., fingerstick glucose < 80 mg/dL; see B, below).

B. Glucose

1. *Dose:* 25 g (50 mL or 1 ampule) of 50% dextrose in water (D50W) IV.
2. Most patients with neuroglycopenia will begin to respond after several minutes.
3. *Cautions:*
   a. The malnourished patient or the intoxicated patient (including the patient with a history of chronic alcohol use) should be given thiamine 100 mg IV or intramuscularly (IM) prior to glucose administration.
   b. Sulfonylurea (e.g., chlorpropamide)-induced hypoglycemia may not respond quickly to glucose administration. Recurrence of hypoglycemia may also occur because of the long half-life of many of these agents (e.g., chlorpropamide and glyburide).
   c. Glucose should be administered only if absolutely necessary to the patient postresuscitation from cardiac arrest or after a period of severe hypotension. Data indicate that *hyperglycemia* results in a worse neurologic outcome in the setting of anoxic brain injury.

C. Glucagon

1. In rare circumstances, if IV access cannot be obtained, consider IM or subcutaneous (SQ) glucagon.
2. *Dose:* 1 mg per ampule, administer 1 mg IM.
3. *Caution:* glucagon therapy may take 10–15 minutes to resolve symptoms.

D. Additional Therapy

After the mental status has normalized, complex carbohydrates and protein may be administered orally (PO). Alternatively, a

5–10% dextrose in water (D5–10W) IV drip may be started after the initial D50W bolus has been given.

V. DISPOSITION

A. Discharge

Insulin-treated diabetic patients whose hypoglycemia is rapidly reversed without complications can be considered for discharge from the ED. The patient should be sent home only if oral intake can be resumed, and a responsible person is available in the home to monitor for any recurrent hypoglycemic episodes. Prior to discharge, the reason for the hypoglycemic episode must be reasonably determined and adjustments made to prevent recurrence. Close follow-up with the patient's primary physician must be ensured.

B. Admit

1. Patients in whom the cause of hypoglycemia is undetermined (admit for further monitoring and evaluation).

2. Patients who have suffered injury, cardiac complications, or neurologic complications secondary to their hypoglycemia.

3. Depending on clinical circumstances, admission is also reasonable for patients whose hypoglycemia is secondary to either oral agents or a long-acting insulin preparation.

VI. PEARLS AND PITFALLS

A. Replete thiamine stores in any alcoholic or malnourished patient *prior* to administering large doses of IV glucose.

B. Teach family members of patients who take insulin about the use of glucagon. Make sure glucagon is available in the home for emergency use.

C. After resolution of the hypoglycemia, talk with the patient about the cause of the event and use the opportunity as a teaching experience. Examples of common causes include insulin or sulfonylurea use and ingestion of large quantities of alcohol, or exercise without any alterations in insulin dose or diet.

D. Consider ordering a pregnancy test in young women with a recent history of frequent hypoglycemia. Hypoglycemia is common in early pregnancy.

E. Consider admitting all elderly patients with sulfonylurea-induced hypoglycemia, especially those taking chlorpropamide.

F. Encourage all diabetic patients to wear a Medic-Alert bracelet or necklace.

G. Have the patient eat some type of complex carbohydrate (e.g., graham crackers and milk) prior to ED discharge.

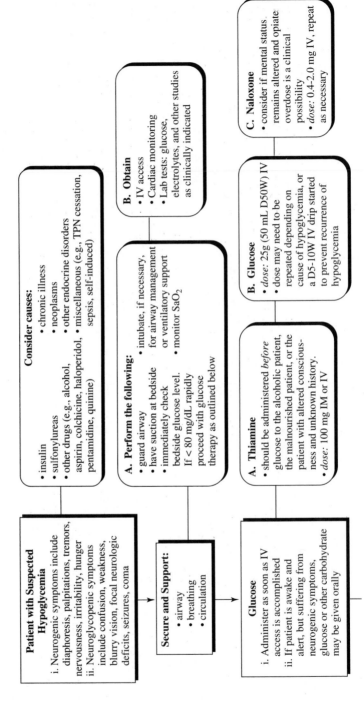

Patient with Suspected Hypoglycemia

i. Neurogenic symptoms include diaphoresis, palpitations, tremors, nervousness, irritability, hunger

ii. Neuroglycopenic symptoms include confusion, weakness, blurry vision, focal neurologic deficits, seizures, coma

Consider causes:
- insulin
- sulfonylureas
- other drugs (e.g., alcohol, aspirin, colchicine, haloperidol, pentamidine, quinine)
- chronic illness
- neoplasms
- other endocrine disorders
- miscellaneous (e.g., TPN cessation, sepsis, self-induced)

Secure and Support:
- airway
- breathing
- circulation

A. Perform the following:
- guard airway
- have suction at bedside
- immediately check bedside glucose level. If < 80 mg/dL rapidly proceed with glucose therapy as outlined below
- intubate, if necessary, for airway management or ventilatory support
- monitor SaO₂

B. Obtain
- IV access
- Cardiac monitoring
- Lab tests: glucose, electrolytes, and other studies as clinically indicated

Glucose

i. Administer as soon as IV access is accomplished

ii. If patient is awake and alert, but suffering from neurogenic symptoms, glucose or other carbohydrate may be given orally

A. Thiamine
- should be administered *before* glucose to the alcoholic patient, the malnourished patient, or the patient with altered consciousness and unknown history.
- *dose:* 100 mg IM or IV

B. Glucose
- *dose:* 25g (50 mL D50W) IV
- dose may need to be repeated depending on cause of hypoglycemia, or a D5-10W IV drip started to prevent recurrence of hypoglycemia

C. Naloxone
- consider if mental status remains altered and opiate overdose is a clinical possibility
- *dose:* 0.4-2.0 mg IV, repeat as necessary

712

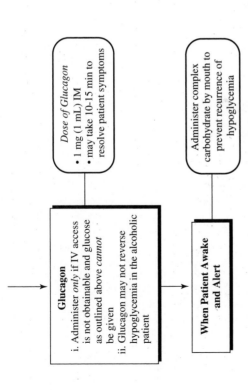

Figure 19–5. Emergency therapy of hypoglycemia.

713

Do *not* do any of the following:

A. Administer glucagon if IV access is present.

B. Administer IV glucagon.

C. Offer patients with impaired consciousness oral intake.

D. Overtreat the hypoglycemia. *Most* patients receiving insulin respond to 25 g (50 mL D50W) of IV glucose.

BIBLIOGRAPHY

Boyle PJ, Schwartz NS, Shah SD, et al: Plasma glucose concentrations at the onset of hypoglycemic symptoms with poorly controlled diabetes and in nondiabetics. N Engl J Med 1988;318:1487–1492.

Cryer PE, Binder C, Bolli GB, et al: Hypoglycemia in IDDM. Diabetes 1989;38:1193–1199.

Cryer PE: Iatrogenic hypoglycemia as a cause of hypoglycemia-associated autonomic failure in IDDM: A vicious cycle. Diabetes 1992;41:255–260.

Slama G, Traynard PY, Desplanque N, et al: The search for an optimized treatment of hypoglycemia. Arch Intern Med 1990;150:589–593.

The DCCT Research Group: Epidemiology of severe hypoglycemia in the diabetes control and complications trial. Am J Med 1991;90:450–459.

MYXEDEMA COMA

"The nightmare of Life-in-Death was she,
Who thicks man's blood with cold."

SAMUEL TAYLOR COLERIDGE

I. ESSENTIAL FACTS

A. Definition

Untreated hypothyroidism that has advanced to the point of multiple organ dysfunction and neurologic impairment is referred to as *myxedema coma.* The disease most commonly presents in elderly individuals as progressive confusion, withdrawal, or "failure to thrive," culminating in stupor or frank coma. A high incidence of suspicion is necessary to correctly diagnose myxedema coma.

B. Epidemiology

1. The prevalence of hypothyroidism is between 0.3% and 1.8%, with females being affected much more commonly than males.

2. Only a small fraction of hypothyroid individuals will remain undiagnosed for a sufficiently long period of time to develop myxedema coma.

3. The elderly patient's predilection for myxedema coma is explained by the incorrect attribution of hypothyroid symp-

toms to "old age" and by the greater likelihood of an intercurrent precipitating illness in older individuals.

4. Even with aggressive therapy, the mortality rate of this condition approaches 50%.

C. Etiology

1. Common causes of *primary thyroid failure* in developed countries are glandular destruction from autoimmune disease, radioiodine therapy, and surgical therapy for thyrotoxicosis.

2. Less common causes of hypothyroidism include infiltrative thyroid disease and metabolic defects in thyroid hormone synthesis.

3. Drugs that may precipitate hypothyroidism include lithium, amiodarone, and iodide-containing compounds.

4. Only 5% of hypothyroidism is secondary to pituitary or hypothalamic failure.

5. Factors leading to obtundation in advanced hypothyroidism include hyponatremia, hypothermia, hypoglycemia, impaired clearance of medications (e.g., sedatives), and impaired cerebral oxygen delivery due to hypoventilation and reduced cardiac output.

6. *Myxedema coma* is usually precipitated by an infection, cardiac event, trauma, cold exposure, new medication, or other serious illness.

II. CLINICAL EVALUATION

A. History

Determine from family, friends, or the patient's medical record whether there is a history of hypothyroidism, thyrotoxicosis, or use of thyroid medication. (Thyrotoxicosis may resolve and progress insidiously to hypothyroidism even without prior radioiodine or surgical treatment.)

B. Symptoms and Signs

Caregivers or the medical record may note clinical findings suspicious for hypothyroidism prior to the patient's presentation: weakness, lethargy, memory impairment, slow speech, dry skin, cold intolerance, constipation, weight gain, and diminished hearing.

C. Physical Examination

1. **Vital Signs.** May be remarkable for hypothermia, bradycardia, hypotension, and a decreased respiratory rate. A core body temperature less than 30°C is not unusual in myxedema coma and predicts a poor outcome.

2. **Skin.** Cool, dry, and sallow in appearance due to anemia, vasoconstriction, and retention of carotene pigments.

3. **HEENT.** Reveals characteristic periorbital edema, coarse hair, and macroglossia (may be severe enough to cause upper-airway obstruction). Eyebrows may be thinned or absent, especially their lateral aspect (though this is a very nonspecific finding).

4. **Neck.** A healed thyroidectomy scar or the small firm goiter of chronic lymphocytic thyroiditis may immediately clarify the diagnosis.

5. **Chest.** Should be carefully examined for signs of pleural effusion, pneumonia, or pulmonary edema.

6. **Heart.** Patient is frequently bradycardic; an S4 may suggest myocardial ischemia, an S3 suggests congestive heart failure, and a rub indicates pericarditis.

7. **Abdomen.** Bowel sounds may be absent, and the abdomen may be tympanitic as a result of paralytic ileus. Search carefully for masses or localized tenderness.

8. **Extremities.** May be remarkable for nonpitting edema.

9. **Reflexes.** May be completely absent. If present, the deep tendon reflexes are usually diminished and exhibit a characteristic delayed relaxation phase.

10. **Neurologic Examination.** The presence of focal neurologic findings is compatible with old cerebrovascular disease or a new stroke as the trigger for the patient's decompensation. Although mental status is generally depressed, the patient may be confused or agitated, a presentation that has been termed "myxedema madness."

In addition to the specific findings above, a careful search should be made for localized infection (often without fever or leukocytosis), abdominal crisis, trauma, or other serious illness that precipitated myxedema coma.

D. Laboratory Studies

1. *Routinely* obtain the following:
   a. Complete blood count (CBC).
   b. Glucose level.
   c. Electrolyte panel.
   d. Blood urea nitrogen (BUN) and creatinine levels.
   e. Arterial blood gas (ABG).
   f. Blood cultures.
   g. Cortisol level.
   h. Chest roentgenogram.
   i. Anion gap.
   j. Urinalysis and urine culture.

    k. Calcium, magnesium, phosphate levels.
    l. Electrocardiogram (ECG).

2. Obtain the following *thyroid studies:*
    a. Total serum thyroxine (T_4).
    b. T_3 resin uptake (T_3RU).
    c. Thyroid-stimulating hormone (TSH).

3. Additional studies *may be required,* depending on clinical circumstances:
    a. Toxicologic screen.
    b. Liver function tests.
    c. Cholesterol level.
    d. Creatinine phosphokinase (CPK).
    e. Amylase/bilirubin levels.
    f. Head computed tomography (CT).
    g. Lumbar puncture.
    h. Serum pregnancy test.

4. *Common laboratory results* that may be present include the following:
    a. *Thyroid Function Results* are unlikely to be available until the patient is admitted to the ICU. The presence of myxedema coma is confirmed by the findings of a low free thyroxine index (FT_4I) and an elevated TSH. The FT_4I is calculated from the total serum thyroxine (T_4) level and the triiodothyronine resin uptake (T_3RU), both of which are usually available within 12–24 hours of the patient's presentation:

$$FT_4I = T_4 \times T_3RU(patient)/T_3RU(control)$$

    A depression of the FT_4I often accompanies serious illness and can be confused with true hypothyroidism. A clue to the presence of this "sick euthyroid" syndrome is the finding of an elevated or high-normal T_3RU despite the low T_4. *In true myxedema coma, the T_4 and T_3RU are both clearly depressed, and the TSH is elevated* (unless the patient is receiving glucocorticoids or dopamine, or has hypothyroidism secondary to pituitary or hypothalamic failure).
    b. Anemia: mild normochromic, normocytic anemia may be present.
    c. *Hyponatremia, hypoglycemia, and hypochloremia* may occur.
    d. *Respiratory acidosis, hypoxemia.*
    e. Bradycardia, low-voltage QRS, nonspecific T-wave changes, and occasionally conduction abnormalities will be seen on the ECG.
    f. *Pulmonary congestion, pleural effusion, or pneumonia* may be seen on the chest film. Enlargement of the cardiac silhouette may be due to chamber dilatation or pericardial effusion.
    g. *Paralytic ileus* may be seen on the abdominal film.

    h. *Elevated creatinine phosphokinase levels, hypercholester-olemia, and elevated cerebrospinal fluid protein* occur with myxedema coma.

III. DIFFERENTIAL DIAGNOSIS

The physician who initially evaluates a patient with advanced hypothyroidism must consider the many possible causes of altered mental status accompanied by dysfunction of major organ systems, especially the cardiac and pulmonary systems. Even if myxedema coma is suspected immediately, the presence of a concurrent illness precipitating the patient's decompensation must be assumed. The finding that most often prompts specific consideration of hypothyroidism is hypothermia. The differential diagnosis of hypothermia includes the following:

A. Cold exposure.

B. Central nervous system disease.

C. Congestive heart failure.

D. Drug-induced.

    1. Barbiturates

    2. Anesthetics.

    3. Alcohol.

    4. Phenothiazines.

E. Uremia.

F. Endocrine disease.

    1. Adrenal insufficiency.

    2. Hypoglycemia.

    3. Hypopituitarism.

    4. Hypothyroidism.

G. Sepsis.

H. Starvation.

IV. THERAPY

Figure 19–6 presents the emergency therapy of myxedma coma.

A. Initial Management

Assess, secure, and support airway, breathing, and circulation as indicated. (See Chapter 1. II.)

    1. Guard the airway, administer supplemental oxygen, establish intravenous (IV) access, monitor both cardiac rhythm and

oxygen saturation (SaO$_2$), obtain vital signs, and check the fingerstick glucose level. Treat hypoglycemia if present with 50 mL of 50% dextrose in water (D50W).

2. Initiate crystalloid resuscitation for hypotension or volume depletion with normal saline (NS) or lactated Ringer's (LR) solution (dextrose may be added as necessary depending on glucose level). Carefully monitor cardiac and pulmonary systems. Do not administer hypotonic fluids. Vasopressor agents should be avoided, if possible, since they may produce arrhythmias in the setting of the rapid thyroid hormone replacement that is to follow (see B, below).

B. Hormone Therapy

1. Blood should be drawn for measurement of the serum T$_4$, T$_3$RU, TSH, and baseline cortisol level after making the clinical diagnosis of myxedema coma.

2. *Thyroid hormone replacement* should then be started immediately.
   a. Levothyroxine, 300-500 µg IV, followed by 50-100 µg IV per day until the patient is able to take oral medications. This is the drug of choice.
   b. Once the patient is able to take oral medications in the ICU, levothyroxine may be given orally in a dose of 100-150 µg/day.
   c. An increase in the body temperature and improvement in mental status are usually seen within 24 hours of beginning levothyroxine therapy.

3. *Glucocorticoid hormone replacement* is begun concurrently with thyroid hormone replacement to correct the relative hypoadrenalism that accompanies advanced hypothyroidism. Complete adrenal failure may be present if the patient's thyroid failure is one component of an autoimmune polyglandular dystruction syndrome.
   a. Hydrocortisone, 100 mg IV every 6 hours for the first 2–3 days of treatment, should be administered.
   b. Glucocorticoid replacement may generally be stopped after 2–3 days.
   c. Definitive evaluation of adrenal function in the ICU should be performed if the patient's condition does not continue to improve rapidly or if the random serum cortisol drawn on presentation is < 20 µg/dL.

C. Therapy of Complications

1. **Hypothermia.** Treat as per new (1994) ACLS guidelines. A core body temperature < 30°C requires active internal rewarming.

2. **Respiratory Failure.** Frequently monitor ABGs and oxygen administration. Mechanical ventilation is often necessary.

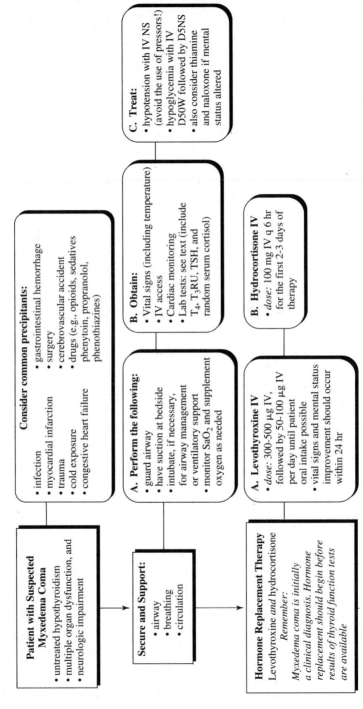

Patient with Suspected Myxedema Coma
- untreated hypothyroidism
- multiple organ dysfunction, and
- neurologic impairment

Consider common precipitants:
- infection
- myocardial infarction
- trauma
- cold exposure
- congestive heart failure
- gastrointestinal hemorrhage
- surgery
- cerebrovascular accident
- drugs (e.g., opioids, sedatives, phenytoin, propranolol, phenothiazines)

Secure and Support:
- airway
- breathing
- circulation

A. Perform the following:
- guard airway
- have suction at bedside
- intubate, if necessary, for airway management or ventilatory support
- monitor SaO₂ and supplement oxygen as needed

B. Obtain:
- Vital signs (including temperature)
- IV access
- Cardiac monitoring
- Lab tests: see text (include T₄, T₃RU, TSH, and random serum cortisol)

C. Treat:
- hypotension with IV NS (avoid the use of pressors!)
- hypoglycemia with IV D50W followed by D5NS
- also consider thiamine and naloxone if mental status altered

Hormone Replacement Therapy
Levothyroxine *and* hydrocortisone
Remember:
Myxedema coma is initially a clinical diagnosis. Hormone replacement should begin before results of thyroid function tests are available

A. Levothyroxine IV
- *dose:* 300–500 μg IV, followed by 50–100 μg IV per day until patient oral intake possible
- vital signs and mental status improvement should occur within 24 hr

B. Hydrocortisone IV
- *dose:* 100 mg IV q 6 hr for the first 2–3 days of therapy

General Supportive Therapy

i. Hypothermia: rewarm as appropriate for body temperature
ii. Respiratory failure: support oxygenation and ventilation as clinically indicated
iii. Hyponatremia: free water restrict patient and avoid hypotonic IV solutions
iv. Ileus and urinary retention: place nasogastric tube and Foley catheter
v. Hypoglycemia: monitor blood sugar and support with dextrose infusions as necessary
vi. Diagnose and treat any precipitating medical or surgical illness

Figure 19–6. Emergency therapy of myxedema coma.

Avoid volume overload due to the impaired cardiac output that accompanies myxedema coma. Central hemodynamic monitoring with a Swan-Ganz catheter may be necessary in the ICU.

3. **Hyponatremia.** Generally responds to free-water restriction. Avoid the administration of hypotonic fluids.

4. **Hypoglycemia.** Treat, as noted under A, above, with IV glucose given as D50W followed by 5% dextrose in NS (D5NS) or LR (D5LR).

5. **Ileus and Urinary Retention.** Treat with a nasogastric tube and Foley catheter, respectively.

D. Identification and Treatment of Precipitating Illness

The patient should be assumed to have a serious infection, abdominal crisis, trauma, medication overdose, or a new neurologic or cardiac event until proven otherwise. Cultures of all possible sites of infection should be performed and consideration given to starting broad-spectrum antibiotics pending culture results. If emergency surgery is required, impaired clearance of anesthetic agents and analgesic medications should be anticipated.

V. DISPOSITION

Although mild hypothyroidism with normal vital signs, a clear sensorium, and no evidence of organ dysfunction is routinely treated on an outpatient basis, *myxedema coma requires hospital admission to an ICU.*

VI. PEARLS AND PITFALLS

A. Start hormone replacement therapy before laboratory confirmation of hypothyroidism is available if there is a reasonable clinical suspicion of myxedema coma.

B. Provide both IV levothyroxine and hydrocortisone replacement.

C. Recognize that thyroid hormone replacement may precipitate an arrhythmia or myocardial ischemia. Continuous electrocardiographic and hemodynamic monitoring should be performed during the first 48–72 hours of treatment.

D. Expect the patient to have a serious intercurrent illness requiring aggressive diagnostic and therapeutic efforts.

Do *not* do any of the following:

A. Assume that a normal temperature and leukocyte count excludes infection in advanced hypothyroidism.

B. Cause water intoxication, drug intoxication, or volume overload during the course of therapy.

C. Use passive external heat sources to rewarm the hypothermic patient whose core body temperature is < 30°C.

D. Use pressor agents unless absolutely necessary.

BIBLIOGRAPHY

Arlot S, Debussche X, Lalau J-D, et al: Myxoedema coma: response of thyroid hormones with oral and intravenous high-dose L-thyroxine treatment. Intens Care Med 1991;17:16–18.

Gavin LA: Thyroid crises. Med Clin N Am 1991;75:179–193.

Mitchell JM: Thyroid disease in the emergency department. Thyroid function tests and hypothyroidism and myxedema coma. Emerg Med Clin N Am 1989;7:885–902.

Myers L, Hays J. Myxedema coma. Crit Care Clin 1991;7:43–56.

Smallridge RC: Metabolic and anatomic thyroid emergencies: A review. Crit Care Med 1992; 20:276–291.

THYROID STORM

> *"Tis a portentous sign*
> *When a man sweats, and at the same*
> *time shivers."*
>
> PLAUTUS

I. ESSENTIAL FACTS

A. Definition

Hyperthyroidism that has advanced sufficiently to cause hyperthermia and altered mental status is referred to as *thyroid storm*. This condition is frequently accompanied by circulatory collapse or an arrhythmia that may be fatal. An abrupt transition from compensated hyperthyroidism to thyroid storm may be caused by an intercurrent medical or surgical illness. In elderly individuals, the diagnosis may be confused by the absence or blunting of the usual symptoms of thyrotoxicosis. Prompt recognition and aggressive treatment of thyroid storm are necessary for an optimal outcome.

B. Epidemiology

1. The prevalence of hyperthyroidism in the community ranges from 0.2% to 1.9%. Hyperthyroidism is usually fairly well tolerated in the interval between onset of symptoms and definitive therapy.
2. Thyroid storm is estimated to occur in < 2% of hyperthyroid individuals.

C. Etiology

1. Hyperthyroidism is caused by any of the following:
   a. Graves' disease: an immunoglobulin binds to the thyroid-

stimulating hormone (TSH) receptor and causes excessive thyroid hormone production and a diffuse goiter. The presence of true exophthalmos, which reflects the ocular pathology frequently associated with Graves' disease, establishes this diagnosis with certainty.

b. Autonomous overproduction of thyroid hormone: one or more hyperfunctioning thyroid nodules may be detected by palpation or radioiodine scanning.

c. Excessive entry of preformed thyroid hormone into the circulation: thyroiditis with massive lysis of colloid or ingestion of exogenous levothyroxine. The thyroid radioactive uptake determination will be suppressed in this category of hyperthyroidism.

2. Regardless of cause, a sufficiently high level of circulating thyroid hormone leads to excessive sympathetic tone and cardiac irritability through induction of beta-adrenergic receptors.

a. Increased sympathetic tone, with accelerated tissue catabolism and futile metabolic cycling, causes excessive heat production.

b. Cutaneous vasodilation and expansion of plasma volume for heat dissipation place additional demands on the heart.

c. Fever, which marks the transition from compensated hyperthyroidism to thyroid storm, is generally associated with circulatory collapse and failure of heat loss mechanisms. Fever may also be due to a serious underlying infection that caused the decompensated hyperthyroid state.

3. Factors that have been reported to *precipitate* thyroid storm include infection, diabetic ketoacidosis, pulmonary embolism, stroke, labor and delivery, trauma, burns, surgery, iodine contained in drugs and dyes, and radioactive iodine given to treat hyperthyroidism.

II. CLINICAL EVALUATION

A. History

A history of previously diagnosed thyrotoxicosis will be obtained in most patients presenting with thyroid storm. Radioactive iodine therapy in the preceding 2–3 weeks followed by massive thyroid necrosis, or discontinuation of antithyroid medication, may be the proximate cause of the patient's condition.

B. Symptoms and Signs

1. Symptoms of *hyperthyroidism* include restlessness, agitation, weakness, weight loss despite increased appetite, heat intolerance, hyperdefecation, diaphoresis, palpitations, dyspnea, diarrhea, and scant menses in premenopausal females. Symptoms of congestive heart failure or arrhythmia frequently dominate the presentation of hyperthyroidism in the elderly.

Apathetic hyperthyroidism, with symptoms of withdrawal, blunted affect, and inanition, may also occur in elderly patients.

2. In *thyroid storm* the following occur:
   a. Fever (temperature > 37.8°C).
   b. Significant tachycardia.
   c. Exaggerated thyrotoxic symptoms.
   d. Organ system dysfunction:
      i. Neurologic: anxiety, restlessness, confusion, psychosis, emotional lability, coma.
      ii. Cardiac: sinus tachycardia, atrial fibrillation, wide-pulse pressure, congestive heart failure.
      iii. Gastrointestinal: weight loss, anorexia, nausea and vomiting, abdominal pain.

C. Physical Examination

1. **Vital Signs.** Tachycardia (irregular tachycardia in atrial fibrillation), widened pulse pressure, and fever (often in excess of 40°C).

2. **Skin.** May be smooth, flushed, diaphoretic, and occasionally jaundiced.

3. **HEENT.** Ocular examination reveals the characteristic stare and lid lag of hyperthyroidism. True exophthalmos, chemosis, or oculomotor defects indicate the presence of Graves' disease.

4. **Neck.** May reveal a diffuse goiter with bruit, a multinodular goiter, or a single thyroid adenoma. Goiter is frequently absent in the elderly.

5. **Chest.** Look for pneumonia (possible precipitant of storm), effusions, and/or pulmonary edema.

6. **Cardiac.** A hyperdynamic apical impulse is common; look for regurgitant or ejection murmers, elevated jugular venous pressure, and gallops.

7. **Gastrointestinal.** May reveal hepatomegaly and tenderness. Note bowel tones and any findings suggestive of a surgical abdomen.

8. **Genitourinary.** Search for infection and check heme content of stool.

9. **Extremities.** Peripheral edema may be present. Graves' dermopathy (pretibial myxedema) is an uncommon but pathognomonic finding of Graves' disease.

10. **Neurologic:** Generally reveals tremor, hyperreflexia, and proximal muscle weakness. Altered mental status ranges from agitation to frank psychosis with terminal apathy and coma.

D. Laboratory Studies

Remember: the diagnosis of thyroid storm is made on the basis of clinical rather than laboratory findings.

1. *Routinely* obtain the following:
   a. Complete blood count (CBC).
   b. Glucose level.
   c. Electrolyte panel.
   d. Blood urea nitrogen (BUN), creatinine levels.
   e. Blood cultures.
   f. Electrocardiogram (ECG).
   g. Chest roentgenogram.
   h. Urinalysis and culture.
   i. Calcium, magnesium, and phosphate levels.

2. *Thyroid studies* are mandatory (however, the results will not be available while the patient is in the ED):
   a. Total serum thyroxine (T_4).
   b. Total serum triiodothyronine (T_3).
   c. Thyroid-stimulating hormone (TSH).
   d. T_3 resin uptake (T_3RU).

3. Additional studies that *may be required,* depending on clinical circumstances, include
   a. Arterial blood gas (ABG).
   b. Amylase, bilirubin levels.
   c. Liver function tests.
   d. Toxicologic screen (e.g., stimulants).
   e. Head computed tomography.
   f. Lumbar puncture.
   g. Abdominal films.

4. Common laboratory results include the following:
   a. *Elevated thyroid studies:* Characteristic abnormalities in hyperthyroidism include an elevated serum total thyroxine (T_4) level, an elevated triiodothyronine resin uptake (T_3RU), and a low serum TSH level. Occasionally, the T_4 level is normal and only the serum total triiodothyronine (T_3) level is elevated ("T_3 toxicosis"). The presence of advanced age, serious intercurrent illness, or glucocorticoid therapy may cause confusion by blunting the expected increases in the serum T_3 and T_4 levels. There is no specific elevation of thyroid hormone levels that separates thyroid storm from uncomplicated thyrotoxicosis.
   b. *Sinus tachycardia, atrial arrhythmias, nonspecific ST- or T-wave changes,* and *increased P-wave and QRS voltages* **may occur.**
   c. *Congestive heart failure,* including pulmonary congestion and cardiomegaly, are frequently present. A *pulmonary infiltrate* would suggest pneumonia as a precipitant of thyroid storm. A substernal goiter may reveal itself as an *upper-mediastinal mass.*
   d. **Laboratory findings may include** *hypercalcemia, abnormal liver function tests,* and *elevated BUN and creatinine levels* reflecting prerenal azotemia.

III. DIFFERENTIAL DIAGNOSIS

The two features that distinguish thyroid storm from compensated hyperthyroidism, fever and altered mental status, are usually caused by infection. Appropriate microbial cultures should be obtained on all patients at the time of presentation. Toxic ingestions, most notably amphetamines, cocaine, and phencyclidine, may mimic the agitation and hyperadrenergic state of thyroid storm. Heat stroke, malignant neuroleptic syndrome, and delirium tremens may elevate the body temperature and reproduce some of the cardiovascular features of thyroid storm. Finally, acute psychosis may not only cause agitation similar to that seen in hyperthyroidism, but may also lead to a transient mild elevation of the T_4 level.

IV. THERAPY

Figure 19-7 presents the emergency therapy of thyroid storm.

A. Initial Management

Assess, secure, and support the airway, breathing, and circulation as indicated. (See Chapter 1. II.)

1. Guard the airway, administer supplemental oxygen, establish intravenous (IV) access, monitor both cardiac rhythm and oxygen saturation (SaO_2), obtain vital signs, and check the fingerstick glucose level. Treat hypoglycemia if present with 50 mL of 50% dextrose in water (D50W).

2. Initiate crystalloid resuscitation for hypotension or volume depletion with normal saline (NS) or lactated Ringer's (LR) solution (dextrose may be added as necessary depending on glucose level). Carefully monitor cardiac and pulmonary systems.

3. Use vasopressor agents (e.g., *dopamine*) if hypotension is not initially responsive to appropriate volume replacement.

B. Block Thyroid Hormone Production

Treatment of thyroid storm should begin with the immediate administration of a thionamide drug (propylthiouracil [PTU] or methimazole) to block new hormone synthesis. Neither of these drugs can be given parenterally. *PTU is preferred over methimazole because of its additional ability to block peripheral T_4 to T_3 conversion.*

1. Propylthiouracil (PTU) 300–400 mg orally (PO) or per nasogastric tube every 6 hours. Some authors recommend starting treatment with a 1-g loading dose; *or*

2. Methimazole 40 mg per rectum (PR) every 6 hours. In patients with unreliable upper-gastrointestinal function, methimazole tablets may be crushed, dissolved in saline, and administered rectally. PTU cannot be administered in this fashion.

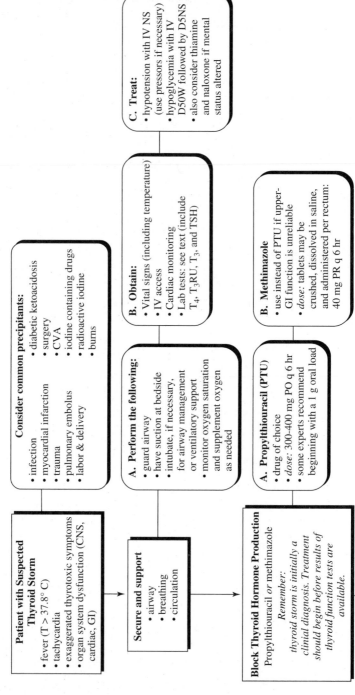

Patient with Suspected Thyroid Storm
- fever (T > 37.8° C)
- tachycardia
- exaggerated thyrotoxic symptoms
- organ system dysfunction (CNS, cardiac, GI)

Consider common precipitants:
- infection
- myocardial infarction
- trauma
- pulmonary embolus
- labor & delivery
- diabetic ketoacidosis
- surgery
- CVA
- iodine containing drugs
- radioactive iodine
- burns

Secure and support
- airway
- breathing
- circulation

A. Perform the following:
- guard airway
- have suction at bedside
- intubate, if necessary, for airway management or ventilatory support
- monitor oxygen saturation and supplement oxygen as needed

B. Obtain:
- Vital signs (including temperature)
- IV access
- Cardiac monitoring
- Lab tests: see text (include T_4, T_3RU, T_3, and TSH)

C. Treat:
- hypotension with IV NS (use pressors if necessary)
- hypoglycemia with IV D50W followed by D5NS
- also consider thiamine and naloxone if mental status altered

Block Thyroid Hormone Production
Propylthiouracil or methimazole
Remember:
thyroid storm is initially a clinical diagnosis. Treatment should begin before results of thyroid function tests are available.

A. Propylthiouracil (PTU)
- drug of choice
- *dose:* 300-400 mg PO q 6 hr
- some experts recommend beginning with a 1 g oral load

B. Methimazole
- use instead of PTU if upper-GI function is unreliable
- *dose:* tablets may be crushed, dissolved in saline, and administered per rectum: 40 mg PR q 6 hr

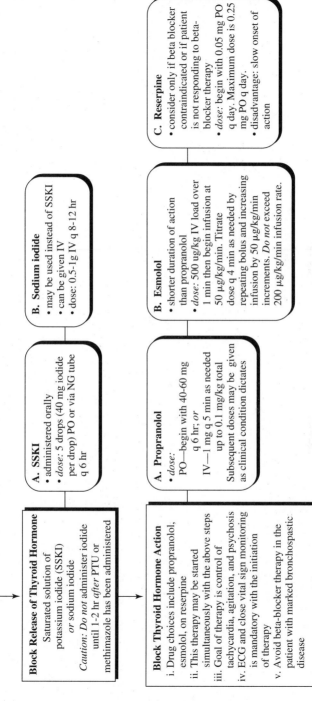

Figure 19–7. Emergency therapy of thyroid storm.

Illustration continued on following page.

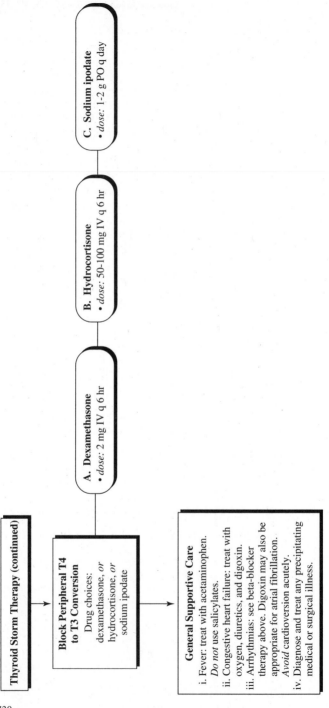

Thyroid Storm Therapy (continued)

Block Peripheral T4 to T3 Conversion
Drug choices: dexamethasone, *or* hydrocortisone, *or* sodium ipodate

A. Dexamethasone
• *dose:* 2 mg IV q 6 hr

B. Hydrocortisone
• *dose:* 50-100 mg IV q 6 hr

C. Sodium ipodate
• *dose:* 1-2 g PO q day

General Supportive Care
i. Fever: treat with acetaminophen. *Do not* use salicylates.
ii. Congestive heart failure: treat with oxygen, diuretics, and digoxin.
iii. Arrhythmias: see beta-blocker therapy above. Digoxin may also be appropriate for atrial fibrillation. *Avoid* cardioversion acutely.
iv. Diagnose and treat any precipitating medical or surgical illness.

Figure 19-7. Continued

C. Block Release of Thyroid Hormone

One to two hours after administering the first dose of thionamide, iodide is given to block the release of stored thyroid hormone. Blockade of intrathyroidal organification by the previously administered thionamide ensures that iodide given therapeutically will not be incorporated into newly synthesized thyroid hormone. Two choices are available: a saturated solution of potassium iodide for oral administration or sodium iodide for intravenous administration.

1. Saturated solution of potassium iodide (SSKI, 40 mg iodide per drop), 5 drops PO or via nasogastric tube every 6 hours; *or*
2. Sodium iodide 0.5–1 g IV every 8–12 hours.

D. Block Hormone Action

Beta-blocker therapy is used to immediately treat neuromuscular and cardiac abnormalities caused by the hyperadrenergic state associated with thyroid storm.

1. Propranolol may be given IV or PO. The dose of propranolol is adjusted to relieve tremor and reduce the heart rate < 100 beats/min.
   a. *Dose:*
      i. Oral: start with 40–60 mg PO every 6 hours.
      ii. Intravenous: 1 mg IV every 5 minutes, up to 0.1 mg/kg total.
   b. If the IV route is chosen, ECG and blood pressure monitoring is mandatory.
   c. Large doses of propranolol may be necessary because of increased metabolism of the drug in the thyrotoxic state.
   d. Use with caution in the presence of bronchospasm or congestive heart failure. Congestive heart failure in thyrotoxicosis is *not* a contraindication to beta blockade because improved diastolic filling, achieved by reduction of the heart rate, may offset the negative inotropic action of the beta blocker.
2. Esmolol: some authors suggest a trial of esmolol, an ultra-short-acting cardioselective beta blocker, to evaluate the overall effect of beta blockade on cardiac performance. If the drug is not tolerated, the IV infusion of esmolol may be terminated with rapid dissipation of the drug's effect.
   Dose. Load with 500 µg/kg IV over 1 minute, then begin infusion at 50 µg/kg/min. If response is inadequate after 4 minutes, the loading dose may be repeated and the infusion increased to 100 µg/kg/min. Subsequent doses are similarly titrated every 4 minutes by repeating the loading dose and changing the infusion by 50-µg/kg/min increments. The infusion should not exceed 200 µg/kg/min.
3. Reserpine has been used to decrease adrenergic activity in the occasional patient who does not respond to beta-blocker therapy.

E. Block Peripheral T₄ to T₃ Conversion

1. Both PTU and propranolol have the beneficial effect of inhibiting conversion of T_4 to the active thyroid hormone T_3 in peripheral target tissues.
2. Glucocorticoids should be used to achieve even more complete inhibition of peripheral conversion. Either dexamethasone or hydrocortisone can be used.
   a. Dexamethasone 2 mg IV every 6 hours. *Or*
   b. Hydrocortisone 50-100 mg IV every 6 hours.
   c. Glucocorticoid administration will also correct the relative adrenal insufficiency caused by accelerated cortisol metabolism in the thyrotoxic state.
3. The radiographic contrast agent sodium ipodate is also a powerful blocker of T_4 to T_3 conversion and may be given. *Dose:* 1-2 g PO per day.
4. Blockers of peripheral conversion may be particularly useful in treating thyroid storm caused by toxic levothyroxine ingestion or by thyroiditis with uncontrolled release of preformed thyroid hormone into the circulation.

F. Additional Therapeutic Considerations

An aggressive effort should be made to diagnose and treat any underlying illness that may have precipitated the patient's decompensation.

1. **Fever**

   a. Obtain blood and other appropriate cultures (e.g., lumbar puncture) as indicated.
   b. Assume infection is present and treat empirically until proven otherwise.
   c. Hyperthermia should be treated with acetaminophen (650 mg PO every 4–6 hours). *Do not* use salicylates because they increase free thyroid hormone levels.
   d. A cooling blanket may be necessary.
   e. Severe hyperthermia has been successfully treated with dantrolene.
   f. Some authors have recommended the use of chlorpromazine (25-50 mg IM every 4-6 hours) and meperidine (25-50 mg IV every 4-6 hours) to suppress shivering thermogenesis.

2. **Congestive Heart Failure.** Treat with oxygen, diuretics, and digoxin. Unsually high doses of digoxin may be eventually required because of hypermetabolism of the drug in this setting.

3. **Arrhythmias.** Atrial fibrillation is classically managed with digoxin. Verapamil or diltiazem have also been successfully used in this setting. Cardioversion should generally not be attempted until the patient is adequately anticoagulated and rendered euthyroid.

4. **Hypotension** and **Hypoglycemia.** Treat as noted under A, above.

V. DISPOSITION

The patient in thyroid storm requires ICU admission. Close ECG and hemodynamic monitoring is mandatory, especially in the elderly. In otherwise uncomplicated cases, glucocorticoid and iodide therapy may be withdrawn over the course of 6-8 days, and the patient may be discharged on 300–450 mg of PTU daily in divided doses every 8 hours with a tapering dose of a beta blocker.

VI. PEARLS AND PITFALLS

A. Thyroid storm is a clinical diagnosis: therapy must be started before the results of thyroid studies are available.

B. Aggressively search for and treat possible precipitating illnesses.

C. The elderly patient may not have classic thyrotoxic symptoms yet still be profoundly hyperthyroid.

D. Perform continuous ECG and hemodynamic monitoring during the first 48–72 hours of treatment.

E. Expect accelerated metabolism of propranolol, digoxin, and other drugs in thyroid storm.

Do *not* do any of the following:

A. Assume that the absence of a palpable goiter in the elderly excludes a diagnosis of thyroid storm.

B. Start iodide therapy until thionamide blockade of new thyroid hormone synthesis has been established for 1–2 hours.

C. Attempt cardioversion for atrial arrhythmias before the patient is chemically euthyroid and therapeutically anticoagulated.

BIBLIOGRAPHY

Gavin LA: Thyroid crises. Med Clin N Am 1991;75:179–193.
Howton JC: Thyroid storm presenting as coma. Ann Emerg Med 1988;17:343–345.
Reasner CA, Isley WL: Thyrotoxicosis in the critically ill. Crit Care Clin 1991;7:57–74.
Smallridge RC: Metabolic and anatomic thyroid emergencies: A review. Crit Care Med 1992; 20:276–291.

20

Neurologic Emergencies

COMA

> *"The land of darkness and the shadow of death."*
>
> JOB 10:21

I. ESSENTIAL FACTS

A. Definition

Coma is an inability to be *aroused* to consciousness.

1. *Consciousness* is a state of *awareness* of oneself and one's environment. Anatomically, arousal is "localized" to the reticular activating system (RAS), an ill-defined network of nuclei and tracts extending throughout the brainstem. Awareness requires both an intact RAS and at least some function in the cerebral cortex.

2. The initial goal in management of a comatose patient is to support the airway, breathing, and circulation, and then to rapidly determine whether the problem lies in failure of the RAS or the cerebral cortex, or is a result of a diffuse toxic or metabolic process affecting both.

3. Coma is not a disease but a symptom of a severe underlying pathologic process; therapeutic and diagnostic efforts need to be initiated simultaneously.

B. Etiology

There are three main causes of coma (Table 20–1):

1. *Diffuse (toxic, metabolic, or infectious) causes.* Alcohol and drug ingestion comprise the majority of these.

2. *Subtentorial (posterior fossa or brainstem) lesions.* Infarction and hemorrhage involving the RAS are most common.

3. *Supratentorial lesions with mass effect.* These act by vertically compressing the RAS.

II. CLINICAL EVALUATION

A. History

All available sources of information must be aggressive-ly pursued, including the patient's family and friends, wit-

Table 20–1. CAUSES OF COMA[a]

	PERCENTAGE OF CASES
Diffuse, toxic, and metabolic causes	50–65
Toxic (drugs, poisons)	25–50
Anoxic ischemia	3–5
Infectious (meningitis, encephalitis)	3–5
Hypoglycemia	3–5
Hepatic coma	3–5
Subarachnoid hemorrhage	2–4
Hyperosmolarity	< 3
Hyponatremia	< 3
Other endocrine disorders	< 3
(Addison's hypopituitarism, myxedema)	
Hypercalcemia	< 1
Uremia	< 3
Postictal (seizures)	< 3
Disorder of temperature regulation	< 3
Nutritional deficiencies	< 1
Hypercarbia	< 1
Structural causes	35–50
Supratentorial	25–30
Hemorrhage	
Intracerebral	8–10
Subdural	3–5
Epidural	< 1
Pituitary apoplexy	< 1
Trauma (contusion or occult)	< 3
Infarction (massive)	< 3
Infectious (abscess)	< 3
Tumor	
Primary	< 1
Metastatic	< 3
Subtentorial	
Infarction	
Pontine or brainstem	10–15
Cerebellar	8–10
Epi-or subdural	< 3
Hemorrhage	< 1
Pontine or brainstem	2–4
Cerebellar	< 3
Tumor	< 1
Abscess	< 1
Demyelination	< 1
Basilar migraine	< 1

[a]Following identification of obvious trauma, drug ingestion, and postarrest anoxia.
From Kellerman A, Saver C: Coma. Chapter 87. In Dugdale D, Eisenberg M (eds): Medical Diagnostics. Philadelphia, WB Saunders, 1992, p. 750.

nesses, paramedic notes, and the patient's belongings. Phone calls can provide *invaluable* information. Ask about trauma, medications, drug or alcohol use, medical conditions (including human immunodeficiency virus [HIV] disease), headache (or other preceding symptoms), and psychiatric disorders.

B. Onset

1. Sudden: consider drug overdose, trauma, intracerebral or posterior fossa hemorrhage.

2. Gradual: more likely in toxic–metabolic disorders, infection, brain tumor, or chronic subdural hematomas.

C. Associated Symptoms

1. A history of headache, head trauma (even if trivial), or visual neglect suggests a supratentorial process. Asymmetrical motor or sensory complaints are supportive.

2. A history of dizziness, diplopia, ataxia, vomiting, or an occipital headache suggests a posterior fossa lesion.

3. A history of confusion, delirium, and/or somnolence progressing to coma suggests a metabolic or infectious cause. Histories of alcohol or drug abuse, epilepsy, depression, or pre-existing renal, hepatic, or endocrine disease are supportive.

D. General Physical Examination

Caution: the head or neck of any unconscious patient should not be moved until the cervical spine has been cleared. Cervical spine immobilization should be accomplished simultaneously with airway support.

1. **Vital Signs.** Ensure the adequacy of the airway, ventilation, and blood pressure, and check the core temperature (hypothermia suggests alcohol or barbiturate overdose, hypothyroidism, or adrenal failure; hyperthermia suggests infection, heat stroke, or neuroleptic malignant syndrome).

2. **Undisturbed Observation.** Observe the respiratory pattern and look for any myoclonic jerks, spontaneous movements, or posturing.

3. **Skin.** Note signs of trauma, stigmata of liver disease, pressure sores, petechiae, purpura, needle tracks, or signs of emboli. "Cherry red" skin (rarely seen) suggests carbon monoxide poisoning or tricyclic antidepressant overdose.

4. **Head.** Ecchymoses behind the ear (Battle's sign), periorbital ecchymoses ("raccoon eyes"), blood in the external auditory canal, hemotympanum, or cerebrospinal fluid (CSF) rhinorrhea or otorrhea suggest basilar skull fracture. Mixed CSF and blood will separate as a "double ring" on filter paper or linen.

5. **Mouth.** Inspect for foreign bodies and remove any dentures. Lateral tongue lacerations suggest a recent seizure.

6. **Breath.** Check for the smell of alcohol, liver disease (musty sweet), uremia (urine), ketoacidosis (fruity), and/or cyanide poisoning (bitter almonds).

7. **Neck.** Rigidity suggests meningitis, trauma, or subarachnoid hemorrhage. *Caution:* do not move the neck until cervical spine injury has been ruled out.

8. **Chest, Abdomen, Heart, Extremities, and Rectum.** Perform a careful examination; note rectal tone and check stool for heme.

E. Directed Neurologic Examination

The immediate goal of the neurologic examination is to rapidly determine the level of neurologic function and, specifically, whether the brainstem has failed focally or because of more global dysfunction (Table 20–2).

1. **Respiration.** Most abnormal respiratory patterns will ultimately necessitate intubation. Observation prior to intubation may be helpful in determining the level of intact neurologic function.

    a. *Cheyne-Stokes respirations* (crescendo-decrescendo breathing with intermittent apneic pauses) is seen with global cortical dysfunction and may occur in toxic–metabolic disorders, congestive heart failure, and stroke, as well as in normal elderly patients.

    b. *Central neurogenic hyperventilation* (rapid deep breathing) suggests dysfunction at the midbrain level.

    c. *Apneustic breathing* (prolonged inspiratory cramp followed by an expiratory pause) implies pontine damage.

    d. *Ataxic breathing* (irregular or agonal) suggests medullary involvement and frequently precedes respiratory arrest.

2. **Optic Fundi.** Observe for papilledema (develops after several hours of increased intracranial pressure), absent venous pulsations (may more accurately reflect acute increased intracranial pressure), subhyaloid hemorrhage, and retinal artery spasm (associated with subarachnoid hemorrhage).

3. **Pupillary Responses.** Record size (in millimeters), reactivity, and equality of both pupils.

Table 20–2. ANATOMIC LOCALIZATION OF NEUROLOGIC SIGNS

EXAMINATION FINDINGS	NEUROANATOMIC SUBSTRATE
Cognition	Cortex
Conscious behaviors	Cortex and reticular activating system
Pupils	Midbrain
Extraocular movements (oculocephalic response)	Brainstem (midbrain to medulla)
Motor responses	Pons or medulla (if flaccid)
Respiration	Medulla (if ataxic)

From Kellerman A, Saver C: Coma. Chapter 87. In Dugdale D, Eisenberg M (eds): Medical Diagnostics. Philadelphia, WB Saunders, 1992, p. 753.

a. *Equal and reactive pupils:* strongly suggests a toxic–metabolic cause if other brainstem reflexes are impaired. Symmetrical cortical processes usually produce small, reactive pupils. Mild anisocoria with symmetrical reactivity is most likely congenital. Asymmetrical reactivity suggests an acute structural process.

b. *Bilaterally unreactive pupils:*

  i. Fixed and dilated: medullary lesion, immediate post-anoxia, hypothermia (< 85°F), anticholinergic drugs (atropine, tricyclics), or glutethamide toxicity.

  ii. Midposition and fixed: midbrain lesion, hypothermia, or barbiturate overdose.

  iii. Pinpoint and fixed: pontine lesion, opioid or anticholinesterase overdose. Reactivity can usually be observed with a magnifying glass.

c. *Unequal pupils:*

  i. Unilateral fixed and dilated pupil: suggests an enlarging supratentorial mass lesion with uncal herniation (the pupiloconstrictor fibers of cranial nerve [CN] III are ipsilaterally compressed by the herniating temporal lobe). The pupil may become ovoid and may be "down and out" with lateral deviation of the eye (associated CN III extraocular muscle palsy).

  ii. Unilateral fixed, small pupil: possible Horner's syndrome secondary to carotid artery dissection or occlusion (the opposite pupil is in midposition and reactive).

4. **Corneal Response.** The corneal reflex is tested by applying a cotton tip lightly to the cornea. A positive response is a bilateral blink with upward deviation of the eyes (Bell's phenomena). The afferent arc of this reflex is CN V; the efferent arc is CN VII. Preservation of this response suggests integrity of the brainstem tegmentum from the midbrain to the low pons. Severe toxic–metabolic disorders can suppress this reflex. Absence of blinking on one side suggests facial nerve dysfunction.

5. **Oculocephalic (Doll's Head) Response (Fig. 20–1).**
Caution: this response should not be tested by moving the head until the cervical spine has been cleared.

a. The oculocephalic response becomes evident only with loss of consciousness and release of the overriding control of the frontal gaze centers.

b. In oculocephalic testing of an unconscious patient with an intact brainstem, the eyes will not move with the head and will appear to be fixed on a distant target. This implies functional integrity of the midbrain tegmentum through the medulla.

c. Failure of this reflex (eyes rotate with the head as though tracking an object moving side to side) can be seen with toxic–metabolic derangements or supratentorial lesions.

CONDITION: OCULAR REFLEXES IN UNCONSCIOUS PATIENTS

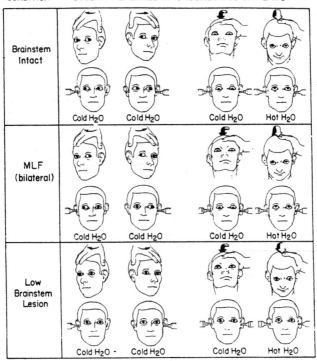

Figure 20–1. Ocular reflexes in unconscious patients. The upper section illustrates the oculocephalic (above) and oculovestibular (below) reflexes in an unconscious patient whose brainstem ocular pathways are intact. Horizontal eye movements are illustrated on the left and vertical eye movements on the right: lateral conjugate eye movements (upper left) to head turning are full and opposite in direction to the movement of the face. A stronger stimulus to lateral deviation is achieved by douching cold water against the tympanic membrane(s). There is tonic conjugate deviation of both eyes toward the stimulus; the eyes usually remain tonically deviated for 1 or more minutes before slowly returning to the midline. Because the patient is unconscious, there is no nystagmus. Extension of the neck in a patient with an intact brainstem produces conjugate deviation of the eyes in the downward direction, and flexion of the neck produces deviation of the eyes upward. Bilateral cold water against the tympanic membrane likewise produces conjugate downward deviation of the eyes, whereas hot water (no warmer than 44°C) causes conjugate upward deviation of the eyes.

In the middle portion of the drawing, the effects of bilateral medial longitudinal fasciculus lesions on oculocephalic and oculovestibular reflexes are shown. The left portion of the drawing illustrates that oculocephalic and oculovestibular stimulation deviates the appropriate eye laterally and brings the eye, which would normally deviate medially, only to the midline, since the medial longitudinal fasciculus, with its connections between the abducens and oculomotor nuclei, is interrupted. Vertical eye movements often remain intact. The lower portion of the drawing illustrates the effects of a low brainstem lesion. On the left, neither oculovestibular nor oculocephalic movements cause lateral deviation of the eyes because the pathways are interrupted between the vestibular nucleus and the abducens area. Likewise, in the right portion of the drawing, neither oculovestibular nor oculocephalic stimulation causes vertical deviation of the eyes. On rare occasions, particularly with low lateral brainstem lesions, oculocephalic responses may be intact even when oculovestibular reflexes are abolished. (From Plum F, Posner JR: Diagnosis of stupor and coma, 3rd ed. Philadelphia, F.A. Davis, 1980.)

Asymmetrical responses suggest brainstem structural lesions.

d. If the cervical spine has not been cleared or if the findings on oculocephalic testing are equivocal, ice-water caloric testing should be performed. After checking for tympanic membrane perforation, the head is elevated to 30 degrees and 50 ml of ice-water is instilled into the external auditory canal. The normal response is conjugate deviation of the eyes to the side of stimulation. Fast nystagmus away from the side of caloric stimulation suggests psychogenic unresponsiveness (an intact cortex is responsible for the fast component).

e. Conjugate eye deviation of the eyes at rest may be caused by cortical or brainstem lesions. Cortically mediated deviation can be overcome with oculocephalic or caloric testing, whereas brainstem-mediated deviation cannot.

f. In the setting of hemiplegia, conjugate gaze deviation away from the hemiplegia suggests a cortical lesion. Deviation ipsilateral to the paretic side suggests a brainstem lesion or nonconvulsive status epilepticus.

g. Except for mild divergence, disconjugate deviation implies a brainstem lesion.

6. **Motor Responses**

a. Abnormal responses should be described as observed. Avoid the words "decorticate" and "decerebrate." Posturing may be subtle and may require noxious stimuli. Pressure applied to the supraorbital ridge or stylomastoid foramen is preferable to a sternal rub because it avoids creating a subcutaneous hematoma.

b. An abnormal but symmetrical response (including bilaterally upgoing toes) may reflect midline structural pathology or a toxic–metabolic state and, thus, has little localizing value.

c. Asymmetrical motor responses suggest a structural lesion.

d. Upper-extremity flexion with lower-extremity extension implies cortical or high-brainstem dysfunction.

e. Extensor posturing of the upper extremities or the upper and lower extremities implies a pathologic process in the deep diencephalon or brainstem.

f. Flaccidity occurs in toxic–metabolic derangements, acute spinal cord injury, or progressive pontine or medullary failure.

F. Clinical Course (Table 20–3)

1. Rostral–caudal progression of neurologic dysfunction is characteristic of supratentorial mass lesions and toxic–metabolic encephalopathy. Midline mass lesions and bilateral lesions may produce few or no focal signs. Laterally placed lesions may demonstrate focal signs early in the clinical course that are

masked by progressive pressure and damage to lower brain centers. Thus, structural lesions can mimic toxic–metabolic coma.

2. The absence of an orderly rostral–caudal progression, especially with impaired oculovestibular and pupillary responses, suggests a subtentorial structural lesion.

3. Toxic encephalopathies can mimic subtentorial lesions: opioid overdose can cause small pupils and apnea resembling medullary damage; anticholinesterase poisoning can cause coma, small pupils, extraocular palsy, and a flaccid quadriparesis similar in presentation to that of pontine hemorrhage.

G. Laboratory Studies and Diagnostic Adjuncts

The necessary laboratory evaluation of the comatose patient depends on the likely cause of the comatose state as determined by history and directed examination.

Table 20–3. TYPICAL SIGNS OF COMA[a]

	HISTORY (PRIOR TO COMA)	PUPILS	OCULO-CEPHALIC RESPONSE AND CALORICS	MOTOR	ROSTRAL TO CAUDAL PRO-GRESSION	BEST TEST
Supratentorial mass lesions	Trauma, headache, focal signs	Unilateral enlargement with CN III dysfunction[b]	Deviate away from hemiplegia; calorics overcome conjugate gaze, or are absent	Focal signs present (early) or flaccid	Present	CT scan
Subtentorial mass lesions	Occipital headache,[b] nausea, vomiting, vertigo, diplopia, ataxia (truncal)	Commonly impaired, often asymmetrical	Deviate toward hemiplegia; calorics[b] fail to overcome disconjugate gaze, or are absent	Signs usually symmetrical or flaccid	Absent	CT scan
Diffuse toxic or metabolic	Confusion, apathy, delirium, somnolence	Preserved despite other brainstem signs[b]	Generally symmetrical or absent	Seizures, myoclonus, possible signs usually symmetrical or flaccid	Often present	Blood chemistries, LP (if infection is suspected)
Psychogenic unresponsiveness	Previous psychiatric history	Intact, normal	Absent, nystagmus with normal calorics[b]	Flaccid or avoidance	None	EEG (if unsure)

[a]Exceptions occur and differentiation may be especially difficult late in clinical course.
[b]Most helpful in differential diagnosis.

Modified from Plum F, and Posner J, The diagnosis of Stupor and Coma, 3rd ed. Philadelphia: F.A. Davis, 1982.

1. *Routinely* obtain the following:
   a. Arterial blood gas (ABG).
   b. Complete blood count (CBC).
   c. Electrolyte panel.
   d. Anion gap.
   e. Blood ethanol level.
   f. Pregnancy test (in females of reproductive age).
   g. Chest roentgenogram.
   h. Electrocardiogram (ECG).
   i. Glucose level.
   j. Blood urea nitrogen (BUN) and creatinine levels.
   k. Calcium, magnesium, and phosphate levels.
   l. Urinalysis.
2. *Consider additional laboratory studies* depending on clinical circumstances:
   a. Blood and urine cultures.
   b. Cervical spine films (anteroposterior, lateral, and odontoid views).
   c. Drug (toxicologic) screens. *Comment:* qualitative tests can be run on blood, urine, and gastric contents. These tests are not very sensitive (0.60–0.70) and do not detect a number of important drugs, and wide variability exists between laboratory results. In addition, detection of one or more drugs on a qualitative test does not guarantee that these agents are responsible for coma, nor does a negative drug screen exclude the diagnosis of drug intoxication.
   d. Specific drug levels. *Comment:* levels of anticonvulsant medications and barbiturates should be obtained in any patient known to be taking these medications. Aspirin and acetaminophen levels should be routinely measured in the overdose patient. A carboxyhemoglobin level is obtained on an ABG specimen and is mandatory when exposure to carbon monoxide is clinically suspected. Methanol and ethylene glycol levels should be considered in the setting of an anion gap acidosis. Drug levels, however, are expensive and should not be ordered without appropriate clinical suspicion (see Chapter 23).
   e. Liver function tests (including total bilirubin, liver enzymes, and prothrombin time).
   f. Measured serum osmolality.
   g. Other metabolic studies (e.g., thyroid function tests, cortisol levels, adrenocorticotropic hormone levels).
   h. Blood type and crossmatch.
3. *Diagnostic adjuncts* include the following:
   a. Computed Tomography
      i. The computed tomography (CT) scan is the radiographic procedure of choice for detecting intracranial mass lesions.
      ii. Resolution depends on the generation of the scanner and the lesion density. High-density intracranial bleeds as small as a few millimeters may be detected. CT has

a sensitivity of 95% and a specificity of 90% for detecting mass lesions in the cerebral hemispheres, diencephalon, and cerebellum.

   iii. Lesions in the midbrain, pons, and medulla are more easily missed owing to interference from adjacent bone, although fine posterior fossa cuts may permit detection of up to 85% of these lesions. Magnetic resonance imaging (MRI) provides better anatomic resolution, but acute hemorrhage (< 7 days) may appear isointense to surrounding brain on both T_1- and T_2-weighted images.

   iv. CT has a sensitivity of approximately 90–95% for detecting acute subarachnoid hemorrhage; lumbar puncture is indicated if the head CT is negative and subarachnoid hemorrhage is still suspected.

   v. Subacute and chronic subdural hematomas may evolve through an isodense phase and thus be detected only by the presence of mass effect. Additionally, an acute subdural hematoma in the setting of a hematocrit of < 23% may appear isodense. Contrast administration is helpful in confirming the diagnosis.

   vi. CT is *not* helpful in detecting toxic–metabolic coma, meningitis, many causes of encephalitis (except frontotemporal hemorrhage in herpes simplex virus encephalitis), small subtentorial lesions, brainstem (nonhemorrhagic) infarction, pituitary apoplexy, and meningeal carcinomatosis.

b. Lumbar Puncture

   i. The lumbar puncture is essential in the evaluation of suspected meningitis or encephalitis and is the most sensitive test for subarachnoid hemorrhage. This test should be strongly considered in any patient with coma, fever, and no evidence of an intracranial mass effect.

   ii. An emergent CT scan should be obtained prior to a lumbar puncture in any of the following clinical situations: papilledema, focally abnormal neurologic examination, depressed level of consciousness, and/or known or suspected HIV infection. Lumbar puncture in the setting of increased intracranial pressure may precipitate herniation.

   iii. Papilledema is a relatively late sign of increased intracranial pressure and may be absent acutely. Venous pulsations in the optic discs are difficult to identify but their presence virtually ensures normal pressure.

   iv. In a patient suspected of having meningitis, blood cultures should be obtained and antibiotic therapy should be instituted immediately (prior to CT scanning, if indicated, and lumbar puncture). Positive CSF cultures may be obtained from a lumbar puncture done ≤ 6 hours after starting antibiotics.

   v. Preexisting blood in the CSF can be distinguished from a traumatic tap by the presence of xanthochromia, no decrease in erythrocytes between the first and fourth samples, or a final-sample erythrocyte count of $> 1000/mm^3$.

vi. CSF protein level, glucose level, and cell count may be normal with a brain tumor or abscess, although the opening pressure is commonly elevated.

vii. Specific additional studies on CSF may include glutamine level (elevated in hepatic encephalopathy), creatine kinase level (BB fraction elevated in anoxic encephalopathy 48–72 hours after onset), viral studies, fungal antigens, and cytology (in suspected carcinomatous meningoencephalitis).

viii. Most complications of lumbar puncture develop within 12 hours.

c. Electroencephalography

i. The electroencephalogram (EEG) is cumbersome to obtain and has little place in the emergent evaluation of coma of unknown cause.

ii. The EEG is much less helpful than the CT scan in discriminating structural from metabolic lesions.

iii. Metabolic disease most commonly produces symmetrical and diffuse slowing, although triphasic waves (not specific for hepatic encephalopathy) and periodic lateralized epileptiform discharges can be seen.

iv. The most useful role for encephalography is in distinguishing repetitive or subclinical seizure activity and in confirming brain death. Seizures, however, rarely cause coma without overt convulsions.

v. Coma can be readily differentiated from psychogenic unresponsiveness by obtaining an EEG; however, most cases can be distinguished on clinical grounds.

vi. Severe toxic or metabolic encephalopathy and hypothermia can produce an isoelectric EEG and must be excluded prior to a diagnosis of brain death.

d. Roentgenography. When readily available, CT scanning has largely replaced roentgenography in the evaluation of suspected intracranial mass lesions after head trauma.

e. Angiography

i. Angiography is rarely indicated for the early evaluation of the comatose patient.

ii. Angiography is sensitive (95%) but less specific (85%) than CT for detecting mass lesions and is much more hazardous to perform.

iii. The primary utility of angiography in coma is in locating aneurysms and confirming vascular spasm.

III. DIFFERENTIAL DIAGNOSIS

The differential diagnosis for the patient presenting with an altered level of consciousness or actual coma is presented below (also see Table 20–1).

A. Cerebrovascular disease (e.g., intracranial hemorrhage, cerebral infarction, subarachnoid hemorrhage)

B. Electrolyte abnormalities (e.g., hyper- or hyponatremia, hyper- or hypocalcemia, hyperkalemia, hyper- or hypomagnesemia)

C. Environmental causes (e.g., hypothermia or heat stroke)

D. Hypertensive encephalopathy

E. Hypoxia or carbon dioxide retention

F. Infection (e.g., sepsis, meningitis, encephalitis, brain abscess, HIV infection, or secondary opportunistic infection)

G. Metabolic abnormalities (e.g., hypoglycemia, diabetic ketoacidosis, hyperglycemic hyperosmolar coma, hepatic failure, uremia, myxedema coma, thyroid storm, Wernicke's encephalopathy)

H. Neoplasms (e.g., metastatic or primary brain lesion)

I. Poisoning (alcohol, drugs, other toxins)

J. Postictal state

K. Trauma (e.g., brain contusion, concussion, diffuse axonal injury, intracranial bleed, subdural hematoma, epidural hematoma)

IV. THERAPY

The evaluation and treatment of the comatose patient should be thorough and systematic in every case. Diagnostic and therapeutic measures must be instituted simultaneously. As a general rule, a final diagnosis and/or definitive therapy should be obtained *within 60 minutes of* ED presentation. The emergency therapy of coma is outlined in Figure 20–2.

A. Initial Management

Assess, secure, and support the airway, breathing, circulation, and neurologic status as indicated. (See Chapter 1. II.)

1. Administer supplemental oxygen, immobilize the cervical spine, and protect the airway as necessary. Endotracheal intubation may be necessary for definitive airway protection or to allow for hyperventilation in the setting of increased intracranial pressure.

2. Obtain vital signs, establish intravenous (IV) access, check the fingerstick glucose level, and order appropriate laboratory studies (see II, above). Monitor both cardiac rhythm and oxygen saturation (SaO_2).

3. Treat hypotension with IV crystalloid. If clinical examination indicates pulmonary vascular congestion, support blood pressure as necessary with dopamine.

4. Perform a directed neurologic examination: assess pupillary activity, level of consciousness, and any lateralized deficits.

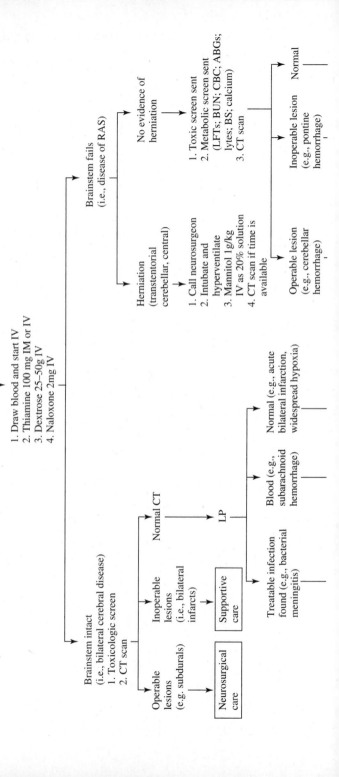

Secure and support airway, breathing, and circulation

1. Draw blood and start IV
2. Thiamine 100 mg IM or IV
3. Dextrose 25–50g IV
4. Naloxone 2mg IV

Brainstem fails (i.e., disease of RAS)

Herniation (transtentorial cerebellar, central)
1. Call neurosurgeon
2. Intubate and hyperventilate
3. Mannitol 1g/kg IV as 20% solution
4. CT scan if time is available

- Operable lesion (e.g., cerebellar hemorrhage)

No evidence of herniation
1. Toxic screen sent
2. Metabolic screen sent (LFTs; BUN; CBC; ABGs; lytes; BS; calcium)
3. CT scan

- Inoperable lesion (e.g., pontine hemorrhage)
- Normal

Brainstem intact (i.e., bilateral cerebral disease)
1. Toxicologic screen
2. CT scan

Operable lesions (e.g. subdurals) → Neurosurgical care

Inoperable lesions (i.e., bilateral infarcts) → Supportive care

Normal CT → LP

- Treatable infection found (e.g., bacterial meningitis)
- Blood (e.g., subarachnoid hemorrhage)
- Normal (e.g., acute bilateral infarction, widespread hypoxia)

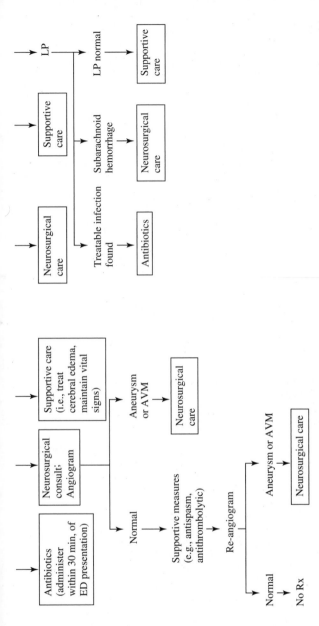

Figure 20-2. Diagnosis and treatment protocol in the comatose patient. LP, lumbar puncture; LFTs, liver function tests; ABGs, arterial blood gases; BS, blood sugar; AVM, arteriovenous malformation. (Adapted from Samuels MA, Aquino TM: Coma and other alterations of consciousness. In Samuels MA (ed): Manual of Neurologic Therapeutics. 3rd Ed. Boston, Little, Brown, 1986, p. 13.)

Thiamine, glucose, and naloxone should be *routinely* administered to the patient with an altered level of consciousness or frank coma:

a. Thiamine is administered to treat potential Wernicke's encephalopathy. Thiamine deficiency may occur in chronic ethanol users, malnourished patients, patients with unusual diets, or patients treated with total parenteral nutrition. Thiamine should be administered *before* glucose in these settings.

   Dose: 100 mg intramuscularly (IM) or IV. In classic Wernicke's encephalopathy 100 mg IV, IM, or orally (PO) should be administered daily until symptoms completely resolve and the patient has an adequate oral intake.

b. Glucose is administered to treat hypoglycemia. If time allows, an immediate fingerstick glucose measurement should be obtained *before* administering parenteral glucose; if the fingerstick glucose level is ≥ 80 mg/dL, parenteral glucose is *unnecessary.*

   Dose: 1–2 ampules (25 g of glucose per 50-mL ampule) of 50% dextrose in water (D50W) IV. This dose may be repeated as necessary, or the patient subsequently started on a dextrose containing IV infusion (either 5% or 10% dextrose [D5 or D10]). *Caution:* hyperglycemia may worsen the neurologic outcome in the resuscitated cardiac arrest patient and should be avoided, if possible, in the setting of cerebral hypoperfusion.

c. Naloxone is given to reverse opioids.

   Dose: 0.4–2 mg IV. Much larger doses (≥ 10 mg) may be required when poisoning occurs with codeine, propoxyphene, pentazocine, and/or fentanyl derivatives. With naloxone, the clinical effects of opioid reversal may be as short as 15–20 minutes and subsequent doses are commonly necessary. Alternatively, after the patient's initial response, a continuous naloxone infusion may be utilized by administering two-thirds of the initially effective bolus dose per hour. *Caution:* in the pregnant patient the dosage of naloxone should be titrated carefully to avoid precipitation of opioid withdrawal in the fetus.

d. Other antidotes should be administered as appropriate in the setting of a known toxin exposure (e.g., flumazenil for benzodiazepine overdose; amyl nitrite, sodium nitrite, and sodium thiosulfate for cyanide poisoning; atropine for cholinergic poisoning; see Chapter 23).

5. General supportive measures include the following:

a. Place a Foley catheter and nasogastric tube (place the nasogastric tube orally instead of nasally in the patient with significant midface injury, suspected basilar skull fracture, or a significant coagulopathy).

b. Protect the eyes from desiccation and injury.

c. Do not leave the patient alone in the ED. Keep the guardrails up on the patient's stretcher.

     d. If the patient requires further studies outside of the ED, he/she should be accompanied by appropriate physician and/or nursing personnel.

B. Control of Ongoing Seizure Activity

    See also Seizures, later in this chapter.

1. Assess, secure, and support the airway, breathing, oxygenation, and circulation as outlined previously.

2. Consider the possibility of thiamine depletion and hypoglycemia; treat as necessary (see IV. A. 4, above). Consider the possibility of magnesium depletion and replace if appropriate (e.g., give 1–2 g magnesium sulfate IV over 20 minutes).

3. Benzodiazepines are the initial drugs of choice for ongoing seizure activity: lorazepam (0.1 mg/kg IV, given no faster than 2 mg/min, total adult dose 4–8 mg) or diazepam (0.15–0.25 mg/kg IV, given no faster than 2–5 mg/min, total adult dose 10–20 mg).

4. Additional drugs may include phenytoin (18 mg/kg IV load [15 mg/kg in the elderly] no faster than 50 mg/min) and/or phenobarbital (10–20 mg/kg IV, no faster than 100 mg/min).

5. Frequently monitor core body temperature and prevent and/or manage hyperthermia as required.

C. Management of Hypo- or Hyperthermia, if Present

1. *Hypothermia* is defined as a core body temperature < 35°C. Wet clothing should be removed and further external heat loss prevented. The rewarming method of choice depends on the patient's body temperature:

    a. For core temperatures of 34–36°C passive external rewarming (blankets) and active external rewarming (hot water bottles, heating pads, radiant heat sources, warming beds) are the methods of choice.

    b. For a core temperature of 30–34°C initiate passive external rewarming with *active external rewarming of truncal body areas only* (i.e., neck, armpits, and groin). Warmed IV fluids and warmed humidified oxygen should additionally be used.

    c. For core temperatures < 30°C active internal rewarming is appropriate: administer warm IV fluids and warm humidified oxygen, and initiate one or more of the following (depending on ED provider's expertise and institution capability): warmed peritoneal lavage, warmed gastric lavage, warmed bladder lavage, esophageal rewarming tubes, and/or extracorporeal rewarming (via heart–lung bypass). *Handle the patient very gently to avoid precipitating ventricular fibrillation!*

2. *Hyperthermia* is an abnormally high core body temperature. Extreme body temperatures are those > 40°C (104°F) in the adult patient.

    a. Hyperthermia should be treated with external cooling: cooling blankets, tepid sponge baths, and/or mist spray with electric fan convection. The core body temperature must be closely monitored. Acetaminophen (650 mg PO or per rectum [PR] every 4 hours) is also reasonable, but its effectiveness depends on the clinical situation. Chlorpromazine (25 mg IM every 6–8 hours) may reduce shivering.

    b. In severe cases, cold baths, intubation, and muscle paralysis with pancuronium (0.1 mg/kg IV) should be considered. Treatment with dantrolene (1–2 mg/kg IV every 6 hours; do not exceed 10 mg/kg/day) may be beneficial but has not been adequately studied to date. Dantrolene can cause hypotension and hepatotoxicity.

D. Management of Increased Intracranial Pressure

Increased intracranial pressure is a potentially life-threatening emergency in need of urgent therapy. Beware of the patient with progressive neurologic deterioration in the ED, or other findings suggestive of impending herniation (e.g., increasingly severe headache, deterioration in level of consciousness, unequal pupils, lateralized motor deficit, or Cushing's reflex [elevated blood pressure with reflex bradycardia]). Consult a neurosurgeon emergently and proceed with the following:

1. Secure and support the airway, breathing, oxygenation, and vital signs as above.

2. Elevate head of bed by 30 degrees (unless contraindicated because of suspected spinal injury or hypotension).

3. Ensure a neutral neck position to allow for optimal venous drainage from the head. If a cervical collar is in place, make sure it is not compressing the jugular veins.

4. Endotracheally intubate the patient and hyperventilate to a PCO_2 of 25–30 mmHg. Hyperventilation decreases intracranial blood volume and intracranial pressure; it is the most effective emergency technique available to the ED physician in this setting.

5. Medications:

    a. Mannitol (1 g/kg as a 20% solution IV over 10–20 minutes) may be given in consultation with a neurosurgeon. Mannitol causes intravascular hyperosmolarity, shrinks brain volume, and reduces intracranial pressure. It should not be used in the setting of cardiac or renal failure.

    b. Furosemide (40–80 mg IV in adults) may also be given in consultation with a neurosurgeon. Medically induced diuresis may assist in reducing intracranial pressure. It should not be administered to the hemodynamically unstable patient.

    c. Decadron (10–20 mg IV push, followed by 4 mg IV, PO, or IM every 6 hours) is helpful if the elevation in intracranial pressure is secondary to a tumor or brain abscess. Decadron is not helpful in acute head injury.

6. If hemodynamic status allows, minimize IV fluid infusion rates to prevent overhydration and worsening cerebral edema.

E. Management of Infection

Meningitis, brain abscess, and/or sepsis mandate emergent antibiotic administration. When meningitis is suspected clinically (meningeal signs/symptoms or fever with an altered mental status), *antibiotic therapy should be started within 30 minutes of the patient's ED presentation.* Ideally, blood cultures and lumbar puncture should be obtained before beginning antibiotics; if there is a delay in obtaining CSF for any reason (e.g., difficult lumbar puncture or head CT deemed clinically necessary before the lumbar puncture) do *not* delay antibiotic administration (see Meningitis/Encephalitis in Chapter 15).

F. Other Definitive Care

By this time the patient's airway and breathing should be secure, oxygenation optimized, unstable vital signs (blood pressure and temperature) appropriately treated, seizures controlled, and neurologic catastrophes (e.g., impending herniation, meningitis) identified and appropriate management instituted. Further definitive care depends on the cause or causes of the comatose state. The reader should refer to the relevant chapter dealing with the identified disorder for further recommendations on specific management.

V. DISPOSITION

The patient with a persistently altered mental status or true coma requires hospital admission (usually to the ICU) for continued diagnosis and therapy.

VI. PEARLS AND PITFALLS

Aside from the wide array of possible causes delineated in Table 20–1, three other states of "apparent unconsciousness" should be considered.

A. *"Locked-in syndrome":* intact arousal and alertness with an inability to act volitionally. It is usually due to brainstem infarction. Voluntary vertical and, occasionally, horizontal eye movements as well as voluntary pupillary accomodation are preserved. Ask the patient to focus on an object several feet away and then several inches in front of his or her face. Pupillary constriction on near gaze (on several trials) implies consciousness.

B. *Severe neuromuscular blockade:* the inability to initiate any voluntary activity may be seen in severe acute inflammatory demyelinating polyneuropathy (Guillain–Barré syndrome), myasthenic crisis, and botulism. Pupillary reactivity is spared in the former two but may be very sluggish in botulism.

C. *Psychogenic unresponsiveness:* a prior history of psychiatric illness may be found. *Vigorous noxious stimulation is counterproductive and rarely helpful.* Observation of behavior (yawning, swallowing, licking of the lips), normal oculocephalic or caloric reflexes, and a normal EEG may be helpful in unclear cases. Often, a strong suggestion that the condition will resolve will afford the patient a graceful way to "regain consciousness."

BIBLIOGRAPHY

Plum F, Posner J: The Diagnosis of Stupor and Coma, 3rd ed. Philadelphia, FA Davis, 1980.
Sacco R, VanGool R, Mohr JP, Hauser WA: Nontraumatic coma: Glasgow Coma Score and coma etiology as predictors of 2-week outcome. Arch Neurol 1990;47:1181–1184.
Samuels, A: Disorders of Consciousness. Chapter 1. In Johnson R (ed): Current Therapy in Neurologic Disease—3. Philadelphia, BC Decker, 1990.
Simon HB: Hyperthermia. N Engl J Med 1993;329(7):483–487.

STROKE

". . .these things that we suffer all come from the brain, when it is not healthy. . ."

HIPPOCRATES

I. ESSENTIAL FACTS

A. Definitions

The World Health Organization (WHO) defines *stroke* as "rapidly developing clinical signs of focal (or global) disturbance of cerebral function, with symptoms lasting longer than 24 hours or leading to death, with no apparent cause other than of vascular origin." *Transient ischemic attacks* (TIAs) are acute episodes of focal loss of cerebral function (including focal visual loss) lasting < 24 hours attributed to a temporarily inadequate blood supply.

B. Pathophysiology

The common pathologic processes that result in a TIA or stroke are occlusion (Fig. 20–3) and hemorrhage of the vasculature of the brain.

1. Occlusive causes may include
   a. Large-vessel thrombosis secondary to carotid or intracranial athero-occlusive disease, hypercoagulable states, vascular dissection, arteritis, and/or vasospasm.
   b. Small-vessel thrombosis secondary to hypertension and arteriosclerosis (with resultant small areas of cerebral

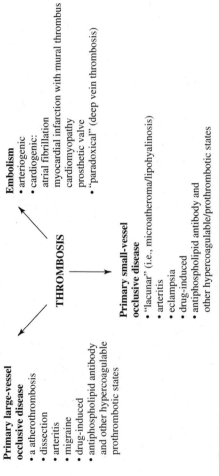

Primary large-vessel occlusive disease
- a atherothrombosis
- dissection
- arteritis
- migraine
- drug-induced
- antiphospholipid antibody and other hypercoagulable prothrombotic states

THROMBOSIS

Primary small-vessel occlusive disease
- "lacunar" (i.e., microatheroma/lipohyalinosis)
- arteritis
- eclampsia
- drug-induced
- antiphospholipid antibody and other hypercoagulable/prothrombotic states

Embolism
- arteriogenic
- cardiogenic:
  atrial fibrillation
  myocardial infarction with mural thrombus
  cardiomyopathy
  prosthetic valve
- "paradoxical" (deep vein thrombosis)

Figure 20–3. The three major pathophysiologic mechanisms underlying the occurrence of stroke. Thrombosis plays an integral role in each mechanism. (From Rothrock and Hart, Antithrombotic therapy in cerebrovascular disease. Ann Intern Med 1991;115:885–895.)

ischemic infarction termed *cerebral lacunae*), hypercoagulable states, arteritis, and/or eclampsia.

c. Emboli of cardiogenic, arterioarterial (e.g., aortic, carotid, or posterior circulation atheromatous plaques), or "paradoxical" (e.g., from a venous source, which subsequently reaches the arterial system via an atrial-septal defect) origin.

d. Inadequate blood flow to border zones between vascular territories (*watersheds*). Watershed infarcts may occur as a complication of hypotension from any cause. More global ischemia/injury may also occur in patients after profound hypotensive episodes (e.g., cardiopulmonary arrest).

2. Hemorrhagic causes may include hypertension, aneurysmal subarachnoid hemorrhage (SAH), ruptured arteriovenous malformation (AVM), amyloid angiopathy, hemorrhagic metastases, venous infarction (which is usually hemorrhagic), sympathomimetic drugs, arteritis, and/or bleeding diatheses.

C. Epidemiology

Stroke is the third leading cause of death in the United States. Approximately 500,000 new cases are diagnosed annually. Because stroke incidence rises exponentially with age, the relative importance of stroke prevention and treatment will increase as the population ages. Risk factors include the following:

1. Older age.

2. Hypertension: relative risk is 4.

3. Smoking: relative risk is 4 (the relative risk among hypertensive smokers is 20).

4. Diabetes mellitus.

5. Elevated serum cholesterol: increased risk for ischemic, but not hemorrhagic, stroke.

6. Obesity, physical inactivity.

7. Oral contraceptives: increased risk is controversial and is based on studies in which patients used preparations containing > 50 μg of estrogen per tablet. Combined smoking and the use of oral contraceptives significantly increases stroke risk.

8. Cardiac disease, including nonvalvular and valvular atrial fibrillation, cardiomyopathy with a thrombus, large anterior myocardial infarction, congenital heart disease, prosthetic or infected heart valves, ventricular aneurysm, mitral valve prolapse with myxomatous changes, or atrial myxoma.

II. CLINICAL EVALUATION

A. History

1. Obtain a detailed account of the patient's exact symptoms, their rapidity of onset and time to maximal intensity, and the patient's activity at the time.

2. Inquire about other associated symptoms (e.g., visual or olfactory aura, headache, aphasia, and palpitations). Headache occurs in approximately 25% of patients, especially in hemorrhagic and embolic strokes. Positive phenomena (e.g., visual aura, involuntary movements, loss of consciousness, and/or incontinence) are rare in stroke and suggest an alternate diagnosis.

3. Accurately determine past neurologic, medical, and surgical history. Determine medication use, drug abuse, pregnancy probability, and any history of recent infections or trauma.

B. Physical Examination

1. **Vital Signs.** Note pulse, blood pressure (BP), respiratory rate, and temperature. Cerebrovascular events often occur in the setting of hypertension or hypotension. Note BP in both arms (asymmetry may suggest subclavian stenosis).

2. **HEENT.** Temporal artery tenderness in elderly patients may suggest temporal arteritis.

3. **Neck.** Examine for nuchal rigidity secondary to subarachnoid hemorrhage or meningitis.

4. **Lungs.** Listen for adequacy of air flow and forcefulness of cough. Carefully auscultate for wheezes, rales, and rhonchi.

5. **Cardiovascular System.** Murmurs, extra heart sounds, rhythm irregularity, and/or an opening snap suggest predisposing heart disease. Auscultate for bruits along the course of the subclavian artery, at the subclavian–vertebral junction, at the angle of the jaw, and over the mastoids and orbits. Absence of a carotid bruit, however, does not rule out carotid artery stenosis.

6. **Extremities.** Examine for stigmata of endocarditis (e.g., splinter hemorrhages, Janeway lesions, Osler's nodes), hemorrhagic diatheses, and/or vaculitis.

7. **Neurologic Function.** Attempt to determine the general vascular territory of the deficit(s) and whether they are cortical or subcortical. Carefully evaluate the following:
   a. Mental status, including level of consciousness, orientation, memory, naming, speech (pronunciation and word choice), understanding, repetition, reading, writing, and copying designs.
   b. Cranial nerves II–XII, including fundoscopic examination and visual field assessment.
   c. Motor function, including muscle bulk, tone, strength, and fine motor control. Pronator drift suggests cortical dysfunction.
   d. Deep tendon reflexes (DTRs): these are hypoactive on the affected side initially; later, they become hyperactive. Describe plantar responses (Babinski's reflex) as flexor (down) or extensor (up).

    e. Sensory perception, including pain, temperature, light touch, and vibration (or position). Test for parietal lobe integrity by providing bilateral simultaneous stimulation. Rhomberg's sign is a position sense test.

    f. Cerebellar function, including balance, heel-to-shin testing, finger-to-nose testing, and gait (if the patient is safely ambulatory).

C. Laboratory Studies

1. Minimally obtain the following:

    a. *Complete blood count (CBC)* including platelet count to evaluate for anemia, infection, erythrocytosis, polycythemia, and/or thrombocytopenia.

    b. *Electrolytes, glucose, blood urea nitrogen (BUN), and creatinine levels.* Remember, hypoglycemia may mimic an acute stroke.

    c. *Prothrombin time* (PT) and *partial thromboplastin time* (PTT).

    d. *Pregnancy test* (in females of reproductive age).

    e. *Chest roentgenogram:* evaluate for heart size, infiltrates, congestive heart failure, and any lesions suggestive of malignancy.

    f. *Electrocardiogram* (ECG): look carefully for an arrhythmia, ventricular hypertrophy, acute ischemia, and old or recent myocardial infarction. Both SAH and ischemic stroke can cause "peaked" T waves, QT-interval changes, and other T-wave and ST-segment changes.

    g. *Noncontrast head computed tomography* (CT):

       i. The primary goal of acute imaging is to rule out hemorrhage and mass effect. Acute hemorrhage will produce an area of increased density; infarction produces an area of decreased density.

      ii. Areas of ischemia and/or edema are not usually seen for at least 24–48 hours after symptom onset. Repeat imaging in 7–10 days may help define the final vascular distribution of the stroke.

     iii. The sensitivity of noncontrast CT in acute SAH is 90–95%. If the CT is negative and the diagnosis of SAH clinically suspected, lumbar puncture is indicated.

     iv. Magnetic resonance imaging (MRI) is preferred over CT in the evaluation of brainstem stroke, subacute hematoma (age 10–20 days), demyelinating diseases, and AVMs.

2. Additional studies are frequently indicated, depending on clinical circumstances. Consider one or more of the following as necessary:

    a. *Erythrocyte sedimentation rate (ESR):* mandatory in any patient ≥ age 50 with headache or transient visual loss to rule out temporal arteritis. An elevated ESR may also suggest another vasculitic or occult inflammatory/ neoplastic process.

b. *Carotid artery Doppler (duplex) sonography:* appropriate noninvasive study in any patient with either a real or suspected anterior circulation TIA or acute stroke syndrome to evaluate for high-grade carotid stenosis that may benefit from surgical intervention (carotid endarterectomy) in appropriate candidates.

c. *Lumbar puncture (LP):* mandatory when meningitis is suspected or when SAH is suspected and the head CT is either negative or equivocal. A head CT should be obtained *prior to* the LP whenever intracranial hypertension or a mass lesion is clinically suspected (e.g., papilledema, focal neurologic examination, significantly altered mental status, or known or suspected human immunodeficiency virus [HIV] infection).

d. *Echocardiography:* used to evaluate the patient for a cardiac source of emboli. The yield in patients without clinical evidence of heart disease is low (< 3%).

   i. Transthoracic echocardiography should be considered in the evaluation of young patients with stroke without an obvious cause; in those without risk factors for, or arteriographic evidence of, primary arterial disease; and in patients with clinical evidence of cardiac disease.

   ii. Transesophageal echocardiography should be considered if patient management would be altered by the identification of minor embolic sources (e.g., a patent foramen ovale, mitral valve prolapse, atrial septal defect) or by detection of a left atrial thrombus in the setting of atrial fibrillation.

e. *Cholesterol level with fractionation (especially HDL cholesterol and LDL to HDL cholesterol ratio):* important in subsequent risk factor reduction for the prevention of secondary stroke (this test is more appropriately ordered by the referral physician; cholesterol fractionation should only be done after an overnight fast).

f. *Angiography:* may be ordered selectively by the consultant neurologist and/or neurosurgeon to identify the location and size of cerebral aneurysms and AVMs, to evaluate suspected symptomatic carotid stenosis or dissection, or to further evaluate suspected subclavian "steal" syndrome (subclavian stenosis with ipsilateral vertebral artery flow reversal).

g. *Magnetic resonance angiography:* noninvasively defines both extra- and intracranial vasculature. At present, artifact from disturbed flow results in underestimation of true stenosis. With improved technology, "one-shot" MRI evaluation of cerebral ischemia and vessel patency may ultimately replace CT and angiography in evaluation of acute ischemic strokes.

h. *Secondary studies* should be ordered as indicated: examples include VDRL (or RPR), Lyme disease titer, urine toxicology screen, antithrombin III level, protein S and C levels, anticardiolipin antibody, blood cultures (in suspected bacterial endocarditis), and/or hemoglobin electrophoresis.

III. DIFFERENTIAL DIAGNOSIS

The distinguishing characteristics of cerebrovascular causes of stroke (including TIA, thrombosis, hemorrhage, embolism, and SAH) are listed in Table 20–4. Other phenomena may mimic stroke but have a fundamentally different pathology. One in ten patients clinically diagnosed as having a "stroke" will be suffering from another disorder and ultimately will have a different prognosis. Alternate causes include the following:

A. Hypotension from acute blood or volume loss, myocardial infarction, hypersensitive carotid sinus, or arrhythmia.

B. Migrainous accompaniments may result in focal neurologic deficits without an accompanying headache. A family history of migraine sometimes is helpful.

C. Labyrinthine disorders, including acoustic neuroma, Meniere's disease, benign positional vertigo, and vestibular neuronitis.

D. Postictal (Todd's) paralysis may occur after an unwitnessed seizure. The patient will usually have a prior history of seizures.

E. Infection, including meningitis, brain abscess, encephalitis, neurosyphilis, and opportunistic infections in immunocompromised patients.

F. Intoxication from barbiturates, alcohol, opioids, and benzodiazepines.

G. Metabolic derangements, including diabetes (hypo- or hyperglycemia), myxedema coma, thyroid storm, and other electrolyte abnormalities (e.g., hyponatremia, hypernatremia, hypercalcemia, hypo- or hypermagnesemia).

H. Subdural or epidural hematomas: up to 50% of patients give no history of a fall or significant trauma.

I. Demyelinating diseases, including multiple sclerosis and optic neuritis. Patients are usually < age 40 and the onset of symptoms is often rapidly progressive rather than abrupt.

J. Previous strokes may be "unmasked" by systemic illness. The CT scan will demonstrate a well-demarcated infarct in the appropriate territory. Prognosis for improvement in this setting is good.

Table 20–4. DIFFERENTIAL DIAGNOSIS OF STROKE

	HISTORY	COURSE	EXAMINATION
Transient Ischemic Attacks (TIAs)	Sudden awareness that portion of normal neurologic function is impaired. Accounts for 60–75% of stroke-like occurrences. Major strokes may follow TIAs or develop from same episode.	Attacks come on suddenly, last from a few seconds to 24 hr, are repetitive, and occur days, weeks or months apart.	*Vertebrobasilar:* Dizziness, ataxia, visual field defect, diplopia, mono-, hemi-, or quadriparesis or sensory disturbance, drop attacks. *Carotid-middle cerebral:* Dysphagia, mono- or hemiparesis, confusion, visual defect (amaurosis fugax).
Cerebral Thrombosis	Patients are 40–70 years old, often have history of atherosclerosis. The stroke is usually sudden, often occurs during sleep. Event is not related to activity. In 80% of cases, the stroke is preceded by one or more minor signs (TIAs, headache, etc.). Because such episodes rarely precede hemorrhage or embolus, their presence is of great help in securing the diagnosis of cerebral thrombosis.	Maximal damage may be immediately apparent; common is stepwise fluctuating deficit. Recovery takes days to months.	Exam varies according to size and location of infarction. Involves internal carotid or vertebrobasilar systems.
Cerebral hemorrhage	Patients are 40–60 years old. Hypertension nearly always present, often in association with atherosclerosis. Headache, nausea, and vomiting often precede deficit. Tends to occur during exercise and during waking hours.	Rapid and steady progression to neurologic deficit or death. Delayed recovery.	Exam varies according to size and location of hemorrhage. Sites include putamen and external capsule (45–60%), cerebral white matter (20–30%), thalamus (10–15%), cerebellum (8–10%) and pons (3–10%).
Cerebral Embolism	As most emboli come from heart, history is often given of valvular heart disease, chronic atrial fibrillation, cardiac surgery. Stroke is sudden, usually unassociated with prodrome or activity.	Sudden onset of maximal deficit. Recovery tends to be rapid.	Exam varies according to size and location: Often in distribution of middle cerebral artery.
Subarachnoid Hemorrhage	Sudden development of excruciating headache, stiff neck, nausea.	Patient becomes confused, stuporous, comatose within hours. Most survive initial episode (> 90%) but incidence of recurrence high (48 deaths/100 patients in 6 months).	Exam is most often normal, save for sensorium. Nonlocalizing or bilateral neurologic findings. Funduscopic exam revealing subhyaloid hemorrhage is diagnostic but uncommonly found.

Table continued on following page

Table 20–4. DIFFERENTIAL DIAGNOSIS OF STROKE *(Continued)*

	ASSOCIATED FINDINGS	LABORATORY	CAUSE	ADDITIONAL COMMENTS
TIAs	67% of patients are hypertensive.	As indicated. Conditions that increase blood viscosity and lead to sludging may be detected, such as consumption coagulopathy, thrombocytosis, dysproteinemia	Mechanism is probably a complete cessation of blood flow, which occurs locally. Microembolism may be associated, particularly when multiple episodes of different pattern are noted.	Between attacks, a neurologic exam is normal. During the episode, symptoms and signs are indistinguishable from evolving infarction. The risk of stroke in a patient with TIA is 12% in the first year.
Cerebral Thrombosis	Evidence of atherosclerosis may be noted. Convulsions are frequent.	CT; other studies as indicated (see text).	Thrombosis or occlusion of a cerebral artery as a result of arteriosclerosis.	The single most common cause of stroke. Thrombosis includes: Reversible ischemic neurologic deficits that resemble TIAs, but signs persist beyond 24 hr, stroke-in-evolution that results in a persistent neurologic deficit; completed stroke.
Cerebral Hemorrhage	Hypertension as noted. Convulsions are rare.	CT; other studies as indicated (see text).	Degeneration of arteries from hypertension results in hyaline thickening of wall, disruption of elastica and microaneurysm formation. These rupture to cause hemorrhage.	Accounts for about 25% of strokes. Prognosis is grave, with 70–75% patients dying in 1–30 days.
Cerebral Embolism	Heart disease: Mitral stenosis, SBE, atrial fibrillation, myxoma, cardiac surgery. Evidence of other embolic phenomena.	CT; other studies as indicated (see text).	In most cases fragment breaks away from thrombus within heart. Can also be from fat, tumor cells, air or vegetations in endocarditis.	Anticoagulation is important in preventing further emboli, and in general is instituted after 48 hours, assuming LP and CT scan are negative for hemorrhage (see text).
Subarachnoid Hemorrhage	None	CT. If negative, then LP. LP: Invariably reveals grossly bloody CSF, under increased pressure (usually > 25,000 red cells). CT demonstrates blood, and aneurysms > 2 cm diameter.	Result from rupture of saccular aneurysm, a defect in arterial wall that occurs at site of arterial branching or bifurcation, particularly in circle of Willis.	Surgery is the treatment of choice in suitable patients who have accessible lesions. Initial efforts are made to prevent and treat the major complications; vasospasm and recurrent hemorrhage.

CT, Computed tomography.
LP, Lumber puncture.

IV. THERAPY

The goals of the ED physician in the acute TIA or stroke patient are to secure oxygenation and vital signs, exclude nonvascular causes of the patient's signs and symptoms, define the type (i.e., ischemic versus hemorrhagic) and vascular territory of the TIA or stroke, expedite appropriate specialist consultation, minimize the extent of secondary damage, and assist in the prevention of recurrent cerebrovascular events.

A. Transient Ischemic Attack

The risk of stroke after a noncardioembolic TIA or a small completed stroke is about 12% in the first year and 7% per year thereafter. This is seven times the risk in an age-matched population of people without TIA.

1. *Assess, secure, and support the airway, breathing, and circulation as necessary.* Do not attempt to lower BP in the hypertensive TIA patient in the ED. Thickened small perforating (internal capsule, brainstem) vessels or stenotic large vessels may require a slightly elevated "pressure head" to maintain patency. Acceptable upper blood pressure limits are a systolic BP of 190 mm Hg and a distolic BP of 100-110 mm Hg.

2. *Obtain a history, perform a physical examination, and obtain relevant laboratory studies as outlined in II, above.* In the patient with anterior (i.e., carotid artery) circulation symptoms or signs within the previous 10 days, also order an urgent carotid artery Doppler study to evaluate for the presence and extent of stenosis.

3. *Consult a neurologist to assist in further diagnosis and optimal management of the TIA patient.* Prevention of recurrent TIA or stroke may include antiplatelet therapy, anticoagulation, or selected carotid artery surgery in appropriate candidates.
   a. Antiplatelet therapy may include one of the following:
      i. *Aspirin* (recommended doses vary from 325 mg/day to 1200 mg/day): the optimal dose is uncertain at this time. Smaller doses (e.g., as low as 75 mg/day) may be as effective as the above, but further studies are needed.
      ii. *Ticlopidine* (250 mg PO bid with food): this is the most effective antiplatelet agent currently available. In a recent study, ticlopidine was demonstrated superior to aspirin in both men and women for stroke prevention after either a TIA or minor stroke. Disadvantages include increased side effects (including diarrhea [20%], rash [14%], and severe but reversible neutropenia [<1%]) and increased cost ($1.13 per tablet). Patients placed on ticlopidine should have a CBC and neutrophil count every 2 weeks for the first 3 months of therapy.

b. Anticoagulation: *Caution:* head CT is mandatory to rule out intracranial hemorrhage prior to administration of either heparin or warfarin.

　i. *Heparin:* consider in the setting of crescendo TIAs (i.e., attacks of TIAs of increasing frequency or severity), TIAs in the patient on antiplatelet therapy (especially if the antiplatelet agent has already been "advanced" from aspirin to ticlopidine), TIAs from a suspected or confirmed cardioembolic source, or TIAs in the vascular territory of known high-grade carotid artery stenosis while awaiting surgical therapy in appropriate candidates.

- Avoid a heparin bolus. Adjust the continuous infusion to maintain the PTT at 2–2.5 times control.
- Short-term risks of anticoagulation with heparin are low (1–4%) and include hemorrhage, thrombocytopenia, thrombosis, and, rarely, the cholesterol emboli syndrome.
- Heparin should be followed by antiplatelet therapy (unless antiplatelet therapy has already been proven ineffective) or warfarin.

　ii. *Warfarin:* initiate therapy with heparin as outlined above. Warfarin may be started after admission and the dose adjusted to maintain an INR (International Normalized Ratio) of 2–3. Warfarin anticoagulation carries a 1–2.5% annual risk of serious bleeding complications and requires close follow-up and frequent monitoring.

c. Surgical therapy: carotid endarterectomy is beneficial and superior to medical therapy in patients with a TIA or minor stroke in the cerebral hemisphere or retina supplied by a carotid artery with ≥ 70% stenosis (as demonstrated by angiography). This presumes that the patient is otherwise a good surgical candidate and the surgery is performed by an experienced neurosurgeon at a center with a combined perioperative stroke and mortality rate ≤ 5.8%.

4. *Assist the neurologist and/or the patient's primary care physician in risk factor reduction.* This may include addressing such issues as smoking cessation, hypertension education (and eventual gradual outpatient control), weight reduction, regular exercise, and lowering of elevated cholesterol levels.

B. Acute Stroke

1. *Assess, secure, and support the airway, breathing, and circulation as necessary.* (See Chapter 1. II.) Administer isotonic saline to maintain euvolemia. Hyperglycemia should be avoided.

2. *Obtain a history, perform a physical examination, and obtain relevant laboratory studies as outlined in II, above.*

3. *Do not attempt to lower BP in the hypertensive acute stroke patient unless severe persistent hypertension is present.* Check the BP in both arms and obtain repeated measurements over time before even considering treating hypertension. *Gradual and careful control* of severe hypertension in the setting of actual or suspected stroke is indicated under the following circumstances:

    a. Acute and significant congestive heart failure.
    b. Thoracic aortic dissection (consult cardiothoracic surgery; also see Chapter 13).
    c. Renal failure.
    d. Hypertensive encephalopathy.
    e. Occlusive stroke *if* the diastolic BP is > 120–130 mmHg. *Caution:* urgently consult a neurologist; slowly lower the diastolic BP to 120 mmHg. Do *not* overcorrect!
    f. Intracerebral hemorrhage *if* the systolic BP is > 220 mmHg or the diastolic BP is > 120 mmHg. *Caution:* urgently consult a neurosurgeon and consider gradual reduction in BP over the next 24 hours to just below these threshold treatment levels. Do *not* overcorrect!
    g. SAH *if* the systolic BP is > 180 mmHg. *Caution:* urgently consult a neurosurgeon and see the section on SAH later in this chapter. Do *not* overcorrect! BP frequently responds to appropriate pain control and patient sedation.

4. *Consult the appropriate service if not done earlier (e.g., neurology and/or neurosurgery) and arrange for hospitalization.*

5. *In consultation with the neurologist, consider anticoagulation in appropriate candidates.*

    a. Consider anticoagulation with *heparin* in patients with acute or fluctuating vertebrobasilar TIA, cardioembolic stroke after 48 hours (see c, below), acute (< 48 hours) ischemic stroke with fluctuating or progressing symptoms and limited deficit, or small completed strokes when evaluation of the carotid artery reveals ≥ 70% carotid artery stenosis on the symptomatic side.
    b. Recent studies of *thrombolytic therapy* have shown *no* clear benefit and a discouragingly high incidence of intracerebral hemorrhage. There may be a future role for intravenous (IV) tissue plasminogen activator (t-PA) in hyperacute (i.e., < 6 hours) stroke, but further studies are needed. At the present time, such therapy is experimental and should only be undertaken in the setting of a well designed clinical trial.
    c. *Delay anticoagulation* for 48 hours after embolic stroke; and do not begin anticoagulation until a repeat CT at 48 hours excludes spontaneous hemorrhagic transformation (hemorrhage is often clinically silent and is most likely to occur in elderly patients and/or after large infarcts).
    d. Do *not* administer heparin to patients with large completed strokes or intracranial hemorrhage.

6. *In consultation with a neurologist, consider antiplatelet therapy in appropriate candidates.*

   a. Antiplatelet agents may reduce the risk of recurrent stroke or other serious vascular events by 25%.
   b. *Ticlopidine* appears to be more efficacious than *aspirin,* but is more expensive and has a greater risk for side effects (see IV. A. 3, above).
   c. Dosage of aspirin and ticlopidine (see IV. A. 3, above).

7. *Additional treatments* include the following:

   a. Steroids, while of no proven benefit in cerebral infarction, should be considered, in combination with hyperventilation (to a PCO_2 of 25 mmHg) and osmotic agents (e.g., mannitol) in managing increased intracranial pressure with impending herniation. *Dose:* dexamethasone 10 mg IV or intramuscularly (IM) initially, followed by 4 mg IV or IM every 4–6 hours. The dose of mannitol in the management of increased intracranial pressure is 0.75–1.0 g/kg IV bolus, followed by 0.25–0.5 g/kg IV every 3–5 hours (adjust to maintain serum osmolarity between 305–315 mosmol/L).
   b. Surgery: a prospective study showed no benefit to extracranial–intracranial bypass grafting for occlusive carotid disease.

V. DISPOSITION

Disposition decisions should be made in consultation with a neurologist.

A. Discharge

1. Consider discharging a reliable, otherwise well patient with a small (i.e., lacunar), completed stroke > 48 hours old in whom close follow-up can be arranged.

2. Consider discharging the patient with an isolated TIA for further outpatient evaluation if *all* of the following conditions apply:

   a. The patient is reliable and does not live alone;
   b. The patient is otherwise well;
   c. Symptoms have completely resolved and the neurologic examination is now completely normal;
   d. Carotid artery sonography/duplex evaluation reveals < 70% occlusion;
   e. There is no evidence for a cardioembolic source of the TIA or the need for anticoagulation with heparin;
   f. Antiplatelet therapy (with either aspirin or ticlopidine) is prescribed at the time of discharge;
   g. Close outpatient follow-up is arranged.

B. Admit

The following patients should be admitted.

1. Patients with an isolated TIA who do not meet all of the above TIA discharge criteria or those with more than one or crescendo TIAs.

2. Patients with an acute stroke.

VI. PEARLS AND PITFALLS

A. Obtain a noncontrast head CT scan on all patients presenting with a focal neurologic deficit of a suspected central cause.

B. Obtain urgent neurologic/neurosurgical consultation in any patient with significantly altered mentation or in any patient whose neurologic status is deteriorating.

C. Perform and carefully document a thorough neurologic examination.

D. Frequently reassess the patient throughout the ED stay.

E. Provide maintenance fluids to avoid dehydration (e.g., normal saline IV).

F. Avoid hyperglycemia in the acute stroke patient.

Do *not* do any of the following:

A. Treat hypertension in the acute stroke patient unless it is persistent or severe, and treatment is clearly necessary (remember, acute hypertension therapy can precipitate occlusion of a critically stenosed vessel and extend the infarct).

B. Administer anticoagulation with heparin or warfarin prior to excluding intracranial hemorrhage with a noncontrast CT.

C. Administer hypotonic solutions (e.g., 5% dextrose in water) because these can worsen cerebral edema.

BIBLIOGRAPHY

Bonita R, Marmot M, Poulter N, et al. Stroke octet (multiple review articles). Lancet 1992; 339: 342–347, 400–405, 473–477, 533–539, 589–594, 721–727 and 791–793.

Cerebral Embolism Study Group: Cardioembolic stroke, early anticoagulation, and brain hemorrhage. Arch Intern Med 1987;147:636–640.

Hass W, Easton J, Adams H, et al: A randomized trial comparing ticlopidine hydrochloride with aspirin for the prevention of stroke in high-risk patients. N Engl J Med 1989;321:501–507.

Haynes RB, Taylor DW, Sackett DL, et al: Prevention of functional impairment by endarterectomy for symptomatic high-grade carotid stenosis. JAMA 1994;271:1256–1259.

Rothrock J, Hart R: Antithrombotic therapy in cerebrovascular disease. Ann Intern Med 1991; 115:885–895.

Taliaferro EH: TIA and stroke admissions. In Critical Decisions in Emergency Medicine. Vol. 8. American College of Emergency Physicians, 1993.

SEIZURES

*The fit makes the patient fall down senseless; and without
his will or consciousness presently every muscle is put in action, as if
all the powers
of the body were exerted to free itself from some great violence.*

WILLIAM HEBERDEN (1710–1801)

I. ESSENTIAL FACTS

A. Definition

A *seizure* is a paroxysmal excessive neuronal discharge leading
to focal or generalized manifestations. *Status epilepticus* is a
seizure lasting > 30 minutes or intermittent seizures lasting > 30
minutes from which the patient does not regain consciousness.

B. Seizure Classification (Table 20–5)

1. Generalized (seizures are bilaterally symmetrical and without
   focal onset)
   a. Absence
       i. Typical (petit mal)
       ii. Atypical
   b. Tonic and/or clonic (grand mal)
   c. Myoclonic/atonic

Table 20–5. PRESENTATION OF GENERALIZED AND FOCAL SEIZURES

GENERALIZED	FOCAL
History	
Idiopathic: Onset frequently occurs in childhood. May have history of birth distress or trauma. Often no antecedent history. *Metabolic:* Patient may have history of diabetes, thyroid disease, renal disease, drug ingestion, or alcoholism.	Patient may report antecedent or immediate head trauma or may have history of hypertension, extracranial vascular disease, or known neoplasm.
Signs and Symptoms	
Sudden loss of consciousness followed by tonic stiffening, then clonic or tonic-clonic activity.	*Motor:* Independent nonvoluntary motor activity. May be simple (single muscle) or complex (group of muscles).
An aura may precede the seizure.	*Sensory:* Dysesthesias, visual disturbances.
Tongue-biting or incontinence may occur. Postictal confusion and amnesia for the period of seizure and preceding events usually occur. Postictal phase varies in duration and can last up to 2 hr.	*Psychomotor:* Repetitive behavioral automatisms or absence (brief loss of awareness due to temporal lobe discharge).

2. Partial (seizures begin focally)
   a. Simple partial seizures (consciousness not impaired; may include motor, sensory, autonomic, or psychic signs/symptoms)
   b. Complex partial seizures (consciousness impaired)
   c. Partial seizures with secondary generalization

C. Epidemiology

1. Approximately 2.5 million people in the United States have epilepsy (1% of the population).

2. The yearly incidence of new-onset seizures is 40/100,000.
   a. Seizure rates are highest in the < 5 years and > 60 years age groups.
   b. Partial seizures are more common than generalized seizures.

D. Etiology

1. Genetic: typical absence, juvenile myoclonic epilepsy, other myoclonic epilepsies, and hereditary neurocutaneous disorders (e.g., neurofibromatosis and tuberous sclerosis)

2. Congenital anomalies: intrauterine infections and chromosomal disorders

3. Antenatal/perinatal insults: maternal infection or drug use, birth trauma, and asphyxia

4. Central nervous system (CNS) infections: meningitis, encephalitis, brain abscess, and opportunistic infections

5. Toxins: alcohol, drugs (including toxic levels of anticonvulsants, isoniazid, anticholinergic agents, and cyclic antidepressants), cocaine, phencyclidine (PCP), heavy metals (e.g., lead, mercury, and chromium), and carbon monoxide

6. Metabolic disorders: uremia, hepatic disease, endocrinopathies, electrolyte disorders, deficiency states, inborn errors of metabolism, hypoxemia, hypoglycemia, and pyridoxine deficiency

7. Trauma (especially with cortical damage): postconcussion (acute or delayed), subdural or epidural hematoma, and anoxia/hypoxia

8. Vascular disease: stroke, hemorrhage, arteriovenous malformations (AVMs), hypertensive encephalopathy

9. Tumor: primary or metastatic disease

10. Withdrawal states: after abrupt discontinuation of alcohol, benzodiazepines, barbiturates, or anticonvulsants

11. Immunologic: connective tissue disease (e.g., systemic lupus erythematosus, vasculitis), serum sickness

II. CLINICAL EVALUATION

A. History

1. Obtain a careful description of the event from the patient and bystanders, including the following: character of the episode, onset (what was the patient doing?), and duration. What was the patient like immediately after the event (e.g., lethargic, confused)? Did the patient suffer any injury during the episode?

2. Inquire about other health problems, trauma history, medical history, other concomitant complaints, and use of medications, alcohol, or other drugs (e.g., cocaine).

3. Is there a family history of seizures?

4. If the patient has a known seizure disorder, inquire about usual seizure pattern, frequency of occurrence, and compliance with antiseizure medications. Seizures may increase in frequency in the setting of lack of sleep, fever, occult infection, medication noncompliance, or other drug use (e.g., alcohol).

B. Physical Examination

Vital signs and a complete head-to-toe physical examination are required to adequately evaluate the patient and to rule out injury.

C. Laboratory Studies

Studies obtained depend on the clinical situation:

1. In patients with a known seizure disorder, a normal physical examination, and a typical seizure for them, consider obtaining only a fingerstick glucose and relevant anticonvulsant drug levels.

2. In patients with a new-onset seizure, consider obtaining electrolytes, glucose, blood urea nitrogen (BUN), and creatinine levels, a complete blood count (CBC), calcium and magnesium levels, pregnancy test, liver function tests, oxygen saturation (SaO_2) ($\pm$ arterial blood gas), urinalysis, and urine toxicologic screen.

D. Cranial Imaging

Patients with any of the following should receive neuroimaging (computed tomography [CT] or magnetic resonance imaging [MRI]) acutely: new-onset seizure, persistent global or focal neurologic deficit, recent history of head trauma, and/or sudden change in usual seizure pattern.

E. Electroencephalography

The neurology consultant may request electroencephalography (EEG) in the patient as an outpatient procedure or after admission. A normal study does not exclude the diagnosis of epilepsy ($\leq 25\%$ of patients with seizure disorders have a normal EEG).

III. DIFFERENTIAL DIAGNOSIS

Conditions that may present with "seizure" activity include the following:

A. Symptomatic seizure secondary to infection or a toxic–metabolic disturbance (e.g., hypoglycemia, uremia, cocaine use).

B. Cardiac disease, including arrhythmias and other causes of cardiovascular syncope. Patients with true syncope may experience abnormal body movements secondary to cerebral hypoperfusion, but mental status should be at normal baseline immediately after the syncopal event (see Chapter 10).

C. Migraine: a history of visual auras preceding an episode of altered sensorium may occur in complicated migraine.

D. Sleep disorders (e.g., narcolepsy, benign nocturnal myoclonus): findings may include a history of cataplexy (sudden collapse while standing *without* loss of consciousness), a positive family history, and/or "paralysis" at the onset or end of sleep.

E. Transient ischemic attacks.

F. Psychiatric disorders, including hyperventilation syndromes, panic attacks, episodic dyscontrol syndrome, fugue states, and pseudoseizures.

IV. THERAPY

A. Initial Management

Assess, secure, and support the airway, breathing, and circulation as necessary. (See the "ABCs" in Chapter 1. II.)

1. Administer supplemental oxygen and protect the airway. Immobilize the cervical spine if acute trauma is suspected.

2. If the patient is actively seizing, do not force anything (including an oropharyngeal airway) into the patient's mouth. A nasopharyngeal airway, however, can be placed during a seizure. The patient should be in the Trendelenburg position to help prevent aspiration. Have suction on and at the bedside, and protect the patient from self-harm. Oxygen saturation and cardiac rhythm should be monitored.

3. Obtain vital signs, establish intravenous (IV) access, check the fingerstick glucose level, and obtain appropriate laboratory values (see II, above).

4. Perform a complete physical examination after airway and vital signs are appropriately stabilized.

5. *Caution:* the patient can be harmed by overtreatment of a completed seizure with aggressive anticonvulsant therapy. *Remember:* most seizures are brief and self-limited. Securing the ABCs and protecting the patient from aspiration and

Status Epilepticus

- Continuous seizure ≥ 30 min or
- Recurrent seizures without return to preictal state between each

or

Prolonged Generalized Seizure

(even if patient is not in actual status, a prolonged seizure [> 5 min] should also be treated as outlined)

↓

- Guard airway, have suction at bedside, ensure oxygenation
- Place nasopharyngeal airway if required
- Vital signs (including temp.); consider arterial blood gas
- Monitor cardiac rhythm and SaO_2

↓

- Obtain IV access, draw blood, check fingerstick glucose, and initiate IV crystalloid
- Send labs: glucose, electrolytes, BUN, creatinine, CBC, calcium, magnesium, phosphate, alcohol level, anticonvulsant drug levels, liver function tests, PT/PTT, toxicology screen
  Consider: serum pregnancy test, blood cultures
- Administer: 100 mg thiamine IV; 25 g dextrose IV (50 mL of D5OW); 1–2 g magnesium sulfate IV (for patient with suspected alcohol history or malnourished; do *not* give if known renal insufficiency; larger magnesium doses necessary in eclampsia)
- Administer: IV antibiotics if infection suspected (e.g., meningitis)

↓

TIME SINCE DIAGNOSIS

0-5 min.

6-9 min.

10-30 min.

- Lorazepam 0.1 mg/kg IV (≤ 2 mg/min; total dose 4–8 mg)

  or

  Diazepam 0.15–0.25 mg/kg IV (≤ 5 mg/min; maximum total adult dose is 20 mg),

  then
- Phenytoin 15–20 mg/kg IV load (15 mg/kg in the elderly). Administer no faster than 50 mg/min. Monitor blood pressure and cardiac rhythm carefully. If patient already on phenytoin, then administer only 9 mg/kg load. *Caution:* phenytoin cannot be given with glucose/dextrose containing solutions.
- Consider nasogastric tube and Foley catheter

$\longrightarrow$

IF SEIZURE PERSISTS:
31-59 min.

- Endotracheal intubation (if not done earlier, must be done now)
- Phenobarbital 20 mg/kg IV (100 mg/min; if seizure controlled before total dose given, decrease the rate of infusion)
- Consider lidocaine (100 mg IV bolus)

$\longrightarrow$

IF SEIZURE PERSISTS:
60 min.

- Diazepam IV infusion 4–8 mg/hr (50 mg in 500 mL NS or D5W at 40 mL/hr-4 mg/hr). Change IV solution q 6 hr

  or

  Pentobarbital anesthesia (5 mg/kg IV load at 25 mg/min, followed by 2.5 mg/kg/min; adjust dose as necessary to achieve "burst suppression" on EEG. EEG monitoring necessary;

  or

  Paraldehyde (0.1–0.15 mL/kg mixed 1:1 with mineral oil and administered PR via Foley catheter). Alternatively, chloral hydrate (30 mg/kg) may also be given PR.

$\longrightarrow$

IF SEIZURE PERSISTS:
61-80 min.

- General anesthesia and neuromuscular blockade. Continuous EEG monitoring mandatory.

Figure 20–4. Emergency medical therapy for a prolonged seizure or status epilepticus.

self-harm are usually the only immediate interventions required.

B. Status Epilepticus

A prolonged generalized seizure (e.g., > 5 minutes duration), requires aggressive medical intervention. The longer the seizure persists, the harder it is to ultimately control. Common causes of status epilepticus (see I.A. above) include withdrawal from anticonvulsants (21%), cerebrovascular disease (21%), alcohol-related causes (18%), metabolic disorders (13%), hemorrhage (7%), infections (4%), hypotension (4%), tumors (3%), anoxia (2%), and miscellaneous causes (7%).

Emergent drug therapy may include the following (Fig. 20–4):

1. Oxygen, thiamine, and glucose. Also consider *magnesium* (e.g., malnourished patients, history of alcohol abuse, eclampsia) and early use of antibiotics (in the patient with suspected sepsis, brain abscess, or meningitis).

2. Benzodiazepines. Lorazepam is preferred over diazepam by many authorities because of its longer antiseizure activity.

3. Phenytoin. Administer phenytoin, even if the seizure is controlled with the above, to provide long-term anticonvulsant activity. It should be administered in normal saline because dextrose or glucose-containing solutions will cause precipitation. Both blood pressure and continuous electrocardiographic monitoring are required, especially in the elderly and patients with cardiovascular disease.

4. Phenobarbital. This agent may cause significant sedation and respiratory suppression, especially in combination with benzodiazepines. For this reason, endotracheal intubation is appropriate *prior to* IV phenobarbital, and phenobarbital should generally be used only if the seizure persists despite interventions 1–3, above. Some patients may also benefit from IV lidocaine.

5. Miscellaneous drugs for persistent seizure activity:
   a. A continuous diazepam intravenous infusion should be considered. Diazepam readily precipitates out of solution; IV tubing should be as short as possible and the solution changed every 6 hours.
   b. Pentobarbital coma should only be initiated in the setting of continuous EEG monitoring. The dose should be adjusted as necessary to achieve "burst suppression" on the EEG. Subsequently, at 2–4-hour intervals, the infusion rate is decreased and the patient and EEG observed for signs of seizure recurrence. When no seizure activity is observed, the pentobarbital may be slowly tapered over the next 12–24 hours. Both blood pressure and electrocardiogram must be monitored closely.
   c. Paraldehyde, if available, may be given either IV or rectally

(PR) for refractory status epilepticus. Chloral hydrate may also be administered rectally.

d. On rare occasions, general anesthesia with halothane and neuromuscular blockade (e.g., pancuronium) are ultimately required. Continuous EEG monitoring is mandatory to confirm actual seizure elimination.

C. General Principles of Anticonvulsant Drug Therapy

1. Monotherapy
   a. The doses of each anticonvulsant should be gradually increased until either seizures are controlled or signs of toxicity appear.
   b. If necessary, a second anticonvulsant can be added to achieve a therapeutic concentration. The first drug should then be slowly tapered and eliminated if possible.
2. Treat the patient, not the anticonvulsant level.
   a. A breakthrough seizure with an anticonvulsant level in the "therapeutic" range may necessitate only a slightly higher dose.
   b. Signs of toxicity may occur at any anticonvulsant level; some patients may tolerate levels above the therapeutic range in order to prevent seizures.
3. CNS concentrations of anticonvulsants are proportional to the free plasma concentrations of the drugs. Most anticonvulsant levels measure the total (i.e., free and protein bound) concentration. The total concentration may not reflect the free fraction under conditions that alter protein binding (e.g., malnutrition, renal disease) or in the presence of some other drugs. Occasionally, both free and total levels should be measured.
4. Anticonvulsants are chosen according to the type of seizure (Table 20–6).
   a. Partial seizures (either simple or complex, with or without secondary generalization): phenytoin = carbamazepine = valproate > phenobarbital or primidone.
   b. Primary generalized tonic–clonic seizures: phenytoin = carbamazepine = valproate > phenobarbital or primidone.
   c. Typical absence seizures (must be EEG confirmed): ethosuximide > valproate.
   d. Atypical absence, tonic, or myoclonic seizures: valproate > valproate + clonazepam > phenytoin.

D. Special Issues

1. Treatment of a first seizure:
   a. Attempt to identify any treatable cause of a new-onset symptomatic seizure. Neurology consultation is appropriate.
   b. Consider the risk of adverse consequences of anticonvulsant medication use versus the risk(s) of a seizure recurrence.
      i. Adverse effects of anticonvulsant medications occur in ≤ 6% of patients.

Table 20-6. ANTICONVULSANT MEDICATIONS

ANTICONVULSANT MEDICATION	INDICATIONS	DOSAGE FORMS	LOADING DOSE	MAINTENANCE DOSE ADULT (MG/D)	THERAPEUTIC LEVEL (μG/ML)	SIDE EFFECTS	
						MAJOR	RARE/ IDIOSYNCRATIC
Phenytoin	GTC Complex partial Simple partial	IV: 50 mg/mL PO: 30 mg, 100 mg (sustained release capsules); 50 mg (chewable tablet). 125 mg/5 mL suspension.	IV: 18–20 mg/kg no faster than 50 mg/min in the adult. PO: 500 mg q 4 hr × 2.	300 mg/D in two divided doses or qhs.	10–20	Gum hyperplasia (10–30%) Cognitive disturbance Ataxia (if toxic) Rash (2–10%) GI upset	Pseudo-lymphoma Hepatotoxicity Peripheral neuropathy Folate deficiency Drug-induced lupus
Carbamazepine	Complex partial Simple partial GTC	100 mg chewable tablet; 200 mg tablet. 100 mg/5 mL suspension.	Rapid loading not appropriate.	Begin with 200 mg bid and increase by 200 mg per week to 800–1200 mg/D in 3–4 divided doses.	4–12 (trough levels)	GI upset Ataxia Fatigue	Myelosuppression (reversible in ~1:5000; irreversible in ~1:50,000) Stevens-Johnson syndrome
Valproic Acid	Atypical & absence GTC Myolonic Atonic Tonic Partial	125 mg, 250 mg, 500 mg (delayed release tablets). 125 mg (sprinkle capsule). Syrup: 250 mg/5 mL.	Rapid loading not appropriate.	Begin with 10–15 mg/kg/D in 2–3 divided doses; increase by 5–10 mg/kg/D in weekly intervals until levels are therapeutic.	50–100	GI upset Drowsiness Rash Headache	Tremor Weight gain Pancreatitis Hepatotoxicity Thrombocytopenia

774

Drug	Indications	Formulation	Dosing	Therapeutic level	Dose-related side effects	Idiosyncratic side effects
Phenobarbital	GTC Complex partial	IV: 60 mg/mL or 130 mg/mL. PO: 15 mg, 30 mg, 60 mg, and 100 mg tablets.	60–250 mg/D in 2 divided doses. IV: in adults 10 mg/kg IV no faster than 60 mg/min. May repeat dose in 30 min.	15–35	Sedation Hyperactivity in children (30%) Ataxia	Aplastic anemia Agranulocytosis Rash Hepatotoxicity
Ethosuximide	Typical absence	250 mg capsules. Syrup: 250 mg/5 mL.	Begin with 250 mg bid and increase by 250 mg q 4–7 days until 750–1000 mg per day in 2–3 divided doses. Rapid loading not appropriate.	40–100	GI upset Ataxia Sedation Hiccups	Pancytopenia Hepatotoxicity Rash
Clonazepam	Second line adjunctive drug for: Atonic Myoclonic Atypical absence Primary GTC	0.5 mg, 1 mg, and 2 mg tablets.	Initial daily dose should not exceed 1.5 mg per day in 3 divided doses. May increase daily dose by 0.5–1.0 mg q 3 days as needed. Do not exceed 15–20 mg/D. Rapid loading not appropriate.	Not helpful.	Ataxia Drooling Drowsiness	Blood dyscrasias

GTC, Generalized tonic-clonic seizure.
Common dose-related side effects of the above medications may include ataxia, somnolence, diplopia (with nystagmus in all directions), slurred speech, paradoxical increase in seizure frequency.

ii. Recurrence risk in 1 year after a single seizure if the workup is negative is 25% in children and ≤ 50% in adults.

c. Avoid diagnosing a patient with epilepsy until a thorough workup is complete: the consequences of this diagnosis on a person's employability, social activities, insurability, and driving may be significant.

2. Withdrawal seizures (e.g., from alcohol, barbiturates, or benzodiazepines) (also see Chapter 23).

a. These usually occur between 1 and 7 days after abstention. They also occur after significant reduction in alcohol intake.

b. Seizures tend to be primary generalized tonic–clonic convulsions. Focal or partial complex seizures should not be assumed to be secondary to withdrawal.

c. There is no clear role for prophylactic or long-term anticonvulsant therapy. Phenytoin or phenobarbital may be necessary for control of severe or protracted seizures. Benzodiazepines given for symptomatic withdrawal may have some protective effect. In some cases, seizure control may necessitate replacement of the original drug (e.g., a continuous infusion of ethanol, phenobarbital, or benzodiazepine).

d. Most patients with a first-time seizure in the setting of alcohol withdrawal should have a thorough evaluation for an alternate diagnosis (i.e., workup should include a head CT, lumbar puncture, and, depending on circumstances, EEG).

e. Replacement of magnesium and calcium with the relevant deficient electrolyte is appropriate and may be helpful in preventing alcohol withdrawal seizures.

3. Pseudoseizures are very difficult to diagnose with confidence, especially in the ED. Many patients have true epilepsy as well.

a. Historical features, such as a lack of incontinence or tongue trauma (despite multiple convulsions) and/or a history of childhood sexual abuse, are suggestive but not diagnostic.

b. A serum prolactin level obtained within 20 minutes of an apparent generalized convulsion that lasted for > 30 seconds is sometimes useful. In most patients with true seizures, the prolactin level will be several-fold higher immediately after the seizure than a baseline level measured 1–2 hours later. This test is not helpful, however, in simple partial and partial complex "seizures" and may not be valid after prolonged convulsions.

V. DISPOSITION

A. Discharge

1. Patients evaluated after one of their usual seizures may be discharged to home provided their anticonvulsant level(s) are appropriate, their mental status has returned to normal, they are

otherwise well, no other condition mandating hospitalization has been identified, and follow-up has been arranged.

2. The neurology consultant may decide not to admit a patient with a new-onset single seizure. Further workup as an outpatient, however, is appropriate only if *all* of the following conditions apply:
   a. Physical examination is normal.
   b. Head CT is unremarkable.
   c. No other condition mandating hospitalization has been found.
   d. Home situation is adequate, including the availability of close observation by a reliable family member or friend.
   e. The patient is reliable.
   f. Follow-up has been arranged.

3. Discharge instructions should include the following:
   a. Anticonvulsant levels should be checked in 4–5 days. Trough (predose) levels should be used for carbamazepine and valproate.
   b. Inform the patient of any local or state laws with respect to motor vehicle driving restrictions. Document this discussion in the medical record.
   c. Patients should also be told to not engage in any activity that would increase the risk of injury or death should a seizure recur (e.g., climbing ladders, taking a bath, swimming, engaging in hazardous activities).
   d. Reproductive-age women should have a pregnancy test prior to starting anticonvulsant therapy. The potential for teratogenicity with any anticonvulsant must be weighed against the deleterious effects of generalized convulsions on the mother and fetus. The overall incidence of fetal malformations in children born to women with epilepsy is 3–6%. This represents a 2–3-fold increased risk and probably reflects both genetic factors and drug effect(s).

B. Admit

The following situations necessitate hospitalization:

1. Status epilepticus (ICU admission is required).

2. Known seizure disorder if:
   a. Three or more seizures have occurred in a 24-hour period.
   b. The patient is significantly subtherapeutic on an anticonvulsant that cannot be loaded (e.g., carbamazepine, valproate).

3. Most patients with new onset seizures

BIBLIOGRAPHY

Drugs for Epilepsy. Med Let 1989;31:1–4.
Fernandez RJ, Samuels MA: Epilepsy. In Samuels MA (ed): Manual of Neurology (4th Ed) Boston: Little, Brown, 1991, pp. 82–118.

Jagoda A, Riggio S: Refractory status epilepticus in adults. Ann Emerg Med 1993; 22:1337–1348.

Treiman DM. The role of benzodiazepines in the management of status epilepticus. Neurology 1990;40(Supp 2):32–42.

Working Group on Status Epilepticus: Treatment of convulsive status epilepticus. JAMA 1993; 270:854–859.

SUBARACHNOID HEMORRHAGE

"For most diagnoses all that is needed is an ounce of knowledge, an ounce of intelligence, and a pound of thoroughness!"

ANONYMOUS

I. ESSENTIAL FACTS

A. Definition

Subarachnoid hemorrhage (SAH) is bleeding into the space beneath the arachnoid covering of the brain.

1. In primary SAH, rupture occurs directly from the blood vessels as they course through this space.

2. Secondary SAH results from extension of blood into the subarachnoid space from a deeper parenchymal source.

B. Epidemiology

1. Primary SAH accounts for 10% of all strokes in the United States annually.

2. Approximately 28,000 new cases of SAH are diagnosed yearly in this country.
   a. Approximately 10,000 (36%) of these patients die before reaching neurosurgical care. Of those surviving, another 8000 (28%) subsequently die or are left with significant disability.
   b. Approximately 10,000 patients (36%) are able to return to a productive life.

3. Associated conditions include polycystic kidney disease, fibromuscular dysplasia, connective tissue disorders, coarctation of the aorta, and a positive family history.

4. Risk factors include
   a. Smoking: relative risk is 2.9 (increasing risk with heavier smoking).
   b. Alcohol use: relative risk is 2.2 if > 2 drinks/day (risk significantly increased with binge drinking).
   c. Hypertension.
   d. Pregnancy/parturition.
   e. Valsalva maneuvers (e.g., weight lifting).
   f. Sexual intercourse.

C. Etiology (Table 20–7)

1. Trauma is the most common cause of *all types* of SAH.

2. Aneurysms account for 70–80% of *primary SAH* and result from an abnormal dilatation of a blood vessel wall. Most intracranial aneurysms are saccular and arise at bifurcation points of vessels that form the circle of Willis. Multiple aneurysms are found in 15–20% of cases. The peak age of rupture is 40–50 years. Less common aneurysm types include arteriosclerotic (fusiform), mycotic (bacterial), and traumatic aneurysms.

3. Arteriovenous malformations (AVMs) are the cause of 5–10% of SAH. They are congenital vascular anomalies in which the capillary bed connecting the arterial and venous systems develops abnormally. Most are supratentorial and are located on or near the cortical surface. The peak age of hemorrhage is 15–20 years. With advancing age the likelihood becomes progressively greater that an SAH is due to aneurysmal rupture rather than an AVM.

4. The remaining 10–20% of SAHs are composed of patients with radiographic or cerebrospinal fluid (CSF) signs of SAH but a normal angiogram. "Occult" aneurysms or perimesencephalic hemorrhage (rupture of small surface vessels on the brainstem adjacent to the basal cisterns) are the presumed cause in these cases.

II. CLINICAL EVALUATION

A. History

1. Headache is the cardinal feature of SAH and is usually *sudden, explosive,* and *global.* The episode will often be described as "the worst headache of my life." Headache is present in almost all (range 86–97%) patients. The patient is often aware of exactly what he or she was doing at the moment of onset.
   a. Some investigators claim that the proportion of SAH among patients with sudden, explosive headache is about 25%.

Table 20–7. CAUSES OF SUBARACHNOID HEMORRHAGE

Traumatic
Spontaneous
  Primary (directly within subarachnoid space)
    Congenital blood vessel abnormalities
      Aneurysm
      Arteriovenous malformation
    Unknown
  Secondary (extension of parenchymal hemorrhage)
    Hypertension
    Blood dyscrasia or anticoagulant therapy
    Neoplasm
    Arteriopathy

From Day AL, and Saleman M, Am Fam Practice Journal v40, July 1989, p. 95.

Table 20–8. SIGNS AND SYMPTOMS OF
SUBARACHNOID HEMORRHAGE

Headache
Alteration of consciousness
Autonomic disturbances
  Fever
  Vomiting
  ECG changes
Meningeal irritation
Presence of focal neurologic deficit
  Early: reflects amount and site of initial hemorrhage
  Late: consequences of rebleeding or delayed vasospasm
Seizures

From Day AL, and Saleman M, Am Fam Practice Journal v40, July 1989, p. 99.

Nearly 1% of all nontraumatic significant headaches are caused by SAH.

b. Approximately 40–50% of patients will have experienced a similar headache ("sentinel bleed") in the days or weeks preceding the SAH.

c. The mortality among patients presenting with SAH who have a history suggestive of a prior warning leak is three times higher than that of patients diagnosed at the time of the initial headache. Significant mortality and morbidity can be avoided if these patients can be identified and treated at the time of the "warning leak" headache.

d. Any patient presenting with a headache of sudden onset, a sudden change in a chronic headache pattern, or unexplained neurologic symptoms or signs consistent with SAH should be aggressively evaluated.

B. Symptoms

Associated symptoms (Table 20–8) will be present in approximately two-thirds of patients with SAH. They include nausea and vomiting (70%), transient loss of consciousness (50%), meningismus or neck pain (30%), coma (20%), motor/sensory deficits (15–20%), and visual disturbances (e.g., blurred or decreased vision and visual field defects) (15%). *Caution:* Neck stiffness, meningismus, and photophobia can take hours to develop. If the patient is seen acutely, the absence of these symptoms should not be used to exclude the possibility of SAH.

C. Signs

Signs of SAH (Table 20–8) can be separated into those of early and late onset.

1. Many patients with SAH who present with headache will be otherwise entirely normal in the several hours after presentation. By contrast, most patients with hypertensive hemorrhage or ruptured AVM will have some focal neurologic deficit.

2. Early signs include
    a. Visual deficits (due to ophthalmic artery aneurysm).
    b. Cranial nerve palsies: Most commonly CN III (with or without pupillary sparing), IV, or VI. Lower cranial nerve palsies may be seen with vertebrobasilar aneurysms.
    c. Subhyaloid hemorrhage: small, smooth, round hemorrhage usually located near the optic nerve head on fundoscopic examination (11–33% of patients). Reflects elevated venous pressure within the optic nerve sheath. *This finding is nearly pathognomonic of SAH.*
    d. Focal motor deficits due to mass effect from a hematoma.
    e. Cardiac disturbances, including subendocardial ischemia, infarction, and arrhythmias, which reflect a massive rise in circulating catecholamines. Potentially malignant arrhythmias (atrioventricular dissociation, idioventricular rhythms, ventricular tachycardia) occur in 20–40% of patients, usually within the first 48 hours.
    f. Hypertension (30%).
    g. Low-grade fever (5–10%).

3. Late signs include
    a. Sudden or progressive obtundation: most often due to rebleeding, hydrocephalus, or hyponatremia.
    b. Focal neurologic deficits: usually secondary to vasospasm or hematoma.
    c. Seizures: may potentiate rebleeding secondary to hypertension and increased intracranial pressure.
    d. Pulmonary edema: may be an early or late complication and may reflect elevated cardiac filling pressures or neurogenic disruption of pulmonary capillary tight-junctions.

D. Physical Examination

The directed physical examination is dictated by the severity of the patient's initial clinical presentation.

1. Obtunded or deteriorating patients require rapid assessment while the airway, breathing, and circulation are stabilized, blood samples are collected, and emergent head computed tomography (CT) scanning is arranged.
    a. Examination should include assessment of nuchal rigidity and level of consciousness, fundoscopic findings, pupillary size and reactivity, oculocephalic responses (in the absence of neck injury), gag reflex, motor tone, reactivity to pain, and deep tendon reflexes (including plantar responses).
    b. Initial blood work as outlined below should be obtained before the patient goes for CT scanning.
    c. If the diagnosis of SAH is strongly suspected, a neurosurgery consultant should be notified while arranging for emergency neuroimaging.

2. Patients with only headache or mild focal deficits should be examined expeditiously but with careful attention to blood

pressure, temperature, fundoscopic findings, visual fields, cranial nerves, motor and sensory findings, deep tendon reflexes, and plantar responses.

E. Laboratory Studies

1. Initial ED studies include
   a. Complete blood count (CBC) with platelets.
   b. Electrolyte panel.
   c. Glucose level.
   d. Blood urea nitrogen (BUN) and creatinine levels.
   e. Prothrombin time/partial thromboplastin time (PT/PTT).
   f. Blood type and cross match.
   g. Electrocardiography (ECG).
   h. Portable chest roentgenogram.
   i. Calcium, magnesium, and phosphate levels.
2. Computed tomography is the initial procedure of choice for the diagnosis of SAH.
   a. Sensitivity for detection of subarachnoid blood is time dependent: 0–24 hours = 95%, 1–5 days = 90%, 5–7 days = 80%, > 1 week = 50%.
   b. In addition to helping distinguish subarachnoid from primary intraparenchymal hemorrhage, CT is useful in identifying hydrocephalus and in localizing the site of the aneurysm (if there is an associated hematoma).
   c. Some centers use contrast infusion CT studies to better delineate aneurysm location. These studies serve as a complement to angiographic evaluation.
3. Lumbar puncture should be performed if SAH is suspected but the CT scan is negative. Absence of blood by CSF examination virtually excludes the diagnosis of SAH.
   a. Examination by spectrophotometry of centrifuged CSF collected at least 12 hours after headache onset is the only definitive way to distinguish SAH-associated xanthochromia from a traumatic tap (see reference by Vermeulen and van Gijn. Also, see VI below).
   b. Lumbar puncture carries with it a small risk of precipitating rebleeding by increasing the transmural pressure across the aneurysm wall.
4. Magnetic resonance imaging is of little use acutely but may identify subpial collections of hemosiderin in patients evaluated several days to weeks after the SAH. Magnetic resonance angiography and T_2-weighted spin-echo studies may identify the aneurysm but, at this time, the technology is not sufficiently advanced to replace angiography.
5. The following specialized studies will be pursued by the admitting neurosurgeon in the patient with subarachnoid hemorrhage:
   a. Cerebral angiography is the study of choice for identifying aneurysm location and for diagnosis of cerebral vasospasm. The site of hemorrhage is identified in 85% of SAHs.

    b. Transcranial doppler may be helpful in the early diagnosis of cerebral vasospasm. Increases in flow velocity suggestive of evolving vasospasm often precede clinical ischemic symptoms and permit early intervention prior to the onset of neurologic deficits.

III. DIFFERENTIAL DIAGNOSIS

The differential diagnosis of primary SAH includes the following:

A. Primary intracerebral hemorrhage with secondary extension into the subarachnoid space.

  1. Hypertensive hemorrhage.

  2. Venous infarction secondary to venous sinus thrombosis.

  3. Hemorrhagic tumors
    a. Primary central nervous system (CNS) tumors (e.g., pituitary adenoma with apoplexy, glioblastoma multiforme).
    b. Metastatic tumors with a tendency to bleed (e.g., melanoma, renal cell carcinoma, choriocarcinoma).

  4. Blood dyscrasias (anticoagulant therapy, disseminated intravascular coagulation, thrombocytopenia).

  5. Amyloid angiopathy: amyloid deposition within the vessel walls of elderly patients results in friability and lobar intraparenchymal hemorrhage, which is usually located in the polar subcortical regions. May be associated with Alzheimer's dementia.

B. Meningitis and ruptured brain abscess. If diagnosis is delayed, the CSF may take on inflammatory characteristics, with elevated leukocyte counts and a low glucose level. Fever, nuchal rigidity, and leukocytosis may be seen in either process.

C. "Thunderclap" migraine with a negative CT scan and a traumatic lumbar puncture (see VI below).

IV. THERAPY

A. **Initial Management**
Secure and support airway, breathing, and circulation as required (see Chapter 1. II).

  1. Guard the airway, have suction on and at the bedside, and provide supplemental oxygen. Endotracheal intubation may be necessary. Keep the patient NPO.

  2. Continuously monitor oxygen saturation (SaO_2) and cardiac rhythm.

  3. Simultaneously with the above, supporting ED staff should obtain vital signs, intravenous (IV) access, fingerstick glucose

level, ECG, and appropriate laboratory values (see II, above). See figure 20-5.

4. Consult a neurosurgeon urgently.

5. Monitor blood pressure carefully.

   a. Hypertension is frequently only transient and will respond to bedrest, necessary analgesia, and sedation.

   b. Ideally, patients should eventually have their blood pressure maintained at pre-SAH levels (e.g., previously normotensive patients should have *persistent* postbleed hypertension gradually reduced to normotensive levels). Any necessary reductions in blood pressure in the severely hypertensive patient, however, should be done very slowly and in a controlled fashion; discuss with the neurosurgeon before specifically treating hypertension with an antihypertensive agent. Under no circumstances should the patient ever become hypotensive.

   c. To carefully monitor blood pressure and fluid status, an arterial line and central venous pressure catheter (or Swan–Ganz catheter) should be placed in either the ED or the ICU after admission.

B. General Measures

1. Keep the patient at bedrest in a quiet, darkened room with the head of the bed elevated 30 degrees.

2. Headache pain should be treated with opioids (e.g., dilaudid 1–2 mg subcutaneously/intravenously (SQ/IV) every 4–6 hours). Consider phenobarbital (30–60 mg IV every 8 hours) for anxiety. Avoid oversedation as this may compromise serial neurologic assessments.

3. The risk of vasospasm is clearly reduced by administering nimodipine (60 mg orally [PO] or via nasogastric tube [after extraction from the capsules] every 4 hours for 21 days). Side effects include a mild antihypertensive effect and occasional headaches. Acute colonic pseudo-obstruction has been reported rarely.

4. Seizures should be appropriately treated with anticonvulsants, including a loading dose of phenytoin (15–20 mg/kg IV, no faster than 50 mg/min). Use of *prophylactic* anticonvulsants, prior to any seizure event, is controversial. Discuss with the neurosurgeon.

5. Some authors advocate dexamethasone (10 mg IV load, then 4 mg IV every 6 hours), although its effect on cerebral edema secondary to SAH is controversial. Discuss with the neurosurgeon.

6. Antifibrinolytic agents such as epsilon-aminocaproic acid (Amicar) are effective in stabilizing aneurysmal clot. Several studies show no improvement in morbidity or mortality, however, and this therapy is associated with an increased risk

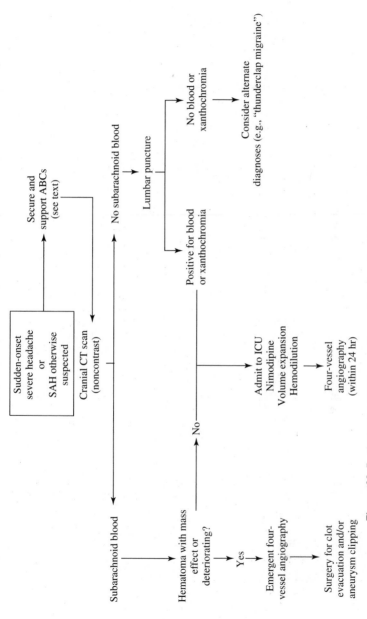

Figure 20–5. Evaluation and therapy of suspected subarachnoid hemorrhage (also see text).

785

of ischemic complications. Discuss with the neurosurgeon (some neurosurgeons advocate administering epsilon-aminocaproic acid [1.5 g/hr IV] until the time of aneurysmal surgery, but discontinuing the drug immediately if clinical signs of ischemia or radiographic or Doppler evidence of vasospasm develops).

7. The risk of vasospasm can be reduced with gentle volume expansion (to a pulmonary artery occlusive pressure of 12–18 mmHg or CVP of 10–12 mmHg) and hemodilution (to a hematocrit of 33–35%). Discuss with the neurosurgeon. Care must be taken to avoid pulmonary edema, compromised oxygenation, or hypertension.

C. Definitive Therapy: Timing of Aneurysm Surgery

1. Early surgery (within 48–96 hours post-SAH) is advocated because successful clip placement virtually eliminates the risk of rebleeding and permits more aggressive treatment of vasospasm with hypertensive therapy than would be safe with an unclipped aneurysm. Risks of early surgery include higher surgical morbidity in medically unstable patients, a possible increased risk of inducing vasospasm, and a greater risk of brain injury during retraction of edematous, friable brain.

2. Late surgery (>10–14 days post-SAH) is advocated by those who believe that preoperative status should be optimized and brain swelling should be allowed to resolve. The risks of delaying surgery are that the patient passes through the window of highest risk for both rebleeding and vasospasm while awaiting definitive therapy.

D. Complications

Complications of SAH are listed in Table 20–9.

Table 20–9. CAUSES OF NEUROLOGIC DETERIORATION, DISABILITY, OR DEATH AFTER ANEURYSMAL SUBARACHNOID HEMORRHAGE

Neurologic complications
  Intraparenchymal hematoma
  Subdural hematoma
  Seizures[a]
  Hydrocephalus[a]
  Cerebral edema[a]
  Increased intracranial pressure[a]
Recurrent hemorrhage[a]
Vasospasm–ischemic stroke
Medical complications
  Hyper- or hyponatremia[a]
  Hypoxia[a]

Atelectasis/pneumonia[a]
Sepsis[a]
Myocardial infarction
Cardiac arrhythmias
Cardiac failure
Gastrointestinal hemorrhage
Complications of surgery or anesthesia[a]
Complications of medical therapy[a]
  Antihypertensive drugs
  Sedatives/analgesics
  Corticosteroids
  Antifibrinolytic drugs

[a]Most frequent causes of neurologic decline at 1 week after SAH and important alternative diagnoses in patients with suspected vasospasm.

From Mafenson HC, Caraccio TR, and Greensher J. Conn's Current Therapy, Rabel RE, ed. W.B. Saunders 1992, p. 1103.

V. DISPOSITION

All patients with SAH require ICU admission and urgent neurosurgical consultation.

VI. PEARLS AND PITFALLS

Xanthochromia must be distinguished from traumatic lumbar puncture:

A. Contrary to popular belief, visually inspecting spun-down CSF for xanthochromia and noting decline in the number of erythrocytes from the first to the last collected tube of CSF are not always reliable in distinguishing SAH from a traumatic lumbar puncture.

B. The potential pitfall in performing lumbar puncture in the first 12 hours lies in confusing "angio-negative SAH" with "thunderclap" migraine and a traumatic tap. Xanthochromia (resulting from the breakdown products of erythrocytes in the CSF) may not be present until 12 hours after the bleed. Lumbar punctures done after an initial traumatic tap will not help clarify this matter as blood from the traumatic tap may also produce xanthochromia.

C. Because of the above, some authors recommend delaying the LP in the stable patient suspected of SAH, whose head CT is negative, until 12 hours after the onset of symptoms. This is a controversial subject and clinical judgment should take precedence.

D. Xanthochromia will persist 12 hours to 2 weeks after the bleeding in all patients with true SAH. At 3 weeks xanthochromia will still be present in 70%, and at 4 weeks it can be found in 40%.

BIBLIOGRAPHY

Jane JA, Kussell NF, Turner JC, Winn HR: The natural history of aneurysms and arteriovenous malformations. J Neurosurg 1985;62:321–323.

Longstreth WT, Nelson LM, Koepsell TD, van Belle G: Cigarette smoking, alcohol use and subarachnoid hemorrhage. Stroke 1992;23:1242–1249.

Ostergaard JR: Headache as a warning sign of impending aneurysmal subarachnoid hemorrhage. Cephalgia 1991;11:53–55.

Van Gijn J: Subarachnoid hemorrhage. Lancet 1992;339:653–655.

Vermeulen M, Van Gijn J: The diagnosis of subarachnoid hemorrhage. J Neurol Neurosurg Psychiatry 1990;53:365–372.

21

Hematologic And Oncologic Emergencies

ANEMIA

"Blood is a very special juice."
JOHANN WOLFGANG VON GOETHE

I. ESSENTIAL FACTS

A. Definition

1. *Anemia* is an abnormal reduction in the circulating erythrocyte mass. In clinical practice, the circulating erythrocyte mass is assessed by the patient's hemoglobin level (normal female: 12–16 g/dL; normal male: 13.5–18 g/dL) and hematocrit (normal female: 38–48%; normal male: 40–52%).

   Note: the hemoglobin level and hematocrit may *not* accurately reflect the erythrocyte mass in the setting of significantly altered plasma volume. For example, dehydration may *elevate* the patient's hemoglobin level/hematocrit without affecting the true erythrocyte mass, and marked plasma volume expansion, such as occurs in pregnancy, may *reduce* the patient's hemoglobin level/hematocrit without affecting the true erythrocyte mass.

2. The normal erythrocyte mass is higher in males than in females; it is not affected in the adult patient by age, race, or ethnic background.

3. Anemia is a sign of an underlying disease process. It has three primary causes:

   a. Erythrocyte loss from hemorrhage.
   b. Erythrocyte destruction from hemolysis.
   c. Inadequate erythrocyte production in the bone marrow.

B. Etiology

1. The most common causes of anemia are
   a. Acute blood loss (25% of cases).
   b. Iron-deficiency anemia (25%).
   c. Anemia associated with chronic inflammatory disorders (25%).
   d. Hemolysis (10%).
   e. Megaloblastic anemia (10%).
   f. Bone marrow failure (5%).

2. Risk factors for anemia include poor diet (e.g., iron, folate, vitamin B_{12} deficiency), chronic diseases, malignancy, medications (e.g., aspirin), and/or a family history of hemoglobinopathy or chronic hemolytic anemia.

II. CLINICAL EVALUATION

A. History

A carefully obtained history in the anemic patient is essential. Inquire about external blood loss (e.g., epistaxis, hematemesis, hematuria, hematochezia, melena, oropharyngeal bleeding, vaginal bleeding), possible internal bleeding (e.g., thoracic, abdominal, retroperitoneal, soft tissue, intra-articular), prior medical/surgical history, trauma history, prior diagnosis of a bleeding diathesis, nutritional status, drug and alcohol use, medication use, and pertinent family history.

B. Symptoms

Symptoms tend to be nonspecific and may include exertional dyspnea or chest discomfort, fatigue, headache, lethargy, palpitations, and/or weakness. The patient's symptoms are generally more pronounced in the setting of a rapidly progressive anemia, especially in individuals with cardiac disease.

C. Signs

Nonspecific physical signs may include pallor, postural hypotension, tachycardia, tachypnea, and a systolic murmur. Other findings can provide clues to the cause of the anemia such as jaundice (hemolysis), hepatosplenomegaly (hemolysis, marrow infiltration), ecchymoses (blood loss), heme-positive stools (blood loss and iron deficiency), and/or neurologic findings (e.g., impaired vibratory and positional sense, ataxia, paresthesias, and mental status changes with vitamin B_{12} deficiency and megaloblastic anemia).

D. Physical Examination

Obtain vital signs and examine the skin, HEENT and neck, chest, heart, abdomen (include a rectal examination and stool heme test), extremities, and neurologic system. If supine vital signs are normal, check for orthostatic changes. Perform a pelvic examination in females.

E. Laboratory Studies

1. *Minimally* obtain the following:
   a. Complete blood count (CBC), including hemoglobin level, hematocrit, erythrocyte indices, leukocyte count, and platelet count.

    b. Peripheral blood smear evaluation for morphologic abnormalities:

      i. Basophilic stippling: possible lead poisoning.

      ii. Hypochromia: iron deficiency.

      iii. Macrocytosis: vitamin B_{12} deficiency, folic acid deficiency, medications, alcohol abuse, hypothyroidism, myelodysplastic syndrome.

      iv. Microcytosis: iron deficiency (*note:* the mean corpuscular volume [MCV] may be normal in early iron deficiency anemia), thalassemia, anemia of chronic disease, sideroblastic anemia, and lead poisoning.

      v. Neutrophil hypersegmentation: vitamin B_{12} deficiency.

      vi. Nucleated erythrocytes: bone marrow disorders such as the myeloproliferative syndrome or infiltration of the bone marrow by cancer.

      vii. Schistocytes: hemolysis caused by disseminated intravascular coagulation (DIC), prosthetic heart valves, or thrombotic thrombocytopenic purpura (TTP).

      viii. Sickle cells: sickle cell anemia.

      ix. Spherocytes: congenital spherocytosis or autoimmune hemolytic anemia.

      x. Target cells: liver disease, hemoglobinopathy.

    c. Reticulocyte count and reticulocyte index

reticulocyte index =

$$\frac{\text{reticuloctye count } (\%) \times \text{patient hematocrit}/45}{\text{shift factor}}$$

where the shift factor is 2.0 for anemia of moderate severity.

2. *Secondary* laboratory tests to further evaluate the suspected cause of anemia are appropriate, although they are unlikely to be immediately available in the ED:

    a. Microcytic or normocytic anemia: obtain serum iron, total iron binding capacity, and serum ferritin.

    b. Macrocytic or normocytic anemia: obtain vitamin B_{12} level, folate, and erythrocyte folate.

    c. Suspected hemolysis (anemia with a reticulocyte index > 3.0%): obtain unconjugated bilirubin, serum haptoglobin, serum lactate dehydrogenase, and direct and indirect Coomb's test (*note:* the direct Coomb's test detects IgG and the third component of complement [C3] on the surface of the erythrocytes; the indirect Coomb's test measures antibody titers in the serum).

3. *Additional* studies may include one or more of the following, depending on clinical circumstances:

    a. Bilirubin level.

    b. Blood type and crossmatch.

    c. Chest roentgenogram.

    d. Electrocardiogram (ECG).

    e. Electrolyte panel, BUN, and creatinine levels.

    f. Liver function tests.

    g. Prothrombin time/partial thromboplastin time (PT/PTT).

    h. Pregnancy test (serum or urine).

    i. Urinalysis.

III. DIFFERENTIAL DIAGNOSIS

A. Erythrocyte Loss from Hemorrhage

Reticulocytosis may not develop for several days after acute blood loss; once reticulocytosis occurs, it will persist until the anemia is corrected or iron stores are depleted, at which time the MCV will also decline.

1. Epistaxis.
2. Gastrointestinal.
3. Genitourinary.
4. Intra-abdominal.
5. Intra-articular.
6. Intrathoracic.
7. Oropharyngeal.
8. Retroperitoneal.
9. Skin/bone/soft tissue.
10. Trauma.
11. Vaginal.

B. Erythrocyte Destruction from Hemolysis

Patients will often present with a family history of hemolytic anemia or evidence of jaundice, scleral icterus, and/or splenomegaly on physical examination; laboratory examination demonstrates an elevated reticulocyte index.

1. **Hereditary Hemolytic Anemias**

    a. Elliptocytosis and pyropoikilocytosis.

    b. Glucose-6-phosphate dehydrogenase deficiency. This is the most common of the erythrocyte enzymopathies. It is a sex-linked deficiency (more common in males) affecting individuals of Mediterranean, African, and Chinese origin. Hemolytic episodes may occur after exposure to oxidant drugs (e.g., antimalarial drugs, sulfonamides), infections, or fava beans.

    c. Pyruvate kinase deficiency.

    d. Sickle cell syndromes.

    e. Spherocytosis.

    f. Unstable hemoglobinopathies.

2. **Acquired Hemolytic Anemias**

    a. Autoimmune hemolytic anemia.

    b. DIC.

    c. Drug-induced hemolytic anemia.
    d. Liver disease.
    e. Paroxysmal nocturnal hemoglobinuria.
    f. Traumatic hemolysis (e.g., prosthetic heart valves).

C. Inadequate Erythrocyte Production in the Bone Marrow

Bone marrow failure is confirmed by a low reticulocyte index. Once the patient has been found to have a hypoproliferative anemia, the MCV provides a clue to the cause.

1. Low MCV (< 82 fL)

    a. Anemia of chronic disease.
    b. Iron deficiency.
    c. Lead poisoning.
    d. Sideroblastic anemia (usually hereditary).
    e. Thalassemia (alpha-thalassemia trait, beta-thalassemia trait).

2. Normal MCV (82–98 fL)

    a. Anemia of chronic disease (infection, human immunodeficiency virus, malignancy, rheumatic diseases).
    b. Endocrinopathy (Addison's disease, hypopituitarism, hypothyroidism).
    c. Iron deficiency (early).
    d. Renal failure.
    e. Primary bone marrow disorders (aplastic anemia, leukemia, infiltrative disorders).
    f. Sideroblastic anemia (usually acquired).

3. Elevated MCV (> 98 fL; megaloblastic anemia)

    a. Alcoholism.
    b. Drugs (e.g., azathioprine, hydroxyurea, methotrexate, sulfasalazine, trimethoprim, zidovudine [AZT]).
    c. Folic acid deficiency.
    d. Liver disease.
    e. Myelodysplasia.
    f. Vitamin B_{12} deficiency.

IV. THERAPY

In the ED, anemia *may* be the initial manifestation of a potentially life-threatening disorder in need of urgent intervention. The treatment goals of the ED physician are to ensure adequate patient oxygenation and ventilation, to stabilize hemodynamic parameters as necessary, to initiate an appropriate diagnostic workup and early consultation with respect to the cause of the anemia, and to arrange for necessary definitive care and a reasonable disposition.

A. Initial Management

Assess, secure, and support the airway, breathing, and circulation as indicated. In the setting of acute and significant blood loss, or in the unstable patient with a severe and symptomatic anemia, resuscitate as necessary and appropriate (see Chapter 1. II and Hypovolemic Shock in Chapter 12).

B. Red Blood Cell Transfusion

Transfusion is appropriate under the following circumstances (also see Blood Component Therapy, later in this chapter):

1. To prevent or treat shock from major blood loss due to trauma or severe hemorrhage.

2. To improve the oxygen-carrying capacity of blood in a symptomatic anemic patient.
    a. Patient age, severity of symptoms, cause of the anemia, and underlying medical condition are important considerations *prior to* transfusion.
    b. Adequate oxygenation is usually ensured with a hemoglobin of 7 g/dL, but patients with advanced age, significant cardiovascular disease, pulmonary disease, or cerebrovascular insufficiency may require a higher hemoglobin.

C. Appropriate Diagnostic Workup

1. Obtain a directed history and perform a physical examination (see II, above).

2. Obtain necessary laboratory values (see II. E, above).

3. Depending on clinical situation (e.g., severity and likely cause of the anemia), consider needed consultation (e.g., internal medicine, hematology/oncology).

D. Definitive Care

Note: definitive therapy of anemia requires treatment of the underlying disease process. Therapeutic interventions for some commonly encountered anemias are outlined below:

1. **Iron Deficiency**.
    a. Causes include menstruation, occult bleeding (usually from the gastrointestinal tract), malabsorption, increased iron requirements (infancy, lactation, pregnancy), pulmonary hemosiderosis, and chronic intravascular hemolysis (with loss of iron in the urine).
    b. Therapy:
        i. Search for the cause of iron loss and treat as necessary.
        ii. Replace iron: ferrous sulfate (300 mg PO tid).
            • Hemoglobin level should increase by 2 g/dL in 4 weeks (failure to do so suggests an initial erroneous

794 / HEMATOLOGIC AND ONCOLOGIC EMERGENCIES

diagnosis, continued occult bleeding, inflammatory block, other deficiency [e.g., folate, vitamin B_{12}], noncompliance, or malabsorption).

- Oral replacement therapy should continue for 6 months after hemoglobin has returned to normal to replenish iron stores.
- Side effects of oral iron include nausea, epigastric discomfort, constipation, and/or diarrhea. Side effects may be minimized by prescribing a liquid preparation and gradually increasing the dose over time or by having the patient take the iron orally with food (although the latter decreases iron absorption).
- Parenteral iron may be administered to patients with severe malabsorption, large iron requirements that cannot be met orally, or intolerance of oral preparations. Parenteral iron does not correct the anemia more rapidly than oral iron and is associated with increased side effects.

2. **Folic Acid Deficiency**

   a. Causes include poor dietary intake, alcohol abuse, malabsorption (e.g., inflammatory bowel disease), drugs (e.g., methotrexate, oral contraceptives, pentamidine, phenytoin, sulfasalazine, trimethoprim), and increased requirements (e.g., pregnancy, chronic blood loss, hemolytic anemia, some malignancies).

   b. Therapy
      i. Search for the cause of folate deficiency, evaluate for simultaneous vitamin B_{12} deficiency (see below), and treat as necessary.
      ii. Replace folate: folic acid (1 mg PO daily).

3. **Vitamin B_{12} Deficiency**

   a. Causes include gastrectomy, gastrointestinal bacterial overgrowth, ileal disease or resection, inadequate diet, intestinal parasites, pancreatic insufficiency, and pernicious anemia.

   b. Therapy
      i. Search for the cause of vitamin B_{12} deficiency, evaluate for simultaneous folate deficiency (see above), and treat as necessary.
      ii. Carefully evaluate for neurologic dysfunction (may occur in the absence of anemia).
      iii. Replace vitamin B_{12}: cyanocobalamin (1000 μg IM daily for 7 days, then weekly for 1–2 months, and then monthly). Reticulocytosis should occur within 1 week and the hemoglobin level should rise over the next 2–3 months.

4. **Anemia of Chronic Disease**

   a. Causes include alcoholic liver disease, autoimmune disorders, chronic infections, congestive heart failure, diabetes mellitus, inflammatory diseases, malignancies, and severe renal disease.

   b. Therapy: correct the underlying cause. Erythropoietin may be used to treat the anemia of chronic renal failure, but it is generally not administered in the ED.

5. **Aplastic Anemia**. This anemia is usually associated with leukopenia and thrombocytopenia.

   a. Patients with newly diagnosed aplastic anemia should *not* be transfused unless the anemia is so severe as to be imminently life-threatening (urgently consult a hematologist for advice; diagnosis is confirmed by bone marrow biopsy).

   b. Immediately stop any possible offending toxin or drug.

   c. Pursue appropriate transfer to a bone marrow transplant center.

6. **Hemolytic Anemia**

   a. Causes: see III. B, above.

   b. Therapy

     i. Stop all potentially offending drugs.

     ii. Consider glucocorticoids for the initial treatment of suspected autoimmune hemolysis (consult a hematologist): prednisone (begin with 1–2 mg/kg/day PO). Splenectomy is indicated in those patients who fail to respond to corticosteroids or in those who require continued high doses of corticosteroids. Other treatment options may include intravenous immunoglobulin or cytotoxic drug therapy.

     iii. Patients with microangiopathic hemolytic anemia due to DIC, TTP, or the hemolytic uremic syndrome (HUS) need urgent hospitalization for specialized care and monitoring.

     iv. Individuals with persistent hemolysis should receive folic acid replacement. Iron stores should also be periodically monitored.

V. DISPOSITION

A. Discharge

Patients with an identified anemia may be discharged from the ED if *all* of the following conditions are met:

1. Vital signs are normal and at the patient's baseline (including orthostatic vital signs).
2. There is no evidence of significant ongoing hemorrhage.
3. The anemia is well tolerated and not severe.
4. Cardiorespiratory and neurologic systems are stable and at the patient's baseline.
5. The patient is reliable.
6. Adequate follow-up is arranged.

B. Admit

Patients who do not meet all of the discharge criteria above, and most patients with acute significant blood loss, will require hospitalization for continued vital sign support and evaluation/treatment.

VI. PEARLS AND PITFALLS

A. Administer oxygen to the symptomatic anemic patient in the ED, and monitor both the patient's oxygen saturation and cardiac rhythm.

B. An erythrocyte transfusion is appropriate in the significantly symptomatic anemic patient.

C. Search carefully for acute or chronic blood loss and support hemodynamic status as clinically indicated.

D. Before beginning iron replacement, order appropriate iron studies, explain potential side effects of iron replacement therapy to the patient, and emphasize the need for continued compliance and follow-up.

E. Serum ferritin is an acute-phase reactant and may be elevated in patients with an inflammatory condition or infection (though in this setting a serum ferritin ≤ 50 ng/mL is still probably indicative of iron deficiency). Serum iron and total iron binding capacity should also be measured.

F. Provide iron supplementation to patients receiving erythropoietin in the setting of chronic renal failure.

G. In the patient with suspected vitamin B_{12} deficiency, carefully document the neurologic examination and simultaneously evaluate for folic acid deficiency (with an erythrocyte folic acid level). Ensure that iron stores are also adequate.

H. Administer packed erythrocytes slowly when transfusing patients with severe anemia and known cardiac dysfunction. Diuretics may be intermittently necessary to maintain an optimal volume status.

I. Blood products should be irradiated prior to transfusing patients with aplastic anemia, leukemia, myelodysplasia, or any other condition with prolonged leukopenia. If the patient is a bone marrow transplant candidate, the blood products should also be screened for cytomegalovirus (CMV); all blood products should be CMV-negative until the patient's CMV status has been determined.

J. Arrange for prompt follow-up for all anemic patients discharged from the ED.

Do *not* do any of the following:

A. Empirically treat megaloblastic anemia with folic acid alone (the anemia of vitamin B_{12} deficiency may respond to folic acid, with continued progression of the neurologic abnormalities).

B. Transfuse a patient with aplastic anemia unless faced with a life-threatening condition (discuss with a hematologist or a bone marrow transplant referral center consultant prior to transfusion).

BIBLIOGRAPHY

Beissner RS, Trowbridge AA: Clinical assessment of anemia. Postgrad Med 1986;80(6):83–95.
Beutler E: The common anemias. JAMA 1988;259:2433–2437.
Hillman RS, Finch CA: The Red Cell Manual. 5th ed. Philadelphia, FA Davis, 1985.

SICKLE CELL DISEASE

> *"There are certain pathological processes and conditions,*
> *one characteristic element of which consists in a*
> *distinct and well marked periodicity in their recurrence."*
>
> ELISHA BARTLETT (1804–1855)

I. ESSENTIAL FACTS

A. Definitions

1. *Sickle cell disease* is a hemolytic anemia resulting from the inheritance of a structurally abnormal hemoglobin, hemoglobin S (Hgb S: valine is substituted for glutamic acid at the sixth position of the beta globulin chain of the hemoglobin molecule). The abnormal Hgb S polymerizes under conditions of reduced pH, low PO_2, low temperature, and/or dehydration with subsequent distortion of the erythrocyte, obstructed capillary blood flow, and cell membrane injury.

2. Sickle genotypes include the following (*note:* sickle cell disease is associated with the homozygous condition, sickle cell anemia, or with the heterozygous conditions sickle-beta thalassemia and sickle-hemoglobin S-C):

   a. Sickle cell trait: individuals heterozygous for the Hgb S gene (Hgb S-A); occurs in approximately 8% of blacks.

      i. The relative high frequency of sickle cell trait is due to the survival advantage of the heterozygote under the selective pressure of *Falciparum* malaria in Africa.

      ii. Patients with sickle cell trait are usually asymptomatic, although painless hematuria and isosthenuria may occur.

   b. Sickle cell anemia: individuals homozygous for the Hgb S gene (Hgb S-S); occurs in 0.15% of black newborns.

   c. Sickle-beta thalassemia (Hgb S-beta thal): most commonly seen in patients of Mediterranean descent; it is generally a milder disease than Hgb S-S or Hgb S-C.

d. Sickle-hemoglobin C (Hgb S-C): occurs in 1:2600 blacks. Disease is of intermediate severity between Hgb S-S and Hgb S-beta thal. Hemoglobin C results from the substitution of lysine for glutamic acid at position six of the beta globulin chain of the hemoglobin molecule.

B. Mortality

The median age of death for patients with sickle cell anemia (Hgb S-S) in a recent study was 42 years for males and 48 years for females (with 50% of patients surviving beyond the 5th decade). An increased risk of early death was seen in individuals with the acute chest syndrome, renal failure, seizures, a baseline leukocyte count > 15,000/μL, and/or a low level of fetal hemoglobin.

II. CLINICAL EVALUATION

A. History

Most individuals presenting to the ED with a symptomatic sickle cell condition are well aware of their disease and its manifestations, especially their typical pattern of painful crisis. Determine the following: precipitating events (e.g., altitude change, dehydration, activity change, cold exposure, illness), usual presenting symptoms, current presenting symptoms, symptoms of infection, trauma history, past medical and surgical history, medication use, circumstances of last ED visit, family history, and oral intake/hydration status.

B. Symptoms and Signs

Patients with sickle cell disease may present to the ED with one or more of the following clinical conditions:

1. Acute pain crisis (vaso-occlusive crisis): acute pain is the most frequent presentation of sickle cell disease in the ED. The pain is due to vascular occlusion of small vessels by sickled erythrocytes. Crises tend to be relatively consistent in nature in any one patient; if there is a change from the usual pattern, other complications need to be excluded. Approximately one-third of sickle cell patients suffer a painful crisis every few years, one-third suffer one to five episodes per year, and ≤ 5% suffer > 40 crises per year.
   a. Bone crisis: skeletal pain occurs more commonly in the extremities than in the axial skeleton.
   b. Chest crisis ("acute chest syndrome"): acute chest pain, frequently pleuritic in nature. May be accompanied by nonproductive cough, dyspnea, hyperventilation, pulmonary infiltrates, and/or hemoptysis (this latter suggests pulmonary infarction).
   c. Abdominal crisis: acute, steady abdominal pain without significant tenderness to palpation or peritoneal findings.

    d. Joint crisis: mono- or oligoarticular pain, with or without a small effusion.

2. Priapism: a painful, prolonged penile erection that ultimately occurs in ≤ 10–40% of males with sickle cell disease. Priapism may be associated with subsequent erectile dysfunction or impotence.

3. Stroke (including transient ischemic attack [TIA], cerebrovascular accident [CVA], and subarachnoid hemorrhage [SAH]): happens in ≥ 10% of sickle patients. TIAs and CVAs frequently occur in the pediatric ages (mean CVA age onset is 10 years); adult patients may suffer an SAH.

4. Aplastic crisis: defined by a sudden drop in the patient's usual hemoglobin level accompanied by a decreased reticulocyte count. It is more common in the pediatric sickle cell patient. Symptoms are those of profound anemia: dyspnea, fatigue, and/or pallor. The aplastic crisis is often associated with viral infections (especially parvovirus B19), folate deficiency, and/or toxins or drugs that inhibit hematopoiesis.

5. Sequestration crisis: occurs when a large proportion of the erythrocyte mass pools in the spleen. Most patients are ≤ 5 years old. Symptoms and signs include tachycardia, dyspnea, abdominal pain, splenic enlargement, falling hematocrit, and prominent reticulocytosis. Infection is a common precipitant. Early recognition and treatment of a major sequestration crisis are critical to prevent hypovolemic shock.

6. Infection: this is the leading cause of hospitalization and death in patients with sickle cell anemia. Sickle cell disease results in immunocompromise, including impaired or absent splenic function with an increased infection risk to encapsulated bacteria (e.g., *Streptococcus pneumoniae, Hemophilus influenzae,* and *Salmonella* spp.).

7. Other miscellaneous complications associated with sickle cell disease include avascular necrosis (most commonly of the hips and shoulders), cholelithiasis, chronic pain behavior, depression, eye conditions (posthyphema complications, proliferative retinopathy, retinal detachment, retinal holes, vitreous hemorrhage), flank pain with renal papillary necrosis, increased pregnancy-related complications, leg ulcers, nephropathy, sickle cell lung disease (a type of chronic obstructive lung disease), and symptoms and signs related to anemia and/or hemolysis.

C. Directed Physical Examination

1. **Vital Signs.** Note tachycardia, postural vital signs, respiratory rate, and temperature.

2. **Skin.** Note jaundice, skin ulcers (pretibial usually), and any evidence of trauma or infection.

3. **HEENT.** Evaluate the oral mucosa for pallor and hydration status; check the conjunctiva for jaundice. Examine the fundi for proliferative retinopathy. Look for evidence of infection (e.g., otitis media, sinusitis, dental abscess).

4. **Neck.** Note suppleness and presence of nodes.

5. **Chest.** Examine for wheezes, rales, and rhonchi.

6. **Heart.** Note degree of tachycardia and listen for murmurs, rubs, or gallops.

7. **Abdomen.** Evaluate for distention, bowel sounds, tenderness, localized peritoneal irritation, and masses. The liver may be enlarged; the spleen is palpable only in the pediatric patient.

8. **Extremities.** Note clubbing, cyanosis, edema, joint pain, and/or inflammation.

9. **Nervous System.** Note mental status and perform a screening examination.

D. Laboratory Studies

1. *Routinely* obtain the following:
   a. Complete blood count. The hemoglobin level is typically 6–9 g/dL, with a mean corpuscular volume (MCV) frequently > 90 fL secondary to reticulocytosis. If the hemoglobin level is < 6 g/dL, exclude aplastic crisis. Leukocytosis is common, probably as a consequence of demargination and a chronically active marrow; but a leukocyte count > 20,000/μL, especially with a left-shifted differential, is suggestive of infection. The peripheral smear may reveal sickled cells, Howell-Jolly bodies (due to functional asplenism), or target cells (in Hgb S-C disease and Hgb S-beta thal).
   b. Reticulocyte count. Usually is 5–30% (mean: 12%). A low reticulocyte count occurs in aplastic crisis.

2. One or more of the following *may be indicated,* depending on clinical circumstances:
   a. Arterial blood gas: appropriate in the dyspneic patient.
   b. Blood cultures: obtain if the patient is febrile or toxic.
   c. Chest roentgenogram: necessary if the patient has a fever or pulmonary symptoms/signs.
   d. Electrocardiogram: obtain in the patient with chest or pulmonary symptoms.
   e. Electrolyte panel, glucose, blood urea nitrogen (BUN), and creatinine levels.
   f. Head computed tomography: appropriate in the patient with an abnormal neurologic examination.
   g. Hemoglobin electrophoresis: reasonable if the diagnosis has not been established or if a variant such as Hgb S-C disease needs to be excluded.

    h. Lumbar puncture: when meningitis or subarachnoid hemorrhage are diagnostic possibilities.

    i. Pregnancy test.

    j. Shoulder and/or hip roentgenograms: obtain if a new pain localizes to either of these areas. Further evaluation for aseptic necrosis may require a bone scan or magnetic resonance imaging scan.

    k. Ultrasound: may be helpful in individuals with abdominal pain.

    l. Urinalysis: obtain in patients with urinary tract symptoms or fever.

III. DIFFERENTIAL DIAGNOSIS

Patients with sickle cell disease can present with a variety of painful complaints that may be caused by conditions other than sickle cell-induced vaso-occlusion (Table 21–1).

IV. THERAPY

A. First-Line Therapy

1. Administer oxygen (begin with 2–5 L/min via nasal cannula) and maintain oxyhemoglobin saturation ≥ 95%.

2. Initiate intravenous (IV) hydration. In severely hypovolemic patients replace volume deficits with normal saline (NS) as required, then change the hydration fluid to 5% dextrose in 0.45% NS (D5 ½ NS) at 200–300 mL/hr. This hypotonic solution is theoretically advantageous: increasing intracellular volume may reduce the concentration of Hgb S and thereby decrease sickling.

Table 21–1. DIFFERENTIAL DIAGNOSIS OF SICKLE CELL DISEASE

SYMPTOM	LABORATORY FINDINGS	RULE OUT
Chest pain	Infiltrate on chest roentgenogram	Pneumonia Pulmonary embolism Pulmonary infarction Bone marrow emboli
Right-upper-quadrant abdominal pain	Elevated bilirubin level	Cholelithiasis Cholecystitis Hepatic infarction Hepatitis
Flank pain	Hematuria	Renal infarction Pyelonephritis
Confusion, central nervous system findings		Cerebral infarction Meningitis Subarachnoid hemorrhage Transient ischemic attack

3. Rapidly perform a directed physical examination and obtain appropriate laboratory values (see II, above). Evaluate the patient carefully for aplastic crisis, infection, priapism, pulmonary infarction, sequestration crisis, stroke, and/or worsening chronic hemolytic anemia.

4. Promptly administer analgesics for pain control. Many EDs appropriately use pain protocols and treatment plans.
   a. Reasonable parenteral opioid regimens include the following:
      i. Morphine sulfate (bolus plus infusion): 5 mg bolus IV (plus diphenhydramine 50 mg IV) followed by 5 mg/hr continuous morphine infusion. Supplemental doses of morphine ("rescue" doses) may be given hourly for persistent pain. The hourly "rescue" doses may be increased by 10–20% every several hours if required. The continuous infusion may also be adjusted upward every 2–3 hours as necessary. For patients with good pain control within 4–6 hours, and who are otherwise appropriate for hospital discharge (see V, below), oral controlled-release morphine (e.g., MS Contin) should be started 1 hour before stopping the IV infusion. *Or*
      ii. Morphine sulfate (bolus only): 4–10 mg IV load, followed by 2–6 mg IV bolus hourly as needed. *Or*
      iii. Hydromorphone 1–3 mg IV, followed by 1–2 mg IV hourly as needed. *Caution:* with any of the above, initially re-evaluate patients every 15 minutes for pain control, vital signs, and oversedation (e.g., systolic blood pressure < 100 mmHg, respiratory rate < 10–12/min, or pulse < 60 beats/min).
   b. Antiemetics (e.g., hydroxyzine 25–50 mg intramuscularly [IM], or promethazine 25 mg IM or IV) may be added to the above regimens as indicated.
   c. Some patients in vaso-occlusive crisis benefit from ketorolac (30–60 mg IM).

5. Administer appropriate antibiotics to patients with an identified infection or those who are febrile (T > 38.3°C) after obtaining necessary cultures as clinically indicated.

6. Provide oral folic acid supplementation (1 mg daily).

B. Second-Line Therapy

1. Transfusion therapy and urgent hematology consultation are indicated in the following situations:
   a. Acute CVA or TIA (goal: reduce Hgb S to < 30% of circulating hemoglobin).
   b. Acute or chronic hypoxia.
   c. Acute priapism unresponsive to hydration and analgesia (also consult urology).
   d. Acute progressive lung disease (pulmonary infarctions).

    e. Acute splenic or hepatic sequestration crisis.

    f. Aplastic crisis.

    g. Severe anemia with resultant physiologic compromise (e.g., angina, cerebral dysfunction, moderate to severe dyspnea, high-output cardiac failure, profound fatigue).

2. Partial-exchange transfusion, in which a proportion of the patient's red cells are exchanged with normal red cells, is indicated in the following situations (again, consult a hematologist):

    a. Acute chest syndrome that fails to improve within 4 days of hospitalization.

    b. After a patient has had a CVA (the risk of recurrence is reduced with partial-exchange transfusion).

    c. Before radiographic contrast injection (especially intra-arterial contrast).

    d. In patients who require general anesthesia for surgery.

    e. Pregnancy, at 28 weeks gestation.

    f. Severe pain crises (those lasting > 7 days) or those requiring recurrent hospitalizations despite appropriate conservative therapy.

    g. To assist skin ulcer healing.

3. Transfusion has *no role* in the management of an acute uncomplicated pain crisis or in the treatment of the sickle patient's chronic, stable, steady state anemia. Complications from transfusion include alloimmunization, hepatitis, iron overload, and potential human immunodeficiency virus infection.

V. DISPOSITION

A. Discharge

Patients with sickle cell disease who present to the ED with an acute pain crisis may be discharged to home if *all* of the following conditions apply:

1. Vital signs are at the patient's baseline.

2. Pain is adequately controlled.

3. The patient can take oral liquids and medications well.

4. Infection has been excluded.

5. Follow-up has been arranged.

It is appropriate to prescribe the following medications at the time of discharge: an oral opioid (limited amount), an antiemetic, folic acid, and a stool softener.

B. Admit

Patients with any of the conditions listed in Table 21–2 should be hospitalized for continued care.

Table 21–2. INDICATIONS FOR HOSPITAL ADMISSION IN SICKLE CELL DISEASE

Infectious Complications

Sepsis
Meningitis
Pyelonephritis
Febrile infant
Febrile seizures
Osteomyelitis
Pneumonia with multilobar infiltrate, high fever, hemoptysis, or severe chest pain

Vaso-occlusive Complications

Refractory pain crisis
Refractory priapism
Acute dactylitis

Anemic Complications

Symptomatic anemia requiring transfusion
Aplastic crisis requiring transfusion
Acute sequestration syndromes
Symptomatic hypoxia

Other Acute Events

Acute persistent neurologic deficit
Acute pulmonary embolus
Sequestration syndromes
Pulmonary edema
Acute vision loss

Obstetric Complications

Pain crisis
Pyelonephritis
Toxemia
Thrombophlebitis

From Pollack CV, Emergencies in sickle cell disease. Emerg Med Clin N Am 1993;11(2):376.

VI. PEARLS AND PITFALLS

A. Administer supplemental oxygen and appropriate hydration as indicated to patients with sickle cell disease.

B. Provide adequate analgesia, but avoid opioid abuse.

C. Diligently evaluate the patient for infection.

D. Consider aseptic necrosis or osteomyelitis in those individuals with prolonged bone pain.

E. Arrange for appropriate follow-up with a primary care provider at the time of the patient's ED discharge.

F. Encourage genetic and prenatal counseling in those families with a history of sickle cell disease.

Do *not* do any of the following:

A. Transfuse blood in the ED in an attempt to shorten the duration of an acute pain crisis.

B. Discharge the patient if there is evidence of infection.

BIBLIOGRAPHY

Brookoff D, Polomano R: Treating sickle cell pain like cancer pain. Ann Intern Med 1992;116: 364–368.

Platt OS, Brambilla DJ, Rosse WF, et al. Mortality in sickle cell disease: life expectancy and risk factors for early death. N Engl J Med 1994;330(23):1639–1644.

Pollack CV, Jr: Emergencies in sickle cell disease. Emerg Med Clin N Am 1993;11(2): 365–378.

Samuels-Reid JH: Common problems in sickle cell disease. Am Fam Phys 1994;49(6): 1477–1486.

BLEEDING DISORDERS

"Only my blood speaks to you in my veins."

WILLIAM SHAKESPEARE

I. ESSENTIAL FACTS

A. Definition

A *bleeding disorder* is the clinical manifestation(s) of an altered hemostatic mechanism. The disorder may be secondary to an abnormality in either primary or secondary hemostasis:

1. Disorders of *primary hemostasis* involve increased fragility of small blood vessels (e.g., vasculitis), an abnormal number of platelets, or abnormally functioning platelets. Clinical manifestations may include mucous membrane bleeding (including epistaxis and gingival bleeding), petechiae, and/or superficial purpura.

2. Disorders of *secondary hemostasis* involve decreased activity of one or more clotting factors (i.e., a coagulation disorder). Clinical manifestations may include delayed, recurrent oozing from wounds and/or hematoma formation (including intramuscular hemorrhage, visceral bleeding, and hemarthoses).

3. A disorder in either primary or secondary hemostasis may result in menorrhagia or gastrointestinal hemorrhage.

A bleeding disorder can be either congenital or acquired. Most patients with inherited defects manifest their bleeding disorder in childhood and frequently have a family history of bleeding; acquired defects are usually noted in adults and are generally associated with an underlying disease. Some patients have abnormalities in both primary and secondary hemostasis.

B. Epidemiology

1. Bleeding disorders affect approximately 30–50 per 100,000 people.

2. Risk factors for a bleeding disorder include
   a. Alcohol abuse.
   b. Anticoagulant use.

   c. Autoimmune disorders.

   d. Aspirin use.

   e. Chemotherapy.

   f. Other drugs.

   g. Infection.

   h. Inherited disorders, including

      i. *Hemophilia A:* an X-linked recessive disorder with deficient activity of factor VIII.

      ii. *Hemophilia B* (Christmas disease): an X-linked recessive disorder with deficient activity of factor IX. It is one-seventh as common as hemophilia A.

      iii. *von Willebrand's disease:* this is the most common congenital hemostatic disorder; it is characterized by a deficiency in von Willebrand factor with resultant decreased platelet function and a variable decrease in factor VIII activity. Several subtypes of the disease have been described, with most generally inherited in an autosomal dominant manner.

   i. Liver disease.

   j. Malignancy.

   k. Renal failure.

   l. Vitamin K deficiency (secondary to broad-spectrum antibiotics, warfarin [Coumadin], poor nutrition).

II. CLINICAL EVALUATION

A. History

The following specific details should be determined:

1. Type of bleeding, including epistaxis, petechiae (small dot hemorrhages on the lower extremities or palate), purpura (many petechiae or larger superficial hemorrhages), bleeding during menses, bleeding after dental extraction or other procedures, generalized oozing, gastrointestinal hemorrhage, and/or bleeding into soft tissues or joints.

2. Onset of the bleeding problem (e.g., life-long history versus recent onset of bleeding difficulties).

3. Nature of the inciting event: spontaneous versus post-traumatic hemorrhage.

4. Family history of bleeding.

5. Underlying systemic illness, particularly cancer, liver disease, and/or renal disease.

6. Medications used, including antibiotics, anticoagulants, nonsteroidal anti-inflammatory drugs, and/or aspirin.

7. Alcohol and/or other drug use.

B. Symptoms

1. Platelet Disorders. Bleeding from gums, epistaxis, hematuria, or prolonged bleeding immediately after trauma (including dental extractions).

2. Coagulation Disorders. Extended or delayed bleeding after trauma. Patients with hemophilia usually present with deep visceral bleeding, particularly hemarthroses or bleeding into muscle.

C. Physical Examination

1. **Vital Signs.** Note pulse, blood pressure, respiratory rate, and temperature.

2. **Skin.** Observe for petechiae, purpura, ecchymoses, and spider angiomata.

3. **HEENT.** Look for conjunctival hemorrhage, petechiae on the palate, and oozing from nasal mucosa or gums.

4. **Neck.** Check for suppleness and nodes.

5. **Chest and Heart.** Auscultate lungs and precordium carefully.

6. **Abdomen.** Look for the presence of hepatomegaly, spleno-megaly, and/or ascites.

7. **Rectum.** Gently palpate for masses and check stool for heme.

8. **Extremities.** Examine joints for stiffness or swelling consistent with hemarthroses, and evaluate for joint deformity consistent with previous hemarthroses. Petechiae on the lower extremities are often seen with thrombocytopenia.

D. Laboratory Studies

In the patient with a bleeding disorder a complete blood count (CBC), and blood urea nitrogen (BUN) and creatinine levels should be obtained. A blood type and crossmatch is appropriate if the clinical situation indicates a transfusion will be necessary. The cause of the bleeding disorder can usually be determined quickly in the ED with the following studies (also see Table 21–3):

1. **Platelet Count** (normal: 150,000–300,000/μL): the risk of bleeding increases after trauma or surgery when the platelet count is <50,000/μL. Spontaneous bleeding rarely occurs until the platelet count is <20,000/μL unless there is an underlying vascular defect.

2. **Bleeding Time** (normal: 3.5–9.5 minutes): this assesses platelet function, requires experienced personnel to perform, and is most useful in patients who have mucosal bleeding despite a normal platelet count. The bleeding time is prolonged with functional platelet disorders, von Willebrand's disease (may also be normal in this setting), aspirin use, and when the platelet count is <100,000/μL.

3. **Prothrombin Time** (PT; normal 11–14 seconds): this measures clotting initiated by the extrinsic (factor VII) and common pathways (factors V, X, thrombin, and fibrinogen). A clinically important factor deficiency prolongs the PT by

Table 21–3. COMMON HEMOSTATIC DISORDERS AND ASSOCIATED LABORATORY ABNORMALITIES

CONDITION	ABNORMAL TESTS	NORMAL TESTS
Vitamin K deficiency	PT (PTT sometimes also abnormal)	Platelets, PTT, TT
Liver disease		Fibrinogen, platelets, TT
Early	PT, PTT	
Chronic	Fibrinogen, FDP, PT, PTT, TT	
Disseminated intravascular coagulation	Fibrinogen, FDP, platelets, PT, PTT, TT	
Heparin contamination	PTT, TT	PT
Lupus anticoagulant	PTT (PTT does not correct with a 1:1 mix)	Platelets, PT, TT

more than 3 seconds as compared to a control in most laboratories.

a. Isolated prolongation of the PT may be caused by early liver disease, early warfarin effect, fat malabsorption with vitamin K deficiency, and factor VII deficiency.

b. The PT is used to guide warfarin therapy because of its reproducibility. However, the thromboplastin tissue factor reagent used in the test differs from laboratory to laboratory. In order to standardize the PT among institutions, each batch of tissue factor is compared to a standard tissue factor provided by the World Health Organization (WHO). From this value is obtained an *international normalized ratio (INR)*, which is defined as the PT ratio that would have been obtained if WHO international reference thromboplastin had been used. The INR is useful in the management of patients who are chronically anticoagulated with warfarin.

4. **Partial Thromboplastin Time** (PTT; normal 20–40 seconds): the PTT measures clotting initiated by the intrinsic pathway (kallikrein, kininogen, and factors VIII, IX, XI, XII) and common pathway (factors V, X, thrombin, and fibrinogen). The PTT is an effective screening test for all clotting factors except VII and XIII; it is generally prolonged if factor levels are < 20% of normal. Clinically important factor deficiencies usually prolong the PTT by 8–12 seconds beyond control.

a. The PTT is clinically useful for monitoring anticoagulation with heparin. Isolated prolongation of the PTT is often due to hemophilia A, hemophilia B, or severe von Willebrand's disease.

b. Isolated prolongation of the PTT also occurs with deficiency of prekallikrein, kininogen, and the "lupus anticoagulant."

None of these conditions, however, is associated with clinical bleeding.

5. **Other Laboratory Tests.** The following are occasionally helpful, depending on the clinical situation:
   a. Thrombin time (TT): assesses abnormalities of fibrin formation and detects heparin contamination.
   b. Fibrinogen levels: decreased in disseminated intravascular coagulation (DIC) or afibrinogenemia.
   c. Fibrin degradation products (FDP): elevated in DIC.
   d. Clot stability test: evaluates the function of factor XIII. Patients who have a bleeding diathesis, but normal screening tests, may have depressed factor XIII levels and an abnormal clot stability test.

III. DIFFERENTIAL DIAGNOSIS

A. Causes of Thrombocytopenia

1. Decreased marrow production (decreased bone marrow megakaryocytes) related to
   a. Alcohol use.
   b. Disorders associated with defective myelopoiesis (e.g., aplastic anemia, Fanconi's syndrome, myelodysplasia, paroxysmal nocturnal hemoglobinuria).
   c. Disorders associated with marrow invasion (e.g., infection, leukemia, metastatic carcinoma).
   d. Drug use (e.g., chemotherapeutic agents, ethanol, estrogens, thiazide diuretics, trimethoprim-sulfamethoxazole).
   e. Viral infection.

2. Increased peripheral platelet destruction (normal to increased number of megakaryocytes in the bone marrow).
   a. Immune-mediated destruction:
      i. Drug-induced immune thrombocytopenic purpura (e.g., gold, heparin, quinidine, quinine, rifampin, sulfonamides).
      ii. Idiopathic thrombocytopenic purpura (ITP).
      iii. Neonatal alloimmune purpura.
      iv. Post-transfusion purpura.
   b. Nonimmunologic destruction:
      i. Disseminated intravascular coagulation (DIC).
      ii. Hemolytic uremic syndrome (HUS): characterized by renal dysfunction, hemolytic anemia, and thrombocytopenia.
      iii. Hypersplenism.
      iv. Thrombotic thrombocytopenic purpura (TTP): characterized by neurologic abnormalities, hemolytic anemia, thrombocytopenia, ± fever, ± renal dysfunction.

3. Congenital thrombocytopenia related to
   a. Fanconi's anemia.

     b. May-Hegglin anomaly.

     c. Wiskott-Aldrich syndrome.

B. Platelet Dysfunction

1. Aspirin use.

2. Multiple myeloma with paraproteinemia.

3. Myeloproliferative disorders.

4. Uremia.

5. von Willebrand's disease.

C. Coagulation Factor Deficiencies

1. Acquired deficiencies: Vitamin K deficiency (resulting in decreased levels of factors II, VII, IX, and X) is the most common cause of an acquired coagulation factor deficiency. The most common causes include dietary insufficiency (e.g., in the setting of alcohol abuse), biliary tract obstruction, liver disease, warfarin use, and/or broad-spectrum antibiotics.

2. Circulating anticoagulants (often seen in the rheumatic diseases).

3. Consumptive coagulopathy (e.g., DIC, massive transfusion).

4. Hemophilia A.

5. Hemophilia B.

6. von Willebrand's disease (variable decrease in factor VIII activity).

IV. THERAPY

A. Initial Management

Assess, secure, and support the airway, breathing, and circulation as indicated.

In the setting of acute and significant internal or external blood loss, resuscitate as necessary and appropriate (see Chapter 1. II and Hypovolemic Shock in Chapter 12).

B. Correction of the Abnormality Responsible for the Bleeding Diathesis

Therapy of a bleeding disorder in an emergency frequently requires immediate action before the cause of the disorder is determined; the laboratory evaluation will help determine which blood products should be used to correct the defect.

1. **Treatment of Thrombocytopenia**

    a. Transfusion with platelets is indicated in patients with a platelet count of < 50,000/μL if *any* of the following conditions apply: the patient is actively bleeding, is at risk of bleeding secondary to recent trauma, or requires operative intervention or an invasive procedure. Platelet transfusion is also appropriate in the nonbleeding, nontraumatized patient who has a platelet count of < 10,000/μL to prevent spontaneous bleeding.

b. Generally 6–10 units of platelets are transfused (see Blood Component Therapy later in this chapter). One hour and 24 hours after the platelet infusion, the platelet count should be rechecked to determine the adequacy of the response to the transfusion.

2. Treatment of Platelet Dysfunction

a. Most episodes of platelet dysfunction are probably secondary to aspirin or other drug use. Stop the aspirin; it will take up to 7 days for the bleeding time to return to normal. Platelet transfusion may temporarily reverse the deficit prior to surgery or an invasive procedure.

b. Patients with von Willebrand's disease are treated as follows:

    i. 1-Desamino-8-D-arginine-vasopressin (DDAVP): used in patients with mild to moderate von Willebrand's disease.

    Dose: 0.3 μg/kg IV; may repeat in 12 and 24 hours. Tachyphylaxis develops when additional doses are given. *Caution:* do not use DDAVP in patients with known type IIB von Willebrand's disease (characterized by enhanced interaction between von Willebrand's factor and platelets) because it may worsen thrombocytopenia.

    ii. Cryoprecipate: administration of this blood product will usually normalize the bleeding time.

    Dose: infuse 1–2 units of cryoprecipitate per 10 kg body weight. Repeat the infusion in 12 hours if the bleeding continues, and daily for 5–10 days in the event of surgery or trauma.

3. Treatment of Congenital Coagulation Factor Disorders

a. Hemophilia A: patients with bleeding due to hemophilia A can be corrected in three ways, with the method chosen dependent on the source and/or severity of bleeding:

    i. Mild hemophilia/mild mucosal bleeding: DDAVP in the doses used for von Willebrand's disease may control bleeding.

    ii. Moderate or severe hemophilia: factor VIII concentrate is used to raise factor VIII activity to 50% of normal. (*Note:* in the setting of life-threatening hemorrhage [e.g., intracranial, retroperitoneal, or retropharyngeal bleeding], major surgery, or potential airway compromise, factor VIII activity should be raised to 100% of normal.) Use the following formula to calculate the initial dose:

$$\text{Dose (units)} = (\text{desired \% activity} - \text{initial \% activity}) \times (\text{weight in kg})/2$$

Recombinant factor VIII should be used wherever possible because of the increased risk of viral transmission with factor VIII concentrates obtained from pooled plasma.

iii. Cryoprecipitate may be used to replace factor VIII when recombinant factor VIII is not available. The same dose should be used as described above for von Willebrand's disease.

b. Hemophilia B: DDAVP is *not* effective. Fresh frozen plasma (FFP; 5–6 units) may be used for mild bleeding. Prothrombin-complex concentrate is used for severe bleeding (consult a hematologist for appropriate dosing).

4. **Treatment of Acquired Coagulation Factor Disorders**

a. Vitamin K deficiency: patients should receive vitamin K when deficiency is suspected.

Dose: Vitamin K 10 mg subcutaneously (SQ), intramuscularly (IM), or intravenously (IV) every day for 3 days. (*Caution:* if given IV infuse no faster than 1 mg/min.) Patients who have uncontrolled bleeding should receive FFP (4 units IV). Subsequent FFP administration may be required, depending on the monitored PT and evidence of continued bleeding.

b. Bleeding due to liver disease: Vitamin K should be given but is not as likely to be effective. FFP may transiently improve hemostasis. Monitor the platelet count and administer platelet transfusions if clinically appropriate.

5. **Disseminated Intravascular Coagulation**
Optimal therapy depends on treatment of the underlying disease process. Judicious use of blood products, including platelets, FFP, and cryoprecipitate to replace fibrinogen, may be of temporary benefit; consult a hematologist urgently.

V. DISPOSITION

A. Discharge

Consider discharging the patient to home if *all* of the following conditions apply:

1. Bleeding was only minor and is now controlled.
2. Vital signs are normal and stable.
3. The hematocrit is stable and acceptable.
4. The underlying condition does not require hospitalization.
5. The patient is reliable.
6. Follow-up has been arranged.

B. Admit

Patients who do not fit all of the above discharge criteria, and any patient with potentially serious bleeding, should be admitted for observation and continued therapy.

VI. PEARLS AND PITFALLS

A. Initial therapy of the patient with a bleeding disorder should focus on aggressive assessment and support of the patient's airway, breathing, and circulation.

B. A patient with known hemophilia and a potentially life-threatening bleed (e.g., central nervous system, retroperitoneal, retropharyngeal) will require an initial IV dose of 50 units/kg of factor VIII.

C. A patient anticoagulated with warfarin (Coumadin) who develops significant bleeding can usually have the coagulopathy controlled with 4–5 units of FFP. A small dose of vitamin K (5–10 mg SQ, IM, or IV) will partially reverse the warfarin effect. Vitamin K 20–30 mg IV or SQ will completely reverse the effect and make the patient refractory to subsequent anticoagulation with warfarin for weeks.

D. Broad-spectrum antibiotics may prolong the PT. Vitamin K may be used to correct the abnormality in this setting.

E. The patient with a coagulapathy in the setting of liver disease should also be given vitamin K (10 mg SQ or IM each day for 3 days).

Do *not* do any of the following:

A. Give DDAVP to patients with potential or known type IIB von Willebrand's disease or to patients with severe hemophilia.

B. Give DDAVP more than two or three times, as tachyphylaxis will develop.

BIBLIOGRAPHY

Bachmann F: Diagnostic approach to mild bleeding disorders. Semin Hematol 1980; 17:292–305.

Brettler DB, Levine PH: Factor concentrates for treatment of hemophilia: which one to choose? Blood 1989;73:2067–2073.

Colman RW, et al: Hemostasis and Thrombosis. Philadelphia, JB Lippincott, 1987.

Johanos AM: Hemostasis and coagulopathies. Chapter 42. In Markovchick VJ, et al (eds): Emergency Medicine Secrets. Philadelphia, Hanley & Belfus, 1993.

BLOOD COMPONENT THERAPY

> *"The blood is the life."*
> DEUTERONOMY 12:23

I. ESSENTIAL FACTS

A. *Blood component therapy* is the replacement of essential blood constituents in response to certain medical conditions (e.g., severe symptomatic anemia). Unfortunately, blood product administration has definite associated risks, and complications can be life-threatening. Therefore, the risks and benefits of transfusion must always be weighed, and, if possible, discussed with the patient before the administration of blood products.

B. *Blood products* are usually collected, separated, stored, and then subsequently distributed from a central source. Indications for transfusion and the products available may differ from center to center. The indications and methods of transfusion presented below are general guidelines.

II. RED BLOOD CELL TRANSFUSION

A. Indications

1. To prevent or treat shock from major blood loss due to trauma or severe hemorrhage.

2. To improve the oxygen-carrying capacity of blood in a symptomatic anemic patient.
   a. Patient age, severity of symptoms, cause of the anemia, and underlying medical condition are important considerations prior to transfusion.
   b. Adequate oxygenation is usually ensured with a hemoglobin level of 7 g/dL, but patients with advanced age, significant cardiovascular disease, pulmonary disease, or cerebrovascular insufficiency may require a higher hemoglobin level.

B. Type and Crossmatch Procedures

Samples of the patient's blood to be used for typing purposes should be carefully labeled by the person obtaining the patient's blood immediately *before* that blood is drawn. After arrival at the blood bank, several tests are performed to ensure maximal blood product compatibility between the donor blood and the recipient. In a patient with compromised vital signs secondary to blood loss, maintenance of volume status with crystalloid is appropriate while awaiting the red cells.

1. **Universal Donor Blood.** Type O-negative blood (low-titer type-O if whole blood is being used) is indicated in critical

situations where *immediate* blood transfusion is necessary and there is not sufficient time for type-specific blood, complete type and crossmatched blood, or autotransfusion procedures.

2. **Type-Specific Blood.** Blood that has undergone an abbreviated type and crossmatch procedure that requires 10–20 minutes of blood bank time. It is the appropriate blood bank order when red blood cells are required in an emergent situation. Type-specific blood is ABO and Rh typed at the blood bank and is usually saline-immediate-spin crossmatched (donor cells are mixed with recipient serum to confirm ABO compatibility).

3. **Complete Type and Crossmatching.** This involves ABO typing, Rh typing, antibody screening, and the saline-immediate-spin crossmatch. Complete type and crossmatching requires 30–45 minutes of blood bank time (even more time will be required if antibodies are found). A type and crossmatch dedicates a certain number of units to a given patient for a given period of time (generally 48 hours). It is the appropriate blood bank order when red cells are required, but the patient's clinical status is stable enough to allow for the time needed to adequately perform the complete type and crossmatch. (*Note:* if blood is not needed currently, but *may* be needed an uncertain time in the near future, the appropriate blood bank order is a *type and screen.* A type and screen involves ABO typing, Rh typing, and antibody screening. In this circumstance, no units are dedicated to the patient until needed, at which time the blood bank quickly performs a saline-immediate-spin crossmatch [which requires only 5–10 minutes] and makes the requested number of units available).

C. Available Red Cell Products

1. **Whole Blood.** One unit of whole blood has a volume of approximately 500 mL and a hematocrit of 35–40%. It is unavailable as a transfusion option in many blood bank systems.

   a. "Whole blood" contains essentially no granulocytes or platelets after 24 hours of refrigerated storage; the whole blood may also be deficient in coagulation factors, depending on how long it has been stored (factors V and VIII decay the fastest).

   b. Whole blood or modified whole blood is rarely used. Its main indication is in the setting of massive hemorrhage where both oxygen-carrying capacity and volume need rapid replacement (even in this setting, the use of crystalloid and packed red cells is often more appropriate and convenient).

2. **Packed Red Cells.** One unit of packed red cells has a volume of 325 mL and a hematocrit of 55–65%. This is the most common red blood cell product used to increase oxygen-

carrying capacity. In general, one unit transfused should increase the patient's hemoglobin level by 1 g/dL.

3. **Leukocyte-Poor Red Cells.** These are the appropriate blood component when red cell transfusion is required in the following categories of patients: those who have had two or more previous nonhemolytic febrile transfusion reactions, those who are at risk for cytomegalovirus (CMV) transmission, or those who may require multiple and repeated transfusions over time (to decrease the incidence of alloimmunization).

4. **Washed Red Cells.** These are the appropriate blood component when red cell transfusion is required in patients who have had, or who are known to be at risk for, urticarial or anaphylactic transfusion reactions (which are usually due to antibodies to donor plasma proteins).

D. Transfusion Procedure

1. Inquire about any prior history of a transfusion reaction and the nature of that reaction.

2. Carefully confirm the identity of the patient as well as the appropriately typed and matched blood product with standard identification procedures and record same (*remember:* a clerical error is the most common reason for a potentially life-threatening hemolytic transfusion reaction!).

3. Blood products should be administered through an 18-ga or larger intravenous (IV) catheter. A standard 170-μm filter (present in most transfusion tubing kits) should be utilized in all transfusions.

4. The only fluid that should run along with the blood product is normal saline. Hypotonic solutions may cause hemolysis; lactated Ringer's solution contains calcium and may lead to clotting.

5. The patient should be monitored regularly during the transfusion and observed for any untoward reaction.

6. The rate of transfusion should be as fast as the patient's clinical status allows: patients in shock require rapid blood product administration, hypovolemic patients also tolerate fairly rapid administration, but individuals with cardiac dysfunction need to be transfused more slowly (packed red cell units must always be administered in < 4 hours, however, to minimize the risks of bacterial contamination).

E. Potential Complications

1. **Acute Hemolytic Reaction.** This is the most dangerous consequence of a mismatched transfusion. It is usually a consequence of a clerical error, and it is due to recipient antibodies against the transfused red cells, which result in rapid intravascular hemolysis of the transfused cells.

    a. **Signs and Symptoms.** Fever, chills, restlessness, anxiety, flushing, chest or back pain, tachycardia, and tachypnea. Shock may occur. In an unconscious patient, hypotension or bleeding may be the only manifestation. Extravascular hemolysis is usually due to Rh incompatibility and is associated with malaise and fever; shock and renal failure are uncommon with Rh incompatibility.

    b. **Management**

        i. Immediately stop the transfusion!

        ii. Replace all IV tubing.

        iii. Support the patient's airway, breathing, and circulation as required with oxygen and IV crystalloid (use pressors if necessary).

        iv. Check for any clerical error.

        v. Notify the blood bank immediately and send them the following: the remainder of the unused unit and two samples of the patient's blood (one sample in a red-topped tube, the other sample in an ethylenediaminetetraacetic acid [EDTA] tube).

        vi. Obtain samples of the patient's blood for the following laboratory tests: complete blood count (CBC) (with platelets), electrolyte panel, blood urea nitrogen (BUN), creatinine, bilirubin, prothrombin time (PT), partial thromboplastin time (PTT), thrombin time, fibrinogen, and fibrinogen degradation products.

        vii. Place a Foley catheter, examine a freshly voided urine specimen for free hemoglobin, and maintain a urine output $\geq$ 1-2 mL/kg/hr with aggressive IV hydration (supplemented with mannitol [25–50 g IV] or furosemide [20–40 mg or more IV] if necessary). Hemodynamic monitoring may be required in the unstable patient.

        viii. Alkalinize the urine to enhance free hemoglobin excretion.

        ix. Consult a nephrologist and hematologist.

2. **Febrile Reaction.** This is the most common transfusion reaction (estimated incidence of 1–3%). It is caused by pre-existing recipient antibodies to donor leukocyte and platelet antigens. Signs and symptoms, besides fever and chills, may include chest pain, cough, dyspnea, headache, hypotension, myalgias, tachycardia, and/or vomiting. Initial treatment should include stopping the transfusion and *ruling out* a life-threatening hemolytic transfusion reaction as outlined under II. E. 1, above. After a hemolytic transfusion reaction has been ruled out, management should be symptomatic and may include acetaminophen (650–1000 mg orally [PO] or rectally [PR]) and diphenhydramine (50 mg intramuscularly [IM] or IV). If recurrent febrile reactions are a problem, consider utilizing leukocyte-poor red cells, premedication with acetaminophen and diphenhydramine, and/or the use of a leukocyte filter.

3. **Allergic Reactions.** These reactions are due to the interaction of antibodies to plasma proteins. The most common manifestation of this reaction is urticaria. The transfusion does not need to be stopped, but diphenhydramine (25–50 mg IM or IV) should be administered. An actual anaphylactic reaction may occur and is generally due to IgA deficiency (incidence 1:650) in the recipient. An anaphylactic reaction should be treated by stopping the transfusion and administering epinephrine (0.3–0.5 mg subcutaneously [SQ], IM, or, in severe cases, starting an epinephrine IV infusion [2-10 μg/min IV]), corticosteroids (125 mg Solu-Medrol IV), and inhaled beta agonists for wheezing.

   Individuals known to be IgA deficient or who have had a prior anaphylactic reaction to a red cell transfusion should receive washed red cells in the future.

4. **Alloimmunization.** This results from the development of antibodies against donor antigens, which may result in hemolytic or nonhemolytic transfusion reactions and a decreased red cell increment in subsequent transfusions.

5. **Delayed Hemolytic Transfusion Reactions.** These may occur up to several weeks after a transfusion and are due to an undectable level of antibody in the recipient to the donor's cells that results in an amnestic immune response. Patients may present with a rising bilirubin level and a fall in their hemoglobin level with a positive Coomb's test. These reactions may be serious and should be treated similarly to acute hemolytic reactions.

6. **Graft Versus Host Disease (GVHD).** This occurs as a consequence of donor T lymphocytes engrafting, multiplying, and attacking a severely immunocompromised recipient. Signs and symptoms (which usually occur within 1 week) may include bone marrow suppression, erythematous maculopapular skin rash, fever, gastrointestinal complaints (anorexia, nausea, vomiting, diarrhea), and liver abnormalities (including abnormal liver function tests and hepatomegaly). Death may result. The best treatment of GVHD is its prevention by gamma irradiation of all cellular blood components prior to transfusion in at-risk patients (e.g., patients with leukemia, lymphoma, or other significant immunocompromised disease states).

7. **Infections.** Despite extremely careful modern blood bank procedures, a small but definite risk of human immunodeficiency virus (HIV), hepatitis B and C, and/or syphilis transmission remains when a blood product is transfused. Blood may also become contaminated during handling, leading to transfusion of endotoxin and bacteria. Other agents that may be transmitted via blood transfusion include non-A-non-B-non-C hepatitis, CMV, Epstein-Barr virus, malaria, babesiosis, and trypanosomiasis.

8. **Massive Transfusion.** A massive transfusion is defined as the replacement of one or more patient blood volumes (about 10 units). Such a transfusion requirement may occur in the setting of trauma or significant gastrointestinal hemorrhage. The complications associated with massive transfusion are outlined below:

a. Bleeding is due to depletion of platelets and coagulation factors. The platelet count, PT, and PTT should be checked regularly (i.e., after every 4–5 units transfused). Replacement of platelets depends on the circumstances (see III, below); coagulation factors should be replaced when the PT or PTT is > 1.5 times control in the setting of recent or ongoing bleeding.

b. Hypothermia may occur in the setting of transfused refrigerated blood; cardiac arrhythmias may result. Efficient blood warmers should be utilized when multiple units are to be transfused.

c. Citrate intoxication occurs most commonly in patients with a massive, rapid transfusion or in those with significant liver disease. Hypocalcemia, tetany, hypomagnesemia, and/or cardiac irritability may result. The patient's ionized calcium and the QT-interval on the electrocardiogram (ECG) (QT prolongation occurs with hypocalcemia) should be monitored periodically. Symptomatic hypocalcemia should be treated as necessary with calcium chloride (1–10 mL of a 10% solution IV).

d. Other electrolyte abnormalities may include hyperkalemia (stored blood has a potassium concentration ≤ 20 mEq/L) and acidosis, though these are relatively rare. Serum electrolytes should be periodically monitored and abnormalities treated as clinically indicated.

e. Miscellaneous problems may include volume overload, congestive heart failure, and noncardiogenic pulmonary edema.

III. PLATELET TRANSFUSIONS

A. Indications

1. Platelets are generally transfused to prevent or control bleeding due to thrombocytopenia unassociated with immune-mediated thrombocytopenia.

2. Patients who are not bleeding can usually maintain hemostasis if the platelet count is ≥ 10,000/μL. Most clinicians recommend a platelet transfusion if the count is below this level in the nonbleeding patient.

3. Patients actively bleeding, or those who require surgery or an invasive procedure, need to maintain a platelet count ≥ 50,000/μL. Patients who have a low platelet count because of a consumptive coagulopathy may require platelet support until the underlying cause is corrected.

B. Available Platelet Products

1. **Random-Donor Platelets.** Platelet concentrates are prepared by centrifuging whole blood. One unit of platelets contains about 5×10^{10} platelets in 50 mL plasma and will generally increase the patient's platelet count by 5000–10,000/µL. When a platelet transfusion is needed, the usual order is for 4–10 units. Patients with a fever, a consumptive process, or a previous transfusion may have a smaller than expected increment to the transfusion.

2. **Single-Donor Random Platelets.** These are obtained by pheresis of a single volunteer donor. Single-donor platelets usually provide a yield similar to 6–10 units of platelets with a decreased risk of alloimmunization.

3. **Human Leukocyte Antigen (HLA)-Matched Platelets.** These are rarely used in the ED. They are obtained by pheresis of an HLA-matched donor for those patients who have become alloimmunized and fail to respond to random-donor platelets. They should not be used if the donor is also a potential bone marrow donor.

C. Administration

Platelet transfusions should be matched for ABO and Rh compatibility to decrease alloimmunization, but crossmatch procedures are not used. Like red cells, platelets should be administered through a filter to eliminate microaggregates. If patients chill with platelet administration, special filters may also be employed to remove the leukocytes.

D. Potential Complications

Complications are similar to those associated with red cell transfusions; hemolytic transfusion reactions do not occur.

IV. PLASMA TRANSFUSION

Plasma component factors that might be utilized in the ED include fresh frozen plasma and cryoprecipitate.

A. Fresh Frozen Plasma (FFP)

1. One unit of FFP contains all clotting factors and has a volume of 200–250 mL. It is obtained by freezing (at $-18°C$) the plasma separated from a unit of whole blood within 8 hours of that unit's collection.

2. FFP may be used to treat clinically significant bleeding, or to prevent excessive hemorrhage prior to surgery or an invasive procedure, in the setting of a coagulopathy (i.e., PT or PTT > 1.5 times control). The coagulopathy may be secondary to any of the following: an unknown coagulation factor deficiency (e.g., V, VIII, IX, XI), liver disease, warfarin use, heparin use,

a massive blood transfusion, or disseminated intravascular coagulation (DIC). FFP may also be utilized in the setting of a therapeutic plasma exchange.

3. A unit of FFP will generally increase clotting factors by 2–3%, and the usual starting dose is 2 units. FFP must be ABO compatible with the patient, should be used within 2–6 hours of thawing, and must be administered through a blood transfusion filter.

4. FFP may cause allergic reactions and has the same risk of disease transmission as whole blood.

B. Cryoprecipitate

1. Cryoprecipitate is prepared by slowly thawing a unit of FFP at 1–6°C and collecting the white proteinaceous precipitate that forms. It is rich in fibrinogen and also contains factor VIII:C, factor VIII, von Willebrand's factor, and factor XIII.

2. It may be used in the treatment of patients with hemophilia or von Willebrand's disease, or in those individuals who are hypofibrinogenemic as a consequence of a congenital deficiency, liver disease, or a consumptive coagulopathy.

3. Cryoprecipitate should be thawed like FFP and administered through a blood filter. ABO compatibility is desirable but not mandatory.

   Dosing.
   a. In hypofibrinogenemia: empirically administer 1 unit of cryoprecipitate for every 5 kg body weight.
   b. In von Willebrand's disease: standard dose is 1 unit of cryoprecipitate per 10 kg of body weight.
   c. In hemophilia A:
      number of units of cryoprecipitate = [(plasma volume in mL × % increase in factor VIII needed) / 100] / 80

4. Viral transmission is a risk with cryoprecipitate administration.

V. PEARLS AND PITFALLS

A. Meticulously follow identification procedures and correctly label specimens in all circumstances and especially when blood is drawn for type and crossmatch purposes.

B. Meticulously identify the patient and the blood for that patient, and double check both before starting any transfusion procedure.

C. Use component therapy rather than whole blood.

D. Use irradiated blood products in patients who are leukopenic or who are otherwise at risk for GVHD (consult a hematologist when in doubt).

E. Immediately stop a transfusion when a hemolytic transfusion reaction is suspected.

F. A transfusion may be continued and symptomatic treatment initiated in the setting of an urticarial reaction.

G. Use low-titer O-negative blood only when mandated by a critical life-threatening hemorrhage or profound and imminently life-threatening anemia.

H. Periodically check platelets, coagulation factors, ionized calcium, and the ECG in massively transfused patients. Rewarm blood components prior to administration in this setting.

I. Consider utilizing FFP to temporarily correct the PT in patients who are on warfarin, rather than vitamin K, because of the difficulty in restoring adequate therapeutic anticoagulation after vitamin K is given.

Do *not* do any of the following:

A. Transfuse red cells in otherwise healthy anemic patients who only complain of fatigue when their hemoglobin level is > 7 g/dL.

B. Transfuse red cells when crystalloid could be utilized for vital sign support.

C. Transfuse platelets in patients with autoimmune thrombocytopenia.

D. Transfuse platelets in a nonbleeding surgical patient when the platelet count is ≥ 50,000/µL.

E. Transfuse plasma for the purposes of volume expansion or as a nutritional supplement.

BIBLIOGRAPHY

Development Task Force of the College of American Pathologists: Practice parameter for the use of fresh-frozen plasma, cryoprecipitate, and platelets. JAMA 1994;271(10): 777–781.

Labadie LL: Transfusion therapy in the emergency department. Emerg Med Clin N Am 1993; 11(21):379–406.

Masouredis SP, Nusbacher J, Murphy S, et al: Preservation and clinical use of blood and blood components. In Williams WJ, Beutler E, Erslev AJ, et al (eds): Hematology, 4th ed. New York, McGraw-Hill, 1990, pp. 1628–1673.

Mollison PL: Blood Transfusion in Clinical Medicine, 8th ed. Philadelphia, JB Lippincott, 1989.

EPIDURAL SPINAL CORD COMPRESSION

*"To learn how to treat disease,
one must learn how to recognize it."*

JEAN MARTIN CHARCOT (1825–1893)

I. ESSENTIAL FACTS

A. Definition

Epidural spinal cord compression is compression of the spinal cord and/or the cauda equina by an extrinsic mass in the epidural space. This mass is usually secondary to metastatic cancer of the vertebral body; occasionally, epidural compression may arise from tumor extension through the intravertebral space to the paravertebral space. Intramedullary or leptomeningeal metastases may also occur. *Spinal cord compression is a true neurologic emergency that may cause sensory abnormalities, bowel and bladder dysfunction, and/or paralysis.*

B. Epidemiology

1. Epidural cord compression occurs in approximately 5% of patients who die of cancer (about 20,000 patients per year in the United States).
2. Breast, lung, and prostate cancer account for 50% of cases. Other responsible malignancies include lymphoma, multiple myeloma, melanoma, and renal cell carcinoma. In children, the most common responsible malignancies are sarcoma, neuroblastoma, and lymphoma.
3. The involved regions of the spinal cord include
   a. Thoracic spine (most common site: 60% of cases).
   b. Lumbosacral spine (25%).
   c. Cervical spine (15%).

II. CLINICAL EVALUATION

A. History

1. Determine whether there is a current or prior history of cancer, back complaints, neurologic complaints, trauma, other health problems, medication use, and drug allergies.
2. Thoroughly inquire about back pain, other pain, muscle weakness, sensory abnormalities, and bowel/bladder/sexual dysfunction.

B. Symptoms

1. Pain: in 95% of adult patients the initial symptom is pain (which may be spinal, radicular, or referred).
   a. Cancer-related back pain tends to be insidious in nature and progressive in severity. It usually precedes sensory and autonomic dysfunction by weeks to months.
   b. Radicular pain may be intermittent and is easily confused with other visceral ailments (e.g., pleurisy).
   c. Referred pain may occur in an area removed from the involved region of the spinal cord (e.g., an L1 lesion may cause pain in the iliac crests).

d. An electric shock-like sensation shooting down the body with neck flexion (Lhermitte's sign) may be due to an epidural lesion in the cervical spine.

2. Distinguishing degenerative spinal disease from epidural compression can be difficult:

   a. Pain from degenerative disease tends to be localized to the low lumbar and/or cervical spine, is stable and well known to the patient, and is improved by recumbency.

   b. Pain from epidural compression is usually progressive, frequently involves the thoracic spine, tends to be well localized, improves during the course of the day and is worse at night, is aggravated by coughing or sneezing, and is worse with recumbency (e.g., bedrest).

3. Neurologic complaints may include sensory dysfunction (including dysesthesia, hypesthesia, numbness, and tingling; and/or abnormalities of proprioception, temperature, and vibration), motor complaints (weakness progressing to paralysis), and/or autonomic dysfunction (early complaints of constipation, urinary hesitancy, and incomplete bladder emptying may progress to urinary retention, incontinence [bowel or bladder], and sphincter abnormalities). The location of the tumor determines the neurologic deficit.

C. Physical Examination

1. Obtain vital signs and perform a directed skin, HEENT, neck, back, chest, heart, abdominal, genital, rectal, and extremity examination.

2. Perform a careful neurologic examination. Early in the course of epidural cord compression, pain may be elicited by percussion over the spine. Since most epidural lesions are dorsal, the cortical spinal tracts, posterior columns, and spinocerebellar tracts are commonly affected, resulting in motor weakness, spasticity, and hyperactive reflexes. The specific deficits depend on the location of the lesion(s):

   a. Cervical and thoracic spine:

      i. Spasticity and hyperactive reflexes are early signs of myelopathy.

      ii. Plantar responses may be abnormal (i.e., upgoing toes).

      iii. Proprioception and vibratory senses in the feet may be abnormal.

      iv. Weakness progressing to paraplegia or quadraplegia is a late finding.

      v. A palpable bladder may be present; incontinence is a late finding.

   b. T12-L1:

      i. Sphincter dysfunction may occur.

      ii. Perineal sensory loss may result in absent bulbocavernosus and cremasteric reflexes.

c. Below L1:
   i. Cauda equina syndrome may occur secondary to the involvement of multiple nerve roots, with resultant saddle anesthesia, decreased sphincter tone, sensory abnormalities, bilateral sciatica, lower-extremity flaccid motor weakness, and/or bowel/bladder/sexual dysfunction. Motor and sensory loss may be asymmetric.
   ii. Reflexes may be diminished. Plantar reflexes are normal.
   Caution: a completely normal neurologic examination does not rule out early epidural spinal cord compression.

D. Diagnostic Evaluation

1. **Laboratory Studies**
   There are no laboratory studies that assist in the diagnosis. Cerebrospinal fluid findings are nonspecific, and a lumbar puncture should *not* be performed unless meningitis is strongly suspected (lumbar puncture may worsen the neurologic deficit in the setting of epidural compression).

2. **Radiographic Studies**
   a. **Roentgenography.** This study reveals metastatic spinal disease in 85% of patients with epidural compression, particularly in individuals with breast or lung cancer. Abnormalities seen may include lytic lesions, blastic lesions, vertebral body collapse, eroded pedicles, or soft tissue masses. Roentgenograms are less likely to be abnormal in individuals with lymphoma or a pediatric neoplasm.
   b. **Radionuclide Bone Scanning.** This study is more sensitive but less specific than plain roentgenography, and it may not detect lesions due to multiple myeloma. A bone scan is reasonable in patients at risk for spinal metastatic disease who have a normal neurologic examination and unremarkable plain films.
   c. **Spinal Computed Tomography (CT).** This is more sensitive and specific than either plain roentgenography or radionuclide bone scanning in distinguishing malignant from benign vertebral disease. Spinal CT alone, however, is not very sensitive in detecting epidural involvement.
   d. **CT-Myelography.** Until recently, this was the imaging study of choice to confirm epidural spinal cord compression. CT-myelography should be performed in a patient suspected of epidural compression when magnetic resonance imaging (MRI) is unavailable or the patient cannot tolerate MRI (e.g., because of a cardiac pacemaker).
   e. **MRI.** A total-spine MRI is the study of choice, when available, to detect epidural compression. It is as good or better than myelography in this setting; contrast-enhanced

MRI is superior in detecting leptomeningeal masses. MRI is also the study of choice to detect vertebral metastases and paravertebral masses.

III. DIFFERENTIAL DIAGNOSIS

The many causes of back pain include degenerative joint disease, infections, herniated lumbar disc, Paget's disease, trauma, and visceral referred pain (see Chapter 3 for a more extensive differential diagnosis). *In any patient with cancer and back pain, epidural cord compression must be excluded because of the devastating consequences associated with undiagnosed and untreated cord compression!*

IV. THERAPY

A. Corticosteroids

1. Corticosteroids should be promptly given to the patient with either confirmed epidural spinal cord compression or those in whom the diagnosis is strongly suspected clinically while awaiting diagnostic imaging.

2. Dexamethasone is the steroid of choice:

   Dose: 10–100 mg IV initially, followed by 4–24 mg four times per day. The larger doses (i.e., 100 mg IV followed by 24 mg IV every 6 hours) should be used in patients with rapidly progressive or significant neurologic abnormalities, the smaller doses for patients with no or only mild neurologic impairment. Dexamethasone will subsequently be slowly tapered over the course of radiotherapy.

B. Consultation

A neurosurgeon, oncologist, and radiation oncologist should be consulted immediately.

C. Definitive Care

1. Radiotherapy is generally the definitive treatment of choice, and patient outcome correlates with neurologic status at the time of diagnosis. More than 80% of ambulatory patients prior to initiation of therapy will remain ambulatory after radiotherapy; unfortunately, only 10% of paraplegic patients will regain ambulatory function with treatment.

2. Surgical intervention with laminectomy followed by radiotherapy is associated with an increase in morbidity. Neurosurgical intervention (i.e., anterior decompression with spinal stabilization), however, is appropriate in the following patient circumstances:
   a. The diagnosis of the lesion is in doubt or the patient is without a prior tissue diagnosis.

b. Epidural cord compression is occurring in a previously irradiated field.

c. Progressive neurologic deterioration is occurring during the course of radiotherapy despite high-dose corticosteroids.

d. Spinal instability.

e. Radioresistant tumors.

f. Intractable pain.

V. DISPOSITION

Patients with suspected or confirmed epidural spinal cord compression should be hospitalized.

VI. PEARLS AND PITFALLS

A. Consider epidural spinal cord compression in any patient with a history of cancer and back pain.

B. Consider epidural spinal cord compression in any cancer patient with unexplained, atypical, or apparently referred pain.

C. Begin dexamethasone as soon as possible if cord compression is clinically suspected—even before definitive diagnostic imaging.

D. Total-spine MRI should be performed in suspected epidural cord compression.

E. Consult a neurosurgeon and radiation oncologist early.

F. A patient being treated for known epidural cord compression who presents with worsening symptoms should receive the maximum dexamethasone dose; a neurosurgeon should be immediately consulted.

Do *not* do any of the following:

A. Exclude the possibility of epidural cord compression on the basis of normal spinal roentgenograms.

B. Exclude the possibility of cord compression because of prior radiotherapy for same.

C. Discharge the patient if there is any neurologic deficit.

BIBLIOGRAPHY

Byrne T: Spinal cord compression from epidural metastases. N Engl J Med 1992;327: 614–619.
Maguire WM: Mechanical complications of cancer. Emerg Med Clin N Am 1993;11(2): 421–430.
Wilson JK, Masaryk TJ: Neurologic emergencies in the cancer patient. Semin Oncol 1989;16: 490–503.

Superior Vena Cava Syndrome

> *"Symptoms, then, are in reality nothing but the cry from suffering organs."*
>
> Jean Martin Charcot

I. ESSENTIAL FACTS

A. Definition

The *superior vena cava* (SVC) *syndrome* is caused by the partial obstruction of blood flow through the superior vena cava. Impaired blood return to the right side of the heart results in elevated venous pressure in the head, neck, upper extremities, and thorax, leading to facial and upper-extremity edema, tracheal edema, potential airway compromise, pericardial effusion, and/or pleural effusions. Impaired cardiac output may also cause headache, decreased visual acuity, altered consciousness, and central nervous system (CNS) damage.

B. Etiology

1. Four pathophysiologic events may cause the SVC syndrome: compression, invasion, thrombosis, or fibrosis.

2. In > 80% of patients extrinsic compression of the SVC is caused by a mediastinal malignancy, most commonly bronchogenic carcinoma or lymphoma. The SVC syndrome occurs in 3–8% of patients with lung cancer or lymphoma.

II. CLINICAL EVALUATION

A. History

1. Inquire about the presence and duration of facial and upper-extremity swelling, chest pain, dyspnea, cough, headache, and neurologic complaints.

2. Determine whether the patient has a current or prior history of cancer, tuberculosis, thyroid disease, sarcoidosis, indwelling subclavian catheter, and/or aortic aneurysm.

B. Symptoms and Signs

1. Patients often present with edema of the face, neck, upper extremities, and/or upper thorax. Dyspnea is frequent and is more severe in the supine position.

2. Additional symptoms may include cough, dizziness, dysphagia, headache, hoarseness, mental status changes, seizures, syncope, and/or visual complaints.

3. Signs may include tachypnea, distended neck and upper-extremity veins, facial swelling, plethora, and cyanosis.

Engorged collateral circulation may result in dilated superficial veins of the chest, neck, or sublingual area. Stridor is rare but when present requires emergent evaluation and treatment. Confusion and disorientation are both consistent with elevated intracranial pressure.

C. Physical Examination

1. **General.** Quickly note degree of patient distress and any evidence of airway compromise requiring immediate intervention.

2. **Vital Signs.** Note tachycardia, tachypnea, blood pressure, temperature, and oxygen saturation.

3. **Skin.** Check for prominent superficial veins on the chest, neck, and upper extremities.

4. **HEENT.** Evaluate for facial swelling and/or plethora.

5. **Neck.** Note suppleness, nodes, jugular venous distention, stridor, and any palpable thyroid abnormalities.

6. **Lymph Nodes.** Evaluate for prominent supraclavicular, cervical, or axillary adenopathy that may be appropriate for tissue biopsy in a patient without a prior cancer diagnosis.

7. **Chest.** Note wheezes, rales, and/or rhonchi. Carefully evaluate for pleural effusions.

8. **Heart.** Listen for murmurs, rubs, and/or gallops.

9. **Abdomen.** Note distention, bowel sounds, tenderness, masses, and/or findings of localized peritoneal irritation. Note whether stool is heme positive.

10. **Extremities.** Evaluate for clubbing, cyanosis, and edema.

11. **Central Nervous System.** Note mental status and perform a thorough neurologic examination.

D. Laboratory Studies

1. The following are appropriate initially:
   a. Arterial blood gas (ABG).
   b. Complete blood count (CBC) with platelets.
   c. Electrolyte panel.
   d. Glucose, blood urea nitrogen, and creatinine levels.
   e. Calcium, magnesium, and phosphate.
   f. Prothrombin time/partial thromboplastin time (PT/PTT).
   g. Electrocardiogram (ECG).
   h. Chest roentgenogram.
   i. Urinalysis.
2. Additional imaging studies include the following:
   a. Chest computed tomography (CT) is the imaging modality of choice in the patient with suspected SVC syndrome to further evaluate the mediastinum.

    b. Head CT is also appropriate if the neurologic examination is abnormal to evaluate for possible concomitant intracranial metastases.

    c. Angiography, radionuclide venography, or Doppler examination may determine the location of the obstruction. These studies are generally not required, however, as the chest CT is usually definitive.

III. DIFFERENTIAL DIAGNOSIS

A. Malignancy (e.g., bronchogenic carcinoma, lymphoma) is the most frequent cause of the SVC syndrome (80–97% of patients).

B. Other causes may include aortic aneurysm, benign cysts, central venous lines, fibrosis, goiter, histoplasmosis, sarcoidosis, thrombi, trauma, tuberculosis, and vasculitides.

C. Conditions that may mimic the SVC syndrome include pericardial tamponade, congestive heart failure, and/or large pleural effusions. Unlike the SVC syndrome, these disorders do not usually present with upper-extremity edema.

IV. THERAPY

Note: The treatment priorities of the ED physician are to support airway, vital signs, and mental status (death from the SVC syndrome occurs secondary to either airway obstruction or increased intracranial pressure); to appropriately diagnose the SVC syndrome and initiate urgent consultant involvement; and to facilitate initiation of definitive care. Most patients presenting with the SVC syndrome are *not* at imminent risk for death; tissue biopsy of the suspected lesion causing the syndrome should precede radiotherapy (or chemotherapy) in most circumstances.

A. Initial Management

Secure and support airway, breathing, and circulation.

1. Guard the airway, have suction on and at the bedside, and provide supplemental oxygen. *Elevate the head of the bed to help alleviate cerebral edema.*

    a. Quickly assess the patient's gag reflex, cough, and breathing.

    b. Intubation is appropriate if

       i. The patient is unable to protect the airway.

       ii. The patient has inadequate spontaneous ventilations.

       iii. Oxygenation is inadequate (< 90% hemoglobin saturation despite 100% oxygen supplementation).

       iv. The patient's airway is in imminent risk of obstruction secondary to severe edema.

       v. Hyperventilation (PCO_2 25–30 mmHg) is required to emergently reduce increased intracranial pressure.

    Caution: endotracheal intubation may be extremely difficult because of distorted head/neck/airway anatomy from soft tissue swelling. Fiberoptic-guided intubation may be necessary.

2. *Simultaneously* with the above, supporting ED staff should obtain vital signs, intravenous (IV) access (upper-extremity swelling may mandate obtaining IV access in the lower extremities), a chest film, ECG, and appropriate laboratory values (see II, above).

3. *Hypotension* (systolic blood pressure [BP] < 90 mmHg) should be treated initially with normal saline (NS) or lactated Ringer's (LR) infusion; monitor pulmonary status and cardiac function closely.

   a. Use pressors if severe head/neck/upper-extremity swelling or clinical evidence of pulmonary edema (cardiogenic or non-cardiogenic) contraindicates further fluid administration in the hypotensive patient. In most instances dopamine will be the drug of choice (*dose:* begin with 2-5 µg/kg/min IV and adjust infusion as necessary for systolic BP of 95–100 mmHg).

   b. *Caution:* if the patient is hemodynamically stable, *do not* aggressively infuse crystalloid.

B. Confirmation of the Diagnosis of the SVC Syndrome

1. Arrange for chest CT (see II. D. 2, above).

2. Obtain appropriate consultation (e.g., oncologist, radiation oncologist, pulmonary specialist, thoracic surgeon).

C. Adjunctive Medical Therapy

1. *Diuretics* are appropriate in the hemodynamically stable patient with dyspnea or mental status changes and may provide temporary symptomatic relief. Consider furosemide (20-40 mg IV).

2. The role of *corticosteroids* is controversial, but patients with clinical evidence of increased intracranial pressure may benefit. Consider dexamethasone (10 mg IV every 6 hours).

D. Definitive Care

Optimal definitive treatment of the SVC syndrome will occur outside of the ED, after the cause of the syndrome has been accurately determined. Since most cases are secondary to malignancy, this ultimately requires tissue biopsy *prior to* radiation or chemotherapy.

1. **Radiotherapy.** Radiotherapy is the treatment of choice for the SVC syndrome due to most malignancies. Many patients respond within 72 hours, and ≥ 90% of patients will respond to radiotherapy within 3 weeks.

2. **Chemotherapy.** Chemotherapy is very effective when the SVC syndrome is secondary to small cell lung cancer or

lymphoma. In this setting, chemotherapeutic agents should *not* be administered into high-pressure upper-extremity veins.

3. **Surgery.** Surgery is most likely to benefit patients with acute onset of severe symptoms and concomitant signs of rapidly progressive airway obstruction or significant cerebral edema, nonmalignant causes of the SVC syndrome, or malignancies resistant to radiation or chemotherapy.

4. **Anticoagulation.** When the SVC syndrome is secondary to thrombosis (e.g., associated with an indwelling central venous catheter), anticoagulation with heparin is indicated. If a central venous catheter is present and symptoms/signs do not improve within several days, the indwelling line should be removed.

V. DISPOSITION

A. Discharge

Patients with a previously diagnosed malignancy who present with only *mild symptoms* of the SVC syndrome may be discharged to home if *all* of the following conditions apply:

1. There is absolutely no evidence of airway compromise, dyspnea, or increased intracranial pressure.
2. Vital signs are normal.
3. Patient is reliable and has an adequate home situation.
4. Consultation with an oncologist has been made.
5. Follow-up is arranged within 24 hours.

B. Admit

Patients who do not have a tissue diagnosis or who have evidence of rapidly progressive symptoms should be hospitalized for evaluation and definitive care.

VI. PEARLS AND PITFALLS

A. Temporizing measures to provide symptomatic relief of the SVC syndrome in the ED include oxygen supplementation, necessary airway and vital sign support, elevation of the head of the bed, and administration of diuretics.

B. Ninety percent of cases of the SVC syndrome are caused by malignancy. A tissue diagnosis of the causative malignancy needs to be established promptly. Appropriate consultation should be obtained urgently to facilitate this process prior to initiation of radiation or chemotherapy.

C. In patients who have a known malignancy but who also have an indwelling central venous catheter, catheter-associated thrombosis as a cause of the SVC syndrome should be considered. Any central venous catheter, including cardiac pacemakers, may cause SVC obstruction.

BIBLIOGRAPHY

Helms SR, Carlson MD: Cardiovascular Emergencies. Semin Oncol 1989;16:463–470.
Maguire WM: Mechanical complications of cancer. Emerg Med Clin N Am 1993;11(2): 421–430.
Nieto AF, Doty DB: Superior vena cava obstruction: Clinical syndrome, etiology, and treatment. Curr Probl Cancer 1986;10:443–484.
Yaholom J: Superior vena cava syndrome in DeVita V, Hellman S, Rosenberg S (eds): Cancer, Principles and Practice of Oncology, 3rd Ed. Philadelphia, JB Lippincott, 1989.

22

Rheumatologic Emergencies

*"The rheumatism is a common name for
many aches and pains, which have yet got no peculiar appellation,
though owing to very different causes."*

WILLIAM HEBERDEN (1710–1801)

EVALUATION OF THE PATIENT WITH ARTHRITIS

I. INTRODUCTION

Patients may present to the ED with a variety of conditions causing the chief complaint of "joint pain."

A. *Arthritis* occurs when structures within the joint capsule (e.g., synovium, articular cartilage, menisci) are inflamed or injured. Under these circumstances, the joint discomfort is secondary to an abnormality within the joint itself (articular cause).

B. Joint pain may also arise from an abnormality *outside* of the joint, including dysfunction of structures around the joint (periarticular causes; see Table 22–1), or from structures completely removed from the joint area (referred pain; see Table 22–2).

C. To distinguish among articular, periarticular, and referred causes of joint pain, a careful history and physical examination are mandatory. This chapter will address the *articular* causes of joint discomfort.

Table 22-1. PERIARTICULAR CAUSES OF JOINT PAIN

Bursitis	Muscle strain
Fasciitis	Myofascial pain
Ligament sprain	Tendinitis

Table 22-2. REFERRED CAUSES OF JOINT PAIN

Nerve entrapment	Tumors
Osteomyelitis	Vasculopathy
Radiculopathy	

II. CLINICAL EVALUATION

A. History

The history should include a thorough inquiry into the patient's presenting complaint (including trauma history), other active medical problems, past medical and surgical history, medication use, and allergies. In further assessing the patient's joint pain, the following five questions are important in arriving at a final diagnosis:

1. *Is the arthritis inflammatory or noninflammatory?*
    a. Joint pain and stiffness are typically worse with rest and upon awakening in patients with inflammatory conditions. The stiffness persists for at least 30 minutes after rising and usually lasts much longer. Joint complaints generally improve with activity (except in inflammatory arthritis secondary to infection or crystal deposition, in which any joint activity is extremely painful).
    b. Patients with noninflammatory conditions have minimal morning stiffness (< 15 minutes), and pain is most prominent with movement of the affected joint(s).
    c. Documentation of an inflammatory arthritis often requires arthrocentesis and synovial fluid analysis (see II. C, below).

2. *Is the condition acute or chronic?*
    a. Acute arthritis implies a rapid onset and duration < 8 weeks. Important causes of acute monoarticular arthritis include infection, crystal deposition (e.g., gout and pseudogout), and trauma. *Nongonococcal bacterial infections are the most worrisome and significant causes of acute monoarthritis in the ED;* they can result in the destruction of articular cartilage in as little as 1–2 days.
    b. Arthritis that has been present for ≥ 8 weeks is termed *chronic.*

3. *What is the pattern of joint involvement?*
    a. The pattern of joint involvement is useful in limiting the

differential diagnosis. Tables 22–3 to 22–5 list the most common causes of arthritis by their pattern: monoarticular (one joint), pauciarticular (two to five joints), or polyarticular (six or more joints).

b. Recognition of either of two additional disease patterns, episodic and migratory, is also helpful in making the diagnosis (Table 22–6).

4. *Are there associated systemic features?* The patient's arthritis may be the most prominent manifestation of a systemic disease. Inquire about symptoms and signs referrable to other organ systems, especially the skin, eyes, heart, and gastrointestinal and genitourinary systems. Systemic features will be

Table 22–3. CAUSES OF MONOARTHRITIS

INFLAMMATORY	NONINFLAMMATORY
Infection	Trauma/fracture
	Osteoarthritis
Neisseria gonorrhoeae	Avascular necrosis
Other bacteria	Synovial neoplasm
Endocarditis	
Tuberculosis	
Fungi	
Lyme disease	
Crystals	
Urate (gout)	
Calcium pyrophosphate	
Hydroxyapatite	
Spondyloarthropathy	
Ankylosing spondylitis	
Reiter's syndrome	
Psoriatic arthritis	
Miscellaneous	
Palindromic rheumatism	

Table 22–4. CAUSES OF PAUCIARTHRITIS

INFLAMMATORY	NONINFLAMMATORY
Infection	Osteoarthritis
Endocarditis	
Neisseria gonorrhoeae	
Rheumatic fever	
Lyme disease	
Crystals	
Polymyalgia rheumatica	
Spondyloarthropathy	
Sarcoidosis	

Table 22–5. CAUSES OF POLYARTHRITIS

INFLAMMATORY	NONINFLAMMATORY
Viral infection	Primary osteoarthritis
Human parvovirus B19	Fibromyalgia
Hepatitis B	
Rubella	
Serum sickness	
Antibiotics	
Rheumatoid arthritis	
Systemic lupus erythematosus	
Other connective-tissue diseases	
Scleroderma	
Polymyositis	
Mixed connective-tissue disease	

Table 22–6. EPISODIC AND MIGRATORY ARTHRIDITIES

EPISODIC	MIGRATORY
Crystal-induced arthritis	Rheumatic fever
Palindromic rheumatism	*Neisseria gonorrhoeae*
Reiter's syndrome	
Lyme arthritis	

discussed in greater detail with the individual conditions presented later.

5. *Do patient demographics narrow the differential diagnosis?* Patient characteristics, such as age, race, sex, and lifestyle, frequently assist in sorting out the diagnostic possibilities. This will be discussed in greater detail with the individual conditions.

B. Physical Examination

1. **Vital Signs.** Note pulse, blood pressure, respiratory rate, and temperature.

2. **Skin.** Examine carefully for rashes, recent needle sticks, and/or evidence of trauma. Subtle psoriatic patches may sometimes be seen between the buttocks or behind the ears. Look at the nails carefully for pitting (psoriasis) or splinter hemorrhages (endocarditis). Erythema nodosum may suggest inflammatory bowel disease, Behçet's syndrome, or sarcoidosis. *Keratoderma blennorrhagicum* (pustular psoriasis associated with Reiter's syndrome) often affects the palms of the hands and/or the soles of the feet.

3. **HEENT.** Closely examine the eyes and the oropharynx. Anterior uveitis is associated with the inflammatory spondy-

loarthopathies. Mouth ulcers may be seen in Behcet's syndrome, systemic lupus erythematosus, and Reiter's syndrome.

4. **Neck.** Look for tenderness, nodes, and thyroid abnormalities.

5. **Chest.** Listen for breath sounds, wheezes, rales, and rhonchi.

6. **Heart.** Evaluate for murmurs, rubs, and/or gallops.

7. **Abdomen.** Listen for bowel sounds. Examine for tenderness, organomegaly, or masses.

8. **Genitourinary.** Evaluate carefully for infection.

9. **Musculoskeletal.** All joints should be briefly examined and then a focus made on the painful joint(s). Note any swelling, tenderness, limitation of motion, and deformity. Allow the joint to be moved passively and actively, and palpate periarticular structures. Resisted range of motion will often accentuate a tendinitis or a muscle strain. *Remember:* a patient presenting with a very painful monoarthritis who will *not* allow joint movement probably has "bugs, blood, or crystals" (BBC) in that joint. Carefully evaluate neurovascular status.

C. Arthrocentesis and Synovial Fluid Analysis

1. Analysis of synovial fluid is an important adjunct to the history and physical examination in a patient with joint inflammation. Arthrocentesis will confirm the presence or absence of joint inflammation and is critical in the evaluation of joint infection and crystal-induced arthritis. The presence of fat droplets in the synovial fluid may suggest an undetected fracture.

2. Materials required for arthrocentesis include 1–2% lidocaine, sterile gloves, 10% povidone-iodine solution, syringes and needles, and necessary sterile drapes. After explaining the procedure to the patient and obtaining written consent, locate and mark the appropriate point of entry into the joint space. Cleanse the skin, drape the area, and anesthetize the skin and subcutaneous tissues with 1–2% lidocaine using a 25-gauge needle. Next, in a strictly sterile manner, attach the needle to an appropriately sized syringe and aspirate the joint fluid (a 22-gauge needle, at a minimum, should be used to aspirate fluid from a joint; if infection is suspected, use an 18-gauge needle).

3. In the ED, the following joints are those that require aspiration most frequently:
    a. Shoulder (Fig. 22–1): approach either anteriorly or posteriorly. *Anteriorly:* the joint is entered just lateral to the inferior edge of the coracoid process, with the needle directed medially and dorsally. Avoid the medial side of the coracoid process because of the presence of the thoracoacromial artery. *Posteriorly:* the needle is inserted approximately 1 cm inferior to the posterior tip of the acromion and directed in an anteromedial direction.

   b. Wrist (Fig. 22–2): flex the wrist slightly and approach the joint from the dorsal aspect just distal to either the radius or the ulna. The radial side is best entered just ulnar to the thumb extensor tendon at the edge of the distal radius; the ulnar side is entered at any point distal to the ulna, with the needle directed slightly radially.

   c. Knee (Fig. 22–3): this is the joint most commonly requiring aspiration. The best approach is medially, just below the patella, halfway between the patella's superior and inferior poles. Keep the needle parallel to the undersurface of the patella during aspiration. Applying

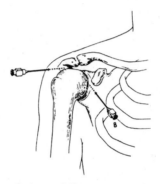

Figure 22–1. Injection of subacromial bursa or supraspinatus; **B,** anterior approach for injection of glenohumeral joint. (Illustration provided by Dr. D. Neustadt. From Rodman G, Schumacher HR (eds): Primer on the Rheumatic Diseases. 8th Ed. Arthritis Foundation, 1983.)

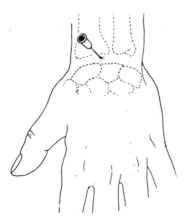

Figure 22–2. Arthrocentesis of the wrist (radial approach). (Illustration provided by Dr. D. Neustadt. From Rodman G, Schumacher HR (eds): Primer on the Rheumatic Diseases. 8th Ed. Arthritis Foundation, 1983.)

pressure to the suprapatellar area is helpful in maximizing the available fluid for removal. The quadriceps muscle needs to be relaxed in order to easily enter the joint and aspirate fluid.

    d. Ankle (Fig. 22–4): approach at a point just medial to the tibialis anterior tendon and lateral to the medial malleolus. Plantar flex the joint slightly; direct the needle posterolaterally.

4. Analyze the synovial fluid:

    a. Routine studies should include a cell count and

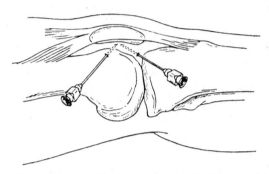

Figure 22–3. Arthrocentesis of knee (medial approach). (Illustration provided by Dr. D. Neustadt. From Rodman G, Schumacher HR (eds): Primer on the Rheumatic Diseases. 8th Ed. Arthritis Foundation, 1983.)

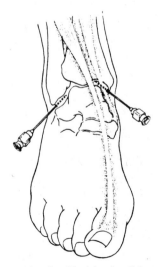

Figure 22–4. Arthrocentesis of ankle joint (medial and lateral approaches). (Illustration provided by Dr. D. Neustadt. From Rodman G, Schumacher HR (eds): Primer on the Rheumatic Diseases. 8th Ed. Arthritis Foundation, 1983.)

Table 22–7. SYNOVIAL FLUID ANALYSIS

CLASSIFICATION	CLARITY	LEUKOCYTE COUNT (CELLS/µL)	% POLYS
Normal	Transparent	< 200	< 25
Noninflammatory	Transparent	< 2000	< 25
Inflammatory	Translucent	< 75,000	> 50
Septic	Opaque	> 75,000	> 75

differential, crystal analysis, Gram stain, and culture.

b. At the bedside, one should be able to read newsprint through noninflammatory fluid in a glass tube (a plastic syringe makes the fluid look more translucent and more inflammatory).

c. Table 22–7 presents a classification of synovial fluid by clarity, leukocyte count, and percentage of neutrophils. (*Caution:* an "inflammatory" fluid may be infected; not all septic joints, have synovial fluid with "septic" characteristics.)

D. Other Laboratory Studies

1. Examination of joint fluid as outlined above is the most important test in the patient with new-onset arthritis.

2. The need for other tests (e.g., CBC, erythrocyte sedimentation rate [ESR], serum uric acid, blood cultures, rheumatoid factor) should be individualized and dictated by the clinical situation.

3. Roentgenograms are frequently *unhelpful* in the absence of trauma, and a normal film does not rule out arthritis.

INFECTIOUS CAUSES OF ARTHRITIS

I. NONGONOCOCCAL SEPTIC ARTHRITIS

A. Patient Demographics

1. May occur at any age.

2. High-risk groups include immunocompromised patients, injection drug users, and patients with underlying arthritic conditions (especially rheumatoid arthritis).

3. *Caution:* patients with rheumatoid arthritis and a septic joint have a significant mortality rate. *Any rheumatoid arthritis patient who presents with a joint inflamed out of proportion to his/her overall disease activity has an infected joint until proven otherwise.*

4. Prompt diagnosis is mandatory! Cartilage damage begins to occur within 24–48 hours of onset.

B. Systemic Features

Symptoms commonly include fever, chills, and malaise. Joint pain is intense, the patient resists any movement of the affected joint, and the surrounding area is usually warm and erythematous.

C. Joint Pattern

1. Usually a monoarthritis (rarely a pauciarthritis of subacute onset).

2. The principal joints involved are the knee (50% of cases), followed by the hip, shoulder, wrist, ankle, and elbow. Small joints are almost never affected by a hematogenously spread infection.

3. Injection drug users may have axial joint involvement (e.g., sacroiliac, spine, sternoclavicular).

D. Organisms

1. *Staphylococcus aureus* most common (60% of cases).

2. *Streptococcus sp.* (25%).

3. Gram-negative organisms (15%).

4. Injection drug users may have atypical gram-negative organisms (including *Pseudomonas*).

E. Laboratory Studies

Minimally, obtain the following:

1. Arthrocentesis. Send for Gram stain, cell count, crystal analysis, and culture. Synovial fluid leukocyte counts in this setting are generally 20,000–100,000 cells/μL, with a neutrophil predominance.

2. Blood cultures.

3. CBC.

4. Electrolyte panel; glucose, BUN, and creatinine levels.

5. ESR. An elevated ESR can be followed over time to help confirm adequate therapy. A normal ESR, however, does *not* rule out a septic joint!

6. Urinalysis and culture.

7. Roentgenography of the affected joint. Usually normal unless infection has been present for ≥ 2 weeks.

F. Therapy

1. **Arthrocentesis.** Frequent joint aspirations (at least daily) are indicated. Surgical drainage is necessary for a septic hip, a

septic joint with a prosthesis, or when loculations prevent adequate needle aspiration. Consult an orthopedist early for *any* septic joint.

2. **Intravenous (IV) Antibiotics.** Drugs of choice depend on the Gram stain, but should always include adequate coverage for *S. aureus.* Reasonable initial choices include
   a. Nafcillin (1 g IV every 4 hours) or a first-generation cephalosporin (e.g., cefazolin 1–2 g IV every 8 hours); and
   b. Gentamicin (3–5 mg/kg/day, divided, every 8 hours IV) or ciprofloxacin (400 mg IV every 12 hours).

3. Immobilize the joint.

G. Disposition

Hospital admission is required.

II. DISSEMINATED GONOCOCCAL INFECTION

A. Patient Demographics

1. Typically seen in the sexually active, young, urban population; but overall occurs in < 1% of patients who contract gonorrhea. Gonococcal arthritis is the leading cause of septic arthritis in young persons in the United States.

2. Patients with recurrent disease may have a deficiency in one of the terminal complement components (C5–C8).

B. Systemic Features

1. Fever, anorexia, and skin lesions (usually small in number [5–30 lesions]; painful or asymptomatic; vesicular, pustular, or maculopapular; located on the trunk and/or extremities) occur 1 day to 2 months after sexual acquisition of *N. gonorrhoeae.*

2. Joint symptoms are initially migratory pauciarthralgias. Tenosynovitis (tendon sheath inflammation) is also common in the early stages.

3. Fewer than 25% of patients have local genitourinary symptoms.

C. Joint Pattern

1. Up to 50% of patients develop purulent synovitis.

2. The most commonly affected joints are the knees, ankles, wrists, and/or elbows, in a mono- or pauciarticular pattern.

D. Laboratory Studies

Minimally, obtain the following:

1. Arthrocentesis of the affected joint. Send for Gram stain, cell count, crystal analysis, and culture.

2. Blood cultures.

3. CBC.

4. Electrolyte panel; glucose, BUN, and creatinine levels.

5. Urinalysis and culture.

6. Pregnancy test.

7. Cultures of the genitourinary tract (for chlamydia and gonorrhea) and rectum (for gonorrhea).

8. Also consider an oropharyngeal culture in patients with symptoms in this area or a history of oral sex.

9. RPR.

Note: culture yield varies with the site and is highest from the genitourinary tract (75% positive culture rate), followed by the synovial fluid (60%), and blood (24%).

E. Therapy

1. **Arthocentesis.** Patients with high synovial fluid leukocyte counts may benefit from daily joint aspiration and irrigation.

2. **IV Antibiotics.** The patient should be simultaneously treated for gonorrhea and chlamydia:
   a. Ceftriaxone (1 g IV daily) or ceftizoxime (1 g IV every 8 hours) or cefotaxime (1 g IV every 8 hours); and
   b. Doxycycline (100 mg PO or IV bid) or ofloxacin (300 mg PO bid); in pregnant patients use erythromycin (500 mg PO every 6 hours).

3. Consider joint immobilization.

F. Disposition

Hospital admission is initially required. After an inpatient clinical response, the patient may be discharged to complete a 7–10-day total course of antibiotic therapy (reasonable discharge antibiotics include cefixime [400 mg PO bid] or ciprofloxacin [500 mg PO bid]; *and* doxycycline [100 mg PO bid]).

III. INFECTIVE ENDOCARDITIS

Infective endocarditis is also discussed in Chapter 15.

A. Patient Demographics

1. Bacterial endocarditis should be considered in any patient with joint complaints who uses injection drugs, has valvular heart disease, or has a prosthetic heart valve.

2. Overall, 40% of patients with endocarditis have musculoskeletal manifestations; in many, these are the patient's presenting complaints.

B. Systemic Features

1. Fever, chills, and anorexia are frequent.

2. Most patients (85%) have a cardiac murmur, but the absence of a murmur does not exclude the diagnosis. A new or changing murmur is a key finding but is seen in only a minority of patients.

3. Approximately 50% of patients have cutaneous manifestations, including petechiae (most common skin finding; may be seen in the extremities, conjunctiva, buccal mucosa, and/or palate), Osler's nodes (small, painful nodules usually on finger or toe pads), Janeway lesions (hemorrhagic, flat, painless macular plaques; usually on palms or soles), and/or splinter hemorrhages (subungual, linear, reddish-brown streaks).

4. Other manifestations *may* include Roth's spots (oval, pale, peripherally hemorrhagic fundoscopic lesions usually found near the optic disc), splenomegaly, pulmonary symptoms (cough, pleurisy, pneumonia), congestive heart failure, arrhythmias, and/or neurologic symptoms/signs (secondary to meningitis, subarachnoid hemorrhage, brain abscess, or stroke).

C. Joint Pattern

1. The most common musculoskeletal symptom is inflammatory back pain.

2. The typical joint pattern is a mono- or pauciarticular arthritis. Both axial (spinal, sacroiliac, sternoclavicular, and/or acromioclavicular) and peripheral joints (usually large joints of the upper and lower extremities) may be involved.

D. Laboratory Studies

Minimally, obtain the following:

1. Arthrocentesis of inflamed joints. The synovial fluid from involved joints is inflammatory, but in only rare cases is it actually septic (most of the musculoskeletal manifestations are secondary to immune complex deposition).

2. Blood cultures (a minimum of three).

3. CBC.

4. Chest roentgenogram.

5. Electrolyte panel; glucose, BUN, and creatinine levels.

6. ECG.

7. ESR. An elevated ESR can be followed over time to help confirm adequate therapy. A normal ESR does *not* rule out endocarditis!

8. Pregnancy test (mandatory in reproductive-age females).

9. Urinalysis and culture. The urine sediment is frequently abnormal.

E. Therapy

See Infective Endocarditis in Chapter 15 for specific therapy.

F. Disposition

Hospitalization is required.

IV. LYME DISEASE

Lyme disease is also discussed in Chapter 15.

A. Patient Demographics

1. Caused by the spirochete *Borrelia burgdorferi*. It is the most frequently reported arthropod-borne disease in the United States, with highest incidence in the Northeast, upper Midwest, and northern California.

2. Most cases have their onset between May and August.

3. Only 25% of patients recall a tick bite.

B. Systemic Features

1. In 70% of patients, the initial manifestation is a rash (erythema migrans), characterized by a concentric, erythematous, expanding lesion usually found in the groin or axilla. Secondary skin lesions may develop in ≤ 50% of patients.

2. Low-grade fever, malaise, myalgias, arthralgias, headache, and neck stiffness are also common initial manifestations.

3. Other findings may include neurologic complaints (aseptic meningitis, cranial neuropathies [including Bell's palsy: may be bilateral], radiculoneuropathy, and meningoencephalitis) and cardiac abnormalities (atrioventricular blocks; sometimes ventricular dysfunction).

C. Joint Pattern

A relapsing and remitting arthritis may follow the neurologic and cardiac abnormalities described above. The typical joint pattern is mono- or pauciarticular affecting the large joints (especially the knees). Large effusions are frequent.

D. Laboratory Studies

The diagnosis depends on the clinical presentation of the patient combined with a reasonable probability of tick exposure from an endemic area. Serologic tests for antibodies to *B. burgdorferi* provide adjunctive confirmation but by themselves do not prove the diagnosis.

E. Therapy

See Lyme Disease in Chapter 15 for specific therapy.

CRYSTAL-ASSOCIATED ARTHRITIS

I. URATE GOUT

A. Patient Demographics

1. The typical patient is a middle-aged male, often overweight and hypertensive. Women are usually not affected until after menopause. Prevalence is high in South Sea Islanders and Filipinos.

2. Most patients have insufficient renal uric acid clearance; a minority have a partial enzymatic defect and overproduce uric acid.

3. Alcohol impairs renal handling of uric acid and increases production. Thiazide diuretics, furosemide, and cyclosporine elevate uric acid levels by interfering with renal elimination.

4. Patients with renal insufficiency have elevated uric acid levels.

5. Surgery or medical illness may provoke an attack.

B. Systemic Features

Patients often awaken at night or in the early morning with severe pain, tenderness, and erythema in the affected joint(s). A low-grade fever may be present. With long-standing hyperuricemia, tophi (painless, firm, soft tissue deposits of chalky sodium urate) may be present over the helix of the ear, olecranon area, fingers, and toes. Some patients have a history of nephrolithiasis.

C. Joint Pattern

Gout is usually a mono- or pauciarthritis. The most common areas affected are the first metatarsophalangeal joint, ankle, and/or knee. Involvement of the small joints of the hand or the wrist is less common. Most attacks are self-limited and last < 10 days.

D. Laboratory Studies

Minimally, obtain the following:

1. Arthrocentesis of inflamed joint. Send for Gram stain, cell count, crystal analysis, and culture. *Note:* in a patient with a prior history of gout, and with classic joint involvement, arthrocentesis may not be necessary.

2. Consider a serum uric acid level. Remember, however, that an elevated uric acid level does not prove gout, and some patients with an acute attack have a normal serum uric acid level.

E. Therapy

1. Nonsteroidal anti-inflammatory drugs (NSAIDs) are the usual agents of choice. They should be given at maximum dosage for

1–2 days, and then the dose lowered, but not stopped. Possible regimens include the following:

  a. Indomethacin 50 mg PO every 6 hours for 2 days, then 50 mg PO every 8 hours for 3 days, then 25 mg PO every 8 hours for 2–3 days.

  b. Naproxen 750 mg PO to start, then 250 mg PO every 8 hours until attack has completely subsided.

2. Colchicine is effective, but toxicities limit its usefulness. Colchicine is contraindicated in the patient with significant gastrointestinal, renal, or cardiac disease.

   Dose:

   • Oral: 0.5–1.2 mg PO to start, then 0.5–0.6 mg PO every 1–2 hours until gouty pain ceases or nausea, vomiting, or diarrhea develop. The cumulative dosage should not exceed 7–8 mg for the attack.

   • Intravenous (this route is not recommended as it may cause myelosuppression, myopathy, and neuropathy): 2 mg IV to start, followed by 0.5 mg IV every 6 hours as needed (do not exceed 4 mg for a treatment course or within a 24-hour time period).

3. Corticosteroids are appropriate in the patient for whom NSAIDs and colchicine are contraindicated or for refractory attacks:

   a. Prednisone 40-60 mg PO every morning until an adequate response, then tapered gradually over 10–14 days. *Or*

   b. Triamcinolone (Aristospan) intra-articular (IA) injection: 20–40 mg IA for large joints, 15–20 mg IA for medium-sized joints. *Or*

   c. Corticotropin (ACTH) 40-80 units IM or IV every day for 2 to 3 days.

F. Follow-up

Follow-up with a primary care physician or rheumatologist is necessary to address chronic treatment issues.

II. CALCIUM PYROPHOSPHATE GOUT (PSEUDOGOUT)

A. Patient Demographics

1. Attacks of calcium pyrophosphate gout typically occur in elderly patients and may be provoked by surgery or medical illness.

2. The cause is idiopathic in most cases.

3. In some patients, the underlying cause is hypercalcemia, hypomagnesemia, hypothyroidism, or hemochromatosis.

B. Systemic Features

During the acute attack there may be fever, joint erythema, and tenderness similar to urate gout, though usually not of the same intensity.

C. Joint Pattern

Pseudogout is a mono- or pauciarticular arthritis. The knee is most commonly affected, followed by other large joints. Involvement of the first metatarsophalangeal joint is *uncommon*. Attacks last a few days to a few weeks.

D. Laboratory Studies

1. Arthrocentesis of the inflamed joint. Send for Gram stain, cell count, crystal analysis, and culture. The most helpful finding is the presence of weakly birefringent rhomboidal crystals in the synovial fluid.
2. Roentgenography. If obtained, films frequently reveal linear calcification of the intra-articular cartilage (chondrocalcinosis).
3. Other studies. Once the diagnosis of calcium pyrophosphate gout is made, consider checking iron studies, thyroid stimulating hormone, and serum calcium, magnesium, and phosphate to evaluate for a treatable underlying metabolic condition.

E. Therapy

Intra-articular corticosteroids or oral NSAIDs are effective for treatment. See Gout, earlier in this chapter.

SPONDYLOARTHROPATHIES

I. ANKYLOSING SPONDYLITIS

A. Patient Demographics

1. Most patients are 20–40 years old; the male to female ratio is approximately 4:1.
2. The family history is frequently positive for a spondyloarthropathy given the association of these conditions with human leukocyte antigen (HLA)-B27 (> 90% of patients).
3. Arthritis of the axial skeleton indistinguishable from ankylosing spondylitis may occur in > 5% of patients with inflammatory bowel disease; the arthritis may precede the onset of bowel disease by several years.

B. Systemic Features

1. Commonly include nonpainful oral ulcers, episodic uveitis, and/or enthesopathy (inflammation of the muscular or tendinous attachments to bone, including the Achilles tendon, plantar fascia, and intercostal muscles).
2. Less common features may include cardiac abnormalities (atrioventricular blocks, aortic regurgitation), neurologic emer-

gencies (cauda equina syndrome, cord compression with fractures—see below), amyloidosis, and pulmonary fibrosis (rarely).

C. Joint Pattern

1. The axial skeleton is most commonly involved, especially the sacroiliac joints.
   a. Low back and buttock ache: worse on awakening, improves through the course of the day and with activity.
   b. The sacroiliac joints may be tender with palpation or stress (forced abduction and external rotation of the hip places pressure on the contralateral sacroiliac joint).
   c. Limited lumbar spinal motion in all three planes. The Schober test is used to assess lumbar motion: a horizontal line is drawn on the upright patient at the L5-S1 area and a second line is drawn 10 cm cephalad. With forward flexion the distance between these two lines should increase to ≥ 15 cm in the normal patient; failure to do so indicates limited spinal mobility.

2. Appendicular skeletal manifestations:
   a. Large joints (especially the hips) are usually affected in a pauciarticular pattern.
   b. Peripheral joint involvement is seen in 20–30% of patients, especially women.

D. Laboratory Studies

1. Roentgenography of the sacroiliac joints is the most important test to confirm sacroiliitis.

2. Other relevant laboratory studies may include a CBC (anemia not uncommon) and ESR or C-reactive protein (usually elevated). HLA-B27 testing is not usually necessary.

E. Therapy

1. NSAIDs are the therapeutic agents of choice. Drugs with long half-lives help to ensure compliance. Possibilities include
   a. Piroxicam 20 mg PO daily.
   b. Indomethacin SR 75 mg PO bid.
   c. Nabumetone 1500 mg PO daily.
   d. Naproxen 500 PO bid.
   e. Diclofenac 75 mg PO bid.

Patients with ankylosing spondylitis typically have marked improvement with one of these agents within a few days and often with the first dose.

F. Ankylosing Spondylitis Emergencies

1. **Spinal Fracture.** Patients with long-standing ankylosing spondylitis are at risk for spinal fracture, instability, and

potential spinal cord injury after even minor trauma. Hyper-extension is the usual mechanism.

a. The most common sites of injury are the C5-C6 and C6-C7 segments, although any spinal segment can be involved.

b. Any patient with advanced ankylosing spondylitis should be evaluated for fracture and possible cord injury when he/she complains of constant localized spine pain. Evaluation should begin with appropriate immobilization and spinal roentgenography. Tomography, bone scanning, and/or computed tomography scans may be required for adequate visualization of the involved area.

c. Early consultation with an orthopedist and/or neurosurgeon is appropriate.

2. **Cauda Equina Syndrome**

a. Impingement on the nerves of the cauda equina results in symptoms of buttock pain, bowel and bladder dysfunction, saddle anesthesia, and/or leg weakness.

b. Magnetic resonance imaging (MRI) is the preferred imaging modality. Urgent neurosurgical consultation is mandatory.

G. Disposition/Follow-Up

1. Ankylosing spondylitis emergencies, as outlined above, require urgent consultation and hospitalization.

2. Patients not requiring hospitalization should be referred for continuing care to monitor response to treatment, allow for further education about the disease (including complications), and ensure optimal physical therapy.

3. The patient with uveitis requires an ophthalmology consult.

II. REITER'S SYNDROME (REACTIVE ARTHRITIS)

A. Patient Demographics

1. Reiter's syndrome is one of the most common causes of inflammatory arthritis in young males in North America. Most patients are 20–40 years old; the male to female ratio is approximately 5:1.

2. More than 80% of patients are HLA-B27 positive.

3. Reiter's syndrome generally is preceded by infection with one or more of the following organisms: *Chlamydia trachomatis, Salmonella, Shigella, Campylobacter,* or *Yersenia.* It may also occur in association with human immunodeficiency virus (HIV) infection.

B. Systemic Features

The patient has a pauciarthritis and one or more of the following: episodic uveitis, conjunctivitis, painless oral ulcers, enthesopathy, keratoderma blennorrhagicum (pustular psoriasis on the palms and soles), circinate balanitis (shallow, painless, erythematous ulcers in a circular distribution on the glans penis), hyperkeratosis under the fingernails, diarrhea, and/or urethritis/cervicitis.

C. Joint Pattern

1. Pauciarthritis affecting large peripheral joints (with considerable effusion).

2. Inflammatory low back pain is a frequent complaint. If a sacroiliitis is present, it is often asymmetrical.

3. Enthesopathic involvement of the Achilles tendon and plantar fascia is also common.

D. Laboratory Studies

Reiter's syndrome is a clinical rather than a laboratory diagnosis. The CBC may reveal anemia and an elevated leukocyte count; the ESR is also frequently elevated. Culture for gonorrhea, chlamydia, and HIV testing are warranted in selected cases.

E. Therapy

NSAIDs are appropriate for initial treatment and should be dosed as described for ankylosing spondylitis, above.

F. Follow-Up

Referral for monitoring of disease activity and consideration of second-line agents such as sulfasalazine and methotrexate is warranted. Most patients with Reiter's syndrome will have episodic attacks and will need ongoing care. The patient with uveitis requires an ophthalmology consult.

III. PSORIATIC ARTHRITIS

A. Patient Demographics

1. Approximately 7% of patients with psoriasis have an inflammatory arthritis; the male to female ratio is 1:1.

2. Psoriatic spondylitis is associated with HLA-B27; peripheral arthritis is not.

3. Like Reiter's syndrome, psoriatic arthritis may be associated with HIV infection.

B. Systemic Features

Psoriasis is the main distinguishing feature, although it may be missed if not diligently searched for (plaques are sometimes only evident behind the ears, on the scalp, in the umbilicus, or between the buttocks).

C. Joint Pattern

A variety of patterns may occur: a pauciarthritis (affecting hands, feet, knees, ankles, hips, and wrists in an asymmetrical pattern); a distal interphalangeal joint predominant form (often includes severe nail changes); arthritis mutilans (with severe destruction of hand joints); or a rheumatoid arthritis-like pattern. Psoriatic spondylitis may accompany any of these. Patients with psoriatic arthritis may also suffer from swelling and tenderness of the digits between the interphalangeal joints ("sausage digits") similar to the other spondyloarthropathies.

D. Laboratory Studies

There are no "diagnostic" tests. The CBC may reveal anemia; the ESR is frequently elevated and may be useful in assessing adequacy of therapy. HIV testing may be warranted in selected cases. If the patient's arthritic presentation is polyarticular, rheumatoid arthritis is a consideration.

E. Therapy

In the ED, NSAIDs should be used for initial therapy (see Ankylosing Spondylitis, above).

F. Disposition/Follow-Up

Most of these patients will have a chronic arthritis. Follow-up is mandatory for monitoring response to treatment.

MISCELLANEOUS RHEUMATOLOGIC DISEASES

I. RHEUMATOID ARTHRITIS

A. Patient Demographics

1. The prevalence of rheumatoid arthritis (RA) in the United States is approximately 1%. Prevalence of the disease increases with age up to the 7th decade.
2. Women are affected two to three times more often than men.
3. The cause remains undetermined. There is a relationship between rheumatoid arthritis and the HLA-DR4 gene (found in 60–80% of patients).

B. Systemic Features

Rheumatoid arthritis is a systemic disease. Fatigue, weight loss, fatigability, and low-grade fever may occur. Approximately 50% of patients develop extra-articular disease that may involve the skin (e.g., rheumatoid nodules, ulcers, palpable purpura, alopecia), eyes (e.g., episcleritis, scleritis, keratoconjunctivitis sicca), lungs (e.g., pleural effusion, pleuritis, rheumatoid nodules, interstitial fibrosis), heart (e.g., pericarditis, myocarditis, valvulitis, conduction defects), gastrointestinal system (e.g., hepatomegaly, visceral perforation), nervous system (e.g., cervical myelopathy, neuropathies), muscles (myopathy), and/or blood vessels (vasculitis).

C. Joint Pattern

The disease may initially present as a mono- or pauciarthritis, but is usually a symmetrical polyarthritis affecting the small joints of the hands and feet. It does *not* affect the distal interphalangeal joints.

D. Laboratory Studies

Obtain a CBC, ESR, and rheumatoid factor; consider an antinuclear antibody (ANA) test because systemic lupus erythematosus may also present with a polyarthritis. Rheumatoid factor is positive in up to 75% of patients (but may not appear for up to 1 year after the onset of symptoms). The 25% of patients who are rheumatoid factor seronegative usually have a less severe course.

E. Therapy

The initial treatment goal is to control joint pain and inflammation. An NSAID should be prescribed for this purpose. Low-dose corticosteroids (prednisone 5–10 mg PO every AM) can be used in severe initial presentations; consultation with internal medicine or rheumatology is appropriate.

F. RA Emergencies

1. **Rheumatoid Vasculitis.** Usually occurs in a patient with long-standing severe disease even though the rheumatoid arthritis may be otherwise quiescent.
   a. Manifestations may include gangrene of the digits, intestinal bleeding or perforation, mononeuritis multiplex, and/or renal dysfunction (rarely).
   b. These patients require rheumatologic consultation for early institution of immunosuppressive therapy. Admission is frequently necessary.

2. **C1-C2 Subluxation.** Inflammatory changes may result in instability of the C1-C2 articulation and extensive pannus formation.
   a. Complications may include a variety of neurologic symptoms and serious potential sequelae. Patients can complain of shocks down the back with flexion of the neck, "drop" attacks, loss of sphincter control, paresthesias, and/or focal weakness. Some of these symptoms may be due to vertebral artery impingement.
   b. Immediate cervical spine immobilization (including a hard

cervical collar), cervical radiographs (anteroposterior, lateral, odontoid, and obliques), and neurosurgical/orthopedic consultation are appropriate. Cervical spine MRI has emerged as a useful tool to document the degree of subluxation and cord impingement.

3. **Septic Arthritis.** Individuals with a septic joint have significant mortality (20% if one joint is affected and > 50% if more than one joint is septic).

    a. The infected joint may go "unnoticed" by the patient secondary to immunosuppressive therapy and the presumption that the involved joint is only a rheumatoid arthritis flare.

    b. Inflammation of one joint out of proportion to the other joints or out of proportion to overall disease activity is always suggestive of a septic joint.

    c. Adequate therapy requires arthrocentesis and drainage, orthopedic consultation, IV antibiotics, and hospitalization. Consider arthroscopic lavage of the involved joint(s) in the operating room.

G. Disposition/Follow-Up

1. Patients with a rheumatoid arthritis emergency, as outlined above, require urgent consultation and hospitalization.

2. Patents not requiring admission should be referred for ongoing care. The patient requires ongoing education about his/her disease, including the possible need for second-line drug use (e.g., auranofin, chloroquine, hydroxychloroquine, or methotrexate).

II. SYSTEMIC LUPUS ERYTHEMATOSUS

A. Patient Demographics

1. The cause of systemic lupus erythematosus (SLE) is unknown.

2. Most patients are 20–40 years old at the time of disease onset; the female to male ratio is approximately 9:1. SLE is more common in blacks.

3. Several medications may cause a drug-induced lupus, including anticonvulsants, beta blockers, hydralazine, isoniazid, methyldopa, penicillamine, phenothiazines, procainamide, and quinidine (many of these agents are more likely to cause a positive ANA test than an actual SLE-like syndrome).

B. Systemic Features

May include dysfunction in one or more of the following areas:

1. **Skin.** The classic "butterfly" rash is an erythematous, maculopapular eruption on the malar region of the face that spares the nasolabial folds. Other skin findings may include

alopecia (occurs in the majority of patients during active disease), maculopapular rashes with a fine scale (frequently evident between the joints of the hands), discoid lupus (a scarring rash typically affecting the face, scalp, and extremities), urticaria, verrucae, angioedema, and/or livedo reticularis (seen on the extremities, frequently over the knees; more common in patients with underlying anticardiolipin antibodies). Exposure to ultraviolet light worsens most SLE-associated rashes. Raynaud's phenomenon is seen in ≥ 25% of patients.

2. **Pulmonary.** May include pleuritis, lupus pneumonitis, alveolar hemorrhage, and/or pulmonary hypertension.

3. **Cardiac.** May include pericarditis, arrhythmias, conduction disturbances, ischemia (from coronary arteritis or atherosclerosis), and/or congestive heart failure.

4. **Gastrointestinal.** Abdominal complaints may occur from vasculitis, peritonitis, and/or pancreatitis.

5. **Nervous System.** May include psychosis and/or seizures.

6. **Renal.** Proteinuria, urinary casts; may include a rapidly progressive glomerulonephritis.

7. **Hematologic.** Hemolytic anemia, leukopenia, lymphopenia, and/or thrombocytopenia.

8. **Miscellaneous.** Fevers, weight loss, fatigue, and anorexia are common. Patients with anticardiolipin antibodies are at risk for venous and arterial thrombosis.

C. Joint Pattern

1. Arthralgias are common.

2. Most patients have a nonerosive, nondeforming arthritis that is usually symmetrical and often migratory. The joints most frequently affected are the proximal interphalangeal, metacarpophalangeal, wrist, and knee joints.

3. Tenosynovitis may occur and can result in rupture of the patellar or Achilles tendons.

4. Avascular necrosis (principally of the hips, knees, shoulders, and/or ankles, in that order) may occur as a complication of steroid therapy.

D. Laboratory Studies

1. In patients with *suspected* SLE, *minimally* obtain the following:
   a. CBC with platelets.
   b. Electrolyte panel; glucose, BUN, and creatinine levels.
   c. Urinalysis.
   d. ESR.
   e. ANA. Positive in > 95% of patients with SLE.

f. Other autoantibody titers. A negative anti-SSA antibody test combined with a negative ANA test rules out SLE (except in the very rare individual who may have a complement-deficiency state; this can be evaluated by obtaining a CH_{50}, which is usually extremely low or unmeasurable in this situation). An antihistone antibody is useful in patients with suspected drug-induced lupus (positive in > 80% of such patients).

2. In patients with *established* SLE, presenting with suspected exacerbation of disease activity, consider obtaining the following:
   a. CBC with platelets.
   b. Electrolyte panel; glucose, BUN, and creatinine levels.
   c. Urinalysis.
   d. ESR.
   e. CH_{50}.
   f. Double-stranded DNA. If an old chart is available, compare results of the above studies with prior baseline data. Elevation in double-stranded DNA and ESR combined with decreased complement activity (i.e., decreased CH_{50}) confirm increased disease activity.

E. Initial Outpatient Therapy

SLE is a disease of exacerbations and remissions. In the absence of life-threatening disease (see below), patients with mild arthritis or serositis can frequently be treated with an NSAID. Moderate symptoms will usually respond to corticosteroids (prednisone 20–60 mg/day in divided doses). Most of the rashes of SLE respond to topical corticosteroids or low-dose systemic therapy.

F. SLE Emergencies

1. Potential *life-threatening complications* of SLE include glomerulonephritis with rapidly rising creatinine, central nervous system lupus (psychosis, seizures, or stroke), marked thrombocytopenia, vasculitis, and severe hemolytic anemia.

2. These patients need aggressive evaluation, consultation (internal medicine and/or rheumatology), rapid initiation of treatment (usually with high-dose corticosteroids), and hospitalization.

3. The possibility of a serious concomitant infection should be considered in any patient with SLE who is being treated with chronic immunosuppressive therapy.

G. Disposition

1. The patient with a severe flare of SLE (e.g., high fever; significant anorexia; severe arthritis, serositis, and/or myositis) should be admitted for institution of therapy and close monitoring of response.

2. Life-threatening disease as described above also mandates admission.

H. Follow-Up

For patients not requiring admission, referral to a rheumatologist or an internist familiar with SLE for disease monitoring and dosing of corticosteroids and/or other immunosuppressive medication is appropriate. Patients with discoid lupus should be referred to a dermatologist; those with mild nephritis should see a rheumatologist and/or nephrologist.

III. OSTEOARTHRITIS

A. Patient Demographics

1. Osteoarthritis is the most common joint disease.
2. It is characterized by progressive articular cartilage loss, bony remodeling, subchondral bone thickening, and osteophyte development.
3. Idiopathic (primary) disease occurs without a known predisposing factor; most patients are > 60 years old. Secondary disease occurs because of an underlying joint insult, including trauma, metabolic disease, avascular necrosis, and congenital abnormalities.

B. Systemic Features

There are few systemic features of primary osteoarthritis. The metabolic causes of osteoarthritis (e.g., hemochromatosis, Wilson's disease, Paget's disease, diabetes mellitus, acromegaly) may have a variety of systemic features that will not be discussed here.

C. Joint Pattern

1. Primary disease most commonly affects the distal and proximal interphalangeal joints of the hands, the metacarpophalangeal joints of the thumbs, hips, knees, the spine, and the first metatarsophalangeal joints of the great toes.
2. Involvement of other joints (e.g., shoulders, elbows, wrists; especially if involved in a symmetrical pattern) suggests a possible underlying metabolic abnormality.
3. Knee pain is a frequent presenting complaint in the ED. Patients can develop effusions after mild trauma or overuse. The arthritic complaints are usually noninflammatory (i.e., pain with use, relief with rest, morning stiffness < 30 minutes).

D. Laboratory Studies

If arthrocentesis is performed, the synovial fluid is usually noninflammatory. Roentgenograms typically reveal some combination of joint space narrowing, subchondral sclerosis, subchondral cysts, and osteophytes.

E. Therapy

1. Salicylates or other NSAIDs are the drugs of choice. NSAIDs should not be prescribed to the patient with underlying renal disease, active peptic ulcer disease, a prior history of significant gastrointestinal bleeding, or a history of NSAID intolerance.

2. Patients intolerant of NSAIDs may benefit from acetaminophen (650 mg PO every 4–6 hours) for analgesia.

3. Intra-articular corticosteroids (triamcinolone) may occasionally be used to provide both pain relief and improved joint motion. The dose for the knee is 20-40 mg (Aristospan). Intra-articular injections should not be repeated more often than every 4–6 months.

F. Disposition/Follow-Up

Referral is appropriate for continuation of therapy and close monitoring for potential NSAID side effects/toxicities. Patients also benefit from physical therapy (range of motion and strengthening exercises) and involvement in nonimpact-loading aerobic conditioning exercises (e.g., swimming, walking, stationary bicycling).

IV. TEMPORAL ARTERITIS (GIANT CELL ARTERITIS)

A. Patient Demographics

1. Temporal arteritis is a vasculitis generally involving the arteries of the head and neck. *The ophthalmic artery may be affected with resultant sudden and irreversible loss of vision.*

2. Patients are ≥ 50 years old, women are affected more frequently than men, and it occurs more commonly in whites.

B. Systemic Features

1. Symptoms are usually of gradual onset and most commonly include headaches (65% of patients; frequently located in the temple area), polymyalgia rheumatica (50% of patients; characterized by aching and morning stiffness in two of the following three areas: neck, shoulder girdle, and/or hips), fever (40% of patients), jaw claudication (40% of patients; defined as pain with chewing), and fatigue.

2. Partial or complete visual loss may develop in approximately 20% of patients.

3. Other less common complaints may include upper- or lower-extremity claudication, abnormal pulses, acute hearing loss, hemiparesis, brainstem strokes, and/or acute myocardial infarction.

C. Laboratory Studies

1. CBC (normocytic anemia and thrombocytosis are usually present).

2. ESR (usually > 50 mm/hr; but may be normal in 1-2% of patients).

3. Referral for temporal artery biopsy is necessary for diagnostic confirmation (see below).

D. Therapy

Any patient ≥ 50 years old reasonably suspected of having temporal arteritis (e.g., recent onset of headaches, episodic visual abnormalities, or jaw caludication; ± an elevated ESR) should be started on prednisone (45-60 mg PO every day in two divided doses) as soon as possible. Arrangements should then be made for diagnostic confirmation with a temporal artery biopsy (usually performed by ophthalmology). A delay of ≤ 1 week between initiation of corticosteroid therapy and temporal artery biopsy will not affect the biopsy results.

E. Disposition/Follow-Up

Urgent referral is appropriate to both ophthalmology and rheumatology (or an internist experienced in treating temporal arteritis) for continuing care.

BIBLIOGRAPHY

Baker DG, Schumacher HR Jr: Acute monoarthritis. N Engl J Med 1993;329(14):1013–1020.

Bland JH: Rheumatoid subluxation of the cervical spine. J Rheumatol 1990;17:134–137.

Espinoza LR, Aguilar JL, Berman A, et al: Rheumatic manifestations associated with human immunodeficiency virus infection. Arthritis Rheum 1989;32:1615–1622.

Esterhal JL, Gelb I: Adult septic arthritis. Orthop Clin N Am 1991;22:503–514.

Fernandez-Herlihy L: Temporal arteritis: clinical aids to diagnosis. J Rheumatol 1988; 15:1797–1801.

Gardner GC, Weisman MH: Pyarthrosis in patients with rheumatoid arthritis: a report of 13 cases and a review of the literature from the past 40 years. Am J Med 1990;88:503–511.

Graham B, Van Peteghem PK: Fractures of the spine in ankylosing spondylitis: diagnosis, treatment, and complications. Spine 1989;14:803–807.

Hamerman D: The biology of osteoarthritis. N Eng J Med 1989;320:1322–1329.

Mills JA: Systemic lupus erythematosus. N Engl J Med 1994;330:1871–1879.

Puig JG, Michian AD, Jimenez ML, et al: Female gout: clinical spectrum and uric acid metabolism. Arch Intern Med 1991;151:726–732.

Roberts WN, Liang MH, Stern SH: Colchicine in acute gout. JAMA 1987;257:1920–1922.

23

Toxicologic Emergencies

STANDARD THERAPY OF THE POISONED/ OVERDOSE PATIENT

> *"Poisons and medicine are oftentimes
> the same substance given with different intents."*
> PETER MERE LATHAM (1789–1875)

I. ESSENTIAL FACTS

A. Definitions

1. A *poison* (or *toxin*) is a substance that is capable of causing damage to bodily structure and/or function. *Poisoning* occurs when exposure (e.g., inhalation, ingestion, injection, dermal contact) to a toxin results in harmful effects on a biologic system.

2. Overdose is defined as an excessive exposure (intentional or unintentional) to a chemical substance. Overdose may or may not result in poisoning.

B. Epidemiology

1. On the basis of data collected by the American Association of Poison Control Centers (AAPCC), an estimated 4.3 million poisoning cases occurred in the United States in 1993.

2. The AAPCC determined the following:
   a. 90.3% of poisonings occurred in the home.
   b. 56% occurred in children < 6 years of age.
   c. 86.3% of poisonings were accidental; 10.9% were intentional. Accidental poisonings exceeded intentional poisonings in every age group.
   d. In 93.2% of cases only a single substance was implicated.
   e. Of the 626 poisoning fatalities reported, 83% of the adult deaths (≥ 19 years of age) were intentional.
   f. 75% of poison exposures were ingestions.

C. Patients in Whom Poisoning or Drug Overdose Should be Suspected

1. The patient with an *altered level of consciousness,* including *coma.*

2. The young patient with a *life-threatening arrhythmia.*

3. The *trauma patient.*

4. The patient with a *bizarre* or *puzzling* clinical presentation.

D. Mortality

1. The leading agents to cause poisoning deaths are analgesics, antidepressants, stimulants and street drugs, sedative/hypnotics/antipsychotics, cardiovascular drugs, and alcohols.

2. With proper toxicologically oriented treatment the mortality of patients with *drug-induced coma* should be < 1%.

II. CLINICAL EVALUATION

Important: evaluation of the patient should take place *simultaneously* with treatment as outlined more thoroughly in IV, below.

A. History

1. Attempt to obtain an accurate history. Important information may be gathered from the patient, family, ambulance/police personnel, witnesses, Medic Alert/medical information bracelets, pill containers in the patient's clothing, pill containers at the scene, and the medical record.

2. Seek out answers to the following five questions: *who* was exposed; *what* were they exposed to (and how much?); *when* did the exposure occur; *where* did it occur (could there be other victims?); and *why* did this happen (e.g., intentional versus accidental exposure)?

3. Be suspicious of information as well: on average 50% of poisoning/overdose information is inaccurate. Presume the worst possible scenario and be prepared to manage it.

B. Symptoms and Signs

An enormous variety of symptoms and signs are possible. Depending on the drug or toxin, any organ system in the body may be affected. Table 23–1 lists some of the more frequently encountered agents involved in poisonings/overdoses and their associated clinical syndromes (toxidromes).

C. Cautions

Before proceeding with the physical examination:

1. If there is *any* historical or physical evidence of trauma and/or the patient has neck pain, an altered mental status, *or* an abnormal neurologic examination, then the cervical spine *must* be appropriately immobilized.

2. If the patient has an altered level of consciousness and there are no contraindications to such positioning (e.g., head

Table 23–1. TOXICOLOGIC SYNDROMES (TOXIDROMES)

Toxin	Vital Signs	Mental Status	Symptoms	Clinical Findings	Lab Findings
Acetaminophen	Normal	Normal	Anorexia, nausea, vomiting	RUQ tenderness Jaundice	Abnormal LFTs
Amphetamines	Hypertension, tachycardia, hyperthermia	Hyperactive, agitated, toxic psychosis	Hyperalertness	Mydriasis, hyperactive bowel sounds, flush, diaphoresis	—
Anticholinergics	Tachycardia, hypotension, hypertension, hyperthermia	Altered (agitation, lethargy to coma)	Blurred vision, confusion	Dry mucous membranes, mydriasis, diminished bowel sounds, urinary retention	ECG abnormalities, widened QRS complex
Arsenic (acute)	Hypotension, tachycardia, hyperthermia	Alert to comatose	Abdominal pain, vomiting, diarrhea, dysphagia	Dehydration, hair loss	Renal failure, abnormal abdominal x-ray, dysrhythmias
Arsenic (chronic)	Normal	Normal to encephalopathic	Abdominal pain, diarrhea	Melanosis, hyperkeratosis, sensory-motor neuropathy, hair loss, Mee's line, skin cancer	Leukopenia, thrombocytopenia, proteinuria, hematuria, abnormal LFTs
Barbiturates	Hypoventilation, hypotension, hypothermia	Altered (lethargy to coma)	Intoxication	Disconjugate eye movement, hyporeflexia, bullae	Abnormal ABGs
Beta blockers	Hypotension, bradycardia	Altered (lethargy to coma)	Confusion, dizziness	Cyanosis, seizures	Hypoglycemia, ECG abnormalities
Botulism	Hypoventilation	Normal unless hypoxic	Blurred vision, dysphagia, sore throat, diarrhea	Ophthalmoplegia, mydriasis, ptosis	Normal Multiple patients with common or varied symptoms
Carbon monoxide	Often normal	Altered (lethargy to coma)	Headache, dizziness, confusion, nausea, vomiting	Seizures	Elevated carboxyhemoglobin, ECG abnormalities Multiple patients with commonor varied symptoms
Clonidine	Hypotension, hypertension, bradycardia, hypoventilation	Altered (lethargy to coma)	Dizziness, confusion	Miosis	Normal
Cocaine	Hypertension, tachycardia, hyperthermia	Altered (anxiety, agitation, delirium)	Hallucinations	Mydriasis, tremor, perforated nasal septum, diaphrosis, seizures	ECG abnormalities, increased CPK
Cyclic antidepressants	Tachycardia, hypotension, hyperthermia	Altered (lethargy to coma)	Confusion, dizziness	Mydriasis, dry mucous membranes, distended bladder, flush, seizures	Prolonged QRS complex, cardiac dysrhythmias

Table 23–1. TOXICOLOGIC SYNDROMES (TOXIDROMES) Continued

TOXIN	VITAL SIGNS	MENTAL STATUS	SYMPTOMS	CLINICAL FINDINGS	LAB FINDINGS
Digitalis	Hypotension, bradycardia	Normal to altered	Nausea, vomiting, anorexia, visual disturbances, confusion	None	Hyperkalemia, ECG abnormalities, increased digoxin level
Disulfiram/ Ethanol	Hypotension, tachycardia	Normal	Nausea, vomiting, headache, vertigo	Flush, diaphoresis, tender abdomen	Abnormal ECG (ventricular arrhythmias)
Ethylene glycol	Tachypnea	Altered (lethargy to coma)	Intoxication	—	Anion gap acidosis, osmolar gap, crystalluria, hypocalcemia.QTc prolongation, renal failure
Iron	Hypotension (late), tachycardia (late)	Normal unless hypotensive, lethargy	Nausea, vomiting, diarrhea, abdominal pain, hematemesis	Tender abdomen	Hyperglycemia (child.), leukocytosis (child.), heme + stool/vomit, metabolic acidosis, ECG and x-ray abnormalities
Isoniazid	Often normal	Normal or altered (lethargy to coma)	Nausea, vomiting	Seizures, peripheral neuropathy?	Anion gap, metabolic acidosis, abnormal LFTs
Isopropyl alcohol	Hypotension, hypoventilation	Altered (lethargy to coma)	Intoxication	Hyporeflexia, breath odor of acetone	Ketonemia, ketonuria, no glycosuria
Lead	Hypertension, hyperthermia	Altered (lethargy to coma)	Irritability, abdominal pain, nausea, vomiting, constipation	Tender abdomen, peripheral neuropathy, seizures	Anemia, basophilic stippling, radiopaque material on abdominal x-ray
Lithium	Hypotension (late)	Altered (lethargy to coma)	Diarrhea, confusion	Weakness, tremor, ataxia, myoclonus, seizures	Leukocytosis (chronic therapy), ECG abnormalities, renal abnormalities
Meperidine	Hypotension, bradycardia, hypoventilation, hypothermia	Altered (lethargy to coma)	Intoxication	Mydriasis, absent bowel sounds, seizures	Abnormal ABGs
Mercury	Hypotension (late)	Altered (psychiatric disturbances)	Salivation, diarrhea, abdominal pain	Stomatitis, ataxia, tremor	Proteinuria, renal failure
Methanol	Hyperventilation, hypotension	Altered (lethargy to coma)	Blurred vision, abdominal pain, intoxication	Hyperemic disks	Anion gap metabolic acidosis, increased osmolar gap

Table continued on following page

Table 23–1. TOXICOLOGIC SYNDROMES (TOXIDROMES) Continued

Toxin	Vital Signs	Mental Status	Symptoms	Clinical Findings	Lab Findings
Opioids	Hypotension, bradycardia, hypoventilation, hypothermia	Altered (lethargy to coma)	Intoxication	Miosis, absent bowel sounds	Abnormal ABGs
Organo-phosphates/ carbamates	Bradycardia/ tachycardia, hypotension, hyperventilation/ hypoventilation	Altered (lethargy to coma)	Diarrhea, abdominal pain, blurred vision, vomiting	Salivation, diaphoresis, lacrimation, urination, defecation, miosis, seizures	Abnormal RBC & plasma cholinesterase activity
Phencyclidine	Hypertension, tachycardia, hyperthermia	Altered (agitation, lethargy to coma)	Hallucinations	Miosis, diaphoresis, myoclonus, blank stare, nystagmus, seizures	Myoglobinuria, leukocytosis, increased CPK
Phenothiazines	Hypotension, tachycardia, hypothermia/ hyperthermia	Altered (lethargy to coma)	Dizziness	Miosis/ mydriasis, decreased bowel sounds, tremor	Abnormal ECG, abnormal KUB
Salicylates	Hyperventilation, hyperthermia	Altered (agitation, lethargy to coma)	Tinnitus, nausea, vomiting, confusion	Diaphoresis, tender abdomen	Anion gap metabolic acidosis, respiratory alkalosis, abnormal LFTs & coagulation studies
Sedative-hypnotics	Hypotension, hypoventilation, hypothermia	Altered (lethargy to coma)	Intoxication	Hyporeflexia, bullae	Abnormal ABGs
Theophylline	Tachycardia, hypotension, hyperventilation, hyperthermia	Altered (agitation, lethargy to coma)	Nausea, vomiting, diaphoresis, confusion	Diaphoresis, tremor, seizures	Hypokalemia, hyperglycemia, metabolic acidosis, abnormal ECG

From Goldfrank LR, et al: Goldfrank's Toxicologic Emergencies. 4th ed. East Norwalk, CT, Appleton & Lange, 1990, pp. 66–67.

trauma, pulmonary edema), the airway must be initially protected by placing the patient in the Trendelenburg position with the left side dependent. Suction should be available at the bedside.

D. Physical Examination

The directed physical examination should minimally include the following:

1. **Vital Signs.** Note pulse, blood pressure, respiratory rate, and temperature. A "fifth" vital sign should be oxygen saturation (SaO_2), continuously obtained with a pulse oximeter.

2. **Skin.** Note flushing or pallor, diaphoresis or dryness, any signs of recent needle sticks, and/or evidence of trauma.

3. **HEENT.** Evaluate pupil size and reactivity; closely examine the oropharynx, and check the patient's gag reflex.

4. **Neck.** Look for tenderness or evidence of trauma.

5. **Chest.** Assess air-flow, wheezing, symmetry of breath sounds, and rales or rhonchi. Determine the effectiveness of the patient's cough.

6. **Heart.** Listen for murmurs, rubs, and/or gallops.

7. **Abdomen.** Listen for bowel sounds. Examine for tenderness, organomegaly, masses, or evidence of pregnancy.

8. **Neurologic Examination.** A thorough neurologic examination is mandatory, with special emphasis on determining the patient's level of consciousness, pupillary responses, other cranial nerve functions, motor responses, and reflexes.

Note: the poisoned patient can have rapid and dramatic changes in his/her clinical status with time. Examination (especially with respect to airway, breathing, circulation, and neurologic status) must be repeated frequently throughout the patient's ED stay.

E. Monitoring

Continuous monitoring in the ED should routinely include the following:

1. Vital signs.
2. Cardiac monitoring.
3. SaO_2 monitoring.

F. Laboratory Studies

The laboratory evaluation of the poisoned patient will be dependent on the likely agent(s) to which the patient was exposed and the overall clinical problem with which the patient presents. In trivial exposures, laboratory evaluation *may not* be necessary.

1. *Routinely* obtain the following:
   a. Complete blood count (CBC).
   b. Electrolyte panel.
   c. Anion gap.
   d. Glucose level.
   e. Blood urea nitrogen (BUN) and creatinine levels.
   f. Electrocardiogram.
   g. Pregnancy test.
   h. Acetaminophen level.

Note: the causes of an elevated anion gap include alcohol, toluene, methanol, uremia, diabetic ketoacidosis, paraldehyde, iron, isoniazid, lactic acidosis, ethylene glycol, salicylates, and strychnine. The mnemonic is "AT MUD PILES."

2. If the patient has an altered level of consciousness consider *also* obtaining the following studies:
   a. Arterial blood gas (ABG).
   b. Measured serum osmolality.
   c. Calcium, magnesium, and phosphorus levels.
   d. Urinalysis.
   e. Ethanol level.
   f. Chest roentgenography.

   Note: serum osmolality can be calculated as

   Serum osmolality = 2 (Na) + BUN/2.8 + glucose/18

   where Na is in mEq/L, and BUN and glucose are in mg/dL. If the measured serum osmolality differs from the calculated serum osmolality by more than 10 mOsm/kg, then suspect the presence of unmeasured osmotically active solutes (e.g., acetone, isopropyl alcohol, ethanol, ethylene glycol, mannitol, methanol).

3. *Additional studies to consider,* depending on clinical circumstances, may include one or more of the following:
   a. Abdominal films (see F. 6, below)
   b. Blood and urine cultures.
   c. Cervical spine films (anteroposterior, lateral, and odontoid views).
   d. Head computed tomography (CT).
   e. Liver function tests (LFTs)
   f. Lumbar puncture.
   g. Prothrombin time/partial thromboplastin time (PT/PTT).
   h. Relevant drug levels (see F. 4, below).
   i. Toxicologic screens (see F. 5, below).

4. Occasionally *drug levels/quantitative tests* are helpful. Consult with the laboratory on the best specimen to obtain (e.g., serum, whole blood, ABG). They are useful and should be obtained in the following exposures:
   a. Acetaminophen.
   b. Carbamazepine.
   c. Carboxyhemoglobin (ABG specimen for carbon monoxide exposure).
   d. Erythrocyte cholinesterase and pseudocholinesterase (insecticide exposure).
   e. Digoxin.
   f. Ethanol.
   g. Ethylene glycol.
   h. Heavy metals.
   i. Isopropyl alcohol.
   j. Iron.
   k. Lithium.
   l. Methanol.
   m. Methemoglobin (caused by exposure to aromatic nitro and amino compounds).
   n. Paraquat.
   o. Phenobarbital.

p. Phenytoin.
q. Quinidine.
r. Salicylate.
s. Theophylline.

5. *Toxicologic screens* (may require blood, gastric, and/or urine samples) are expensive, seldom provide information of much help in the immediate management of the patient, and are ordered too frequently. Minimize their use. In particular, consider general "tox" screens only when:
   a. A patient has severe clinical or biochemical abnormalities possibly secondary to a drug or poison.
   b. A patient has seizures, coma, or a head injury and there is suspicion of a drug ingestion.
   c. One must differentiate functional psychosis from a drug effect.
   d. One must differentiate hypoxic brain death from a prolonged drug effect.
   e. A patient presents with a confusing clinical picture, a-typical symptoms or signs, and historical clues are lacking.

   Remember: a "negative" toxicologic screen does not exclude an exposure to a substance not tested for.

6. Some drugs/poisons *may be radiopaque* (e.g., chloral hydrate, heavy metals, iodide, psychotropic medications, sodium, and enteric-coated tablets). Obtaining an abdominal film is occasionally useful in the patient's clinical evaluation. A normal abdominal film, however, does not rule out exposure to one or more of these agents.

III. DIFFERENTIAL DIAGNOSIS

A. Table 23–1 lists some frequently encountered toxidromes.

B. If the patient is presenting with an altered level of consciousness or coma, the differential diagnosis, in addition to poisoning/overdose, includes

1. Hypoxia or carbon dioxide retention.

2. Trauma (e.g., brain contusion, concussion, diffuse axonal injury, intracranial bleed, subdural hematoma, epidural hematoma).

3. Cerebrovascular disease (e.g., intracranial hemorrhage, cerebral infarction, subarachnoid hemorrhage).

4. Infection (e.g., sepsis, meningitis, encephalitis, brain abscess, human immunodeficiency virus [HIV] infection or secondary opportunistic infection).

5. Hypertensive encephalopathy.

6. Neoplasms (e.g., metastatic or primary brain lesion).

7. Postictal state.

8. Metabolic abnormalities (e.g., hypoglycemia, diabetic ketoacidosis, hyperglycemic hyperosmolar coma, hepatic failure, uremia, myxedema coma, thyroid storm, Wernicke's encephalopathy).

9. Electrolyte abnormalities (e.g., hyper- or hyponatremia, hyper- or hypocalcemia, hyperkalemia, hyper- or hypomagnesemia).

10. Environmental causes (e.g., hypothermia or heat stroke).

IV. THERAPY

The treatment of the poisoned patient should be thorough and systematic in every case. The following six therapeutic steps are a framework within which poisoning care occurs (Fig. 23–1). In many cases these therapeutic "steps" will need to take place simultaneously. Depending on the exposure, some of the later steps (e.g., enhancing elimination) may not be applicable.

A. **Step 1.** *Assess, secure, and support the airway, breathing, circulation, and neurologic status (the "ABCs") as indicated.* (Also see Chapter 1. II.)

1. Administer supplemental oxygen, protect the airway as necessary, and immobilize the cervical spine if trauma is suspected.
   a. Endotracheal intubation is appropriate when gastric lavage is to be performed in the patient with altered mentation or an inadequate cough or gag reflex; also strongly consider intubation in the early management of a patient with a significant ingestion of a rapidly acting sedative, hypnotic, or convulsant agent (e.g., cyclic antidepressant) even if the airway is initially adequate.
   b. The poisoned patient with altered mentation should be placed in the Trendelenburg position with the left side dependent. This is also the correct position in which to perform gastric lavage.

2. Obtain vital signs, establish intravenous (IV) access, check the fingerstick glucose level if mental status is altered, and order appropriate laboratory studies (see II, above). Monitor both cardiac rhythm and SaO_2.

3. Treat hypotension initially with IV crystalloid; monitor pulmonary status and cardiac function closely.
   a. If the clinical examination indicates pulmonary vascular congestion, support blood pressure as necessary with dopamine (begin with 2–5 µg/kg/min IV and adjust as necessary for a systolic blood pressure of 95–100 mmHg).
   b. In cyclic antidepressant overdoses, norepinephrine is depleted and the pressor of choice is probably norepinephrine (0.5-30 µg/min IV).

    c. If a pure alpha agonist is desired, use phenylephrine (administer 0.1-0.5 mg IV slowly, followed by 40-180 µg/min IV infusion).

    d. *Caution:* if the patient is hemodynamically stable, do not aggressively administer crystalloids. Both pulmonary edema and cerebral edema are significant complications to be avoided in the poisoned patient.

4. The patient with altered mentation should receive thiamine (100 mg IM or IV), glucose (25 g IV if the fingerstick glucose is < 80 mg/dL), and naloxone (0.4-2 mg or more IV). See Step 3, below.

5. Control ongoing seizure activity (also see Chapter 20).

    a. Consider the possibility of magnesium depletion and replace if appropriate (e.g., 1-2 g magnesium sulfate IV over 20 minutes; larger doses are needed in the pregnant patient with eclampsia).

    b. Benzodiazepines are the initial drugs of choice: lorazepam (0.1 mg/kg IV, given no faster than 2 mg/min, total adult dose 4-8 mg) or diazepam (0.15-0.25 mg/kg IV, given no faster than 2-5 mg/min, total adult dose 10-20 mg).

    c. Additional drugs may include phenytoin (18 mg/kg IV load [15 mg/kg in the elderly] no faster than 50 mg/min) and/or phenobarbital (10-20 mg/kg IV, no faster than 100 mg/min). Intubation should be accomplished prior to phenobarbital administration.

6. Provide general supportive care as necessary. Do not leave the patient with significantly altered mentation in the ED room alone. Keep the guardrails up on the patient's stretcher; soft restraints are reasonable to prevent self-harm.

7. Cautions

    a. Most early poisoning deaths are secondary to a failure to adequately support and secure the patient's airway, breathing, circulation, and neurologic status. The need for meticulous care in these areas can not be overemphasized. Aggressive use of airway protection techniques, including "prophylactic" intubation, will save lives!

    b. Hypoventilation and/or hypoxia may not be apparent clinically. Presume the overdose patient is hypoxic until proven otherwise. Cardiac monitoring and pulse oximetry should be *routine* in any poisoned patient who has the slightest alteration in consciousness or who is *at risk* for same.

    c. Emesis should never be induced in the patient with a depressed level of consciousness, poor cough reflex, abnormal gag reflex, or who is at risk for the rapid development of these (e.g., cyclic antidepressant overdose).

    d. Do not perform gastric lavage without first intubating the patient with a depressed level of consciousness (even if the cough and gag reflex are normal).

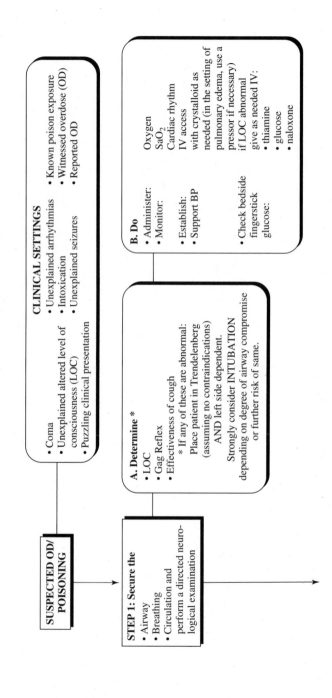

CLINICAL SETTINGS

- Coma
- Unexplained altered level of consciousness (LOC)
- Puzzling clinical presentation
- Unexplained arrhythmias
- Intoxication
- Unexplained seizures
- Known poison exposure
- Witnessed overdose (OD)
- Reported OD

SUSPECTED OD/ POISONING

STEP 1: Secure the
- Airway
- Breathing
- Circulation and perform a directed neurological examination

A. Determine *
- LOC
- Gag Reflex
- Effectiveness of cough
  * If any of these are abnormal: Place patient in Trendelenberg (assuming no contraindications) AND left side dependent.
  Strongly consider INTUBATION depending on degree of airway compromise or further risk of same.

B. Do
- Administer:
- Monitor:
  - Oxygen
  - SaO$_2$
  - Cardiac rhythm
- Establish:
- Support BP
  - IV access with crystalloid as needed (in the setting of pulmonary edema, use a pressor if necessary
- Check bedside fingerstick glucose:
  - if LOC abnormal give as needed IV:
    - thiamine
    - glucose
    - naloxone

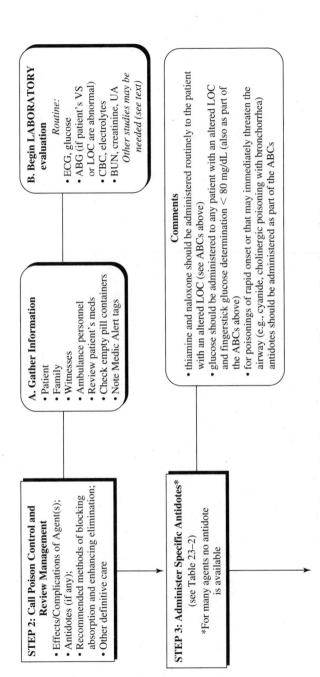

STEP 2: Call Poison Control and Review Management
- Effects/Complications of Agent(s);
- Antidotes (if any);
- Recommended methods of blocking absorption and enhancing elimination; Other definitive care

A. Gather Information
- Patient
- Family
- Witnesses
- Ambulance personnel
- Review patient's meds
- Check empty pill containers
- Note Medic Alert tags

B. Begin LABORATORY evaluation

Routine:
- ECG, glucose
- ABG (if patient's VS or LOC are abnormal)
- CBC, electrolytes
- BUN, creatinine, UA
  Other studies may be needed (see text)

STEP 3: Administer Specific Antidotes*
(see Table 23–2)
*For many agents no antidote is available

Comments
- thiamine and naloxone should be administered routinely to the patient with an altered LOC (see ABCs above)
- glucose should be administered to any patient with an altered LOC and fingerstick glucose determination < 80 mg/dL (also as part of the ABCs above)
- for poisonings of rapid onset or that may immediately threaten the airway (e.g., cyanide, cholinergic poisoning with bronchorrhea) antidotes should be administered as part of the ABCs

Figure 23–1. Emergency therapy of the poisoned/overdose patient.

871

C. Inhalational Exposure

- Administer 100% oxygen via non-rebreather mask.

B. Dermal Exposure

- Remove clothing.
- In most instances rinse with water for 30 min minimum.
- Certain *industrial* exposures may demand special care: review with Poison Control.

A. Ocular Exposure

- Saline or water irrigation for 20 min minimum.
- *Alkali* exposure may require hours of irrigation!
- Clean face/eyelashes/eyebrows.

D. Gastrointestinal Exposure (75% of poisonings are ingestions)

- Gastric Lavage and Activated Charcoal: method of choice for a suspected life-threatening ingestion, especially when the patient presents within 1-2 hr of ingestion.
- Activated Charcoal Only: suspected non-life-threatening ingestion > 1–2 hr post-ingestion. (Many experts recommend activated charcoal only, even in the serious ingestion, when the patient presents > 1-2 hr after ingestion).
- See text for a discussion of Ipecac Induced Emesis and Whole Bowel Irrigation.
- Do *not* Perform Gastric Emptying Procedure IF: ingestion is a caustic substance (especially alkali) or if ingested substance is a low viscosity petroleum distillate (see text).

STEP 4: Block Absorption

- Perform simultaneously with the above steps!
- Care of the airway takes priority over blocking absorption.
- When using lavage and charcoal, some experts recommend putting charcoal down the orogastric tube first, then lavaging, then repeating charcoal administration.
- Charcoal is:
  i. Not effective for: iron, caustics (mineral acids and inorganic alkali), electrolytes, or hydrocarbons.
  ii. Probably not effective for alcohols (including methanol, ethanol, and ethylene glycol).
  iii. Not indicated in the patient who is an acetaminophen overdose when the patient presents ≥ 4 hr post-ingestion.

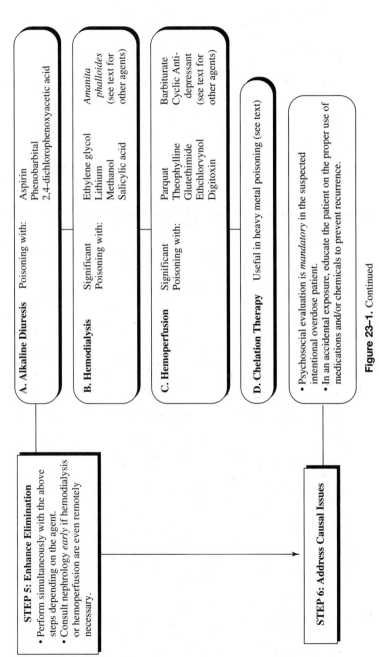

STEP 5: Enhance Elimination
- Perform simultaneously with the above steps depending on the agent.
- Consult nephrology *early* if hemodialysis or hemoperfusion are even remotely necessary.

A. Alkaline Diuresis   Poisoning with:

Aspirin
Phenobarbital
2,4-dichlorophenoxyacetic acid

B. Hemodialysis   Significant Poisoning with:

Ethylene glycol
Lithium
Methanol
Salicylic acid

Amanita phalloides (see text for other agents)

C. Hemoperfusion   Significant Poisoning with:

Parquat
Theophylline
Glutethimide
Ethchlorvynol
Digitoxin

Barbiturate
Cyclic Anti-depressant (see text for other agents)

D. Chelation Therapy   Useful in heavy metal poisoning (see text)

- Psychosocial evaluation is *mandatory* in the suspected intentional overdose patient.
- In an accidental exposure, educate the patient on the proper use of medications and/or chemicals to prevent recurrence.

STEP 6: Address Causal Issues

Figure 23–1. Continued

873

B. **STEP 2.** *Rapidly obtain a history, complete the directed physical examination* (as outlined in II, above), *and call Poison Control to review the current treatment recommendations for the suspected exposure.* The following management issues should be determined in consultation with poison control for each of the agents to which the patient was exposed:

1. Complications/effects of the agent(s).

2. Antidotes (if any) and their dosage.

3. Recommended techniques for blocking absorption and enhancing elimination.

4. Other recommended definitive care.

C. **STEP 3.** *Give specific antidotes.*

1. Depending on the exposure, administering available antidote(s) should frequently occur *simultaneously* with the above steps. For poisonings known to have a very rapid onset (e.g., cyanide) or that quickly compromise the airway (e.g., organophosphate poisoning with bronchorrhea) the administration of the appropriate antidote should be part of the ABCs.

2. For the patient with an altered level of consciousness, thiamine, glucose, and naloxone should also be *routinely* administered as part of the ABCs (step 1 above).
   Naloxone is given to reverse opioids. The usual dose is 0.4-2 mg IV. Much larger doses (> 10 mg) may be required when poisoning occurs with codeine, propoxyphene, pentazocine, or certain fentanyl derivatives. The clinical effects of narcotic reversal with naloxone may be as short as 15-20 minutes and subsequent doses are commonly necessary. Alternatively, after the patient's initial response, a continuous naloxone infusion may be utilized by administering two-thirds of the initially effective bolus dose per hour. *Caution:* in the pregnant patient, the dosage of naloxone must be titrated carefully to avoid precipitation of narcotic withdrawal in the fetus.

3. The use of some other commonly used antidotes in poison management is outlined in Table 23–2.

4. Unfortunately, most drugs/toxins *will not* have a specific antidote.

D. **STEP 4.** *Block absorption.* Depending on exposure, blocking absorption should frequently take place *simultaneously* with the above steps.

1. *Ocular.* Immediately treat with saline or water irrigation for at least 20 minutes (eyelids retracted). Make every effort to remove the substance from the face, eyebrows, and eyelashes. "Neutralizing" chemicals should *not* be used. Alkali eye contamination is a true ophthalmologic emergency: hours

Table 23–2. SOME COMMONLY USED ANTIDOTES IN POISONING/ OVERDOSE MANAGEMENT (DOSES FOR ADULTS)

Toxin	Antidote	Antidote Administration
Acetaminophen	N-Acetylcysteine	140 mg/kg PO loading dose, then 70 mg/kg PO q 4 hr for 17 doses. Repeat a dose if patient vomits within 1 hr of its administration.
Anticholinergic agents (examples include: antihistamines, antiparkinsonian drugs, antipsychotic agents, atropine)	Physostigmine	Use only if necessary to manage coma, convulsions, dysrhythmias, or delirium. Dose is 1–2 mg IV over 5 min; effect lasts 20–60 min. May repeat dose; do not exceed 6 mg over time.
Benzodiazepines	Flumazenil	0.2 mg IV over 30 sec. If no response in 30 sec give 0.3 mg IV over 30 sec. Subsequent doses of 0.5 mg IV may be given, each over 30 sec and one minute between doses, to a total of 3–5 mg.
Beta blockers	Glucagon	50–150 µg/kg IV over 1 min, followed by a continuous infusion of 1–5 mg/hr titrated to vital signs.
Calcium channel blockers, hydrofluoric acid, fluorides	Calcium (calcium chloride for calcium channel blocker overdose; calcium gluconate for hydrofluoric acid or fluoride exposure)	*For calcium-channel-blocker overdose:* give 1 g calcium chloride IV over 5 min. Continuously monitor cardiac rhythm. *For hydrofluoric acid burns:* infiltrate each square cm of dermis and SQ tissue with 0.5 mL of 10% calcium gluconate as needed for pain control. A calcium gel may also be applied to the burn surface. *For PO fluoride ingestion:* give 10 g calcium gluconate in 250 mL water PO. Maximum dose is 30 g/day.
Cyanide	Amyl nitrite, sodium nitrite, and sodium thiosulfate	Inhale amyl nitrite ampule for 30 sec of every min, give 100% O_2 between amyl nitrite inhalations. Use a new ampule q 3 min and continue until sodium nitrite can be given IV. Sodium nitrite dose is 300 mg IV (10 mL of a 3% solution) at a rate of 2.5–5 mL/min. Then administer 12.5 g of sodium thiosulfate IV.
Cyclic antidepressants	Sodium bicarbonate	1–3 mEq/kg IV as necessary to maintain blood pH at 7.50. Alkalinization results in increased protein binding of cyclic antidepressant and minimizes the amount of free drug available. Useful in the management of cyclic antidepressant induced cardiac arrhythmias or hypotension.
Digitalis glycosides	Digoxin-specific antibody fragments	Milligrams of digoxin ingested divided by 0.6 = number of vials required. If amount ingested is unknown, but life-threatening dysrhythmias are present, give 20 vials. If 6 hr postingestion dig level is available, the number of vials to administer is = (dig level in ng/mL × 5.6 × wt in kg) divided by 600.
Iron	Deferoxamine mesylate	15 mg/kg/hr IV; or 90 mg/kg IM (maximum of 1 g per injection) q 8 hr. Maximum dose is 6 g in 24 hr. Use only IV route for life-threatening exposures. During therapy, monitor urine output, urine color, and iron levels.
Methanol, ethylene glycol	Ethanol	Loading dose is 10.0 mL/kg of 10% EtOH in D5W solution IV over 30 min. Also begin a maintenance dose of 0.66–1.30 mL/kg/hr IV of 10% solution. Maintain blood ethanol concentration at 100–150 mg/dL. Watch glucose and sodium levels closely. If patient is being dialyzed, add 91 mL/hr to maintenance dose.
Isoniazid, hydrazine, monomethylhydrazine mushrooms	Pyridoxine	*Unknown amount ingested:* give 5 g IV over 5 min. *Known amount ingested:* give 1 gram pyridoxine IV every 5 min for every gram ingested. An overdose of pyridoxine may result in neuropathy.
Organophosphate or carbamate insecticides	Atropine	Begin with 2 mg IV test dose. Then administer 2–4 mg IV q 10–15 min as needed until cessation of secretions occurs. For organophosphate insecticide poisoning, pralidoxime chloride (1–2 g IV q 6 hr) should be administered after initial treatment with atropine.

Adapted from Desforges p. 1679; and Mofenson et al p. 1111.

of eye irrigation may be necessary depending on the substance and the measured eye pH. Consultation with ophthalmology is mandatory for significant alkali eye exposures.

2. *Dermal.* Remove contaminated clothing and dust off all dry material. Rinse the skin with water for at least 30 minutes. Remember to thoroughly rinse hair, navel, and fingernails. Avoid forceful flushing in a shower because this may cause deeper penetration of the toxin into the skin. Alkalis can require hours of irrigation. Be very cautious to isolate clothing and avoid concomitant staff member exposure. *Caution:* certain industrial dermal exposures must be treated differently, as noted below:

   a. Elemental metals (including sodium, potassium, and lithium) may explode on exposure to water. Irrigate with oil; use no water.

   b. Mustard gas: wash with oil, kerosene, or gasoline; then wash with soap and water.

   c. Oil-based compounds (e.g., pesticides) should be washed off with green soap or shampoo, followed by water irrigation.

   d. With unusual industrial exposures (e.g., chromic acid, alkyl mercury, phenol, phosphorus, elemental metals, hydrofluoric acid) call Poison Control immediately for specific recommendations on proper dermal decontamination.

3. *Inhalational.* Remove the patient from the exposed environment and administer 100% oxygen. (*Note:* the only exception to this rule is the patient who has been exposed to paraquat or diquat, where high concentrations of oxygen may result in pulmonary fibrosis.)

4. *Gastrointestinal (GI) Exposures.* Most poisonings involve oral ingestion; GI decontamination is an appropriate consideration. Multiple techniques for GI decontamination are available: gastric lavage, activated charcoal alone or with gastric lavage, ipecac-induced emesis, and whole-bowel irrigation. The technical aspects of performing each of these methods are presented in Table 23–3. The best technique to use is fraught with controversy at this time and may be quite variable between different EDs. *The rational use of GI decontamination should take into account the agent ingested, the time since ingestion, and the agent's known rapidity of absorption from the GI tract.*

   a. Gastric lavage with activated charcoal is the GI decontamination procedure of choice in the ED for the patient with a suspected life-threatening overdose when the patient presents within 1-2 hours of toxic ingestion. Gastric lavage is appropriate *several to many hours* after ingestion in *any* of the following circumstances:

      i. Significant overdose has occurred with an agent

Table 23-3. GASTROINTESTINAL (GI) DECONTAMINATION PROCEDURES: TECHNICAL ASPECTS

Gastrointestinal Lavage

Indications

GI lavage is the decontamination procedure of choice (combined with activated charcoal) when the patient has suffered a life-threatening ingestion (especially when the patient presents within 1–2 hr of ingestion) or when an acute ingestion results in an altered level of consciousness (after first securing the airway).

Procedure

1. Assess and secure the airway. If the patient has a depressed level of consciousness (or is at significant risk for same during the procedure), an inadequate gag reflex, or an inadequate cough reflex, endotracheal intubation (with a cuffed endotracheal tube) is necessary before lavage. Supplemental oxygen should be supplied as necessary. Continuous SaO_2 monitoring is appropriate *throughout* the procedure.
2. Place the patient in the Trendelenburg position, left side dependent.
3. Have suction on and at the bedside.
4. Place soft restraints (minimal) on the patient's extremities: this will help prevent the patient from removing the orogastric tube once placed.
5. Use a 36-French size, or larger, orogastric tube (adult patients); and *premeasure* the correct length the tube should be inserted by noting the distance from the patient's nose to the midepigastrium on the tube (with tape).
6. Place an endoscopy bite block in the patient's mouth.
7. Gently, but firmly, place the orogastric tube into the mouth, and advance it into the pharynx, esophagus, and stomach. Confirm tube placement by injecting 50 mL of air into the tube and auscultating bubbling over the epigastrium. If the patient coughs, is stridorous, or cannot speak (if alert), the tube is in the trachea and must be withdrawn immediately.
8. Before commencing with lavage, attach the tube to suction and "vacuum" the stomach contents as empty as possible.
9. Begin gastric lavage with 200 mL aliquots of fluid (tap water or saline), removing each aliquot (generally via gravity into a bag on the floor using a "Y" tubing set-up) before introducing the next. The stomach should be manually massaged through the abdominal wall as each aliquot is being drained. In the smaller adult patient, the pediatric patient, or when large lavage volumes are used, warmed normal saline is the lavage fluid of choice.
10. Once the lavage fluid is clear, continue for another 2–3 L.
11. When the lavage is completed, administer an activated charcoal slurry (1 g/kg; see below) down the orogastric tube. (Many poison experts recommend introducing the charcoal slurry at the *start* of the lavage, completing lavage, and then repeating the administration of charcoal).
12. Clamp the tube, withdraw it, and continue to protect the patient's airway.

Contraindications

Alkali ingestion, aliphatic hydrocarbon ingestion (e.g., gasoline, kerosene, mineral spirits), hematemesis, insignificant and nontoxic ingestions.

Activated Charcoal

Activated charcoal should be used in most toxic ingestions. The surface area of commercially available activated charcoals is 900 to 1200 m^2/g, with an adsorptive capacity of about 500–1000 mg of drug per gram of charcoal. (*Depending on the ingested substance,* many poison experts recommend using *only* activated charcoal [without lavage] when the patient presents more than 1–2 hr after ingestion.)

Procedure

1. If the charcoal comes in a powdered form, it should be mixed with 4–8 parts water or cathartic. Sorbitol (mix with 2 mL/kg of 70% solution) is the cathartic of choice because of its rapid onset of action. Catharsis should *not* be used in the presence of ileus (absent bowel sounds), bowel obstruction, or suspected bowel perforation; or in the setting of known and significant electrolyte disturbance, small children, or hypovolemic adults. If the charcoal comes in a container already combined with sorbitol or water, thoroughly mix the solution before giving it to the patient. (*Note:* the charcoal

Table continued on following page

frequently settles into a "block" in the bottom of the container; it may be necessary to cut open the container with scissors and pour the mixture into a basin to manually break up the block and resuspend the charcoal into solution before the mixture is ready for administration).

2. If an orogastric tube has been placed for lavage purposes (see above), the charcoal slurry may be placed down the tube. In the awake, alert, cooperative patient, the charcoal slurry may be sipped from a closed container through a large straw. Alternatively, a nasogastric tube can be placed and the charcoal slurry administered down the nasogastric tube (the slurry may have to be further diluted with normal saline to prevent clogging of the small lumen of the nasogastric tube).

3. Dosage of activated charcoal: 1 g per kilogram body weight (approximately 50–100 g).

4. If the patient vomits, the dose of charcoal should be repeated. Sometimes an antiemetic (e.g., metoclopramide 5–10 mg IV) is necessary.

5. Repetitive dosing of charcoal (0.5–1.0 g/kg every 2–4 hr) is controversial. Do *not* add a cathartic to the repetitive charcoal doses. Repeat doses may be useful for toxins with biliary/gastric secretion (e.g., phencyclidine) or recirculating metabolites (e.g., phenobarbital, phenytoin, theophylline).

Cautions

1. Charcoal is *not* effective in the following toxic ingestions:
   a. Caustics (mineral acids, inorganic alkali).
   b. Electrolytes (sodium, potassium, magnesium).
   c. Ethanol.
   d. Methanol.
   e. Ethylene glycol.
   f. Hydrocarbons.
   g. Iron, lead, lithium, mercury.

2. In acetaminophen overdoses, charcoal will bind the antidote acetylcysteine and should not be used in the late-presenting patient ($\geq$ 4 hr) when antidote delivery is crucial.

Contraindications

Charcoal should not be used after caustic acid or alkali ingestions.

Ipecac-Induced Emesis

Indications

1. An awake and alert patient with good airway protective reflexes who presents within 30–45 min of a non-life-threatening, nonsedating ingestion.

2. In most circumstances, ipecac is appropriate first-aid treatment of accidental ingestions in the home, but its use is currently very limited in modern ED poison management.

Procedure

1. Obtain the patient's history and assess the cough and gag reflex to determine if he/she is a candidate for ipecac-induced emesis.

2. The adult patient should be given 30 mL (2 tblsp) of ipecac syrup PO. Follow its administration with two to three glasses of plain water. Repeat the dose if vomiting does not occur within 20–30 min. If no effect is observed after the second dose proceed with gastric lavage.

Contraindications

1. *Never* use ipecac if one of the following rapidly acting convulsants has been ingested:
   a. Amphetamines.
   b. Camphor.
   c. Chlordane.
   d. Cocaine.
   e. Cyclic antidepressants.
   f. Isoniazid.
   g. Lindane.
   h. Nicotine.
   i. Strychnine.

2. *Never* use ipecac in the already-vomiting patient; or the patient with an abnormal gag reflex, depressed level of consciousness, marked hypertension, hematemesis, or

Table 23–3. GASTROINTESTINAL (GI) DECONTAMINATION
PROCEDURES: TECHNICAL ASPECTS *Continued*

significant cardiovascular or cerebrovascular disease. Ipecac should also not be used when an oral antidote is crucial in the management of the overdose, or when the patient is in the third trimester of pregnancy.

3. Do not use ipecac when the ingested substance is a hydrocarbon, caustic acid, or alkali.

Whole-Bowel Irrigation

Indications

The role of whole-bowel irrigation in toxic ingestions is uncertain. It should be considered, however, in the setting of massive ingestions (especially in the late-presenting patient), ingestions of toxins not well adsorbed by charcoal (e.g., iron, lithium, lead), or after the ingestion of drug packets (e.g., cocaine "body packers").

Procedure

1. Polyethylene glycol lavage-electrolyte solution (Golytley, CoLyte) is given either orally (awake and alert patient with good airway protective mechanisms), by nasogastric tube, or by lavage tube. The adult dose is 2 L/hr, and it is administered for 4–6 hr or until the rectal effluent becomes clear.
2. It may be necessary to administer an antiemetic to the patient (e.g., metoclopramide 5–10 mg IV).

Contraindications

Whole-bowel irrigation should not be used in the setting of ileus or suspected GI tract obstruction or perforation.

---

    known to decrease gut motility (e.g., anticholinergic agent, cyclic antidepressant).
  ii. Significant overdose has occurred with an agent slowly absorbed fom the GI tract (e.g., carbamazepine).
 iii. Clinical evidence indicates that significant drug persists in the stomach and is still available for removal (e.g., roentgenograms showing multiple iron tablets in the stomach).
 iv. Clinical evidence indicates that a drug concretion or "bezoar" has formed (drugs known to form concretions include barbiturates, glutethimide, iron, meprobamate, and salicylates). Concretion formation may require prolonged lavage and/or endoscopic-assisted removal.

  b. Activated charcoal should be used in almost all overdose situations (though some substances are known not to be bound by charcoal, and charcoal may compromise the use of some oral antidotes—see Table 23–3).
    i. More than 1–2 hours postingestion, many authorities suggest administering activated charcoal *only* and dispensing with gastric lavage (except for specific circumstances as outlined in 4a, above).
    ii. In controlled experiments, activated charcoal is as effective as gastric lavage or ipecac-induced emesis at any time (except for agents known not to be absorbed by activated charcoal). The longer the time from

ingestion to GI decontamination, the more activated charcoal *exceeds* either ipecac-induced emesis or gastric lavage in efficacy.

iii. In the early postingestion period, gastric lavage and activated charcoal combined are more effective than either one alone.

c. Ipecac-induced emesis is reasonable for home use in the awake and alert patient with a non-life-threatening, nonsedating ingestion. In the ED, however, its use should be limited to the treatment of a completely awake and alert patient with a non-life-threatening and nonsedating ingestion who presents within 30–45 minutes of exposure (see Table 23–3).

d. Whole-bowel irrigation should be considered in the setting of massive ingestions (especially in the late-presenting patient), ingestions of toxins not adsorbed by charcoal (e.g., iron, lithium, lead), or after the ingestion of drug packets (e.g., "body packers").

e. *Caution:* GI decontamination as outlined above should *not* be performed in the patient who has ingested a caustic substance (especially alkali) or a low-viscosity petroleum distillate (e.g., gasoline, kerosene, lighter fluid). *It is* appropriate, however, to lavage a hydrocarbon ingestion *after first protecting the airway with a cuffed endotracheal tube* when the hydrocarbon or its additives is/are a significant absorbable toxin (e.g., **c**amphor, **h**alogenated hydrocarbon, **a**romatic hydrocarbon) or contains an associated poison of significant toxicity (e.g., heavy **m**etal, **p**esticide [note the mnemonic "CHAMP"]).

f. *Controversies* in determining the best method of gastrointestinal decontamination include the following:

   i. Controlled studies using animals or human volunteers are difficult to apply to the clinical setting.

   ii. Prospective studies using real patients are limited and plagued by multiple variables difficult or impossible to control (e.g., time of poison ingestion, specific poison ingested, patient factors).

   iii. Different poisons/drugs may, in and of themselves, effect the efficacy of a given GI decontamination regimen (e.g., the poison may effect GI motility/transit time). Therefore, a GI decontamination procedure that works for one agent may not be the procedure of choice for another agent.

   iv. *There is no controlled, prospective data that indicates any method of GI decontamination in human beings decreases mortality in the setting of an oral poison ingestion.*

E. **STEP 5.** *Enhance elimination.* There are multiple methods to enhance the elimination of certain toxic compounds from the body, the most useful of which include the following: alkaline diuresis, hemodialysis, hemoperfusion, and chelation. These four methods are discussed in more detail below. Orally administered activated charcoal ("gastrointestinal dialysis") will enhance the elimination of salicylates, theophylline, digoxin, benzodiazepines, carbamazepine, and phenytoin—its use has been described in IV. D, above.

1. *Alkaline Diuresis*

   a. Useful in aspirin, phenobarbital, and 2,4-dichlorophenoxyacetic acid overdoses.
   b. *Techniques* to alkalinize the urine:
      i. Bolus therapy: 1-2 mEq/kg sodium bicarbonate IV over 30-60 minutes, repeated as necessary until the desired urine and serum pHs are obtained; *or*
      ii. Continuous infusion therapy: add 2 ampules of sodium bicarbonate (50 mEq per ampule) to 1 L of 5% dextrose in water (D5W) and infuse at twice maintenance rates (in the volume-depleted patient, it is appropriate to add 1.5 ampules of sodium bicarbonate to 1 L of 0.45% normal saline and run at 20 mL/kg for the first 30-60 minutes of treatment).

   The goal of urinary alkalinization is to achieve a urine pH ≥ 8.0 while maintaining blood pH ≤ 7.50.

   c. *Cautions:* hydration status must be closely followed; serum potassium should be checked frequently and kept within normal limits.

2. *Hemodialysis*

   a. Hemodialysis utilizes a semipermeable membrane to remove certain elements from the body by virtue of differences in their rates of diffusion across that membrane.
   b. Hemodialysis is indicated immediately for the treatment of significant poisonings with any of the following (consult a nephrologist urgently):
      i. Ethylene glycol.
      ii. Lithium.
      iii. Methanol.
      iv. Salicylic acid
      v. *Amanita phalloides* mushrooms.
   c. The following toxins may also be removed from the body by hemodialysis, and its use may be necessary depending on the extent of exposure to these agents:
      i. Acetaminophen.
      ii. Arsenic (trivalent).
      iii. Bromide.
      iv. Chloral hydrate (as tri-chloroethanol).
      v. Ethanol.
      vi. Isopropyl alcohol.
   d. Complications of hemodialysis include access site diffi-

culties, hypotension, bleeding, infection, electrolyte and osmotic imbalances, and air embolism.

3. *Hemoperfusion*

   a. Hemoperfusion passes blood through a cartridge containing carbon and/or activated charcoal to remove adsorbable toxins from the blood.
   b. It is indicated immediately if intoxication is significant for paraquat or theophylline. (Theophylline is also dialyzable, but hemoperfusion is the preferred method of removal in the significantly poisoned patient.)
   c. It also should be considered if supportive measures are unsuccessful or if prolonged coma is anticipated for:
      i. Amitriptyline.
      ii. Chloral hydrate.
      iii. Chlorophenothane (DDT).
      iv. Digitoxin.
      v. Digoxin.
      vi. Ethchlorvynol.
      vii. Glutethimide.
      viii. Methaqualone.
      ix. Methotrexate.
      x. Methophenobarbital.
      xi. Nortriptyline.
      xii. Pentobarbital.
      xiii. Phenobarbital.
      xiv. Phenytoin.
   d. Complications of hemoperfusion include access site difficulties, hypotension, bleeding, thrombocytopenia, leukopenia, hypoglycemia, and/or hypocalcemia.

4. *Chelation Therapy*

   a. Chelation therapy is useful in heavy-metal poisoning. The metal is tightly bound into the chelator's ring and then eliminated from the body via the kidneys.
   b. Chelating agents include the following (for the exact dosing, administration, and cautions in the use of these agents consult a toxicology text):
      i. *Calcium disodium edetate (EDTA):* used in acute lead poisoning. It will also chelate cadmium, chromium, cobalt, copper, magnesium, nickel, selenium, tellurium, tungsten, uranium, vanadium, and zinc.
      ii. *Dimercaprol (BAL):* initial chelator of choice in acute lead poisoning. It will also chelate antimony, arsenic, bismuth, chromates, copper, gold, mercury, and nickel.
      iii. *d-Penicillamine:* useful in the chelation of iron, arsenic, cadmium, chromates, cobalt, copper, lead, mercury, nickel, and zinc.
      iv. *Deferoxamine mesylate:* chelator of choice in symp-

tomatic iron poisoning or when serum iron levels are > 350 μg/dL.

F. **STEP 6.** *Address Causal Issues*

1. Many poisonings in adults are intentional.

2. Psychosocial evaluation (via a medical social worker and/or the psychiatry consultant) is *mandatory* in the suspected intentional overdose patient. It is also appropriate in the setting of drug abuse, alcohol abuse, in the patient with a prior psychiatric history, the homeless patient, the handicapped patient, the parent with dependent minors, and the elderly patient.

3. Patients at high risk of repeat overdose include the elderly, adolescents, college students, patients with a prior history of a suicide attempt or a known psychiatric history, patients suffering significant stressful life events, and the clinically depressed patient.

4. In the setting of accidental exposure, every effort should be made to instruct and educate the patient in the proper use of medications or chemicals so as to prevent recurrence of the event. In work-related exposures, contact the relevant governmental agency (e.g., public health department) as appropriate.

V. DISPOSITION

A. Discharge

1. The patient who is completely asymptomatic and who has received thorough evaluation, treatment, and appropriate ED observation may be discharged. The exact length of time the patient must be observed, even if asymptomatic, will vary with the agent to which the patient was exposed. It is crucial that, before discharge, step 6, above, be completed. Prior to discharge, medical follow-up must be arranged and documented.

2. The intoxicated patient must be held until they are medically cleared and clinically no longer pose a danger to themselves or others. Reasonable transportation from the ED should also be arranged.

3. The ED physician has an obligation to detain a patient, with force if necessary, if the patient has been potentially exposed to a mind-altering drug until the patient is medically and psychosocially clear. An "against medical advice" discharge is *not* an option in this circumstance.

B. Admit

1. In general, it is safest to have a low threshhold to admit the poisoned patient. Any of the following parameters mandate

admission: persistent vital-sign abnormalities, altered mentation, the patient remains symptomatic from the exposure, other significant co-morbid conditions are present, the patient needs continued treatment (e.g., acetylcysteine administration in the acetaminophen overdose), and/or there is potential for delayed toxicity.

2. The decision to admit the patient to a general medical floor, a telemetry unit, or the ICU must be based on the toxin to which the patient was exposed, clinical findings in the ED, and the recognized potential for further deterioration. The patient with an altered mental status, oxygenation or ventilation abnormalities, significant vital sign abnormalities (including temperature), significant co-morbid conditions, significant electrolyte abnormalities, or who has a cardiac rhythm abnormality should be admitted to the ICU.

VI. PEARLS AND PITFALLS

A. The highest priority in the poisoned patient is the support and management of the patient's airway, breathing, circulation, and neurologic status.

B. Routinely and aggressively monitor the patient's cardiac rhythm and SaO_2.

C. Routinely administer thiamine, glucose, and naloxone to the ED patient who presents with an altered level of consciousness.

D. Suspect concomitant drug exposure, trauma, significant electrolyte or glucose abnormality, and/or infection in the clinically intoxicated patient.

E. Be alert and able to manage the many complications that occur in the poisoned patient:

1. Airway compromise.

2. Arrhythmias.

3. Aspiration.

4. Bowel perforation.

5. Cerebral edema.

6. Electrolyte disturbances.

7. Hematemesis.

8. Hyperthermia.

9. Hypotension.

10. Hypothermia.

11. Hypoventilation.

12. Hypoxia.

13. Ileus.

14. Injury.

15. Pulmonary edema (cardiogenic and noncardiogenic).

16. Seizures.

17. Shock.

18. Trauma.

F. Obtain a psychosocial evaluation in all known or potential intentional exposures.

Do *not* do any of the following:

A. Completely believe the history.

B. Presume the asymptomatic toxin exposure is benign.

C. Lavage the patient without first protecting the airway.

D. Fail to identify the cyclic antidepressant overdose, aspirin overdose, acetaminophen overdose, or carbon monoxide exposure.

E. Fail to identify other substances with significant delayed toxicity: antitumor drugs, carbon tetrachloride, colchicine, digoxin, ethylene glycol, heavy metals, methanol, mushrooms, some narcotics (e.g., diphenoxylate), aspirin, and slow-release preparations.

BIBLIOGRAPHY

Bayer MJ, Klatzko MD, Kulig KW: The poisoned patient. Patient Care 1990; June 15: 176-207.

Goldfrank LR, Flomenbaum NE, Lewin NA, et al (eds): Goldfrank's Toxicologic Emergencies. 4th Ed. East Norwalk, CT, Appleton & Lange, 1990.

Ilano AL, Raffin TA: Management of carbon monoxide poisoning. Chest 1990;97:165–169.

Kellermann AL, Fign SD, LoGerfo JP, Copass MK: Impact of drug screening in suspected overdose. Ann Emerg Med 1987;16(11):1206–1216.

Kulig K: Initial management of ingestions of toxic substances. N Engl J Med 1992;326(25): 1677–1681.

Litovitz TL, Clark LR, Soloway RA: 1993 Annual Report of the American Association of Poison Control Centers Toxic Exposure Surveillance System. Am J Emerg Med 1994; 12(5):546.

Merigian KS, Woodard M, Hedges JR, et al: Prospective evaluation of gastric emptying in the self-poisoned patient. Am J Emerg Med 1990;8(6):479–483.

Perrone J, Hoffman RS, Goldfrank LR: Special considerations in gastrointestinal decontamination. Emerg Med Clin N Am 1994;12(2):285–299.

MANAGEMENT OF SPECIFIC POISONINGS

I. ACETAMINOPHEN (APAP)

A. General Considerations

1. Acetaminophen is a common antipyretic and analgesic agent present in many prescription and nonprescription medications (Table 23–4). Poisoning with APAP results in centri-

Table 23–4. ACETAMINOPHEN-CONTAINING COMPOUNDS

Actifed Plus	Datril	Sine-Aid
Allerest	Dristan	Sine-Off
Anacin-3	Esgic	Sinutab
Benadryl Plus	Excedrin	TheraFlu
Bromo-Seltzer	Fioricet	Tylenol
Comtrex	Midrin	Tylox
Congesprin	Nyquil	Triaminicin
Contac Jr.	Panadol	Tussagesic
Coricidin	Percocet	Vanquish
Cotylenol	Percogesic	Vicodin
Darvocet-N	Phenaphen	Wygesic

From Done AK, Pediatrics 1960;26:800.

lobularhepatic necrosis; acute renal failure may uncommonly occur.

2. The antidote for APAP poisoning is N-acetylcysteine (NAC).

B. Pharmacodynamics

1. APAP is rapidly absorbed from the gastrointestinal tract. Peak plasma levels occur 30–120 minutes after a therapeutic dose. Delayed gastric emptying slows absorption.

2. The serum half-life ($t_{1/2}$) of APAP is normally 2 hours; it increases to ≥ 8 hours in a toxic ingestion or liver failure.

3. After absorption, APAP is metabolized in the adult liver and renally excreted. Four percent of any given dose is converted into a toxic intermediate via the P-450 cytochrome oxidase system. This intermediate requires conjugation with glutathione for detoxification. In an APAP overdose, glutathione depletion occurs, the toxic intermediate accumulates, and hepatic damage ensues. The antidote NAC substitutes for glutathione and prevents accumulation of the toxic intermediate.

4. Ingestion of >140 mg/kg in children or 7.5 g in adults may result in liver damage.

5. When the time of acute APAP ingestion is known, the acetaminophen nomogram can be used to predict toxicity and the need for NAC antidote therapy (Fig. 23–2).
   a. Therapeutic intervention using the nomogram should be based on APAP levels obtained at least 4 hours postingestion. Before that time, the nomogram may *underestimate* potential toxicity.
   b. Table 23–5 lists drugs that induce the cytochrome P-450 system, thereby facilitating production of the toxic intermediate. If the APAP overdose patient is taking any of these medications, hepatic toxicity may occur at serum levels *less* than predicted by the nomogram.

Table 23–5. SOME DRUGS THAT MAY POTENTIATE APAP TOXICITY

Antihistamines	Griseofulvin
Barbiturates	Meprobamate
Carbamazepine	Phenytoin
Glutethimide	Rifampin

C. Clinical Presentation

The clinical presentation of APAP overdose is given in Table 23–6.

Table 23–6. CLINICAL STAGES OF ACETAMINOPHEN TOXICITY

STAGE	HOURS POSTINGESTION	SIGNS AND SYMPTOMS
I	2–24 hr	None or anorexia, nausea, vomiting, diaphoresis, malaise
II	24–48 hr	Asymptomatic. Elevated AST, ALT, bilirubin, PT
III	48–72 hr	Hepatic necrosis, jaundice, bleeding, encephalopathy/coma, seizures, electrolyte disturbances, secondary renal failure, myocardial necrosis, arrhythmias

From Rumack BH, Matthew H: Pediatrics 1975;55:873.

D. Management

1. As in all overdose situations, the initial management priority is *support of the patient's airway, breathing, circulation, and neurologic status* (see Standard Therapy of the Poisoned/Overdose Patient, IV. A, earlier in this chapter). If mental status or vital signs are altered, suspect another toxin or other significant medical condition in the APAP-poisoned patient.

2. *Gastric emptying* is appropriate for an acute APAP ingestion. Its efficacy declines, however, the longer the time interval between ingestion and treatment.

   a. Ipecac-induced emesis may be considered when the patient presents within 30 minutes of ingestion. After this time, its efficacy at preventing absorption significantly declines. In the late-presenting patient, ipecac is contraindicated because it interferes with the administration of NAC antidote therapy.

   b. Gastric lavage should be performed if the patient presents within 2 hours of ingestion, if the timing of ingestion is uncertain, if the patient has an altered level of consciousness; *or* in cases of suspected polydrug overdose.

   c. The use of charcoal in APAP overdose management remains a matter of debate and is variable between institutions. Activated charcoal will bind APAP, but it also (to a much lesser extent) binds the antidote NAC. A reasonable

Estimating potential for hepatotoxicity: The following nomogram has been developed to estimate the probability that plasma levels in relation to intervals post ingestion will result in hepatotoxicity:

1. If the acetaminophen level determined at least 4 hours following an overdose falls above the broken line, administer the entire course of acetylcysteine treatment.

2. If the acetaminophen level, determined at least 4 hours following an overdose, falls below the broken line, acetylcysteine treatment is not necessary or if already initiated may be discontinued.

*Adapted from Rumack and Matthew; *Pediatrics* 55:871-876, 1975

Cautions For Use of This Chart:
1. The time coordinates refer to time post-ingestion.
2. Serum levels drawn before 4 hours may not represent peak levels.
3. The graph relates only to plasma levels following a single acute overdose ingestion.

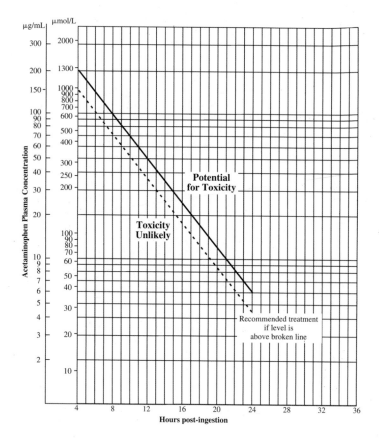

4. The broken line, which represents a 25% allowance below the solid line, is included to allow for possible errors in acetaminophen plasma assays and estimated time from ingestion of an overdose.

Figure 23–2. Nomogram: Plasma or serum acetaminophen concentration versus time post-acetaminophen ingestion. *(From Management of Acetaminophen Overdose. McNeil Consumer Products Co., 1986),* in Goldfrank et al: Acetaminophen. Chapter 22. In Goldfrank L et al (eds): Goldfrank's Toxicologic Emergencies. 4th Ed. Norwalk, CT, Appleton & Lange, 1990, p. 254.

approach is to use activated charcoal if the patient presents within 4 hours of ingestion, or in the setting of a multi-drug overdose. If the time of ingestion is uncertain, or known to be ≥ 4 hours prior to patient presentation, then activated charcoal should *not* be used.

3. *Laboratory evaluation* should minimally include a CBC, electrolyte panel, glucose, BUN, creatinine, APAP level, salicylate level, and liver function tests (AST, ALT, bilirubin, PT), and pregnancy test.

4. *Antidote therapy with N-acetylcysteine:*
    a. Use the nomogram when the patient's APAP level is known to decide on the need for NAC. NAC should be routinely given to the APAP-overdose patient when *any* of the following conditions apply:
        i. The patient's APAP level is in the toxic range per the nomogram.
        ii. The time of ingestion is unknown or > 24 hours prior to presentation and the APAP level is >10 µg/mL.
        iii. The APAP level is borderline toxic and the patient has ingested other drugs that induce the cytochrome P-450 system (see Table 23–5).
        iv. An APAP level is not available.
        v. The patient presents < 4 hours after ingestion and a stat APAP level within that time is > 300 µg/mL.
    b. Antidotal efficacy declines with time. NAC is maximally effective if given within 8 hours of ingestion, and therapy is still beneficial within 24 hours of ingestion. Twenty-four hours or more postingestion the efficacy of NAC is uncertain, but it is appropriate if serum APAP levels are still measurable.
    c. *Dose:* 140 mg/kg PO loading dose, followed by 70 mg/kg PO every 4 hours for 17 additional doses (72 hours of antidote therapy). If charcoal was used for gastric decontamination, consider increasing the NAC loading dose to 190 mg/kg. NAC may be diluted 1:3 with water, juice, or carbonated beverage to mask its taste. When vomiting occurs within 1 hour of NAC administration, the dose should be repeated. A nasogastric or duodenal tube should be employed if vomiting NAC is a persistent problem. Metoclopramide (Reglan) 10 mg IV may be used to combat vomiting. There are essentially no known contraindications to the use of NAC.

5. *Disposition:* hospitalization is mandatory for NAC therapy and hepatic function monitoring in the known or potentially toxic APAP ingestion.

BIBLIOGRAPHY

Anker AL, Smilkstein MJ: Acetaminophen: concepts and controversies. Emerg Med Clin N Am 1994;12(2):335–349.

Flanagan RJ, Meredith TJ: Use of N-acetylcysteine in clinical toxicology. Am J Med 1991;
91:131S–139S.
Janes J, Routledge PA: Recent developments in the management of paracetamol (acetaminophen) poisoning. Drug Saf 1992;7:170–177.

II. ANTICHOLINERGIC AGENTS

A. General Considerations

1. Many different substances produce anticholinergic effects (Table 23–7).

2. The antidote for severe anticholinergic poisoning is physostigmine. This antidote may produce significant side effects, however, and its use should be limited to the life-threatening situation.

B. Pharmacodynamics

Anticholinergic agents produce their toxic effects via cholinergic/muscarinic receptor blockade. Such receptors are present in the central nervous system (CNS); the salivary, lacrimal, and sweat glands; pupils; tracheobronchial tree; cardiac conduction system; and GI and genitourinary tracts.

C. Clinical Presentation

1. CNS muscarinic blockade may produce the following: agitation, anxiety, delirium, hallucinations (e.g., "lilliputian" hallucinations: seeing "little people"), psychosis, seizures and myoclonus, pyramidal signs (e.g., hyperreflexia, up-going toes,

Table 23–7. AGENTS WITH ANTICHOLINERGIC PROPERTIES

Nonprescription medications	Antihistamines
Soporifics (Nytol, Sominex, SleepEze, Unisom, etc.)	Decongestants (brompheniramine, diphenhydramine, hydroxyzine, etc.)
Decongestants (Actifed, Allerest, Benadryl, Chlorpheniramine, Contac, Dristan, Sinutab, etc.)	Phenothiazines (Promethazine [Phenergan] etc.)
Analgesic compounds (Excedrin-PM, etc.)	H₂-Blockers (cimetidine [Tagamet], famotidine [Pepcid], ranitidine [Zantac], etc.)
Antiemetics (Dramamine)	Antidepressants (Doxepin [Sinequan] etc.)
Phenothiazines (Chlorpromazine [Thorazine], fluphenazine [Prolixin], perphenazine [Trilafon], thioridazine [Mellaril], thiothixene [Navane], trifluoperazine [Stelazine], etc.)	Belladonna alkaloids (atropine, glycopyrrolate [Robinul], etc.)
Antiparkinson drugs (benztropine [Cogentin], procyclidine [Kemadrin], trihexyphenidyl [Artane])	Mydriatics (atropine, cyclopentolate [Cyclogyl], homatropine, tropicamide [Mydriacyl], etc.)
Heterocyclic antidepressants (amitriptyline [Elavil], desipramine [Norpramin], doxepin [Sinequan], imipramine [Tofranil], nortriptyline [Pamelor], protriptyline [Vivactil], etc.)	Plants
	Fungi (*Amanita* sp.)
	Jimson weed *(Datura)*
	Deadly nightshade *(Atropa belladonna)*
	Potato eyes, leaves, and sprouts
	Tomato vines

clonus), and/or medullary paralysis, with apnea, coma, and death.

2. Peripheral muscarinic blockade may produce the following: decreased glandular secretion (sweat, saliva, tears, mucus), mydriasis, tachycardia, hyperthermia, ileus and gastric atony, urinary retention, hypotension, and shock.

3. Some anticholinergics (especially phenothiazines and cyclic antidepressants) are cardiotoxins and may produce the following: vagolysis with tachycardia, decreased conduction velocity with re-entrant arrhythmias, and direct myocardial depression. The ECG may show prolongation of the QRS, PR, and/or QT_c intervals.

4. The mnemonic for the signs of acute poisoning is

   "Hot as a Hare,

   Blind as a Bat,

   Dry as a Bone,

   Red as a Beet, and

   Mad as a Hatter."

5. Chronic anticholinergic poisoning (e.g., the patient treated with an antidepressant drug or antiparkinson drug) may present with central symptoms only, including agitation, confusion, and cognitive impairment.

D. Management

1. As in all overdose situations, the initial management priority is *support of the patient's airway, breathing, circulation, and neurologic status* (see Standard Therapy of the Poisoned/Overdose Patient, IV. A, earlier in this chapter). The cardiac rhythm and SaO_2 should be continuously monitored; vital signs and neurologic status must be closely followed.

2. *Gastric emptying* is appropriate in the setting of an ingestion and should include lavage and administration of activated charcoal and a cathartic. Gastric atony from anticholinergic effects may increase the accessibility of unabsorbed toxin to gastric lavage and/or activated charcoal many hours postingestion. Ipecac should not be used because of the risk of anticholinergic-induced mental status changes and seizures.

3. *Laboratory evaluation* should minimally include a CBC; elecrolyte panel; glucose, BUN, and creatinine levels; ECG; and toxicologic screen.

4. *Antidote therapy with physostigmine:*
   a. Physostigmine is an acetylcholinesterase inhibitor; it antagonizes the effects of both central and peripheral cholinergic blockade.
   b. *Cautions:* physostigmine may cause seizures, bradycardia, bronchorrhea, muscle weakness, and exacerbations of

Table 23–8. CLINICAL PRESENTATION AND MANAGEMENT OF ANTICHOLINERGIC POISONING

CLINICAL FINDINGS	MANAGEMENT
Central Anticholinergic Syndrome	
Agitation/delirium	Supportive care
Psychosis/hallucinations	Physostigmine only if absolutely necessary
Seizures/myoclonus	Support airway and oxygenation
	Diazepam 5–10 mg given slowly (2 mg/min) IV
	Phenytoin 18–20 mg/kg IV (no faster than 50 mg/min; monitor cardiac rhythm) is a possible adjunct
	Physostigmine if refractory to standard management of seizures
Medullary paralysis/apnea/coma	Intubation and mechanical ventilator support
	Physostigmine
Peripheral Anticholinergic Syndrome	
Cardiovascular	
Supraventricular arrhythmias	Propanalol 0.1 mg/kg IV in 1.0-mg increments as pulse and BP allow
	Physostigmine if above is insufficient
Ventricular arrhythmias	Lidocaine 1 mg/kg IV bolus, followed by 2–4 mg/min infusion
	Propanalol as above
	Phenytoin 1 g IV (no faster than 50 mg/min) is a possible adjunct
	Synchronized DC countershock if patient is unstable
Hypotension/shock	IV crystalloid or colloid support
	Pressor agents (dopamine, norepinephrine, or phenylephrine) if necessary
	Consider physostigmine
Hyperthermia	Acetaminophen, cooling blanket, mist spray with fan convection
Urinary retention	Foley catheter
Ileus/gastric atony	NPO, observation; consider nasogastric tube (especially if patient vomiting)
Dry mucosa/dry eyes/mydriasis	Supportive care

airway reactivity. It should be used only if absolutely necessary to combat the effects of a life-threatening anticholinergic poisoning (e.g., intractable seizures, coma, or symptomatic supraventricular tachycardias). Physostigmine should *not* be used in the setting of cardiac conduction disturbances or a cyclic antidepressant overdose (it has caused asystole in this setting).

   c. *Dose:* 2 mg given slowly (over 5 minutes) IV in the adult patient. Clinical effect lasts 20-60 minutes; repeat doses may be necessary. Total dose should not exceed 6 mg over time.

5. *Additional care* should be provided as in Table 23–8 above. Anticipate the potential for mental status deterioration, seizures, airway compromise, apnea, cardiac arrhythmias, and/or shock.

6. *Disposition:* the symptomatic patient with anticholinergic poisoning must be closely monitored until symptoms and signs (e.g., mental status changes, tachycardia) have completely resolved. This may necessitate hospital admission to a telemetry unit or ICU bed. Intentional overdoses require psychiatric evaluation.

BIBLIOGRAPHY

Delaney KA: Anticholinergics. Chapter 130. In Rosen et al (eds): Emergency Medicine: Concepts and Clinical Practice. 3rd Ed. St. Louis, CV Mosby, 1992, pp. 2534–2540.
Schneck HJ, Rupreht J: Central anticholinergic syndrome (CAS) in anesthesia and intensive care. Acta Anaesthesiol Belg 1989;40:219–228.
Vanderhoff BT, Mosser KH: Jimson weed toxicity: management of anticholinergic plant ingestion. Am Fam Phys 1992;46:526–530.

III. ANTICONVULSANTS

The anticonvulsant drugs (ACDs) are used in the treatment of a variety of conditions, including epilepsy, chronic pain syndromes, and mood disorders. Patients with these diagnoses are at a higher risk of attempted suicide than the general population, and these drugs are increasingly seen in suicidal attempts. Inadvertent poisonings also occur.

PHENYTOIN

A. General Considerations

Phenytoin is the most commonly prescribed ACD. It facilitates sodium extrusion from neurons and thereby stabilizes threshold hyperexcitability. Toxic doses produce CNS stimulation, probably via cerebellar inhibition. The more common side effects of the drug are cerebellar signs and symptoms.

B. Pharmacodynamics

1. Phenytoin is rapidly absorbed from the small intestine. Peak blood levels occur 2–12 hours after ingestion depending on dose and dosage form. It is highly protein bound, and tissue levels are not saturated for 7–14 days. Once tissue levels are saturated, small increases in dosage may cause large increases in blood levels.

2. The amount of "free" phenytoin (non-protein-bound phenytoin) determines the drug's pharmacologic activity. "Free" phenytoin increases substantially in the setting of decreased serum albumin, increased serum bilirubin, or uremia.

3. Detoxification occurs in the liver, largely via parahydroxylation. Patients may vary considerably in their ability to metabolize phenytoin. Most of the drug is excreted in the bile as inactive metabolites, which are reabsorbed and then excreted in the urine.

4. Multiple drugs may affect phenytoin's metabolism (Table 23–9).

5. Plasma $t_{1/2}$ is about 22 hours (range: 7–42 hours). Optimum therapeutic serum levels are 10–20 µg/mL, and mild nystagmus is normal in the therapeutic range.

6. Doses of 2–5 g are potentially lethal.

C. Clinical Presentation

1. Signs and symptoms of toxicity may include the following:
   a. *CNS effects:* nystagmus, ataxia, dysarthria, confusion, tremor, hyperreflexia, lethargy, dystonic posturing, seizures; rarely stupor or coma.
      i. Levels < 30 µg/mL rarely produce findings other than nystagmus.
      ii. Ataxia is common with levels > 30 µg/mL.
      iii. At levels > 40 µg/mL, lethargy and dysarthria are prominent (chronic users may be asymptomatic, however, even with levels of 50 µg/mL).
   b. *Cardiovascular effects:* decreased refractory period and increased conduction velocity (class IB antiarrhythmic), altered automaticity, hypotension, and circulatory collapse.
   c. *Hematologic effects:* eosinophilia, macrocytosis, megaloblastic anemia, and sometimes pancytopenia.
   d. *Miscellaneous effects:* nausea, vomiting, myositis, hepatitis, renal failure.

Table 23–9. COMMON DRUG INTERACTIONS WITH PHENYTOIN

↑ PHENYTOIN LEVELS	↓ PHENYTOIN LEVELS	EITHER ↑ OR ↓ PHENYTOIN LEVELS	↑ SEIZURES WITH PHENYTOIN	EFFICACY IMPAIRED BY PHENYTOIN
Acute ethanol ingestion	Chronic ethanol ingestion	Phenobarbital	Cyclic antidepressants	Steroids
Benzodiazepines	Carbamazepine	Valproic acid		Cardiac glycosides
Warfarin	Molindone			Tetracyclines
Disulfiram	Calcium-containing antacids			Furosemide
Estrogens and oral contraceptives				Quinidine
H₂ blockers				Rifampin
Isoniazid				Theophylline
Phenothiazines				
Sulfonamides				
Trazodone				
Salicylates				

D. Management

1. As in all overdose situations, the initial management priority is *support of the patient's airway, breathing, circulation, and neurologic status* (see Standard Therapy of the Poisoned/ Overdose Patient, IV. A, earlier in this chapter). The cardiac rhythm and SaO_2 should be continuously monitored; vital signs and neurologic status must be closely followed.

2. *Gastric emptying* is appropriate in the setting of an acute ingestion and should include gastric lavage, and administration of activated charcoal and a cathartic. Multiple-dose activated charcoal is effective and should be considered in the setting of a life-threatening ingestion.

3. *Laboratory evaluation* should minimally include a CBC; electrolyte panel; glucose, BUN, and creatinine levels; ECG; and phenytoin plasma level. A repeat phenytoin level should be obtained at least several hours after the initial level to evaluate for continued drug absorption.

4. *Additional care:*
   a. Seizures should be managed with airway and breathing support, diazepam, and phenobarbital (if necessary).
   b. Do not administer medications that can displace phenytoin from protein and exacerbate its toxicity (e.g., chlorothiazide, phenylbutazone, salicylates, and/or sulfonamides).
   c. Provide meticulous supportive care and guard against secondary complications: patient self-injury, aspiration, infection, electrolyte disturbance, GI hemorrhage.
   d. Patients with a seizure disorder should not restart phenytoin therapy after an overdose until therapeutic levels (10-20 µg/mL) are again present and the cause of the overdose has been corrected.

5. *Disposition:* admit patients with moderate to severe toxicity, rising blood levels in the ED, and/or suicidal ideation. Patients with accidentally induced mild toxicity (e.g., blood level 30 µg/mL and gait disturbance) should also be admitted if there is no responsible friend or relative to observe and care for the patient at home.

BIBLIOGRAPHY

Larsen JR, Larsen LS: Clinical features and management of poisoning due to phenytoin. Med Toxicol Adverse Drug Exp 1989;4:229–245.

Mellick LB, Morgan JA, Mellick GA: Presentations of acute phenytoin overdose. Am J Emerg Med 1989;7:61–67.

Wyte CD, Berk WA: Severe oral phenytoin overdose does not cause cardiovascular morbidity. Ann Emerg Med 1991;20:508–512.

CARBAMAZEPINE (TEGRETOL)

A. General Considerations

This iminostilbene derivative is structurally like the cyclic antidepressants, and it has similar toxicities in an overdose situation (including alpha-adrenergic blockade, anticholinergic effects, and quinidine-like cardiotoxicity). Carbamazepine (CBZ) is increasingly used as an alternative to lithium in the treatment of bipolar affective disorder; it is also effective in the treatment of pain syndromes and epilepsy.

B. Pharmacodynamics

1. GI absorption of CBZ is slow, with peak levels occurring 4–5 hours after ingestion. It is 76% bound to albumin.

2. The drug is hepatically metabolized, and the $t_{1/2}$ is variable: 12–17 hours in chronic users and 25–65 hours in first-time users.

3. Therapeutic serum levels are 4–12 µg/mL.

4. CBZ *decreases* the $t_{1/2}$ of phenytoin, warfarin, tetracycline, and theophylline. Breakthrough vaginal bleeding can occur when used in combination with oral contraceptives.

5. Life-threatening toxicity may occur after acute ingestion of ≥ 10 g.

C. Clinical Presentation

1. Signs and symptoms of toxicity may include the following:
   a. *CNS effects:* drowsiness, confusion, ataxia, dizziness, diplopia, nystagmus, mydriasis, extrapyramidal movements, seizures, coma.
   b. *Cardiovascular effects:* tachycardia, heart failure, collapse, shock, arrhythmias (including atrioventricular (AV) block).
   c. *Hematologic effects:* thrombocytopenia, agranulocytosis, aplastic anemia.
   d. *Miscellaneous effects:* nausea and vomiting, hepatitis, Lyell's or Stevens-Johnson syndrome, the syndrome of inappropriate anti-diuretic hormone secretion (SIADH), and the adult respiratory distress syndrome (ARDS).

2. Signs and symptoms appear 1–3 hours post overdose. Neurologic and cardiovascular complications are the most worrisome toxicities.

D. Management

1. As in all overdose situations, the initial management priority is *support of the patient's airway, breathing, circulation, and neurologic status* (see Standard Therapy of the Poisoned/Overdose Patient, IV. A, earlier in this chapter). The cardiac rhythm and SaO_2 should be continuously monitored; vital signs and neurologic status must be closely followed. If a pressor agent is required for blood pressure support, phenylephrine may have advantages over dopamine or norepinephrine because of the alpha-blocking and arrhythmogenic potential of CBZ.

2. *Gastric emptying* is appropriate and should include gastric lavage and administration of activated charcoal and a cathartic even if the patient presents many hours after ingestion. Multiple-dose activated charcoal is effective and should be considered in a life-threatening ingestion.

3. *Laboratory evaluation* should minimally include a CBC; electrolyte panel; glucose, BUN, and creatinine levels; ECG, and a CBZ level. Because of CBZ's slow GI absorption, a repeat level several hours after the first level should be checked.

4. *Additional care:*
   a. Seizures should be managed with diazepam and phenobarbital.
   b. Cardiac toxicity should be managed similarly to the cyclic antidepressant poisoned patient (see X. Cyclic Antidepressants later in this chapter).
   c. Hemoperfusion should be considered in patients with status epilepticus or significant cardiac toxicity, or in patients with very high serum levels. Hemodialysis is indicated in severe poisoning associated with renal failure.

5. *Disposition:* admit patients with CNS symptoms or signs, persistent CBZ-induced vital-sign abnormalities, CBZ levels ≥ 20 µg/mL, rising CBZ levels, CBZ-induced ECG changes, and/or suicidal ideation. Admitted patients should minimally have continuous cardiac monitoring.

BIBLIOGRAPHY

Fisher RS, Cysyk B: A fatal overdose of carbamazepine: case report and review of literature. *J Toxicol Clin Toxicol* 1988;26:477–486.

Kasarskis EJ, Kuo CS, et al: Carbamazepine-induced cardiac dysfunction. Characterization of two distinct clinical syndromes. *Arch Intern Med* 1992;152:186–191.

Sethna M, Solomon G, Cedarbaum J, Kutt H: Successful treatment of massive carbamazepine overdose. *Epilepsia* 1989;30:71–73.

VALPROIC ACID

A. General Considerations

This carboxylic acid (dipropylacetic acid) is gaining increasing popularity in the treatment of epilepsy, migraine headaches, and mood disorders. Its mechanism of action remains unclear but may be related to increasing GABA bioavailability in the brain. Valproate is available as the simple sodium salt (Depakene) or as divalproex sodium (Depakote).

B. Pharmacodynamics

1. Valproic acid (VPA) is rapidly absorbed from the GI tract. Peak plasma levels occur 1–4 hours after ingestion. Food in the gut will delay absorption.

2. Plasma $t_{1/2}$ ranges from 6 to 16 hours. The use of enzyme-

inducing drugs (such as other ACDs) may promote faster metabolism and a shorter $t_{1/2}$.

3. Metabolism is dependent on hepatic glucuronidation and mitochondrial beta oxidation. The drug is eliminated in the urine as a ketometabolite, which may lead to a positive urine test for ketones.

4. The therapeutic level is variable but is generally considered to be 50–100 µg/mL.

5. The usual dose is 15–60 mg/kg/day; some patients may tolerate doses up to 100 mg/kg/day with much higher plasma levels. In this range, VPA is 90% protein bound. Protein binding decreases with higher VPA levels, use of other highly protein-bound drugs, or in the presence of other fatty acids. Free VPA may more accurately reflect the drug's CNS bioavailability.

C. Clinical Presentation

Toxicities include

1. Drowsiness, lethargy, coma (all enhanced by combination with alcohol); tremor, ataxia, nystagmus, diplopia, dysarthria, and cerebral edema.

2. Nausea and vomiting.

3. Hepatitis with hyperammonemia and coagulopathy—rare, but may be fatal.

4. Platelet dysfunction.

5. Unpredictably enhanced toxicity of barbiturate, salicylate, carbamazepine, phenytoin, warfarin, or other hepatically metabolized drugs.

6. Renal failure.

D. Management

1. As in all overdose situations, the initial management priority is *support of the patient's airway, breathing, circulation, and neurologic status* (see Standard Therapy of the Poisoned/Overdose Patient, IV. A, earlier in this chapter). The cardiac rhythm and SaO_2 should be continuously monitored; vital signs and neurologic status must be closely followed.

2. *Gastric emptying* is appropriate and should include gastric lavage and administration of activated charcoal and a cathartic. Multiple-dose activated charcoal should be considered in the setting of a life-threatening ingestion. Although VPA is rapidly absorbed from the GI tract, the presence of food in the gut will significantly slow absorption and make VPA accessible to lavage hours into the ingestion.

3. *Laboratory evaluation* should minimally include a CBC;

Table 23–10. COMMONLY USED ANTIPSYCHOTIC AGENTS

GENERIC NAME	TRADE NAME	SEDATION	EXTRA-PYRAMIDAL	ANTI-CHOLINERGIC	HYPOTENSION
Chlorpromazine	Thorazine	3+	2+	2+	3+
Thioridazine	Mellaril	3+	1+	3+	2+
Perphenazine	Trilafon	2+	3+	1+	1+
Prochlorperazine	Compazine	2+	3+	1+	1+
Fluphenazine	Prolixin	1+	3+	1+	1+
Trifluoperazine	Stelazine	1+	3+	1+	1+
Thiothixene	Navane	1+	2+	2+	2+
Haloperidol	Haldol	1+	3+	1+	1+

electrolyte panel; glucose, BUN, and creatinine levels; ECG; liver function tests; PT/PTT; and a VPA level.

4. *Additional care* is largely supportive and should include the appropriate management of thrombocytopenia, coagulopathy, coma, and/or significant hepatic dysfunction. The role of hemodialysis and hemoperfusion in the life-threatening VPA overdose is uncertain.

5. *Disposition:* admit all patients with CNS effects, persistent vital-sign abnormalities, and/or suicidal ideation. The asymptomatic VPA overdose patient should be observed in the ED for a minimum of 6 hours and a nontoxic VPA level rechecked after that time before being considered for discharge.

BIBLIOGRAPHY

Dupuis RE, Lichtman SN, Pollack GM: Acute valproic acid overdose. Clinical course and pharmacokinetic disposition of valproic acid and metabolites. Drug Saf 1990;5:65–71.
Khoo SH, Leyland MJ: Cerebral edema following acute sodium valproate overdose. J Toxicol Clin Toxicol 1992;30:209–14.

IV. ANTIPSYCHOTIC AGENTS (INCLUDING PHENOTHIAZINES AND HALOPERIDOL)

A. General Considerations

1. The phenothiazines are major tranquilizers frequently used in the treatment of psychosis. Haloperidol is a butyrophenone neuroleptic with many of the same antidopaminergic effects as the phenothiazines but with fewer anticholinergic toxicities (Table 23–10).

2. Additional structural classes of antipsychotics include dibenzoxazepines (e.g., loxapine), diphenylbutylpiperidines (e.g., pimozide), indoles (e.g., molindone), and thioxanthenes (e.g., thiothixene).

3. These agents are frequently overdosed, often in combination with other drugs such as sedatives, cyclic antidepressants, lithium, and alcohol.

B. Pharmacodynamics

1. Phenothiazines are readily absorbed from the gut or parenterally. Absorption may be delayed secondary to anticholinergic effects.

2. Peak plasma levels occur 2–4 hours after oral administration.

3. Hepatic metabolism occurs, with about 50% of an absorbed dose enterohepatically recirculated; the other 50% is eliminated by urinary excretion.

4. The phenothiazines cause varying degrees of central anticholinergic and antidopaminergic effects. These agents also produce peripheral anticholinergic effects, alpha-adrenergic blockade, direct (quinidine-like) myocardial toxicity, and lowered seizure threshold.

C. Clinical Presentation

1. *CNS effects:* confusion, lethargy, ataxia, slurred speech, seizures (especially with loxapine). In severe cases, coma and respiratory depression may occur. Sometimes, paradoxical agitation and delirium are seen.

2. *Peripheral anticholinergic effects:* mydriasis, hyperthermia, ileus, flushed skin, anhidrosis, urinary retention, tachycardia.

3. *Cardiovascular effects:* hypotension, ECG interval prolongation (PR, QRS, QT_c), tachycardias (including ventricular arrhythmias), or bradycardias (including heart block and asystole).

4. *Movement disorders:* acute dystonia (e.g., oculogyric crisis; torticollis; jaw, lip, and tongue spasm), parkinsonism, akathisia, and tardive dyskinesia (this latter occurs months to years after the use of these agents).

5. *Miscellaneous:* hypothermia, hyperthermia, leukopenia, agranulocytosis, hemolytic anemia, gynecomastia, galactorrhea.

D. Management

1. As in all overdose situations, the initial management priority is *support of the patient's airway, breathing, circulation, and neurologic status* (see Standard Therapy of the Poisoned/ Overdose Patient, IV. A, earlier in this chapter). The cardiac rhythm and SaO_2 should be continuously monitored; vital signs and neurologic status must be followed closely. Vasopressor agents (e.g., phenylephrine or norepinephrine) may be required for hypotension unresponsive to appropriate fluid resuscitation.

2. *Gastric emptying* should occur in the setting of an acute ingestion. Aggressive use of activated charcoal is almost always appropriate: enterohepatic recirculation of phenothiazines makes these agents accessible to charcoal removal *many hours* postingestion. Gastric lavage (after securing the airway

as necessary) combined with activated charcoal administration is reasonable when the patient presents within several hours of ingestion or when the patient is comatose: neuroleptic-induced gastric atony may increase the accessibility of unabsorbed toxin to gastric removal many hours after ingestion. Ipecac should not be used because of the risk of drug-induced mental status changes and/or seizures.

3. *Laboratory evaluation* should minimally include a CBC; electrolyte panel; glucose, BUN, and creatinine levels; ECG, urinalysis, and toxicologic screening. Quantitative neuroleptic drug levels are not useful in management. Additional studies that should be considered, depending on patient presentation, include ABGs, chest and abdominal roentgenography (phenothiazines are radiopaque); pregnancy test; creatinine phosphokinase (CPK), calcium, magnesium, and phosphate levels; and/or liver function tests.

4. *Additional care* (Table 23–11)

   a. Seizures should be managed with diazepam, phenytoin, and/or phenobarbital as necessary (see Standard Therapy of the Poisoned/Overdose Patient, earlier in this chapter).

   b. An ECG is mandatory. Carefully evaluate for prolongations of QT_c and QRS intervals, as these may herald the onset of ventricular arrhythmias. Prophylactic phenytoin administration (10-18 mg/kg IV at 25-50 mg/min) may prevent these. Alternatively, some experts recommend IV sodium bicarbonate (begin with 1-2 mEq/kg IV) to raise the serum pH to 7.50 when QRS widening occurs. Symptomatic ventricular arrhythmias or bradycardias may be treated by usual ACLS protocols (see Chapter 13). Class Ia antiarrhythmics (procainamide, quinidine, disopyramide) and beta blockers are contraindicated.

   c. Dystonic reactions (e.g., oculogyric crisis, spasmodic torticollis) are often relieved by diphenhydramine (25-mg increments IV, not to exceed 100 mg over 4 hours) or benztropine (1-2 mg IM or IV, repeated if necessary).

   d. Neuroleptic malignant syndrome, a rare and potentially fatal syndrome, is characterized by hypertonic skeletal muscle activity, altered mentation, hyperthermia, and fluctuating autonomic nervous system activity in the setting of neuroleptic medication use. The mainstays of therapy are appropriate attention to the patient's airway, breathing, circulation, and neurologic status; vital-sign support; benzodiazepine sedation for muscle rigidity and agitation, electrolyte management, evaluation and treatment for concomitant infection, and treatment of hyperthermia. Adjunctive medications that are believed useful in the management of the hyperthermia and muscle rigidity of the neuroleptic malignant syndrome include dantrolene (1-2 mg/kg IV every 6 hours, not to exceed 10 mg/kg per day) and bromocriptine (7.5-60 mg/kg/day PO or via a nasogastric tube in divided doses every 8 hours). Muscle paralysis

Table 23–11. ANTIPSYCHOTIC DRUG OVERDOSE: MANIFESTATIONS AND TREATMENT

Toxic Effect	Manifestations	Treatment
Anticholinergic		
Central	Agitation, disorientation, delirium	Supportive care
	Hallucinations, coma, seizures	Diazepam (and phenytoin for status epilepticus Physostigmine (for life-threatening symptoms)
Peripheral	Tachyarrythmias Mydriasis Dry (No sweat, saliva) Urinary retention, ileus Hyperthermia	Supportive care; physostigmine (for life-threatening symptoms); See text for adjuncts
Antidopaminergic (altered dopaminergic–cholinergic receptor balance)	Extrapyramidal reactions Dystonias (including oculogyric and buccolingual crises, torticollis, and opisthotonus) Parkinsonism Akathisia (restlessness and muscle discomfort)	Diphenhydramine 50 mg IM or IV; or Benztropine 2 mg IM or IV
Increased dopaminergic receptor sensitivity because of chronic blockade	Tardive dyskinesia	*Caution:* anticholinergics exacerbate
Alpha-adrenergic blockade	Vasodilation Hypotension	IV fluids Phenylephrine or norepinephrine if necessary
Quinidine-like myocardial toxicity	Increased QT_c, QRS, PR intervals Myocardial depression Arrhythmias	Supportive care; ?phenytoin or sodium bicarbonate Follow ACLS guidelines, but avoid type Ia antiarrhythmic agents

after intubation is sometimes necessary for muscle hyperactivity control (use pancuronium). Myoglobinuria is a complication of this syndrome and should be managed as appropriate.

e. *Disposition:* completely asymptomatic patients must be observed and monitored in the ED for a *minimum* of 6 hours. If at any time ECG abnormalities are detected, telemetry admission and at least 24 hours of continuous cardiac monitoring is indicated. Significantly symptomatic patients (e.g., profound mental status changes, arrhythmias) require ICU admission.

BIBLIOGRAPHY

Gratz SS, Levinson DF, Simpson GM: The treatment and management of neuroleptic malignant syndrome. Prog Neuropsychopharmacol Biol Psychiatry 1992;16:425–434.

Li C, Gefter WB: Acute pulmonary edema induced by overdosage of phenothiazines. Chest 1992;101:102–104.

V. BARBITURATES

A. General Considerations

1. Barbiturates are sedative-hypnotic agents that reversibly depress excitable tissues, including the CNS, skeletal muscle, and smooth muscle. In severe overdoses, cardiac muscle may also be affected.

2. In the 1950s and 1960s barbiturates were responsible for the majority of deaths caused by drug ingestion. With the availability of safer, nonbarbiturate sedatives (e.g., benzodiazepines), barbiturates are much less frequently prescribed today. The exception is phenobarbital, which is still a commonly prescribed anticonvulsant.

3. Over the past three decades, the outcomes from an acute barbiturate ingestion have significantly improved through the use of aggressive supportive measures. There is no antidote.

B. Pharmacodynamics

1. Barbiturates are absorbed rapidly from the GI tract. The presence of food decreases absorption.

2. Traditionally, barbiturates have been divided into three classes on the basis of their duration of action: short-acting barbiturates, whose duration of action is generally < 3 hours (e.g., pentobarbital and secobarbital); intermediate-acting barbiturates, whose duration of action is 3–6 hours (e.g., amobarbital); and long-acting barbiturates, whose duration of action is > 6 hours and whose $t_{1/2}$ is generally > 40 hours (e.g., mephobarbital, metharbital, phenobarbital, and primidone) (Table 23–12).

3. The shorter-acting agents are almost completely metabolized in the liver, with the inactive metabolites subsequently renally excreted. The longer-acting agents are renally excreted and have only limited liver metabolism.

Table 23–12. PHARMACODYNAMICS OF COMMON BARBITURATES

	Long-Acting	Intermediate	Short-Acting	
Detoxification	Renal excretion	Hepatic/renal	Hepatic	
Drug	Phenobarbital (Luminal)	Amobarbital (Amytal)	Secobarbital (Seconal)	Pentobarbital (Nembutal)
Hypnotic dose (mg)	100–200	50–200	100–200	50–100
Duration (hr)	6	3–6	3	3
Plasma $t_{1/2}$ (hr)	24–96	14–42	20–28	21–42
Fatal dose (g)	5	?	3	3

Adapted from Goldfrank L, Osborn H: The barbiturate overdose. Hosp Phys, Sept. 1977, p. 30.

C. Clinical Presentation

Signs and symptoms of barbiturate poisoning include

1. CNS depression and coma: in severe overdoses, the pupils may appear fixed and dilated; brainstem reflexes may be absent; the patient may be areflexic; and the toes upgoing.

2. Respiratory depression: this occurs early and may progress through Cheyne-Stokes respirations to apnea, resulting in acute respiratory acidosis and hypoxemia. Aspiration pneumonitis is a common complication.

3. Hypotension, hypothermia, and shock: medullary vasomotor centers, myocardium, and vascular smooth muscle are depressed. Acute renal failure may be a subsequent complication.

4. Skin bullae: these lesions, especially interdigital, are reported in 6% of cases but are not diagnostic.

D. Management

1. As in all overdose situations, the initial management priority is *support of the patient's airway, breathing, circulation, and neurologic status* (see Standard Therapy of the Poisoned/ Overdose Patient, IV. A, earlier in this chapter). Continuously monitor the patient's SaO_2 and cardiac rhythm; vitals signs and neurologic status must be closely followed. Invasive hemodynamic monitoring (e.g., Swan-Ganz catheterization) may be necessary to help manage volume status and vasopressor use.

2. *Gastric emptying* is mandatory and should include gastric lavage and administration of activated charcoal and a cathartic. Use multiple-dose activated charcoal in the setting of a life-threatening ingestion. Phenobarbital undergoes enterohepatic recirculation and is accessible to charcoal "GI dialysis" many hours into the ingestion. The possibility of coingestants (e.g., ethanol) is always a consideration.

3. *Laboratory evaluation* should minimally include an ABG level; ECG; CBC; electrolyte panel, glucose, BUN, and creatinine levels, urinalysis; ethanol level; chest roentgenogram, general toxicologic screen, and a barbiturate level (if possible). Plasma levels do not accurately reflect CNS levels, however, and serum levels do not account for acquired tolerance or the additive effects of other drug(s) such as ethanol.

4. *Enhanced elimination:*
   a. Alkaline diuresis may be useful with a long-acting barbiturate overdose (e.g., phenobarbital). See Standard Therapy of the Poisoned/Overdose Patient, IV. E. 1, earlier in this chapter.
   b. Hemodialysis should be considered in the setting of renal or hepatic failure, significant electrolyte/acid–base disturbance, shock, or hypothermia; 6 hours of hemodialysis

removes as much phenobarbital as 24 hours of alkaline diuresis.

    c. Charcoal hemoperfusion should be considered in the management of a severe phenobarbital overdose unresponsive to other therapies.

5. *Additional supportive care:*

    a. Aspiration should be managed with aggressive pulmonary toilet; gastric decompression should occur with a nasogastric tube. Antibiotics are indicated if a pneumonia subsequently develops. Corticosteroids are not indicated.

    b. Hypothermia should be managed as appropriate.

6. *Disposition:* asymptomatic patients who have ingested short-acting barbiturates should be monitored in the ED for at least 6 hours; those who have ingested long-acting barbiturates should be monitored for at least 10 hours. Patients with persistent mental-status changes, vital-sign abnormalities, rising barbiturate levels, or moderate to severe toxicity must be admitted for continuous cardiorespiratory monitoring and appropriate supportive care. Suicidal patients must always be admitted.

BIBLIOGRAPHY

deBoer WB, Kendall PA, Breheny FX: Alpha coma and barbiturate poisoning. Anaesth Intens Care 1989;17:503–504.

Lindberg MC, Cunningham A, Lindberg NH: Acute phenobarbital intoxication. South Med J 1992;85:803–807.

VI. BENZODIAZEPINES

A. General Considerations

1. Benzodiazepines (BZPs) are commonly prescribed for the treatment of anxiety, muscle spasm, and convulsive disorders (Table 23–13). They are also frequently abused and overdosed. Fortunately, even with large benzodiazepine-only ingestions, there are few reported fatalities.

2. The antidote for benzodiazepine overdose is flumazenil.

Table 23–13. COMMONLY USED BENZODIAZEPINES

DRUG	ONSET	HALF-LIFE ($T_{1/2}$) (HR)
Alprazolam (Xanax)	Intermediate–fast	12–15
Chlorazepate (Tranxene)	Fast	50–200
Chlordiazepoxide (Librium)	Intermediate (60–90 min)	10–30
Clonazepam (Klonopin)	Fast	18–50
Diazepam (Valium)	Very fast (45 min)	20–80
Flurazepam (Dalmane)	Intermediate	>100
Lorazepam (Ativan)	Intermediate	10–20
Oxazepam (Serax)	Slow	5–10
Prazepam (Centrax)	Slowest	50–200
Temazepam (Restoril)	Fast	10–15
Triazolam (Halcion)	Fast	2–3

B. Pharmacodynamics

1. BZPs are rapidly and completely absorbed from the gastrointestinal tract.

2. The metabolism of the different BZPs varies; except for oxazepam and temazepam, BZPs have from one to five *active* metabolites.

3. Age and hepatic disease will increase the elimination $t_{1/2}$.

C. Clinical Presentation

1. The severity of findings varies directly with the amount of drug ingested. Signs of BZP overdose include ataxia, dysarthria, lethargy, nystagmus, muscle weakness, and hypotonia.

2. Coma, respiratory depression, and hypotension are more common if BZPs are ingested in combination with other sedative-hypnotics such as ethanol, barbiturates, cyclic antidepressants, and/or opioids. These signs are clues that a polydrug ingestion has likely occurred.

D. Management

1. As in all overdose situations, the initial management priority is *support of the patient's airway, breathing, circulation, and neurologic status* (see Standard Therapy of the Poisoned/ Overdose Patient, IV. A, earlier in this chapter). Continuously monitor SaO_2; vital signs and neurologic status should be closely followed.

2. *Gastric emptying* is appropriate in the setting of an acute ingestion, but the technique employed should be individualized to the clinical circumstances. Gastric lavage is less effective the longer the time interval between ingestion and presentation. Activated charcoal and cathartic administration, however, is reasonable even in the late-presenting patient. The presence of coingestants is always a consideration. Do not use ipecac.

3. *Laboratory evaluation* should minimally include a CBC; electrolyte panel; glucose, BUN, and creatinine levels; ECG; and ethanol level. Commonly used toxicologic screens identify only about 25% of the available benzodiazepines in use today.

4. *Antidote therapy with flumazenil:*
   a. This BZP partial agonist/competitive antagonist has reversed coma and ventilatory depression in severely poisoned patients. It may also reverse cardiovascular depression. Its $t_{1/2}$ is only about 20 minutes.
   b. *Dose:* 0.2 mg IV over 30 seconds. If no response in 30 seconds, give 0.3 mg IV over 30 seconds. Subsequent doses of 0.5 mg IV may be given, each over 30 seconds and 1 minute between doses, to a total of 3-5 mg. After an initial response, resedation should be treated every 20 minutes, as needed. If resedation does not occur within 2 hours of a 1-mg dose, it is unlikely to occur later.

   c. *Cautions:* If there is no response to a total dose of 5 mg over time, then BZPs are *not* the major cause of the patient's sedation. Flumazenil administration may result in seizures. It is contraindicated in the BZP-allergic patient or one who takes BZPs for a potentially life-threatening condition (e.g., epilepsy). It is not recommended in the setting of a concomitant cyclic antidepressant overdose. It may complicate further management of the BZP-dependent patient and may cause withdrawal syndromes.

5. *Disposition:* patients must remain monitored in the ED until mental status remains normal even without the use of flumazenil. Large overdoses, polydrug overdoses, and those requiring large or repeat doses of flumazenil should be admitted for continuous cardiorespiratory monitoring. The suicidal patient must always be admitted.

BIBLIOGRAPHY

Gaudreault P, Guay J, et al: Benzodiazepine poisoning. Clinical and pharmacological considerations and treatment. Drug Saf 1991;6;47–265.

Spivey WH: Flumazenil and seizures: analysis of 43 cases. Clin Ther 1992;14:292–305.

Weinbroum A, Halpern P, Geller E: The use of flumazenil in the management of acute drug poisoning—a review. Intens Care Med 1991;17:S32–S38.

VII. CALCIUM CHANNEL BLOCKERS

A. General Considerations

1. Calcium channel blockers are commonly used medications in the treatment of hypertension, coronary artery disease, migraine headaches, cerebrovascular vasospasm, and cardiac arrhythmias (Table 23–14).

2. Overdose with this class is on the increase owing to patterns of prescription. Of the available agents, overdose with verapamil is the most life-threatening.

3. Although calcium chloride is commonly listed as an antidote, its effectiveness is limited.

Table 23–14. THE CALCIUM CHANNEL BLOCKERS

DRUG	NEGATIVE INOTROPIC EFFECTS
Amlodipine	−
Diltiazem	+
Felodipine	−
Isradipine	Least
Nicardipine	+/−
Nimodipine	+/−
Nifedipine	+/−
Verapamil	Most

B. Pharmacodynamics

1. These drugs selectively antagonize slow calcium-entry channels in cardiac and vascular smooth muscle.

2. Onset of action is within 10 minutes, and peak blood levels occur 30 minutes after ingestion. Calcium channel blockers are rapidly absorbed from the GI tract and are highly protein bound.

3. Hepatic metabolism produces inactive metabolites, which are then renally excreted.

4. The $t_{1/2}$ is about 2 hours; however, "XL," "LA," "CD," or "SR" preparations have their onset of action after about 6 hours and remain in the serum for up to 24 hours.

5. These agents do not alter serum calcium concentrations.

6. Concomitant use of beta-blocking drugs or digoxin will exacerbate the cardiac effects of the calcium channel blockers.

C. Clinical Presentation

1. Signs and symptoms include dizziness, nervousness, fatigue, generalized weakness, palpitations, flushing, heart failure with generalized edema, nausea and vomiting, hypotension and/or shock.

2. Cardiac arrhythmias include bradycardia and/or AV nodal block. Bundle branch block may also occur.

3. Renal function may be impaired.

D. Management

1. As in all overdose situations, the initial management priority is *support of the patient's airway, breathing, circulation, and neurologic status* (see Standard Therapy of the Poisoned/ Overdose Patient, IV. A, earlier in this chapter). Hypotension should be treated with rapid volume infusion. Vasopressors may be given adjunctively and are mandatory in the patient unresponsive to appropriate volume resuscitation. Infusions of dopamine, norepinephrine, and/or epinephrine have been used successfully. Continuously monitor the cardiac rhythm, SaO_2, blood pressure, urine output, and fluid balance.

2. *Gastric emptying* is appropriate in the setting of an acute ingestion, but the technique employed should be individualized to the clinical circumstances. Calcium channel blockers are rapidly absorbed from the GI tract. Gastric lavage and administration of activated charcoal and a cathartic should be used within the first hour after ingestion. Gastric lavage is less effective the longer the time interval between ingestion and presentation. In the late-presenting patient, consider dispensing with lavage and administering only activated charcoal with cathartic. If a sustained-release preparation has been

ingested, charcoal and cathartic use is mandatory and effective. Ipecac is not recommended in the management of an acute ingestion.

3. *Laboratory evaluation* should minimally include a CBC; electrolyte panel; glucose, BUN, and creatinine levels; ECG; and chest roentgenogram.

4. *Antidote therapy with calcium chloride:*
   a. Calcium chloride is indicated in the treatment of brady-cardia, AV block, and/or hypotension in the setting of a calcium channel blocker overdose, but its effectiveness is limited.
   b. *Dose:* 1 g IV over 5 minutes. Dose may be repeated as necessary, but do not exceed a total of 4 g IV over time. Alternatively, a continuous calcium chloride infusion (20-50 mg/kg per hour) may be started after the initial 1-g bolus.

5. *Additional care:*
   a. Bradycardia or high-degree AV block should be treated with atropine, isoproterenol, and cardiac pacing as necessary. Isoproterenol may exacerbate hypotension, however, and an epinephrine infusion (2-10 µg/min IV) is theoretically a better agent in this setting. High-dose glucagon (3.5-5 g IV) may also be effective; but its duration of action is only 15 minutes (a continuous infusion is frequently necessary at 1–5 mg/hr).
   b. Heart failure will require the use of inotropic agents (e.g., dopamine and/or dobutamine).
   c. The action of neuromuscular blocking agents may be potentiated in the setting of a calcium-channel-blocker overdose.

6. *Disposition:* the asymptomatic patient must be observed in the ED for a minimum of 6 hours (even longer if a sustained-release preparation was ingested) before being medically cleared. All symptomatic patients must be admitted for continuous cardiorespiratory monitoring. Suicidal patients must always be admitted.

BIBLIOGRAPHY

Kerns W II, Kline J, Ford MD: β-blocker and calcium channel blocker toxicity. Emerg Med Clin N Am 1994;12(2):365–390.

Pearigen PD, Benowitz NL: Poisoning due to calcium antagonists. Experience with verapamil, diltiazem and nifedipine. Drug Saf 1991;6:408–430.

Ramoska EA, Spiller HA, Myers A: Calcium channel blocker toxicity. Ann Emerg Med 1990; 19:649–653.

VIII. CARBON MONOXIDE

A. General Considerations

1. Carbon monoxide (CO) is the product of incomplete combustion of organic fuels. Common sources include

internal-combustion engine exhaust, smoke from fires (e.g., buildings, charcoal, "Sterno"), and poorly maintained furnaces.

2. It is colorless, odorless, tasteless, nonirritating, and heavier than air.

3. It remains one of the leading causes of poisoning deaths in the United States. The diagnosis of CO poisoning is based on the history and physical examination and confirmed by measuring carboxyhemoglobin (COHb) concentration in the blood (ABG sample). COHb is usually < 3% in nonsmokers; it can be up to 10-11% in smokers who inhale. Symptoms are usually present when the COHb level has reached 20%.

4. The antidote for CO poisoning is 100% oxygen; hyperbaric oxygen treatment is also frequently necessary.

B. Pharmacodynamics

1. Absorption is directly related to the concentration of the gas in air, duration of exposure, and the patient's minute ventilation. Toxicity is further dependent on COHb and is enhanced by anemia or a high metabolic rate.

2. The affinity of hemoglobin for CO is 220 times greater than it is for oxygen. COHb shifts the oxyhemoglobin dissociation curve to the left, further decreasing the availability of oxygen to the tissues. Inspiration of 0.1% CO at room air results in a 50% decrease in blood oxygen-carrying capacity.

3. CO directly binds with cytochromes, inhibiting oxidation-reduction at the cellular level.

4. The lungs excrete CO. At room air, COHb has a $t_{1/2}$ of 4-5 hours. While breathing 100% oxygen at atmospheric pressure, the $t_{1/2}$ is reduced to 60 minutes; in a hyperbaric chamber at 2-3 atmospheres of pressure, the $t_{1/2}$ is about 23 minutes.

C. Clinical Presentation

1. The signs and symptoms of CO poisoning are related to hypoxia of the most susceptible organs, the brain and heart (Table 23–15). Correlation of signs and symptoms with CO levels, however, is only approximate: the manifestations of CO poisoning may be variable and do not necessarily follow any progression. Loss of consciousness can occur without warning!

2. The "classic" sign of cherry-red mucosae and/or nail bed lunulae is almost never present (< 15% of patients).

3. *Cautions:*
   a. A low or undetectable COHb level does *not* exclude the diagnosis. Tissue concentrations may still be significant after blood concentrations have decreased, frequently

Table 23-15. SIGNS AND SYMPTOMS OF CARBON MONOXIDE POISONING

SIGNS AND SYMPTOMS	% COHb SATURATION
Asymptomatic	< 10
Tightness across forehead; possibly slight headache, dilatation of cutaneous blood vessels	10–20
Headache; throbbing in temples	20–30
Severe headache, weakness, dizziness, dimmed vision, nausea and vomiting, collapse	30–40
As above, with greater possibility of collapse or syncope; increased respiration and pulse	40–50
Syncope, increased respiration and pulse; coma with intermittent convulsions; Cheyne-Stokes respiration	50–60
Coma with intermittent convulsions, depressed cardiac function and respiration, possible death	60–70
Weak pulse and slowed respiration; respiratory failure and death	> 70%

From Goodman LS, Gilman A (eds): The Pharmacological Basis of Therapeutics, 4th ed. New York, Collier-MacMillan, 1970, p. 930.

secondary to the administration of oxygen or a delay in checking levels. *Comatose patients suspected of CO poisoning have responded dramatically to hyperbaric oxygen therapy despite undetectable COHb measurements!*

b. In the absence of respiratory embarrassment, the PaO_2 is *normal* in patients with CO poisoning: the calculated COHb saturation can be grossly inaccurate and should not be used for diagnosis or treatment.

D. Management

1. As in all overdose situations, the initial management priority is *support of the patient's airway, breathing, circulation, and neurologic status* (see Standard Therapy of the Poisoned/ Overdose Patient, IV. A, earlier in this chapter). Initiate immediate treatment with 100% oxygen via a tight-fitting nonrebreather mask. The unconscious or uncooperative patient should be given 100% oxygen via endotracheal tube. Continuously monitor the cardiac rhythm, vital signs, and neurologic status.

2. *Laboratory evaluation* should minimally include an ABG, COHb concentration (on the ABG sample), ECG, CBC, chest roentgenogram, routine blood chemistries, and pregnancy test.

3. *Enhanced elimination with hyperbaric oxygen (HBO) therapy:*

   a. HBO is indicated at 2-3 atmospheres of pressure in any of the following categories of CO poisoned patient (early consultation with the nearest HBO chamber personnel is appropriate):

      i. Unconscious or history of same (regardless of COHb level).

      ii. Any neurologic or neuropsychiatric impairment (regardless of COHb level).

     iii. Acute ECG abnormalities (regardless of COHb level).

     iv. COHb level ≥ 25%.

      v. Any symptomatic pregnant patient (regardless of COHb level).

     vi. Any asymptomatic pregnant patient if COHb level is ≥ 15%.

    vii. Young child whose COHb level is ≥ 15%.

   viii. Metabolic acidosis in the setting of CO exposure.

  b. Serial treatments may benefit those who remain unconscious.

  c. The complications of HBO therapy include ear discomfort, tympanic membrane injury, deficits in visual acuity, and oxygen toxicity (CNS and/or lungs).

4. *Disposition:*

  a. Consider discharging patients who meet *all* of the following conditions:

      i. Suffered only minimal symptoms (e.g., headache, dizziness) prior to therapy.

     ii. Are completely asymptomatic after treatment with 100% oxygen therapy.

    iii. COHb levels are < 5% after treatment with 100% oxygen therapy.

    iv. Have normal vital signs, ECG, ABG levels, and physical examination at time of discharge.

  b. Patients who do not satisfy all of the above should be admitted for continued monitoring and 100% oxygen therapy. Most experts would admit a patient (even if asymptomatic) whose COHb level at any time was ≥ 25%. Delayed complications of CO poisoning are many (e.g., personality changes, apraxia, disorientation, incontinence, and parkinsonism). HBO therapy is useful in the prevention of delayed complications; repeated treatments in the hyperbaric chamber may be required.

BIBLIOGRAPHY

Gorman DF, Runciman WB: Carbon monoxide poisoning. Anesth Intens Care 1991; 19:506–511.

Ilano AL, Raffin TA: Management of carbon monoxide poisoning. Chest 1990;97:165–169.

Tomaszewski CA, Thom SR: Use of hyperbaric oxygen in toxicology. Emerg Med Clin N Am 1994;12(2):437–460.

IX. COCAINE

A. General Considerations

1. Cocaine is a local anesthetic and CNS stimulant. It is an alkaloid obtained from the evergreen shrub *Erythroxylum coca,* which is extensively cultivated in the Andean highlands of South America.

a. The alkaloid is extracted from the leaves and crystallized as the hydrochloride salt ("street" cocaine).

b. Freebase cocaine is more heat stable and volatile than the hydrochloride salt and is better suited for smoking (or injecting). Respiratory absorption of the drug is rapid and complete, yielding higher blood and brain levels and a more intense high or "rush."

c. Crack, like freebase cocaine, produces a more rapid and intense euphoria than does "street" cocaine. It comes in solid "rocks" and is smoked in a pipe. All forms of cocaine are addictive, especially crack.

2. The use of various forms of cocaine has increased dramatically. Over 40 million Americans have tried it, and approximately 6.2 million individuals use it regularly. Many consider crack addiction to be this country's most serious drug problem.

3. Street names for cocaine include "coke," "snow," "toot," "blow," "nose candy," "flake," and "rock."

4. Routes of administration may include any of the following:
   a. Nasal insufflation: "snorting," "tooting."
   b. Intravenous: "firing up," "shooting up," "mainlining."
   c. Smoking crack or freebase.
   d. Applying to mucous membranes.

5. "Dosage:" the lethal dose of cocaine is estimated to be 1–2 g, but varies, depending on mode of use, purity of the product, and the individual patient.
   a. One "line" of coke = 25 mg (12.5 mg cocaine, assuming 50% purity).
   b. One coke spoon = approximately 5–10 mg.
   c. One "hit" of freebase = approximately 67 mg.

6. "Body packers," "mules," or "runners" attempt to smuggle the drug by swallowing large packets of cocaine. If one or more of these packets ruptures internally, a massive cocaine overdose swiftly occurs.

B. Pharmacodynamics

1. Despite local vasoconstriction, cocaine is rapidly absorbed from all mucous membranes and the GI tract. Toxicity results when absorption exceeds the rate of detoxification and excretion.

2. Cocaine is hydrolyzed by plasma cholinesterase and hepatic enzymes. People with inherently low levels of cholinesterase metabolize cocaine (as well as succinylcholine) slowly.

3. Cocaine and its metabolites are excreted in the urine and can be detected there 5 minutes after IV administration. Urine tests for cocaine may remain positive for days. About 10% of cocaine is excreted unchanged in the urine.

4. The distributional $t_{1/2}$ is 20–40 minutes and corresponds to the drug's psychological effects. The mean plasma $t_{1/2}$ is 2.8 hours.

5. Cocaine facilitates release and blocks the reuptake of cate-cholamine neurotransmitters (e.g., norepinephrine and dopa-mine) by nerve terminals at the synaptic cleft.

C. Clinical Presentation

1. Clinical findings are varied and depend on the drug's purity and dosage. Table 23–16 outlines the common clinical symptoms and signs. Generally, the signs progress (downward in the table). In most reactions, progression is not extensive and begins to abate within 20 minutes. In severe reactions, rapid acceleration of signs and symptoms occurs, and death may result in minutes. Most cocaine deaths occur before the patient reaches the hospital.

2. The clinical presentation may be complicated by other concomitantly abused drugs or one of the substances fre-

Table 23–16. COCAINE REACTIONS

PHASE	CNS SIGNS AND SYMPTOMS	CARDIOVASCULAR/RESPIRATORY SIGNS AND SYMPTOMS
Phase I: Early stimulation	Euphoria Elation, good humor Talkative, garrulous Excited, flighty Restless, irritable Stereopathy, bruxism Nausea, vertigo Headache, cold sweats Tremor (nonintention) Twitching face/fingers Generalized tics Preconvulsive tonic–clonic jerks Pseudohallucinations Paranoid psychosis Mydriasis Hyperthermia Sense of impending doom	Tachycardia (may be preceded by reflex bradycardia) Hypertension Skin pallor Tachypnea Premature ventricular contractions
Phase II: Advanced stimulation	Decreased response to stimuli Deep tendon reflexes increased Tonic/clonic seizures Encephalopathy CNS hemorrhage Malignant hyperthermia	Tachycardia Hypertension High-output congestive heart failure Ventricular arrhythmias Cardiogenic shock Hypoxia/cyanosis Irregular respirations (Cheyne-Stokes) Cardiorespiratory collapse
Phase III: Depressive	Flaccid paralysis Coma with pupils fixed and dilated Medullary paralysis with loss of vital support functions Death	Ventricular fibrillation Cardiopulmonary failure Pulmonary edema Cardiac arrest

Modified from Gay GR: Ann Emerg Med 1982;11:562.

Table 23–17. AGENTS COMMONLY USED TO ADULTERATE COCAINE

To Add Weight	To Add Taste	To Add Effect
Glucose	Lidocaine	Amphetamines
Lactose	Procaine	Caffeine
Mannitol	Tetracaine	Phencyclidine
		Ephedrine
		Quinine

quently added to cocaine by the patient's supplier (Table 23–17).

D. Management

1. As in all overdose situations, the initial management priority is *support of the patient's airway, breathing, circulation, and neurologic status* (see Standard Therapy of the Poisoned/Overdose Patient, IV. A, earlier in this chapter). Continuously monitor SaO_2 and the cardiac rhythm; closely follow vital signs and the clinical examination.
2. *Gastric decontamination* with aggressive use of activated charcoal is appropriate in the acute ingestion. Lavage may also be reasonable, but ipecac should not be used. If cocaine packets are in either the vagina or rectum ("body stuffers"), they should be removed carefully under direct visualization. "Body packers" should be treated with whole-bowel irrigation.
3. *Specific management* depends on the severity of the patient's presentation.
   a. For mild reactions with normal vital signs, "ART" therapy is effective:
      i. *Acceptance* (caring intervention).
      ii. *Reduction* of stimulation.
      iii. *Talking* down the patient (reassurance).
   b. A short-acting benzodiazepine (e.g., midazolam: 2 mg given slowly IV, followed by 1 mg IV every 3-5 minutes as necessary) may be used to sedate the patient with increased anxiety and/or muscle spasm.
   c. For seizures, support/secure the airway and use diazepam (begin with 5-10 mg given slowly IV) or lorazepam (2-4 mg IV, no faster than 2 mg/min; maintains anticonvulsant levels in the CNS for a longer time than diazepam), and/or a short-acting barbiturate (e.g., pentobarbital, begin with 100 mg IV in a 70-kg patient, followed by smaller doses as needed up to 200-500 mg total). For status epilepticus, treat with diazepam or lorazepam followed by phenobarbital (100 mg/min IV up to a total dose of 20 mg/kg if necessary) (see Chapter 20).
   d. Hyperthermia should be managed by cooling blankets, or mist spray and large fan convection. Intubation and muscle

paralysis may also be required. Treatment with dantrolene (1-2 mg/kg IV every 6 hours; do not exceed 10 mg/kg/day; can cause hypotension and hepatotoxicity) may be beneficial but has been inadequately studied in this setting.

e. Sinus tachycardia and hypertension are generally self-limited and can be managed by sedation, control of hyperthermia, and observation. Moderate to severe and persistent hypertension, however, will require specific therapy. Consider *one* of the following agents:

 i. Sodium nitroprusside (begin with 0.5 µg/kg/min IV and titrate as necessary).

 ii. Nitroglycerin (begin with 5 µg/min IV and increase in 5-10-µg/min increments every 3-5 minutes as necessary).

 iii. Phentolamine (begin with 5 mg IV bolus, followed by continuous IV infusion of 0.2-0.5 mg/min).

 iv. Labetalol (20 mg IV over 2 minutes, followed by 40-80 mg IV bolus every 5 minutes as needed till the desired effect is achieved; maximum dose is 300 mg over time).

 Isolated beta-blocker therapy (e.g., propranolol alone) should be avoided because of the theoretical risk of "unopposed" alpha-adrenergic activity and paradoxical worsening of hypertension. If a beta blocker is necessary for tachycardia management, use labetalol as per above, or combine a short-acting beta blocker (e.g., esmolol) with a vasodilating agent (e.g., sodium nitroprusside).

f. Treat symptomatic ventricular ectopy or arrhythmias as per Advanced Cardiac Life Support (ACLS) guidelines (e.g., lidocaine 1 mg/kg IV, followed by 2-4 mg/min continuous infusion). Labetalol may be added if necessary.

4. *Complications:*

a. Complications of cocaine abuse include stroke (vasospastic, subarachnoid hemorrhage, or other intracranial hemorrhage), myocardial infarction, arrhythmias, pneumothorax/pneumomediastinum/pneumopericardium, visceral ischemia, trauma, nasal septal perforation, and infections associated with injection drug use.

b. "Body packers" are at imminent risk of fatal cocaine overdose if the packet(s) should rupture in the GI tract. Abdominal roentgenograms may show the number, size, and location of the packets. Whole-bowel irrigation and hospitalization are indicated (see Standard Therapy of the Poisoned/Overdose Patient, earlier in this chapter). Surgery is necessary in cases of obstruction or intestinal ischemia.

5. *Disposition:* patients with mild cocaine intoxication should be observed in the ED for 3-6 hours. They may be discharged after that time if completely asymptomatic. The possibility of "hidden" cocaine in the vagina or rectum must be considered before discharge. Referral for drug abuse counseling and

treatment should be made. Moderate to severely poisoned patients or those with significant complications should be admitted for continuous cardiorespiratory monitoring and appropriate supportive care. "Body packers" must remain in the ICU till all packets have been safely passed.

BIBLIOGRAPHY

Mueller PD, Benowitz NL, Olson KR: Cocaine. Emerg Med Clin N Am 1990;8:481–493.
Olshaker JS: Cocaine chest pain. Emerg Med Clin N Am 1994;12(2):391–398.

X. CYCLIC ANTIDEPRESSANTS

A. General Considerations

1. Cyclic antidepressants (CAs) are used in the treatment of major depression, chronic pain, insomnia, and enuresis.
2. A variety of agents are available, most of which are classified according to the ringed structure of the central portion of the molecule:
   a. Tricyclic: desipramine, nortriptyline, protriptyline (all secondary amines); amitriptyline, doxepin, imipramine, trimipramine (all tertiary amines); amoxapine (a dibenzoxazepine).
   b. Tetracyclic: maprotiline.
   c. Triazolopyridine: trazodone.
   d. Bicyclic: fluoxetine (Prozac).
3. Overdose with one of the tricyclic or tetracyclic agents listed above is a true *medical emergency.* There is large patient to patient variability in the lethal dose, but in general: ingestions of < 20 mg/kg cause few fatalities; 35 mg/kg is the approximate median lethal dose; and death is likely with overdoses > 50 mg/kg.
   a. Excessive ingestion of tricyclic/tetracyclic antidepressants is one of the leading causes of hospitalization and death from prescription drug overdose.
   b. Rapid progression of symptoms and signs may occur in the ED (e.g., mild lethargy may proceed to frank coma with ventricular arrhythmias within 30 minutes of ED arrival; most complications occur within 6 hours of ingestion).
   c. The tricyclic agents cause complex central and peripheral adrenergic and cholinergic receptor effects and direct quinidine-like cardiotoxicity.
   d. Maprotilene overdose results in an increased incidence of seizures.
   e. Amoxapine overdose has few cardiovascular effects, but a high incidence of CNS toxicity and seizures.
4. Fortunately, the newer cyclic antidepressants differ in their clinical effects from the older agents when taken in overdose:
   a. Trazodone: no cardiac effects and few CNS effects. May cause significant hypotension.

b. Fluoxetine: few overdoses have been reported; fairly benign agent when taken in overdose (nausea and vomiting are common, rarely may cause seizures). This is the most commonly prescribed antidepressant in the United States.

5. Although there is no true antidote for CA poisoning, *alkalinization therapy is beneficial in patient management* (maintaining blood pH at 7.5 through hyperventilation and/or sodium bicarbonate infusion). Its mechanism of action is unclear, but alkalinization may increase protein binding of the CA and decrease the amount of free drug available for toxicity. The sodium in sodium bicarbonate may also be beneficial in reversing CA-induced blockade of sodium channels.

B. Pharmacodynamics

1. In overdose, CAs are *initially* absorbed rapidly; but as drug levels rise absorption occurs very slowly secondary to anticholinergic-induced gastric atony.

2. Once absorbed, most of the CA is tissue/plasma protein bound. Tissue levels may be 200 times greater than plasma levels; thus, toxicity may occur at "therapeutic" blood levels.

3. CAs undergo extensive first-pass hepatic metabolism. Subsequent biliary excretion or secretion into the stomach occurs and the drug is then reabsorbed in the gut (enterohepatic recirculation). Final excretion occurs in the urine.

4. Toxicity in the setting of overdose is not completely understood, but the following do occur (does not apply to trazodone or fluoxetine): anticholinergic effects (e.g., mental status changes, seizures, tachycardias); impaired synaptic reuptake of norepinephrine (e.g., hypertension, arrhythmias); quinidine-like cardiac toxicity (conduction disturbances, myocardial depression); peripheral alpha-adrenergic blockade (e.g., hypotension); and inhibited central sympathetic reflexes.

C. Clinical Presentation

Table 23–18 presents the toxic effects of CAs.

D. Management

1. As in all overdose situations, the initial management priority is *support of the patient's airway, breathing, circulation, and neurologic status* (see Standard Therapy of the Poisoned/Overdose Patient, IV. A, earlier in this chapter).

a. The patient with an inadequate airway or ventilation should be emergently intubated and mechanically ventilated. Even if the patient has a good gag and cough reflex on presentation, if there are mental status changes or a history of significant ingestion, *early intubation is appropriate.* Signs and symptoms (e.g., seizures, coma, life-threatening arrhythmias) can progress quickly in the CA-overdose

Table 23–18. TOXIC EFFECTS OF THE CYCLIC ANTIDEPRESSANTS

EFFECT	MECHANISM	SITE	SIGNS/SYMPTOMS
Atropine-like	Anticholinergic	*Muscarinic receptors* Central	Anxiety-agitation Delirium-hallucinations Myoclonus-seizures
		Peripheral	Dilated pupils Hyperpyrexia Tachyarrhythmias Urinary retention Dry secretions Ileus
Cocaine-like	Block norepinephrine reuptake	*Adrenergic receptors* Central α	Psychomotor activation
		Peripheral (α and β)	↑ Cardiac contractility Tachyarrhythmias (supraventricular and ventricular) Hypertension
Reserpine-like	Catecholamine depletion	Central	Obtundation Coma
		Peripheral	↓ Cardiac ouput ⎤ "Cardiovascular Hypotension ⎟ collapse" Shock ⎦
Phenothiazine-like	α-Adrenergic blockade	*α Adrenergic receptors* Central	Sedation
		Peripheral	Vasodilatation Hypotension
Quinidine-like	Membrane stabilization	Myocardium	Decreased contractility and falling cardiac output
		Conduction pathways	↑ Refractory periods ↓ Conduction ⎡Esp. His bundle ⎣Not AV node ↑ Automaticity; arrhythmias
		ECG ⎡↑ PR ⎤ ⎢↑QRS⎥ ⎣↑QT ⎦	Conduction disturbances —AV block —Bundle branch block —Intraventricular re-entrant rhythm

patient. Early intubation will also facilitate blood alkalinization through the use of purposeful hyperventilation.

  b. Continuously monitor the patient's SaO_2 and cardiac rhythm; vital signs and neurologic status must be followed closely.

  c. Hypotension or shock should initially be treated with blood alkalinization (see D. 4. a, below) and cautious volume resuscitation. Both ARDS and cardiogenic pulmonary edema are risks in the CA-overdose patient, and *excessive crystalloid administration must be avoided.* Early invasive hemodynamic monitoring (e.g., Swan-Ganz catheterization) should be considered in the hemodynamically unstable patient. Norepinephrine (or phenylephrine) is appropriate when a vasopressor is required.

d. Manage seizures with airway control, blood alkalinization (see D. 4. a, below), diazepam, ± phenytoin, ± phenobarbital.

2. *Gastric emptying* should include gastric lavage and administration of activated charcoal and a cathartic up to 12 or more hours after ingestion. If mental status is altered (even if the patient has a good cough and gag reflex), prophylactic intubation with a cuffed endotracheal tube should occur before gastric emptying (see D. 1. a, above). Ipecac should not be used.

a. Many experts recommend the following procedural sequence: empty the stomach by attaching the orogastric tube to suction ("vacuum" the stomach), administer activated charcoal (1 g/kg) via the orogastric tube, perform large-volume gastric lavage till clear, then repeat charcoal administration with cathartic.

b. After lavage and activated charcoal administration as per 2. a, above, repeat doses of activated charcoal (without cathartic) are recommended every 4-8 hours until a charcoal stool is produced (avoid gastric distention, however, in the setting of drug-induced anticholinergic effects). Multiple-dose activated charcoal may be effective in binding CAs and reducing drug $t_{1/2}$ by adsorption of gastric secreted and enterohepatically recirculated drug.

3. *Laboratory evaluation* should minimally include an ABG; ECG; CBC; electrolyte panel; glucose, BUN, and creatinine levels; urinalysis; chest roentgenogram, toxicologic screen, and cyclic antidepressant drug level.

a. The ECG should be evaluated carefully, and serial ECGs are appropriate.

i. A QRS duration ≥ 0.10 second is a sign of severe toxicity and correlates approximately with a plasma drug level ≥ 1000 ng/mL. *This is the most important interval to inspect on the serial ECGs.*

ii. Abnormal QT_c prolongation may be useful in predicting *potential* for arrhythmia; although, it is usually elevated above baseline in the presence of CAs, and it may be difficult to measure because of tachycardia and slurring of the T wave into the P and U waves. QT_c prolongation does *not* correlate with plasma CA concentration.

iii. The terminal 0.04 second of the frontal plane QRS vector > 120 degrees is a marker for CA exposure, but it does not correlate with toxicity.

b. CA drug levels are useful in confirming drug ingestion, but "therapeutic" levels do not rule out serious toxicity in the setting of overdose.

4. *Additional care* (Table 23–19):

a. Alkalinization of the blood to a pH of 7.5 should be utilized for patients with any of the following: coma, seizures,

Table 23–19. MANAGEMENT OF TOXICITY IN CYCLIC ANTIDEPRESSANT OVERDOSE

CLINICAL SIGNS (IN APPROXIMATE ORDER OF APPEARANCE)	TREATMENT (IN ORDER OF PREFERENCE)	COMPLICATIONS OF TREATMENT	COMMENTS
CNS			
Agitation, delirium, hallucinations	Supportive care and meticulous attention to airway, SaO$_2$, and cardiac monitoring		Do not use physostigmine to manage these anticholinergic induced effects
Myoclonic jerks (these are common, do not confuse with seizures)	Conservative/supportive care		Myoclonic jerks may herald the onset of seizures
Seizures	1.a) Support airway and oxygenation		
	1.b) Diazepam 5–10 mg IV	CNS depression	Effective and drug of choice
	1.c) Blood alkalinization (hyperventilation and/or sodium bicarbonate)	Hypokalemia	
	2. Phenytoin 15 mg/kg IV, no faster than 50 mg/min	Hypotension, bradycardia, conduction defects	Must administer slowly
	3. Phenobarbital 10–20 mg/kg IV no faster than 100 mg/min	CNS depression Hypotension	Use only if seizures persist despite earlier measures; intubation necessary now if not done already
Coma	1. Meticulous supportive care, SaO$_2$ and cardiac monitoring		Coma usually lasts 24 hr Physostigmine may improve mental status, but increases seizure risk and cardiac conduction problems and is not recommended
	2. Blood alkalinization will not change mental status, but is appropriate for other expected concomitant complications	May cause hypokalemia	
Respiratory			
Depression/apnea	Intubation with cuffed endotracheal tube and assisted ventilation Meticulous supportive care with continuous monitoring of SaO$_2$ and cardiac rhythm		

Table 23–19. MANAGEMENT OF TOXICITY IN CYCLIC
ANTIDEPRESSANT OVERDOSE *Continued*

CLINICAL SIGNS (IN APPROXIMATE ORDER OF APPEARANCE)	TREATMENT (IN ORDER OF PREFERENCE)	COMPLICATIONS OF TREATMENT	COMMENTS
Aspiration	Meticulous airway control and support; aggressive suctioning		Early intubation with a cuffed endotracheal tube should help prevent Do not begin antibiotics unless the patient develops signs of infection (e.g., fever, leukocytosis, infiltrates on chest film)
ARDS	Support of oxygenation and ventilation with intubation and mechanical ventilation; fluid restriction; PEEP		
Cardiovascular			
Supraventricular Tachyarrhythmias Sinus tachycardia Atrial tachycardia Atrial fibrillation Atrial flutter Junctional tachycardia (supraventricular tachycardia with a widened QRS often closely simulates ventricular tachycardia)	1. Blood alkalinization and appropriate supportive care (ensure normal serum potassium and magnesium) 2. Follow ACLS guidelines, but avoid beta blockers because of the risk of hypotension, and conduction blocks 3. Physostigmine (2 mg IV over 5 min); clinical effect will last from 20–30 min, repeat doses may be necessary	Hypokalemia Seizures, other cholinergic toxicity, asystole	Generally, treatment beyond blood alkalinization unnecessary unless rate not tolerated because of myocardial ischemia or hypotension Dose very carefully and use only as a therapy of "last resort" for a life-threatening situation unresponsive to ACLS guidelines
Conduction Blocks			

1° AVB
2° AVB
  Mobitz I
  Mobitz II
3° AVB
Intraventricular Blocks
QRS > 100 msec
Bundle branch blocks (usually
right > left)
Fascicular blocks
Combinations of the above
	1. Blood alkalinization and appropriate supportive care (ensure normal serum potassium and magnesium)
	2. Follow ACLS guidelines: pace as appropriate
	3. Phenytoin (15 mg/kg IV, no faster than 50 mg/min)
		Hypokalemia
		
		Use remains controversial; may increase the risk of ventricular tachycardia
			Mobitz II usually short-lived, but may progress to 3° AVB

Table continued on following page

Table 23–19. MANAGEMENT OF TOXICITY IN CYCLIC ANTIDEPRESSANT OVERDOSE *Continued*

CLINICAL SIGNS (IN APPROXIMATE ORDER OF APPEARANCE)	TREATMENT (IN ORDER OF PREFERENCE)	COMPLICATIONS OF TREATMENT	COMMENTS
Ventricular Arrhythmias			
PVCs Ventricular tachycardia	1. Blood alkalinization and appropriate supportive care (ensure normal serum potassium and magnesium)	Hypokalemia	
	2. Follow ACLS guidelines: but beta blockers and type Ia antiarrhythmics (e.g., procainamide, quinidine) are contraindicated		Dose lidocaine carefully: may cause CNS toxicity and seizures
	3. Phenytoin (15 mg/kg IV, no faster than 50 mg/min)	Use remains controversial	
Ventricular fibrillation	Defibrillation and proceed with ACLS guidelines for cardiopulmonary arrest management, including use of blood alkalinization (pH 7.5)		Beta blockers and type Ia antiarrhythmics are contraindicated
Asystole	Manage as per ACLS guidelines, including blood alkalinization (pH 7.5)		Final common arrhythmia in severe fatal overdose Though atropine is generally contraindicated in CA overdose, it should be used per ACLS guidelines if asystole occurs
Hypotension	1. Blood alkalinization	Hypokalemia	Effective; safe
	2. Judicious crystalloid infusion and careful monitoring	Congestive heart failure, worsened ARDS	
	3. Pressor support with norepinephrine (begin at 2 µg/min IV and titrate as necessary)	Infiltration of peripheral IV will cause tissue necrosis	Preferred route of administration is via central line
	4. Intra-aortic balloon pump		Use not reported

tachycardia, conduction defects, ventricular arrhythmias, and/or hypotension. Alkalinization may be achieved via hyperventilation (see 1. a, above) or sodium bicarbonate (1-2 mEq/kg IV over several minutes, titrated to pH and repeated as necessary). Follow serum electrolytes (e.g., potassium, sodium) regularly, and maintain in the normal range.

b. Phenytoin (15-20 mg/kg IV, no faster than 50 mg/min) is frequently used in the management of ventricular arrhythmias and conduction defects in the CA-overdose patient. It is also appropriate in the management of seizures (see 1. d, above). Its use in arrhythmia prophylaxis is controversial but favored at some institutions; its effectiveness in this regard has been inadequately studied in humans. In the dog model, ventricular tachycardia is increased when phenytoin is used prophylactically.

c. ARDS may occur, especially in the severe CA overdose. Frequency of ARDS increases dramatically in the setting of a polydrug ingestion. Manage appropriately with intubation, mechanical ventilation, fluid restriction, and positive end expiratory pressure (PEEP).

d. Cardiac pacing is appropriate in the setting of symptomatic bradycardias and heart blocks.

e. Physostigmine *should be avoided* in the CA-overdose patient. Though older literature recommended its routine use to reverse the anticholinergic effects of CA poisoning, this drug *increases* the risk of bradycardias, asystole, and seizures.

f. Contraindicated drugs include disopyramide, procainamide, quinidine, and beta blockers.

5. *Disposition:*

a. If the patient shows *absolutely no signs* of toxicity during 6 hours of continuous monitoring in the ED (QRS duration must remain < 0.10 second throughout this time), and appropriate gastric emptying has been accomplished (including the use of activated charcoal), the patient is medically cleared and psychiatric consultation/disposition should be obtained.

b. If *at any time* during the patient's ED stay signs or symptoms occur (e.g., altered mental status, QRS duration ≥ 0.10 second, conduction defects, seizures, hypotension, anticholinergic effects) admission to the ICU is mandated. The cardiac rhythm should be monitored for 24 hours *after* all signs of toxicity are absent (delayed cardiac arrest has occurred in the CA-overdose patient).

BIBLIOGRAPHY

Buchman AL, Dauer J, Geiderman J: The use of vasoactive agents in the treatment of refractory hypotension seen in tricyclic antidepressant overdose. J Clin Psychopharmacol 1990; 10:409–413.

Ellison DW, Pentel PR: Clinical features and consequences of seizures due to cyclic antidepressant overdose. Am J Emerg Med 1989;7:5–10.

Groleau G, Jotte R, Barish R: The electrocardiographic manifestations of cyclic antidepressant therapy and overdose: a review. J Emerg Med 1990;8:597–605.

Pimentel L, Trommer L: Cyclic antidepressant overdoses, a review. Emerg Med Clin N Am 1994;12(2):533–547.

XI. DIGITALIS

A. General Considerations

1. Digitalis is a cardiac glycoside obtained from the leaf of the foxglove plant (*Digitalis purpurea*). Many other plants are also known to contain digitalis-like glycosides (e.g., lily of the valley [*Convallaria majalis*] and common oleander [*Nerium oleander*]).

2. Digoxin is the most common digitalis preparation in the United States; it is frequently used in the treatment of congestive heart failure and supraventricular tachycardias (especially atrial fibrillation and atrial flutter).

3. Up to 30% of medical patients taking a digitalis preparation exhibit some element of toxicity at the time of hospital admission. Chronic and inadvertent intoxication is a more common cause of poisoning than an acute overdose; it should be considered in any patient prescribed a digitalis preparation.

4. The mortality rate in the setting of massive poisoning *before* the availability of antidote therapy was as high as 50%.

5. The antidote for digoxin poisoning is digoxin-specific Fab antibody fragments (Digibind).

B. Pharmacodynamics

1. About 50-80% of an oral dose of digoxin is rapidly absorbed from the GI tract. Antacids and food will delay absorption.

2. Peak serum levels occur within several hours of ingestion, but maximum clinical effect and/or toxicity is delayed for 3-6 hours or longer. The $t_{1/2}$ is 30-40 hours, but considerable variability exists.

3. Most of the drug (60-80%) is eliminated unchanged in the urine; a smaller fraction is excreted in the bile. Enterohepatic recirculation of digoxin occurs.

4. Overdose with digoxin results in poisoning of the sodium-potassium adenosine triphosphatase pump.

C. Clinical Presentation

1. *Noncardiac toxicities:*
   a. CNS effects: drowsiness, confusion, disorientation, headache, hallucinations, toxic psychosis.
   b. GI effects: anorexia, nausea, vomiting, abdominal pain, diarrhea.

    c. Visual effects: blurring, scotomas, flashes of light or sparks, halos, abnormal color perception, photophobia.

    d. Miscellaneous effects: fatigue, malaise, weakness.

2. *Cardiac toxicities/arrhythmias:*

    a. Ventricular premature contractions (PVCs) (including multifocal PVCs and bigeminy).

    b. Tachycardias: nonparoxysmal junctional tachycardia, atrial tachycardia with AV block, ventricular tachycardia, fascicular tachycardia (tachycardia with a right-bundle-branch block morphology but QRS duration < 0.12 second), and ventricular fibrillation.

    c. Atrial fibrillation with a slow and regular ventricular response.

    d. Bradycardias and blocks: sinoatrial arrest, sinoatrial block, second-degree AV block (usually Mobitz type I [Wenkebach]), third-degree AV block.

3. Hyperkalemia: correlates with the degree of poisoning and with morbidity/mortality.

4. Digitalis toxicities are more severe in the setting of hypoxia, acid–base disturbances, significant myocardial disease, and/or concomitant electrolyte abnormalities (e.g., hypokalemia, hypomagnesemia, hypercalcemia).

D. Management

1. As in all overdose situations, the initial management priority is *support of the patient's airway, breathing, circulation, and neurologic status* (see Standard Therapy of the Poisoned/Overdose Patient, IV. A, earlier in this chapter). Continuously monitor the patient's cardiac rhythm and SaO_2.

2. *Gastric emptying* is appropriate in the setting of an acute ingestion. Digoxin is rapidly absorbed from the GI tract. Gastric lavage and administration of activated charcoal and a cathartic should be used within the first 1-2 hours after ingestion. The longer the time interval between oral overdose and presentation, however, the less effective gastric lavage is. Vagal stimulation during lavage may worsen arrhythmias if significant absorption has already occurred. In the late-presenting patient, dispense with lavage and administer only activated charcoal with cathartic. Repeat doses of charcoal (0.5-1 g/kg without cathartic every 2-4 hours) will improve digoxin elimination. Ipecac is not recommended in the management of an acute ingestion.

3. *Laboratory evaluation* should minimally include a CBC; electrolyte panel; glucose, BUN, and creatinine levels; ECG; digoxin level; calcium, magnesium, and phosphate levels, and a chest roentgenogram.

4. *Antidote therapy with digoxin-specific antibody, Fab fragments:*

    a. Clinical response to antibody therapy begins within 20-30 minutes of administration. Antibody is effective in poisonings with digoxin, digitoxin, or plants that contain a digitalis glycoside (e.g., common oleander).

b. Indications: the presence of *any* of the following mandates antibody therapy:

   i. Digitalis-induced potentially life-threatening arrhythmias (e.g., ventricular tachycardia, ventricular fibrillation, progressive bradycardias unresponsive to atropine, high-degree AV block).

   ii. Digitalis-associated hyperkalemia (> 5.5 mEq/L in the setting of an acute overdose).

   iii. An acute ingestion with shock or significant pump failure.

c. Consider antibody therapy, even in the absence of symptoms, in the patient with a history of an acute massive ingestion (> 10 mg in the adult), or a steady-state digoxin level > 10 ng/mL.

d. *Dose:* one vial = 40 mg of dig-Fab; one vial binds 0.6 mg digoxin or digitoxin. It is administered IV over 15-30 minutes. In a critical situation (e.g., digoxin-associated ventricular fibrillation) the antibody may be given as a bolus.

   i. If amount ingested is known:

$$\text{Vials of dig-Fab needed} = [\text{Amount ingested (in mg)} \times 0.8]/(0.6).$$

   ii. If a steady state serum level is available:

$$\text{Vials of dig-Fab needed} = [\text{Steady-state level (ng/mL)} \times 5.6 \text{ L/kg} \times \text{weight (kg)}]/600.$$

   iii. When no estimate of the amount ingested can be made and steady-state serum levels are not yet available, then initial dose should be 20 vials.

e. *Cautions:* adverse effects occur in fewer than 1% of patients, but may include hypokalemia after rapid reversal of digoxin-associated hyperkalemia; worsened congestive heart failure; rapid atrial fibrillation; pruritis and/or facial swelling. Digoxin-specific antibody is expensive (one vial: $323).

5. *Additional care:*

a. Maintain patient oxygenation.

b. Correct electrolyte abnormalities known to exacerbate digoxin toxicity (e.g., hypokalemia, hypomagnesemia, and/or hypercalcemia).

c. Symptomatic hyperkalemia should *not* be treated with IV calcium chloride (calcium will worsen digoxin toxicity). Digoxin-specific antibody is the treatment of choice (see D. 4, above); glucose/insulin and bicarbonate may also be used if necessary.

d. Bradycardias and heart block should be treated as per ACLS recommendations with atropine (0.5-1.0 mg IV every 3-5 minutes as needed to maximum dose of 0.04 mg/kg), ± pacing. Digoxin-specific antibody is appropriate when bradycardias do not respond to atropine or when high-grade AV block is present (see D. 4, above).

  e. Ventricular arrhythmias: phenytoin (15 mg/kg IV, no faster than 25-50 mg/min) and lidocaine (1 mg/kg IV followed by a continuous infusion of 2-4 mg/min) are the antiarrhythmic drugs of choice. Magnesium sulfate (1-2 g IV over 1-2 minutes followed by 2 g/hr IV for 4-5 hours) may also be beneficial. Cardioversion of unstable ventricular tachycardia is potentially dangerous in the setting of digitalis toxicity; it should be done only if absolutely necessary after a minimum of 200 mg of phenytoin has been administered: use low energies (e.g., begin with 5-10 Joules). Ventricular arrhythmias mandate digoxin-specific antibody therapy (see D. 4, above). *Contraindicated* drugs in this setting include quinidine, disopyramide, and procainamide.

  f. Hemodialysis is not effective at removing digoxin, but it is indicated in the management of severe acid–base or electrolyte disturbances complicated by renal insufficiency.

6. *Disposition:*

  a. The completely asymptomatic patient with a trivial ingestion must be monitored in the ED for 4-6 hours. If throughout that time the patient remains symptom/sign free, has no electrocardiographic abnormalities, and has serial digoxin levels that are neither rising nor in the toxic range, the patient may be medically cleared. Appropriate psychosocial evaluation and disposition should then be obtained.

  b. All patients with signs or symptoms of digoxin toxicity, or whose serum levels are > 2 ng/mL in the setting of an acute ingestion, must be admitted to the ICU for meticulous monitoring and continuation of definitive care.

BIBLIOGRAPHY

Lewin LA, Goldfrank LR, Howland JA, Kirstein RH: Digitalis. Chapter 35. In Goldfrank LR, et al (eds). Goldfrank's Toxicologic Emergencies. 4th Ed. East Norwalk, CT, Appleton & Lange, 1990, pp. 359–364.

Smith TW: Review of clinical experience with digoxin immune Fab (Ovine). Am J Emerg Med 1991;9:1–6 (suppl. 1).

Woolf AD, Wenger T, Smith TW, Lovejoy FH, Jr: The use of digoxin-specific Fab fragments for severe dititalis intoxication in children. N Engl J Med 1992;326:1739–1744.

XII. ETHANOL

A. General Considerations

1. Ethanol is a CNS depressant and systemic toxin.

2. It is the most commonly abused drug in the United States, and it plays a major role in 50% of accidental deaths and 10% of all fatalities.

3. Twelve percent of all U.S. health care dollars are spent on alcohol-related illness.

B. Pharmacodynamics

1. Ethanol is rapidly absorbed from the gastrointestinal tract. Food will delay absorption.

2. An acute ingestion of 1 mL/kg of 100% ethanol will raise the blood level by 100-130 mg/dL; serum osmolality increases by 23 mOsm/L for every 100-mg/dL increase in the blood ethanol level.

3. A blood alcohol level (BAL) of 80–100 mg/dL is generally considered intoxicating, although judgment and fine motor skills are compromised at lower levels. A BAL > 400 mg/dL is potentially fatal.

4. Metabolism is primarily hepatic and generally follows fixed-rate (zero-order) kinetics.
   a. In intoxicated *nontolerant* individuals: BALs decrease by 15-20 mg/dL/hr.
   b. In intoxicated *tolerant* individuals: BALs may decrease by 30-40 mg/dL/hr.

5. The lethal dose of ethanol is reported to be 5-8 g/kg in adults and 3 g/kg in children, but there is considerable individual variability.

C. Clinical Presentation

1. Signs of common drunkenness include ataxia, dysarthria, and nystagmus. Ethanol may also produce an agitated state. Either of these conditions can progress to stupor and coma with respiratory depression. The awake patient frequently has an increased pain threshold, which may mask other significant injuries/illnesses (e.g., head and spinal trauma, compartment syndromes, and/or an acute abdominal catastrophe).

2. Other alcohol-related patient presentations include
   a. *Alcoholic ketoacidosis:* an elevated anion-gap-type acidosis. Usually occurs in the setting of binge drinking, inadequate nutritional intake, and nausea/vomiting.
   b. *Wernicke's encephalopathy:* a thiamine-deficient state characterized by confusion, ataxia, and varying degrees of ophthalmoplegia.
   c. *Korsakoff's psychosis:* an irreversible chronic psychosis characterized by disorientation, amnesia, and confabulation.
   d. *Infection:* including pneumonia, cellulitis, meningitis, and/or hepatitis. Alcoholics suffer from a relative immunodeficiency.
   e. *Trauma.*

D. Management

1. As in all overdose situations, the initial management priority is *support of the patient's airway, breathing, circulation, and*

neurologic status (see Standard Therapy of the Poisoned/ Overdose Patient, IV. A, earlier in this chapter). Rapidly evaluate for possible concomitant head and/or spinal trauma. The patient with a potential cervical spine injury must be appropriately immobilized (hard cervical collar, head supported, patient attached to a backboard, and suction on and at the bedside).

2. In the setting of an altered mental status, and assuming no other contraindications, position the patient in Trendelenburg with the left side dependent. Carefully guard against aspiration.

3. Administer 100-200 mg thiamine IM or IV (in the awake and alert patient thiamine may be given PO). If the mental status is altered, quickly assess the bedside fingerstick glucose level. Administer parenteral glucose (25-50 g 50% dextrose in water [D50W] IV) if necessary. Dextrose containing solutions should only be given *after* thiamine replacement. Naloxone should be given if a concomitant opioid exposure is suspected.

4. *Gastric emptying* with gastric lavage may be indicated after securing the airway in the patient who presents within 1 hour of an acute ethanol overdose, or when other significant coingestants are suspected. Ethanol is rapidly absorbed from the GI tract, however, and it is not readily accessible to gastric emptying procedures. Ethanol is not well bound by charcoal. Ipecac use is not appropriate.

5. *Laboratory evaluation* in the intoxicated patient with a significantly altered level of consciousness should minimally include CBC; electrolyte panel; glucose, BUN, and creatinine levels; ABG; ECG; ethanol level; calcium, magnesium, and phosphate levels; and urinalysis.

6. Use physical restraints as necessary to prevent patient self-injury.

7. Perform a complete head-to-toe physical examination in search of occult trauma, infection, and/or other serious medical conditions.

8. *Disposition:* continuously observe the patient in the ED until the mental status has cleared. If the mental status does not improve with time an emergent head CT scan is indicated. The patient without significant medical or traumatic complications may be discharged to home when *completely awake, alert, and safely ambulatory.* Preferably, the patient should be discharged to a capable family member or friend. Patients with BALs in the legally intoxicated range for the particular locale (e.g., $\geq$ 100 mg/dL in most states) must not be allowed to drive home from the ED. Referral for drug counseling and therapy is appropriate at the time of ED discharge.

E. Alcohol Withdrawal

Also see Seizures in Chapter 20.

1. The withdrawal syndrome generally occurs 1–3 days after abstaining from ethanol or after decreasing the usual level of chronic ethanol consumption.

2. Stages of ethanol withdrawal:
   a. *"The shakes:"* onset in 6-8 hours; characterized by anxiety, nausea, and tremors.
   b. *Hallucinations:* onset in 0-24 hours; hallucinations may be visual, visual and auditory, tactile, and/or olfactory.
   c. *Seizures:* onset in 7-48 hours and grand mal in type (usually limited in number and duration).
   d. *Delirium tremens (DTs):* occurs in approximately 5% of untreated withdrawal patients. The onset is in 3-5 days; signs and symptoms include altered mentation, motor hyperactivity, and autonomic hyperactivity.

3. *Management of acute ethanol withdrawal:*
   a. Evaluate for other concomitant illnesses and trauma. Fever ≥ 38.2°C mandates investigation (sputum, blood, urine, and CSF cultures, as indicated) and should not simply be ascribed to ethanol withdrawal.
   b. Administer thiamine, folic acid, and multivitamins.
   c. Evaluate for and treat as necessary hypoglycemia, nutritional deficiencies, and any serious electrolyte abnormalities (including hyponatremia, hypokalemia, hypocalcemia, and hypomagnesemia).
   d. Administer an appropriate ethanol "substitute" for adequate control of the patient's withdrawal signs and symptoms. Benzodiazepines are the most commonly used agents for this purpose (Table 23–20); they also simultaneously act as anticonvulsants. The substitute drug is used to sedate the patient and then is gradually tapered as clinical status allows (generally over 3–5 days). Anticholinergic agents (e.g., diphenhydramine, benztropine, trihexyphenidyl) may be used as adjuncts, but only after

Table 23–20. PARENTERAL BENZODIAZEPINE MANAGEMENT OF ETHANOL WITHDRAWAL FOR HOSPITALIZED PATIENTS

DRUG	DOSING REGIMEN
Diazepam or	Initially 5–10 mg given slowly IV; follow with 5 mg IV every 15 minutes until patient sedated; then 5–15 mg IV every 2–6 hours carefully titrated as necessary.
Lorazepam	2-mg increments IV every 15–20 minutes until patient sedated; then 2 mg IV every 4 hours carefully titrated as necessary. Lorazepam is the preferred drug in elderly patients or in patients with renal or hepatic disease.

primary sympathetic and neurologic symptoms are controlled with an ethanol substitute.

   e. Atenolol (50-100 mg/day PO) may be used in combination with benzodiazepines to manage mild to moderate ethanol withdrawal. It shortens the duration of the withdrawal syndrome, but it should not be used in patients with a history of heart failure or reactive airways disease. Its use has been inadequately studied in severe ethanol withdrawal.

   f. Phenytoin is *not* an acceptable substitute, and neuroleptics (e.g., haloperidol and the phenothiazines) should be avoided because they lower the seizure threshold.

   g. *Disposition:* the patient in active ethanol withdrawal should be admitted if *any* of the following conditions apply:

     i. History of prior moderate to major withdrawal symptoms or complications.

     ii. Altered mental status.

     iii. Focal, recurrent, or prolonged seizures.

     iv. Significant vital-sign abnormality.

     v. History of prior delirium tremens.

     vi. Currently in delirium tremens.

     vii. Significant comorbid medical or surgical condition (including major electrolyte abnormality).

BIBLIOGRAPHY

Charness ME, Simon RP, Greenberg DA: Ethanol and the nervous system. N Engl J Med 1989; 321:442–454.

Duffens K, Marx JA: Alcoholic ketoacidosis—a review. J Emerg Med 1987;5:399–406.

Wrenn KD, Slovis CM, et al: The syndrome of alcoholic ketoacidosis. Am J Med 1991; 91:119–128.

XIII. OTHER ALCOHOLS

ETHYLENE GLYCOL

A. General Considerations

1. Ethylene glycol (EG) is the main ingredient in antifreezes, coolants, and de-icers. It tastes sweet and is usually dyed blue-green.

2. Like methanol, propylene glycol, and isopropyl alcohol, it may be ingested by the patient as a substitute for ethanol.

3. EG poisoning (and/or methanol poisoning) should be suspected in the patient with a combined anion-gap acidosis and an elevated osmolal gap (> 10 mOsm/L).

4. The antidote for EG poisoning is ethanol.

B. Pharmacodynamics

1. EG is rapidly absorbed from the stomach and distributed throughout the body.

2. Alcohol dehydrogenase metabolizes EG to glyoxylic acid, which is subsequently oxidized to oxalic acid. There is a variable latent period (4-12 hours) between ingestion and toxicity that corresponds to the biotransformation of nontoxic EG into its toxic metabolic byproducts. The metabolic byproducts cause severe anion-gap metabolic acidosis, CNS depression, cardiovascular dysfunction, hypocalcemia, and renal failure. Deposition of oxalate crystals can occur in any vital organ and cause significant dysfunction.

3. The antidote ethanol inhibits the metabolism of EG.

4. The lethal dose of EG is 1-2 mL/kg.

C. Clinical Manifestations

1. The earliest manifestation is inebriation *without* the characteristic odor of ethanol on the breath. Headache, nausea/vomiting, and CNS depression may subsequently occur.

2. Congestive heart failure, pulmonary edema, and/or cardiac arrhythmias may ensue after 12-24 hours.

3. Renal dysfunction is often locally painful and may present as acute tubular necrosis secondary to oxaluria 24-72 hours after ingestion.

4. Diagnostic evidence of ethylene glycol poisoning includes the presence of a severe anion-gap acidosis with urinary oxalate crystals and an osmolal gap. Oxalate chelation may result in profound hypocalcemia.
   a. In EG poisoning, the fundoscopic examination is normal (unlike methanol poisoning).
   b. Detection of EG in the blood is diagnostic.
   c. Serum osmolality will increase by 19 mOsm/kg for each 100 mg/dL of EG in the blood.

D. Management

1. As in all overdose situations, the initial management priority is *support of the patient's airway, breathing, circulation, and neurologic status* (see Standard Therapy of the Poisoned/Overdose Patient, IV. A. earlier in this chapter). The patient's SaO_2 and cardiac rhythm should be monitored continuously; vital signs, neurologic status, and urine output should be closely followed.

2. *Gastric emptying* with lavage followed by activated charcoal and cathartic administration is appropriate in the patient presenting within 4 hours of ingestion. Most authorities believe, however, that charcoal binds EG poorly or not at all.

3. *Laboratory evaluation* should minimally include ABGs; CBC; electrolyte panel; glucose, BUN, and creatinine levels; ECG; urinalysis; serum osmolality; EG level; ethanol level; and serum calcium, magnesium, and phosphate levels.

4. *Antidote therapy with ethanol:*
   a. Ethanol loading dose: 10.0 mL/kg of 10% ethanol in D5W IV over 30 minutes.
   b. Maintenance infusion: begin with 1.5 mL/kg/hr IV (10% ethanol) at the same time as the above loading dose; titrate as necessary to a serum ethanol level of 100-150 mg/dL. Because ethanol is removed during dialysis, double the maintenance infusion dose during dialysis.
   c. *Caution:* during IV ethanol therapy monitor the patient's serum glucose and ethanol levels frequently.

5. *Enhance elimination with hemodialysis.* Hemodialysis is indicated in patients with *any* of the following:
   a. Symptomatic poisoning.
   b. Significant metabolic acidosis.
   c. Significant renal dysfunction.
   d. Pulmonary edema.
   e. Serum EG levels > 25 mg/dL.

   (*Note:* some authorities recommend hemodialysis in *every* case of confirmed EG poisoning regardless of the above—consult a nephrologist early!)

6. *Additional care:*
   a. Pyridoxine (50 mg IM every 6 hours) may promote metabolism of glyoxylic acid to glycine instead of to oxalic acid. Thiamine (100-200 mg IM or IV) should also be administered.
   b. Moderate to severe metabolic acidosis (pH < 7.2) should be treated with sodium bicarbonate. Large doses may be required repeatedly. Follow both acid–base status and serum potassium levels closely during bicarbonate therapy.
   c. Symptomatic hypocalcemia (tetany or cardiac dysfunction) is treated with IV calcium gluconate. Treating *asymptomatic* hypocalcemia may exacerbate calcium oxalate precipitation and is not indicated.

7. *Disposition:* patients suffering from EG poisoning must be admitted to the ICU.

BIBLIOGRAPHY

Burkhart KK, Kulig KW: The other alcohols. Methanol, ethylene glycol, and isopropanol. Emerg Med Clin N Am 1990;8:913–928.
Saladino R, Shannon M: Accidental and intentional poisonings with ethylene glycol in infancy: diagnostic clues and management. Pediatr Emerg Care 1991;7:93–96.

Isopropyl Alcohol

A. General Considerations

1. Isopropyl alcohol is the second most commonly ingested alcohol after ethanol. It is found in rubbing alcohol, antifreeze, industrial solvents, disinfectants, window-cleaning solutions, and skin and hair products.

2. Patients known to ingest this agent include chronic alcoholics, suicidal individuals, and children. Toxicity may also occur in children (through inhalational and perhaps dermal absorption) when sponge bathing with rubbing alcohol is used to control pediatric fever.

3. Ingestion of isopropyl alcohol causes an osmolal gap; but, unlike ethylene glycol and methanol, anion-gap metabolic acidosis does not occur. There is no antidote for isopropyl alcohol poisoning.

B. Pharmacodynamics

1. Isopropyl alcohol is rapidly absorbed from the GI tract; peak effect occurs 2 hours postingestion.

2. Fifty to eighty percent of an ingested dose is slowly metabolized by hepatic alcohol dehydrogenase to acetone, which is subsequently eliminated by the lungs and kidneys. Unlike ethylene glycol and methanol, however, it is the parent compound (not acetone) that is responsible for toxicity.

3. 100 mg/dL of isopropyl alcohol will raise serum osmolality by 17.6 mOsm/L.

4. Isopropyl alcohol is twice as potent as ethanol; it acts as a CNS and cardiac depressant.

5. The lethal dose is variable, but is generally reported as 2-4 mL/kg.

C. Clinical Presentation

1. *CNS effects:* dizziness, headache, rapid inebriation, lethargy, ataxia, coma.

2. *GI effects:* nausea, vomiting, gastritis, abdominal pain, hematemesis.

3. *Cardiovascular effects:* hypotension, myocardial depression.

4. *Miscellaneous effects:* fruity acetone breath odor, ketonuria, ketonemia, osmolal gap.

D. Management

1. As in all overdose situations, the initial management priority is *support of the patient's airway, breathing, circulation, and neurologic status* (see Standard Therapy of the Poisoned/ Overdose Patient, IV. A, earlier in this chapter). The patient's SaO_2 and cardiac rhythm should be monitored continuously; vital signs and neurologic examination should be closely followed. Hypotension indicates a severe overdose: treat with fluids, ± vasopressors (e.g., dopamine), + hemodialysis (see D. 4, below).

2. *Gastric emptying* with lavage is appropriate if the patient presents within 2 hours of ingestion; the rapid absorption of

this agent makes gastric decontamination unhelpful after that time. Activated charcoal binds isopropyl alcohol poorly, but it is reasonable if a polydrug ingestion has occurred.

3. *Laboratory evaluation* should minimally include an ABG ; CBC; electrolyte panel; glucose, BUN, and creatinine levels; ECG; urinalysis; serum osmolality; isopropyl alcohol level; ethanol level; and serum ketones.

4. *Enhanced elimination with hemodialysis.* Hemodialysis is effective at removing isopropyl alcohol, but its indications in this setting are not universally agreed upon; consult a nephrologist. Consider hemodialysis in the isopropyl alcohol poisoned patient if any of the following is present:
   a. Coma.
   b. Hypotension.
   c. Isopropyl alcohol level > 400 mg/dL.

5. *Additional care:*
   a. Meticulous supportive care is the mainstay of therapy.
   b. Administer thiamine (100-200 mg IM or IV).
   c. Consider the possibility of a coingestant.
   d. Manage gastritis with an H_2 blocker (e.g., cimetidine [150 mg IV loading dose followed by 37.5 mg/hr continuous IV infusion] or ranitidine [50 mg IV every 6-8 hours]) and evaluate for GI hemorrhage.

6. *Disposition:* awake and alert patients must be observed in the ED for 6 hours before being medically cleared for psychosocial disposition. The patient with an altered mental status should be hospitalized. A moderate to severely depressed level of consciousness or vital-sign compromise mandates ICU admission.

BIBLIOGRAPHY

Corrado CF Jr; Toxic alcohol ingestions. Lesson 24. In Critical Decisions in Emergency Medicine. Vol. 6: Focus on Chemical and Environmental Emergencies. Little NE (editor-in-chief). American College of Emergency Physicians, 1991, pp. 177–186.
Goldfrank LR, Flomenbaum NE, Lewin NA, Howland MA: Methanol, ethylene gycol, and isopropanol. Chapter 47. In Goldfrank LR et al (eds): Goldfrank's Toxicologic Emergencies. 4th Ed. Appleton & Lange. East Norwalk, CT, 1990, pp. 481–492.

METHANOL

A. General Considerations

1. Methanol (wood alcohol) is widely available as a solvent, as a solid burning alcohol ("Sterno"), and as an additive to many substances (e.g., windshield wiper fluid, fuel substitutes, gasoline antifreeze). It (and/or benzene) may be used to denature ethanol and make it unfit for consumption in paint thinners and cleaners.

2. Accidental ingestion of methanol or denatured alcohol may occur because it is less expensive than alcoholic beverages, or

as a result of improperly made home-brewed "moonshine" (cases may be seen in clusters). Methanol can also be absorbed from the skin or via the respiratory tract.

3. Methanol poisoning (and/or ethylene glycol poisoning) should be suspected in any patient with a combined anion-gap metabolic acidosis and an elevated osmolal gap.

4. The antidote for methanol poisoning is ethanol.

B. Pharmacodynamics

1. Methanol is readily absorbed from the GI tract (starting in the stomach) and distributed throughout the body.

2. The toxic effects of methanol occur secondary to its hepatic metabolites. Alcohol dehydrogenase converts methanol to formaldehyde, which is subsequently oxidized to formic acid. The latent period between ingestion of methanol and toxic symptoms (12-24 hours) corresponds to this period of hepatic biotransformation.

3. Administration of ethanol, whose metabolism by alcohol dehydrogenase is faster and preferential, can reduce the metabolism of methanol. Methanol can then be renally excreted, or hemodialyzed in the unoxidized state.

4. Methanol poisoning frequently produces an osmolal gap: 100 mg/dL of methanol increases serum osmolality by 33.7 mOsm/L.

5. Serum methanol levels ≥ 20 mg/dL are serious and demand immediate and aggressive therapy.

C. Clinical Presentation

1. Symptoms may be latent for 8-36 hours after ingestion, and they may be further delayed in cases of concomitant or subsequent ethanol ingestion.

2. Major signs and symptoms of methanolism include headache; dizziness; vomiting; back, flank, or abdominal pain; elevated pancreatic amylase; visual changes (see C. 3, below); and CNS dysfunction (from restlessness to coma). Inebriation is not prominent unless ethanol or another two-carbon alcohol has been ingested.

3. Prominent visual symptoms include visual blurring, poor acuity, halo or tunnel vision, photophobia, and/or seeing "snowfields" or a "snowstorm." Funduscopic findings of methanol poisoning include retinal edema and blurred disc margins with hyperemia.

4. A severe anion-gap metabolic acidosis is usually present.

5. Ingestion of as little as 4 mL of methanol can lead to blindness, and 80–150 mL can be fatal.

D. Management

1. As in all overdose situations, the initial management priority is *support of the patient's airway, breathing, circulation, and neurologic status* (see Standard Therapy of the Poisoned/ Overdose Patient, IV. A, earlier in this chapter). The cardiac rhythm should be continuously monitored. Maintain a generous urine output throughout therapy.

2. *Gastric emptying* with lavage is indicated if the patient presents within several hours of ingestion. Activated charcoal does not bind methanol well. Ipecac is not indicated.

3. *Laboratory evaluation* should minimally include a CBC; electrolyte panel; glucose, BUN, and creatinine levels; anion gap; ECG; ABG level; urinalysis; serum osmolality; methanol level; ethanol and serum calcium, magnesium, and phosphate levels.

4. *Antidote therapy with ethanol:*
   a. Ethanol loading dose: 10.0 mL/kg of 10% ethanol in D5W IV over 30 minutes.
   b. Maintenance infusion: begin with 1.5 mL/kg/hr IV (10% ethanol) at the same time as the above loading dose; titrate as necessary to a serum ethanol level of 100-150 mg/dL. Double the maintenance infusion during dialysis. Ethanol antidote therapy should be continued until the patient's blood methanol level is 0.
   c. *Caution:* during IV ethanol therapy monitor the patient's serum glucose and ethanol levels frequently.

5. *Enhance elimination with hemodialysis.* Hemodialysis in the treatment of methanol poisoning is indicated in patients with *any* of the following:
   a. Metabolic acidosis.
   b. Visual symptoms.
   c. Renal dysfunction.
   d. Blood methanol level > 20-25 mg/dL.
   e. History of ingestion $\geq$ 40 mL by an adult.

6. *Additional care:*
   a. Administer 100-200 mg thiamine IM or IV.
   b. Ensure a normal serum glucose level throughout therapy.
   c. Moderate to severe metabolic acidosis (pH < 7.2) should be treated with IV sodium bicarbonate. Massive doses may be required. Follow both acid–base status and serum potassium levels closely during bicarbonate therapy.
   d. Administer folinic acid (1 mg/kg IV every 4 hours) to increase the metabolism of formate.
   e. 4-Methylpyrazole (an inhibitor of alcohol dehydrogenase) appears to be a very promising antidote for methanol poisoning, but it is not yet available in the United States.

7. *Disposition:* the methanol poisoned patient should be admitted to the ICU for continued definitive care (e.g., hemodialysis, acid–base management, electrolyte management).

BIBLIOGRAPHY

Burkhart KK, Kulig KW: The other alcohols. Methanol, ethylene glycol, and isopropanol. Emerg Med Clin N Am 1990;8:913–928.

Liesivuori J, Savolainen H: Methanol and formic acid toxicity: biochemical mechanisms. Pharmacol Toxicol 1991;69:157–163.

Palmisano J, Gruver C, Adams ND: Absence of anion gap metabolic acidosis in severe methanol poisoning: a case report and review of the literature. Am J Kidney Dis 1987; 9:441–444.

XIV. LITHIUM

A. General Considerations

1. Lithium (Li^+) is a mainstay medication in the therapy of bipolar affective disorder; it acts by competing with sodium at neuronal and other receptors in the body.

2. It is available most commonly as lithium carbonate. Lithium citrate comes as a liquid preparation but is more irritating to the gut.

3. Lithium is a potentially lethal drug when taken in overdose, with a mortality rate as high as 15%.

B. Pharmacodynamics

1. Lithium is rapidly absorbed from the GI tract; peak plasma levels occur 2-4 hours after ingestion.

2. The $t_{1/2}$ is 6-12 hours, but because of tissue storage via the Na^+–K^+ transport system, lithium remains in the body for 10-14 days. Its volume of distribution is essentially that of Na^+, and the toxicities of lithium are potentiated by Na^+ loss (e.g., fever, diarrhea, diuresis).

3. Therapeutic lithium levels are generally 0.6-1.5 mEq/L. Toxic effects are most commonly seen with levels $\geq$ 1.6 mEq/L but may also be seen in the therapeutic range. Severe toxicities are expected with levels $\geq$ 2-3 mEq/L.

4. Serum levels may not accurately reflect body stores, especially in chronic users.

C. Clinical Presentation

1. *CNS toxicities*: see Table 23–21.

2. *GI toxicities:* nausea, vomiting, and diarrhea.

3. *Renal toxicities:* decreased renal concentrating capacity and polyuria (nephrogenic diabetes insipidus), interstitial nephritis, hypernatremia.

4. *Cardiovascular effects:* arrhythmias (particularly ventricular), ST depression, T-wave changes, and rarely, cardiovascular collapse.

5. *Miscellaneous:* hypercalcemia, hyperparathyroidism, goiter, nonketotic hyperglycemia, and neutrophilia.

Table 23–21. NEUROLOGIC TOXICITIES OF LITHIUM

Serum Li⁺ Level (mEq/L)	Neurologic Signs and Symptoms
< 1.5	Lethargy, fatigue, weakness, memory and concentration difficulties, fine tremor
1.5–2.0	Coarse tremor, ataxia, dysarthria, visual disturbances, hyperreflexia, hypertonia, fasciculations, extrapyramidal syndromes, confusion
3.0–5.0	Seizures, coma, flaccidity, irreversible brain injury
≥ 5.0–7.0	Death

D. Management

1. As in all overdose situations, the initial management priority is *support of the patient's airway, breathing, circulation, and neurologic status* (see Standard Therapy of the Poisoned/Overdose Patient, IV. A, earlier in this chapter). The patient's SaO_2 and cardiac rhythm must be continuously monitored; closely follow vital signs, neurologic status, and urine output.

2. *Gastric emptying* with lavage is appropriate in the patient who presents within the first several hours of ingestion. Activated charcoal is not effective in binding lithium. Ipecac is not indicated.

3. *Laboratory evaluation* should minimally include a CBC; electrolyte panel; glucose, BUN, and creatinine levels; ECG; urinalysis; serum osmolality; lithium level; and serum calcium, magnesium, and phosphate levels.

4. *Enhance elimination with hemodialysis.* Hemodialysis is indicated in any of the following patient situations:

   a. Moderate or severe CNS symptoms (e.g., seizures, obtundation), regardless of serum level.

   b. Cardiac arrhythmias, regardless of serum level.

   c. Serum levels ≥ 3.5 mEq/L, even if asymptomatic.

   d. Patients with renal insufficiency and levels ≥ 2.0 mEq/L. After dialysis, serum lithium levels should be monitored every 2-4 hours. Rebound is common, and repeat dialysis is frequently necessary. Dialysis should be repeated until lithium levels remain below 1.0 mEq/L.

5. *Additional care:*

   a. Seizures should be initially treated with diazepam, ± phenytoin, ± phenobarbital.

   b. Diuretics acting on the ascending limb of the loop of Henle or the distal tubule may worsen lithium toxicity and are contraindicated (e.g., furosemide, ethacrynic acid, or thiazides).

   c. Neuroleptics may potentiate lithium toxicity.

   d. If diabetes insipidus ensues, urinary losses should be matched with IV fluids isotonic with the urine, and serum electrolyte abnormalities further managed as appropriate.

6. *Disposition:*

a. Patients with minimal to mild toxicity should remain monitored in the ED until signs and symptoms have abated and repeat serum levels remain in the therapeutic range. At that point they are medically cleared and psychiatric consultation for further disposition should be obtained.

b. Patients with moderate to severe toxicity must be admitted to a monitored bed for continued definitive care (e.g., dialysis, rhythm management, electrolyte management).

BIBLIOGRAPHY

Hauger RL, O'Connor KA, et al: Lithium toxicity: when is hemodialysis necessary? Acta Psychiatr Scand 1990;81:515–517.

Simard M, Gumbiner B, et al: Lithium carbonate intoxication: a case report and review of the literature. Arch Intern Med 1989;149:36–46.

Smith SW, Ling LJ, Halstenson CE: Whole bowel irrigation as a treatment for acute lithium overdose. Ann Emerg Med 1991;20:536–539.

XV. MONOAMINE OXIDASE INHIBITORS

A. General Considerations

1. Monoamine oxidase inhibitors (MAOIs) were introduced in the late 1950s and gained great popularity in the 1960s for the therapy of endogenous depression. Their use has declined since the introduction of less toxic agents. Four drugs of this class are currently in use: phenelzine (Nardil), isocarboxazid (Marplan), tranylcypromine (Parnate), and selegiline (Eldepryl).

2. They irreversibly bind monoamine oxidase and prevent the degradation of monoamines (e.g., dopamine, norepinephrine, epinephrine, and serotonin).

3. Usual daily doses are 10-60 mg. Overdoses as small as 2-3 mg/kg result in severe toxicity and have been fatal.

4. Transient hypertensive crises are seen when these drugs are taken with foods containing tyramine (e.g., aged cheeses, red wines, yeast and meat extracts, smoked/pickled meats or fish, Italian broad beans). A single dose of meperidine with MAOIs results in rapid, severe, and potentially life-threatening reactions (hyperthermia, muscle rigidity, hypotension, coma, and death). Serious drug interactions have also occurred with many other agents, including amphetamines, clomipramine, cocaine, dextromethorphan, fluoxetine, and L-tryptophan.

B. Pharmacodynamics

1. MAOIs are readily absorbed from the GI tract, hepatically metabolized, and the inactive metabolites excreted in the urine.

2. Peak plasma levels occur about 2½ hours after ingestion. Plasma $t_{1/2}$ is approximately 3 hours.

3. Phenelzine and tranylcypromine are metabolized to amphet-amines, causing presynaptic norepinephrine release. This "autopotentiation" may underlie the toxicities of these drugs.

4. Postsynaptic norepinephrine release in the CNS and cardiac tissue is blunted, with a subsequent decrease in norepineph-rine's synaptic uptake and re-release. This biphasic availabil-ity is analogous to bretylium and may explain the late CNS and cardiac depression seen with MAOI overdose.

5. Phenelzine and isocarboxazid also block histamine degrada-tion.

C. Clinical Presentation

1. The primary toxicities are secondary to CNS and peripheral sympathetic excitation (Table 23–22).

2. Additional findings may include peaked T waves on the ECG in the absence of hyperkalemia; rhabdomyolysis, acute myocardial infarction, and/or prolonged coma.

3. Patients are generally asymptomatic for 6-12 hours, with the development of worsening symptoms and signs over the next 12-24 hours.

D. Management

1. As in all overdose situations, the initial management priority is *support of the patient's airway, breathing, circulation, and neurologic status* (see Standard Therapy of the Poisoned/Overdose Patient, IV. A, earlier in this chapter). The patient's SaO_2 and cardiac rhythm should be continuously monitored; vital signs and neurologic status must be followed closely. If vasopressors become necessary for blood pressure support, they must be used cautiously and at reduced dosages; norepinephrine is the preferred drug in this setting.

2. *Gastric emptying* with lavage, activated charcoal, and cathar-tic should be accomplished as rapidly as possible. Ipecac is not appropriate.

3. *Laboratory evaluation* should minimally include a CBC; electrolyte panel; glucose, BUN, and creatinine levels; ECG;

Table 23–22. THE SPECTRUM OF MAOI TOXICITIES

TOXICITY	SIGNS AND SYMPTOMS
Mild	Neuromuscular/psychomotor agitation and hyperactivity
Moderate	Altered mental status, hyperthermia, hypertension, tachycardia, tachypnea, hyperglycemia, leukocytosis
Severe	Hyperpyrexia, seizures (tonic–clonic or myoclonic); coma; CNS, cardiovas-cular and respiratory depression; rigidity alternating with flaccidity

Table 23–23. SUGGESTED MANAGEMENT OF PHYSIOLOGIC ABNORMALITIES RESULTING FROM MAOI OVERDOSE

ABNORMALITY	TREATMENT OPTIONS
Neuromuscular irritability/seizures	Diazepam, barbiturates, phenytoin, pancuronium
Hyperthermia	Acetaminophen, external cooling, pancuronium, dantrolene, bromocriptine
Hypertension	Phentolamine, nitroprusside, beta blockers (use cautiously)
Hypotension	Volume, norepinephrine
Supraventricular tachyarrhythmias	Propanolol, digoxin, verapamil
Ventricular tachyarrhythmias	Lidocaine, procainamide, phenytoin, beta blockers
Bradyarrhythmias	Pacing, atropine, isoproterenol, epinephrine

Adapted from Linden CH, et al: Ann Emerg Med 1984;131:1142.

Table 23–24. THERAPEUTIC AGENTS THAT MAY COMPLICATE MAOI OVERDOSE MANAGEMENT

AVOID	USE WITH CAUTION AND/OR REDUCE DOSAGE
Alpha methyldopa	Atropine
Bretylium	Beta blockers
Clonidine	Digoxin
Ganglionic blockers	Dopamine
Guanethidine	Epinephrine
Nonbarbiturate sedative-hypnotics	Isoproterenol
Oral antihypertensive agents	Norepinephrine
Salicylates	Phenothiazines
Succinylcholine	Verapamil

ABG; urinalysis; and calcium, magnesium, and phosphate levels. "Toxic" levels of MAOIs are not defined; there is no clinical utility in checking plasma levels.

4. *Additional care* (Tables 23–23 and 23–24):

   a. CNS irritability, muscle irritability, or seizures should be treated with diazepam and/or phenobarbital. Phenytoin may be added if necessary but is of uncertain benefit in this setting. If muscle paralysis is required, intubate the patient and use pancuronium (0.1 mg/kg IV). Succinylcholine should not be used. The seizing patient who requires muscle paralysis after antiseizure medications should have electroencephalographic monitoring to evaluate seizure activity and treatment efficacy. Other sedative-hypnotics and opioids should not be used because of potential interactions with MAOIs and exaggerated CNS/ cardiovascular depression.

   b. Hyperthermia: any degree of temperature elevation should be aggressively treated with appropriate cooling measures (e.g., cooling blanket, tepid sponge baths, mist spray with fan convection) and acetaminophen. Neuromuscular blockade (intubation and pancuronium) may be required to relieve muscle rigidity. Severe hyperthermia has been reported following MAOI overdose and may require management with dantrolene (1-2 mg/kg IV every 6 hours; not to exceed 10 mg/kg/day) and bromocriptine (5 mg PO initially followed by 2.5 mg PO every 8 hours). The use of these latter agents in this setting, however, has been inadequately studied.

   c. Severe hypertension should be managed with an alpha blocker (e.g., phentolamine [5 mg IV bolus followed by continuous infusion of 0.2-0.5 mg/min] or with sodium nitroprusside [0.25-10.0 µg/kg/min IV]). Oral antihypertensives are difficult to titrate, have prolonged durations of action, and should not be used. Ganglionic blockers and centrally acting alpha-adrenergic agents (e.g., clonidine, alpha methyldopa, guanethidine) are unpredictable in MAOI overdose, and their use should be avoided. Beta blockers may help in managing MAOI-induced hypertension if excessive cardiac stimulation is present; otherwise, they can *increase* hypertension because of unopposed alpha-adrenergic stimulation.

   d. Cardiac arrhythmias in this setting are difficult to treat. Symptomatic bradycardias should preferably be managed with cardiac pacing. If atropine, isoproterenol, and/or epinephrine are used their dosages should be reduced. Stable ventricular tachycardias should be treated with lidocaine or procainamide. Bretylium is contraindicated because its effects are similar to those of MAOIs.

   e. Urinary acidification is *not* recommended. It only increases excretion of unmetabolized MAOIs by 8%, and it may precipitate urinary myoglobin. Dialysis may improve symptoms, but it does not decrease the time until resolution of toxicity.

5. *Disposition:* all MAOI overdoses should be admitted to the ICU for *at least* 24 hours of continuous monitoring.

BIBLIOGRAPHY

Linden CH, Rumack BH, Strehlke C: Monoamine oxidase inhibitor overdose. Ann Emerg Med. 1984;13:1137–1144.

Rudorfer MV: Monoamine oxidase inhibitors: reversible and irreversible. Psychopharmacol Bull 1992;28:45–57.

XVI. OPIOIDS

A. General Considerations

1. Opium is an air-dried milky exudate obtained from the opium poppy (*Papaver somniferum* or its variety *album*). Opiates are natural derivatives of opium, including codeine, heroin, and morphine. *Opioid* refers to drugs with opium-like activity,

including the natural opium derivatives, semisynthetic derivatives, and synthetic agents (Table 23–25). *Narcotic* is a nonspecific term that refers to any agent capable of producing insensibility or stupor. In common practice, the term *narcotic* is used interchangeably with the term *opioid*.

Table 23–25. COMMONLY USED OPIOIDS

DRUG	PRODUCT NAME	DOSE EQUIVALENT TO 10 MG OF MORPHINE	COMMENTS
Opium Derivatives			
Morphine		10 mg	
Codeine		120 mg	Lower abuse/addiction potential
Tincture of opium	Paregoric	16–25 mL	Used in various antidiarrheals with lower abuse/addiction potential; accidental poisonings in children do occur
Semisynthetic			
Diacetyl morphine	Heroin	3 mg	Street names: "smack," "horse"
Hydromorphone	Dilaudid	1.5 mg	Street name: "legal heroin"
Oxycodone	Percodan, Tylox, Percocet	10 mg	Oral compounds containing aspirin, acetaminophen, phenacetin, and/or caffeine; abuse potential
Hydrocodone	Vicodin, Hycodan	10 mg	Found in many abused cough/cold remedies
Synthetic			
Meperidine	Demerol	75–100 mg	IV use associated with greater dependency and more severe withdrawal than for heroin; metabolite is epileptogenic
Methadone	Dolophine	10 mg	Used in heroin withdrawal/maintenance programs
Butorphanol	Stadol	2 mg	Agonist-antagonist
Levorphanol	Levo-Dromoran	2 mg	
Pentazocine	Talwin	50 mg	Lower, but real, abuse/addiction potential; IV use includes "T's and blues" (pentazocine and tripelennamine, an antihistamine; also combined with heroin or paregoric as "blue velvet")
Propoxyphene	Darvon, Darvocet	240 mg	Low analgesic efficacy and addiction potential; may cause cardiac conduction delays; often compounded with acetaminophen, which may cause hepatic necrosis yielding hypoglycemia, etc.
Diphenoxylate	Lomotil	40 mg	Combined opioid and atropinic
Fentanyl	Sublimaze	100–125 µg	Often used in combination with the butyrophenone droperidol for anesthesia

2. Overdose with these drugs causes a syndrome of miotic pupils (meperidine may cause dilated pupils), depressed level of consciousness, and ventilatory embarrassment.

3. The antidote for an opioid overdose is naloxone.

4. Addiction is dependent on relative potency of the opioids, mode of use, duration and frequency of use, degree of receptor agonism, and other variables. Addiction is defined by
   a. Tolerance: requirement of successively higher doses to produce the same effects.
   b. Obsessive–compulsive drug seeking and using behaviors.
   c. Physical dependence, resulting in withdrawal symptoms upon drug discontinuance.

B. Pharmacodynamics

1. Analgesia, sedation, and euphoria are a result of opioid binding to specific CNS receptors similar to that of endogenous enkephalin and beta-endorphin peptides.

2. Additional effects include ventilatory depression; miosis (mydriasis with meperidine); hypotension; stimulation of the chemoemetic trigger zone; histamine release (not with fentanyl); and GI, genitourinary, and biliary smooth muscle spasm (less with meperidine). Smooth muscle spasm may result in delayed gastric emptying, constipation, urinary retention, and biliary colic.

C. Clinical Presentation

1. The "classic" patient with an opioid overdose is characterized by lethargy or coma, pinpoint pupils, and ventilatory depression. (*Reminder:* pinpoint pupils may also be seen in poisoning with anticholinesterases [e.g., organophosphorous insecticides], parasympathomimetics [e.g., bethanechol], sympatholytics [e.g., ergot alkaloids, clonidine], chloral hydrate, barbiturates, nicotine, and some mushrooms.)

2. Additional findings may include acute pulmonary edema, needle "tracks," sclerosed/thrombosed veins, and/or cutaneous abscesses. Absence of "tracks" may only mean that either accidental or suicidal overdose has occurred by "snorting" or oral ingestion.

3. Propoxyphene overdose may present with early drowsiness, vertigo, nausea, and vomiting. Convulsions and pulmonary edema are common, and patients with a large overdose may suffer a rapid collapse and sudden death. Less frequently, delusions, hallucinations, dysphoria, disorientation, headache, abdominal pain, and rash occur. The course of the overdose may be prolonged.

4. Complications of opioid abuse are multiple and include acute pulmonary edema, pneumonia (e.g., aspiration or from septic

emboli), pulmonary fibrosis, tuberculosis, bacterial endocarditis, meningitis, epidural abscess, transverse myelitis, hepatitis, cardiac arrhythmias, stroke, trauma, compartment syndromes, cellulitis, septic arthritis, osteomyelitis, renal insufficiency, sexually transmitted diseases, and human immunodeficiency virus (HIV) infection.

D. Management

1. As in all overdose situations, the initial management priority is *support of the patient's airway, breathing, circulation, and neurologic status* (see Standard Therapy of the Poisoned/Overdose Patient, IV. A, earlier in this chapter). Early and appropriate use of naloxone (see below) may reverse respiratory depression and obviate the need for intubation. SaO_2 and cardiac rhythm should be continuously monitored. Airway status, vital signs, and mental status must be followed closely.

2. *Gastric emptying* with lavage, activated charcoal, and cathartic is appropriate in the setting of a significant opioid ingestion. Opioid-induced delayed gastric emptying makes GI decontamination reasonable even in the late-presenting patient. The possibility of polydrug ingestions is also a consideration. Gastric emptying is obviously ineffectual in the setting of injection drug use.

3. *Laboratory evaluation* should minimally include a CBC; electrolyte panel; glucose, BUN, and creatinine levels; ECG; chest roentgenogram; ABG; urinalysis; and pregnancy test (in reproductive-age females). A toxicologic screen is reasonable in the uncommunicative or seriously ill patient; some synthetic high-potency opioids (e.g., fentanyl) are not detected on routine toxicologic screens. Consider the posibility of concomitant acetaminophen and/or salicylate ingestion.

4. *Antidote therapy with naloxone:*
   a. Naloxone is an extremely safe, specific, nontoxic agent for the treatment of opioid overdose.
   b. *Dose:* begin with 0.1-2.0 mg IV and repeat as necessary for reversal of respiratory depression and/or markedly depressed level of consciousness (begin with the 2-mg dose in critical situations). In the pregnant patient, administer the minimal amount of naloxone necessary to reverse the mother's respiratory depression; avoid precipitating frank withdrawal in either mother or fetus. In the setting of a serious propoxyphene or pentazocine overdose, the use of up to 16-20 mg of IV naloxone may be necessary.
   c. The mean $t_{1/2}$ of naloxone is 64 minutes, and the clinical effects last only 15-30 minutes. Repeat doses are commonly needed, and close patient observation is mandatory. A continuous naloxone infusion is frequently useful: two-thirds of the bolus dose that was needed for reversal

of respiratory depression should be infused per hour IV (an additional minibolus may be required 20-30 minutes after the infusion is started).

5. *Additional care:*

   a. The patient presenting with an altered level of consciousness should also be given thiamine (100-200 mg IM or IV) and glucose (25-50 g D50W IV if the fingerstick glucose level is < 80 mg/dL).

   b. Pulmonary edema/ARDS is treated with oxygen to maintain an appropriate SaO_2. In cases of continued hypoxia and/or acidosis, ventilator therapy with adequate $FiO_2 \pm PEEP$ is indicated. Digitalis, diuretics, phlebotomy, and/or tourniquets are *not* indicated. Diuretic administration for opioid-induced pulmonary edema can result in significant hypotension.

   c. Carefully evaluate the patient for the possibility of traumatic, pulmonary, cardiac, or infectious disease complications.

6. *Disposition:* the patient who has suffered a parenteral opioid overdose must be observed in the ED for a minimum of 6 hours after initial stabilization with naloxone. If repeat doses of naloxone are required over that time period, then ICU admission is mandated for 12-24 hours of monitoring. All significant oral opioid overdoses and individuals with pulmonary edema should be admitted to the ICU.

E. Opioid Withdrawal

1. An abstinence syndrome occurs when chronic opioid use is discontinued. Though unpleasant, it is not associated with any mortality in the absence of other significant medical condition(s). Symptoms generally begin 12-14 hours after last use and begin to diminish by 72 hours.

2. Symptoms and signs may include lacrimation, rhinorrhea, sweating, yawning, restlessness, insomnia, mydriasis, piloerection, muscle twitching, myalgia, arthralgia, abdominal pain, tachycardia, hypertension, tachypnea, fever, anorexia, nausea, severe akathisia, vomiting, diarrhea, dehydration, hyperglycemia, and hypotension.

3. *Therapy:*

   a. Opioids should generally not be prescribed by the ED physician for purposes of tapered withdrawal management of the addict.

   b. Clonidine may be prescribed to ameliorate many of the withdrawal symptoms. Different regimens are used, and optimal dosing will vary between patients. Consider starting with 6 µg/kg per day in two or three divided doses for 5 days, then taper slowly. The patient must be informed of the risks of hypotension with clonidine therapy, the need for a slow clonidine taper, and the risks of marked sedation and hypotension if further opioids are used while the patient is taking clonidine.

c. Medical social work consultation and referral to a detoxification center are appropriate.

BIBLIOGRAPHY

Challoner KR, McCarron MM, Newton EJ: Pentazocine (Talwin) intoxication: report of 57 cases. J Emerg Med 1990;8:67–74.

Ford M, Hoffman RS, Goldfrank LR: Opioids and designer drugs. Emerg Med Clin N Am 1990; 8:495–511.

Ling W, Wesson DR: Drugs of abuse—opiates. West J Med 1990;152:565–572.

Martin M, Hecker J, et al: China white epidemic: an eastern United States emergency department experience. Ann Emerg Med 1991;20:158–164.

Schug SA, Zech D, Grond S: Adverse effects of systemic opioid analgesics. Drug Saf 1992; 7:200–213.

XVII. SALICYLATES

A. General Considerations

1. Aspirin (acetylsalicylic acid), is present in numerous over-the-counter and prescription medications (Table 23–26).

2. The maximum adult therapeutic dose of aspirin is 650 mg PO every 4 hours. Therapeutic drug levels for chronic inflammatory conditions (e.g., rheumatoid arthritis) are 15-30 mg/dL. Tinnitus occurs with blood levels > 30 mg/dL.

3. Salicylate poisoning in adults occurs either intentionally as an acute suicide attempt, or more subtly as an accidental overdose from taking increased amounts over time for "therapeutic" reasons. The former is generally readily identified and treated, with mortality rates ≤ 2% with appropriate therapy. The latter can be difficult to identify; and, in one series, had a mortality rate of 25%, largely secondary to delays in diagnosis and treatment.

4. Oil of wintergreen (methyl salicylate) is an especially dangerous formulation, containing 7.8 g of salicylate (equivalent to 21 adult aspirin tablets) per teaspoon (5 mL). One to two teaspoons of oil of wintergreen is a potentially lethal dose of salicylate in the young child.

Table 23–26. COMMON SALICYLATE-CONTAINING PREPARATIONS

Alka-Seltzer	Congespirin	Goody's Powders
Anacin	Darvon Compound	Midol
APC	Dristan	Percodan
Ascriptin	Easprin	Phenaphen
Aspergum	Ecotrin	St. Joseph's
BC Powders	Empirin	Sine-Aid
Bromo-Seltzer	Fiorinal	Sine-Off
Bufferin	4-Way Cold Tablets	Vanquish

Table 23–27. SALICYLATE POISONING: TOXIC DOSE, SIGNS, AND SYMPTOMS

TOXICITY CATEGORY	APPROXIMATE DOSE	SIGNS AND SYMPTOMS
Asymptomatic	<< 100 mg/kg	Subjective complaints only; no objective evidence of toxicity
Mild	100–200 mg/kg	Hyperventilation, nausea, vomiting, lethargy, tinnitus
Moderate	200–300 mg/kg	Hyperventilation, vomiting, sweating, hyperthermia, vertigo, agitation and hallucinations or lethargy/stupor
Severe	300–400 mg/kg	Hyperventilation, seizures, coma, shock

5. The common over-the-counter preparation Excedrin contains salicymide, acetaminophen, and caffeine. Salicymide does not cause salicylate poisoning. Excedrin Extra-Strength, however, does contain salicylate in place of salicymide.

B. Pharmacodynamics

1. Aspirin is absorbed from the stomach and upper small bowel. Many factors can delay absorption, including food, pylorospasm, enteric-coated preparations, anticholinergic agents, opioids, ileus, or aspirin concretions ("bezoars").

2. Hydrolysis of aspirin to *salicylic acid* occurs during absorption and first-pass hepatic metabolism. Salicylic acid is responsible for both the therapeutic and toxic effects of aspirin.

3. In an overdose, salicylates uncouple oxidative phosphorylation, resulting in a hypermetabolic state, increased use of glucose, abnormal carbohydrate metabolism, CNS effects, renal potassium wasting, and significant acid–base disturbances.

4. Salicylic acid undergoes hepatic conjugation along several pathways, and the various metabolites are excreted and secreted into the urine.

5. The $t_{1/2}$ of a therapeutic dose is 2-4 hours; the $t_{1/2}$ of a toxic dose may be 15-30 hours.

C. Clinical Presentation

1. Symptoms and signs of salicylate toxicity are presented in Table 23–27.

2. Miscellaneous effects include hearing loss, hypocalcemia, tetany, other electrolyte abnormalities (hyper- or hyponatremia, hypokalemia), hypoglycemia, anion-gap metabolic acidosis (see below), noncardiogenic pulmonary edema, GI hemorrhage, acute renal failure, platelet dysfunction, and coagulopathy (prolonged PT).

3. Acid–base disturbances are common in salicylate poisoning (Fig. 23–3).

   a. In the pediatric age group, the usual acid–base disturbance consists of an initial respiratory alkalosis rapidly progressing to a metabolic acidosis. In adults, mixed acid–base disturbances are more frequent.

   b. Acidosis is particularly deleterious because it increases the nonionized fraction of salicylate and enhances its passage into the cerebrospinal fluid (CSF): the severity of salicylate poisoning correlates best with critical brain levels of the drug.

4. The Done nomogram (Fig. 23–4) relates serum salicylate level to severity of intoxication in the setting of an *acute* ingestion. Before applying the nomogram to any clinical case, note the following:

   a. The nomogram is valid only for a single acute salicylate ingestion in a patient with normal renal function. It does not apply to cases of chronic salicylism, ingestion of enteric-coated tablets, or ingestion of oil of wintergreen.

   b. The time elapsed since ingestion must be known (at least 6 hours must have elapsed since ingestion before the nomogram is applicable).

   c. Ensure that the units reported by the toxicology laboratory correspond to the units used in the nomogram (mg/dL).

   d. Never rely solely on a single salicylate level to evaluate toxicity. The symptomatic patient must be presumed toxic irrespective of the level obtained, and two or more levels should be checked 3-6 hours apart to evaluate for continued absorption, efficacy of therapy, and need for hemodialysis.

D. Management

1. As in all overdose situations, the initial management priority is *support of the patient's airway, breathing, circulation, and neurologic status* (see Standard Therapy of the Poisoned/ Overdose Patient, IV. A, earlier in this chapter).

   a. An inadequate airway or ventilatory depression requires intubation and mechanical ventilation.

   b. Almost all salicylate poisoned patients are volume depleted and are at risk for *hypoglycemia;* dextrose-containing crystalloid solutions (initially 5% dextrose in normal saline or lactated Ringer's solution) should be empirically administered and the infusion rate adjusted to ensure a generous urine output (2-3 mL/kg/hr).

   c. Hypotension should be treated initially with volume. Vasopressors (e.g., dopamine or norepinephrine) may be required adjunctively. The development of noncardiogenic pulmonary edema is an ever-present risk in the seriously poisoned patient. Invasive hemodynamic monitoring may be necessary.

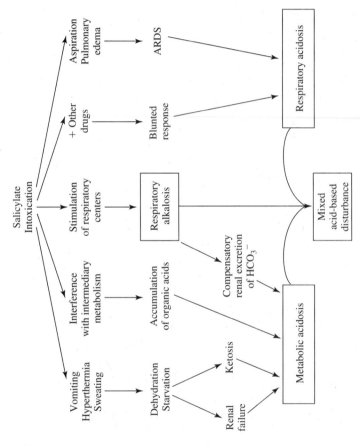

Figure 23-3. Pathophysiology of acid–base disturbances in salicylate intoxication.

953

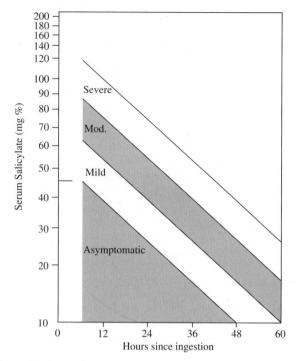

Figure 23–4. Done nomogram. (From Done AK: Pediatrics 1960;26:800.)

    d. The patient with an altered mental status should receive thiamine, glucose, and naloxone. Seizures should be managed with airway control, diazepam, ± phenytoin, ± phenobarbital.

2. *Gastric emptying* is mandatory in the setting of an acute ingestion, even in the late presenting patient.

    a. Gastric lavage, activated charcoal, and a cathartic should be used. Consider repeat administration of charcoal (repeat doses should not contain a cathartic) every 4 hours until a charcoal stool is produced. Ipecac is not recommended.

    b. Suspected aspirin concretions may be demonstrated by barium swallow roentgenography. Their removal may be facilitated by one or more of the following techniques:

        i. Whole-bowel irrigation (see Table 23–3).

        ii. Endoscopic mechanical disruption and removal.

3. Continuously monitor the cardiac rhythm and SaO_2; closely follow vital signs, neurologic status, urine output (with bladder catheterization), and fluid balance. Blood glucose level, acid–base status, and electrolytes should be checked hourly in seriously ill patients.

4. *Laboratory evaluation* should minimally include a CBC; electrolyte panel; glucose, BUN, and creatinine levels;

salicylate level; acetaminophen level; ABG; chest roentgenogram; ECG; urinalysis; PT/PTT; and platelet count. Enteric-coated tablets may be apparent on an abdominal film.

5. *Enhanced elimination with alkalinization:*
   a. Alkalinization of the plasma is recommended to minimize CSF–brain salicylate levels; alkalinization of the urine will markedly enhance renal salicylate elimination.
   b. Alkalinization is appropriate in patients with any of the following:
      i. Symptomatic patients.
      ii. Salicylate levels ≥ 35 mg/dL.
      iii. Already present acid–base disturbances.
      iv. Patients with rapidly rising salicylate levels.
   c. Goals of alkalinization are to maintain serum pH ≤ 7.50 while attempting to maintain a urine pH of 7.5-8.0.
   d. *Technique:* Initiate alkalinization by administering 1-2 mEq/kg sodium bicarbonate IV over 30-60 minutes. Follow with repeat doses as needed, or use a continuous bicarbonate infusion (e.g., add 1-3 ampules of sodium bicarbonate [50 mEq per ampule] to 1 L D5W and begin infusion at 200 mL/hr). Titrate to the desired serum and urine pH. The concentration and administration rate of a continuous bicarbonate infusion will depend on the severity of the acidosis, severity of the overdose, and the presence of other concomitant electrolyte abnormalities (e.g., hypernatremia or hyponatremia).
   e. *Cautions:*
      i. Actual alkalinization of the urine in severe salicylate poisoning is often difficult secondary to coexistent severe potassium depletion. In the patient with normal renal function, potassium chloride or acetate (begin with 20-40 mEq/L) should be added to the maintenance or bicarbonate infusion. Adjust the dose as necessary to maintain serum potassium in the normal range. In severe salicylate poisoning extremely large doses of potassium chloride are needed.
      ii. Overly aggressive alkalinization may lead to sodium overload, severe metabolic alkalosis, and exacerbation of the potassium deficit. Urine pH should be followed but *not* solely used to assess therapy. Serial measurement of arterial pH is mandatory.
      iii. Do *not* use the carbonic anhydrase inhibitor acetazolamide (Diamox) for alkalinization.

6. *Enhanced elimination with hemodialysis:*
   a. Hemodialysis may be life-saving in severe salicylate poisoning.
   b. Hemodialysis is indicated when any of the following conditions applies:
      i. Severe toxicity is predicted by the Done nomogram (e.g., salicylate level >120 mg/dL at 6 hr).
      ii. Renal failure.

Table 23–28. SUMMARY OF SALICYLATE OVERDOSE MANAGEMENT

TOXIC MANIFESTATION	PATHOPHYSIOLOGY	TREATMENT	COMMENTS
Metabolic acidosis	Interference with intermediary metabolism Ketosis Renal failure Renal HCO_3- excretion	*For severe acidosis:* IV $NaHCO_3-$ (1–2 mEq/kg infused over 30–60 min; repeat as necessary) *To decrease brain salicylate:* Continuous infusion of $NaHCO_3-$ containing solutions (1–3 mEq/kg/L IV fluids)	Acidosis increases salicylate toxicity by increasing CSF–brain levels. Keep blood pH < 7.50; serum K^+ should be maintained in the normal range
Respiratory alkalosis	Stimulation of respiratory centers by salicylates	None If tetany, consider 5 mL of 10% $CaCl_2$ IV	Alkalosis may be exacerbated by $NaHCO_3$ therapy
Respiratory acidosis	Aspiration ARDS Other drugs Very high salicylate levels	Intubation and ventilatory therapy Adequate FiO_2 PEEP	More common in adults
Volume (saline) depletion	Vomiting Decreased intake Renal losses	Volume repletion with isotonic solutions; solutions should contain glucose (D5)	↑ BUN, normal creatinine UNa < 20
Renal failure	*Acute tubular necrosis* Shock, ischemia, fluid–electrolyte and acid-base disturbance	Careful management of fluid–electrolytes, especially K^+ Dialysis	↑ BUN, creatinine UNa > 40
Hypernatremia (water depletion)	Hyperventilation Sweating	1. Volume (saline) repletion first 2. See therapy of hypernatremia in Chapter 17	Moderate to severe Correct hypernatremia slowly (administer ½ of free water deficit in first 24 hr; correct remaining deficit over next 1–2 days)
Hyponatremia (water excess)	1. Inappropriate water intake or fluid management 2. Salicylate-induced inappropriate ADH	1. Restriction of free water intake 2. *If severe:* a. Hypertonic saline (3%) b. Furosemide diuresis 3. See therapy of hyponatremia in Chapter 17	Correct hyponatremia slowly (no faster than 2.5 mEq/L per hr; no more than 20 mEq/L in 24 hr)

      iii. Pulmonary edema (cardiogenic or noncardiogenic).
      iv. Coma.
      v. Severe acid-base and/or electrolyte abnormalities despite appropriate therapy.
      vi. Hepatic compromise.
      vii. Coagulopathy.
  7. *Additional care* (Table 23–28):
    a. Hypoglycemia is a significant contributor to morbidity and mortality in salicylate poisoning. All crystalloid infusions

Table 23–28. SUMMARY OF SALICYLATE OVERDOSE MANAGEMENT *Continued*

Toxic Manifestation	Pathophysiology	Treatment	Comments
Hypokalemia	Loss of K^+ with large amounts of organic acids in urine Initial K^+ may be "normal" due to acidosis (like DKA)	Add KCl (20–40 mEq/L) to IV solutions in the patient with normal renal function	See therapy of hypokalemia in Chapter 17
Tetany	Due to alkalosis with ↓ ionized Ca^{2+} (normal serum Ca^{+2})	Treat especially if seizures: 5 ml of 10% $CaCl_2$ IV	Tetany may be exacerbated by bicarbonate therapy
CNS dysfunction Seizures Coma	CNS toxicity of salicylates Also fluid-electrolyte, acid-base, and glucose disturbances	1. $CaCl_2$ as above for seizures due to alkalosis 2. Diazepam, 0.1 mg/kg	Treat ↓ Na^+, K^+, glucose, hypoxia, and acidosis as above
Hyperglycemia (adults)	Stimulation of hepatic gluconeogenesis		Glucosuria commonly present
Hypoglycemia (infants)	?	1. Use D5–D10 containing IV solutions 2. May need push doses of D50W	Hypoglycemia and ketoacidosis have been reported in a nondiabetic adult
ARDS "Pulmonary edema"	Salicylate-induced ARDS Shock Aspiration	1. Careful fluid-electrolyte management 2. Ventilator therapy with adequate FiO_2 and PEEP	"Pulmonary edema" similar to heroin, propoxyphene, methadone
Hyperthermia	Uncoupling of oxidative phosphorylation with ↑ heat production	Cool H_2O sponging Cooling mattress; spray mist water with electric fan convection	
Disorders of hemostasis	↓ Prothrombin and factor VII Platelet dysfunction	Vitamin K, fresh frozen plasma if patient actively bleeding	Bleeding problems uncommon
Rhabdomyolysis and myoglobinuria	Associated with hyperthermia	*Prevent ATN* IV hydration; maintain good urine output. Once well hydrated may consider diureses with furosemide and/or mannitol.	

should have dextrose added (5 g/dL minimum). Monitor serum glucose levels regularly.

    b. Hyperthermia should be treated with necessary cooling measures (cooling blankets, tepid sponge baths, mist spray and convection fans). Acetaminophen is unlikely to be of help.

    c. Coagulopathy (prolonged PT) should be treated with vitamin K administration (10-40 mg [rarely up to 50 mg]

IM or IV. If vitamin K must be given IV, administer very cautiously and no faster than 1 mg/min). The actively bleeding patient should be given fresh frozen plasma.

d. Tetany in the setting of hyperventilation can be treated with 10% calcium chloride (5 mL) administered slowly IV.

8. *Disposition:*

   a. The persistently asymptomatic patient with repeated nontoxic and nonrising salicylate levels over time may be medically cleared and referred for psychiatric evaluation.

   b. Patients with persistent symptoms, rising salicylate levels, toxic levels, continued vital-sign abnormalities, acid–base disturbances, or other evidence of moderate to severe toxicity should be admitted to the ICU for the continuation of definitive care. The possibility of chronic salicylism must be considered and appropriately managed in the symptomatic patient with nontoxic blood levels.

BIBLIOGRAPHY

Durnas C, Cusack BJ: Salicylate intoxication in the elderly. Recognition and recommendations on how to prevent it. Drugs Aging 1992;2:20–34.

Keller RE, Schwab RA, Kronzolok EP: Contribution of sorbitol combined with activated charcoal in prevention of salicylate absorption. Ann Emerg Med 1990;19:654–656.

Yip L, Dart RC, Gabow PA: Concepts and controversies in salicylate toxicity. Emerg Med Clin N Am 1994;12(2):351–364.

XVIII. STIMULANTS

A. General Considerations

1. This class of drugs includes amphetamines (e.g., methamphetamine, dexedrine), methylphenidate (Ritalin), and some decongestants and diet pills (e.g., phenylpropanolamine, phenylephrine, caffeine). The management of cocaine poisoning has been presented earlier in this chapter.

2. Overdose with these agents produces psychomotor agitation that may progress to a heat stroke-like syndrome with hypertension and other sympathomimetic effects.

3. Drugs in this class may be ingested, smoked, snorted, or injected, depending on the drug.

B. Clinical Presentation

1. The patient may be initially agitated, tremulous, flushed, perspiring, and delirious, with tachycardia, mydriasis, and hypertension. Hyperreflexia, muscular twitching, and vivid, threatening visual hallucinations are seen with higher doses. Dry mouth, nausea and vomiting, and abdominal cramps may occur.

2. With severe poisoning, seizures, severe hyperthermia, and coma may occur.

3. Complications may include CNS vasculitis producing a stroke-like syndrome; hemorrhagic and nonhemorrhagic cerebrovascular accidents; heat-stroke-like syndrome with coagulopathy, rhabdomyolysis, and the many complications related to injection drug use (endocarditis, hepatitis, HIV infection).

C. Management

1. As in all overdose situations, the initial management priority is *support of the patient's airway, breathing, circulation, and neurologic status* (see Standard Therapy of the Poisoned/Overdose Patient, IV. A, earlier in this chapter). Continuously monitor the cardiac rhythm and vital signs.

2. *Gastric emptying* for an acute ingestion should include lavage and administration of activated charcoal and a cathartic. Gastric emptying is not helpful when the stimulant has been administered parenterally. The possibility of coingestants (e.g., ethanol) is a consideration. Aggressive supportive care, as outlined below, takes priority over gastric emptying.

3. *Laboratory evaluation* should minimally include a CBC; electrolyte panel; glucose, BUN, and creatinine levels; ECG; and toxicologic screen.

4. *Supportive care:*
   a. Treat hyperactivity, agitation, and/or anxiety by placing the patient in a quiet room with minimal stimulation. A short-acting benzodiazepine (e.g., midazolam 2 mg given slowly IV, followed by 1 mg IV every 3-5 minutes as necessary) may be used for sedation. Alternative agents to consider include diazepam (5-10 mg given slowly IV), or in severe cases haloperidol (2-5 mg IV every 20 minutes as necessary).
   b. For seizures, manage the airway as necessary and administer diazepam (5-10 mg given slowly IV). For status epilepticus treat with diazepam followed by phenytoin (15-20 mg/kg IV no faster than 50 mg/min) and/or phenobarbital (20 mg/kg IV no faster than 100 mg/min) (see Chapter 20).
   c. Hyperthermia should be treated with external cooling: cooling blankets, tepid sponge baths, mist spray with electric fan convection. Core body temperature must be closely monitored. In severe cases, iced baths and intubation/muscle paralysis with pancuronium should be considered. Treatment with dantrolene (1-2 mg/kg IV every 6 hours; do not exceed 10 mg/kg/day; can cause hypotension and hepatotoxicity) may be beneficial but has been inadequately studied in this setting.
   d. Moderate to severe hypertension requires treatment. Drugs to consider include sodium nitroprusside (begin at 0.5 μg/kg/min IV) or phentolamine (5-mg bolus IV, followed

by a continuous infusion 0.2-0.5 mg/min). Isolated beta-blocker therapy (e.g., propranolol alone) should be avoided because of the theoretical risk of "unopposed" alpha-adrenergic activity and paradoxical worsening of hypertension.

e. Treat symptomatic ventricular ectopy or arrrhythmias per ACLS guidlines (see Chapter 13). Lidocaine may lower the seizure threshold. Some experts prefer beta-blocker therapy for symptomatic ventricular ectopy or ventricular tachycardia. Consider the short-acting agent esmolol (500 μg/kg IV load, followed by 50-100 μg/kg/min) and be prepared to add a vasodilator as outlined above if paradoxical hypertension occurs.

5. *Disposition:* patients must be managed and observed in the ED for *at least 1 hour after* symptoms/signs have completely resolved and vital signs have normalized. Once medically clear, psychosocial evaluation should be accomplished. Moderate to severe poisoning (e.g., persistent mental status changes, vital-sign abnormalities, rhabdomyolysis, other significant comorbid conditions) will require hospitalization, frequently to the ICU for continued definitive care.

BIBLIOGRAPHY

Aaron CK: Sympathomimetics. Emerg Med Clin N Am 1990;8:513–526.
Lake CR, Gallant S, et al: Adverse drug effects attributed to phenylpropanolamine: a review of 142 case reports. Am J Med 1990;89:195–208.

XIX. THEOPHYLLINE

A. General Considerations

1. Theophylline has been used since 1937 in the treatment of asthma and other chronic obstructive pulmonary diseases. Accidental poisonings may occur in children, and adults occasionally take deliberate overdoses.

2. The most common cause of toxicity in all age groups is iatrogenic, which occurs because of large individual differences in plasma clearance and serum $t_{1/2}$.

B. Pharmacodynamics

1. Various theophylline and derivative preparations vary widely in their equivalents of anhydrous theophylline and in their bioavailability (Table 23–29).

2. After absorption from the gut or IV administration, about 50% of theophylline is reversibly protein bound. Thereafter, the plasma theophylline concentration curve follows two phases: *rapid distribution* (30-45 minutes) and *slow elimination* ($t_{1/2}$ of 3-13 hours).

3. Hepatic microsomal enzymes determine 90% of theophyl-

Table 23-29. THEOPHYLLINE-CONTAINING PREPARATIONS

% Equivalents of
ANHYDROUS THEOPHYLLINE

100%	***Theophylline***
	Aerolate Primatene
	Bronkodyl Quibron
	Bronkotabs Slo-Phyllin
	Elixophyllin Theo-Dur
	Marax
79%	***Aminophylline (ethylenediamine theophylline)***
	Aminophylline
	Mudrane
60%	***Oxtriphylline (choline theophylline)***
	Choledyl
51%	***Theophylline sodium glycinate***
	Asbron G
48%	***Theophylline calcium salicylate***
	Quadrinal

Table 23-30. FACTORS AFFECTING THEOPHYLLINE PLASMA CLEARANCE AND SERUM HALF-LIFE

↓ Clearance/ ↑ $T_{1/2}$ (↓ Maintenance Dose Required)	↑ Clearance/ ↓ $T_{1/2}$ (↑ Maintenance Dose Required)
Premature neonates	Children
Liver disease	Smokers (tobacco, marijuana)
Congestive heart failure	High-protein–low-carbohydrate diets
Pulmonary disease	Charcoal-broiled foods
Obesity	Lithium carbonate
Dietary methylxanthines (tea, coffee)	Phenytoin
H_2 blockers (e.g., cimetidine, ranitidine)	Carbamazepine
Quinolone antibiotics (e.g., ciprofloxacin)	Rifampin
Oral contraceptives	
Beta blockers	
Allopurinol (high dose)	
Macrolide antibiotics (e.g., erythromycin, azithromycin, clarithromycin, clindamycin)	
? Thiabendazole	

line's clearance. Many factors are known to influence the clearance rate (Table 23–30).

4. At lower serum levels, a 1-mg/kg IV bolus will raise the serum level 2 µg/mL. At higher levels, hepatic enzymes become saturated; at levels >10 µg/mL, the same bolus will produce a greater rise in serum theophylline level.

5. Theophylline produces smooth-muscle relaxation and weak bronchodilation. It reduces pulmonary vascular resistance,

increasing perfusion of hypoventilated areas of lung early in the course of treatment. Like xanthine derivatives, it causes CNS stimulation (and lowers the seizure threshold), coronary vasodilatation, diuresis, and cardiac and skeletal muscle stimulation (including enhanced diaphragmatic contractility).

C. Clinical Presentation

Table 23–31 presents the toxicities of theophylline by serum level.

1. Signs and symptoms of early theophylline toxicity (nausea, vomiting, headache, tremor, sinus tachycardia) *do not* necessarily precede serious toxic effects. Patients may accumulate levels > 50 µg/mL without any signs or symptoms of toxicity and then suddenly develop seizures, serious arrhythmias, or cardiopulmonary arrest.

2. Alternatively, serious signs of toxicity may occur at serum levels 20-50 µg/mL (but not < 20 µg/mL). Monitoring serum levels is imperative!

3. Many oral theophylline preparations contain multiple other ingredients (e.g., ephedrine, barbiturates, hydroxyzine, and potassium iodide) that may contribute to toxicity and complicate the clinical picture.

4. Slow- or sustained-release preparations often are in a waxy matrix that continues to release theophylline and may form drug bezoars.

D. Management

1. As in all overdose situations, the initial management priority is *support of the patient's airway, breathing, circulation, and*

Table 23–31. SERUM THEOPHYLLINE LEVELS AND TOXICITY

SERUM LEVEL (µG/ML)	TOXICITY
0–5	No toxicity; little or no therapeutic effect
5–10	No toxicity; slight improvement in pulmonary symptoms/signs
10–20	Therapeutic window
15–25	*GI toxic effects:* nausea, vomiting, abdominal cramps, occasionally hematemesis
25–35	*CNS toxic effects:* headache, akathisia, agitation, tremor, delirium, hallucinations
35–50	*Cardiovascular toxic effects:* sinus tachycardia, hypertension, and arrhythmias (including supraventricular tachycardia, PVCs)
>50	*Serious/fatal toxic effects:* seizures, coma, cerebral edema, hypotension and shock, hyperthermia, severe cardiac arrhythmias (including ventricular tachycardia, ventricular fibrillation, and asystole) apnea, cardiopulmonary arrest

neurologic status (see Standard Therapy of the Poisoned/ Overdose Patient, IV. A, earlier in this chapter).

    a. Continuously monitor the patient's SaO_2 and cardiac rhythm; vital signs and neurologic status must be closely followed.

    b. Hypotension or shock should be treated with volume resuscitation. Vasopressors (e.g., dopamine) should be utilized if hypoperfusion/hypotension does not respond to fluid therapy.

    c. Manage seizures with airway control and diazepam, ± phenytoin, ± phenobarbital. The seizures caused by theophylline are notably resistant to conventional therapies and may only respond to rapid lowering of serum levels by hemoperfusion. General anesthesia with neuromuscular blockade may be needed to control seizure activity and prevent rhabdomyolysis (see Chapter 20).

2. *Gastric emptying* should include gastric lavage and administration of activated charcoal and a cathartic. Multiple-dose activated charcoal is effective at reducing theophylline blood levels ("GI dialysis") even in the setting of an iatrogenic *IV overdose.*

3. *Laboratory evaluation* should minimally include an ABG; ECG; CBC; electrolyte panel; glucose, BUN, and creatinine levels; urinalysis; and theophylline level. Repeat theophylline levels over time are mandatory.

4. *Enhanced elimination with charcoal hemoperfusion:*

    a. Hemoperfusion is indicated under any of the following circumstances:

       i. Serum levels ≥ 80 µg/mL after an acute ingestion, even when asymptomatic.

      ii. Serum levels ≥ 60 µg/mL after a chronic ingestion, even when asymptomatic.

     iii. Serum levels > 50 µg/mL complicated by serious signs or symptoms (e.g., seizures, arrhythmias).

     iv. Serum levels ≥ 40 µg/mL in patients < 6 months or > 60 years of age; or when the patient has concomitant significant cardiopulmonary disease.

    b. Peritoneal (1.3 mL/min) and hemodialysis (24.3 mL/min) clearances of theophylline are well below normal healthy adult clearance (about 50 mL/min) and hemoperfusion clearances (100-150 mL/min). Therefore, hemodialysis should be considered only when acute renal failure and severe acid–base, electrolyte, or volume disturbances complicate theophylline intoxication.

5. *Additional care:*

    a. Supraventricular arrhythmias should be managed according to ACLS guidelines. Meticulous management of hypoxia, acid–base status, and electrolyte abnormalities (e.g., hypokalemia) is mandatory. Adenosine, diltiazem, and verapamil are the drugs of choice. A beta blocker (e.g., propranolol, esmolol) may be used in the absence of active obstructive pulmonary disease. Avoid digoxin.

b. Ventricular tachyarrhythmias should also be managed according to ACLS guidelines. A beta blocker (e.g., propranolol, esmolol) may be used in the absence of active obstructive pulmonary disease. As above, meticulous management of hypoxia, acid–base status, and electrolyte abnormalities is crucial. Rapid lowering of serum theophylline levels with hemoperfusion is indicated.

6. *Disposition:* the theophylline level should be rechecked hourly. Appropriate monitoring and therapy (e.g., repeat doses of activated charcoal, electrolyte management) must be continued until the patient is completely stable and the theophylline level is reduced to < 20 μg/mL. At that time, psychosocial evaluation/disposition should be completed. The patient with moderate to severe signs and symptoms of toxicity, rising serum levels, or repeat levels ≥ 35 μg/mL should be admitted to a monitored bed for continued definitive care. ICU admission is frequently necessary.

BIBLIOGRAPHY

Heath A, Knudsen K: Role of extracorporeal drug removal in acute theophylline poisoning. A review. Med Toxicol Adverse Drug Exp 1987;2:294–308.

Paloucek FP, Rodvold KA: Evaluation of theophylline overdoses and toxicities. Ann Emerg Med 1988;17:135–144.

Sessler CN: Theophylline toxicity: clinical features of 116 consecutive cases. Am J Med 1990; 88:567–576.

INDEX

Note: Page numbers in *italics* refer to illustrations; page numbers followed by t refer to tables.

"ABCs," of emergency care, 3

Abdominal aortic aneurysm, abdominal pain in, 34t

Abdominal pain, 29–38
differential diagnosis of, 32, 34t–37t
disposition in, 32–33, 38
from gallstones, 546–547
history in, 30
laboratory studies for, 33t
physical examination in, 31–32
radiologic evaluation of, 33t
types of, 29

Abdominal radiograph(s), indications for, 11t

ABGs (arterial blood gases). See *Arterial blood gas(es) (ABGs)*.

Abortion, septic, 646
spontaneous, 644–646

Abruptio placenta, 647–648

ACE (angiotensin converting enzyme) inhibitor(s), for myocardial infarction, *262*, 268, 274t–275t

Acetaminophen, antidotes to, 875t
compounds containing, 886t
dosage of, 20
poisoning from, 862t, 885–890, 886t, *888–889*, 890t

Acetic acid(s), dosage of, 21t

N-Acetylcysteine, for acetaminophen poisoning, 887, 890

Acid-base disorder(s), 581–593
compensation for, 583–584, 585t
history in, 584–585
in salicylate poisoning, 952, *953*, 956t
laboratory studies in, 586
mixed, 590–592
physical examination in, 585–586
treatment of, 592

Acidosis, lactic, 588
metabolic. See *Metabolic acidosis*.
renal tubular, 587
respiratory, 582, 589

Acoustic neuroma, and vertigo, 83

Acquired immunodeficiency syndrome (AIDS), 359–383
aphthous ulcers in, 379
candidiasis in, 378–379
classification of, 360t
cryptococcal meningitis in, 373
definition of, 359
diarrhea in, 377–379, *381*, 382

Acquired immunodeficiency syndrome (AIDS) *(Continued)*
epidemiology of, 359
laboratory diagnosis of, 361
neurosyphilis in, 373, *375*
oral herpes simplex ulcers in, 376, 379
T-cell count in, 360t, 361, 364
toxoplasmosis in, 373, *375*
treatment of, 361–362
tuberculosis in, *524–525*
with central nervous system symptoms, 370–376
etiology of, 370
laboratory studies in, 371–372
management algorithm for, *374–375*
physical examination in, 370–371
treatment of, 372–373, *374–375*, 376
with gastrointestinal symptoms, 376–382
diagnostic approach to, 377–378
treatment of, 378–379, *380–381*, 382
with respiratory symptoms, 362–370
disposition in, 367, 370
history in, 363
laboratory studies in, 365t, 365–366
management algorithm for, *368–369*
physical examination in, 364
T-cell count in, 364
treatment of, 366–367, *368–369*

Acrodermatitis chronica atrophicans, 447

Activated charcoal, for poisoning, *877–878*, 879–880

Activity restriction(s), in mononucleosis, 467

Acute renal failure (ARF), 593–607
cardiac output in, 602
causes of, 594–596, 595t, 599–601
definition of, 593–594
disposition in, 605–606
epidemiology of, 597
hemodialysis for, 604–605
history in, 597–598
hyperkalemia in, 602–603
hypotension in, 602
hypovolemia in, 602
laboratory studies in, 598–599
life-threatening, 601–603
oliguric, conversion to nonoliguric, 604
physical examination in, 598
postrenal, 595t, 595–596, 601, 603
prerenal, 594–595, 595t, 599–600, 603–604

Acute respiratory distress syndrome (ARDS), in cyclic antidepressant poisoning, 923t, 925
in salicylate poisoning, 957t
Acute respiratory failure (ARF), 289–300
classification of, 290
definition of, 290
disposition in, 298–299
epidemiology of, 290–291
etiology of, 291, 292t, 293
history in, 293
laboratory studies in, 295–296
signs and symptoms of, 294–295
treatment of, 296, 297t, 298
Acute tubular necrosis (ATN), 600
Acyclovir, for genital herpes, 507–508, 508t
for herpes simplex ulcers, in acquired immunodeficiency syndrome, 379
Adenitis, mesenteric, abdominal pain in, 36t
Adenosine, for atrial fibrillation, 220, 222t
for paroxysmal supraventricular tachycardia, 229
for ventricular tachycardia, 236
in diagnosis of atrial flutter, 225
Adrenal crisis, 673–681
definition of, 673
differential diagnosis of, 677
disposition in, 680–681
epidemiology of, 673–674
history in, 674
laboratory studies in, 675–677
physical examination in, 675
signs and symptoms of, 674
treatment of, 677, 678–679, 680
Adrenal function study(ies), in adrenal insufficiency, 676
Adrenocorticotropic hormone (ACTH) stimulation test, 676–677
AIDS (acquired immunodeficiency syndrome). See Acquired immunodeficiency syndrome (AIDS).
Airway, esophageal obturator, 149, 150
nasopharyngeal, 143–144, 144
primary survey of, 7
upper, components of, 139–140
Airway management, in cardiorespiratory arrest, 146
intubation for, 151–163. See also Intubation.
nasopharyngeal airway for, 143–144, 144
oropharyngeal airway for, 144, 144–145
oxygen for, 146, 147t–148t, 148
patient monitoring for, 148
prehospital devices for, 148–149, 150
rescue breathing for, 145–146
surgical, 163–166
Airway obstruction, by foreign bodies, 141–142
causes of, 141
positioning in, 142
signs and symptoms of, 140–141

Albumin, with paracentesis, for ascites, 571
Albuterol, for anaphylactic shock, 175
for asthma, 303, 304t, 306
for chronic obstructive pulmonary disease, 320, 324t
for hyperkalemia, 624
Alcohol, for ethylene glycol poisoning, 935
for methanol poisoning, 959
isopropyl, poisoning from, 935–937
poisoning from, 863t, 929–933
Alcohol ketoacidosis, 930
Alcohol withdrawal, 932t, 932–933
Alkaline diuresis, for barbiturate poisoning, 904
for poisoning, 873, 881
Alkalinization therapy, for cyclic antidepressant poisoning, 919
for salicylate poisoning, 955
Alkalosis, in ventricular fibrillation, 202
metabolic, 582, 589–590, 626
respiratory, 582, 590
Allergic reaction(s), to red blood cell transfusion, 818
Allergic vulvovaginitis, 669
Alloimmunization, 818
Alteplase (tissue plasminogen activator, t-PA), for myocardial infarction, 264–266, 273t
Altovaquone, for Pneumocystis carinii pneumonia, 367
Alveolar hypoventilation, and acute respiratory failure, 291
Amikacin, for pneumonia, 499t
Aminoglycoside(s), for septic shock, 192
Aminophylline, for anaphylactic shock, 175
for asthma, 304t, 307
for chronic obstructive pulmonary disease, 321, 324t
for pulmonary edema, 243
Amitriptyline, for headache, 123t
Amoxicillin, for asthma, 305t
for chronic obstructive pulmonary disease, 325t, 326
for Lyme disease, 449t
for otitis media, 471t
for pneumonia, 498t
for sinusitis, 518t
for vaginosis, 670
Amoxicillin/clavulanate (Augmentin), for animal bites, 390t
for cellulitis, 401t–402t
for otitis media, 471t
for sinusitis, 518t
Amphetamine(s), poisoning from, 862t, 958–960
Amphotericin B, for cryptococcal meningitis, 373
Ampicillin, for diarrhea, 79t
for gallbladder disease, 551
for pneumonia, 498t
for septic shock, 193
for urinary tract infection, 536t
Ampicillin/sulbactam (Unasyn), for cellulitis, 401t–402t

Ampicillin/sulbactam (Unasyn), for cellulitis *(Continued)*
for gallbladder disease, 551
for pancreatitis, 579
Amrinone, for cardiogenic shock, 181
for pulmonary edema, *242*, 243
Amylase level(s), in evaluation of abdominal pain, 33t
in pancreatitis, 575
Analgesic(s), for animal bites, 388
for gallbladder disease, 551
for low back pain, 53–54
for nephrolithiasis, 633
for pancreatitis, 579
for pelvic inflammatory disease, 663–664
for sickle cell crisis, 802
Anaphylactic shock, 171–177. See also
Shock, anaphylactic.
Anaphylaxis, mediators of, 171
Anemia, 788–797
aplastic, 795
definition of, 788
differential diagnosis of, 791–792
disposition in, 795–796
etiology of, 788–789
hemolytic, 795
history in, 789
iron deficiency, 793–794
laboratory studies in, 789–791
physical examination in, 789
signs and symptoms of, 789
treatment of, 792–795
with chronic disease, 794–795
with folic acid deficiency, 794
with vitamin B_{12} deficiency, 794
Anesthesia, for intubation, 158
topical, for nasotracheal intubation,
161–162
translaryngeal, for nasotracheal intubation, 162
Anesthetic(s), for rapid-sequence intubation, 154t
Aneurysm(s), and subarachnoid hemorrhage, 779
aortic, abdominal, pain in, 34t
Aneurysmectomy, for subarachnoid hemorrhage, 786, 786t
Angina, chest pain in, 58t
electrocardiography in, 66–67
unstable, management of, 70
Angiography, coronary artery, in myocardial infarction, 257
in pulmonary embolism, 342
in stroke, 757
Angioplasty, coronary, vs. thrombolytic
therapy, for myocardial infarction,
266–267
Angiotensin converting enzyme (ACE) in-
hibitor(s), for myocardial infarction,
262, 268, 274t–275t
Animal bite(s), 383–393
analgesia for, 388
antimicrobial therapy for, 389–391, 390t
cellulitis from, 401t

Animal bite(s) *(Continued)*
complications of, 386–387
debridement of, 389
disposition in, 392–393
epidemiology of, 384t, 384–387
history in, 387
laboratory studies in, 387–388
local anesthesia for, 388–389
organisms in, 384, 386t
physical examination in, 387
tetanus immunization for, 391
wound care for, 388–389
Anion gap, 583
in mixed acid-base disorders, 591
Anion gap metabolic acidosis, 587–588
and hypokalemia, 626
in diabetic ketoacidosis, 689
Anistreplase (APSAC), for myocardial infarction, 264, 273t
Ankle(s), arthrocentesis of, 839, *839*
Ankylosing spondylitis, 848–850
Antiarrhythmic agent(s), 227t
Antibiotic(s), for animal bites, 390t,
390–391
for asthma, 305t
for chronic obstructive pulmonary disease, 325t, 326
for diarrhea, 78, 79t–80t
for encephalitis, 457, 460, 460t
for food-borne disease, 422
for gallbladder disease, 551
for infectious hemoptysis, 333
for meningitis, 457, 460, 460t
for pancreatitis, 579
for pelvic inflammatory disease, 663,
664t
for pneumonia, 494t–495t, 497,
498t–499t
for respiratory symptoms in acquired immunodeficiency syndrome, 366–367,
369
for septic shock, 192–193
for sinusitis, 517
intravenous, for disseminated gonococcal
arthritis, 843
for nongonococcal septic arthritis, 842
Antibody(ies), monoclonal antiendotoxin,
for septic shock, 193
Anticholinergic agent(s), antidotes to, 875t
for asthma, 305t
for chronic obstructive pulmonary disease, 324t
poisoning from, 862t, 891t, 891–894,
893t
Anticoagulation, for deep venous thrombosis, with pulmonary embolism, 343
for stroke, 763
for superior vena cava syndrome, 832
for transient ischemic attack, 762
Anticonvulsant(s), 773, 774t–775t, 776
for subarachnoid hemorrhage, 784
poisoning from, 894–900, 895t
Antidepressant(s), cyclic. See *Cyclic anti-
depressant(s).*

Antidiarrheal agent(s), for food-borne disease, 422
Antidote(s), in poisoning, 874, 875t
Antiemetic(s), for food-borne disease, 422
  for nephrolithiasis, 633, 636
  for sickle cell crisis, 802
Antifibrinolytic agent(s), for subarachnoid hemorrhage, 784, 786
Antihistamine(s), for anaphylactic shock, 175
  for sinusitis, 519t
Antimotility agent(s), for diarrhea, in acquired immunodeficiency syndrome, 382
Antimycotic(s), azole, for vaginitis, 672
Antiplatelet therapy, for transient ischemic attack, 761
Antipseudomonal penicillin(s), for septic shock, 192–193
Antipsychotic agent(s), poisoning from, 900t, 900–903, 903t
Antitoxin, for botulism, 395
Aortic aneurysm(s), abdominal, pain in, 34t
Aortic dissection, chest pain in, 60t
  electrocardiography in, 67–68
  management of, 70
  thoracic, 283–289. See also *Thoracic aortic dissection.*
Aortic insufficiency, chest pain in, 60t
Aortic stenosis, chest pain in, 59t
Aortography, in thoracic aortic dissection, 286
Aphthous ulcer(s), in acquired immunodeficiency syndrome, 379
Aplastic anemia, 795
Aplastic crisis, in sickle cell disease, 799
Apneuristic respiration, 737
Appendicitis, 540–545
  abdominal pain in, 35t, 36t
  differential diagnosis of, 542, 543t
  disposition in, 544
  history in, 541
  laboratory studies in, 542
  physical examination in, 541t, 541–542
  treatment of, 543
APSAC (anistreplase), for myocardial infarction, 264, 273t
ARDS (acute respiratory distress syndrome). See *Acute respiratory distress syndrome (ARDS).*
ARF (acute renal failure). See *Acute renal failure (ARF).*
ARF (acute respiratory failure). See *Acute respiratory failure (ARF).*
Arrhythmia(s), 210–238. See also specific type(s).
  disposition in, 212
  evaluation of, 210–211
  history in, 211
  in cyclic antidepressant poisoning, 923t–924t
  in digitalis poisoning, 927, 929
  in monoamine oxidase inhibitor poisoning, 945

Arrhythmia(s) *(Continued)*
  in myocardial infarction, *262*
  in shock, 168
  laboratory studies in, 211
  treatment of, 211–212, 227t
  unstable, 7
Arsenic, poisoning from, 862t
Arterial blood gas(es) (ABGs), in acquired immunodeficiency syndrome, with respiratory symptoms, 366
  in acute respiratory failure, 295
  in asthma, 302–303
  in chronic obstructive pulmonary disease, 319
  in pulmonary embolism, 340–341
  in spontaneous pneumothorax, 353
  indications for, 11t
Arteriovenous malformation(s) (AVMs), and subarachnoid hemorrhage, 779
Arteritis, giant cell, 858–859
  temporal, 858–859
    headache in, 112t
Arthritis, crystal-associated, 846–848
  episodic, 836t
  from infective endocarditis, 843–845
  history in, 834–836, 835t–836t
  in Lyme disease, 446, 449–450, 845
  infectious, 840–845
    disseminated gonococcal, 842–843
    nongonococcal, 840–842
  migratory, 836t
  physical examination in, 836–837
  psoriatic, 851–852
  reactive, 850–851
  rheumatoid, 852–854
  synovial fluid analysis in, 837–840, *838–839*, 840t
Arthrocentesis, 837–840, *838–839*, 840t
  for nongonococcal septic arthritis, 841–842
  in pseudogout, 848
Ascites, definition of, 562
  differential diagnosis of, 567–568
  treatment of, 570–571
Aspiration, in cyclic antidepressant poisoning, 923t
Aspirin, dosage of, 20.21t
  for myocardial infarction, 273t
  for pericarditis, 281
  for transient ischemic attack, 761
Asthma, 300–315
  adjunctive therapy for, *310–311*
  definition of, 300
  differential diagnosis of, 303
  disposition in, 314–315
  epidemiology of, 300
  exacerbating factors in, 300–301
  first-line therapy for, 303, 305t–306t, 306–307
  history in, 301
  laboratory studies in, 302–303
  monitoring in, 302
  physical examination in, 301–302
  pulmonary function tests in, 302

Asthma *(Continued)*
  second-line therapy for, 307
  signs and symptoms of, 301
  third-line therapy for, 307, *309*, 312
Asystole, 204–206, *205*
  in cyclic antidepressant poisoning, 924t
Ataxic respiration, 737
Atenolol, for alcohol withdrawal, 933
  for myocardial infarction, 268, 274t
ATN (acute tubular necrosis), 600
Atrial fibrillation, 217–219, 223
  beta blockers for, 219, 222t–223t
  bretylium for, *221*
  calcium channel blockers for, 218–219, *220*, 222t
  definition of, 217
  differential diagnosis of, 218
  digoxin for, 219, 222t
  diltiazem for, 222t
  esmolol for, 223t
  etiology of, 218
  lidocaine for, *220–221*
  metoprolol for, 223t
  procainamide for, *220–221*
  propranolol for, 222t
  synchronized cardioversion for, 218, 219t
  treatment of, 218–219, 219t, *220–221*, 222t–223t, 223
Atrial flutter, 223–227, 225t, 227t
  adenosine for, 225
  beta blockers for, 226
  calcium channel blockers for, 226
  definition of, 223–224
  diagnostic maneuvers for, 224–226, 225t
  differential diagnosis of, 224
  digoxin for, 226
  diltiazem for, 226
  esmolol for, 226
  etiology of, 224
  propranolol for, 226
  treatment of, 222t–223t, 226–227, 227t
  verapamil for, 226
Atrial tachycardia, multifocal, 230–231
  paroxysmal, 229–230
Atrioventricular block, 231–233
  in cyclic antidepressant poisoning, 923t
Atrophic vaginitis, 669
Atropine, for asystole, *205*
  for chronic obstructive pulmonary disease, 324t
  for myocardial infarction, *262*, 270, 275t
  for sinus bradycardia, 214, *215*, 216t
  for ventricular fibrillation, 202t
AVM(s) (arteriovenous malformations), and subarachnoid hemorrhage, 779
Azithromycin, for chronic obstructive pulmonary disease, 325t, 326
  for pneumonia, 498t
  for sinusitis, 518t
  for urinary tract infection, 537t
Azole antimycotic(s), for vaginitis, 672
AZT (zidovudine), for acquired immunodeficiency syndrome, 361
Aztreonam, for urinary tract infection, 538t

Back pain. See *Low back pain.*
Bacteremia, definition of, 189
Bacterial meningitis. See *Meningitis.*
Bacterial pericarditis, 278
Bacterial peritonitis, spontaneous. See *Spontaneous bacterial peritonitis (SBP).*
Bacterial pneumonia, causative organisms in, 486t
Bacterial vaginitis, 666–667
Bacterial vaginosis, 670, 671t
Balloon pump, intra-aortic, for myocardial infarction, 275
Balloon tamponade, for gastrointestinal bleeding, 560
Barbiturate(s), poisoning from, 862t, 904t, 904–906
Bedside spirometry, in chronic obstructive pulmonary disease, 319
Benign positional vertigo, 85
Benzodiazepine(s), antidotes to, 875t
  for alcohol withdrawal, 932t
  for asthma, 305t, *311*
  for seizures, *771*, 772
    from poisoning, 869
    in acquired immunodeficiency syndrome, 373
    in coma, 749
  poisoning from, 906t, 906–908
Benzodiazepine antagonist(s), dosage of, 27
Beta agonist(s), for asthma, 303, 304t, 306, 307, *308*, *309*
  for chronic obstructive pulmonary disease, 320, *322*, 324t
Beta blocker(s), antidotes to, 875t
  for atrial fibrillation, 219, 222t–223t
  for atrial flutter, 226
  for headache, 122t
  for myocardial infarction, *262*, 267–268
  for sinus tachycardia, 217
  for thoracic aortic dissection, 287–288
  poisoning from, 862t
Beta-human chorionic gonadotropin (hCG), in ectopic pregnancy, 653–654
Bicarbonate. See *Sodium bicarbonate.*
Biliary colic, abdominal pain in, 34t
  definition of, 545
Biliary tract stone(s). See *Gallstone(s).*
Bilirubin level(s), in pancreatitis, 575
Bite(s). See *Animal bite(s).*
Bleeding. See specific type(s).
Bleeding disorder(s), 805–813
  definition of, 805
  differential diagnosis of, 809–810
  disposition in, 812–813
  epidemiology of, 805–806
  history in, 806
  laboratory studies in, 807–809, 808t
  physical examination in, 807
  signs and symptoms of, 806–807
  treatment of, 810–812
Blood component(s), transfusion of, 814–822. See also specific blood component(s).

Blood culture(s), in infective endocarditis, 406–407
Blood ethanol level(s), indications for, 11t
Blood gas(es), arterial. See *Arterial blood gas(es) (ABGs)*.
Blood urea nitrogen (BUN), elevated, non-renal causes of, 607
in acute renal failure, 594
in evaluation of abdominal pain, 33t
"Blue bloater," 318
"Body packing," 917
Bone marrow, inadequate erythrocyte production in, 792
Bone scan, in epidural spinal cord compression, 825
Botulism, 393–396, 862t
Bradycardia, sinus, 213–214, *215*, 216t
Breakthrough bleeding, from oral contraceptives, 650
Bretylium, for arrhythmias, 227t
for atrial fibrillation, *221*
for ventricular fibrillation, *201*, 202t
for ventricular tachycardia, 236
Bronchodilator(s), for anaphylactic shock, 175
Bronchoscopy, for hemoptysis, 335
BUN (blood urea nitrogen). See *Blood urea nitrogen (BUN)*.
Butoconazole (Femstat), for vulvovaginal candidiasis, 671t
Butorphanol (Stadol), dosage of, 25t

C1-C2 subluxation, in rheumatoid arthritis, 853–854
Calcitonin, for hypercalcemia, 610–611
Calcium apatite crystal(s), 629
Calcium channel antagonist(s), for migraine, 117
Calcium channel blocker(s), antidotes to, 875t
for atrial fibrillation, 218–219, *220*, 222t
for atrial flutter, 226
for headache, 123t, 124t
poisoning from, 908t, 908–910
Calcium chloride, for calcium channel blocker poisoning, 910
for hyperkalemia, in acute renal failure, 602
Calcium disodium edetate, for chelation therapy, 882
Calcium gluconate, for hyperkalemia, 623
for hypocalcemia, 614
Calcium oxalate crystal(s), 629
Calcium phosphate crystal(s), 629
Calcium pyrophosphate gout, 847–848
Calculus (calculi), renal. See *Nephrolithiasis*.
Caloric testing, limited, 90–91
Cancer, epidural spinal cord compression from, 822–827
Candidiasis, oral, in acquired immunodeficiency syndrome, 378–379
vulvovaginal, 667, 667t, 671t
Cannula(s), nasal, for oxygen delivery, 147t

Capnocytophaga caninoris, from animal bites, 384
Captopril, for hypertensive urgency, 251t
for myocardial infarction, 260t
Carbamazepine (Tegretol), for seizures, 774t
poisoning from, 896–898
Carbon dioxide detector(s), colorimetric end-tidal, 152
Carbon monoxide poisoning, 862t, 910–913, 912t
Carboxylic acid(s), dosage of, 21t
Cardiac arrest, 198–209
complications of, 197
definition of, 194–195
etiology of, 195, 195t
from asystole, 204–206, *205*
from pulseless electrical activity, 206, *207–208*
from ventricular fibrillation, 197–200, *200*, 200t, 202–203. See also *Ventricular fibrillation*.
postresuscitative care in, 206–209, 209t
treatment of, 195–197
Cardiac arrhythmia(s), 210–238. See also *Arrhythmia(s)*.
Cardiac catheterization, with coronary artery angiography, in myocardial infarction, 257
Cardiac disease, dyspnea in, 98t
Cardiac enzyme(s), in chest pain, 68
in myocardial infarction, 257
Cardiac massage, for hypovolemic shock, 188
Cardiac output, in acute renal failure, 602
Cardiac tamponade, in cardiogenic shock, treatment of, 183
with pericarditis, 282
Cardiogenic shock, 177–184. See also *Shock, cardiogenic*.
Cardiopulmonary resuscitation (CPR), 196
Cardiorespiratory arrest, airway management in, 146
Cardiovascular hypertensive emergency, 246, 250t
Cardiovascular triad, in shock, 168–169
Carotid artery Doppler ultrasonography, in stroke, 757
Carotid endarterectomy, for transient ischemic attack, 762
Carotid sinus massage, in evaluation of syncope, 133
in evaluation of vertigo, 90
Cat bite(s), 385
Catecholamine crisis, 246, 250t
Cauda equina syndrome, 825, 850
Cavernous sinus thrombophlebitis, 517
CBC (complete blood count). See *Complete blood count (CBC)*.
Cefazolin, for cellulitis, 401t
Cefotetan, for gallbladder disease, 551
Cefoxitin, for septic shock, 192
Ceftriaxone, for cellulitis, 401t
for chlamydia, 503t

Ceftriaxone *(Continued)*
  for diarrhea, 79t
  for gonorrhea, 503t
  for Lyme disease, 449t
Cefuroxime, for animal bites, 390t
  for asthma, 305t
  for cellulitis, 401t
  for chronic obstructive pulmonary disease, 325t
  for otitis media, 471t
Cellulitis, 396–398, *399*, 400, 401t–402t
  orbital, 397, 517
Central nervous system (CNS) hypertensive emergency, 246, 250t
Central venous catheterization, in shock, 170
Cephalexin, for animal bites, 390t
Cephalosporin(s), for encephalitis, 460t
  for epiglottitis, 414
  for meningitis, 460t
  for pelvic inflammatory disease, 664t
  for pneumonia, 498t
  for septic shock, 192
  for urinary tract infection, 536t–538t
Cerebellar hemorrhage/infarction, and vertigo, 83
Cerebral embolism, 759t–760t
Cerebral hemorrhage, 759t–760t
Cerebral thrombosis, 759t–760t
Cerebrovascular accident (CVA). See *Stroke.*
Cervical carcinoma, 649
Cervical polyp(s), 648
Cervicitis, mucopurulent, 501–503
Charcoal, activated, for poisoning, *877–878*, 879–880
Chart(s), documentation in, 16–19
Chelation therapy, for poisoning, *873*, 882–883
Chemical pleurodesis, for spontaneous pneumothorax, 356
Chemotherapy, for superior vena cava syndrome, 831
Chest pain, 56–72
  cardiac enzymes in, 68
  definition of, 56
  disposition in, 72
  echocardiography in, 68
  electrocardiography in, 66–67
  etiology of, 56, 57t–63t
  gastrointestinal studies in, 68–69
  history in, 57, 64–65
  in myocardial infarction, 58t, 253
  management of, 69–71
  physical examination in, 65–66
  radiography in, 67–68
  ventilation/perfusion scan in, 68
Chest radiograph(s), indications for, 11t
Chest wall, disease of, dyspnea in, 98t
Cheyne-Stokes respiration, 737
CHF (congestive heart failure). See *Congestive heart failure (CHF).*
Chlamydia, 501–506, 503t
  cultures for, 107

Chlamydia, extragenital, 505
Chlamydial pneumonia, 489t
Chloramphenicol, for cellulitis, 401t
  for diarrhea, 79t
Chlorpheniramine (Chlor-Trimaton), for sinusitis, 519t
Chlorpromazine (Thorazine), for headache, 120t
Cholangitis, abdominal pain in, 34t
  definition of, 546
  history in, 547
  treatment of, 552
Cholecystitis, abdominal pain in, 34t
  chest pain in, 63t
  complications of, 546
  definition of, 545
  history in, 547
  treatment of, 552
Choledocholithiasis, definition of, 545
Cholesterol level(s), in stroke, 757
Choline magnesium trisalicylate (Trilisate), dosage of, 21t
Chronic obstructive pulmonary disease (COPD), 316–328
  adjunctive therapy for, 326
  definition of, 316
  differential diagnosis of, 319
  disposition in, 327–328
  epidemiology of, 316–317
  exacerbating factors in, 317
  first-line therapy for, 319–320, *322*, 324t–325t
  history in, 317
  laboratory studies in, 319
  monitoring in, 318–319
  physical examination in, 318
  risk factors for, 317
  second-line therapy for, 320–321, *323*, 324t
  signs and symptoms of, 317–318
  third-line therapy for, 321, *323*, 324t, 325–326
Ciprofloxacin, for cellulitis, 401t
  for diarrhea, 79t–80t
    in acquired immunodeficiency syndrome, 379
  for otitis media, 471t
  for pneumonia, 499t
  for urinary tract infection, 536t–538t
Cirrhosis, definition of, 562
Clarithromycin, for pneumonia, 498t
  for sinusitis, 518t
Clindamycin, for pelvic inflammatory disease, 664t
  for pneumonia, 499t
  for vaginosis, 670, 671t
Clonazepam, for seizures, 775t
Clonidine, for hypertensive urgency, 251t
  for opioid withdrawal, 949–950
  poisoning from, 862t
Clotrimazole (Gyne-lotrimin, Mycelex), for vulvovaginal candidiasis, 671t
Cluster headache, 111t
  treatment of, 124t, 125, 126t

CNS (central nervous system) hypertensive emergency, 246, 250t
Coagulation factor disorder(s), 810–812
Coagulopathy, in salicylate poisoning, 957–958
COBRA (Consolidated Omnibus Budget Reconciliation Act), criteria for patient transfer, 15–16
Cocaine, poisoning from, 862t, 913–918, 915t–916t
Codeine, dosage of, 24t
Colchicine, for gout, 847
Colic, biliary, abdominal pain in, 34t
  definition of, 545
Colorimetric end-tidal carbon dioxide detector(s), 152
Coma, 734–752
  clinical course of, 740–741, 741t
  control of seizures in, 749
  definition of, 734
  differential diagnosis of, 744–745
  drug screens in, 742
  etiology of, 734, 735t
  history in, 734–735
  hyperglycemic hyperosmolar, 699–707. See also *Hyperglycemic hyperosmolar coma (HHC).*
  hyperthermia in, 749–750
  hypothermia in, 749
  infection in, 751
  intracranial pressure in, 750–751
  laboratory studies in, 741–744
  motor responses in, 740, 741t
  myxedema, 714–723. See also *Myxedema coma.*
  neurologic examination in, 737t, 737–740
  physical examination in, 736–737
  respiration in, 737
  symptoms associated with, 736
  treatment of, 745–751, *746–747*
    in cyclic antidepressant poisoning, 922t
Complete blood count (CBC), in sickle cell disease, 800
  indications for, 12t
Computed tomography (CT), contrast-enhanced, in pancreatitis, 576–577
  in acquired immunodeficiency syndrome with central nervous system symptoms, 372
  in coma, 742–743
  in epidural spinal cord compression, 825
  in headache, 114
  in stroke, 756
  in subarachnoid hemorrhage, 782
  in thoracic aortic dissection, 286
Congestive heart failure (CHF), 238–245
  clinical features of, 239–240
  definition of, 238
  differential diagnosis of, 240
  disposition in, 244–245
  etiology of, 238–239

Congestive heart failure (CHF) *(Continued)*
  gradual-onset, 244
  laboratory studies in, 240
  treatment of, 240–244, 241t, *242*
    with pulmonary edema, 241–244, *242*
    without pulmonary edema, 244
Conjunctivitis, gonococcal, 504
Conscious sedation-analgesia, 26–28
Consolidated Omnibus Budget Reconciliation Act (COBRA), criteria for patient transfer, 15–16
Consultation, 10, 13–14
Continuous positive airway pressure (CPAP), 147t
Contraceptive(s), breakthrough bleeding from, 650
Contrast venography, in deep venous thrombosis, 339
Contrast-enhanced computed tomography, in pancreatitis, 576–577
COPD (chronic obstructive pulmonary disease), 316–328. See also *Chronic obstructive pulmonary disease (COPD).*
Corneal response(s), in coma, 738
Coronary angioplasty, vs. thrombolytic therapy, for myocardial infarction, 266–267
Coronary artery angiography, in myocardial infarction, 257
Corticosteroid(s), for anaphylactic shock, 176
  for asthma, 304t, 306, *308*
  for chronic obstructive pulmonary disease, 320–321, *323*, 324t
  for epidural spinal cord compression, 826
  for gout, 847
  for *Pneumocystis carinii* pneumonia, 367, *369*
  for septic shock, 193
  for sinusitis, 517, 519t
  for status migrainosis, 125
  intra-articular, for osteoarthritis, 858
CPAP (continuous positive airway pressure), 147t
CPR (cardiopulmonary resuscitation), 196
Creatinine, elevated, nonrenal causes of, 607
  in evaluation of abdominal pain, 33t
Cricothyrotomy, 165–166
  needle, 163–165
Critically ill patient(s), laboratory studies in, 10, 11t–13t
Crossmatching, for red blood cell transfusion, 814–815
Crotamiton (Eurax), for scabies, 474t
Cryoprecipitate, transfusion of, 821
Cryptococcal meningitis, in acquired immunodeficiency syndrome, 373
Crystal-associated arthritis, 846–848
Crystalloid(s), for acute renal failure, 602
  for nephrolithiasis, 633
  for septic shock, 192
  restriction of, in hypovolemic shock, 188

CT (computed tomography). See *Computed tomography (CT)*.

Culdocentesis, in ectopic pregnancy, 655, 655t

CVA (cerebrovascular accident). See *Stroke*.

Cyanide, antidotes to, 875t

Cyanosis, 140

Cyclic antidepressant(s), antidotes to, 875t
  for headache, 123t
  poisoning from, 862t, 918–925, 920t, 922t–924t

Cyproheptadine, for headache, 123t

Cyst(s), ovarian, ruptured, abdominal pain in, 37t

Cystine crystal(s), 630

Cystitis, clinical evaluation in, 534–535
  etiology of, 533
  laboratory studies in, 535
  treatment of, 536t–538t

Dantrolene, for hyperthermia, in coma, 750

Dapsone, for *Pneumocystis carinii* pneumonia, 367

DDAVP
  (1-desamino-8-D-arginine-vasopressin), for von Willebrand's disease, 811

DDC (dideoxycytidine, zalcitabine), for acquired immunodeficiency syndrome, 362

DDI (didanosine), for acquired immunodeficiency syndrome, 361

DeBakey system, for classification of thoracic aortic dissection, 283, *284*

Decadron, for increased intracranial pressure, 750

Deep tendon reflex(es), in stroke, 755

Deep venous thrombosis (DVT), with pulmonary embolism, 337–350
  arterial blood gases in, 340–341
  contrast venography in, 339
  definition of, 337–338
  differential diagnosis of, 342
  disposition in, 349
  electrocardiography in, 341
  epidemiology of, 338
  history in, 338
  impedance plethysmography in, 340
  inferior vena cava barriers for, 348–349
  laboratory studies in, 342
  pulmonary angiography in, 342
  pulmonary scintigraphy in, 341, 341t
  radioiodinated fibrinogen in, 340
  risk factors for, 338, 339t
  signs and symptoms of, 338–339, 340t
  surgical embolectomy for, 349
  treatment of, 342–343, *344–347*, 348–349
  ultrasonography in, 339–340
  ventilation-perfusion scanning in, 341, 341t

Defasciculation, in orotracheal intubation, 157

Definitive care, 4, 10, 13–14

1-Desamino-8-D-arginine-vasopressin (DDAVP), for von Willebrand's disease, 811

Desferoxamine mesylate, for chelation therapy, 882–883

Dexamethasone, for adrenal crisis, *679*, 680
  for asthma, 304t, 307
  for epidural spinal cord compression, 826
  for headache, 120t, 126t
  for stroke, 764
  for subarachnoid hemorrhage, 784
  for thyroid storm, *730*, 732

DHE (dihydroergotamine), for headache, 120t, 125, 126t

Diabetes mellitus, definition of, 682

Diabetic ketoacidosis, abdominal pain in, 34t
  anion gap metabolic acidosis in, 689
  differential diagnosis of, 690

Diabetic ketoacidosis (DKA), 687–699
  definition of, 687
  disposition in, 697–698
  epidemiology of, 687–688
  history in, 688
  laboratory studies in, 689
  physical examination in, 688
  signs and symptoms of, 688
  treatment of, 690–691, *692–695*, 696–697, 699

Dialysis. See *Hemodialysis*.

Diaphoresis, in airway obstruction, 140

Diarrhea, 73–81
  antibiotics for, 78, 79t–80t
  differential diagnosis of, 75, 76t–77t
  disposition in, 79, 81
  history in, 73–74
  infectious, 76t
    in acquired immunodeficiency syndrome, 377–379, *381*, 382
  laboratory studies in, 75
  medications associated with, 75t
  osmotic, 76t
  physical examination in, 74
  radiologic evaluation of, 75
  rehydration solutions for, 78
  secretory, 76t
  treatment of, 78, 79t–80t

Diazepam (Valium), for asthma, 305t
  for seizures, *771*, 772
    in coma, 749
  for vertigo, 93

Diazoxide, for hypertensive emergency, 249t

Diclofenac sodium (Voltaren), dosage of, 21t

Dicloxacillin, for animal bites, 390t
  for cellulitis, 401t

Didanosine (DDI), for acquired immunodeficiency syndrome, 361

Dideoxycytidine (zalcitabine, DDC), for acquired immunodeficiency syndrome, 362
Diffusion limitation, and acute respiratory failure, 293
Diflunisal (Dolobid), dosage of, 21t
   for headache, 122t
Digitalis, antidotes to, 875t
   poisoning from, 863t, 926–929
Digoxin, for atrial fibrillation, 219, 222t
   for atrial flutter, 226
   for pulmonary edema, *242*, 243
   for torsades de pointes, 237t
Dihydroergotamine (DHE), for headache, 120t, 125, 126t
Diltiazem, for atrial fibrillation, 222t
   for atrial flutter, 226
   for paroxysmal supraventricular tachycardia, 229
Dimenhydrinate (Dramamine), for vertigo, 94
Dimercaprol, for chelation therapy, 882
Diphenhydramine (Benadryl), for anaphylactic shock, 175
   for sinusitis, 519t
Disability(ies), primary survey of, 8
Disc herniation, 47
Discharge, to home, criteria for, 14–15
Discharge instruction(s), documentation of, 18
Disequilibrium, 86
Disposition, 4, 14–16
Disseminated gonococcal arthritis, 842–843
Disulfiram, poisoning from, 863t
Diuresis, alkaline, for barbiturate poisoning, 904
   for poisoning, *873*, 881
Diuretic(s), for chronic obstructive pulmonary disease, 325t, 326
   for hyperkalemia, 624
Diverticulitis, abdominal pain in, 36t
Dix-Hallpike maneuver, 90, *91*
Dizziness, 82–95
   causes of, 82–86
   definition of, 82
DKA (diabetic ketoacidosis). See *Diabetic ketoacidosis (DKA).*
Dobutamine, for cardiogenic shock, 181
   for myocardial infarction, 261t
   for pulmonary edema, *242*, 243
   postresuscitative, after cardiac arrest, 208
Documentation, 16–19
   of discharge instructions, 18
   of vital signs, 17
Dog bite(s), 385
Doll's head response, 738, *739*, 740, 741t
Done nomogram, for salicylate poisoning, 952, *954*
Dopamine, for acute renal failure, 604
   for cardiogenic shock, 180
   for myocardial infarction, 261t
   for poisoning, 868
   for pulmonary edema, *242*

Dopamine *(Continued)*
   for septic shock, 192
      for sinus bradycardia, 214, *215*, 216t
      postresuscitative, after cardiac arrest, 208
Doppler ultrasonography, carotid artery, in stroke, 757
   in deep venous thrombosis, 339
Doxycycline, for animal bites, 390t
   for chlamydia, 503t
   for chronic obstructive pulmonary disease, 325t, 326
   for gonorrhea, 503t
   for Lyme disease, 448, 449t
   for pelvic inflammatory disease, 664t
   for pneumonia, 498t
   for syphilis, 511
   for urinary tract infection, 537t
Drug screen(s), 866–867
   in coma, 742
Duodenal ulcer(s), abdominal pain in, 35t
   perforated, chest pain in, 63t
DVT (deep venous thrombosis). See *Deep venous thrombosis (DVT).*
Dyspepsia, abdominal pain in, 35t
Dyspnea, 96–104
   causes of, 96–97, 98t
   definition of, 96
   disposition in, 102–103
   epidemiology of, 96
   history in, 97, 99–100
   laboratory studies in, 99
   physical examination in, 97, 99
   treatment of, 100–101, *101–102*
Dysuria, 104–109
   definition of, 104
   differential diagnosis of, 105
   etiology of, 105
   history in, 105–106
   physical examination in, 106–107
   urine examination in, 107–109

EBV (Epstein-Barr virus), and mononucleosis, 464, *465*
ECG (electrocardiography). See *Electrocardiography (ECG).*
Echocardiography, in chest pain, 68
   in evaluation of syncope, 132–133
   in myocardial infarction, 257
   in pericarditis, 280
   in stroke, 757
   transesophageal, in thoracic aortic dissection, 286
Eclampsia, 250t
Ectopic pregnancy, 651–660
   abdominal pain in, 37t
   definition of, 651
   differential diagnosis of, 655–656
   disposition in, 660
   epidemiology of, 652
   history in, 652
   laboratory studies in, 653–655
   physical examination in, 653
   signs and symptoms of, 652

Ectopic pregnancy *(Continued)*
  treatment of, 656–657, *658–659*, 660
  vaginal bleeding in, 643–644
EEG (electroencephalography). See *Electroencephalography (EEG)*.
Eikenella corrodens, from animal bites, 384
Elderly person(s), infective endocarditis in, 407
Electrical activity, pulseless, 206, *207–208*
Electrocardiography (ECG), in angina, 66–67
  in antipsychotic poisoning, 902
  in aortic dissection, 67–68
  in cardiogenic shock, 178
  in chest pain, 66–67
  in cyclic antidepressant poisoning, 921
  in hyperkalemia, 622
  in myocardial infarction, 67, 255–256, 256t
  in pericarditis, 280
  in pneumothorax, 68
  in pulmonary embolism, 67, 341
  in shock, 173
  in stroke, 756
  in syncope, 132
  signal-averaged, 133
Electroencephalography (EEG), in coma, 744
  in seizures, 768
Electrolyte(s), in adrenal insufficiency, 675–676
  in evaluation of abdominal pain, 33t
  in evaluation of syncope, 132
Electrolyte panel, indications for, 12t
Electrophysiologic (EPS) testing, in evaluation of syncope, 133–134
ELISA (enzyme-linked immunosorbent assay), 361
Embolectomy, for deep venous thrombosis, 349
Embolism, cerebral, 759t–760t
  pulmonary. See *Pulmonary embolism*.
Emergency care, "ABCs" of, 3
Emergency medicine, definition of, 1
  scope of, 1–2
Emergent condition(s), definition of, 3
Encephalitis, definition of, 453
  differential diagnosis of, 457
  disposition in, 461–462
  etiology of, 453–454
  history in, 456
  lumbar puncture in, 456–457
  signs and symptoms of, 456
  treatment of, 457, *458–459*, 460t, 460–461
Encephalopathy, hepatic, definition of, 562
  laboratory studies in, 565
  treatment of, 569–570
  hypertensive, 250t
  in Lyme disease, 447
  Wernicke's, 930

Endarterectomy, carotid, for transient ischemic attack, 762
Endocarditis, infective, 402–409. See also *Infective endocarditis (IE)*.
Endometrial carcinoma, 649
Endotracheal intubation, 151–163. See also *Intubation*.
Endotracheal tube(s), 153
End-tidal carbon dioxide detector(s), colorimetric, 152
Enolic acid(s), dosage of, 22t
Enteritis, regional, abdominal pain in, 36t
Enzyme(s), cardiac, in myocardial infarction, 257
Enzyme-linked immunosorbent assay (ELISA), 361
Epidural spinal cord compression, 822–827
Epiglottitis, 409–415
  definition of, 409
  differential diagnosis of, 411
  epidemiology of, 409=410
  history in, 410
  laboratory studies in, 411
  physical examination in, 410–411
  signs and symptoms of, 410
  treatment of, *412–413*, 414
Epinephrine, for anaphylactic shock, 174–175
  for asthma, 304t, 307, *309*
  for asystole, *205*
  for pulseless electrical activity, *207*
  for sinus bradycardia, 214, *215*, 216t
  for ventricular fibrillation, 199, *200–201*, 202t
EPS (electrophysiologic) testing. See *Electrophysiologic (EPS) testing*.
Epstein-Barr virus (EBV), and mononucleosis, 464, *465*
Ergot alkaloid(s), for migraine, 116
Ergotamine (Cafergot, Ergostat), for headache, 121t, 124t
Erythema nigrans, in Lyme disease, 444, 445t, 446, 448
Erythrocyte(s), destruction of, from hemolysis, 791–792
  hemorrhagic loss of, 791
  inadequate production of, 792
Erythrocyte sedimentation rate (ESR), in headache, 113
  in stroke, 756–757
Erythromycin, for animal bites, 390t
  for asthma, 305t
  for cellulitis, 401t
  for diarrhea, 79t
  for pneumonia, 498t
  for streptococcal pharyngitis, 481
  for urinary tract infection, 537t
Esmolol, for atrial fibrillation, 223t
  for atrial flutter, 226
  for hypertensive emergency, 249t
  for myocardial infarction, 268, 274t
  for paroxysmal atrial tachycardia, 230

Esmolol *(Continued)*
   for paroxysmal supraventricular tachy-
      cardia, 229
   for thoracic aortic dissection, 287
   for thyroid storm, *729*, 731
Esophageal electrode(s), in diagnosis of
   atrial flutter, 226
Esophageal obturator airway, 149, *150*
Esophageal varices, hemorrhage of,
   559–560
Esophagitis, chest pain in, 62t
Esophagus, rupture of, management of, 71
ESR (erythrocyte sedimentation rate). See
   Erythrocyte sedimentation rate (ESR).
Estrogen cream, for atrophic vaginitis, 671t
Ethambutol, for tuberculosis, 528t, 529
Ethanol, for ethylene glycol poisoning, 935
   for methanol poisoning, 939
   poisoning from, 863t, 929–933
Ethanol ketoacidosis, 930
Ethanol level(s), indications for, 11t
Ethanol withdrawal, 932t, 932–933
Ethosuximide, for seizures, 775t
Ethylene glycol, antidotes to, 875t
   poisoning from, 863t, 933–935
Etidronate, for hypercalcemia, 612
Etodolac (Lodine), dosage of, 21t
Euvolemic hyponatremia, 618
Exigent condition(s), definition of, 2–3
Eye(s), poisons in, *872*, 874, 876

Faber test, 42
Factor VIII, for coagulation factor disor-
   ders, 811–812
Felon, 427, *427–428*
Femoral stretch test, 42
Fenamic acid(s), dosage of, 22t
Fenoprofen (Nalfon), dosage of, 21t
Fentanyl (Sublimaze), dosage of, 25t, 27
   for rapid-sequence intubation, 154t
Fever, from red blood cell transfusion, 817
Fibrillation, atrial. See *Atrial fibrillation*.
Fibrinogen, radioiodinated, in deep venous
   thrombosis, 340
Fibroid(s), uterine, 648
Fistula test, 91
Fitz-Hugh-Curtis syndrome, 505
   abdominal pain in, 35t
Flow-volume loop(s), in dyspnea, 100
Fluconazole (Diflucan), for oral candidiasis,
   379
   for vulvovaginal candidiasis, 671t
Fluid replacement therapy. See *Volume re-
   placement therapy*.
Flumazenil, dosage of, 27
   for benzodiazepine poisoning, 907–908
Fluoxetine, for headache, 123t
Flurbiprofen (Ansaid), dosage of, 21t
Folic acid, deficiency of, 794
Food-borne disease(s), 415–423
   causes of, 417, 418t–421t
   definition of, 415
   disposition in, 422

Food-borne disease(s) *(Continued)*
   epidemiology of, 415–416
   history in, 416
   laboratory studies in, 417
   pathogenesis of, 416
   physical examination in, 417
   symptoms of, 417
   treatment of, 420–422
Foreign body(ies), airway obstruction by,
   141–142
Foscarnet, for genital herpes, 508, 508t
   for infectious diarrhea, in acquired
      immunodeficiency syndrome, 379
Fracture(s), spinal, from ankylosing
   spondylitis, 849–850
Free thyroxine index (FT$_4$I), 717
Free water deficit, calculation of, 617
Fresh frozen plasma, transfusion of,
   820–821
FT$_4$I (free thyroxine index), 717
Furosemide, for acute renal failure, 604
   for ascites, 570
   for chronic obstructive pulmonary dis-
      ease, 325t
   for hypertensive emergency, 249t
   for hyponatremia, 620
   for increased intracranial pressure, 750
   for myocardial infarction, *262*, 269
   for pulmonary edema, *242*, 243

Gallbladder disease, 545–549, *550*,
   551–553
   differential diagnosis of, 549
   disposition in, 552
   history in, 546–547
   imaging procedures for, 548
   laboratory studies in, 547–548
   physical examination in, 547
   treatment of, 549, 550t, 551–552
Gallium nitrate, for hypercalcemia, 612
Gallstone(s), classification of, 546
   history in, 546–547
Gallstone pancreatitis, definition of, 546
Ganciclovir, for infectious diarrhea, in acquired immunodeficiency syndrome,
   379
Ganglionitis, geniculate, and vertigo, 83
Gastric aspirate, in gastrointestinal bleeding, 556
Gastric lavage, for poisoning, 876,
   877–878
Gastric ulcer(s), abdominal pain in, 35t
Gastrointestinal bleeding, 553–561
   definition of, 553–554
   differential diagnosis of, 556–557
   disposition in, 560–561
   epidemiology of, 554
   gastric aspirate in, 556
   history in, 554–555
   in acquired immunodeficiency syndrome,
      377
   laboratory studies in, 555–556
   physical examination in, 555

Gastrointestinal bleeding *(Continued)*
  role of consultants in, 558–559
  treatment of, 557–560
Geniculate ganglionitis, and vertigo, 83
Genital herpes, 506–509, 508t, 670
Gentamicin, for infective endocarditis,
  408t
  for pelvic inflammatory disease, 664t
  for pneumonia, 499t
  for septic shock, 192
  for urinary tract infection, 538t
Giant cell arteritis, 858–859
  headache in, 112t
Glomerular disease, 600–601
Glucagon, for hypoglycemia, 710, *713*
  for hypotension, in anaphylactic shock,
  176
Glucocorticoid(s), for hypercalcemia, 611
  for myxedema coma, 719
Glucose, for coma, 748
  for hyperkalemia, 624
    in acute renal failure, 603
  for hypoglycemia, 710, *712*
  in evaluation of abdominal pain, 33t
Gonococcal arthritis, 842–843
Gonococcal conjunctivitis, 504
Gonococcal pharyngitis, 504
Gonorrhea, 501–506, 503t
  cultures for, 107
Gout, calcium pyrophosphate, 847–848
  urate, 846–847
Graft versus host disease (GVHD), from
  red blood cell transfusion, 818
Granulomatous disease(s), and hypercalcemia, 609
GVHD (graft versus host disease), from
  red blood cell transfusion, 818

Haloperidol (Haldol), poisoning from, 900t,
  900–903, 903t
Hand infection(s), 423–429. See also specific type(s).
hCG (human chorionic gonadotropin), in
  ectopic pregnancy, 653–654
Head tilt–chin lift, for airway obstruction,
  142
Headache, 109–127
  classification of, 114–115
  cluster, 111t
    treatment of, 124t, 125, 126t
  disposition in, 127
  epidemiology of, 109
  history in, 110, 113, *113*
  laboratory studies in, 113–114
  migraine, classification of, 114
    treatment of, 116–117, *118–119*,
    120t–121t
  muscle contraction, 111t
    classification of, 114–115
  pathophysiology of, 109–110
  physical examination in, 113
  primary, 111t
  psychogenic, 111t

Headache *(Continued)*
  secondary, 110, 112t
    classification of, 115
  temporal pattern in, *113*
  tension, 111t
    classification of, 114–115
    treatment of, 115–117, *118–119*,
    120t–124t, 125, 126t
Heimlich maneuver, 142
Hematocrit, in evaluation of abdominal
  pain, 33t
Hemodialysis, for acute renal failure,
  604–605
  for barbiturate poisoning, 904–905
  for ethylene glycol poisoning, 935
  for hypercalcemia, 611
  for isopropyl alcohol poisoning, 937
  for lithium poisoning, 941
  for methanol poisoning, 939
  for poisoning, *873*, 881–882
  for salicylate poisoning, 955–956
Hemodynamic instability, in myocardial infarction, *263*, 270–272
Hemolysis, erythrocyte destruction from,
  791–792
  laboratory studies for, 790
Hemolytic anemia, 795
Hemolytic reaction, from red blood cell
  transfusion, 816–817
  delayed, 818
Hemoperfusion, for poisoning, *873*, 882
  for theophylline poisoning, 963
Hemophilia. See *Bleeding disorder(s).*
Hemophilus influenzae pneumonia, 488t,
  491t
Hemoptysis, 329–337
  definition of, 329
  differential diagnosis of, 332–333, 336
  etiology of, 329
  history in, 329–330
  laboratory studies in, 331–332
  physical examination in, 330–331
  treatment of, 333, *334*, 335–336
Hemorrhage, cerebellar, and vertigo, 83
  cerebral, 759t–760t
  erythrocyte loss in, 791
  gastrointestinal. See *Gastrointestinal
    bleeding.*
  of esophageal varices, 559–560
  postpartum, 648
  subarachnoid, 759t–760t. See also *Sub-
    arachnoid hemorrhage (SAH).*
Hemorrhagic shock. See *Shock, hypovolemic.*
Hemostasis, disorders of. See *Bleeding dis-
  order(s).*
Henderson-Hasselbach equation, 582
Heparin, for deep venous thrombosis, with
  pulmonary embolism, 343
  for myocardial infarction, *261*, 267,
  273t–274t
  for stroke, 763
  for transient ischemic attack, 762

Hepatic encephalopathy. See *Encephalopathy, hepatic.*
Hepatic failure, 561–573
  clinical features of, 563
  definition of, 562–563
  differential diagnosis of, 566–568
  disposition in, 572–573
  history in, 563–564
  initial management of, 568
  laboratory studies in, 565–566
  mortality in, 563
  physical examination in, 564–565
  role of consultants in, 572
  signs and symptoms of, 564
Hepatitis, abdominal pain in, 35t
  from isoniazid, 531
  viral, 429–443. See also *Viral hepatitis.*
Hepatobiliary scintigraphy (HIDA scan), 548
Hepatorenal syndrome, 571
Hepatotoxiity, in acetaminophen poisoning, *888*
Hepatotrophic virus(es), 430–432
Hernia(s), hiatal, chest pain in, 62t
  inguinal, abdominal pain in, 37t
Herpes simplex virus (HSV), genital infections from, 506–509, 508t, 670
  oral ulcers from, in acquired immunodeficiency syndrome, 376, 379
Herpetic whitlow, 425–427
Heterophil-negative mononucleosis, 466t
HHC (hyperglycemic hyperosmolar coma). See *Hyperglycemic hyperosmolar coma (HHC).*
Hiatal hernia, chest pain in, 62t
HIDA scan (hepatobiliary scintigraphy), 548
Histamine H_2 blockers, for gastrointestinal bleeding, 559
History, in evaluation of abdominal pain, 30
HLA (human leukocyte antigen)–matched platelet(s), transfusion of, 820
Home, discharge to, criteria for, 14–15
Hormone(s), for myxedema coma, 719, *720*
HSV (herpes simplex virus). See *Herpes simplex virus (HSV).*
Human bite(s), 385
  cellulitis from, 402t
Human chorionic gonadotropin (hCG), in ectopic pregnancy, 653–654
Human immunodeficiency virus (HIV). See *Acquired immunodeficiency syndrome (AIDS).*
Human leukocyte antigen (HLA)–matched platelet(s), transfusion of, 820
Hydatiform mole, 646–647
Hydralazine, for hypertensive emergency, 249t
Hydrazine, antidotes to, 875t
Hydrocodone with acetaminophen (Vicodin), dosage of, 24t
Hydrocortisone, for adrenal crisis, 677, *679*, 680
  for asthma, 304t, 306

Hydrocortisone *(Continued)*
  for myxedema coma, 719, *720*
  for thyroid storm, *730*, 732
Hydromorphone (Dilaudid), dosage of, 24t, 25t
  for sickle cell crisis, 802
Hydroxyzine (Vistaril), for anaphylactic shock, 175
  for nephrolithiasis, 633
Hyperbaric oxygen therapy, for carbon monoxide poisoning, 912–913
Hypercalcemia, 608–612
Hyperglycemia, definition of, 682
  without ketosis, 681–687
    disposition in, 686
    history in, 682
    laboratory studies in, 683
    physical examination in, 682–683
    treatment of, 683, *684–685*, 686
Hyperglycemic hyperosmolar coma (HHC), 699–707
  definition of, 699
  differential diagnosis of, 701
  epidemiology of, 699–700
  history in, 700
  laboratory studies in, 700–701
  physical examination in, 700
  signs and symptoms of, 700
  treatment of, 702, *703–705*, 706
Hyperkalemia, 621–625
  in acute renal failure, 602–603
  in diabetic ketoacidosis, 689
Hypernatremia, 615–617
  in diabetic ketoacidosis, 689
  in hyperglycemic hyperosmolar coma, 701
  in salicylate poisoning, 956t
Hyperosmolar coma, hyperglycemic. See *Hyperglycemic hyperosmolar coma (HHC).*
Hypertension, headache in, 112t
  in acute stroke, 763
  in cocaine poisoning, 917
  in monoamine oxidase inhibitor poisoning, 945
  in stimulant poisoning, 959–960
  in stroke, 763
  in subarachnoid hemorrhage, 784
  portal, 562
  pulmonary, chest pain in, 61t
Hypertensive emergency, 245–252
  definition of, 245–246
  disposition in, 250–251
  history in, 246
  physical examination in, 247
  treatment of, 247, *248*, 249t–250t
Hypertensive encephalopathy, 250t
Hypertensive urgency, 246, 248–250, 251t
Hyperthermia, in coma, 749–750
  in monoamine oxidase inhibitor poisoning, 944–945
  in salicylate poisoning, 957, 957t
  in stimulant poisoning, 959
Hypertonic hyponatremia, 618

Hypertonic saline, for hypovolemic shock, 187–188
Hypervolemic hyponatremia, 619
Hypocalcemia, 612–615
Hypoglycemia, 707–714
  definition of, 707–708
  differential diagnosis of, 709–710
  disposition in, 711
  epidemiology of, 708
  etiology of, 708
  history in, 708–709
  in salicylate poisoning, 957t
  laboratory studies in, 709
  physical examination in, 709
  signs and symptoms of, 709
  treatment of, 710–711, 712–713, 714
Hypokalemia, 625–628
  in salicylate poisoning, 957t
  in ventricular fibrillation, 203
Hypomagnesemia, in ventricular fibrillation, 203
Hyponatremia, 618–621
  in salicylate poisoning, 956t
Hypoparathyroidism, and hypocalcemia, 613
Hypotension, in acute renal failure, 602
  in anaphylactic shock, 175–176
  in cyclic antidepressant poisoning, 924t
  in superior vena cava syndrome, 831
Hypothermia, in coma, 749
Hypotonic hyponatremia, 618
Hypoventilation, alveolar, and acute respiratory failure, 291
Hypovolemia, in acute renal failure, 602
Hypovolemic hyponatremia, 618
Hypovolemic shock, 184–188. See also Shock, hypovolemic.

IBD (inflammatory bowel disease), diarrhea in, 77t
Ibuprofen, dosage of, 21t
  for headache, 122t
IE (infective endocarditis). See Infective endocarditis (IE).
Imidazole(s), for vulvovaginal candidiasis, 670, 671t, 672
Imipenem, for cellulitis, 401t
  for gallbladder disease, 551
  for pancreatitis, 579
  for pneumonia, 499t
  for septic shock, 192
Immunocompromised patient(s), tuberculosis in, 524–525
Impedance plethysmography, in deep venous thrombosis, 340
Indomethacin, dosage of, 21t
  for gout, 847
  for headache, 122t
  for pericarditis, 281
Infarction, cerebellar, and vertigo, 83
Infection(s), and vertigo, 83
  arthritis from, 840–845
  disseminated gonococcal, 842–843
  from red blood cell transfusion, 818

Infection(s), and vertigo (Continued)
  in coma, 751
  in sickle cell disease, 799
  nongonococcal, 840–842
Infectious diarrhea, 76t
  in acquired immunodeficiency syndrome, 377–379, 381, 382
Infectious mononucleosis, 462–467. See also Mononucleosis.
Infective endocarditis (IE), 402–409
  arthritis from, 843–845
  classification of, 403, 403–404
  definition of, 402
  differential diagnosis of, 407
  epidemiology of, 402–403
  evaluation of, 405
  from injection drug abuse, 403, 403, 407
  history in, 404
  in elderly, 407
  laboratory studies in, 406–407
  native-valve, 403, 403
  prosthetic valve, 403, 407
  signs and symptoms of, 404, 406, 406t
  treatment of, 408, 408t
Inferior vena cava barrier(s), for deep venous thrombosis, 348–349
Inflammatory bowel disease (IBD), diarrhea in, 77t
Influenza virus(es), pneumonia from, 490t, 493t
Inguinal hernia(s), abdominal pain in, 37t
Injection drug abuse, cellulitis from, 397, 401t
  endocarditis from, 403, 403, 407
Insulin, for diabetic ketoacidosis, 691, 693, 696, 699
  for hyperglycemia, without ketosis, 683, 685
  for hyperglycemic hyperosmolar coma, 702, 704, 706
  for hyperkalemia, 624
    in acute renal failure, 603
Interstitial nephritis, 601
Intervertebral disc(s), herniation of, 47
Intestinal ischemia, abdominal pain in, 36t
Intra-aortic balloon pump, for myocardial infarction, 275
Intra-articular corticosteroid(s), for osteoarthritis, 858
Intracranial pressure, in coma, 750–751
  in intubation, 158
Intravenous pyelogram (IVP), in nephrolithiasis, 631–632
Intubation, 151–163
  anesthesia for, 158
  confirmation of, 159, 161
  equipment for, 152–156, 154t–155t, 156
  for chronic obstructive pulmonary disease, 326–327
  in acute respiratory failure, 296
  in asthma, 310, 313–314
  in poisoning, 868
  in trauma patient, 152, 153t
  indications for, 7, 151

Intubation *(Continued)*
  intracranial pressure in, 158
  nasotracheal, 151–152, 161–162
  orotracheal, 151, 156–159, *160*, 161
  rapid-sequence, 153t
    anesthetics for, 154t
    neuromuscular blocking agents for,
      155t, 158
  routes for, 151–152
Iodinated glycerol, for chronic obstructive
    pulmonary disease, 325t
Iodoquinol, for diarrhea, 80t
Ipecac, for acetaminophen poisoning, 887
Ipratropium bromide, for asthma, 305t,
    310, 312–313
  for chronic obstructive pulmonary dis-
    ease, 324t
Iron, antidotes to, 875t
  poisoning from, 863t
Iron deficiency anemia, 793–794
Iron supplement(s), 794
Irritable bowel syndrome, abdominal pain
    in, 36t, 37t
Isoniazid, antidotes to, 875t
  for tuberculosis, 528t, 529, 531
  hepatitis from, 531
  poisoning from, 863t
Isopropyl alcohol, poisoning from, 863t,
    935–937
Isoproterenol, for sinus bradycardia, 216t
Itraconazole (Sporanox), for vulvovagi-
    nal candidiasis, 671t
IVP (intravenous pyelogram), in nephroli-
    thiasis, 631–632

Jarisch-Herxheimer reaction, 511
Jaw thrust, for airway obstruction, 142
Jet-mixing oxygen mask, 147t

Ketamine, for asthma, 306t
  for rapid-sequence intubation, 154t
Ketoacidosis, alcohol, 930
  diabetic. See *Diabetic ketoacidosis
    (DKA)*.
Ketoconazole (Nizoral), for vulvovaginal
    candidiasis, 671t
Ketoprofen (Orudis), dosage of, 21t
Ketorolac (Toradol), dosage of, 21t
  for headache, 120t
  for nephrolithiasis, 633
Kidney(s). See also entries under *Renal*.
  stones, in. See *Nephrolithiasis*.
Knee(s), arthrocentesis of, 838–839, *839*
Korsakoff's psychosis, 930

Labetalol, for hypertensive emergency, 249t
  for hypertensive urgency, 251t
Laboratory study(ies), in critically ill pa-
    tient, 10, 11t–13t
Labyrinthitis, and vertigo, 84
Lactic acidosis, 588
Lactulose, for hepatic encephalopathy, 569
Laryngoscope(s), 153, 155, *156*
Laryngoscopy, in epiglottitis, 411

Larynx, anatomy of, 139
Laser therapy, in hemoptysis, 335
Lateral medullary syndrome, and vertigo,
    83–84
Lead intoxication, abdominal pain in, 34t
Lead poisoning, 863t
Left ventricular failure, signs and symp-
    toms of, 239
Legionella pneumonia, 489t, 492t
Leiomyoma(s), uterine, 648
Leukocyte-poor red cell(s), transfusion of,
    816
Levothyroxine, for myxedema coma, 719,
    720
Lice infestation, 472–475, 474t
Lidocaine, for arrhythmias, 227t
  for atrial fibrillation, *220–221*
  for cluster headache, 125, 126t
  for myocardial infarction, *262*, 269, 275t
  for premature ventricular contractions,
    234
  for ventricular fibrillation, 199, *201*, 202t
  for ventricular tachycardia, 235
Lindane (Kwell), 474t
Lisinopril, for myocardial infarction, 260t
Listeria monocytogenes, and meningitis,
    453
Lithium, for headache, 124t
  poisoning from, 863t, 940–942, 941t
Liver. See also entries under *Hepatic*.
LOC (loss of consciousness), differential
    diagnosis of, 134–135, 135t
"Locked-in syndrome," 751
Lorazepam (Ativan), for asthma, 305t
  for seizures, *771*, 772
  in coma, 749
Loss of consciousness (LOC), differential
    diagnosis of, 134–135, 135t
Low back pain, analgesics for, 53–54
  definition of, 39
  differential diagnosis of, 45–49, 46t
  disposition in, 54–55
  epidemiology of, 40
  genitourinary examination in, 43
  history in, 40–41
  laboratory tests for, 43–45, 44t
  management algorithm in, *51–53*
  muscle relaxants for, 54, 54t
  musculoskeletal, management of,
    53–54
  neurologic examination in, 42–43, 43t
  physical examination in, 41–43
  psychological factors in, 43
  radiologic evaluation of, 44t, 44–45
  referred, 39–40
  treatment of, 49, 53–54
  Waddell's sign in, 43
Lumbar puncture, in coma, 743–746
  in encephalitis, 456–457
  in headache, 114
  in meningitis, 455, 456
  in stroke, 757
  in subarachnoid hemorrhage, 782
  traumatic, vs. xanthochromia, 787

Lumbar spine, radiographs of, indications for, 12t
Lumbar sprain, 45–47
Lyme disease, 443–452
  arthritis from, 446, 449–450, 845
  definition of, 443–444
  disposition in, 451
  encephalopathy in, 447
  epidemiology of, *442*, 444
  erythema nigrans in, 444, 445t, 446, 448
  laboratory studies in, 447–448
  signs and symptoms of, 444–447, 445t
  transmission of, 444
  treatment of, 448–451, 449t

Magnesium sulfate, for asthma, 305t
  for hypertensive emergency, 249t
  for myocardial infarction, *262*, 268–269
  for premature ventricular contractions, 234
  for seizures, *770*
  for torsades de pointes, 237, 237t
  for ventricular fibrillation, *201*, 202t, 203
Magnetic resonance angiography, in stroke, 757
Magnetic resonance imaging (MRI), in epidural spinal cord compression, 825–826
  in subarachnoid hemorrhage, 782
  in thoracic aortic dissection, 286
Malabsorption, diarrhea from, 77t
Malathion, for pediculosis, 474t
Mannitol, for acute renal failure, 604
  for increased intracranial pressure, 750
  for stroke, 764
MAO (monoamine oxidase) inhibitor(s), poisoning from, 942–945, 943t–944t
Mask(s), for oxygen delivery, 147t
Mechanical ventilation, for acute respiratory failure, 296, 297t
  for asthma, *310–311*, 313–314
  for chronic obstructive pulmonary disease, 326–327
  pneumothorax from, 357
Meclizine (Antivert), for vertigo, 94
Meclofenamate, dosage of, 22t
  for headache, 122t
Medical record(s), documentation in, 16–19. See also *Documentation.*
Medication(s), and hypercalcemia, 609
  and vertigo, 85, 89
Mefenamic acid (Ponstel), dosage of, 22t
Meniere's disease, and vertigo, 85
Meningitis, cryptococcal, in acquired immunodeficiency syndrome, 373
  definition of, 453
  disposition in, 461–462
  etiology of, 452–453
  headache in, 112t
  history in, 454, 456
  laboratory studies in, 454–455
  signs and symptoms of, 454, 456
  treatment of, 457, *458–459*, 460t, 460–461

Menometrorrhagia, definition of, 638
Menorrhagia, definition of, 638
Menstruation, vs. abnormal vaginal bleeding, 638
Mental status, in acute respiratory failure, 295
Meperidine (Demerol), dosage of, 24t, 25t
  for gallbladder disease, 551
  for nephrolithiasis, 633
  for pancreatitis, 579
  poisoning from, 863t
Mercury poisoning, 863t
Mesenteric adenitis, abdominal pain in, 36t
Metabolic acidosis, 582, 586–588
  anion gap, 587–588
    and hypokalemia, 626
    in diabetic ketoacidosis, 689
Metabolic alkalosis, 582, 588–589
  and hypokalemia, 626
Metaproterenol, for asthma, 304t, 306
  for chronic obstructive pulmonary disease, 320, 324t
Methanol, antidotes to, 875t
  poisoning from, 863t, 937–939
Methergine, after incomplete abortion, 645
Methimazole, for thyroid storm, 727, *728*
Methohexital, for rapid-sequence intubation, 154t
Methylprednisolone, for asthma, 304t.306
  for chronic obstructive pulmonary disease, 321, 324t
Methylxanthine(s), for asthma, 304t–305t, 307, *309*, 312
  for chronic obstructive pulmonary disease, 321, *323*, 324t
Methysergide, for headache, 123t
Metoclopramide (Reglan), for headache, 120t
Metolazone, for acute renal failure, 604
Metoprolol, for atrial fibrillation, 223t
  for myocardial infarction, 268, 274t
  for sinus tachycardia, 217
  for thoracic aortic dissection, 288
Metronidazole, for diarrhea, 79t
  for hepatic encephalopathy, 569
  for infectious diarrhea, in acquired immunodeficiency syndrome, 379
  for pelvic inflammatory disease, 664t
  for trichomoniasis, 671t, 672
  for vaginosis, 670, 671t
Metrorrhagia, definition of, 638
Mezlocillin, for gallbladder disease, 551
  for pancreatitis, 579
  for septic shock, 192
MI (myocardial infarction). See *Myocardial infarction (MI).*
Miconazole (Monistat), for vulvovaginal candidiasis, 671t
Midazolam, for asthma, 305t
  for cocaine poisoning, 916
  for conscious sedation, 27
  for rapid-sequence intubation, 154t
Middle ear, abnormalities of, and vertigo, 85

Migraine, 111t
  classification of, 114
  treatment of, 116–117, *118–119*, 120t–121t
Migratory arthritis, 836t
Milrinone, for cardiogenic shock, 181
Minocycline, for encephalitis/meningitis prophylaxis, 461
Miscarriage, 644–646
Mithramycin, for hypercalcemia, 611–612
Mitral valve prolapse, chest pain in, 59t
Mobitz atrioventricular block, 232
Monoamine oxidase (MAO) inhibitor(s), poisoning from, 942–945, 943t–944t
Monoarthritis, causes of, 846t
Monoclonal antiendotoxin antibody(ies), for septic shock, 193
Mononucleosis, 462–467
  differential diagnosis of, 464, 466
  disposition in, 467
  epidemiology of, 463
  heterophil-negative, 466t
  history in, 463
  laboratory studies in, 464, *465*
  signs and symptoms of, 463–464
  splenic rupture in, 467
  treatment of, *465*, 466t, 466–467
Morphine, dosage of, 25t
  for myocardial infarction, 259, 273t
  for nephrolithiasis, 633
  for pulmonary edema, 242, *242*
  for sickle cell crisis, 802
Motion sickness, and vertigo, 85
Motor response(s), in coma, 740, 741t
MRI (magnetic resonance imaging). See *Magnetic resonance imaging (MRI)*.
Mucolytic-expectorant(s), for chronic obstructive pulmonary disease, 326
Mucopurulent cervicitis, 501–503
Multifocal atrial tachycardia, 230–231
Muscle contraction headache, 111t
  classification of, 114–115
Muscle relaxant(s), for low back pain, 54, 54t
Musculoskeletal disease, chest pain in, 63t
  low back pain in, management of, 53–54
Mushroom(s), antidotes to, 875t
Mycoplasma pneumonia, 488t, 491t
Myocardial infarction (MI), 195t, 252–277
  abdominal pain in, 35t
  adjunctive therapy for, 267–270
  arrhythmias in, *262*
  chest pain in, 58t, 253
  definition of, 252
  differential diagnosis of, 257–258, *260*
  disposition in, 272
  electrocardiography in, 67
  epidemiology of, 252–253
  first-line therapy for, 258, *260–261*, 274t–275t
  hemodynamic instability in, *263*, 270–272
  initial assessment in, 257
  laboratory studies in, 255–257, 256t

Myocardial infarction (MI) *(Continued)*
  management algorithm for, *260–264*
  pericarditis with, 277–278
  physical examination in, 254–255
  risk factors for, 253
  symptoms of, 253–254
  thrombolytic therapy for, *261*, 264–267
    contraindications to, 265t
    vs. coronary angioplasty, 266–267
  treatment of, 70
    with cardiogenic shock, 182–183
    vs. pericarditis, 281
    vs. thoracic aortic dissection, 286
Myocardial ischemia, 195t
Myoglobinuria, in salicylate poisoning, 957t
Myxedema coma, 714–723
  definition of, 714
  differential diagnosis of, 718
  disposition in, 722
  epidemiology of, 714–715
  etiology of, 715
  history in, 715
  laboratory studies in, 716–718
  physical examination in, 715–716
  signs and symptoms of, 715
  treatment of, 718–719, *720–721*, 722

Nadolol, for headache, 122t
Nafcillin, for cellulitis, 401t
  for infective endocarditis, 408t
Nalbuphine (Nubain), dosage of, 25t
Naloxone, for coma, 748
  for opioid poisoning, 874, 948–949
  for septic shock, 193
Naproxen (Naprosyn, Anaprox), dosage of, 21t–22t
  for headache, 121t, 122t
Nasal cannula(s), for oxygen delivery, 147t
Nasopharyngeal airway(s), 143–144, *144*
Nasotracheal intubation, 151–152, 161–162
Native-valve endocarditis, 403, *403*
Needle cricothyrotomy, 163–165
Neisseria meningitis, 452
Neomycin, for hepatic encephalopathy, 569
Nephritis, interstitial, 601
Nephrolithiasis, 629–637
  analgesics for, 633
  antiemetics for, 633, 636
  classification of, 629–630
  differential diagnosis, 632–633
  disposition in, 636–637
  epidemiology of, 630
  history in, 630
  hydration for, 633
  laboratory studies in, 631–632
  management algorithm for, *634–635*
  physical examination in, 631
  urologic consultation in, 636
Neuralgia, trigeminal, headache in, 112t
Neuroleptic malignant syndrome, 902–903
Neuroma(s), acoustic, and vertigo, 83
Neuromuscular blockade, 751–752

Neuromuscular blocking agent(s), for asthma, 306t, *311*
for rapid-sequence intubation, 155t, 158
Neuromuscular disease, dyspnea in, 98t
Neuronitis, vestibular, and vertigo, 84–85
Neurosyphilis, in acquired immunodeficiency syndrome, 373, *375*
Nifedipine, for headache, 123t
for hypertensive urgency, 251t
Nimodipine, for subarachnoid hemorrhage, 784
Nitrofurantoin, for urinary tract infection, 536t
Nitroglycerin, for cardiogenic shock, 182
for hypertensive emergency, 249t
for myocardial infarction, 258, 259t, 261t, 266
for pulmonary edema, *242*, 243
Nitroprusside, for hypertensive emergency, 249t
for pulmonary edema, *242*, 243
Nongonococcal septic arthritis, 840–842
Nonrebreather reservoir mask(s), for oxygen delivery, 147t
Nonsteroidal anti-inflammatory drug(s) (NSAIDs), dosage of, 20, 21t–22t, 22–23
for ankylosing spondylitis, 849
for gout, 846–847
for migraine, 116, 122t
for osteoarthritis, 858
Nonurgent condition(s), definition of, 3
Norepinephrine, for cardiogenic shock, 180
for hypotension, in anaphylactic shock, 176
for myocardial infarction, 261t
for poisoning, 868
for pulmonary edema, *242*
for septic shock, 192
postresuscitative, after cardiac arrest, 208
Norfloxacin, for urinary tract infection, 536t
Nortriptyline, for headache, 123t
NSAIDs (nonsteroidal anti-inflammatory drugs). See *Nonsteroidal anti-inflammatory drug(s) (NSAIDs).*
Nylen-Barany maneuver, 90, *91*
Nystagmus, in vertigo, 88
Nystatin, for oral candidiasis, 379

Octreotide, for infectious diarrhea, in acquired immunodeficiency syndrome, 379
Oculocephalic response, 738, *739*, 740, 741t
Ofloxacin, for diarrhea, 79t–80t
for pelvic inflammatory disease, 664t
for urinary tract infection, 536t–538t
Oligomenorrhagia, definition of, 638
Oliguric acute renal failure, conversion to nonoliguric acute renal failure, 604
Opioid(s), dosage of, 23–26, 24t–25t
for migraine, 117

Opioid(s) *(Continued)*
poisoning from, 864t, 945–950, 946t
naloxone for, 874
Opioid withdrawal, 949–950
abdominal pain in, 34t
Optic fundus (fundi), in coma, 737
Oral candidiasis, in acquired immunodeficiency syndrome, 378–379
Oral contraceptive(s), breakthrough bleeding from, 650
Oral ulcer(s), from herpes simplex virus, in acquired immunodeficiency syndrome, 376
Orbital cellulitis, 397, 517
Organophosphate(s), antidotes to, 875t
poisoning from, 864t
Oropharyngeal airway(s), *144*, 144–145
Orotracheal intubation, 151, 156–159, *160*, 161
Osmotic diarrhea, 76t
Osteoarthritis, 857–858
Otitis externa, 468–472, *470*, 471t
Otitis media, 468–472, *470*, 471t
Ovarian cyst(s), ruptured, abdominal pain in, 37t
Ovarian torsion, abdominal pain in, 37t
Overdose, definition of, 860
Oxacillin, for infective endocarditis, 408t
Oxycodone (Percocet, Percodan), dosage of, 24t
Oxygen, for airway management, 146, 147t–148t, 148
for asthma, 303, 304t, *308*
for chronic obstructive pulmonary disease, 319, *322*, 324t
for cluster headache, 125, 126t
for myocardial infarction, 259t
for respiratory symptoms in acquired immunodeficiency syndrome, 366
hyperbaric, for carbon monoxide poisoning, 912–913
Oxygen mask(s), 147t
Oxygen tent(s), 147t
Oxymetazoline (Afrin), for sinusitis, 518t

Pacemaker(s), transcutaneous. See *Transcutaneous pacemaker (TCP).*
Packed red cell(s), transfusion of, 815
Pain. See also specific type, e.g., *Chest pain.*
in epidural spinal cord compression, 823–824
in sickle cell crisis, 798–799
Pain management, 19–28, 21t–22t, 24t–25t
for low back pain, 53–54
Palmar-space infection(s), 427
Pamidronate, for hypercalcemia, 612
Pancreatitis, 574–581
adjunctive therapy for, 579–580
analgesics for, 579
chest pain in, 63t
definition of, 574
differential diagnosis of, 578
disposition in, 580

Pancreatitis *(Continued)*
 epidemiology of, 574
 gallstone, definition of, 546
 history in, 574–575
 imaging procedures in, 576–577
 laboratory studies in, 575–576
 physical examination in, 575
 prognosis in, 577, 577t
 treatment of, 578–580
Pancuronium (Pavulon), for asthma, 306t
 for rapid-sequence intubation, 155t
Paracentesis, with albumin therapy, for ascites, 571
Paraldehyde, for seizures, *771*, 772–773
Parasympathetic nervous system, stimulation of, in ventricular fibrillation, 203
Parenteral opioid(s), 25t
Paronychia, 424–425, *424–426*
Paroxysmal atrial tachycardia, 229–230
Paroxysmal supraventricular tachycardia, 228–229
Partial thromboplastin time (PTT), in bleeding disorders, 808
PASG (pneumatic anti-shock garment), 188
Pasteurella multocida, from animal bites, 384
Patient condition(s), ranking of, 2–3
Patient transfer, criteria for, 15–16
Patrick test, 42
Pauciarthritis, causes of, 835t
PCP (*Pneumocystic carinii* pneumonia). See *Pneumocystic carinii* pneumonia (PCP).
Pediculosis, 472–475, 474t
Pelvic inflammatory disease (PID), 661–666
 abdominal pain in, 37t
 analgesics for, 663–664
 complications of, 661
 definition of, 661
 diagnosis of, 662–663
 differential diagnosis of, 663
 disposition in, 665
 history in, 661
 laboratory studies in, 662
 patient education in, 664–665
 physical examination in, 662
 risk factors for, 661
 signs and symptoms of, 661–662
 treatment of, 663–665, 664t
D-Penicillamine, for chelation therapy, 882
Penicillin, antipseudomonal, for septic shock, 192–193
 for animal bites, 390t
 for Lyme disease, 449t
 for neurosyphilis, 373
 for pneumonia, 498t
 for streptococcal pharyngitis, 481
 for syphilis, 511
Pentamidine, for *Pneumocystis carinii* pneumonia, 367
 for *Pneumocystis carinii* pneumonia prophylaxis, 363
Pentobarbital, for seizures, *771*, 772

Percutaneous translaryngeal ventilation, 163–165
Perforated duodenal ulcer(s), chest pain in, 63t
Pericardiocentesis, 280
Pericarditis, 277–282
 chest pain in, 60t
 complications of, 282
 definition of, 277
 differential diagnosis of, 280–281, 281t
 disposition in, 281
 etiology of, 277–278, 278t
 laboratory findings in, 279–280
 physical examination in, 279
 signs and symptoms of, 279
 treatment of, 281
Perihepatitis, abdominal pain in, 35t
Periorbital cellulitis, 397
Peritonitis, abdominal pain in, 34t
 bacterial, spontaneous. See *Spontaneous bacterial peritonitis (SBP)*.
Permethrin, for scabies, 474t
Pharyngitis, gonococcal, 504
 streptococcal, 477–484. See also *Streptococcal pharyngitis*.
Pharynx, anatomy of, 139
Phencyclidine, poisoning from, 864t
Phenobarbital, for seizures, 775t
 in coma, 749
 in acquired immunodeficiency syndrome, 373
Phenothiazine(s), for migraine, 116–117
 poisoning from, 864t, 900t, 900–903, 903t
Phentolamine, for hypertensive emergency, 249t
Phenylephrine, for hypotension, in anaphylactic shock, 176
 for sinusitis, 518t
Phenylpropanolamine, for sinusitis, 518t
Phenylpropionic acid(s), dosage of, 21t
Phenytoin, for cyclic antidepressant poisoning, 925
 for paroxysmal atrial tachycardia, 230
 for seizures, *771*, 772, 774t
 in acquired immunodeficiency syndrome, 373
 in coma, 749
 poisoning from, 894–896, 895t
Pheochromocytoma(s), hypertensive emergency from, 250t
Phosphate, for diabetic ketoacidosis, *695*, 697
 for hypercalcemia, 611
Phosphodiesterase inhibitor(s), for cardiogenic shock, 181
Physical examination, in secondary survey, 9
Physostigmine, for anticholinergic poisoning, 892–893
"Pink puffer," 318
Pinworm, 669
Piperacillin, for pneumonia, 498t
 for septic shock, 193

Piroxicam (Feldene), dosage of, 22t
Placenta previa, 647
Plasma, transfusion of, 820–821
Platelet(s), transfusion of, 819–820
Platelet count, in bleeding disorders, 807
Platelet dysfunction, 810, 811
Plethysmography, impedance, in deep
    venous thrombosis, 340
Pleurisy, chest pain in, 61t
Pleurodesis, chemical, for spontaneous
    pneumothorax, 356
Pneumatic anti-shock garment (PASG), 188
Pneumocystis carinii pneumonia (PCP),
    prophylaxis for, 363
    treatment of, 367, 369
Pneumomediastinum, chest pain in, 61t
Pneumonia, 484–501
    abdominal pain in, 35t
    antibiotics for, 494t–495t, 497, 498t–499t
    chest pain in, 62t
    classification of, 484–485, 485t
    community-acquired, 486t
    definition of, 484
    differential diagnosis of, 497
    disposition in, 499–500
    epidemiologic categories in, 494t–495t
    etiology of, 485t–486t
    history in, 487
    laboratory studies in, 493, 495–497
    mortality in, 485–486
    pathogens in, 486t, 488t–493t
    physical examination in, 487, 491–492
    radiographic evaluation in, 492–493
    supportive care in, 499
Pneumothorax, chest pain in, 61t
    electrocardiography in, 68
    from mechanical ventilation, 357
    management of, 71
    spontaneous, 350–358. See also *Sponta-
      neous pneumothorax.*
    tension, 351, 357
    traumatic, 356
Poison(s), exposure of eyes to, *872*, 874,
    876
    exposure of skin to, *872*, 876
Poisoning. See also specific drugs and sub-
    stances.
    activated charcoal for, *877–878*
    antidotes in, 874, 875t
    chelation therapy for, *873*, 882–883
    complications of, 884–885
    definition of, 860
    differential diagnosis of, 867–868
    disposition in, 883–884
    enhancement of elimination in, 880–883
    epidemiology of, 860–861
    gastric lavage for, 876, *877–878*
    hemodialysis for, 605, *873*, 881–882
    hemoperfusion for, *873*, 882
    history in, 861
    intubation in, 868
    laboratory studies in, 865–867
    management algorithm for, *870–873*
    monitoring in, 865

Poisoning *(Continued)*
    mortality in, 861
    physical examination in, 864–865
    psychosocial evaluation in, 883
    seizure control in, 869
    signs and symptoms of, 861, 862t–864t
    supportive therapy for, 868–869, *870*
    whole-bowel irrigation for, *879*
Polyarthritis, causes of, 836t
Polyp(s), cervical, 648
Porphyria, acute intermittent, abdominal
    pain in, 34t
Portal hypertension, 562
Positional vertigo, 85
Positive-pressure ventilation, 145–146
Post–cardiac injury syndrome, 278
Posterior fossa, tumors of, and vertigo, 84
Postpartum hemorrhage, 648
Postrenal acute renal failure, 595t,
    595–596, 601, 603
Potassium, for hyperglycemic hyperosmolar
    coma, *705*
    for thyroid storm, *729*, 731
    for torsades de pointes, 237t
    for ventricular fibrillation, 203
Potassium replacement therapy, 627–628
    for diabetic ketoacidosis, *694*, 696
PPD (purified protein derivative), in pneu-
    monia, 493
PPD (purified protein derivative) testing,
    527, 530t, 530–531
Prednisone, for gout, 847
    for temporal arteritis, 859
Preeclampsia, 250t
Pregnancy, ectopic. See *Ectopic pregnancy.*
    vaginal bleeding during, 641–642
Pregnancy test(s), in ectopic pregnancy,
    653–654
    indications for, 12t
Prehospital care, definition of, 2
Premature ventricular contraction(s)
    (PVCs), 233–234
Prerenal acute renal failure (ARF),
    594–595,595t, 599–600, 603–604
Presyncope, 82
Primary survey, 7–9
    definition of, 3
Probenecid, for pelvic inflammatory dis-
    ease, 664t
Procainamide, for arrhythmias, 227t
    for atrial fibrillation, *220–221*
    for ventricular fibrillation, *201*
    for ventricular tachycardia, 235–236
Prochlorperazine (Compazine), for head-
    ache, 120t
    for nephrolithiasis, 633
    for vertigo, 93
Prolactin level(s), after seizures, 776
Promethazine (Phenergan), for nephrolithia-
    sis, 633
    for vertigo, 93
Propionic acid(s), dosage of, 21t
Propranolol, for atrial fibrillation, 222t
    for atrial flutter, 226

Propranolol *(Continued)*
  for headache, 122t
  for myocardial infarction, 268, 274t
  for paroxysmal atrial tachycardia, 230
  for paroxysmal supraventricular
    tachycardia, 229
  for thoracic aortic dissection, 288
  for thyroid storm, *729*, 731
Propylthiouracil, for thyroid storm, 727, *728*
Prosthetic valve endocarditis, 403, 407
Prothrombin time, in bleeding disorders,
    807–808
Pseudoephedrine hydrochloride (Sudafed),
    for sinusitis, 518t
Pseudogout, 847–848
Pseudometabolic acidosis, 588
Pseudoseizure(s), 776
Psoriatic arthritis, 851–852
Psychogenic headache, 111t
Psychogenic unresponsiveness, 752
Psychosis, Korsakoff's, 930
PTT (partial thromboplastin time), in
    bleeding disorders, 808
Pulmonary angiography, in pulmonary em-
    bolism, 342
Pulmonary artery catheterization, in shock,
    170
Pulmonary edema, treatment of, with car-
    diogenic shock, 183
  with congestive heart failure, 241–244,
    242
Pulmonary embolism, angiography in, 342
  chest pain in, 62t
  electrocardiography in, 67, 341
  management of, 71
  radiography in, 67
  with deep venous thrombosis, 337–350.
    See also *Deep venous thrombosis
    (DVT), with pulmonary embolism.*
Pulmonary function test(s), in asthma, 302
Pulmonary hypertension, chest pain in, 61t
Pulmonary scintigraphy, in pulmonary
    embolism, 341, 341t
Pulseless electrical activity, 206, *207–208*
Pulseless ventricular tachycardia. See
    Ventricular fibrillation.
Puncture wound(s), cellulitis from, 398
Pupillary response(s), in coma,
    737–738.741t
Purified protein derivative (PPD), in pneu-
    monia, 493
Purified protein derivative (PPD) testing,
    527, 530t, 530–531
PVCs (premature ventricular contractions),
    233–234
Pyelonephritis, abdominal pain in, 35t
  clinical evaluation in, 534–535
  etiology of, 533
  laboratory studies in, 535
  treatment of, 536t–538t
Pyogenic pericarditis, 278
Pyramethamine, for toxoplasmosis, in ac-
    quired immunodeficiency syndrome,
    373

Pyrazinamide, for tuberculosis, 528t,
    529
Pyrethrin(s), for pediculosis, 474t

Quinacrine, for diarrhea, 80t

Rabies prophylaxis, for animal bites, 391,
    392t
Radiation therapy, for epidural spinal cord
    compression, 826
  for superior vena cava syndrome, 831
Radiograph(s), abdominal, indications for,
    11t
  chest, indications for, 11t
  of lumbar spine, indications for, 12t
Radioiodinated fibrinogen, in deep venous
    thrombosis, 340
Rapid-sequence intubation, 153t
  anesthetics for, 154t
  neuromuscular blocking agents for, 155t,
    158
RBC (red blood cells). See *Red blood cell
    (RBCs).*
Reactive arthritis, 850–851
Real-time ultrasonography, in deep venous
    thrombosis, 340
Record(s), documentation in, 16–19. See
    also *Documentation.*
Red blood cell (RBCs), transfusion of,
    814–819
  allergic reaction to, 818
  crossmatching for, 814–815
  for anemia, 793
  graft-versus-host disease from, 818
  hemolytic reaction from, 816–817
    delayed, 818
"Red flag(s)," 6
Reflex(es), in stroke, 755
Regional enteritis, abdominal pain in, 36t
Rehydration solution(s), 78
Reiter's syndrome, 850–851
Renal bicarbonate reclamation, enhanced,
    and metabolic alkalosis, 589
Renal calculi. See *Nephrolithiasis.*
Renal failure, acute. See *Acute renal failure
    (ARF).*
  hypertensive emergency from, 250t
Renal tubular acidosis, 587
Repolarization, early, vs. pericarditis,
    280–281
Rescue breathing, 145–146
Reserpine, for thyroid storm, *729*, 731
Respiration, apneuristic, 737
  ataxic, 737
  Cheyne-Stokes, 737
  in coma, 737
Respiratory acidosis, 582, 589
Respiratory alkalosis, 582, 590
Respiratory disease, dyspnea in, 98t
Respiratory failure, acute, 289–300. See
    also *Acute respiratory failure (ARF).*
Resuscitation, 7–9
  definition of, 3–4
Reticulocyte index, 790

Rh immune globulin (RhoGAM), in ectopic pregnancy, 657, 660
  in threatened abortion, 644
Rhabdomyolysis, in salicylate poisoning, 957t
Rheumatoid arthritis, 852–854
Rheumatoid vasculitis, 853
Rifampin, for encephalitis/meningitis prophylaxis, 461–462
  for infective endocarditis, 408t
  for tuberculosis, 528t, 529
Right ventricular failure, signs and symptoms of, 239

SAH (subarachnoid hemorrhage). See *Subarachnoid hemorrhage (SAH)*.
Salicylate(s), dosage of, 20, 21t
  poisoning from, 864t, 950–958, 951t
    acid-base disorders in, 952, *953*, 956t
    Done nomogram for, 952, *954*
  preparations containing, 950t
Saline, hypertonic, for hypovolemic shock, 187–188
Salsalate (Disalcid), dosage of, 21t
SBP (spontaneous bacterial peritonitis). See *Spontaneous bacterial peritonitis (SBP)*.
Scabies, 474t, 475–476
  definition of, 475
  diagnosis of, 476
  differential diagnosis of, 476
  signs and symptoms of, 475–476
  transmission of, 475
  treatment of, 474t, 476
Schober test, 849
Scintigraphy, hepatobiliary, 548
  pulmonary, in pulmonary embolism, 341, 341t
Scopolamine, for vertigo, 94
Secondary survey, 9–10
  definitions of, 4
Secretory diarrhea, 76t
Sedation, conscious, with analgesia, 26–28
Sedative-hypnotic(s), poisoning from, 864t
Seizure(s), 766–777
  classification of, 766t, 766–767
  definition of, 766
  differential diagnosis of, 769
  disposition in, 776–777
  epidemiology of, 767
  etiology of, 767
  history in, 768
  in acquired immunodeficiency syndrome, 373
  in cocaine poisoning, 916
  in coma, 749
  in cyclic antidepressant poisoning, 922t
  in monoamine oxidase inhibitor poisoning, 944
  in poisoning, 869
  in stimulant poisoning, 959
  in theophylline poisoning, 963
  initial management of, 769, *770*, 772
  laboratory studies in, 768
  physical examination in, 768

Seizure(s) *(Continued)*
  prolactin levels after, 776
  treatment of, 749, *771*, 772, 774t
  vs. syncope, 134–135, 135t
  withdrawal, 776
Sepsis, definition of, 189
Septic abortion, 646
Septic arthritis, 840–845
Septic shock, 189–194. See also *Shock, septic*.
Septic tenosynovitis, 428–429
Sequestration crisis, in sickle cell disease, 799
Serum electrolyte panel, indications for, 12t
Serum osmolarity, in diabetic ketoacidosis, 689–690
  in hyperglycemic hyperosmolar coma, 701
Sexually transmitted disease(s) (STDs), 501–512. See also specific type(s).
  dysuria in, 106
Shock, 167–194
  anaphylactic, 171–177
    definition of, 171
    differential diagnosis of, 173
    disposition in, 176–177
    etiology of, 172t
    incidence of, 172
    laboratory studies in, 173
    mediators of, 171
    signs and symptoms of, 172–173, 173t
    treatment of, 173–176
  cardiogenic, 177–184
    definition of, 177
    diagnosis of, 178–179
    disposition in, 184
    etiology of, 177
    incidence of, 177
    invasive monitoring in, 178
    laboratory studies in, 178
    signs and symptoms of, 177–178
    treatment of, 179–183
  cardiovascular triad in, 168–169
  clinical findings in, 167–168
  definition of, 167
  hypovolemic, 184–188
    classification of, 184t, 184–185
    definition of, 184
    diagnosis of, 185–186
    laboratory studies in, 185
    signs and symptoms of, 185
    treatment of, 186–188
  initial care in, 171
  patient monitoring in, 169–170
  septic, 189–194
    definition of, 189
    diagnosis of, 191
    etiology of, 189–190
    incidence of, 190
    laboratory studies in, 191
    mortality in, 190
    risk factors for, 190
    signs and symptoms of, 190–191
    treatment of, 191–193
  vital signs in, 167–168

Shoulder, arthrocentesis of, 837, *838*
Shunt(s), and acute respiratory failure, 293
Sickle cell crisis, pain in, 798–799, 802
Sickle cell disease, 797–804
  analgesics for, 802
  aplastic crisis in, 799
  definition of, 797
  differential diagnosis of, 801, 801t
  disposition in, 803, 804t
  genetic characteristics of, 797–798
  history in, 798
  infection in, 799
  laboratory studies in, 800–801
  mortality in, 798
  physical examination in, 799–800
  sequestration crisis in, 799
  signs and symptoms of, 798–799
  stroke in, 799
  treatment of, 801–803
Signal-averaged electrocardiography, 133
Sinus bradycardia, 213–214, *215*, 216t
Sinus tachycardia, 214, 216–217
Sinusitis, 512–520
  complications of, 516–517
  definition of, 513
  diagnostic studies in, 516
  differential diagnosis of, 516
  disposition in, 519–520
  epidemiology of, 513
  history in, 513–515
  pathogens in, 514t
  pathophysiology of, 513, 514t
  physical examination in, 515–516
  treatment of, 517, 518t–519t
SIRS (systemic inflammatory response syn-
    drome), 189
Sitting root test, 42
Skin, poisons on, *872*, 876
SLE (systemic lupus erythematosus),
    854–857
Small bowel obstruction, abdominal pain
    in, 36t
Sodium bicarbonate, for acid-base disor-
    ders, 592
  for asystole, *205*
  for diabetic ketoacidosis, *694*, 696–697
  for hyperkalemia, 623
    in acute renal failure, 602
  for pulseless electrical activity, *208*
  for ventricular fibrillation, 199, *201*, 202t
Sodium iodide, for thyroid storm, *729*, 731
Sodium ipodate, for thyroid storm, *730*,
    732
Sodium nitroprusside, for cardiogenic
    shock, 182
  for myocardial infarction, 261t
Sodium polystyrene sulfonate (Kayexalate),
    for hyperkalemia, 624
    in acute renal failure, 603
Specialty consultation, 10, 13–14
Spectinomycin, for urinary tract infection,
    536t
Spinal cord, compression of, 48–49

Spinal cord compression, epidural, 822–827
Spinal fracture, from ankylosing spondyli-
    tis, 849–850
Spinal stenosis, 47–48
Spine, lumbar. See *Lumbar spine*.
Spirometry, bedside, in chronic obstructive
    pulmonary disease, 319
  in dyspnea, 100
Spironolactone, for ascites, 570
Splenic infarction, abdominal pain in, 35t
Splenic rupture, abdominal pain in, 35t
  in mononucleosis, 467
Spondylitis, ankylosing, 848–850
Spondyloarthropathy, 848–852
Spondylolisthesis, 48
Spontaneous abortion, 644–646
Spontaneous bacterial peritonitis (SBP),
    definition of, 562–563
  laboratory studies in, 565–566
  treatment of, 571
Spontaneous pneumothorax, 350–358
  definition of, 350–351
  differential diagnosis of, 354
  disposition in, 357–358
  epidemiology of, 351
  etiology of, 351, 352t
  history in, 352
  laboratory studies in, 353–354
  signs and symptoms of, 353
  treatment of, 354, *355*, 356–357
Sputum test(s), 495–496
  in tuberculosis, 527
Stabilization, definition of, 4
Stanford system, for classification of tho-
    racic aortic dissection, 283, *284*
Staphylococcal pneumonia, 490t, 493t
Status epilepticus, *770–771*, 772–773
Status migrainosis, 125
STDs (sexually transmitted diseases),
    501–512. See *Sexually transmitted dis-
    ease(s) (STDs)*; specific type(s).
Stimulant(s), poisoning from, 958–960
Stomach. See entries under *Gastric* and
    Gastrointestinal.
Straight leg raising test, 42
Streptococcal pharyngitis, 477–484
  diagnosis of, 477
  laboratory studies in, 477
  treatment of, 481, *482–483*
Streptococcal pneumonia, 488t, 491t
  and meningitis, 452
Streptokinase, for deep venous thrombosis,
    348
  for myocardial infarction, 264, 273t
Stridor, in airway obstruction, 140–141
Stroke, 752–765
  acute, 762–764
  definition of, 752
  differential diagnosis of, 758, 759t–760t
  disposition in, 764–765
  epidemiology of, 754
  history in, 754–755
  hypertension control in, 763

Stroke *(Continued)*
  in sickle cell disease, 799
  laboratory studies in, 756–758
  pathophysiology of, 752, *753*, 754
  physical examination in, 755–756
  with transient ischemic attack, 761–762
Struvite crystal(s), 629
Stylet(s), for intubation, 153
Subacute infective endocarditis, 404
Subarachnoid hemorrhage (SAH), 759t–760t, 778–787
  aneurysmectomy for, 786, 786t
  definition of, 778
  differential diagnosis of, 783
  epidemiology of, 778
  etiology of, 779, 779t
  headache in, 112t
  history in, 779–780
  hypertension in, 784
  laboratory studies in, 782–783
  physical examination in, 781–782
  signs and symptoms of, 780t, 780–781
  treatment of, 784–786, *785*
Subclavian steal syndrome, and vertigo, 84
Succinylcholine, for rapid-sequence intubation, 155t
Sulfonylurea(s), for hyperglycemia, without ketosis, 686
Sulindac (Clinoril), dosage of, 21t
  for headache, 122t
Sumatriptan succinate (Imitrex), for headache, 117, 126t
Superior vena cava syndrome, 828–832
Supraventricular tachycardia, paroxysmal, 228–229
Sympathomimetic(s), for chronic obstructive pulmonary disease, 324t
Synchronized cardioversion, for atrial fibrillation, 218, 219t
Syncope, 128–138
  causes of, 129t–130t
  definition of, 128
  diagnostic problems in, 128–129
  differential diagnosis of, 134–135, 135t
  disposition in, 136–137
  epidemiology of, 128
  history in, 130–131
  laboratory studies in, 132–134
  management of, 135–136
  physical examination in, 131–132
  prognosis in, 128
Synovial fluid, analysis of, 837–840, *838–839*, 840t
Syphilis, 509–512
Systemic inflammatory response syndrome (SIRS), 189
Systemic lupus erythematosus (SLE), 854–857

Tachycardia, atrial, multifocal, 230–231
  paroxysmal, 229–230
  sinus, 214, 216–217

Tachycardia *(Continued)*
  supraventricular, paroxysmal, 228–229
  ventricular, 234–236
T-cell count, in acquired immunodeficiency syndrome, 360t, 361, 364
TCP (transcutaneous pacemaker). See *Transcutaneous pacemaker (TCP)*.
TEE (transesophageal echocardiography). See *Transesophageal echocardiography (TEE)*.
Temporal arteritis, 858–859
  headache in, 112t
Tenosynovitis, septic, 428–429
Tension headache, 111t
  classification of, 114–115
Tension pneumothorax, 351, 357
Terbutaline, for asthma, 304t, 307, *309*
  for chronic obstructive pulmonary disease, 320, 324t
Terphenadine (Seldane), for sinusitis, 519t
Tetanus prophylaxis, 520–521, *522*
  for animal bites, 391
Tetany, in salicylate poisoning, 957t
Tetracycline, for animal bites, 390t
  for asthma, 305t
  for pneumonia, 498t
  for syphilis, 511
Theophylline, for asthma, 305t, 312
  for chronic obstructive pulmonary disease, 321, 324t
  poisoning from, 864t, 960–964, 961t–962t
  preparations containing, 961t
Thiamine, for coma, 748
  for ethanol poisoning, 931
  for hypoglycemia, 710, *712*
Thiopental, for rapid-sequence intubation, 154t
Thoracic aortic dissection, 283–289
  classification of, 283, *284*
  definition of, 283
  diagnostic imaging in, 286
  differential diagnosis of, 286–287
  disposition in, 288
  epidemiology of, 284
  history in, 284–285
  laboratory studies in, 285
  physical examination in, 285
  treatment of, 287–288
Thoracostomy, tube, for spontaneous pneumothorax, 356
Thoracotomy, for spontaneous pneumothorax, 356
Thrombocytopenia, 809–810, 810–811
Thrombolytic therapy, for deep venous thrombosis, with pulmonary embolism, 343, 348
  for myocardial infarction, 259t–260t, 267–270
    complications of, 269
    contraindications to, 268t
    vs. coronary angioplasty, 266–267
  for stroke, 763

Thrombophlebitis, cavernous sinus, 517
Thrombosis, cerebral, 759t–760t
Thyroid storm, 723–733
  definition of, 723
  differential diagnosis of, 727
  disposition in, 733
  epidemiology of, 723
  etiology of, 723–724
  history in, 724
  laboratory studies in, 725–726
  physical examination in, 725
  signs and symptoms of, 724–725
  treatment of, 727, *728–730*, 731–733
TIA (transient ischemic attack), 759t–760t, 761–762
Ticarcillin, for pneumonia, 498t
  for septic shock, 192–193
Ticarcillin/clavulanate (Timentin), for gall-bladder disease, 551
  for pancreatitis, 579
Tick bite(s), prophylactic therapy for, 450–451
Ticlopidine, for stroke, 764
  for transient ischemic attack, 761
Tilt table testing, in evaluation of syncope, 133
TIPS (transjugular intrahepatic portosystemic shunt), for gastrointestinal bleeding, 560
Tissue plasminogen activator (t-PA, alteplase), for myocardial infarction, 264–266, 273t
Tobramycin, for pneumonia, 499t
  for septic shock, 192
Tolmetin (Tolectin), dosage of, 21t
Topical anesthesia, for nasotracheal intubation, 161–162
Torsades de pointes, 236–238, 237t
Toxicology screen(s), 866–867
  in coma, 742
  indications for, 13t
Toxoplasmosis, in acquired immunodeficiency syndrome, 373, *375*
t-PA (tissue plasminogen activator, alteplase), for myocardial infarction, 264–266, 273t
Trachea, anatomy of, 139–140
Transcutaneous pacemaker (TCP), for myocardial infarction, 270
  for sinus bradycardia, 214, *215*
Transesophageal echocardiography (TEE), in chest pain, 69
  in thoracic aortic dissection, 286
Transfer, criteria for, 15–16
Transfusion(s). See also specific blood component(s).
  for sickle cell disease, 802–803
  massive, 819
Transient ischemic attack (TIA), 759t–760t, 761–762
Transjugular intrahepatic portosystemic shunt (TIPS), for gastrointestinal bleeding, 560

Translaryngeal anesthesia, for nasotracheal intubation, 162
Translaryngeal ventilation, percutaneous, 163–165
Trauma, and vertigo, 85
  intubation methods in, 152, 153t
  vaginal bleeding from, 649
Traumatic pneumothorax, 356
Triage, definition of, 2
Triamcinolone, for gout, 847
Trichomoniasis, 667, 672
Trigeminal neuralgia, headache in, 112t
Trimethaphan, for hypertensive emergency, 249t
Trimethoprim-sulfamethoxazole, for asthma, 305t
  for chronic obstructive pulmonary disease, 325t, 326
  for diarrhea, 79t–80t
  for infectious diarrhea, in acquired immunodeficiency syndrome, 379
  for otitis media, 471t
  for *Pneumocystis carinii* pneumonia, 367
  for *Pneumocystis carinii* pneumonia prophylaxis, 363
  for pneumonia, 498t
  for sinusitis, 518t
  for urinary tract infection, 536t, 538t
Trousseau's sign, 575
T-tube, for oxygen delivery, 148t
Tube thoracostomy, for spontaneous pneumothorax, 356
Tuberculin skin test (PPD), 493, 527, 530t, 530–531
Tuberculosis, 521–533
  chest radiography in, 527
  definition of, 521
  disposition in, 531–532
  epidemiology of, 523, 526
  infection control in, 529–530
  pathogenesis of, 523, *524–525*
  physical examination in, 526
  prevention of, 530t, 530–531
  purified protein derivative testing in, 527, 530t, 530–531
  signs and symptoms of, 526
  sputum test in, 527
  transmission of, 523
  treatment of, 528t, 528–529
Tuberculous pericarditis, 278
Twenty-four-hour urine evaluation, in nephrolithiasis, 632

Ulcer(s), aphthous, in acquired immunodeficiency syndrome, 379
  duodenal, abdominal pain in, 35t
  perforated, chest pain in, 63t
  from herpes simplex virus, in acquired immunodeficiency syndrome, 376
  gastric, abdominal pain in, 35t
Ultrasonography, Doppler, carotid artery, in stroke, 757
  in deep venous thrombosis, 339–340

Ultrasonography *(Continued)*
 in ectopic pregnancy, 654–655
 in gallbladder disease, 548
 in nephrolithiasis, 632
 in pancreatitis, 576
Unresponsiveness, psychogenic, 752
Unstable angina, management of, 70
Urate gout, 846–847
Uremic pericarditis, 277
Ureteral stone(s), abdominal pain in, 37t
Urethritis, clinical evaluation in, 534–535
 etiology of, 533
 in males, 502
 laboratory studies in, 535
 treatment of, 536t–538t
Urgent condition(s), definition of, 3
Uric acid crystal(s), 629
Urinalysis, in acute renal failure, 599
 in dysuria, 107–109
 in evaluation of abdominal pain, 33t
Urinary tract infection(s) (UTIs), 533–535,
 536t–538t, 537–539, 670
Urine, examination of, in dysuria, 107–109
Urine culture, indications for, 13t
Urokinase, for deep venous thrombosis,
 348
Uterus, leiomyomas of, 648
UTIs (urinary tract infections). See *Urinary
 tract infection(s) (UTIs).*

Vaccination, for viral hepatitis, 440–442,
 441t
Vagal tone, decrease of, maneuvers for,
 225t
Vaginal bleeding, 638–651
 abnormal, vs. normal menstruation, 638
 breakthrough, from oral contraceptives,
 650
 differential diagnosis of, 641–643
 epidemiology of, 638–639
 from hydatiform mole, 646–647
 history in, 639
 hormonal causes of, 650
 in abruptio placenta, 647–648
 in cervical carcinoma, 649
 in cervical polyps, 648
 in ectopic pregnancy, 643–644
 in endometrial carcinoma, 649
 in miscarriage, 644
 in placenta previa, 647
 in postpartum hemorrhage, 648
 in pregnancy, 641–642
 in spontaneous abortion, 644–646
 in systemic disease, 649
 in uterine leiomyomas, 648
 initial management of, 643
 laboratory studies in, 640–641
 physical examination in, 639–640
 traumatic, 649
Vaginitis, 666–673
 definition of, 666
 diagnosis of, 668t, 668–669
 etiology of, 666t, 666–667, 669

Vaginitis *(Continued)*
 history in, 667
 physical examination in, 667–668
Vaginosis, bacterial, 670, 671t
Vagolysis, in orotracheal intubation,
 157–158
Valproic acid, for seizures, 774t
 poisoning from, 898–900
Valsalva maneuver, in vertigo, 90
Valvular decompensation, treatment of,
 with cardiogenic shock, 183
Vancomycin, for cellulitis, 401t
 for diarrhea, 80t
 in acquired immunodeficiency syndrome, 379
 for infective endocarditis, 408t
 for pneumonia, 499t
Varices, esophageal, hemorrhage of,
 559–560
Vasculitis, rheumatoid, 853
Vasodilator(s), for cardiogenic shock,
 181–182
 for hypertensive emergency, 249t
 for myocardial infarction, 272, 275t
 for thoracic aortic dissection, 288
Vasopressin (Pitressin), for gastrointestinal
 bleeding, 559
Vasopressor(s), for cardiogenic shock,
 180–181
 for myocardial infarction, 272, 275t
 for septic shock, 192
Vecuronium, for rapid-sequence intubation,
 155t
Vena cava syndrome, 828–832
Venography, contrast, in deep venous
 thrombosis, 339
Ventilation, in acute respiratory failure, 296
 in pneumonia, 499
 positive-pressure, 145–146
 translaryngeal, percutaneous, 163–165
Ventilation-perfusion (V/Q) mismatch, and
 acute respiratory failure, 291, 293
Ventilation-perfusion (V/Q) scanning, in
 chest pain, 68
 in pulmonary embolism, 341, 341t
Ventricular failure, signs and symptoms of,
 239
Ventricular fibrillation, 197–200, *200*, 200t,
 202–203
 alkalosis in, 202
 clinical evaluation in, 198–199
 hypokalemia in, 203
 hypomagnesemia in, 203
 identification of, 197–198
 refractory, 199–200, 202
 treatment of, 199–200, *200–201*, 202–203
Ventricular tachycardia, 234–236
Venturi mask, 147t
Verapamil, for atrial fibrillation, 222t
 for atrial flutter, 226
 for headache, 123t, 124t
 for paroxysmal supraventricular tachycardia, 229

Vertebrobasilar insufficiency, and vertigo, 84
Vertigo, 82–85
  benign positional, 85
  central, 87t
  disposition in, 94–95
  epidemiology of, 88–89
  history in, 89–90
  laboratory evaluation in, 91–92
  management of, 92–94
  medications causing, 89
  nystagmus in, 88
  peripheral, 87t
  physical examination in, 90
  provocative testing in, 90–91, 91
Vestibular neuronitis, and vertigo, 84–85
Viral hepatitis, 429–443
  definition of, 429
  differential diagnosis of, 436, 438
  disposition in, 442–443
  laboratory studies in, 434–435, 434–436, 437t–438t
  patient education in, 439
  prophylaxis for, 440–442, 441t
  prophylaxis for contacts in, 439
  risk factors for, 432t, 432–433
  signs and symptoms of, 433
  treatment of, 438–439
Viral meningitis. See Meningitis.
Viral pericarditis, 277, 278t
Viral pneumonia, causative organisms in, 486t
Vital sign(s), documentation of, 17
  in acute respiratory failure, 294
Vital signs, in shock, 167–168
Vitamin B$_{12}$, deficiency of, 794
Vitamin D, deficiency of, and hypocalcemia, 613
Vitamin K, deficiency of, 810, 812
Volume replacement therapy, for cardiogenic shock, 179–180
  for diabetic ketoacidosis, 691, 693
  for hypercalcemia, 610
  for hyperglycemia without ketosis, 683, 685
  for hyperglycemic hyperosmolar coma, 702, 704

Volume replacement therapy (Continued)
  for hypernatremia, 616
  for hypovolemic shock, 186–188
  for salicylate poisoning, 952, 956t
  for septic shock, 192
  for sickle cell disease, 801
von Willebrand's disease, 811
V/Q (ventilation-perfusion). See Ventilation-perfusion (V/Q).
Vulvovaginal candidiasis, 667, 667t, 670, 671t, 672
Vulvovaginitis, allergic, 669

Waddell's sign, in low back pain, 43
Wallenberg's syndrome, and vertigo, 83–84
Warfarin, for transient ischemic attack, 762
Washed red cell(s), transfusion of, 816
Water loss, and hypernatremia, 615, 617
Water-related injury(ies), cellulitis from, 397, 401t
WBCs (white blood cells), in evaluation of abdominal pain, 331
Wenckebach atrioventricular block, 232
Wernicke's encephalopathy, 930
White blood cell (WBCs), in evaluation of abdominal pain, 33t
Whitlow, herpetic, 425–427
Whole blood, transfusion of, 815
Whole-bowel irrigation, for poisoning, 879
Withdrawal seizure(s), 776
Wound(s), puncture, cellulitis from, 398
Wrist, arthrocentesis of, 838, 838

Xanthochromia, vs. traumatic lumbar puncture, 787

YAG laser, in hemoptysis, 335

Zalcitabine (dideoxycytidine, DDC), for acquired immunodeficiency syndrome, 362
Zidovudine (AZT), for acquired immunodeficiency syndrome, 361